MASSAGE THERAPY

PRINCIPLES AND PRACTICE

THIRD EDITION

Susan G. Salvo

BEd, LMT, NTS, CI, NCTMB

Co-Owner, Co-Director, and Instructor
Louisiana Institute of Massage Therapy
Lake Charles, Louisiana

SAUNDERS

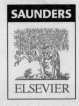

ELSEVIER

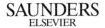

11830 Westline Industrial Drive
St. Louis, Missouri 63146

MASSAGE THERAPY: PRINCIPLES AND PRACTICE,
3rd EDITION   ISBN: 978-1-4160-3652-4

ISBN: 978-1-4160-3652-4

Publishing Director: Linda Duncan
Acquisitions Editor: Kellie White
Developmental Editor: Kim Fons
Publishing Services Manager: Julie Eddy
Project Manager: Andrea Campbell
Designer: Julia Dummitt

Printed in Canada

Last digit is the print number: 9 8 7 6 5 4 3 2 1

There are so many people to thank ...

A retired English teacher who has proofed and edited my grammar,
A friend who has comforted and advised me through good and stormy times,
A wise mentor who has set a sterling example of how to live life and respect others,
A nanny, who has cared for my four youngest children like they were her own grandchildren,
with love and nurturing and pride,

Amazingly, they have one thing in common— they are all the same person.
This book is dedicated to Maggie Woosley—thank you for becoming part of our family.

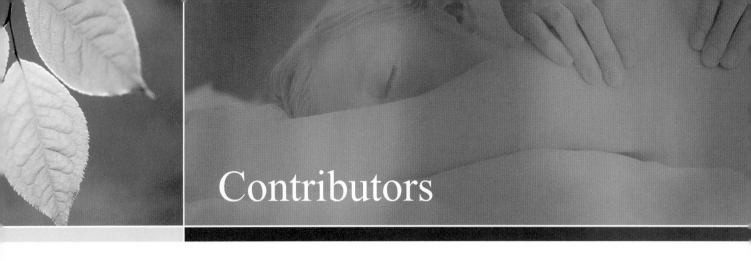

Contributors

MICHAEL A. BREAUX, LMT
Co-owner, Louisiana Institute of Massage Therapy
Lake Charles, Louisiana
Past Chairman, Louisiana State Board of Massage Therapy
Website: http://www.LaMassageSchool.com
Clinical Massage for Sports and Rehabilitation

KARYN CHABOT, DAy, LMT
Sacred Stone Center for Holistic Education and Therapy
Middletown, Rhode Island
Website: http://www.sacredstonehealing.com
Hydrotherapy and Spa Applications and Energy-Based
  Bodywork Therapy: Shiatsu and Ayurveda

RITA S. LeBLEU, LMT, MA
Rhetorical and Interpersonal Communication
DeQuincy, Louisiana
Biographical Sketches

MARIA MATHIAS, BS
Developmental Specialist-Infant Massage Specialist
Department of Pediatrics, Division of Neonatology
University of New Mexico Health Sciences Center
Certified Massage Instructor for the state of New Mexico
Certified Infant Touch and Massage Instructor and Trainer
Co-Founder, International Institute of Infant Massage
Albuquerque, New Mexico
Website: http://www.infantmassageinstitute.com
Infant massage section of Pregnancy and Infant Massage

WAYNE MATHIAS, MS
Recreation Administration
Certified Infant Touch and Massage Instructor and Trainer
Co-Founder, International Institute of Infant Massage
Albuquerque, New Mexico
Website: http://www.infantmassageinstitute.com
Infant massage section of Pregnancy and Infant Massage

HAYLEY A. SALVO
Bachelors in Journalism, Magna Cum Laude
University of Missouri–Columbia
KBIA Radio in Columbia
Biographical Sketches

DIEGO SANCHEZ, Dipl ABT (NCCAOM), CP
  (AOBTA), LMT
Owner, SoHo Shiatsu
New York, New York
Zen Shiatsu Instructor, Dept. of Psychology, Catholic
  University, Montevideo–Uruguay
Website: http://www.sohoshiatsu.com
Energy-Based Bodywork Therapy: Shiatsu and Ayurveda;
  Shiatsu

RALPH R. STEPHENS, BSEd, LMT, NCBTMB
Owner, Ralph Stephens Seminars, LLC
Cedar Rapids, Iowa
Website: http://www.ralphstephens.com
Seated Massage

H. MICHEAL TARVER, PhD
Professor, Department Head of Social Sciences
  and Philosophy
Arkansas Tech University
Russellville, Arkansas
A Historical Perspective of Massage

GEORGIA TETLOW
Energy-Based Bodywork Therapy: Shiatsu and Ayurveda;
  Ayurveda

JEANINE UTZMAN BABINEAUX, PhD, APRN,
  C-FNP
Professor, Graduate Program
College of Nursing
McNeese State University
Massage Physiology: Benefits, Indications,
  Contraindications, and Endangerment Sites

KENNETH G. ZYSK, PhD, DPhil
Associate Professor
Institute for Cross-Cultural and Regional Studies
Department of Asian Studies
University of Copenhagen
Copenhagen, Denmark
Energy-Based Bodywork Therapy: Shiatsu and Ayurveda;
  Ayurveda

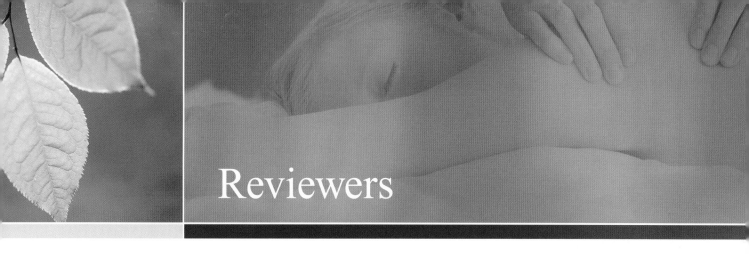

Reviewers

SANDRA KAUFFMAN ANDERSON, BA, LMT, NCTMB
Desert Institute of the Healing Arts
Tucson, Arizona

WILLIAM L. BARRY, LAc, RMT
Phoenix School of Holistic Studies
Houston, Texas

JOANN BOCK, LMT, RPP
Florida School of Massage
Gainesville, Florida

KAREN BROOKS, NTS, LMT
New Mexico School of Natural Therapeutics
Albuquerque, New Mexico

IRIS BURMAN, LMT
Educating Hands School of Massage
Miami, Florida

GLORIA RAY CARPENETO, PhD, MST, NCTMB
Villa Julie College
Baltimore, Maryland

LAUREN M. CHRISTMAN, MFA, LMP
Brian Utting School of Massage
Seattle, Washington

SUNNY COOPER, MS, Dipl ABT (NCCAOM)
Life Circles, Inc.
Ogden, Utah

LEOPOLD D. CORMIER, BS, DC
Austin, Texas

DON CORNWELL, PhD, DOM
New Mexico School of Natural Therapeutics
Albuquerque, New Mexico

NANCY W. DAIL, BA, LMT, NCTMB
Downeast School of Massage
Waldoboro, Maine

PATRICIA MARIE HOLLAND, BS, LMT
Desert Institute of the Healing Arts
Tucson, Arizona

KAMALAPATI S. KHALSA, CSMT
Phoenix Therapeutic Massage College
Phoenix, Arizona

ROBERT KING
Chicago School of Massage Therapy
Chicago, Illinois

GLENN MANCEAUX, PT, DC
Flynn, Manceaux, Arcement Chiropractic and Physical Therapy Clinic
Houma, Louisiana

JIM McKNIGHT, BA, LMT
Delta Junction, Alabama, and Honolulu, Hawaii

CHERIE MONLEZUN
Interim Dean of Education-College of Therapeutic Massage and Clinic Director
Rainstar University of Complementary and Alternative Medicine
Scottsdale, Arizona

CAROLYN A. NELKA, BA, CMT
Catonsville Community College
Catonsville, Maryland

THERESE A. NOVAK, MSN, RN, CS
Iowa Health Center
Iowa, Louisiana

GRANT PARKER, BSc, RMT, DC
Sprott-Shaw Community College
Nanaimo, British Columbia, Canada

MARY L. PUGLIA, MS, PhD
Phoenix Therapeutic Massage College
Phoenix, Arizona

FRANK PUGLIA, MBA, current Arizona teaching
  certificate
Phoenix Therapeutic Massage College
Phoenix, Arizona

JUNE E. SCHNEIDER, NCTMB
Baltimore School of Massage
Baltimore, Maryland

JAN SCHWARTZ, LMT, NCTMB
Desert Institute of the Healing Arts
Tucson, Arizona

DAVE SHAHAN
Colorado Institute of Massage Therapy
The University of Arizona Medical School
Colorado Springs, Colorado, and Tucson, Arizona

VERNON SMITH, PhD, Dipl ABT (NCCAOM),
  Certified Instructor (AOBTA)
Massage Therapy College of Baton Rouge
Baton Rouge, Louisiana

SARI SPIELER, LMT
Seattle, Washington

DONALD R. THIGPEN, DC, BS, LMT
Chiropractic Center for Pain and Rehabilitation
Louisiana Institute of Massage Therapy
Lake Charles, Louisiana

BONNIE THOMPSON, LMT, CNMT, CFT, FT
Colorado Institute of Massage
Colorado Springs, Colorado

DENNIS M. WALKER, MD, FAAOS
Lake Charles Memorial Hospital
Lake Charles, Louisiana

JERRY WEINERT, RN, LMT, NCTMB
Desert Institute of the Healing Arts and Southwest Wellness
  Educators
Tucson, Arizona

PAMELA L. WILSON, OTR/L, NTS, LMT
Healthy Touch
Albuquerque, New Mexico

PAUL WYMAN, BA, CMT
Denver, Colorado

JOHN YATES
West Coast College of Massage Therapy
Vancouver, British Columbia

ROBIN ZILL
The Spa Center, Inc.
Hillsborough, North Carolina

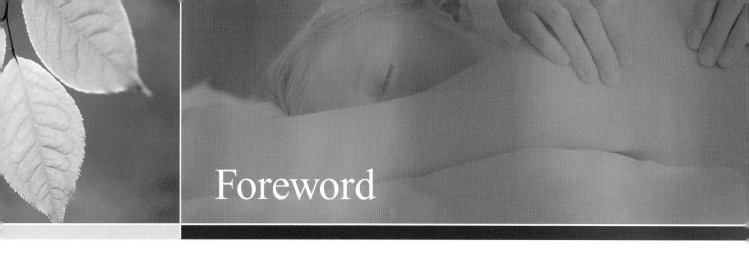

Foreword

Susan Salvo's comprehensive textbook *Massage Therapy: Principles and Practice* presents a body of work that takes its readers through a course of study providing far more than basics. Whether you are a brand new student, just graduated or consider yourself "an old pro" this text has a great deal to offer you. The facts are here; I don't think Susan has left anything out.

In addition she has gathered a store of new developments you need to know about if you are to stay ahead of the forward looking direction bodywork is taking. Known information is presented in a different light. New information has moved on from theory to proven science.

The present lifestyle of Americans has guaranteed low back pain for almost the entire population. Massage therapists will find that the latest work on muscles presented in this text will broaden their practice and attract that most needy clientele, people suffering from muscular pain and dysfunction.

Within my lifetime of 93 years, massage, attitudes toward massage and results from using massage have taken a healthy turn. Once considered a luxury for a wealthy, well traveled group who regularly frequented European "spas," today's massage has spread its wings to shelter anyone in the know. "Knowing" is the property of those who keep up with positive trends.

The conditions that *could* be fostered during the first three years of life determine the body's development for good or that other thing. My mother imported a baby nurse from Hamburg, Germany so for my first three years I was given daily massages and baby exercise. It was from this early foundation that I developed an athlete's body that serves me still.

Fact: American public school children from six to sixteen are the weakest, most tense children in the world. American grade school and college students, unless they are upper level varsity sports material, get criminally limited movement. Most youngsters who do earn that honor are "natural athletes." Athletes of every stamp need body work to *prevent* injuries and insure success. Not many Americans are interested in the condition of their bodies unless they are athletes, dancers, gymnasts and the like. A massage therapist can improve any performance calling for strength, flexibility and stamina. Muscles in the hands of trained body workers will give up spasm causing aches and pains.

Lucky is the therapist who has the wit, will and skill to care for his or her own body. Susan Salvo has provided those tools too and has pointed out that each of us is responsible for what we do with the bodies *we* have made.

It's a new time with new ideas and we have a leader in the field who believes we should each make the most of it. Imagine what will happen when we do.

BONNIE PRUDDEN
Director, Bonnie Prudden Myotherapy® Inc.
PO Box 65240
Tucson, AZ 85728
800-221-4634
http://www.bonnieprudden.com
info@bonnieprudden.com

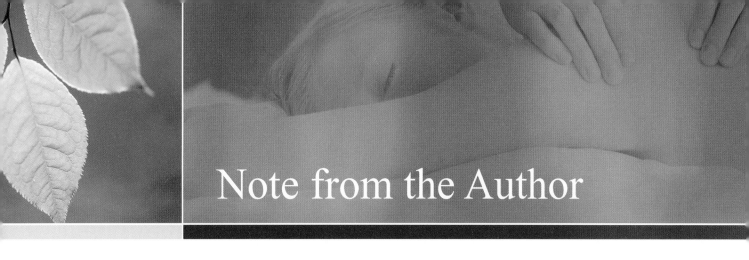

Note from the Author

Massage works miracles. There's the miracle "cure" of working out rotator cuff trigger points just before the big golf game. There's the wonder of de-stressing the harried mother of twins with a scrub, a soak, and a hot stone massage. There's the look of peace as the businessman's brow un-furrows during a session of Asian bodywork. One of my favorite miracles is what massage does to attitude. A first-time client may come in the door with a combination of excitement and apprehension, wearing that "Oooh, I've never done this before" look. But after the massage, he is smiling and saying "Why did I wait so long to try this?" Sometimes the miracle comes from the emotional release of a client who just needs to talk or cry.

As therapists, we not only facilitate and participate in these minor miracles, we too are changed by them.

Most major religions contain stories of miracles. Many of the miracle stories are based on doctrines of love for our fellow man. Touch is often used as a vehicle for the transmission of these miracles. This is true for Judeo-Christian teaching, Buddhism, Islamic belief, Native American lore, and even the old pagan mythologies. Regardless of our personal ideologies, beliefs, and differences, we can all participate in small miracles on a daily basis through the use of touch. Our one common belief is the power of the work itself. And so we go out into the world much like the monks, missionaries, prophets, priests, and priestesses of old to do this work. We are disciples of touch, working little miracles, changing the world one person at a time.

As a teacher, I am always gratified to have someone approach me and say "I've had massages all over the world, and the best massages I've ever received have been from your students." This is another miracle in itself—how can you train someone to be a better therapist than you are yourself? I cannot take the credit; I believe that it is due to the philosophy of my own past instructors. I have had three kinds of teachers in my lifetime:

- those that were in the classroom only to collect a paycheck,

- those that held back certain vital facts so that you could never know as much as they or be as good as they or even make perfect scores on their tests, and
- those that fearlessly held nothing back, that encouraged questions, that challenged me to do my best, that taught with passion.

It is this third type of instructor that I have attempted to emulate. It is this philosophy of sharing knowledge with passion, upon which the creation of this textbook is based. Our school has been used as a testing ground for new theories and techniques. Each new edition of this book is the result of combining:

- tried and true techniques for working on the body,
- the latest in research about massage and pathologies,
- graphic art and photography that say a thousand words,
- simple methods for remembering complicated structures and functions,
- the use of new technologies to enhance learning, and
- a common-sense return to basics when last year's advances turn out to be problematic.

By taking each chapter to the classroom for test runs, we have expanded, modified, reduced, compressed, deleted, and combined, until the finished product is one that is friendly to the eye, meets the needs of the student, reduces the workload of the teacher, and produces massage therapists for the clients of tomorrow.

While no textbook can meet all the needs of every student and every instructor, we've made great efforts to listen to your suggestions and respond to your feedback. We, the authors and editors, remain open to ways of improving this text. Please feel free to contact us with your ideas.

SUSAN G. SALVO
susansalvo@hotmail.com
www.LaMassageSchool.com

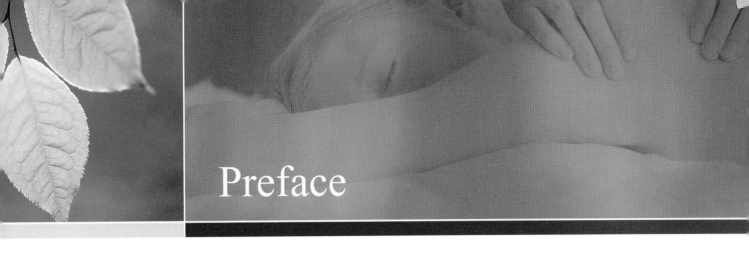

Preface

Massage is multidimensional—it is simultaneously an art and a science—and through learning it you will become a sculptor, a technician, a confidant, a musician, a teacher, an actor, and a healthcare professional. Massage education continues to evolve and educational standards are on the rise. This textbook addresses today's massage education needs by combining the classically accepted ideology of the past with today's new concepts. We use modern educational techniques to bridge the gap between old and new, thus creating the highest-quality educational and reference materials to be found in the field of massage therapy. Our primary aim is to provide the fundamental topics that massage therapy schools must teach students to prepare them for a career in massage therapy.

Who Will Benefit From This Book?

Students will benefit from the user-friendly nature of this book. This text is based on the fusion of massage and anatomical science, focusing on their commonalities. The stunning photography and detailed illustrations provide both instruction and inspiration to the learner, and the format of the book is readable and engaging.

Teachers will appreciate the back-to-basics style that makes the material so teachable. Massage is a very useful and effective health care tool; yet, some authors and instructors, in a well-meaning attempt to elevate the profession to a higher science, have overcomplicated an incredibly simple subject. Massage school is not medical school. Hence, a massage text should be readable and even enjoyable. It's a fact—students learn better when they are enjoying themselves.

Established massage therapists use the text as a method of updating their knowledge, studying for advanced certificate exams, and as a resource, desk reference, and teaching tool for clients.

Organization

This textbook is divided into five units.

In Unit One, we begin with the background work, including the history of massage, establishing the client/therapist relationship, and the massage environment.

In Unit Two, we learn the basics such as hygiene and safety, indications and contraindications, body and table mechanics, Swedish massage, assessment and treatment planning, and how massage is adapted to special populations, such as infants, pregnant women, the elderly, and individuals facing chronic and terminal illnesses.

It is not until Unit Three that we approach anatomy and physiology. By this point, the average student is completely engaged with the subject matter of massage, and expresses anticipation rather than apprehension about the hard sciences.

In Unit Four, we build upon the knowledge of the first three units by teaching more advanced modalities such as hydrotherapy and spa applications, foot reflexology, clinical massage for sports and rehabilitation, seated massage, and Eastern modalities.

Unit Five prepares the therapist for the practical operation of a practice in the business world.

Distinctive Features of This Book

Interweaving massage with the anatomical sciences – The anatomy and physiology chapters explore each body system, explaining the structure and function of the key components in relevant terminology. Woven into the anatomy are associated injures, diseases, and conditions, along with precautions, contraindications, and adaptations for massaging clients who are affected by these problems. The anatomy and physiology chapters are written **from** and **for** a massage therapist's point of view. This book incorporates a general knowledge of anatomical science while focusing on aspects that are most important to the massage practitioner.

Emphasis on the musculoskeletal system – To thoroughly cover the topic of muscles, their origins, insertions, actions, and innervations, we have chosen to divide the skeletal and muscular systems into four chapters. Two cover each system in general and the other two chapters highlight each system by nomenclature, listing each muscle and bone individually with illustrations and important details.

Biographical sketches – We have included biographies and candid interviews with many of the pioneers of massage therapy, both past and present. New biographies focus on individuals who may not be well known on a national level, but are out in communities touching the lives of others through massage.

Self Tests – We want you to pass your tests. Giving you anatomy information and teaching you massage routines is not enough if you cannot pass the licensing exams. We have included self tests at the end of each chapter to assist the student in self-assessment, as well as studying for and taking tests. Yes, there is a skill involved and, if you know and understand that skill, your test-taking ability will improve. We call it becoming "test-wise." Hence, you can use this book as a study guide to prepare for and successfully pass state and/or national examinations. Other study tips include the use of mnemonic devices and an understanding of the prefixes, suffixes, and word roots of anatomical terminology.

New to This Edition

Case Studies – Many chapters include case studies, a study of a person or persons involved in a situation. Each case study will present the student with several questions to ponder. Most often, there is more than one dilemma so the situation must be thought about from several different angles. Each solution has consequences. Often the best solution is the one with the fewest negative consequences. The therapist may be faced with some ethical and moral decisions. Case studies are valuable sources of information, stimulating dialogue between instructors and students, fostering open-mindedness, and promoting acceptance of human fallibility. All of the case studies presented are factual, based on the experiences of real massage therapists.

CASE STUDY:
Client Gifts

Chastity, a massage therapist, had a marriage that was coming to an end. She worked in a contract labor setting for another massage therapist, Jill. To minimize expenses, Chastity was looking for a cheaper apartment. Chastity had had a difficult time with the separation, and the stress was evident to many of her clients. One client, Bill, had questioned her until she had finally divulged her dilemma. That night, Bill talked the problem over with his wife, Marjorie, and then offered to let Chastity stay at their camp on the river, rent free, until she got back on her feet financially. Chastity was so excited to finally get a break. When Jill came in to close the books for the day, Chastity was bubbling over and proceeded to tell her boss about her new living arrangements. Jill was quiet for a moment and then said, "Chastity, we need to talk."

Jill's view was that accepting free rent from a client, especially one of the opposite gender, was an unethical decision. "What will you do if he just shows up and lets himself in unexpectedly?" Jill asked. "What if he asks for legitimate favors? Aren't you going to feel somewhat indebted?"

Jill tried to get Chastity to understand her point of view, but Chastity just became sullen and eventually hostile. "I thought you'd be happy for me," cried Chastity, barely able to hold back the tears.

Despite the fact that Chastity had been a loyal and productive employee for several years, Jill told her that she had to make a choice—find another living arrangement or find a new job.

If you were Chastity, how would you analyze the situation ethically? How would you approach Jill for further dialogue on the subject? What would your decision be in regard to the situation?

If you were Jill, what would you do to put yourself in Chastity's place? What, if any, compromise would you be willing to make?

If Chastity chooses to stay, what kind of dialogue might prevent further similar occurrences?

If Chastity chooses to leave, what kind of references would you give to a prospective employer?

DVD – Included with the book is a bound-in DVD with nearly two hours of video instruction. Five areas will be featured including body mechanics, table mechanics, client intake, treatment planning, and technique. Also included are more than 10 animations allowing the student to view different anatomical structures and physiological functions, such as brain anatomy and function of the heart. A DVD icon will appear in the text whenever a pertinent video clip or animation is available.

GUIDELINES FOR PROPER BODY MECHANICS

(6-11)

New figures – This edition features more than 150 new figures. Most of the new images are from my brother, photographer Chris Salvo, and his lovely partner and wife, Suzanne Salvo, and from illustrators Barbara Cousins and Jeanne Robertson.

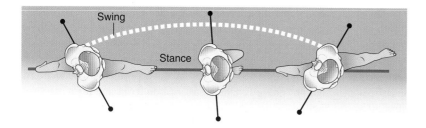

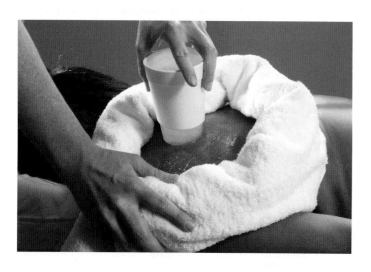

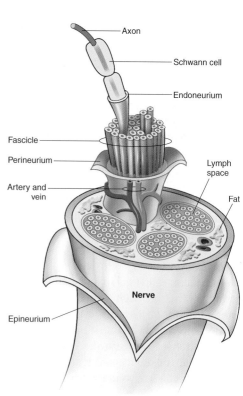

Internet activities – Each chapter includes activities that direct readers to the internet for exploration of material and concepts.

Internet support – Sprinkled throughout the text, you will find Evolve boxes indicating that additional material is available online. The Evolve website for this text has been radically expanded to include crossword puzzles, drag-and-drop exercises, video clips, student tips, a collection of additional graphic images, links to other resources and, because you requested it, a mock national certification exam.

> **evolve** *Log on to your student account from the Evolve website and view the basic strokes demonstration and their variations from this chapter. Use this as you practice at home.* ■

Table Talk – This feature is a place where I share additional information, expound on important concepts, offer suggestions and recommendations, present historical facts, and suggest tips for remembering test material.

TABLE TALK

Perineal massage increases tissue elasticity and decreases the likelihood of tearing the perineum during fetal delivery (stage 2 labor). Because the perineum is located in the genital region, the massage therapist is not permitted to administer perineal treatments. Perineal massage can be self-administered or administered by her husband or birth coach. Perineal massage is most beneficial during the last 6 weeks of pregnancy and during the first and second stage of labor.

Pathologies – We've increased coverage to include more than 200 different pathologies. To simplify the subject, we've also reduced the specifics of each pathology by making the discussions of massage precautions and suggestions more succinct. For greater in-depth instruction, we recommend our companion textbook, *Mosby's Pathology for Massage Therapists* by Susan Salvo and Sandy Anderson.

Nutrition appendix – This new Appendix will include the following topics: basic nutrition principles, nutrients such as vitamins and minerals, and the basic food groups and their recommended daily allowances. This information can be used for client education or as a guide for the therapist as he or she pursues a healthy lifestyle.

Pharmacology appendix – New to this edition is the inclusion of fundamental pharmacology for the massage therapist. When screening clients for the appropriateness of massage, therapists will ask clients about their health. Because much of our population has medical conditions managed by prescription medications, understanding their effects has become increasingly important.

Changes to chapter on Assessment and Planning – We've taken a different approach to this chapter and it now includes:

- a discussion that contrasts and compares SOAP and APIE notes,

- an introduction of a new, simpler method for devising a treatment plan (PPALM),
- techniques for conducting a client interview,
- explanation of HIPAA guidelines, and
- information on medications and how they might affect the massage.

NEW chapter on Pregnancy and Infant Massage – The pregnancy section discusses the discomforts of pregnancy, complications and high-risk factors, treatment guidelines, positioning considerations, and information relating to labor and postpartum. The infant massage section includes a massage routine for infants as well as how to set the environment and screen for precautions and contraindications.

Revamped chapter on Adaptive Massage – This chapter includes new information on implanted devices and updated sections on massage for three of the fastest growing segments of our population: cancer patients, people who are HIV positive, and geriatric clients.

New illustrations for Skeletal and Muscular System chapters – New and larger figures from Joe Muscolino's textbook, *The Muscular System Manual*, make the content in these chapters easier to understand through clear visual representations of anatomy.

NEW chapter on the Reproductive System – This edition includes a chapter dedicated to the male and female reproductive systems.

Expanded material on Hydrotherapy and Spa Applications – Because one third of therapists are now employed in spas, this chapter has been updated to include various types of spas, guidelines for treatment (before, during, and after), underwater massage, more on aromatherapy, and Ayurveda techniques.

New chapter on Foot Reflexology – This chapter includes maps of zones, landmarks, reflexes, basic techniques, treatment guidelines, and a simple routine.

Additional Learning Aids

Key terms and glossary – Key terms are bolded throughout the textbook. They can also be located in the glossary for easy access to definitions.

Mini-Labs – These short lab sessions within chapters are skill-building activities designed so that left-brained and right-brained techniques reinforce each other. Direct student participation enhances the learning process by stimulating creativity and imagination.

MINI-LAB

Spray the back of your hand with tap water. Blow on the damp surface, and describe the sensation as the water evaporates. Speculate how evaporation of water (sweat) from the skin surface can regulate the temperature of the body. Repeat the experiment with alcohol, which evaporates at a lower temperature than water, and compare the results.

Special format for coverage of the musculoskeletal system – Muscles are laid out in a special format, detailing origins, insertion, actions, nerve, and special notes on muscles. Muscle illustrations are large and clearly presented.

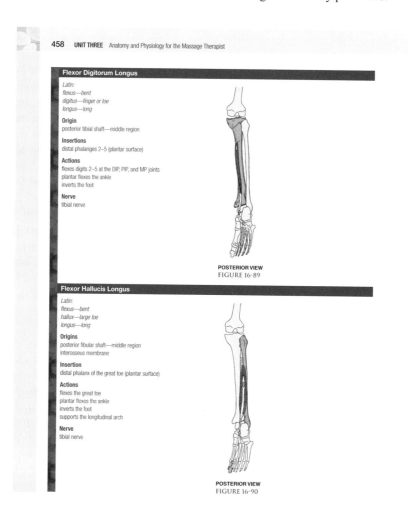

Flexor Digitorum Longus

Latin:
flexus—bent
digitus—finger or toe
longus—long

Origin
posterior tibial shaft—middle region

Insertions
distal phalanges 2–5 (plantar surface)

Actions
flexes digits 2–5 at the DIP, PIP, and MP joints
plantar flexes the ankle
inverts the foot

Nerve
tibial nerve

POSTERIOR VIEW
FIGURE 16-89

Flexor Hallucis Longus

Latin:
flexus—bent
hallux—large toe
longus—long

Origins
posterior fibular shaft—middle region
interosseus membrane

Insertion
distal phalanx of the great toe (plantar surface)

Actions
flexes the great toe
plantar flexes the ankle
inverts the foot
supports the longitudinal arch

Nerve
tibial nerve

POSTERIOR VIEW
FIGURE 16-90

Biographical sketches – We have included biographies and candid interviews with many of the pioneers of massage therapy, both past and present.

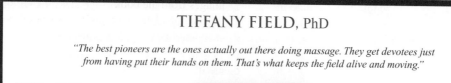

TIFFANY FIELD, PhD

"The best pioneers are the ones actually out there doing massage. They get devotees just from having put their hands on them. That's what keeps the field alive and moving."

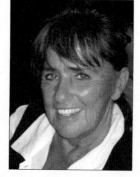

Tiffany Field has always been a woman on the move. As the daughter of an insurance executive and teacher, she lived in 12 different places when she was growing up, but now she has found her home—and her life's calling—on the beach in Hollywood, Florida.

She is not a massage therapist, and she has not developed any particular massage modality; however, her work has dramatically affected the credibility of the profession. Tiffany Field is a professor of pediatrics, psychology, and psychiatry, and she is the director of the University of Miami School of Medicine's

$7.05 billion in annual savings might be realized.

The potential for Field's research and the cost-cutting measures earned her the grant money to explore touch therapy further. Currently, her group is studying the effects of massage on all ages, from cocaine-exposed newborns to arthritic geriatric patients. *Massage Therapy Reduces Anxiety and Enhances EEG Pattern of Alertness and Math Computations* is one of the most recent studies being conducted.

Some of the work being examined at TRI is particularly groundbreaking. Al-

Self Tests – These are included to assist the student in self-assessment, as well as studying for and taking tests. Yes, there is a skill involved, and if you know and understand that skill, your test-taking ability will improve. We call it becoming "test-wise." Hence, you can use this book as a study guide to prepare for and successfully pass state and/or national examinations.

SELF TEST

690   UNIT FOUR A User's Guide to Complementary and Adjunctive Therapies

MATCHING I

Place the letter of the answer next to the term or phrase that best describes it.

A. Aromatherapy	E. Essential oil	I. Sauna
B. Body mask	F. Glow	J. Spa
C. Conduction	G. Herbal wrap	K. Spa tub
D. Cryotherapy	H. Hydrotherapy	L. Vichy shower

_____ 1. The internal and external therapeutic use of water and complementary agents

_____ 2. Place where water therapies are administered

_____ 3. Exchange of heat while the body's surface is in direct contact with the thermal agent

_____ 4. External, therapeutic application of very cold water or ice

_____ 5. Spa treatment in which mud or other products are applied to most of the body

_____ 6. Body wrap in which the sheets have been soaked in herbal tea

_____ 7. Heated pool with high-pressure jets that agitate and circulate water

_____ 8. Dry heat treatment in which the client is in a wood-lined room

_____ 9. Shower taken while client reclines on a special table as jets of water spray from multiple overhead-mounted showerheads

_____ 10. The use of plant-derived essential oils for therapeutic purposes

_____ 11. Concentrated essences of aromatic plants

_____ 12. Term that is synonymous with the word *scrub*

Inspiration – Besides providing intellectual stimulation, one of our goals is to have the book inspire students emotionally and spiritually. This is accomplished through the use of insightful and thought-provoking quotations throughout the book.

> *"Where the spirit does not work with the hand, there is no art."*
> Leonardo da Vinci

Ancillaries

DVD – As mentioned above, the DVD in the back of this textbook contains nearly 2 hours of video showing specific massage techniques, routines, procedures, client interactions and case study video. Several animations are also included.

For Instructors

TEACH – TEACH resources on Evolve and in print will continue to support the instructor's needs. The Lesson Plan Manual is designed to help instructors prepare for classes and will reduce lesson plan preparation time, give new and creative ideas to promote student learning, and help make full use of a rich array of resources.

Evolve – Instructors will also find the following on the Evolve website:
- Testbank in Exam View format with 1200 questions
- Answer keys to self test questions
- Downloadable forms such as PPALM, intake, and student surveys
- Image collection in JPG and PowerPoint, containing all images from the book
- Supplemental collection of images not found in the book
- Teaching tips for each chapter
- Testing and grading information
- Crossword puzzles for handouts
- And much more!

For Students

Evolve – Students will find the following on the Evolve website:
- Client consultation video clips
- Audio glossary
- Image collection (same as instructor site)
- Downloadable forms
- Activities including drag-and-drop exercises, muscle drawing activities, and games
- Mock National Certification Exam
- Web Links

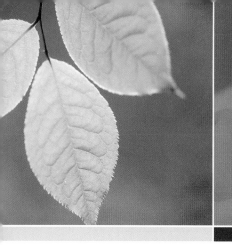

Acknowledgments

I would like to acknowledge the following individuals who assisted me in writing this edition:

Sandra Kauffman Anderson, Jeanene Babineaux, William Barry, Jennifer Behn, Jennifer Breaux, Mike Breaux, Lisa Bunch, Karyn Chabot, Elizabeth Clark, Teena Cole, Jessica Corbello, Barb Cousins, Susie Ogg Cormier, Bill Curet, Tari Dilks, Catherine Dupuis, Trish Ecker, Cindy Ellender, Joey Erwin, Kim Fons, Alice Funk, Tricia Grafelman, Christy Granger, James Hollingshed, Karen Kinslow, Kathie Lea, Rita LeBleu, Maria and Wayne Mathias, Cherie Monlezun, Eric Munn, Joseph Muscolino, Grant Parker, Hayley Salvo, Suzanne and Chris Salvo, Diego Sanchez, Jennifer Schaaf, Randall Short, Ralph Stephens, H. Micheal Tarver, Donald Thigpen, Dennis Walker, Freda Whalen Plues, Kellie White, and Maggie Woosley.

A word of appreciation for Joseph E. Muscolino, DC: Over the years this book has evolved and gained popularity basically due to one element—the teamwork of the editorial staff and contributors. For this third edition, the greatest contribution was the addition of the illustrations in Joe Muscolino's book *The Muscular System Manual*. I was awed when I first picked it up and I highly recommend that it be included in the library of every serious massage therapist. Thank you, Dr. Muscolino.

SUSAN G. SALVO

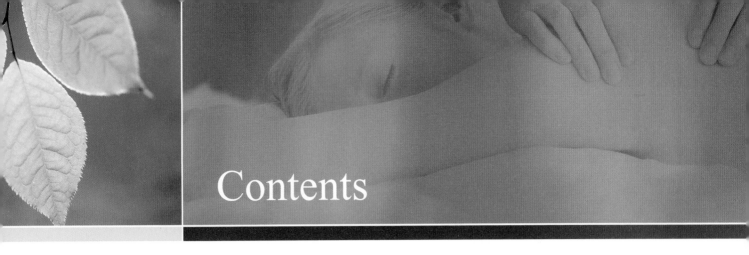

Contents

UNIT ONE

SURVEYING THE TERRITORY: HISTORY, STANDARDS, BOUNDARIES, EQUIPMENT, AND ENVIRONMENT

1 A Historical Perspective of Massage, *3*
   H. Micheal Tarver, PhD

2 The Therapeutic Relationship, *15*

3 Tools of the Trade and the Massage
   Environment, *43*

UNIT TWO

BENEFITS, CONTRAINDICATIONS, SCREENING, TECHNIQUE, AND SPECIAL CONSIDERATIONS FOR THE MASSAGE PRACTITIONER

4 Infection Control, Safety, Health, and
   Hygiene, *63*

5 Massage Physiology: Research, Effects,
   Indications, Contraindications, and
   Endangerment Sites, *81*

6 The Science of Body and Table Mechanics, *107*

7 Swedish Massage Movements and Swedish
   Gymnastics, *141*

8 Assessment and Planning, *191*

9 Pregnancy and Infant Massage, *217*
   Susan G. Salvo, BEd, LMT, NTS, CI, NCTMB
   Maria Mathias, MS
   Wayne Mathias, BS

10 Adaptive Massage, *239*

UNIT THREE

ANATOMY AND PHYSIOLOGY FOR THE MASSAGE THERAPIST

11 Introduction to the Human Body: Cells, Tissues,
   and the Body Compass, *261*

12 Integumentary System, *293*

13 Skeletal System and Joint Movements, *311*

14 Skeletal Nomenclature, *337*

15 Muscular System, *377*

16 Muscular Nomenclature and Kinesiology, *399*

17 Nervous System, *505*

18 Endocrine Glands and Hormones, *541*

19 Circulatory System, *559*

20 Respiratory System, *589*

21 Digestive System, *609*

22 Urinary System, *631*

23 Reproductive System, *645*

UNIT FOUR

A USER'S GUIDE TO COMPLEMENTARY AND ADJUNCTIVE THERAPIES

24 Hydrotherapy and Spa Applications, *665*

25 Foot Reflexology, *695*

26 Clinical Massage for Sports and
   Rehabilitation, *711*
   Susan G. Salvo, BEd, LMT, NTS, CI, NCTMB
   Michael A. Breaux, LMT

27 Seated Massage, *739*
   Ralph R. Stephens, BSEd, LMT, NCTMB

28 Eastern Massage Therapies: Shiatsu,
   Acupressure, Ayurveda, Thai Massage,
   and Polarity, *753*
   *Diego Sanchez, Dipl ABT (NCCAOM), CP (AOBTA),
      LMT*
   Kenneth G. Zysk, PhD, DPhil
   Georgia Tetlow
   Susan G. Salvo, BEd, LMT, NTS, CI, NCTMB

UNIT FIVE
BUSINESS PRACTICES

29 The Business of Massage, *791*

APPENDICES

Appendix A
The National Certification Board for Therapeutic Massage and Bodywork Code of Ethics, *825*

Appendix B
The National Certification Board for Therapeutic Massage and Bodywork Standards of Practice, *826*

Appendix C
Common Abbreviations, Symbols, Prescriptive Directions, Medical Terminology, Pathologies, Modalities, and Findings, *828*

Appendix D
Nutrition, *830*

Appendix E
Pharmacology, *837*

GLOSSARY, *849*

ILLUSTRATION CREDITS, *866*

INDEX, *868*

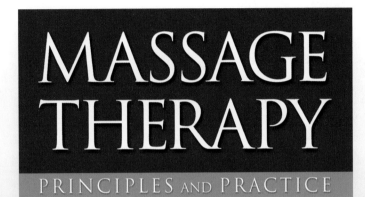

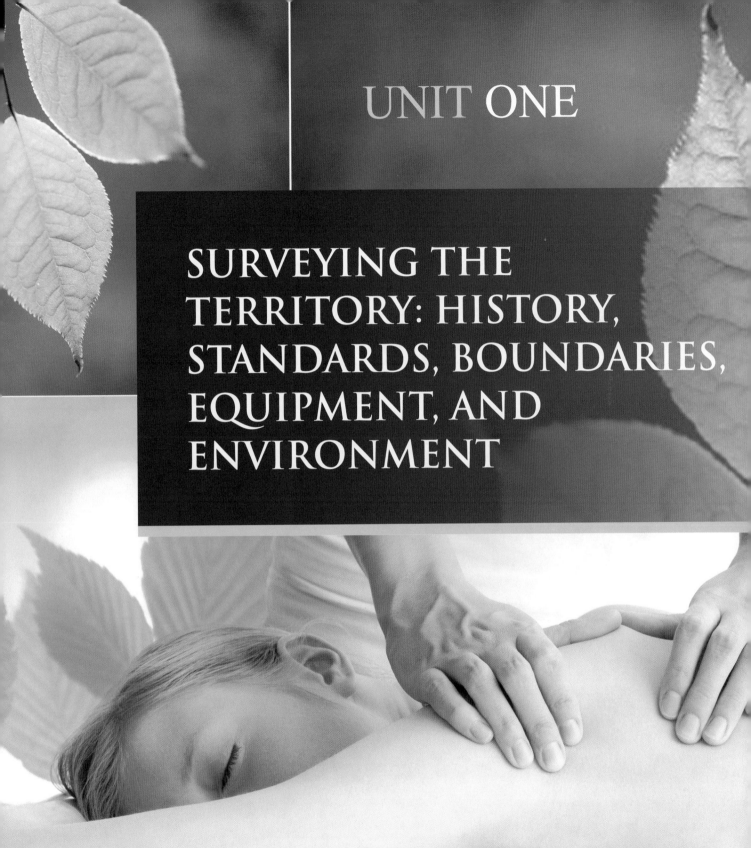

UNIT ONE

SURVEYING THE TERRITORY: HISTORY, STANDARDS, BOUNDARIES, EQUIPMENT, AND ENVIRONMENT

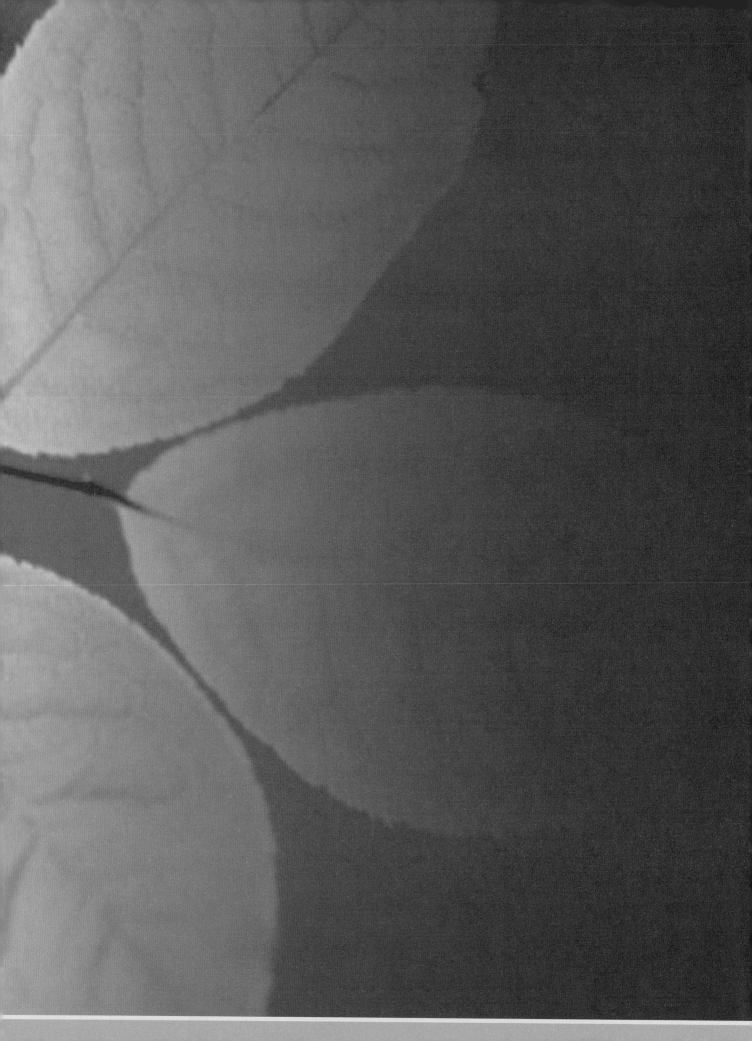

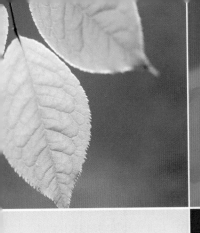

A Historical Perspective of Massage

H. Micheal Tarver, PhD

"Travel is fatal to prejudice, bigotry, and narrow-mindedness."
—Mark Twain

STUDENT OBJECTIVES

After completing this chapter, the student should be able to:

- Define the term massage
- Name major figures in the development of medicine and specifically in massage therapy
- Discuss the ancient views and uses of massage that incorporate both Eastern and Western cultures
- Explain the role of the European Renaissance and Enlightenment on the professionalism of massage therapy
- Distinguish the contributions of Pehr Henrik Ling from those of later physicians and therapists
- Reconstruct the development of therapeutic massage that incorporates the various massage styles
- Integrate recent developments in the field of therapeutic massage into the original framework of Pehr Ling and his students

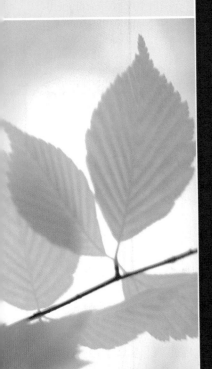

INTRODUCTION

Massage can be defined as a systematic and scientific manipulation of the soft tissues of the body for the purpose of obtaining or maintaining health. The history of massage and healing touch is long and complex, with more than 75 different types of massage and *bodywork,* a generic term used to describe massage and its various forms. Archaeological and historical evidence indicates that massage and healing touch have been practiced for thousands of years in all regions of the globe. Massage is instinctive. It is a natural response to rub our aches and pains, whether or not we are familiar with the medical knowledge behind these actions. In modern health care, massage has taken on an important role. It has been shown beneficial to reduce stress, enhance blood circulation, decrease pain, promote sleep, reduce swelling, enhance relaxation, and increase oxygen capacity of the blood. Massage has also been recognized as a nondrug treatment for cancer and postoperative pain.

In this chapter, we will briefly examine the history of massage from its earliest records to the present (Figure 1-1). The goals of this chapter are to provide the massage therapist with the information necessary to illustrate the path taken in the development of the profession and to instill in the therapist a sense of connection with those who preceded him or her. Some names will be familiar, and others will be quite foreign. You need not memorize every name mentioned in the following pages, although some are important enough that you should know them (ask your instructor). What the names, with their different nations of origin, tell us is that the development of massage therapy was a global endeavor; people from around the world contributed to the knowledge base that transformed massage from folk remedy to medical treatment. It should be noted that from the beginning of this chapter, the word *massage* is used to refer to soft tissue manipulation, even though the term did not come into use until the middle of the nineteenth century. The origin of the word massage is unclear, but it can be traced to numerous sources: the Hebrew word *mashesh,* the Greek roots *masso* and *massin,* the Latin root *massa,* the Arabic root *mass'h,* the Sanskrit word *makeh,* and the French word *masser.*

THE PREHISTORIC WORLD

In prehistoric times (i.e., before written records), evidence supports the position that several groups around the world practiced massage. Archaeologists have found artifacts that depict the use of massage in many world cultures. Although no direct prehistoric evidence verifies the use of massage for medical reasons, the indirect evidence clearly implies that it was used in this manner. For example, European cave paintings (c. 15,000 BC) depict what appears to be the use of healing touch. In this period, extensive pictorial records show the use of massage.

> *"Time is a great teacher, but unfortunately it kills all its pupils."*
> Hector Berlioz

evolve Log on to the Evolve Massage Therapy: Principles and Practice, 3e, website at http://evolve.elsevier.com and register for student resources that accompany this text. Select a password or passcode to use each time you log on to the site. Once the registration process is complete, peruse all the course materials at your disposal. ■

THE ANCIENT WORLD

In the ancient East, a concern with illness has been documented in China for several millennia, and records have revealed that the practice of massage goes back as early as 3000 BC. However, in the period between the second century BC (200 to 101 BC) and the first century AD (AD 1 to 100), Chinese medicine began to take on its basic shape. Manuscripts found in

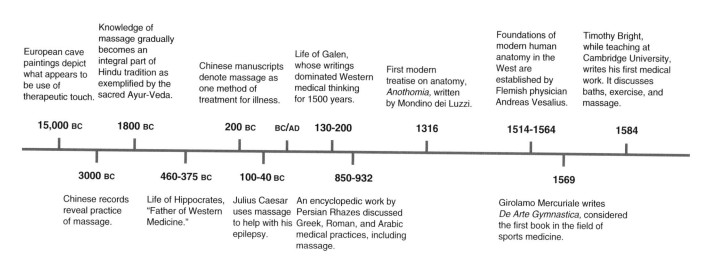

FIGURE 1-1 Massage time line.

China dating from the second century BC discuss massage as one of the various methods of treatment for illnesses. However, acupuncture was not mentioned in Chinese medical writings until 90 BC.

Using their knowledge of massage and later acupuncture, the Chinese developed a style of massage that they termed *amma, amna,* or *anmo.* **Amma** is regarded as the precursor to all other therapies, manual and energetic—the grandparent of all massage techniques. The Chinese had developed the art of massage so well that they were the first to train and employ massage therapists who were blind.

As early as the first century AD, various schools of medical thought had been founded and had already begun to produce diverging ideas. These various ideas and beliefs were compiled under the name of the mythical Yellow Emperor and became the classic scripture of traditional Chinese medicine, the *Huang-ti nei-ching.* Although the exact date of the original writing of the work is unknown, it was already in its present form by approximately the first century BC. The work, commonly known as *Nei Ching,* contained descriptions of healing touch procedures and their uses. Some debate is ongoing over the actual date of this work, with some historians arguing that it was written around 2760 BC. By AD 700, a Chinese ministry of health and a public health system were established.

By the sixth century AD, techniques and use of massage were well established in China and had found their way into Japan. In general, the Japanese methods of massage were basically the same as those of the Chinese. In Japan, we see shiatsu, literally meaning finger pressure; it is considered a component of amma. *Shiatsu* is a Japanese modality based on the Asian concept that the body has a series of energy points, or *tsubo.* Numerous tsubo points are along the body, each with different purposes. The shiatsu practitioner massages tsubo points to bring balance between mind and body. As with the Chinese, the medieval Japanese employed blind massage therapists.

TABLE TALK

In the Pergamon Museum in Berlin, a 2000-year-old alabaster relief depicts a massage treatment.

In addition to the Chinese and Japanese, other Asian cultures practiced massage. On the Indian subcontinent, the practice of massage has also existed for more than 3000 years. Knowledge of massage had probably been brought to India from China, and it gradually became an integral part of Hindu tradition, as exemplified by the inclusion of massage in the sacred practice of **Ayur-Veda** (c. 1800 BC). The Ayur-Veda, literally meaning *code of life,* deals with rebirth, renunciation, salvation, the soul, the purpose of life, the maintenance of mental health, and the prevention and treatment of diseases. As for medicine, the most important Ayurvedic texts are the *Samhitas.* A later work, the *Manav Dharma Shastra* (c. 300 BC), also mentions massage. In addition to the previously mentioned Eastern cultures, the Polynesians have also been documented as practicing therapeutic massage.

The concept of health and medicine in the West began to take shape during the seventh and sixth centuries BC. During that time, the legendary Greek physician Æsculapius **(Asclepius)** evolved into a god who was responsible for the emerging medical profession. His holy snake and staff still remain the symbol of the medical profession. Around 500 BC, the various ideas of healing and treatments in Greece merged into a *techne iatriche,* or healing science. During this process, two individuals, Iccus and Herodicus, concerned themselves with exercise and the use of gymnastics.

Among the followers of this new science was **Hippocrates of Cos** (460 to 375 BC) (Figure 1-2). With his emphasis on the individual patient and his belief that the healer should

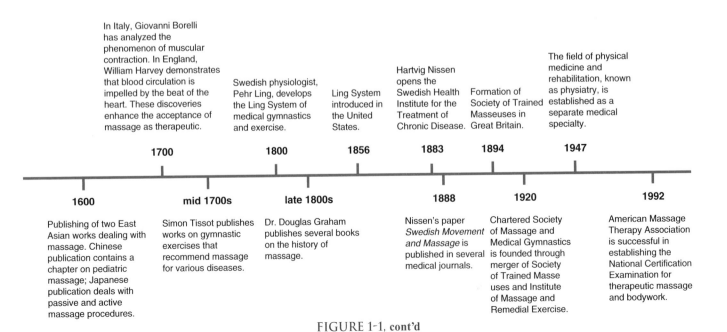

FIGURE 1-1, cont'd

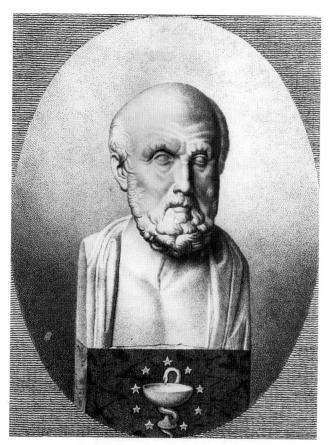

FIGURE 1-2 Hippocrates of Cos.

take care to avoid causing any additional harm to the patient, Hippocrates is generally recognized as the father of modern Western medicine. Although we know little about him, Hippocrates is reputed to have been a fine clinician, a founder of a medical school, and the author of numerous books, although most of the works attributed to him were written by other members of the Hippocratic school. These works are collectively known as the *Corpus Hippocraticum,* which summarized much of what was known about disease and medicine in the ancient world. During the four centuries after the development of the *techne iatriche,* several debates occurred within the healing profession, one of which placed great stock in the value of therapeutic massage. In his essay *On Joints,* Hippocrates wrote, "*μολλ ων ευπειρον σει του ιητρον, αταρ ση και ανατριψιος* " ("The physician must be skilled in many things and particularly friction," section IX, lines 25-26). Hippocrates also noted that after the reduction of a dislocated shoulder, the friction should be done with soft, gentle hands (section IX, lines 31-33). Obviously, Hippocrates was a proponent of massage.

During the transitional period between Greek and Roman dominance in the ancient world, a few individuals helped pass on the medical knowledge of the Greeks and incorporated it into Roman medicine. One such individual was **Aulus Celsus,** who is regarded by many researchers to be the first important medical historian. His *De Medicina* is an outstanding account of Roman medicine, and it bridges the gap between his times and those of Hippocrates. During this

period, massage had gained such acceptance that Julius Caesar (c. 100 to 44 BC) used it to help his epilepsy.

A group of Greek physicians residing in Rome, known as the Methodists, supported a simplistic view of healing and restricted their treatments to bathing, diet, massage, and a few drugs. The earlier practitioners and other groups recognized the importance of touch. The founder of this school of thought was **Asclepiades**. Among his many contributions to Roman medicine was a treatise on friction (massage) and exercise. Although the work is no longer in existence, Aulus Aurelius Cornelius Celsus (c. 25 BC to AD 50) cited it in his writings on friction.

A later follower of Hippocratic medicine was **Galen of Pergamon** (c. AD 130 to 200). Galen was a Roman physician who studied medicine in Alexandria (Egypt) and became the personal physician to the Roman emperor Marcus Aurelius. In at least 100 treatises, Galen combined and unified Greek knowledge of anatomy and medicine; his system continued to dominate medicine throughout the Middle Ages and until relatively recent times. Among his many works, Galen's *De Sanitate Tuenda* considers exercise, the use of baths, and massage. After the Roman Empire divided into eastern and western halves, the decline in learning was much more rapid and severe in the Roman West than in the Greek East (Byzantium).

Farther east of the Romans, the ancient Slavs reportedly used massage. In the Americas, the Mayas and Inca have been documented as practicing joint manipulation and massage. The Inca also used the application of heat in their treatments of joint disorders through the use of the leaves of the chilca bush. They had a higher success rate for *trepanation,* a surgical procedure involving the removal of a segment of the skull, in 2000 BC than the Europeans did in AD 1800. In addition, records indicate that the Cherokees and Navajos used massage in their treatments of colic and to ease labor pains.

*"People and places always have a past
and their identity dissolves unless they
recognize they have a history."*
Nathaniel Hawthorne

THE MIDDLE AGES

After the collapse of the Roman Empire (AD 476), Western medicine experienced a period of decline. In reality, it was only because of the writing efforts of a large number of Western physicians (e.g., Oribasius, Alexander of Tralles) that the ancient medical knowledge of the Greeks and Romans was preserved. After the decline of the Roman Empire, the Hippocratic-Galenic tradition survived in the Greek-speaking East. Then after the fall of Alexandria (AD 642), knowledge of Greek medicine spread throughout the Arabic world.

After the expansion of the Islamic world in the seventh and eighth centuries, the comprehensive body of Greco-Roman medical doctrine was adopted, together with extensive Persian and Hindu medical knowledge. One such example of this synthesis of knowledge was an encyclopedic work (*Kitabu'l Hawi Fi't-Tibb*) by the Persian physician **Rhazes**

(Abu Bakr Muhammad ibn Zakariya al-Razi) (c. AD 850 to 932), which discussed Greek, Roman, and Arabic medical practices, including massage. Another important work was by the Persian physician Abu-Ali al-Husayn ibn-Sina (AD 980 to 1037), generally known as **Avicenna**. He authored numerous medical books that remained the standard until the seventeenth century. His *Canon of Medicine* was an especially famous medical text, one that compiled the theoretical and practical medical knowledge of the time. The work illustrates the tremendous influence of Galen on the medical knowledge of the era; the text makes numerous references to the use of massage. In fact, by the end of the ninth century, almost all of Galen's lengthy medical texts had been translated into Arabic. Apparently the Islamic physicians of the European Middle Ages were more interested in developing and commenting on the truths learned from the Greeks and Romans than they were in discovering new knowledge. The Muslims simply incorporated Greco-Roman medical knowledge into the Islamic framework. Through Latin translations of these Arabic authors, most of the knowledge of Greek medicine was revived in the Christian West (i.e., Europe).

For the most part, Western medical practitioners of the Middle Ages abandoned massage in favor of other treatments. Massage did, however, remain an important procedure for folk healers and midwives, and its procedures were passed on as a healing art form. Subsequently, no early compilation of these techniques and procedures was undertaken.

During the course of the later Middle Ages, the collection, preservation, and transmission of classical medical knowledge occurred. After the twelfth century, medieval medical knowledge in the West expanded, thanks in part to the existing works by the Muslims, who had earlier translated Greek and Latin medical texts into Arabic. By the thirteenth century, medical knowledge had advanced to the point that three major European centers (Montpelier, Paris, and Bologna) were offering degrees in medicine. In 1316, Mondino dei Luzzi wrote *Anothomia,* the first modern treatise on anatomy.

With the revival of classical Greek learning during the Renaissance, Western medicine was revitalized by new translations of old Greek and Latin texts. Among the newly revived texts was Aulus Celsus's *De Medicina,* which came into circulation again, thanks to the newly invented printing press.

"Books are the DNA of civilization."
Anonymous

THE EUROPEAN RENAISSANCE AND ENLIGHTENMENT

The **Renaissance** (c. 1250-1550) was an exciting period in the history of medicine and medical treatments. The word *renaissance* means rebirth, and the Flemish physician, **Andreas Vesalius** (1514-1564) established the foundations of modern human anatomy (in the West) during this time. His *De Humani Corporis Fabrica* (1543) is considered one of the most important studies in the history of medicine. In addition, the Swiss physician Philippus von Hohenheim (1493-1541), better known as **Paracelsus**, laid the foundations of chemical pharmacology, as opposed to herbal remedies. New surgical procedures were also established, particularly those by the French military surgeon **Ambroise Paré** (c. 1510-1590). In addition to inventing several surgical instruments, Paré was among the earliest modern physicians to discuss the therapeutic effects of massage, especially in orthopedic surgery cases. Paré even went so far as to classify various types of massage movements.

> **evolve** *Log on to the Evolve website to see illustrations of Galen of Pergamon and Ambroise Paré.* ■

Two other notable Renaissance physicians were **Girolamo Mercuriale** (1530-1606) and **Timothy Bright** (c. 1551-1615). Mercuriale spent several years in Rome examining the manuscripts of the ancient writers. His extensive knowledge of the attitudes of the Greeks and Romans toward diet, exercise, and their effects on health and disease is evident in *De Arte Gymnastica* (1569), considered to be the first book in the field of sports medicine. The work compiled the history of gymnastics up to that time, synthesizing all that had been written on the use of exercise (for both the purpose of health and the treatment of disease). Bright's first medical work (c. 1584) was divided into two parts, *Hygienina on Restoring Health* and *Therapeutica on Restoring Health.* In this work, Bright discussed baths, exercise, and massage, and he began teaching his ideas to students at Cambridge University in Cambridge, England.

Around the sixteenth century we see two important East Asian works that dealt with massage. The Chinese published *Chen-chiu ta-ch'eng,* which contained a chapter on pediatric massage, and the Japanese published *San-tsai-tou-hoei,* which mentioned both passive and active massage procedures.

By the end of the seventeenth century, Western medicine had experienced a revolution in both ideas and knowledge. In Italy, **Giovanni Alfonso Borelli** (1608-1679) carried out extensive anatomical dissections and had analyzed the phenomenon of muscular contraction. In England, **William Harvey** (1578-1657) had demonstrated that blood circulation in animals is impelled by the beat of the heart through arteries and veins (Figure 1-3). This discovery enhanced the acceptance of massage as a therapeutic measure. Another crucial development during the seventeenth century was the realization of the necessity to compile complete clinical descriptions of disease, generally at bedsides, and to develop specific remedies for each specific disease. In this area, the English physician Thomas Sydenham (1624-1689) was most prominent. At the same time these scientific advances were being made, massage was reemerging as a therapy that was acceptable to the medical profession and as a therapeutic practice for health and disease.

The European Renaissance and Enlightenment era also had an impact on Western medicine. What emerged was an optimistic outlook concerning the role and benefits of the field of medicine. The widely held belief asserted that health

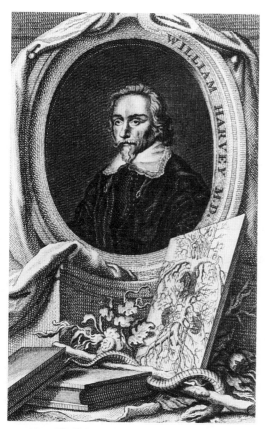

FIGURE 1-3 William Harvey.

was a natural state to be attained and preserved. Within this new philosophy, massage came to be viewed as a popular treatment in Europe. **Simon André Tissot** (1728-1797) published several works on gymnastic exercises that recommended massage for various diseases and gave indications for its use. The eighteenth century also saw the creation of new medical systems that incorporated the anatomical, physiological, and chemical discoveries of the previous 200 years. Some people believed that the gathering and dispensing of this new knowledge would add prestige to the medical profession and help weed out the *quacks.*

THE MODERN ERA

The era of modern massage began in the early nineteenth century when a wide variety of authors were advocating massage and developing their own systems. The most important of these writers was **Pehr Henrik Ling** (1776-1839), a Swedish physiologist and gymnastics instructor. Through his experiences at the University of Lund and the Swedish Royal Central Institute of Gymnastics, Ling developed his own system of medical (or Swedish) gymnastics and exercise, known as the *Ling System, Swedish Movements,* or *Swedish Movement Cure.* The primary focus of Ling's work was on gymnastics applied to the treatment of disease and injury. In this regard, Ling was a proponent of gymnastics, a subject that was promoted more than 2000 years earlier by Herodicus, the teacher of Hippocrates. According to Ling, his **Swedish gymnastics** was a therapeutic system by which we try—by means of influencing movement—to overcome discomfort that has arisen through abnormal conditions.

Ling's system consists of three primary movements: active, passive, and duplicated. *Active movements* were those performed by the patient (e.g., exercise). *Passive movements* were movements of the patient performed by the therapist (e.g., stretching, range of motion). *Duplicated movements* were those performed by the patient with the cooperation of the therapist (e.g., active assistive). As part of duplicated movements, the therapist may oppose (restrain) the patient's movements (active resistive). Other terms used to describe Swedish gymnastics are remedial gymnastics, table stretches, joint mobilizations, and range-of-motion exercises.

Massage was viewed as a component of Ling's overall system. He blended massage with physiology, which was just emerging as a science. Shortly thereafter, the term used to describe this new emphasis was **Swedish massage**. Rightly so, Ling is regarded as the father of Swedish massage. His followers used massage strokes in tandem with the movements described here. Swedish massage and Swedish gymnastics were noted to improve circulation, relieve muscle tension, improve range of motion, and promote general relaxation. This system eventually led to the development of physical therapy as a profession.

From 1813 to 1839, Ling taught these techniques at the Royal Central Institute of Gymnastics in Stockholm, Sweden, which he founded with governmental support. His students were responsible for spreading his ideas throughout the world. Among the more important cities with established schools that were teaching Ling's methods were St. Petersburg, London, Berlin, Dresden, Leipzig, Vienna, Paris, and New York. Within 12 years of his death (1839), 38 institutions in Europe were teaching the Swedish Movements system. Among these students were numerous medical physicians who became convinced of the usefulness of massage and therapeutic exercise in the practice of medicine. Medical physicians could complete Ling's Swedish gymnastics program in 1 year, as compared with 2 to 3 years for nonphysicians. As more physicians trained, massage became more and more acceptable as a traditional medical procedure and practice.

"Where all men think alike, no one thinks very much."
Walter Lippmann

Another key individual in the history of massage was the Dutch physician **Johann Mezger** (1817-1893) (Figure 1-4). Mezger is responsible for making massage a fundamental component of physical rehabilitation. He has also been credited with the introduction of the still-used French terminology to the massage profession (e.g., effleurage, pétrissage, tapotement). The French translated several of the Chinese books on massage, and this effort probably explains why the French terminology for the procedures has become so common in massage texts such as this one. Unlike Pehr Ling, Mezger, being a physician, was much more able than Ling to promote massage using a medical and scientific basis.

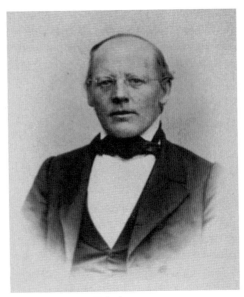

FIGURE 1-4 Johann Mezger.

In this regard, Mezger was quite successful in getting the medical profession to accept massage as a bona fide medical treatment for disease and illness more readily. A significant number of European physicians began to use massage therapy and to publish scientifically its positive results. What occurred was the inclusion of the art of massage in the science of medicine.

Two brothers, **George Henry Taylor** and **Charles Fayette Taylor**, introduced the Swedish Movement system into the United States in 1856. The Taylors had studied the techniques in Europe and returned to the United States, where they opened an orthopedic practice with a specialization in the Swedish Movements. The two physicians published many important works on Ling's system, including the first American textbook on the subject in 1860. A third prominent American follower of the Swedish Movements system was **Douglas O. Graham**. Not only was Dr. Graham a practitioner of the system, but from 1874 to 1925, he also authored several works on the history of massage.

Another prominent practitioner in the United States was **Hartvig Nissen**, who in 1883 opened the Swedish Health Institute for the Treatment of Chronic Diseases by Swedish Movements and Massage (Washington, D.C.). In 1888 Nissen presented the paper *Swedish Movement and Massage,* which was subsequently published in several medical journals. The result of publication was numerous letters from physicians who wanted to know more about Ling's system, and this inquiry led him to publish *Swedish Movement and Massage Treatment* in that same year. Taken together, Nissen's book and Graham's *A Treatise on Massage, Its History, Mode of Application and Effects* (1902) are generally credited with arousing interest in the U.S. medical profession in the benefits of massage.

While the Taylor brothers, Graham, and Nissen were convincing the medical community of the benefits of massage and gymnastics, several other individuals were busy convincing the general public. Among the most famous of these individuals was **John Harvey Kellogg** (1852-1943) of Battle Creek, Michigan. He wrote numerous articles and books on massage and published *Good Health,* a magazine that targeted the general public. Efforts by men such as Kellogg helped popularize massage in the United States.

The end of the nineteenth and beginning of the twentieth centuries witnessed important changes in the use of massage, the most important of which was the development of the field of physical therapy. Physical therapy, which developed from physical education, was responsible for the training of women to work in hospitals, where they used massage and therapeutic exercise to help patients recover.

World War I provided countless opportunities for the use of therapeutic massage, exercise, and other physiotherapeutic methods (electrotherapy and hydrotherapy) in efforts to rehabilitate injured soldiers. During the course of treating war casualties, the earlier ideas of **Just Lucas-Championniere** (1843-1913) were eventually recognized. Dr. Lucas-Championniere advocated the use of massage and passive-motion exercises after injuries, especially fractures.

By the beginning of the twentieth century, massage had begun to be used throughout the West. Once the procedures of massage were accepted, what developed was the profession of massage. In Great Britain, several women who realized the need for the standardization and professionalization of their trade formed *The Society of Trained Masseuses* (1894). The organization was successful in several key areas: establishing a massage curriculum; accrediting massage schools, which had to undergo regular inspections; requiring qualified instructors for the massage classes; and establishing a board certification program. By the end of World War I (1918), the Society had nearly 5000 members.

In 1920 the Society merged with the Institute of Massage and Remedial Exercise, and the new group became known as the *Chartered Society of Massage and Medical Gymnastics.* This new group also took some important steps at professionalism. Among the new membership requirements were physician referrals and the issuance of certificates of competence to persons who passed the required tests. By 1939 the membership in the organization numbered approximately 12,000.

After World War I, medical organizations such as the American Society of Physical Therapy Physicians also formed. In the 1920s and 1930s, programs for physical therapists were becoming standardized, while at the same time physicians were being trained in the field. In 1926 **John S. Coulter** became the first full-time academic physician in physical medicine at the Northwestern University Medical School in Evanston, Illinois. By 1947 the field of physical therapy and rehabilitation was established as a separate medical specialty.

Although many masseurs and masseuses frowned on the encroachment of the medical profession on their art form, the events just described can be viewed with excitement. By the early part of the twentieth century, the Western medical profession had begun to realize what the Chinese and masseurs and masseuses had long preached: Massage had an important place in the treatment of illnesses and diseases. The

PEHR HENRIK LING

Born: 1776; died: 1839. Father of physical therapy and Swedish massage.

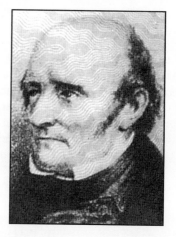

Born in Smaaland, one of the southern provinces of Sweden, Pehr Henrik Ling led an interesting life. After being expelled from school for disciplinary problems, Ling traveled through Europe and eventually returned to Sweden, where he learned fencing (the art of using a sword). In 1804 he accepted a post at the University of Lund, where he taught fencing and gymnastics. At the same time, he studied anatomy and physiology. In his teaching of fencing techniques, he noted that the movements he often wanted his pupils to make were hindered by motions that the student had learned from habit. Ling therefore resolved to teach the movements of the body in a systematic manner. For Ling, this training was important for military concerns, and he viewed fencing as an important part of gymnastics. What he meant was that soldiers could be taught to use weapons and move muscles in ways that were new to them.

At the same time, Ling also developed what is referred to as *Swedish gymnastics,* through which we try—by means of influencing movements—to overcome discomfort that has arisen through abnormal conditions. These gymnastics were composed of only a few stretching movements done by the student alone (active movements), performed by another pupil while the student relaxed (passive movements), or performed by the student with the cooperation of the pupil (duplicated movements such as active assistive and active resistive). In Ling's system, very little, if any, mechanical apparatus was involved.

In 1813 Ling opened the Swedish Royal Central Institute of Gymnastics, where he further developed his own system of medical gymnastics and exercise, known as the *Ling System, Swedish Movements,* or the *Swedish Movement Cure.* The primary focus of Ling's work was on gymnastics applied to the treatment of disease and injury. Massage (later known as Swedish massage) was viewed as a component of Ling's overall system.

Ling was not a physician, and his system of Swedish gymnastics was bitterly opposed by many people within the medical profession during much of his lifetime. However, many of his students were physicians, and these individuals spread his teachings and began to publish success stories of his techniques in respectable medical journals. Ling's influence was so great that, by 1851, 38 schools located throughout Europe were teaching his system of gymnastics and massage.

After years of failing health, Pehr Henrik Ling died in 1839. His legacy is seen today throughout the health professions, especially in the teachings of massage therapy, physical therapy, kinesiology, and gymnastics.

professionalism of medical gymnastics (now called *physical therapy*) simply meant that, in addition to learning the art of massage, the therapist needs also to acquire the scientific background necessary to understand human anatomy and physiology. As this textbook illustrates, the authors and contributors also believe in a well-educated, well-trained massage therapist.

As the health care system in the United States became influenced by biomedicine and technology in the early 1900s, physicians began assigning massage duties to nurses because massage therapy is labor intensive and time consuming. In the 1930s and 1940s, nurses lost interest in massage and abandoned the art. However, a small, dedicated group of therapist kept the art alive until the 1970s, when a new surge of interest developed as part of the fitness craze. This interest continues today.

As technology and medical advances caught up with the profession, a simple massage became decreasingly crucial on its own; it became one procedure in the arsenal of rehabilitation. As a consequence, the British Chartered Society of Massage and Medical Gymnastics changed its name to the Chartered Society of Physiotherapy. In 1943, postgraduates from the College of Swedish Massage in Chicago created the American Association of Masseurs and Masseuses (AAMM). The AAMM changed its name to the American Massage and Therapy Association in 1958 and then again changed its name to the American Massage Therapy Association (AMTA) in 1983. Over time, the AMTA evolved to represent the professional masseurs and masseuses, preferably called *massage therapists.* It is the second largest massage therapist organization, with chapters in all 50 states, and currently has more than 54,000 members in 27 countries.

evolve Log on to the Evolve website and access the course materials for Chapter 1. View the membership pin of the American Association of Masseurs and Masseuses from the 1960s, the current logo of the American Massage Therapy Association, and the current logo of the American Bodywork and Massage Professionals. ■

The Associated Bodywork and Massage Professionals (ABMP) was founded in 1987 as an organization that would include not only massage therapists but also all current and emerging bodywork styles. In 1996 ABMP had 15,000 active members. As of 2006, it has grown to 57,000 members and is currently the largest organization that serves massage therapists. The most significant different between the two

organizations is that AMTA's board is elected and ABMP's board is appointed.

"When you steal from one author, it's plagiarism; if you steal from many, it's research."
Wilson Mizner

NEW METHODS

To date, approximately 75 methods of massage therapy have been classified. Although space limitations prohibit detailed discussions of these procedures, a listing of several styles has been compiled on the *Evolve* website. These styles have been categorized according to their primary approach on the human body, mind, and spirit. Most of these styles were developed in the United States since 1960.

SUMMARY

In the last 25 years, massage has risen in popularity in the United States. Especially important in this rise of popularity are the individuals who are looking for alternative and complementary therapies (e.g., diet, exercise, herbal remedies, acupuncture, acupressure, massage) to supplement their medical treatments and create a positive impact on their health. Massage has been shown to be beneficial for many people.

As a consequence of this increase in popularity, the profession has also grown during this time. In 1988 the AMTA pushed for the development of national certification, which came in 1992 with the independent National Certification Examination for Therapeutic Massage and Bodywork. Massage therapy has become a respected and much-used allied health care profession. According to Eisenberg et al's *Trends in Alternative Medicine Use in the United States, 1990-1997*, massage therapy was the third most prevalent type of alternative and complementary medicine used by adults in the United States in the 1990s. New uses for massage therapy are being discovered daily, with a recent (April 2001) study published in the journal *Archives of Internal Medicine* documenting the effectiveness of massage for chronic back pain. The study also noted that massage was found to be superior to both acupuncture and self-care, over both the short- and long-term.

By no means is this study of massage history complete and exhaustive. A detailed history of massage would take volumes and entail years of research. This chapter should have provided a thorough sense of how the profession developed and in what direction it appears to be headed. More than 75 different varieties of massage and bodywork are available. This chapter has provided a glimpse of how they first began.

evolve

Go to *Chapter Extras* on Evolve for additional illustrations and resources for this chapter. *Extras* for this chapter include:

1. Crossword puzzle (downloadable form)
2. Chinese acupuncture chart (illustration)
3. Comprehensive list of massage methods (text)

MATCHING

Place the letter of the answer next to the term or phrase that best describes it.

A. Active
B. Amma
C. Arte Gymnastica
D. Ayur-Veda
E. Borelli
F. China

G. Harvey, William
H. Hippocrates
I. Ling, Pehr Henrik
J. Massage
K. Mezger, Johann

L. Middle 1900s
M. Nei-ching
N. Passive
O. Swedish gymnastics
P. Swedish massage

_____ 1.   The country in which the first written accounts of therapeutic rubbing (massage) originated

_____ 2.   The original massage technique

_____ 3.   The sacred Indian practice in which massage was included

_____ 4.   The father of modern Western medicine

_____ 5.   Systematic and scientific manipulation of the soft tissues of the body for the purpose of obtaining or maintaining health

_____ 6.   The individual whose efforts led primarily to texts that commonly use French terminology to describe massage strokes

_____ 7.   The classic scripture of traditional Chinese medicine

_____ 8.   Scientist who demonstrated that blood circulation is impelled by the beat of the heart through arteries and veins

_____ 9.   The work generally credited as being the first book in the field of sports medicine

_____ 10. The father of Swedish massage and physical therapy

_____ 11. Along with duplicated and active, the term that describes another movement that used Ling's system of medical gymnastics

_____ 12. Movements performed by the client

_____ 13. When the term *massage* came into use

_____ 14. The person who first analyzed the phenomenon of muscular contraction

_____ 15. Therapeutic system using movement to overcome discomforts that arise from abnormal conditions

_____ 16. A component of Ling's system that blends massage with the science of physiology

INTERNET ACTIVITIES

Visit http://www.amtamassage.org. What sources might be used by a layperson to check the credentials of a massage therapist?

Visit http://massagetherapy.com/careers/stateboards.php. Locate the licensing requirements in the state in which you wish to practice.

Using the websites for both American Bodywork and Massage Professionals at http://www.abmp.com and AMTA at http://www.amtamassage.org, and after reading, contrast and compare memberships to both organizations.

Bibliography

American Massage Therapy Association: *A short history: the American Massage Therapy Association,* 2004. Available at: *http://www.amtamassage.org/about/history.htm*

American Massage Therapy Association: *Advancing the massage therapy profession for 60 Years,* 2006. Available at: *http://www.amtamassage.org/about/history.html*

Basham AL: The practice of medicine in ancient and medieval India. In Leslie C, ed: *Asian medical systems,* Berkeley, Calif, 1976, University of California Press.

Buikstra JE: Diseases of the pre-Columbian Americas. In Kiple KF et al: *The Cambridge world history of human disease,* New York, 1993, Cambridge University Press.

Castiglioni A: *A history of medicine,* New York, 1947, Alfred A Knopf. (Translated by EB Krumbhaar.)

Coulter J: *Physical therapy,* New York, 1932, Paul B Hoeber.

Eisenberg D et al: Trends in alternative medicine use in the United States, 1990-1997: results of a follow-up national survey, *JAMA* 280(18):1569-1575, 1998.

Fryback P, Reinert B: Alternative therapies and control for health in cancer and AIDS, *Clin Nurse Spec* 11(2):64-69, 1997.

Goldberg J et al: The effect of therapeutic massage on H-reflex amplitude in persons with a spinal cord injury, *Phys Ther* 74(8): 728-737, 1994.

Hernandez J: *A history of massage therapy,* 2002. Available at: *http://www.chomg.com/history_of_massage_therapy.html*

Hippocrates: *Hippocrates, vol iii, on wounds in the head, in the surgery, on fractures, on joints, mochlicon,* Cambridge, 1928, Harvard University Press. (Translated by ET Withington.)

Liddel L: *The book of massage: the complete step-by-step guide to Eastern and Western techniques,* New York, 1984, Simon and Schuster.

McMillan M: *Massage and therapeutic exercise,* Philadelphia, 1921, WB Saunders.

Means PA: *Ancient civilizations of the Andes,* New York, 1931, C Scribner's Sons.

Meintz SL: Alternatives and complementary therapies: whatever became of the back rub? *RN* 58(4):49-50+, 1995.

Mulliner MR: *Mechano-therapy: a textbook for students,* Philadelphia, 1929, Lea & Febiger.

Nissen H: *Practical massage in twenty lessons,* Philadelphia, 1905, FA Davis.

Rahman F: *Health and medicine in the Islamic tradition: change and identity,* New York, 1987, Crossroad.

Salmon JW, ed: *Alternative medicine: popular and policy perspectives,* New York, 1984, Tavistock.

Solomon W: What is happening to massage? *Arch Phys Med* 31: 521-523, 1950.

Unschuld PU: History of Chinese medicine. In Kiple KF (ed) et al: *Cambridge world history of human disease,* New York, 1993, Cambridge University Press.

U.S. Department of Health and Human Services: *Acute pain management in adults: operative procedures-quick reference guide for clinicians,* Rockville, Md, 1992, The Department.

U.S. Department of Health and Human Services: *Management of cancer pain: adults-quick reference guide for clinicians,* Rockville, Md, 1994, The Department.

Veith I, Huang T: *Nei ching su wen,* Baltimore, 1949, Williams and Wilkins.

Wanning T: Healing and the mind/body arts: massage, acupuncture, yoga, tai chi, and Feldenkrais, *AAOHN J* 41(7):349-351, 1993.

White J: Touching with intent: therapeutic massage, *Holist Nurs Prac* 2(3):63-67, 1988.

Wide AG: *Handbook of medical and orthopedic gymnastics,* New York, 1905, Funk and Wagnall.

Zyzk KG: *Religious healing in the Veda, with translations and annotations of medical hymns in the Rgveda and the Atharvaveda and renderings from the corresponding ritual texts,* Philadelphia, 1985, American Philosophical Society. (Transactions of the American Philosophical Society, vol 75, p 7.)

Web Resources

The American Massage Therapy Association: A short history: the American Massage Therapy Association. Available at: *http://www.amtamassage.org/about/history.html.* Accessed Nov 1, 2002.

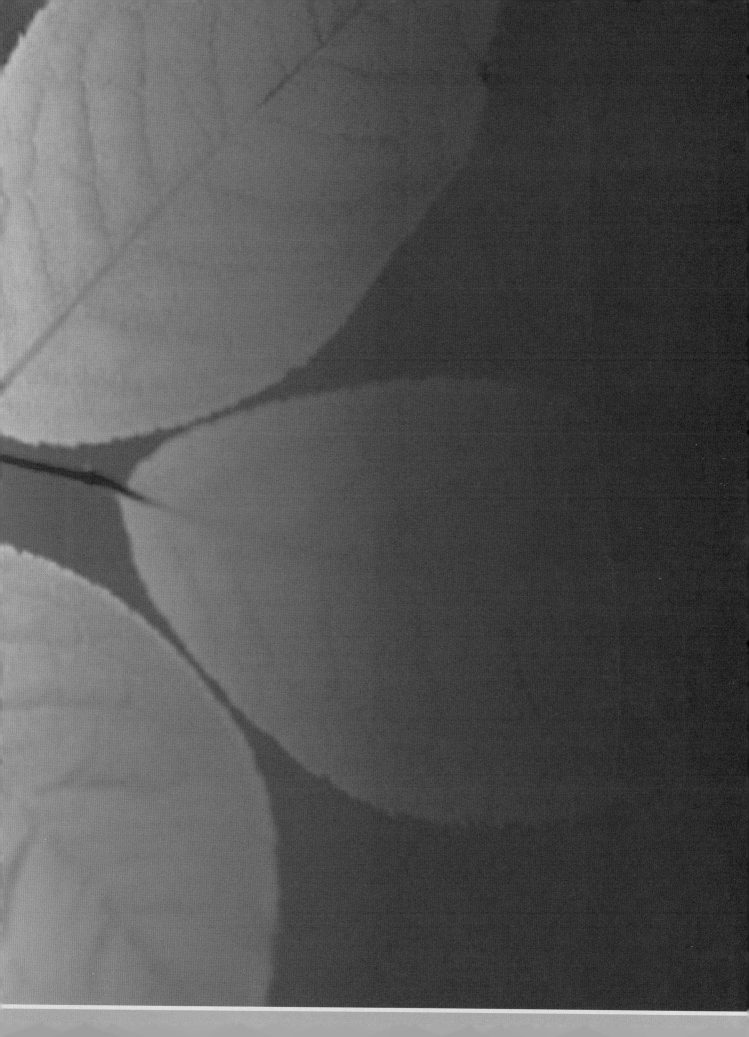

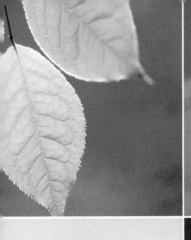

CHAPTER 2

The Therapeutic Relationship

STUDENT OBJECTIVES

After completing this chapter, the student should be able to:

- State all important elements of a therapeutic relationship
- Define appropriate strategies for problem solving
- Contrast and compare legal and ethical issues
- Contrast and compare self-disclosure with confidentiality
- Give the two factors limiting client confidentiality and examples of each
- Define scope of practice, giving what is often permitted and restricted by law
- List principles that constitute NCBTMB's and most regulatory state boards' code of ethics
- Name and discuss the six areas of NCBTMB's standards of practice
- Define boundaries and state their importance in the therapeutic relationship
- Identify characteristics of healthy boundaries
- Point out common mistakes that often lead to crossing boundaries
- Compare and contrast client neglect and client abuse
- Discuss reasons and ways to avoid conflicts of interests
- Compare and contrast transference and countertransference, stating "red flags" of each
- Define dual relationship, identifying reasons they exist and reasons why they are problematic
- State elements of intimacy, contrasting an intimate relationship with a therapeutic relationship
- Define sexual misconduct
- Cite examples of sexual misconduct and guidelines for sexual risk management
- Outline possible consequences of sexual misconduct
- Discuss steps taken when rumors of a fellow therapist's sexual misconduct are revealed

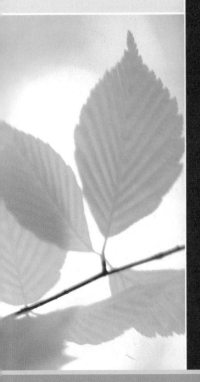

INTRODUCTION

The field of massage therapy can be divided into two major skill areas: (1) hard skills and (2) soft skills. Hard skills include knowledge of anatomy, physiology, pathology, tactile precision (what bony marking is felt), and massage acumen (e.g., how to work on a client's injured hamstring).

Equally, if not more, important are the soft skills of massage therapy. These skills include how to manage the relationship between the client and the therapist, or the therapeutic relationship. This chapter immerses the therapist candidate into the world of the therapeutic relationship. We begin with an overview of the relationship's elements, pausing to examine and acquire good communication skills. Next, we discuss how to resolve problems, because conflicts will arise.

Professionalism is presented as it relates to the therapeutic relationship, comparing legal with ethical issues and self-disclosure with confidentiality (Figure 2-1). This section contains a list of guidelines that a profession establishes to promote consistent professionalism and integrity. These standards apply to all massage therapists in a given jurisdiction and define how the individual therapist relates to the profession as a whole. Although geographically these standards may vary widely, they include many common and vital elements: scope of practice; a code of ethics; standards of practice; and regional, state, or municipal laws. Knowing the laws and standards that govern their profession, abiding by these laws, and adopting these standards are the responsibilities of the student and therapist.

The next area presented is boundaries. As the Robert Frost quotation reminds us, fences (a type of physical boundary) can enhance our relationships with others. Boundaries in all relationships impart a sense of self, a space to be, and a sense of protection. "Our profession has developed a very sophisticated technique for helping people, trial and error," a wise

therapist said to his colleagues. On hearing this statement, one of these colleagues replied, "Yes, and for every error we make, a new rule is created." The student will also find a set of guidelines to assist with ethical decision making. As we explore the topic of boundaries, we will discuss the characteristics of healthy boundaries, working with integrity, and we will outline common mistakes that therapists make within the therapeutic relationship. These mistakes include client neglect and abuse, conflicts of interests, dual relationships, and how to terminate a session appropriately when needed. The inevitable transference and countertransference are also discussed.

Finally, we will explore sexual misconduct, examining the differences between professional and intimate relationship with therapeutic relationships. Sexual risk management and the possibility of encountering a seductive client are outlined. The importance of including this valuable topic in a massage curriculum cannot be overstated. Once the chapter is complete, the therapist candidate will have more to offer his or her clients and the profession.

"The quality of the therapeutic relationship has consistently been shown to be more important than the therapist's clinical outlook."
Kalman Glantz and John Pearce

THERAPEUTIC RELATIONSHIP

Massage is a balance between technical and personal skills, at the heart of which lies the therapeutic relationship. Every time a therapist and a client come together in the context of therapy, this relationship is created. This relationship has a special purpose and goal: to serve the needs and best interests of our clients. This chapter offers guidance in navigating the

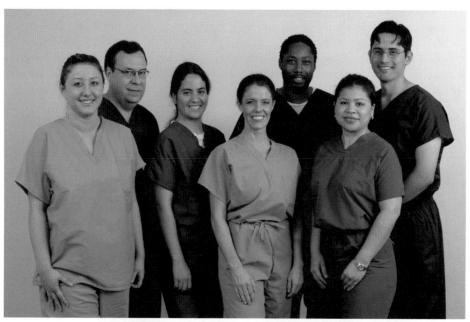

FIGURE 2-1 The massage therapist is a professional.

therapeutic relationship, which involves recognizing what does and does not belong in this experience.

A specific framework and good boundaries define the *therapeutic relationship.* The framework includes the following: communication, trust, client-centered care, compassion, safety, respect, responsibility, structured time, and a power imbalance.

Communication

Open communication must form the basis of the therapeutic relationship. Communication, the exchange of information, permeates every aspect of the therapeutic relationship. It occurs before the first massage, from the initial intake and consultation, to assessing pressure during the massage, to following up after the massage with self-care, subsequent session scheduling, and assessing the massage's effectiveness. The therapist will often use his or her ability to interpret the client's body language as a means of expressing unspoken discomfort felt during the massage.

A client reveals much about him or herself through communication; this information is called self-disclosure and is vital to developing a plan of care for each client. Additionally, boundaries are established and maintained through communication. When a lack of communication exists, ambiguity and resultant conflicts arise. The importance of good, open communication cannot be overstated.

Trust

Trust is the expectation to behave responsibly or honorably. Our clients are often vulnerable people; they come to us in pain or under considerable stress. Because clients are vulnerable, trust, along with open communication, must form the basis of the therapeutic relationship. The client must be assured that the therapist will respect his or her privacy. Trust will grow as a result of continued risk taking from subsequent sessions. The more history of trust we develop with a client, the better outcomes the client can expect. The client-therapist encounter can continue only under conditions of trust in the person and the therapy.

The client must also trust the therapist to do what is in the client's best interest. This concept includes practicing within the therapist's scope of practice and avoiding all opportunities for dual relationships (having more than one relationship with a client) and sexual misconduct. Establishing and maintaining boundaries promote the trust that is necessary for a viable therapeutic relationship.

If the therapist's demeanor, dress, or speech is inconsistent with the professionalism that the client expects, then the client can become alarmed and mistrustful of the competence of care. Trust can be easily upset not only by important issues but also by seemingly insignificant things. For example, if the therapist says that the client can call him or her any time the client needs to yet is not available when contacted, then the statement made is in fact untrue. This careless statement misleads the client, weakens trust, and might damage

the therapeutic relationship. Trust is a key element in establishing and maintaining the therapeutic relationship.

Client-Centered Care

Within any profession, standards are set forth to govern the actions of the individual therapist. This goal is accomplished by having a scope of practice, educational requirements, code of ethics, and standards of practice. These factors may all vary slightly from state to state, but they reflect the same common belief in client-centered care.

When the therapist has a client-centered approach to care, the client feels safe and well attended. The therapist views the client as a partner who shares decision-making power, such as having a voice in the planning process and agreeing with the course of treatment. The therapist should avoid any activity that removes the focus from the client, including conflicts of interest (selling products), dual relationships (turning clients into friends), and sexual misconduct (turning clients into lovers). All of the aforementioned scenarios remove the focus from the client.

Compassion

Compassion is the caring and thoughtful way we relate to our clients. Compassion, often considered as a *feeling,* can be developed into a state of consciousness, a state in which we empathize with our clients, feel close to them, and care about them, all within the context of the therapeutic relationship. Our boundaries, helpful and necessary parameters, are thought by some people to be cold, professional detachment. Compassion is a bridge between the client and the therapist. It can be argued that without compassion, no healing takes place.

Not only is compassion a bridge, but it is also the container for the therapeutic relationship. When being compassionate, the therapist may believe that the whole is greater than the sum of its parts. The therapist may feel the presence of God, nature, or a higher power while in the company of the client, and he or she may see the therapeutic relationship as being a sacred place. Compassion will make a difference in how you deliver the massage; it will help you stay focused on your client.

One story of compassion, offered by a Catholic priest, says much about compassion.

> *"Our job is not to lead people back to the*
> *old days when they trusted [professionals]*
> *and all the other authorities. Nor is our job*
> *to push them toward a premature solution in*
> *hopes of simplifying their lives; and ours."*

> *"We are companions on the journey. Our job is to*
> *suffer these confusing times with them until a new*
> *way emerges. Sometimes we will urge patience.*
> *But year after year, we will stay with them as they*
> *change, all the while we will keep saying, 'I am*
> *a witness that love and compassion works.'"*
> Father Walsh

Safety

The concept of safety in the therapeutic relationship has many aspects, all designed to protect the client from possible or actual harm or injury. First, practicing only within our scope of practice is a safety measure by understanding and respecting the legal parameters of our professional activities. To practice safely, we should also know and comprehend anatomy and physiology, how to address areas near endangerment sites, and how to identify and adapt treatment with regard to contraindications, as well as providing a safe and barrier-free workspace.

Safety and client protection also involve our professional boundaries and show the client that we are clear and careful with boundaries. Through boundaries, we create a sense of safety and security and a relationship that is predictable. Our client knows what to expect, a professional who is above reproach.

Safety also has its roots in communication. Time spent communicating with clients about boundaries and attaining client input regarding treatment planning lets them know that dual relationships are harmful and that we will avoid them because we care about the sanctity of the relationship. Communicating will let the client know that we will protect the therapeutic relationship by doing what is right for the client. While compassionately communicating, the safety of the therapeutic relationship allows the client to reveal more about him or herself. Listening opens the door for clients to feel a deeper sense of safety in the relationship and creates a more profound experience.

Respect

Respect refers to a consideration or thoughtfulness exhibited by words and actions. Respect in the therapeutic relationship has several implications, some of which are discussed in codes of ethics and standards of practice. A therapist must respect the inherent worth of both the client and the therapeutic relationship. Respect is demonstrated through communication during the informed consent process. Here, we explain the *who, how, why,* and *when* of treatment, which allows the client to ask questions and to work toward mutual agreement. We explain to the client the importance of self-disclosure and that all information will be closely guarded. We will inform the client that a breach of confidentiality is both illegal and unethical. Finally, we will let the client know that he or she has the right to refuse any treatment the therapist offers and to expect modifications or termination of treatment.

By having professional boundaries in place, we instill a sense of respect and dignity to our clients, to our profession, and to ourselves. We will also be respectful of client boundaries, valuing not only his or her time spent with us in a therapeutic context but also with regard to his or her personal space. This concept means that touching will take place only during treatment unless the client initiates a hug. Respectful hugs occur when the client is fully dressed, not on the treatment table. We also demonstrate respect for the client when we acknowledge the power differential that is intrinsic to the relationship and do not abuse this power.

Lastly, we show respect to other professions by not performing services for which we are not licensed, such as joint manipulations, prescriptive exercise, or individual counseling, all of which are under the practice of chiropractic, physical or occupational therapy, and psychotherapy, respectively.

Responsibility

Knowing and abiding by the laws and standards that govern the profession are our responsibilities as massage therapists. We possess a professional license and, with it, a professional responsibility and accountability. Being responsible also means refraining from using any substance that would interfere with the ability to make good judgments.

Part of our responsibility is to perform professional activities, which include but are not limited to performing a client intake, conducting assessments, developing a plan of care, obtaining informed consent and agreement of the proposed plan of care, and delivering treatment. Instructing clients on self-care and evaluating the success of the treatment plan, modifying it when needed, are also our responsibilities. We also inform clients as to their responsibilities, some of which are to keep appointments and to pay fees associated with treatments, as indicated by office policy and procedures.

Being a responsible professional also means to inform the client of our professional boundaries, to role model good boundaries, and to maintain them as needed.

Being responsible for our behavior requires periodic self-evaluation, taking inventory of our personal needs and making sure they are met in appropriate ways. The therapeutic relationship is not the place for a therapist to have his or her personal needs met. Doing so sabotages the relationship and opens the door for dual relationships and countertransference (therapist bringing his or her unresolved issues or personal needs into the relationship). We need to be clear about our intentions, focusing on the client and putting his or her needs before our own. Therapeutic progress can be hindered when we use our clients, perhaps unconsciously, to fulfill our own needs. The person in the professional role is held responsible for any negative consequences of his or her actions.

Finally, we have the responsibility to confront a fellow therapist if we hear rumors of unethical or illegal behaviors. If rumors are validated, and if the therapist refuses to be responsible for his or her own actions, the responsible therapist then files a complaint with the proper authorities.

Structured Time

When clients come in for scheduled appointments, the time spent with them is limited and structured. This concept means all attention and focus is on them, that the therapist starts and ends on time, and that nothing interrupts the session. Within the given time frame, anticipated activities occur. The time spent with the client, though limited, should not be rushed. This task may be accomplished by the therapist's relaxed attitude.

Power Differential

Inevitably, a therapeutic relationship will produce a power differential. One person, the client, has a particular need and comes for help to another who is more knowledgeable and skilled, namely the therapist. Sandy Fritz, in her book *Fundaments of Therapeutic Massage* reminds us that clients usually lie down or are seated and the therapist is positioned above them, creating an impression of authority.

This imbalance of power is a natural occurrence in the therapeutic relationship and, in and of itself, is not a problem. Problems may arise when this power is misused to serve the interests of the therapist rather than the client. Any time a power differential exists in a relationship and the person who wields the greater power does not recognize or respect the boundaries of the other, client abuse and client neglect can occur. Nevertheless, the law holds the professional to a higher standard of behavior because of the power differential. The power dynamic between client and therapist does not empower the client to say *no* easily to the therapist.

The therapist must be respectful of the power imbalance and allow it to invoke a sense of reverent power. Reverent power refers to warmth, compassion, and empathy toward the person who is weak or vulnerable. A therapist who develops reverent power uses his or her position to strengthen the client's own internal power and capacity to heal. The therapist uses the power to serve the client.

COLLEGIAL RELATIONSHIPS

The therapeutic relationship goes beyond the one-on-one relationship between therapist and client. It encompasses all professional relationships, including those between health care providers and between the therapist and individuals providing service to the client (e.g., insurance agents). If a physician refers a client to a massage therapist, the therapist must then honor the physician's stricter code of ethics on all accounts, including the preclusion of social contact. The more conservative code of ethics always prevails. Although massage and complementary and alternative therapies encompass many diverse modalities, we must acknowledge a common set of values that serve not only the client but also the entire field. These values include codes of ethics, standards of practice, professional boundaries, and the way in which we conduct ourselves in the therapeutic relationship.

The therapist should relate to any health care approach or treatment plan that acknowledges, respects, and focuses on the needs, expectations, priorities, and satisfaction of the client in the therapeutic relationship.

COMMUNICATION SKILLS

Communication is the act of exchanging information through words, actions, behaviors, body language, and feelings. Communication skills are used in listening, speaking, writing, and assessing nonverbal messages. Communication skills are used in initiating, developing, and maintaining the therapeutic

relationship; greeting the client; explaining and informing the client of services and procedures; collecting and reviewing client information; gaining informed consent; assessing the needs of the client; and developing a treatment plan and room orientation.

Intentions behind communications must be considered because this area gives rise to our behaviors and actions. Even with the clearest intention, delivering a nonverbal signal that may distort or even contradict the intended message is possible. What is seen, what is felt, and what is heard must all match to deliver a congruent, consistent message.

When the client reveals his or her thoughts and feelings, this action is known as *self-disclosure*. The therapist can assist this process by effective communication—hearing what the client is saying, interpreting the message, giving feedback or helpful directions, and performing the massage session according to the information that was received. Communication is vital to the therapeutic relationship. Information is needed to make decisions regarding therapy; this information needs to be clear and concise. Successful communication leads to a satisfied client, one who believes that he or she has been heard.

Good communication skills include:
- Developing effective speaking and listening skills, nonverbal communication techniques, and attitude such that clients believe that time spent with them is not rushed.
- Encouraging clients to ask questions and to participate in the decision-making process.
- Using tact, good judgment, and diplomacy when conducting professional affairs.

Speaking to Clients

Verbal communication is a cooperative effort and includes effective speaking and listening skills, as well as an understanding and use of body language. An effective speaker pauses and asks for periodic feedback to verify that the message he or she intends is the message being received. When asking for feedback, use *open-ended questions*. These questions allow the client to reflect and to clarify his or her own thoughts and feelings and to produce more accurate information. *Closed-ended questions* by comparison are more direct and require a *yes* or *no* response. Once feedback is received, the speaker can make appropriate alterations or corrections (Figure 2-2).

An effective speaker also considers the background or education of the receiver and uses words that the receiver understands. Using anatomical names and medical terminology may be inappropriate for clients who do not have the background or training in these areas.

Listening to Clients

An effective, or active, listener is one who reflects on the other person's message by making a brief statement of the essence of the message in his or her own words. Effective listening is a good way to prevent communication breakdowns assumptions that lead to inappropriate planning, ultimately resulting in client dissatisfaction. Common reflective techniques are paraphrasing, clarifying, and exploring.

Paraphrasing involves stating in your words what you believe the client has said. You may use phrases such as "What I hear you saying is...," "In other words...," "So basically how you feel is...," and so on. The client may acknowledge that you heard correctly, or he or she may resend the message with additional information.

Clarifying involves asking the client for additional information because you are not sure if you understood the intended message. Because they are symbols, words have a wide interpretation from person to person. The meaning of a word such as *pain* varies significantly from one person to another. Is the pain mild, moderate, or severe? Does it occur every day, all day, or only with certain movements or activities? Words such as *a lot, all the time,* and *always* require clarification and feedback to ensure that the therapist understands the client's experience.

Exploring is used to develop a deeper understanding and clearer insight into the client and is demonstrated during the interview discussed in Chapter 8. The therapist assists communication by requesting information through the client intake form. The therapist verbally reviews the completed form to clarify or uncover facts that would be helpful in determining treatment plans and goals, contraindications, and needed referrals.

For the client to believe that the therapist is giving focused attention to receive his or her message, a key ingredient—nonverbal communication—is needed.

> *"No man ever listened himself out of a job."*
> Calvin Coolidge

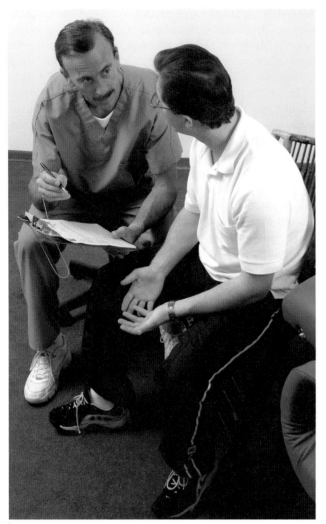

FIGURE 2-2 The massage therapist and the client have a therapeutic relationship.

and misconstrued intentions, which are typically at the root of most ethical dilemmas. Most of us falsely assume that we are listening when we hear. Listening requires focused attention.

Empathy during communication assists the client in revealing more about him or herself. It shows that the therapist is interested in listening. Being empathic requires that the therapist put him or herself in the client's shoes and to understand information from the client's point of view. Listening with empathy requires the therapist to consider the client's words, feelings, and intent. The client will feel a deeper sense of safety if the message is acknowledged. Empathetic listening is the highest form of listening. It takes the most work but reaps the greatest reward.

Effective Listening

A reflective response verifies that the therapist has understood the feelings and content of the client's message and mirrors this understanding back to the client. The client can then correct or modify the listener's perceptions. Unless time is taken to reflect and receive feedback, the therapist may make incorrect

Nonverbal Communication

We communicate with others using five methods: (1) words, (2) tones, (3) gestures, (4) posture, and (5) facial expressions. Because four out of five methods of communicating are nonverbal, body language often gives the therapist more complete information than the spoken word. Nonverbal cues indicate how the client is feeling and his or her internal state. Body language includes the following:

- Facial expressions such as grimaces, frowns, puckers, rapid blinking, and eye contact
- Gestures such as making fists, gripping the table, fidgeting, looking down, and nodding
- Sudden movements such as the toes coming up off the table, buttocks tightening, change in breathing, and lifting of the head
- Sounds such as sighs, grunts, groans, *hmm,* and *uh-huh*
- Posture in relation to others (when one is seated higher than another, or one is standing and one is sitting, usually implying that the higher person is more important or has more power)

In many instances, the client may not tell you that a certain massage move or pressure is too intense or uncomfortable. Body language will communicate his or her unspoken

How Much Do Our Words Really Mean?

Research provided by Dr. Albert Mehrabian, Professor of Psychology at the University of California, Los Angeles, offers his classic statistic on the effectiveness of spoken communication. This model is important to consider factors other than words when conveying a message.

Words we say—7%
How we say them—38%
Body language—55%

discomfort. Look for congruency between what the client says and what his or her body language tells you.

Report your observations. Telling the client what you observe often improves the communication process because what you are observing can be affirmed or denied. Always use personal inquiry over assumed meaning.

Remember that, whether consciously or unconsciously, the client is also reading your body language. The information you project with your body language may affect therapeutic relationships. The client may be distracted if the therapist is speaking in a way that says the client is important but is glancing at the clock and ruffling through papers as if in a hurry. Generally, the strongest message—the message the listener will receive and remember—is the unspoken message because it is perceived to be the most honest (Box 2-1).

The prudent therapist is aware of his or her own body language and uses this information to note discrepancies between the therapist's own emotional and intellectual realities. If the therapist consciously projects an open, caring, professional image through nonverbal body language, then it will strengthen the weight carried by his or her words. When actions match words, the result is an increased feeling of authenticity, comfort, and security for the client.

CONFLICT AND CONFLICT RESOLUTION

When communication is lacking, ambiguity and the resultant conflicts arise. Boundaries become vague, or subservient roles are assumed (see section on Transference and Countertransference). Conflicts may arise interprofessionally with communication between massage colleagues or communication with other health care providers. Some sources of conflicts among physical therapists, chiropractors, or even fellow massage therapists may occur when one professional refers clients to the other, and the professional to whom the client is being referred does not reciprocate. Other potential conflicts include perception of another as an economic threat or as unfair competition.

Conflicts between the client and the therapist often arise when expectations are not met; the therapist is late starting a massage, the therapist does not address problem areas that the client reveal during the massage, or the client cancels an appointment for the third time in a month.

The ability to negotiate and arrive at resolution is part of being a competent, successful therapist and is necessary for having and maintaining healthy relationships. Conflicts that arise provide an invitation to explore resolution options. Creativity must be used because all conflicts will not be resolved using one method. Suggestions for problem solving when conflicts arise are listed here and in Table 2-1.

- Identify and accept the problem.
- Communicate with *I* messages instead of *you* messages; *you* messages can be perceived as blaming the other party.

TABLE 2-1 Healthy and Unhealthy Conflict Resolution Strategies

STRATEGY	ACTION	BY
Fight	Trying to impose one's preferred solution on the other party	Insisting Blaming Criticizing Accusing Shouting
Submit	Lower aspirations and settle for less than one would have liked	Giving in Giving up Agreeing to simply end the conflict Surrendering to what the other wants
Flee	Choose to leave the scene of the conflict	Ceasing to talk Leaving physically, cognitively, and/or emotionally Changing the topic
Freeze	Choose to wait for the other's next move	Waiting Doing nothing
Problem solve	Pursue alternatives that satisfy both sides; develop a win-win strategy	Talking Listening Gathering information Thinking Generating options Resolving

- Have healthy boundaries, which are essential to conflict resolution.
- Look for solutions that are in the best interest of the relationship.
- Be open to a variety of solutions.
- Do not take problems and differences personally.
- Let each party keep his or her respect and dignity.
- Do not deny an adversarial reaction if it is present, but do not assume one either.
- Take full responsibility for your own behavior.
- Communicate clearly about what you want and need; consistently forgoing what you want and need is not conflict resolution.
- Consider the wants and needs of yourself and others as important.
- Separate issues from people.
- Avoid power plays.
- Pick your battles carefully, asking yourself if this issue will matter in 5 or 10 years.
- Save ultimatums for absolute nonnegotiations or late-stage negotiations.
- Do not waste time negotiating nonnegotiables.
- Take time out when angry emotions are running high; step back and look at the problem before reacting.
- Look for the gift or the lesson after the conflict is resolved.

PROFESSIONALISM

Professionalism demonstrates ethical behavior while performing business practices; it is the act of technical competency, reflected in the individual's professional attitude and code of conduct, conveyed to the public. We are fully responsible for what we say and do at all times. The first session is the ideal opportunity to set a professional tone. Because our clients are the most vulnerable of all, open communication must form the basis of the therapeutic relationship.

Professionalism includes not only what people see, or professional image, but also how business is conducted (Box 2-2). The results of our actions and behaviors have a tremendous impact not only on our clientele but also on every person with whom we have a relationship. They have the potential to affect not only our clients but also their families, our colleagues, and the community at large. These aspects of professionalism incorporate confidentiality, scope of practice, codes of ethics, and standards of a professional massage practice. Professionalism needs to be practiced and refined as much as does technique.

Professional Image

Although creating a reputable image clearly serves the individual therapist, it also serves the profession. The massage therapist aspires to hold and maintain a professional image that is credible. Projecting a favorable image includes acting within professional boundaries and demonstrating how the therapist addresses client concerns. It also involves how the therapist is dressed. Wearing a uniform or clothing that separates the

---

BOX 2-2

Qualities of a Professional Massage Therapist

Professional massage therapists have knowledge of techniques and principles that include an understanding of legal and ethical issues. They must also acquire a working knowledge of and tolerance for human nature and individuals' characteristics, given that daily contact with a wide variety of individuals with a host of problems and concerns is a significant part of the work. Courtesy, compassion, and common sense are often cited as the *three Cs* most vital to the success of a massage therapist.

In fact, the first responsibility of a massage therapist is always to provide competent, courteous, and compassionate health care to clients. Other characteristics of a professional massage therapist include:

- Has an aptitude for working with his or her hands
- Is computer literate
- Has good communication skills that include writing, speaking, and listening
- Has and maintains professional boundaries and integrity
- Avoids dual relationships
- Is trustworthy and exhibits a sense of responsibility
- Prepares and maintains client records
- Keeps client information confidential
- Leaves private concerns at home
- Has patience in dealing with others and the ability to work as a member of a team
- Practices with competence and within the scope of his/her training and capabilities
- Projects a favorable professional image
- Possesses expertise that comes through three main sources: technical competence, social validation (through a formal recognition of training and status), and reputation
- Has a relaxed attitude when meeting new people
- Starts and ends each session on time and lets nothing interrupts a session
- Has an understanding of and empathy for others
- Uses appropriate guidelines when releasing information
- Uses tact when resolving conflicts
- Has a willingness to learn new skills and techniques

---

therapist from the client not only makes a statement regarding how we feel about our profession and ourselves, it also helps create a professional atmosphere. In fact, no second chance to make a first impression exists. Additionally, business cards, brochures, and how clients report your work to others constitute professional image.

A therapist may find that evaluating his or her professional image annually is useful. This process should include evaluation from him or herself and other trusted colleagues or mentors. Be open and willing to transform your image, if needed.

LEGAL VERSUS ETHICAL ISSUES

As massage therapists, we examine legal and ethical issues. Knowing the difference and possible consequences are necessary when making decisions during the course of a career.

An issue is *legal* in nature because of the fact that laws, rules, and regulations are associated with it. The primary purpose of laws regarding massage therapy is to protect the public by providing guidelines for obtaining and maintaining licensure. Ideally, laws promote smooth functioning of a society. If laws are broken, then civil or criminal liabilities may occur. On conviction, the therapist may be fined, imprisoned, have his or her license revoked, or suffer other penalties as determined by courts. Laws, rules, and regulations constitute legal issues associated with massage therapy.

The primary purpose of *ethics* is to elevate standards of competence. Ideally, professional ethics build a set of professional values and ideals. If these principles and standards are not followed, then the therapist in violation may be suspended or evicted from the professional society of which he or she is a member, as decided by peers.

SELF-DISCLOSURE AND CONFIDENTIALITY

Beginning at the initial contact and continuing during the course of the therapeutic relationship, clients will reveal their thoughts and feelings to the therapist. Honest and open sharing of these emotions, as well as ideas and insights, is known as **self-disclosure**. As time spent with the therapist progresses, and as the client experiences emotional safety, more of him or herself will be revealed. The therapist must closely protect this information. The safekeeping of this knowledge is called **confidentiality** and is considered the nondisclosure of privileged information; that is, it may not be divulged to a third party. A breach of confidentiality is both illegal and unethical. Self-disclosure and confidentiality are important aspects of the therapeutic relationship.

Confidentiality concerns each client's right to and guarantee of privacy and safety within the therapeutic relationship. This concept means that the client's name, details of his or her treatment, and information shared by the client during sessions are not to be divulged to anyone. Trust is a key element in establishing and maintaining the therapeutic relationship. Anyone who comes to a therapist must be assured that the provider will respect his or her privacy. If the client tells his or her family and friends about the quality of care received, then it is obviously his or her right.

In all social situations, the therapist must do everything in his or her power to protect the confidentiality of the client. Name-dropping is rarely impressive and only reveals us as therapists who do not protect a client's privacy. Telling a third party that someone is a client is never a good idea; doing so risks offending the client. In situations in which the therapist receives a referral from a current client, avoid sharing information regarding the common acquaintance with either client.

The therapist should avoid initiating conversation with a client in a social setting because of the confidentiality factor. Perhaps you might make eye contact, smile, give a nod of courtesy, and allow the client to determine whether to initiate a conversation. Because many social settings exist in which both you and your client may be present, discuss how these situations will be handled beforehand, even as part of the initial visit. Take time to explain that you respect the client's privacy and must ensure confidentiality at all cost.

Respecting confidentiality also means that treatment rooms are in a private setting and should be soundproof so that people standing or passing the room cannot hear talking during the session.

Professional confidentiality is limited by two factors: (1) the therapist's obligation to the law and (2) the therapist's obligation to others.

Regarding the therapist's obligation to the *law,* client records can be subpoenaed by a court of law. Insurance companies require copies of client records before reimbursement is made. The client's written consent must be obtained before the records can be released (see Chapter 8 for more information). Instances when we can legally breach confidentiality include those when a threat to self or others, when suspicion of child or elder abuse, or when a medical emergency exists.

Regarding the therapist's obligation to *others,* releasing his or her records to other health care providers (e.g., physicians, physical or occupational therapists, chiropractors) may be in the client's best interest when working as part of the client's health care team. Our professional experience and opinion may be needed to develop further an overall treatment plan for the mutual client. Again, obtain the client's written consent before releasing the record. Other third-party involvement can include a translator for someone with a language barrier or a relative who has power of attorney for a disabled client.

PROFESSIONAL STANDARDS

In general, professional standards help define and distinguish our profession from other health care professions. As our profession grows, more distinct borders, which give our profession limitations, will be defined. We can call these parameters our professional standards. These standards include the requirements for education and certification, testing and licensing, scope of practice, code of ethics, and standards of practice.

> ### TABLE TALK
>
> The National Certification Test is developed and administered by a private entity, and it is not a state test, even though many states use it for their regulation of massage.

Scope of Practice

Scope of practice is the profession's working parameters. It is often derived from the legal definition of massage and represents professional boundaries and limitations. Scope of practice defines what services that massage therapists can and cannot provide. Being aware of our limits of competency and being clear on our scope of practice ensures us the objectivity to refer a client elsewhere when the need arises. Therapists are required to know and practice only within the scope of practice outlined by the state in which they practice. We need to know what the limits of our skill and our physical abilities are; taking on a client whom we cannot serve well is unethical.

A therapist's scope of practice often restricts professional activities. For example, a massage therapist cannot provide specific information regarding nutrition or perform medical interventions. Massage therapists can neither diagnose nor prescribe medications. Massage therapists cannot provide any other service or therapy that would require a license to practice, such as psychotherapy, chiropractic, acupuncture, physical therapy, or any other branch of medicine, unless we have a license to do so.

As massage therapists, we have a license to touch. What other allowable professional activities can a massage therapist do in addition to massage?

- Encourage clients to pursue a healthy lifestyle (our example is the best teacher).
- Teach preventive measures such as stress-reduction and stress-management techniques, effective breathing techniques, progressive relaxation, and meditation.
- Suggest general dietary modifications when necessary.
- Offer specific recommendations of self-care that are related directly to your service, such as self-massage.
- Perform a general assessment of the client's condition by intake form, interview, and palpation, as well as by consultation with the client's other health care providers.
- Formulate a plan of care based on client assessment.
- Use hydrotherapy and aromatherapy to enhance the benefits of massage.

Code of Ethics

A **code of ethics** is a set of guiding moral principles that governs the individual's course of action. Most licensed health care professions have a code of ethics that members of these professions are expected to follow when working within their scope of practice. Most codes of ethics for massage therapists include governing principles for therapeutic relationships, for professional behavior, for business policies, and for guidance in decision making. These standards of professional conduct help ensure that the welfare of every client remains the priority.

A code of ethics is important to the integrity of any profession. Over time, these codes have evolved and will continue to develop. Ethics within health care fields are concerned with establishing and maintaining proper relationships between individuals coming in for treatment and professionals rendering treatment. Ethics are about relationships. Realizing that clients cannot be unethical is also important. Clients do not have a code of ethics that is tied to their license and professional activities.

Ethics may be a gray area because they reflect our personal values, morals, and principles. Together, our personal

and professional codes of ethics form the basis of all ethical decision making and resultant conduct. Our thoughts, beliefs, and feelings cannot be regulated, but our professional conduct can and is regulated by established professional codes of ethics. When our personal value system conflicts with our professional code of ethics, the professional code of ethics must prevail.

The National Certification Board for Therapeutic Massage and Bodywork (NCBTMB) sets forth both a code of ethics and standards of practice for all certified bodywork practitioners under the organization's purvey. Under examination, the codes of ethics set forth by massage organizations and state licensing boards share the following principles:

- **Confidentiality:** By maintaining client confidentially, we demonstrate honor and respect for each individual.
- **Continuing education:** Through continuing education, therapists stay current with new and developing information and techniques that benefit their clients.
- **Discrimination:** When conducting professional activities, massage therapists cannot discriminate against anyone, specifically regarding race, nationality, gender, religion, or sexual preference.
- **Honesty:** Therapists are required to be honest about their qualifications. Honesty also refers to policing the profession to the extent that we are required to report professional misconduct of a fellow therapist to the proper authorities.
- **Informed consent:** Spending time to inform a client about services and requesting consent to perform those services demonstrate the client participation in the therapeutic relationship.
- **Laws and legislation:** A massage therapist is expected to follow not only the rules and regulations set forth by regulatory agencies but state and local laws as well; this concept is known as the *law of the land*.
- **Professional boundaries:** Avoiding dual relationships and conflicts of interest helps keep the client's highest good as the main focus when conducting professional activities.
- **Quality of care:** The therapist aspires to provide the highest quality of care for each client.
- **Scope of practice:** Therapists are required to know and practice only services stated in their scope of practice outlined by the state in which they practice.
- **Sexual contact:** Therapists are required to avoid initiating or engaging in sexual contact with clients, which includes areas such as proper draping, touching genitalia, and professional attire. Even comments of a sexual nature are prohibited.

NCBTMB's entire code of ethics can be found in Appendix A.

Making Ethical Decisions

When using a code of ethics and standards of practice to help make decisions, some basic guidelines help the therapist maintain the sanctity of the therapeutic relationship.

- Is the decision in the client's best interest?
- Could the decision damage the therapeutic relationship?

- Is the therapist being respectful of the power imbalance and/or the transference (client transferring feelings, thoughts, and behaviors related to someone else onto the therapist) effect?
- Does the decision create a dual relationship, thus injuring the therapeutic relationship?
- Does the decision take us beyond our scope of practice, our training and expertise, or the confines of informed consent?

Some ethical dilemmas are not so much a question of right or wrong but more *which action will do the most good and the least harm.*

In these ambiguous situations, massage therapists may choose to consult an *ethics committee;* these members are specialists who confer with one another; and in some cases professors who teach ethics, to help them make difficult decisions.

Most professions have codes of ethics, and these codes often differ. If another health care provider (e.g., orthopedist, chiropractor, physical or occupational therapist, nurse practitioner) refers a client to a massage therapist, the therapist must honor the stricter code of ethics on all accounts, including the preclusion of social contact. In the cases in which a massage therapist possesses more than one professional license, the profession with the strictest code of ethics would prevail and becomes the standard of conduct for the individual in every therapeutic relationship. In other words, the more conservative code of ethics prevails. To be aware of these guidelines, the therapist may consult the other health care provider or obtain a copy of his or her code of ethics (online or library search).

Standards of Practice

Standards of practice are guiding principles by which members of an organization conduct their day-to-day responsibilities within their scope of practice. Whereas a code of ethics offers guidance for making ethical and moral decisions, the standards are stated in observable and measurable terms. They are statements of enforceable guidelines for professional conduct, as well as actions that will be taken if not followed. The six areas relating to the standards of practice of NCBTMB include the following:

- Professionalism
- Legal and Ethical Requirements
- Confidentiality
- Business Practices
- Roles and Boundaries
- Prevention of Sexual Misconduct

NCBTMB's entire standards of practice can be found in Appendix B.

"In the End, we will conserve only what we love, we will love only what we understand, we will understand only what we are taught."
Baba Dioum (Senegalese conservationist)

BOUNDARIES

In this section, boundaries in the professional arena are outlined. Being aware of boundaries and limitations is crucial to having healthy relationships. If a therapist is unaware of his or her boundaries, then he or she cannot establish or maintain them, and unintentional or intentional abuse is therefore more likely to occur. Boundaries are about safety and protection.

A boundary can be defined as a set of parameters indicating a border or limit. A **boundary,** with regard to relationships, marks or delineates the differences between clients and therapists.

The concept of boundaries has many aspects; they define our personal and professional space, our emotional separateness, our sense of autonomy, how we conduct our business affairs, and how we establish and maintain different kinds of relationships. Boundaries in a family or marital relationship are quite different than those in a therapeutic relationship.

Boundaries clarify each person's role, responsibilities, expectations, and limitations. Boundaries are negotiated and maintained through communication. Communicating with your clients about your professional boundaries and limitations is vital, given that all interactions occur at boundaries—yours and theirs—where you (the therapist) end and where he or she (the client) begins. Through boundaries, healthy relationships are established that are predictable and create a sense of safety and security for clients. Establishing and maintaining respectful boundaries between practitioner and client promotes the trust necessary for a viable therapeutic relationship.

As professionals, we must be sensitive to and respect the rights and boundaries of others. By respecting the boundaries of others, we instill a sense of dignity and respect to our clients, to our profession, and to ourselves.

The irony is that good boundaries cannot be learned from a book; we have to experience them. Hopefully, examples of good boundaries and healthy relationships were role modeled in each person's past. If so, then we know how he or she feels and how safe we feel when we are working with someone who is clear and careful with boundaries. If not, then seek out an individual who personifies healthy boundaries in the context of a therapeutic relationship. Spend time with this person discussing his or her concept of boundaries. A professional counselor may also be helpful in exploring the concept of boundaries.

Given that a vast majority of individuals are visual learners, an image of a boundary may be helpful when creating healthy boundaries. For example, picture being surrounded by a cell's semipermeable membrane. The membrane keeps poisons out, lets nutrients in, and excretes wastes. It also defines the cell's existence by separating it from other cells. Healthy cells have intelligence because they knew whether to be a kidney cell or a brain cell.

Another example is the body's immune system, which functions to maintain the boundary of the body's unique individuality, distinguishing and keeping out what is *not* me.

MOSHE FELDENKRAIS, DSc

Born: May 6, 1904; died: February 9, 1984.

"We settle for so little! As long as we can get by, we let it go at that."

Moshe Feldenkrais's father sold bits of forests, and that was the only ordinary thing about the man. Feldenkrais was reared in the Talmudic tradition and came from a long line of rabbis, some still famous today. Feldenkrais changed his nationality three times before he left home at 13—from Polish to German to Russian. In 1918, at the close of WW I, he left for Turkey, never to see his family again.

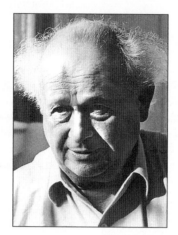

Although Feldenkrais would eventually obtain his doctorate in science and degrees in both mechanical and electrical engineering and proceed to work on the French atomic research program and the British antisubmarine program, he found his passion quite early in life.

As a boy of 16 in Palestine, Feldenkrais was part of a group called the *Haganah,* which means self-defense force. They learned some basic jujitsu, which did not prove successful. At this time in his life, Feldenkrais realized that the only way to learn was to start at the beginning—with the first move.

"And I built this system of defense for any sort of attack where the first movement is not what you think to do, what you decide to do, but what you actually do when you are frightened. And I said, "All right, let's see now, we will train the people so that the end of their first spontaneous movement is where we must start."

Moshe on Moshe on the Martial Arts. From Feldenkrais Journal 12, Issue 2.

Feldenkrais published an instructional book on the subject, which gained him admission to his first judo exhibition. The Japanese minister of education, rather taken by Feldenkrais and what he had accomplished without any formal training, asked him to introduce judo to Europe. Feldenkrais refused, explaining he was unable to devote himself to such an enterprise and continue his university studies at the same time, but the minister was determined. Soon everyone involved agreed that an expert would come to France and work with Feldenkrais when time would allow.

Thus Feldenkrais became the first European to hold a black belt in judo. He was also a fierce soccer player. A soccer injury flared up during the German invasion of France and prompted him to use both his martial arts experience and his engineering and mechanical background to explore the relationship between the nervous system and body function. (A 50/50 chance that surgery would correct the problem was not worth it to Feldenkrais.)

The result of his work is pure genius, but his philosophy became his legacy. He believed in and made a difference to the potential of humankind. He helped men and women become more themselves. He saw the infinite

Characteristics of Healthy Boundaries

The following is a list of healthy boundary characteristics.
- **Awareness and clarity:** The boundary has to be present in the individual's awareness. Becoming self-aware and overcoming prejudices, bigotry, and preferences lead to boundary clarity in the therapeutic relationship. To keep this awareness, the therapist must be able to think clearly at all times. To do so, the therapist should refrain from any mood-altering substances such as recreational drugs or alcohol before and during the process of providing professional services. A conscientious therapist cannot maintain mental and emotional clarity when he or she is impaired or anesthetized.

- **Appropriateness:** The boundary must be appropriate for the setting (personal or professional setting).
- **Congruency:** The boundary must be congruent with the individual's values, goals, and priorities. Boundaries that are incongruent with these important personal elements will be difficult, if not impossible, to maintain.
- **Protective:** The boundary must protect the individual's sense of well-being and integrity. It must also enhance and protect the self-worth of those who encounter our boundaries.
- **Flexibility and adaptability:** The individual should periodically evaluate the appropriateness of boundaries and be willing to create more rigid or flexible boundaries. To have healthy boundaries is to let go of them when necessary.

MOSHE FELDENKRAIS, DSc (*continued*)

possibilities because he, as did Descartes, viewed the human being as a tabula rasa, or clean slate.

"The problem is that much of what we have learned is harmful to our system because it was learned in childhood, when immediate dependence on others distorted our real needs. Long-standing habitual action feels right. Training a body to be perfect in all the possible forms and configurations of its members changes not only the strength and flexibility of the skeleton and muscles, but makes a profound and beneficial change in the self-image and quality of the direction of the self."

From Mind and Body.
Moshe Feldenkrais.

Feldenkrais believed that habitual patterns are imprinted in the nervous system, good or bad, but that verbally directed exercises and manipulation could help the brain and body learn movements that would free bodily limitations and instill our natural birthright, a sense of grace.

Feldenkrais's methods led to what might be considered incredible results. People with multiple sclerosis and cerebral palsy gained a new lease on life, and athletes without any obvious physical limitations sought his therapy.

A typical session consists of an instructor leading a group in various exercises or manipulating an individual through small, repeated movements. This system creates a new awareness or spatial reality, which the brain recognizes as being immediately right or better than the original impeded movement.

The sensations experienced in these sessions bring into focus the tension and stress that make our movement inefficient and prepare us to learn new patterns that permit the body to function at a level much closer to its full human potential. Feldenkrais was big on the concept of learning. He thought it was the gift of life, inextricably tied to personal growth and the key to a healthy body and mind.

"My way of learning, my way of dealing with people is to find out, for that person who wants it, what sort of accomplishment is possible for that person. People can learn to move and walk and stand differently, but they have given up because they think it's too late now, that the growth process has been completed, that they can't learn something new, that they don't have the time or ability. You don't have to go back to being a baby in order to function properly. You can, at any time of your life, rewire yourself, provided I can convince you that there is nothing permanent or compulsive in your system, except what you believe to be so."

From Movement and the Mind.
Moshe Feldenkrais and Will Shutz.

Practitioners worldwide are achieving dramatic results with Functional Integration and Awareness Through Movement. In North America alone, 1500 certified practitioners are listed. Training takes approximately 3 years, and because Feldenkrais believed the only way he could teach his work was through direct experience, graduates leave not only with a diploma and an opportunity for a promising career but also with improved posture, flexibility, coordination, and ease of movement (at any age); freedom from or reduction of pain; profound psychological and emotional growth; improved physical well-being and vitality; and the ability to understand how to learn effectively and enjoyably in any area of life.

Examples of Professional Boundaries

What should our clients expect from us regarding boundaries? First, the therapist will, in his or her own way, model healthy boundaries, such as starting and ending the session on time and not taking telephone calls or allowing other interruptions during the session. Next, the therapist will remain respectful of the client's boundaries. In this way, boundaries are acts not only of self-discipline but also of thoughtfulness and compassion.

The following are examples of professional boundaries. Note that they include issues that may not be covered in NCBTMB's code of ethics or standards of practice. Each item can be used as a topic for discussion, or therapists can use this list to form their own professional conscience regarding their practice. The purpose of the following list is to show the necessity of boundaries and to view them as a means to avoid situations of abuse or neglect to either the client or the therapist.

How Appointments Are Handled

Unlike many other health care providers, few therapists have an office receptionist. Incoming calls are usually handled by telephone with an answer machine. Make sure enough time is allowed between appointments, such as 30 minutes, to return telephone calls and to take care of other items so the work day runs smoothly.

When returning calls and scheduling appointments, let the client know appointment times that are available (i.e., Wednesday at 4 PM) rather than explaining all the reasons the appointment time is unavailable.

Also consider how house calls or out-calls will be handled. For example, you may decide to accept appointments for house calls for clients who have been referred by an existing client or with clients who have a history of treatment at your office.

How Prepared the Therapist Is When the Client Arrives
Clean professional surroundings help clients feel at ease. Having the treatment room ready is another boundary and is an immediate sign of professionalism and caring. This concept involves the restroom as well.

How "No Shows" Are Handled
Most therapists do not charge for missed appointments because they do not want to run the risk of offending a client. However, charging for missed appointments is another example of professional boundaries. An appointment is a contract between the therapist and the client. Enforcing an office policy such as charging full or partial fees if the client fails to call to cancel an appointment within an acceptable time frame shows that we value our time as professionals. Additionally, do we really want to work with a client who does not respect our time?

On the flip side, the same concept is true for the therapist who either forgets or is unable to keep a scheduled appointment. If the therapist does not give adequate notice, he or she must be willing to either give the fees associated with the service to the unlucky client or offer him or her a complimentary session.

How the Therapist Handles Disgruntled Clients
Appropriate steps should be taken when handling a client who is not happy with services rendered. Be willing to listen carefully and sincerely to his or her complaint without interjecting opinions. Once the client has completely stated his or her position, ask, "What would you like for me to do?" Comply within reason. In many instances, the best course of action is to offer a dissatisfied client a refund or gift certificate for a future session, even if no negligence exists on the part of the therapist.

> **evolve** Log on to your Evolve student account. Select the case study for Chapter 2 and, after reading it, write two ways of responding to the problem. Share your essays with your instructor for additional suggestions. ■

Where and When Professional Techniques Are Performed
Social settings are inappropriate places to display professional talents. This concept is not only true for practicing therapists but for students as well. If someone asks you to rub his or her sore neck, and you are not in your office, then you might say, "Right now, I'm not working, and I can do a better job at my office. Why don't we schedule

an appointment for you?" Setting professional boundaries is also about protecting your *off time*. Expecting a massage therapist to work during social time is unfair.

The same concept holds true for professional consultations. Avoid giving professional opinions or advice during social events because the setting is inappropriate. Additionally, you can be held professionally accountable for things said in a social setting that may be contraindicated in that particular person's case; you do not have the necessary information available to you in that setting. Instead, offer the person a business card and request that he or she call you during business hours.

How Physical Contact Is Addressed
Boundaries also involve physical contact. Avoid initiating hugging the client. Mandatory hugs can be intrusive. Letting him or her be in charge of personal space shows respect for the client. The client needs to be fully clothed and not on the massage table while hugging.

During the massage, the therapist must be aware of his or her own body. A client will become uncomfortable if a part of the therapist's body other than the hands, forearms, or elbows touches him or her. When leaning into a client for pressure and leverage, avoid touching the client with your body as you lean, other than the aforementioned body parts. Therapist with large breasts might consider an athletic bra to prevent this potential problem. Additionally, be careful that your garment is not brushing up against the client.

Learning to Say "No"
Practicing healthy professional boundaries also means that we need to let a new client know that we already have enough clients and we would become overextended with any more. It also means refusing to massage a client who exhibits contraindications or who is being sexually inappropriate.

Professional Distance

Professional boundaries create a healthy, professional distance between the client and the therapist. In fact, the distance makes the therapeutic relationship a safe place for the client's experience. Let us consider Chapter 11 of the *Tao Te Ching*:

> *Thirty spokes share the wheel's hub;*
> *It is the center hole that makes it useful.*
> *Shape clay into a vessel;*
> *It is the space within that makes it useful.*
> *Cut doors and windows for a room;*
> *It is the holes which make it useful.*
> *Therefore profit comes from what is there;*
> *Usefulness from what is not there.*
> Lao Tsu

When the space, or distance, is provided for clients to relax and be themselves, healing is more likely to occur. If we fill up the space in the relationship with too much conversation, with our own agendas, or with our own concerns, then the client does not have the opportunity to come out from behind his or her wall (a wall of muscular tension). The professional distance we can provide, similar to the pauses in a symphony, are often the places where peace, sanctity, and oneness are experienced. Providing space is a gift that is not often acknowledged. Professional distance is the gift of the therapeutic relationship, and it demonstrates the importance of protecting it by not entering into dual relationships with our clients (see section on Dual Relationships later in this chapter).

Integrity

Professional boundaries relate directly to the integrity of the therapist. **Integrity** is the whole and undivided integrating of thoughts, values, intentions, and actions. Webster's dictionary defines integrity as the "firm adherence to a code of moral or artistic values." Integrity is central to our work as massage therapists and to our relationships with clients, colleagues, and other health care professionals. In *A Year of Living Consciously,* author Gay Hedricks, Ph.D., defines some guidelines for acting with integrity.

- Do not deny your feelings, but do not wallow in them either.
- Communicate effectively, without assigning blame.
- Tell the whole truth.
- Make commitments selectively, and keep the ones you make.
- Take responsibility for everything you do, and ask others to do the same.

In a healthy therapeutic relationship, a balance exists among safety, care, compassion (existing in a boundary), and risk taking (stretching boundary limits). No formula exists for achieving this balance, but healthy boundaries can provide the foundation on which the therapist builds a relationship with the client. Boundaries are always contextual; they are interpreted in the context of the relationship; boundaries will differ in intimate relationships from therapeutic relationships (Figure 2-3). Having integrity will assist the therapist in having healthy therapeutic relationships.

Boundary Management

Once we step outside the boundaries of the therapeutic relationship, we invite trouble. When we bend our professional boundaries, we encourage others to treat us as nonprofessional. It is helpful to remember that our role is to be massage therapists. This reality does not go away; therefore we must always exhibit professionalism.

Recall that a boundary is a defining border. A massage therapist should know his or her professional boundaries (linked to a scope of practice). The therapist should not only guard boundaries but also be prepared to extend or expand them as bridges (while maintaining his or her integrity) when in contact with individuals or groups of individuals with whom the therapist needs to collaborate.

As boundary managers, massage therapists should know how to overlap boundaries temporarily. This technique is used

Intimate Relationships

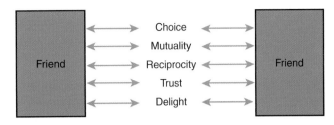

Therapeutic Relationships

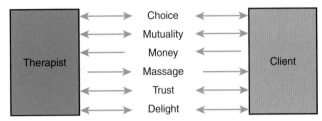

FIGURE 2-3 Intimate versus therapeutic relationships.

when resolving conflict, participating in negotiations, or mediating between groups. When someone crosses the therapist's boundary, he or she is put on alert and prepares for communication or other actions across the border. Conflicts may result.

If established boundaries and the consequences for crossing them are communicated clearly during the initial session, then the therapeutic relationship runs more smoothly, and misunderstandings are reduced or eliminated. During a massage, a sense of oneness and merging often exists. When professional boundaries are clear, it can be wonderfully healing to the client. When they are unclear, it can be destructive or disastrous.

Violation of a boundary can vary greatly and may range from mild issues such as inconsideration or rudeness to the more serious issues of abuse.

Crossing Boundaries: Common Mistakes

Following is a list of some common mistakes therapists make when professional boundaries are crossed. Being forewarned is being forearmed; therefore by examining these pitfalls, you may prevent them.

1. Do not represent yourself as being qualified in a specific modality without proper training and experience. Doing so demonstrates the perils of the *weekend workshop warrior* syndrome; after taking a workshop, the therapist begins too quickly to incorporate the new modality into his or her practice. Yes, practice is necessary to hone a new skill, but caution is required in the time interim between training and certification (Box 2-3). This boundary violation might result in injury to the client. Two examples of this error are working with trigger points and stretching, both passive and active assisted. If done incorrectly, excessive client soreness, bruising, and tissue damage may

occur. Becoming a specialist or an expert in any particular modality does not come overnight. This mistake is an example of client neglect.

2. Playing the psychotherapist, especially when a client experiences an emotional release during a session, is another common error. A separate license is needed to practice individual counseling and psychotherapy. We endanger our clients both mentally and emotionally when we do so. Additionally, playing the psychotherapist shows disrespect for individuals and for the profession of psychotherapy. This mistake is another example of client neglect.

3. Asking a client to be a friend is a boundary violation. This issue is common enough to deserve a lengthy discussion under Dual Relationships. By refraining from moving the therapeutic relationship into a personal friendship, we avoid the dangers of client abuse, client neglect, dual relationships, transference, and countertransference (see following sections).

4. Avoid making comments about a client's appearance. Although a compliment may, at first, seem harmless, if a client has been physically or emotionally abused or traumatized or is a victim or survivor of sexual abuse, then he or she may be on hyper-alert to signs of seduction and misread a careless phrase or gesture. Comments of this

nature may cause further damage or interfere with progress a client has made toward healing of such trauma.

5. Avoid working on a client who clearly presents contraindications. This issue may be a problem if the therapist works in a setting in which refusing a client may be difficult (salon or day spa) or if the massage is part of a spa package. Perhaps the therapist has an overwhelming urge to help and believes the benefits of the massage outweigh the harm it would cause. Refusing to treat a client who is not a good candidate for massage and referring him or her back to his or her primary health care provider would be appropriate in this instance. In some circumstances, the client's best interest is served by saying *no.*

Competency, the ability to do something well, requires continuous study and absorption of new information. Professional competency requires personal accountability, which means that the therapist seriously evaluates his or her knowledge, skill, abilities, and experience before offering professional treatment and is aware of his or her professional limitations in determining when referring to another health care provider is in the client's best interest.

Client Abuse and Client Neglect

When any professional, whether a physician, attorney, minister, or massage therapist, does not recognize or respect the rights and boundaries of the client, the result may be client abuse or client neglect. Additionally, any time a power differential in a relationship exists, client abuse and client neglect can occur.

Client neglect is defined as *unintentional* physical or emotional harm that the client sustains resulting from insensitivity or lack of knowledge on the therapist's part. An example of a neglectful act might be a therapist who mistakes a cyst for a trigger point, causing tissue damage through prolonged pressure. Another example might be a therapist who, rather than providing emotional support for the client, oversteps his or her training, slips into a *counselor* role, and gives unsolicited or untrained advice. In neither of these cases did the therapist intend to harm the client, yet it happened. Negligent treatment is often spawned by ignorance or lack of forethought. Ways to avoid client negligence are (1) staying within your scope of practice, (2) developing a cautious and professional attitude, (3) continuing with your education, and (4) having professional boundaries.

Client abuse is defined as physical or emotional harm that the client sustains from *deliberate* acts of the therapist. An abusive therapist is one who makes a conscious decision to take advantage of a client physically, sexually, financially, or emotionally.

Although rare, physical abuse may include deliberately disregarding the client's request for lighter pressure because the therapist believes that *more pressure is better.* In cases of bruising as a result of physical abuse, the therapist is liable, and the client may elect to file assault and battery charges with the district attorney or file a civil suit for damages.

Sexual abuse may be physical, verbal, or nonverbal, but its intent is to give or receive sexual gratification. This type of abuse is not limited to advances made while the client is receiving a massage. Contact made with a client while not performing professional activities is discouraged because the therapist is always a therapist first. All roles beyond the professional role may satisfy the therapist's needs, but they often serve to harm the client. If both parties want a more intimate relationship, then the NCBTMB recommends discontinuing the client-therapist relationship for a minimum of 6 months before the new relationship is initiated. This type of restriction represents good boundaries and avoids dual relationships.

Financial client abuse is taking advantage of a client's resources. It may be charging more than the standard rate simply because the therapist knows the client is in a high-income bracket. Accepting expensive gifts or access to living quarters for a weekend is financially abusive. A good rule of thumb is to avoid accepting a gift (or a tip) from a client if it exceeds the cost of the massage (e.g., $50.00). Failing to inform new clients about prices or old clients about upcoming price increases is abusive to the client and sabotages the trust of the client-therapist relationship.

Emotional abuse is usually involved in all other types of abusive relationships in which an imbalance of power exists and when the person who wields the greater power does not recognize or respect the boundaries of the other. The therapeutic relationship between a client and the massage therapist is particularly vulnerable to this type of abuse. In relation to the client, the massage therapist has the authoritative position. The client enters into the relationship because the massage therapist has particular skills, knowledge, and abilities. The client may feel close to the therapist because skin-to-skin contact is involved. The client may feel vulnerable both physically and emotionally because he or she is usually lying down and draped, whereas the therapist is standing and clothed. In many instances, when someone removes his or her clothing, he or she may feel emotionally naked and vulnerable. The therapist must have good professional boundaries because of the vulnerability of the client.

Conflicts of Interest: Therapists as Salespersons

When a massage therapist is involved with alleviating pain or discomfort or facilitates a change in behavior, the therapist has the position of power. This imbalance of power is a natural occurrence in the therapeutic relationship and, in and of itself, is not a problem. Problems may arise, however, when this power is misused to serve the interests of the therapist rather than the interests of the client.

Conflicts of interest may arise when a difference exists between the therapist's personal interests and his or her professional obligations. If a conflict of interest arises in the therapeutic relationship, the therapist needs to ask the question and answer honestly, "whose interest am I really serving?"

The most common scenario involving conflicts of interests is when the therapist is selling products. A situation often develops in which the therapist is faced with choosing among the well-being of his or her finances, a duty to provide the best possible care to clients, and the well-being of the therapeutic relationship.

Selling anything to a client other than the professional services for which we have contracted creates a dual relationship, and dual relationships are often problematic. Realize the influence we have over our clients. Furthermore, because of the power differential, is the client really free to refuse the offer? Might the client make the purchase in an attempt to please the therapist? A client may choose not to return to a therapist because the latter is selling a certain product. Perhaps the sales pitch simply feels *funny* to the client. The awkwardness may be so severe that the client chooses to go to a therapist who does not have such requirements.

Suppose a client had an allergic reaction to the supplement or herbal cream that the therapist sold to him or her. What would happen if the client believed that he or she did not gain the benefits he or she was told to expect or the benefits for which he or she had hoped? How would these and other issues be handled? When considering these and many other possibilities, the therapist should use caution or avoid conflicts of interest because they have a way of damaging the therapeutic relationship.

Terminating a Session

Rarely does a massage therapist have to terminate a session because of some inappropriate statement or action by the client. However, if forced to do so, the therapist must be prepared to deal with the situation. Here are some important guidelines when the therapist has made a decision to terminate a massage while in session.
- Remove your hands from the client; step back and toward the door.
- Tell the client that the massage is over.
- Inform the client that you will wait outside while he or she gets dressed.
- Avoid answering questions until the client is dressed and out of the massage room.
- In such cases, asking for full or partial fees would be inappropriate.

If the circumstances leading to the session are extreme, or if the therapist works alone and becomes frightened, either:
- Call someone and stay on the telephone until the client leaves, or
- Lock yourself in a room as a safety measure until the client has left.

Document the events that led to the session termination and what actions were taken. This information can be used as a reference should the situation become libelous. If the situation involved sexual improprieties, then document statements verbatim or describe actions that gave that impression.

Incident Reports

Regardless of how small the incident or unusual the episode, a report should be filled out and retained to document things that happened to a client or to the therapist (Figure 2-4).

INCIDENT REPORT FORM

Date:_____ Client's Name: _____

Time:_____ Therapist's Name: _____

Place:_____

Therapist's Perceptions of Incident:

Actions Taken:

Proposed Resolutions:

_____ _____

Signature of Massage Therapist   Date

Reviewed and Resolved:

Date:_____   Time: _____

Place: _____

Those in attendance:

FIGURE 2-4 A sample incident report form. (Permission is hereby granted to reproduce this form in its entirety, including the copyright notice, for commercial or instructional use but not for resale.)

These reports may involve a client who slips and falls or a client who misplaces belongings. The incident report should include the date, time, and exact location of the occurrence; who was present; and what steps were taken to alleviate the problem. If physical injury was involved, the report should then include the condition of the client when he or she departed from your establishment.

> **evolve** Log on to the Evolve website and access your student account to print out an incident report form for use as mentioned above. ▪

TRANSFERENCE AND COUNTERTRANSFERENCE

Transference and countertransference exhibit themselves in all relationships: therapeutic, personal, and professional. Psychotherapists have long been taught about a phenomenon of personalization that takes place between counselors and their clients. Sigmund Freud was the first to describe it. Even though massage therapists are not counselors, we are involved in a therapeutic relationship and will encounter transference and countertransference and therefore should be trained and prepared to recognize and manage these issues.

As you explore these concepts, remember that transference and countertransference influence relationships in ways that, under certain conditions, may be helpful to everyone concerned. Transference and countertransference are, by their nature, both complex and interrelated. Therapists will remind clients of other people in their lives, past and present. Clients will remind therapists of people in their own lives. Power dynamics, a component of the therapeutic encounter, plays a role. Most transference and countertransference involve its positive expression, which is love. Love serves to equalize power between individuals. Thus the act of loving is connected to power dynamics.

When a client views the therapist as someone other than a health care provider, the result is transference. Conversely, the therapist may experience countertransference if he or she sees the client as something more than a client. Transference can sometimes produce a powerful love (positive transference) or a destructive hatred (negative transference), both of which are based on complete illusion. A painful realization can exist when the individual acts on his or her transference reactions and the bubble finally bursts. Transference can lead disturbed individuals to strange and dangerous behaviors (stalking, assault).

Transference

Transference occurs when the client *transfers* feelings, thoughts, and behaviors related to a significant person in his or her early life (e.g., parents) onto the therapist. In the client's subconscious mind, the therapist assumes a significant role in his or her life. This event may occur when needs that were not being met in the client's personal relationships are now being met in the therapeutic relationship. These needs may be touch needs, the need for attention, listening, validation, and the sense of nurturing that massage can bring. Vulnerability of the client may be enough to bring on feelings of transference. These unconscious feelings are not about the therapist; they are about the client being in touch with old or unresolved feelings and patterns of behavior. Some people refer to transference as a *projection;* you are projecting your own feelings, emotions, or motivations onto another person without realizing it is more about you than it is about the other person. In this case, you may remind your client of his or her mother, with all the irritating things his or her mother did when he or she was growing up.

The client begins to personalize the therapeutic relationship. Instead of seeing the therapist in a professional role, the client's perception is that the therapist is a caring friend, confidant, or possible lover. On some level, clients may resist seeing their therapists as real people, people with flaws. In turn, the therapist may encourage this image by playing it up. Working with or creating transference in therapy can make a therapist look mystical and brilliant. Some disturbed therapists generate positive transference to control and manipulate, artificially inflating their ego. They love the power and think they can handle it.

A relatively common occurrence is for a client, particularly a needy client, to develop a crush on his or her therapist. A client may bring a variety of feelings and pain, both physical and emotional, to the massage table. A therapist who represents the epitome of kindliness, sensitivity, and warmth may inadvertently fill the unmet needs of the client. Seeing his or her therapist as the desirable friend and confidant, a type of person perhaps missing in his or her life, is relatively easy for a needy client.

A therapist must face transference issues and deal with them. Keep in mind that the therapist cannot control how the client thinks. The therapist must recognize transference and reduce the chance of transference becoming problematic. This task is accomplished by developing an awareness of transference. Next, use transference in a way that serves the client toward his or her highest good. This process can be incredibly helpful and have positive influence on the therapeutic process. Realize that successful navigation of these waters requires maturity, integrity, and ethical professionalism. Red-flag signals of possible transference is a client who:

- Frequently asks about your personal life
- Calls you during times you have made clear are for personal time
- Frequently brings you gifts
- Asks for advice in dealing with personal issues
- Frequently asks for more time once the session has ended and is openly disappointed when you do not comply
- Asks you for a date

Countertransference

Countertransference occurs when the therapist brings his or her own unresolved issues or personal needs into the therapeutic relationship. The therapist counters the client's transference, reversing the roles, and tries to get his or her own personal needs met through interactions with the client. Similar to transference, countertransference can stem from unresolved feelings, thoughts, and perceptions about someone from the therapist's past, but not always.

Countertransference can also occur when the therapist has trouble maintaining his or her professional distance and detachment from a client. Detachment is not thinking less of a client but rather thinking of a client less. These feelings may be caused by the attention from transference that triggers the therapist into taking a personal interest in the client or the therapist's playing along and acting on a client's crush.

> *"Attachment is the great fabricator of illusions; reality can be attained only by someone who is detached."*
> Simone Weil

Another example is becoming overly responsible for the client's recovery or feeling offended or irritated when a client expresses criticism of our work instead of being objective. In these and similar situations, boundaries become blurred, which interferes with the ability of the therapist to separate fact from fiction.

Recall that awareness is a characteristic of healthy boundaries. A therapist must be self-aware and avoid bringing his or her emotional baggage into the therapeutic relationship. Therapists must leave personal needs and burdens outside the treatment room and serve only the highest good of each client. The therapeutic relationship needs to be about the client, not about the needs of the therapist; it does not go both ways—it is not a reciprocal relationship.

If countertransference develops unnoticed by the therapist, the result may be emotional and sexual intimacy. Ultimately, the situation damages the therapeutic relationship and removes the focus of healing from the client. In fact, clients are paying us to do what is best for them, to put our needs and desires aside. Red flags of possible countertransference are:

- Having intense feelings toward a client, either positive or negative
- Becoming angry or depressed when a client cancels a scheduled appointment

- Becoming impatient, angry, or depressed when a client is not progressing with treatment
- Being argumentative with a client
- Seeking to or becoming involved in a client's personal life
- Thinking about the client between appointments
- Making excuses for a client's inappropriate behavior
- Giving a particular client additional time during each appointment
- In extreme cases, romantic and sexual fantasizing
- Relaxing professional boundaries

So what can a therapist do if he or she suddenly finds him or herself in this situation?

The massage therapist should take a close look at his or her own needs and examine which ones are not being met. This pattern may repeat itself with other clients if the therapist is not getting his or her needs met from persons outside the therapeutic relationship. Again, the therapist might go to a licensed counselor or colleague who can help identify needs and develop appropriate ways of getting them met.

If the countertransference has progressed, generally the best course of action is to terminate the therapeutic relationship and refer the client to another therapist. This action prevents the dynamic from progressing to an emotional or sexual relationship, which is detrimental to both the client and the therapist. Remember, no good reason exists to have sex with a client. Caution must be taken in this termination of the relationship because the client might feel it as rejection. An open and honest conversation with the client can help lessen the impact of this feeling.

Seductive Client

Some manipulative clients are experts at making the therapist feel special or create situations in which the therapist feels compelled to jump in and rescue the client. These clients are referred to as *seductive* clients because they seem to know just how to throw therapists off balance and create an illusion that a special relationship with them does not count as being inappropriate or unethical. These clients seem to know just the right buttons to push. They are indifferent to the emotional damage they cause.

This pattern of behavior comes from the seductive client's early childhood. The person learns that the best way to get needs met is by seducing others, making them feel needed and special. Seductive clients are actually not asking us to be their lovers. They are revealing how they usually deal with power differentials in relationships. They are showing us how they usually get attention needs met. These signs are indeed red flags of severe transference. This kind of transference is highly volatile, changing quickly from attraction and delight to disappointment and rage. Seductiveness is not about love or sex or affection; it is about dominance, control, selfishness, and aggression.

The therapist who experiences countertransference feels as though a spell has been cast. Much time is spent thinking about the client. An obsession may develop. However, the smallest blunder or *slip of the hand* can turn the therapeutic relationship into a nightmare.

The best way to break the spell is by telling a professional counselor or trusted, mature, unbiased colleague who will give you a good dose of reality.

DUAL RELATIONSHIPS

A therapist needs to work with a professional, objective, and nonjudgmental attitude. Clients need to be able to focus on themselves and avoid taking care of their therapists' needs. These goals may be thwarted when therapists enter into dual relationships with their clients. **Dual relationships** occur when more than one relationship with a client exists.

As might be expected, when a dual relationship occurs, a complex interweaving of roles may exist, and maintaining healthy professional boundaries may be difficult. Treating all clients the same is difficult if some are friends and others are not. Unintentionally, conflicts of interest may arise, boundaries become blurred, and the potential for client abuse is heightened. The therapist cannot promise the client that entering into a dual relationship will have no effect on the therapeutic relationship—no one can make that kind of promise. An emotional bond naturally develops. Assuming a role other than that of therapist will alter the therapeutic relationship, making the task of maintaining boundaries a challenge.

When professional boundaries start to fade, trouble is often around the corner. Remember that the relationship between client and therapist, the essence of a therapeutic relationship, is unequal. A power differential has formed, similar to a parent-child relationship. The client looks up to the therapist to meet his or her needs, to help achieve the goals identified during assessment and planning, whether it is stress relief, pain relief, or just a little TLC.

For the most part, dual relationships are problematic. They can create stress in our lives and shortchange our clients. Strangely, one of the reasons therapists initiate dual relationships is that these relationships seem extremely convenient. The potential friend is right in front of you.

However, with the inevitability of dual relationships, how can they be ethically managed? How can we maintain our professional ethical practices within dual relationships? NCBTMB's standards of practice remind us to avoid relationships that can impair professional judgment. Therefore management of these relationships involves boundaries to help guide us in making decisions and being clear about what role we and they are assuming, not wearing more than one hat at a time (see next section). When our role is that of therapist, be a therapist. When our role is that of friend, be a friend. When our role is that of family member, be a family member.

Remember, maintaining boundaries and ethics is not the client's responsibility. The power differential makes it impossible for a client to be unethical. A professional license denotes professional responsibility, accountability, and adherence to a code of ethics. The person in the professional role is held responsible for any negative consequences of dual relationships.

Most Common Dual Relationship: Friendship

In addition to our roles as therapists, what other roles are possible? Can a therapist become friends with a client? What about a client who becomes a business partner? What if a client becomes romantically or sexually involved with the therapist? Should a therapist rent property or borrow money from a client? Imagining how a romantic, sexual, or business relationship might evolve from the therapeutic relationship is not difficult. Let us explore the most common dual relationship: *friendship.*

If a client becomes a friend, then the therapist now assumes two roles in the client's life. Being exclusive in one single role frequently makes it difficult, if not impossible, for example, to be solely in the role of therapist. Imagine how hard it is *not* to chat with a friend during a massage. Self-disclosure to a client (now friend) will create a different atmosphere during the sessions. In many instances, both the therapist and the client-friend treat scheduled appointments as opportunities to continue developing a personal relationship, a social affair rather than a professional event. The therapist may become careless, not keeping the focus on the client. Whose interest is being served now?

So how does the therapeutic relationship differ from a friendship? In a friendship, the relationship is 50/50; a certain amount of give and take exists between parties. In a friendship, your friend knows as much about you as you know about your friend. This familiarity is not the case in a therapeutic relationship; it is not an equal partnership; a difference in power exists. In a therapeutic relationship, the therapist knows much more about the client than the client knows about the therapist. The therapeutic relationship exists to benefit the client!

Besides, can we really call what develops between a client and a therapist a friendship? Nina McIntosh examines this question in her lovely book, *Educated Heart.* Do we go to their offices, remove our clothing, lie on their desks, get a massage, and pay for their time? This scenario occurs rarely if at all. McIntosh goes so far as to say that we can be social with a client, but we typically do not show what she calls our *lower selves,* the part of us reserved for only those closest to us. This part includes our pettiness, our neediness, our jealousies, our idiosyncrasies, and our quirks. We tend to operate in a professional setting from our *higher selves,* she elaborates, so naturally clients tend to think well of us, better than we really are. The therapist may enjoy this illusion.

Turning clients into friends may also interfere with our relationships with other clients. How would you feel if your male massage therapist was a friend with his client Mary and not with you? If not hurt, you may question his sense of professional boundaries.

Maintaining professional boundaries is difficult with someone with whom we have a close relationship. Despite this fact, friendships with clients routinely develop. How-

ever, as we examine dual relationships in the context of intimacy, we can further illustrate the difference between friendship and professional relationships.

Intimacy

What is an intimate relationship? *Intimacy* is a sensual (an experience of the senses) bond to another in which the following elements exist: choice, mutuality, reciprocity, trust, and delight. This definition of intimacy is generally true for people with whom we are closest, usually family and friends. Briefly looking at these aspects of an intimate relationship, one might say the following:

- The element of *choice* is present in that we can choose to be in the relationship; we cannot be forced into intimacy.
- *Mutuality* goes hand-in-hand with choice; both parties elect to enter and maintain intimacy.
- *Reciprocity* is the knowledge that if I choose to be in the relationship, over time, I will receive as much from the relationship as I give to the relationship.
- *Trust* is the result of continued risk taking. We can choose to trust blindly, without a history of trust, but we are more likely to get hurt.
- Finally, *delight* is the sensual experience that the relationship brings to us because of these first four elements: choice, mutuality, reciprocity, and trust.

The therapeutic relationship, then, is similar to an intimate relationship, with a few important differences (see Figure 2-3). Choice and mutuality exist, or no relationship would exist. Trust is built from the continued risk taking during subsequent sessions. Both parties may experience delight at times because the therapeutic relationship should be pleasurable. Because of these similarities, people sometimes confuse the intimacy of a love relationship with the closeness of the therapeutic relationship.

A key element missing is reciprocity. Recall that the roles are not equal, and therapists do not ask clients to attend to their needs. In intimate relationships, boundaries are let down; dimensions of lives of both parties are shared.

As stated earlier, the therapist is getting paid to be in this relationship; although the fact may be argued that what the client is receiving is worth the money exchanged, the relationship is at best one sided. True, opportunities for closeness and intimacy in therapeutic relationship exist; but with boundaries in place and dual relationship avoided, intimacy will be avoided, and the safety of the therapeutic relationship for the client is protected. The therapist is a caring and compassionate person who can also keep a professional distance from personal involvement with clients.

Self-disclosure to a client outside the therapeutic relationship will create a different atmosphere when the sessions resume. Both parties are often tempted to treat sessions as a time to continue developing a personal relationship rather than maintaining a professional atmosphere. Boundaries begin to crumble, and you become careless about the length of time for the session, or the focus is not kept on the client during the session.

What About Friends Who Become Clients?

What about friends who become clients? Is this arrangement okay? What are possible concerns?

For a therapeutic relationship to occur from a friendship, professional boundaries must be established, just as with all clients. Both parties need to understand their individual positions and responsibilities. The therapist will provide a service for which the client will pay a fee. Just as with all dual relationships, keep the conversation and focus on the client during the massage.

Oddly, people who have friends who are massage therapists might be better off with someone whom they do not know. Remember that the therapeutic relationship is designed to serve the client. A friend may not be willing or able to give the therapist the authority deserved, get the full benefit from the session, or take the work as seriously as he or she would with another therapist who is not also a friend.

While in school, students often ask their friends to be their guinea pigs for practice. The best course of action for them is to realize up front that, after graduation, a fee will be attached. If you know what the fee will be, let them know early on so they will be prepared to pay the requested fee. This time is also a great opportunity for the student to practice being in the role of the therapist with professional boundaries intact, to treat a practice session as he or she would in a professional setting.

Dating Clients

The other potentially awkward dual relationship is moving the therapeutic relationship into a romantic or sexual one. Most codes of ethics, including NCBTMB's, require that a period of 6 months pass between the time the therapist has terminated the client-therapist relationship and begins to pursue a more personal one.

One reason for the delay is to make sure that, if any feelings of transference or countertransference, or both, have occurred (and most likely it has, or the desire for more than a therapeutic relationship would not exist), a span of time occurs for the situation to be evaluated and for reality to set in.

The decision to date or sleep with an ex-client should be considered carefully. Such situations can easily damage the therapist's relationship with other clients, damage reputations, and raise a red flag of its own with the therapist's profession. The best and safest decision is most often to not go out with ex-clients.

Dual Licensure and Dual Roles

In some cases, a licensed massage therapist also holds another professional license to practice in another profession. In these cases, both licensing boards need to be contacted with regard to handling professional situations. In most cases, the person is restricted from wearing *two hats* simultaneously. For example, if acting in the capacity of a licensed mental health counselor, provide only the specific services within that particular

profession's scope of practice. When the massage therapist who is also a licensed counselor gives a massage to his or her counseling client, he or she should provide only the specific services within that particular scope of practice.

Keep in mind that both professions have their independent codes of ethics. The code of ethics for a licensed mental health counselor will be different from the code of ethics for a massage therapist. In cases of an individual's possessing more than one professional license, the profession with the strictest code of ethics prevails and becomes the standard of conduct for the individual in *every* therapeutic relationship.

MINI-LAB

Make a list of five or more situations to create fire drills. These situations can be repeats of past unpleasant experiences or situations that constitute the most uncomfortable or frightening scenarios that might happen to you as a massage therapist. For example, it might be that a client goes into heart failure on the table, you accidentally undrape a client, or someone makes a pass at you.

Act out each situation with a classmate in front of the class. Once the situation is complete, ask the class and/or instructor for other options. Revise the fire drill if necessary. This activity will help you become more prepared to handle difficult situations.

SEXUAL MISCONDUCT

Of all possible boundary violations and breaches in a code of ethics, sexual misconduct is the most devastating. Nothing is so destructive to a therapist or to a client as becoming involved in a game of sexual inappropriateness. The action may be something as innocent as making a comment to a client that was misinterpreted. It may be something as obvious as a male client requesting sexual services. The sensual pleasure inherent in massage is one of its greatest assets, but it is also one of its most obvious liabilities and can lead to situations of abuse, seduction, and exploitation.

Sexual misconduct is defined as any sexual contact between a therapist and a client or any sexualizing of the therapeutic relationship. Given that our profession uses touch as its primary therapeutic tool, therapists need to be prepared for the possibility of their touch being misread. Even though the intention behind our touch is professional and therapeutic, and this is communicated to the client during the informed consent process, the client may experience an emotional or sexual response. The therapist must be aware of the possible impact that his or her touch can have and be willing to take responsibility for how touch affects his or her clients. An ounce of prevention is worth a pound of cure. Ways to avoid situations involving sexual misconduct are listed in the section on Sexual Risk Management.

Given that the therapist is likely to deal with issues, talking about them early is best, such as while you are in school. If we ignore sexual issues, they do not disappear. Through the process of talking about issues, we obtain the *know-how* to make sound decisions. Class discussion regarding sexual issues is important in that students learn not only from a teacher's experience but from their classmates as well. Some of us have blind spots when dealing with these issues and need guidance. The potential for sexual misconduct is in every profession, not just in massage. Sometimes clients are sexually attracted to their therapists; sometimes therapists are sexually attracted to their clients. Therapists need to know that these predicaments can be circumvented and that they are not a victim of themselves or their clients.

William Greenberg, the grievance chairman for the American Massage Therapy Association, states that complaints filed against therapists for sexual misconduct have decreased recently. Greenberg attributes this reduction to the fact that schools are giving more instruction on boundaries in general and sexual boundaries in particular.

Negative Perception of Massage

Some people believe that massage is a euphemism for prostitution. Much of this illusion is perpetuated by movies, television shows, magazines, newspapers, telephone books, and prostitutes who use the term *massage parlor* as a cover for their business activities. In many parts of the country, *massage* and *massage therapist* are presented side by side in lists of services, the former being a form of adult entertainment. Some print media do not separate the two entities—for example, an ad featuring Tootsie's tantric or erotic massage next to a legitimate ad for massage therapy. It is easy to see how people become confused.

To further perpetuate the myth, society sexualizes touch. In fact, sometimes the only way some people are touched is when engaging in sex. Massage is used and often taught as a *foreplay* method in courses intended for couples. Indeed, some massage therapists work out of their homes in what once were bedrooms.

Examples of Sexual Misconduct

This section deals with an array of sexual misconduct examples, ranging from flirting to rape. Boundary violations involving sexual misconduct include:
- Engaging in verbal or physical flirtatious behavior
- Gestures or expressions that are seductive in nature or sexually demeaning
- Looking at a client seductively
- Sexual comments about a client's body or clothing
- Telling sexual jokes
- Failure to ensure privacy through proper draping
- Entering the room before the client is completely draped or dressed
- Conversations about sexual problems, sexual performance, preferences, or fantasies initiated or involving either the therapist or client
- Asking a client for a date

- Unnecessary examination or treatments
- Inappropriate touching of the client's breasts or pelvic area
- Therapist's breast or pelvic area touching a client
- Filming the client without his or her permission
- Masturbation by practitioner or client
- Intercourse
- Rape

Sexual Risk Management

As members of a profession, we are increasingly aware of damage done when boundaries are crossed. Closeness often felt by a client in a therapeutic relationship may lead to misunderstandings and false accusations. We are touching people, sometimes with the gentleness and attentiveness shared with a lover. The therapist may encounter survivors of sexual abuse. These individuals are often hypersensitive to seduction and are more likely than others to misinterpret the therapist's intent. Conversely, some people can easily disassociate and are unable to detect or stop the therapist's inappropriate behavior because they were unable to stop it from happening before. Therapists who are survivors themselves often do not realize that they are being sexually inappropriate with a client.

As with other professions, most complaints are made by female clients against male therapists. With this fact in mind, men are more at risk than women for being accused of sexual misconduct. Although every therapist should be watchful with regard to sexual boundaries, male therapists need to take extra precautions.
- Avoid terms of endearment. One never knows which client might be vulnerable or needy and misread the comment.
- Use anatomical references and clinical terminology.
- When advertising, avoid words such as *release, available any time, open 24 hours a day, my place or yours, total relaxation,* and *full-body massage.*
- When booking an appointment for a new client, ascertain his or her goals for treatment. Note the prospective client's demeanor, tone of voice, and language he or she uses when making the initial appointment. If a prospective client objects to giving you his or her name or telephone number, refuse to schedule the appointment.
- Do not work in a secluded office with clients whom you do not know.
- Do not schedule new clients late in the day or while no one will be in the office.
- Realize the problems associated with a home office. Leading a client through your home to the bedroom area (now a treatment room) can make a client feel uneasy.
- Out-calls deserve special consideration. Screen clients carefully. Perhaps accept out-call requests with people who have been referred by someone you know and trust.
- Avoid sexual signals that you may be inadvertently sending, and avoid sexualizing your work, such as by wearing sexy clothes to work or for one particular client. Short shorts, tank tops, or tops that reveal cleavage should be

avoided. When you start dressing for work as though you are going on a date, you are asking for trouble.

- When work on or near the female breast is merited, the therapist should obtain a separate voluntary consent. Work should be conducted in this area under the sheet and only with members of the same gender as the therapist. If a male therapist is massaging near a female client's breast, ask another female to be present in the room as a safeguard. These precautions greatly reduce the possibility of suspicions of sexual misconduct.

- Be aware of body contact during the massage. Pay attention to the way you lean into your client's body. Be conscious of what part of your body touches the client during strokes, joint manipulations, and stretches.

- If a therapist notices an erection, the most uncomplicated method of handling this situation is to stop massaging the male client. Step back and announce that you need to step out of the room for a few moments, perhaps under the pretense of getting a drink. Stay gone for a few minutes. Knock and reenter the room. If needed, roll the client over and continue the massage. Sometimes just asking him a question that removes him from the current massage experience helps, such as "How's your job going?" or "What is it that you do for a living?" Avoid working on areas that might stimulate this response, such as lower abdomen, inner thighs, and lumbosacral region.

- Approach situations involving sexual behavior with blunt and straightforward statements: "I don't offer sexual services." We have the right to refuse a client who makes us feel unsafe or those who make continued sexual advances once warned.

Consequences of Behavior

Part of understanding boundaries is learning about the consequences when we choose to cross them. Every massage therapist must understand the consequences of inappropriate behavior, particularly sexual misconduct. Behind any sexual misconduct lies a blatant disregard of ethics, morals, and the profession. Becoming sexual with a client, even if it is in a dating situation and not the massage room, is considered to be sexual misconduct. The power dynamic between client and therapist does not empower the client to say *no* easily to the therapist.

If a therapist intentionally or unintentionally sexually violates a client, the realization rarely occurs during the session. Most often, only after the massage does the client have an opportunity to reflect on events and the inappropriateness of the therapist. This being the case, most acts of sexual misconduct by a therapist go unaddressed. The violated client is either silent and blames what happened on him or her, or the client just stops going to the offending therapist.

Inappropriate behavior and sexual misconduct are forms of client abuse and sadistic acts when therapists take advantage of their more powerful positions in the therapeutic relationship to meet their own emotional or sexual needs or for their own personal gain. In these circumstances, the therapist uses the client, often to add some excitement to the therapist's life.

The therapeutic relationship is considered a business arrangement between therapist and client, which benefits the client through healing touch and massage. When a therapist violates the boundaries of the therapeutic relationship, the consequences associated with the violation are often of a corresponding severity. Possible consequences of this type of behavior include loss of income, loss of reputation, loss of marriage, loss of friendships, loss of relationship with peers and colleagues, loss of license, loss of membership in professional organizations, loss of insurance coverage, lawsuits for damages, criminal charges, fines, attorney's fees, court costs, and time in jail.

Both surveys and anecdotal evidence suggest that very little good comes out of these encounters. No way exists to avoid a bad result. If a therapist who crosses the ethical line is out for easy sex, then his or her client feels raped and abused. Then the confused client is likely to feel all the ambivalence and helplessness of an incest victim. In all cases of therapist-client entanglement—every one of them—the therapy the two have been conducting together comes to an end and, in most cases, is replaced by an unstable, unfair, and ultimately unpleasant liaison.

Remember that the therapist is *always* responsible and liable for his or her actions, even if the client initiates the situation. Do not depend on professional liability insurance to cover any damages. Although your insurance company may well provide an attorney to assist in your defense, the policy typically does not cover damages resulting from sexual misconduct.

> *"Our deeds determine us, as much*
> *as we determine our deeds."*
> George Eliot

Sexual Misconduct of a Colleague

If we hear of a fellow therapist who has possibly engaged in sexual misconduct within the therapeutic relationship, then we have a professional responsibility to take action. Empathy and compassion for our colleague in cases of sexual misconduct does not serve the profession.

The first step is to contact the therapist. Let him or her know what is being said so that the therapist has an opportunity to address it. An important step is to approach the therapist, outlining not only the information received but also observations made that directly relate to the misconduct.

If the discovery is made that the therapist in question has been inappropriate and wants to continue the inappropriate relationship with the client, then provide information regarding the professional and legal consequences of such unethical behavior. Suggest that the therapist remove him or herself from the role as therapist, and refer the client to another therapist.

If confrontation does not lead to a change in behavior, with the therapist refusing to act in the best interest of the client, then the next step is to report the situation to the therapist's employer and to file a complaint with the state board that regulates licensure and professional affiliations of which the therapist is a member. Remember that sexual misconduct by a therapist shows disrespect for his or her professional role, is not concerned about boundaries, is indifferent to the emotional damage caused, and shows a lack of concern for the client's well-being.

> **evolve** Log on to your Evolve student account and print out the crossword puzzle for Chapter 2. Use it as a study aid to help you remember important terms and concepts. ■

SUMMARY

This chapter focuses on the therapeutic relationship. When developing an awareness and skill in managing this important aspect of the therapeutic process, we must examine layers upon layers of practice. First, the important elements are reviewed; then communication skills and conflict resolution skills are strengthened. Professionalism, another important aspect of the process, reveals legal and ethical concerns and client confidentiality. Woven into professionalism is scope of practice, a code of ethics, and standards of practice.

Healthy relationships always involve healthy boundaries. Within this concept lie concern over neglect and abuse, conflicts of interests, dual relationships, and transference and countertransference. Crossing of boundaries can also involve sexual misconduct. Learning how to reduce its occurrence with professional behavior and managing risk are hallmarks of a professional.

CASE STUDY:

Scope of Practice

Mike has been working at a chiropractic clinic for 10 years as a massage therapist. Elmer is a patient at the clinic who has been seeing one of the physicians for chiropractic adjustments and Mike for massages for the last 3 years. Elmer comes in with pain in the wrist and proceeds to receive a massage from Mike. The physicians are away from the clinic to attend a chiropractic association meeting; no one is at the clinic except Mike and the office staff.

During the massage, Elmer asks Mike if he has ever had one of the physicians adjust his wrist. Mike replies, "Sure! In this business, you tend to bear weight with your hands, and sometimes the carpal bones become misaligned." Elmer replies, "Well, see if *you* can adjust my wrist. I know you can do it. I trust you. I won't tell anyone." Mike is hesitant but enjoys the compliment. Mike has always wanted to be a physician and have the admiration and respect that go with the title. "Come on," says Elmer, "you know that you know as much about the body as they do." Mike smiles, and grasping Elmer by the right wrist, he pulls down and out and sharply whips the wrist as he has seen his employers do for years. An audible pop is heard, and Elmer's face whitens. "My hand is numb!" he says. "Will this go away? What did you do?"

How might Mike respond to Elmer's inquiry?

Is Mike liable for any damage to Elmer's wrist as a result of his desire to help Elmer?

Should Mike get the office staff involved and document the incident?

How might Mike tell the physicians about the incident when they return?

Is this an ethics issue? Why or why not?

Is this a legal issue? Why or why not?

evolve

Go to *Chapter Extras* on Evolve for additional illustrations and resources for this chapter. *Extras* for this chapter include:

1. The National Certification Board for Therapeutic Massage and Bodywork Code of Ethics (text)
2. The National Certification Board for Therapeutic Massage and Bodywork Standards of Practice (text)
3. Massage practice wheel (illustration)

MATCHING

Place the letter of the answer next to the term or phrase that best describes it.

A. Boundaries	F. Countertransference	K. Licensure
B. Client abuse	G. Dual relationships	L. Scope of practice
C. Client neglect	H. Incident report	M. Standards of practice
D. Code of ethics	I. Integrity	N. Transference
E. Confidentiality	J. Intimacy	

_____ 1. Limits we establish between others and ourselves with regard to various aspects of our lives

_____ 2. An emotional reaction of the therapist that reflects the therapist's inner needs and conflicts

_____ 3. A report to document unusual things that happen to a client during a session

_____ 4. A condition of being whole and undivided

_____ 5. The unconscious tendency of the client to assign to others feelings and attitudes associated with significant people in his or her early life

_____ 6. Nondisclosure of privileged information

_____ 7. A sensual bond to another that involves choice, mutuality, reciprocity, trust, and delight

_____ 8. Relationships that exist in addition to the therapeutic relationship

_____ 9. Unintentional physical or emotional harm that the client sustains resulting from lack of knowledge or insensitivity on the therapist's behalf

_____ 10. A mandatory process to be completed to engage in an occupation that would otherwise be considered unlawful

_____ 11. A list of standards to assist the professional in making good decisions while conducting day-to-day responsibilities within his or her scope of practice

_____ 12. Set of guiding moral principles that govern an individual's course of action

_____ 13. The working parameters of a profession

_____ 14. Physical or emotional harm that the client sustains resulting from deliberate acts of the therapist

INTERNET ACTIVITIES

Visit the United States Department of Veterans Affairs at http://www.va.gov and search for information on *sexual harassment.* Write a short report of the VA's policy on sexual harassment.

Locate the code of ethics for psychologists at http://www.apa.org or social workers at http://www.socialworkers.org. Note similarities and differences in their codes and the NCBTMB's code of ethics for massage therapists located in Appendix A.

Visit http://www.amtamassage.org/about/codeofethics.html, and review the code of ethics for the American Massage Therapy Association. Have any important issues been omitted? If so, which ones?

Bibliography

American Massage Therapy Association: *Credentials used for the massage therapy profession,* 2002. Available at: *http://www.amtamassage.org.*

American Massage Therapy Association: *What are certification, licensing and accreditation?* 2002. Available at: *http://www.amtamassage.org.*

Baron RA: *Psychology,* ed 2, Boston, 1992, Allyn and Bacon.

Baur S: *The intimate hour,* New York, 1997, Houghton Mifflin Company.

Carnes P: *Out of the shadows: understanding sexual addiction,* ed 3, Minneapolis, 2001, Hazelden Publishing & Educational Services.

Dimond B: *The legal aspects of complementary therapy practice: a guide for health care professionals,* New York, 1998, Churchill Livingstone.

Fritz S, Grosenbach MJ, Paholsky K: Ethics and professionalism, *Massage Magazine,* Jan/Feb 1997, p 46.

Fritz S: *Fundamentals of therapeutic massage,* ed 3, St Louis, 2004, Elsevier.

Gill S: Avoid those ticking time bombs: safety or the massage professional, *Massage Bodywork: Nurture Body, Mind, Spirit,* Feb/Mar 2000, p 92.

Hamric AB, Spross JA, Hanson CM: *Advanced practice nursing: an integrative approach,* ed 3, Philadelphia, 2004, Saunders.

Hedricks G: *A year of living consciously: 365 daily inspirations for creating a life of passion and purpose,* New York, 2000, HarperCollins Publishers.

Ignatavicius DD: *Medical-surgical nursing: critical thinking for collaborative care,* ed 5, St Louis, 2005, Elsevier.

Johanson G, Kurtz R: *Grace unfolding, psychotherapy in the spirit of the Tao-te Ching,* New York, 1994, Crown Publishing Group.

Kasl CD: *Women, sex and addiction: a search for love and power,* New York, 1989, Ticknor and Fields.

Kellogg T: *Sex and sexuality: a workshop,* Dallas, 1998, self-published.

Kurtz R: *Body-centered psychotherapy: the Hakomi method,* Mendocino, Calif, 1990, LifeRhythm Books.

McIntosh N: *The educated heart: professional guidelines for massage therapists, bodyworkers, and movement therapists,* ed 2, Baltimore, 2005, Lippincott Williams & Wilkins.

Mehrabian A: *Silent messages: implicit communication of emotions and attitudes,* ed 2, Belmont, Calif, 1980, Wadsworth.

Miller-Keane, O'Toole MT: *Miller-Keane encyclopedia and dictionary of medicine, nursing, and allied health,* ed 7, St Louis, 2005, Elsevier.

National Certification Board for Therapeutic Massage and Bodywork: *Code of ethics and standards of practice,* 2006. Available at: *http://www.ncbtmb.com*

Natural Wellness. *Ethics: therapeutic relationships.* Self-published manual, 2004.

Ogden P: *Boundaries II or somatic psychology,* Boulder, Colo, 1995, Hakomi Integrative Somatics.

Odgen P: *Trauma and the body: a sensorimotor approach to psychotherapy,* New York, 2006, WW Norton & Company.

Roberts B: *Boundaries and the massage therapist: a workshop,* Lake Charles, La, 1999, self-published.

Torres LS: *Basic medical techniques and patient care for radiologic technologists,* ed 4, Philadelphia, 1993, JB Lippincott.

Tsu L: *Tao Te Ching,* New York, 1972, Vintage Books (Translated by Gia-Fu Feng and Jane English).

Webster's new world college dictionary, Springfield, Mass, 1995, G and C Merriam.

Whitfield CL: *Boundaries and relationships: knowing, protecting and enjoying the self,* Deerfield, Fla, 1993, Health Communications.

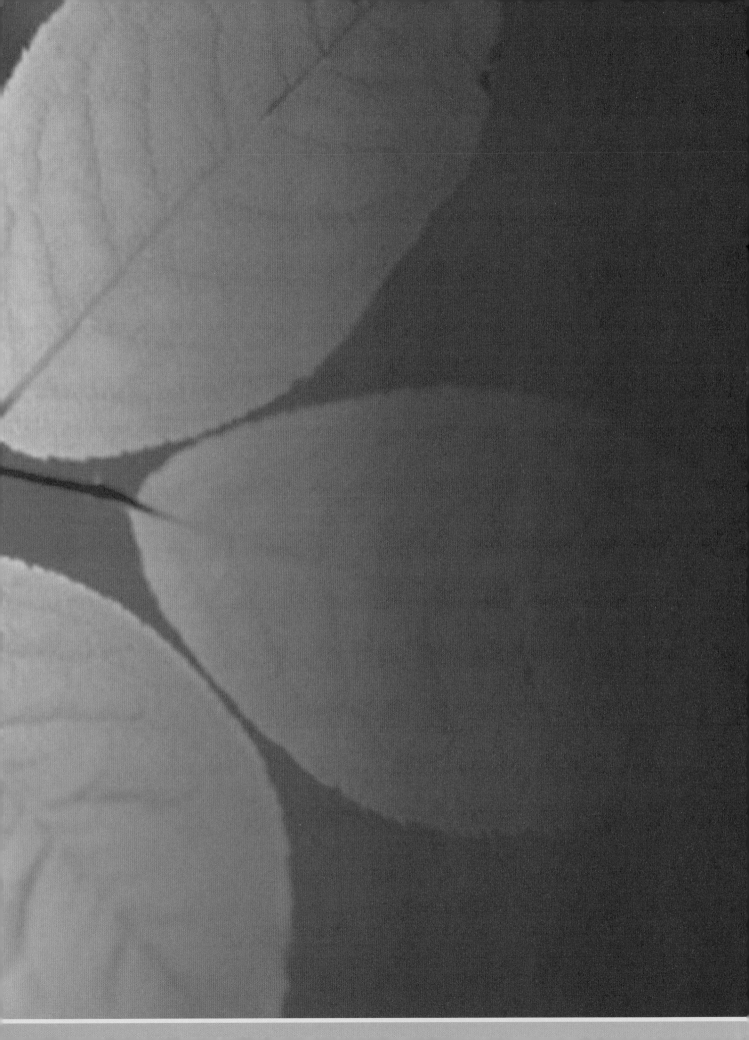

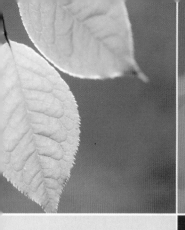

CHAPTER 3

Tools of the Trade and the Massage Environment

"All labor that uplifts humanity has dignity and importance and should be undertaken with painstaking excellence."
—Martin Luther King, Jr.

STUDENT OBJECTIVES

After completing this chapter, the student should be able to:

- Discuss reasons to obtain a massage table from a reputable manufacturer
- Identify and discuss massage table features
- Examine table features such as width, height, length, framing, padding, and fabric
- Discuss table accessories used during the massage
- Apply fabric care to the massage tabletop and table accessories
- Identify conditions or substances that damage vinyl
- Contrast vinyl cleaning and vinyl disinfecting
- Outline desirable features when choosing a massage chair
- Discuss choices of client drape used during the massage
- Explain why clients become chilled during a relaxing massage
- State ways to prevent cross-contamination while using a massage lubricant
- Discuss massage lubricant storage and shelf life
- Create a list of furnishings for the massage room
- Identify guidelines to provide a safe and accessible facility

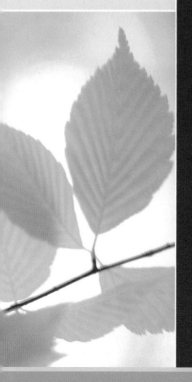

INTRODUCTION

Your career as a massage therapist depends not only on your education and skills training but also on your ability to use wisely the tools of the trade. As with any other skilled artisan, the massage therapist will use tools to express or implement massage. The tools of the massage therapist include the table and related accessories, the lubricants, and the environment where the massage takes place. In this chapter, we will open the therapist's toolbox and examine each instrument. Practical suggestions are included to assist the student in making decisions when choosing equipment and accessories or when designing a room. First, we need to distinguish the difference between a massage room and a massage office.

A massage room, or *massage studio,* is where the therapist performs the massage. It contains the massage table, accessories, lubricants, and other supplies. It may include a Hydrocollator, i.e., a roaster filled with hot stones, or a small freezer filled with cold packs to complement the massage. This chapter will examine the massage room and most of the objects found therein.

The massage office, also known as the *paper office,* is where massage appointments are scheduled, telephone calls are placed, and records are kept. All business-related activities take place in the office. These activities are necessary for your massage practice to run smoothly and efficiently.

Before you start furnishing your massage room, spend time thinking about the image you want to project. Who you are and how you perceive your work will play a role in how your massage room looks and feels. If sports and rehabilitative massage is your forte, your room may look clinical, filled with anatomical charts, medical reference books, and white massage linens. It may also contain a single freestanding locker for clients' garments. A sports massage therapist is more likely to own a portable massage table to be used when his or her services are needed at sports events.

A massage therapist who focuses on wellness and stress reduction will want to create an environment that is warm and relaxing. The walls may be painted in tan colors, with natural or subdued lighting and soothing music playing. A hint of lavender might be detected in the air.

MASSAGE TABLES

The most popular massage tables sold to students are portable tables and account for 90% to 98% of all sales by table manufacturers, with prices ranging from $200 to $600. Portable massage tables are designed to be folded in half and carried from one location to another (Figure 3-1), resembling an oversized suitcase. Some advantages of portable tables are that the therapist is able to make home or office visits, the table can be moved if the therapist is using multiple office locations, and if the massage therapist shares office space with other therapists, he or she can easily move the portable table out of the office. However, the newer sturdy designs have made them a practical choice for a stationary table as well.

Selecting a Table Manufacturer

A massage therapist must feel totally confident in his or her equipment, with the table being the most fundamental piece of equipment. It will most likely be a major expenditure when appropriate accessories are included. Make every effort to obtain professional-grade equipment for the comfort, safety, and security of both the therapist and his or her clients. Purchasing a table package from a reputable, well-established company will accomplish several things. First, these companies tend to provide great customer service. Next, most

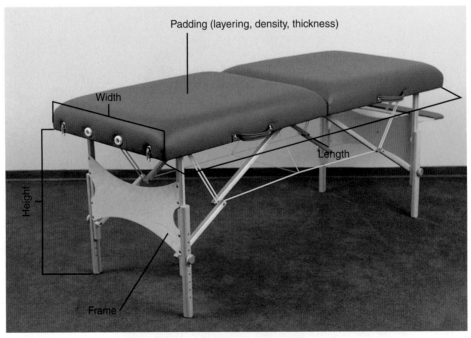

FIGURE 3-1 A typical portable massage table.

established table manufacturers offer a trial period and, if you are not satisfied, will refund your money once the table is returned. Third, these massage product companies offer the best warranties, usually 5 years and up. Last, if the table must be sold as used, their products will be easier to sell and will bring a better price.

TABLE TALK

When the Massage Table Arrives...

When your table arrives, with it will be a packing slip listing the table model, dimensions, color, and manufacturer's address and telephone number. Make a copy of the packing slip and attach it to the bottom of your table with a sheet of adhesive laminate. This information is needed when ordering additional equipment or supplies such as table pads or linens. The original packing slip should be filed away in the unlikely event that the table is lost or stolen.

Massage Table Features

Most manufacturers of massage tables offer many choices on table features such as width, height, length, framing, padding, and fabric. One principle is that the massage table should suit the therapist's body, and the accessories should accommodate the multitude of clients' bodies (wide client: side extensions; tall client: table extender). Let us examine table features.

Width

Most massage tables sold are between 28 and 31 inches wide. In most cases, table width depends on the height of the therapist transporting the table. Short therapists might consider a narrow table because it is easier to lift and carry when folded. Tall therapists do fine with a wide table. Unfortunately, wide tables make reaching across the table and applying pressure difficult for the therapist because of loss of leverage. Another consideration involves clients. Tables less than 28 inches wide often make large-framed clients feel uneasy when lying supine because their arms tend to hang off the sides. Additionally, when performing a side-lying massage on a pregnant client, a wide table is preferred. A practical solution is to employ the use of side extension (see Table Accessories).

Height

All massage tables include an adjustable height range, usually between 22 and 34 inches. Adjustment is achieved, usually in half-inch increments, by lengthening or shortening the four table legs. The optimal working table height is determined by the height of the therapist, his or her style of massage, and client girth. Two generally accepted methods are used to determine individual table height. Take care to relax your shoulders fully to get an accurate measurement.

- Stand by the massage table with arms to your side and make a fist with your hand. With this method, the table height is where the table touches your fist or knuckles (Figure 3-2, *A*).

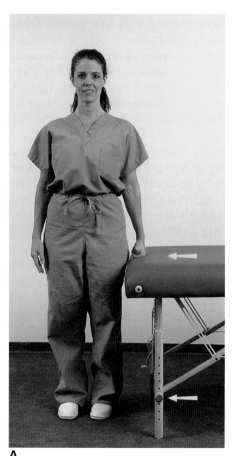 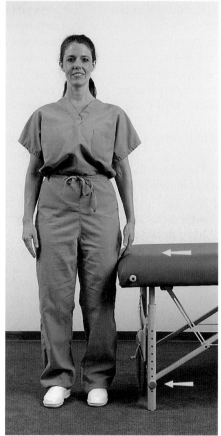

FIGURE 3-2 Two methods of determining the correct height for a massage table. **A**, Hand in a fist touching tabletop. **B**, Hand relaxed with fingertips touching tabletop.

A   **B**

- Stand by the massage table, arms at your side, with wrist and fingers extended. The height where your fingertips slightly brush against the table represents an appropriate table height (Figure 3-2, *B*). Therapists who use deep pressure techniques prefer this table height.

Use a specific table height during a day when several clients are scheduled. Afterward, lie down and note how your body feels. If your arms or shoulders feel achy, the table is too high; you are overcompensating from not being able to use leverage. If your lower back feels stiff, your table is too low; you might be bending your back instead of knees and hips. After massage, the therapist should feel from relaxed to energized. Raise or drop the tabletop until optimal table height is achieved.

Additionally, take into account client girth, which can alter table height by several inches. Remember to let the comfort level of your body dictate an appropriate table height.

Many deep-tissue therapists prefer to adjust their table heights slightly lower than normal to take advantage of their body weight behind downward pressure. Conversely, many therapists who practice Trager, craniosacral therapy, energetic modalities such as Reiki, or polarity often prefer a higher than normal table because it is most comfortable for them.

Length

Most massage tables are either 72 or 73 inches long. Because most therapists use face rests and bolsters, a 6-foot-or-taller client will have ample room because a face rest adds 10 to 12 inches to table length, and a 6- or 8-inch-high bolster will shorten the client's leg length when placed under the knees or ankles.

Frames

Table frames are typically made of either wood or aluminum. The main difference between the two is that wood frames are heavier than metal frames. Aluminum frames have a slight advantage in lateral stability over wooden-frame tables, but this difference probably will not be noticed with a high-quality wooden table.

Small-framed massage therapists often purchase aluminum-frame tables because they are easier to transport than wooden-frame tables. Aluminum tables also have the advantage of quicker leg adjustments. Although the therapist will rarely change table height, clients' torso girth varies enough to make leg adjustability a consideration. This circumstance is especially true when working on the fourth, fifth, or sixth client of the day, when energy conservation and proper body mechanics (or lack thereof) become an issue.

A carbon-fiber frame has made a debut in the massage chair industry as an aluminum alternative. However, the difference in weight is not significant enough to alter a purchase decision. On examination, the amount of carbon fibers in this mostly plastic frame is minuscule. While in use, the carbon-fiber–framed chairs flex and wobble when applying pressure laterally. No advantage is apparent in choosing this product over time-tested aluminum.

Padding

If you ask clients what they remember about being on your massage table, they will often mention table padding. This material adapts to and supports your client's body. When selecting a pad for your massage tabletop, decisions must be made regarding density, thickness, and durability. Let us examine these areas.

- *Density:* Most foam pads are divided into three grades of density: light, medium, and high. High-density foams generally have better *memory*, which is the ability of the foam to return to its original height after its surface has been disturbed. Higher-density foams are heavier and will add weight to your massage table; they are typically used on a table not designed for lighter weights. High-quality tables use medium- to high-density foam because light-density foam does not have enough memory, even when used as a top layer.
- *Loft:* Foam thickness, or loft, typically ranges from 1.5 (firm) to 3 inches (plush). Deep-tissue practitioners traditionally work on tables with firm padding. Using a firm padding prevents loss of the therapist's energy when downward pressure is applied. Thick padding is best for client comfort.
- *Layering systems:* Some tables are padded with a single layer of foam, whereas others are padded with multiple layers. Tables using a *single layer* are preferred by therapist whose focus is on structure and movement when working with clients. The deeper the pressure is, the thinner and simpler the padding system will be. Most therapists us *multiple-layer systems* because these systems are more comfortable for the client than single-layer systems. Dense foams represent the deepest layer, supporting the client's bony framework and preventing the body from bottoming out (detecting the table's wood platform). The upper layers are less dense than the lower layers so as to conform to the body's contours. The softer upper layers better accommodate the therapist when working between the table and the client. Some layering systems are equipped with recessed channels (see Chapter 10). These channels allow comfortable prone positioning for women (reduces pressure on sensitive breast tissue) and create a place where the therapist can reach down the supine-positioned client's back with ease for hand- and career-saving ergonomics.
- *Durability:* In general, table pads will last 4 to 5 years, but do not be surprised if they last 10 years. To discuss foam durability, two factors must come into the equation. First, the type of foam and, second, how often the table is used. Foam padding has a cellular structure that breaks down over time. Some of the newer foam choices, such as AeroCel and UltraCel, are highly resilient and maintain their loftiness four to five times longer than other foams. Additionally, multiple-layer systems usually outlast single-layer systems.

Table Fabric

Table fabric covers the table's foam padding and all table accessories. The most popular fabric choice is vinyl because it is long lasting and easy to clean. Vinyl fabrics also resist oil, perspiration, and makeup stains.

The downside to vinyl is that it can be easily punctured by keys, hairpins, jewelry, and pet claws. Linens have a tendency to slip on a slick vinyl surface, which can be remedied by placing a fitted table pad or fitted sheet beneath massage linens. In addition, the process used to make vinyl is unsafe for the environment, and vinyl contains polyvinyl chloride (PVC), which depletes ozone.

Many table manufactures are offering a vinyl substitute that is as strong and durable as vinyl, if not more so. Ultra leather is an example. It is soft and resists punctures better than vinyl fabrics, but is more expensive.

MINI-LAB

If you are fortunate enough to have table models from different companies displayed at your school, try these tests before you finalize your purchase.

1. *One-Knee Test.* While kneeling down on the table, place your weight on one knee. If you feel the bottom (usually wooden), then padding lacks quality.

2. *The Bounce.* Sit upright on the table and gently bounce up and down. Notice if and how much the table flexes as you land. The ideal table will offer slight resistance as you bounce.

3. *Table Rock.* Grasp the top or bottom of the table and rock it back and forth to check for lateral stability. If the table wobbles, then the table lacks integrity (or knobs need to be tightened).

4. *Ready, Set, Go!* Fold the massage table, and close it securely. Holding it by the handles, lift the table and take about 10 steps. Unfold the table and set it up on its four legs, noticing the ease or difficulties you encounter.

Vinyl Fabric Care

Keep vinyl clean by wiping it down daily with a soft, lint-free towel or an old but clean T-shirt. The worst substances for vinyl are the very things with which one might expect it to come in contact in a massage practice: oils, isopropyl alcohol, and chlorine bleach. Body oils come into contact with vinyl when a protective drape is not used. Vinyl comes into contact with massage oils when it seeps through linens during massage. Both oil types can erode vinyl's protective topcoat, which is specially designed to keep the fabric soft. When the topcoat is damaged by oil, the plasticizers that give it softness, suppleness, and resilience are broken down.

What is used to clean vinyl is more important than how often the vinyl is cleaned. Products that are drying will shorten the fabric's life. If the vinyl needs to be cleaned, use a gentle product such as Simple Green or 409 that is green in color. Avoid vinyl conditioners or protectants because they are unnecessary and will shorten the life of the vinyl by causing it to become dry and brittle, making it susceptible to cracking or splitting.

The other two substances that damage vinyl, isopropyl alcohol and chlorine bleach, are often used in disinfecting (discussed in the following chapter). Disinfect the vinyl only when it comes into contact with unidentifiable substances or body fluids.

Vinyl fabrics are similar to fine wine; they do not like wide temperature ranges. Temperature change is a problem if the massage table is stowed outdoors or in a car. After a home or office visit, put the table indoors. If the vinyl becomes cold, allow it to return to room temperature before it is used for massage. Direct sunlight breaks down vinyl, causing it to become dry and cracked. High temperatures cause vinyl to soften. Again, allow the table to return to room temperature before use. Weight placed on hot vinyl may cause permanent damage by leaving stretch marks in the fabric.

Avoid fabric wear and tear by transporting a portable table in its carrying case. Keeping vinyl unblemished is nearly impossible when moved about—from the massage room to the car, to the client's home or office, back to the car, back to the massage room, and so on. A portable table deserves a carrying case.

*"When the only tool you have is a hammer,
every problem looks like a nail."*
Albert Einstein

Table Accessories

Face Rest

A face rest, or face cradle, allows clients to keep their heads and necks relatively straight while lying prone. See Figure 3-3 for face rest use while the client is in the prone position. It consists of two parts, a crescent-shaped cushion and a frame. The cushion is generally attached to the frame by loop-and-pile fasteners, which enable the cushion to be widened or narrowed, accommodating a range of facial structures. The face rest, which is usually the same fabric as the table, adds approximately 10 to 12 inches to the table's length.

The frame is attached to the table through support rods that insert into grommets at either one end or both ends of the table. Standard face rests allow the head and neck to be in one position—parallel to the tabletop. Adjustable frames allow the neck to be flexed for client comfort and easy access of the posterior head and neck for the therapist. Adjustable frames can be folded down when not in use.

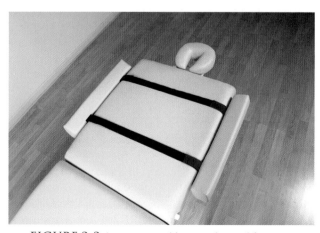

FIGURE 3-3 Arm support side extension and face rest.

Some face rests can be removed from the table and locked into a U shape, allowing clients to lie prone on the floor with comfortable breathing space. Working on the floor may be needed when working with clients such as older adults, who cannot get on and off the table.

Other face rest options include a face hole with plug and the prone pillow. The face hole is an oval opening in the tabletop that allows the client to lay face down. The hole can be closed with a fitted plug when the client is lying supine.

Arm Shelf

The arm shelf, providing a place for arms to rest while a client is in the prone position, is a small platform suspended below the face cradle. See Figure 6-10, *B*, for arm shelf use while the client is in the prone position. Arm shelves that attach to the table frame are more stable than those suspended from the face rest. However, because they are attached, these arm shelves are usable at only one end of the table and cannot be adjusted in height. The arm shelf that is suspended from the face rest may become unclipped or may tilt, swing, or slip, especially if the client presses down on the shelf when turning over. Both models come in a full range of fabrics and colors to match your massage table.

Side Extensions

Side extensions provide a place for the client's arms to rest while in the supine position. They resemble a pair of bolsters connected by wide straps. Also referred to as arm supports, side extensions widen the table (see Figure 3-3) for client comfort; they are also recommended when doing a side-lying massage. Other models slide into grommets located in the sides of the table. Make sure plenty of space in the massage room is available to maneuver around a table with extra width.

Footrest

A footrest is a padded platform covered with table fabric. Having the same width as the table and extending from one end, the footrest attaches by either sliding rods or a locking hinge mechanism. A footrest can increase the length of your massage table by 10 to 12 inches. When it is not

in use, a footrest can either fold down or be slid out of the grommets.

Carrying Case

A carrying case protects table fabric from damage while being transported; it also has padded handles and straps, making the table easier to lift and carry. Most cases have several deep zippered pockets for storage. Many therapists consider a carrying case absolutely necessary if the table is placed in a car for transport. Most cases are made of tough synthetic fabrics such as Cordura nylon.

Table Carts

If you move your table often, a table cart can save your back and shoulders from aches and injury and help conserve your energy. These devices allow the table to be easily rolled instead of lifted and carried. Table carts are attached to a folded table by adjustable quick-clip strap. Once the cart is attached, the table can be easily pushed or pulled. This accessory makes transporting a table easier, but the therapist will still need to lift the table over curbs and up stairs.

Bolsters

Bolsters, or supportive devices, are used to enhance client relaxation by filling the space between the client and the tabletop. A client will relax easily when flexed joints rest on cushions. They are often placed under the client's neck, ankles, and knees (Figure 3-4). These cushions come in a variety of sizes and shapes—tubular, square, rectangular, wedged, and wavy—and can be made of foam or stuffed with feathers or seeds such as buckwheat or flaxseed. The cloth covering the pillows is laundered after each use. Some therapists slide the bolsters under the bottom sheet instead of using individual slipcovers.

A soft, tubular pillow is often used for the neck while the client is in the supine position. The most popular knee and ankle bolsters are 3 × 26 inches, 6 × 26 inches, and 8 × 26 inches. A variety of sizes is recommended to suit individual client needs. Some bolsters can be inflated up to 8 inches. Flat-bottomed bolsters stay in place better than full round

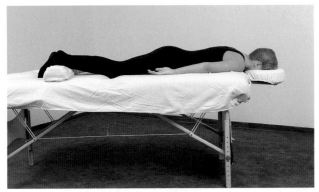
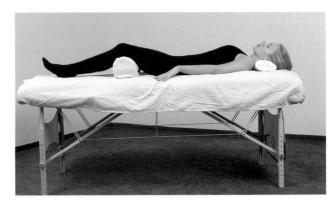

FIGURE 3-4 Bolsters are used to support your client on the massage table.

bolsters. More elaborate cushion systems can be purchased for your practice.

In addition to neck and leg bolsters, keep four to six regular-size bed pillows on hand for client support while in a side-lying position.

A stool can be regarded as a table accessory, an arm shelf. This item is discussed later in this chapter in the section on Furnishing the Massage Room.

EVOLVE *Log on to the Evolve website and, after accessing your student account, view additional images of equipment used by therapists such as bolsters, a stool, and a table cart.* ■

MINI-LAB

Obtain a 3 × 26–inch bolster, a 6 × 26–inch bolster, and an 8 × 26–inch bolster. Lie on your back (supine position) and place the 3 × 26–inch bolster behind your knees for 1 minute. Next, place the 6 × 26–inch bolster behind your knees for 1 minute. Then, place the 8 × 26–inch bolster behind your knees for 1 minute. On a sheet of paper, note the differences you feel in your back, hips, knees, ankles, and feet. Repeat the procedure, but this time lie on your abdomen (prone position) and place the bolsters under your ankles for 1 minute. Again, noting the differences in specific body joints, jot down your findings on a sheet of paper. This exercise will help you understand why bolsters are used in your massage practice and why including several sizes is preferable. One will usually feel more comfortable than the other two, but this will vary from person to person.

MASSAGE CHAIRS

Introduced in the 1980s, chair, or seated, massage has grown in popularity and is found in many settings, from shopping malls and airports to private offices. A massage chair takes up a relatively small amount of space compared with a massage table. Seated massage is performed on the client while he or she is completely clothed. (For more information on seated massage, see Chapter 27.) Many therapists purchase a massage chair after their table purchase and use it as an adjunct to their table work. Some therapists practice solely with a massage chair. The cost of a massage chair is almost the same as a massage table.

Many different massage chairs are on the market today. As is the case when choosing a massage table, different features appeal to different therapists. An important consideration when choosing a massage chair is that the chair be lightweight and simple to set up and take down. The chair should also be sturdy and strong because a wobbly chair makes the person sitting in it feel unsafe. Make sure all the adjustable levers and latches are enclosed completely because exposed ones can pinch therapists' fingers and catch clients' hair. A desktop model is also available.

MASSAGE LINENS

Sheets

Massage linens include a top and bottom sheet for the table, bolster covers, face rest covers, pillowcases, eye pillow covers, and armrest covers. Popular linen fabrics are flannel, cotton, cotton blends, and percale. Most therapists invest in twin sheets sets, fitted and flat sheets and a standard pillowcase. The fitted sheet serves as a bottom sheet; the flat serves as a top drape; the pillow case serves as a bolster cover or drape for the face rest.

White, off-white, or soft pastels suit a soothing environment, and these colors bleach well. Dark colors often reveal oil stains. Be cognizant of the weight and thickness of the sheets. Many inexpensive fabrics such as cotton-polyester blends are transparent and are not appropriate draping material, unless accompanied with a blanket (see below). Whichever fabric you choose, have an alternative cover drape available at the client's request. When using oils as a primary medium, remember that clean linens may appear stained and smell rancid.

Towels

Some therapists use bath-size towels or bath sheets as top drapes. They are thicker and heavier than sheets, provide good client coverage, and provide easy access to the abdomen when a client is supine. Other reasons therapists use towels are easy maneuverability over sheets, and oil stains are less obvious on towels than on sheets.

Blankets

As the body relaxes, blood pressure lowers, circulation returns to the core, and body temperature drops slightly. Have a cotton or woolen blanket to drape over clients if they become chilled. A chilled client will not relax easily. A thoughtful measure is to keep a client from becoming chilled by using a blanket at the start of the session instead of trying to warm a chilled client. Along with warmth, the weight of the blanket adds comfort and a sense of security for the client. Make sure the client blankets are machine washable. The blanket does not replace the top drape. Instead, place the blanket *over* the top drape.

Massage Linen Care

All linens that the client or the therapist touches must be laundered after use. Replace linens whenever they become stained, odorous, or threadbare. Care of contaminated linens will be discussed in the following chapter.

MASSAGE MEDIA

The primary purpose of massage media, which include oils, gels, lotions, creams, butters, and powders, is to reduce friction between the therapist's hands and forearms and the client's skin (Figure 3-5). If insufficient lubricant is used, then

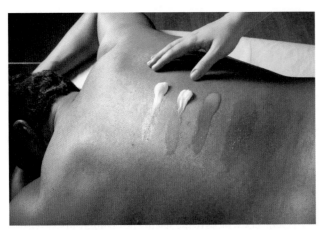

FIGURE 3-5 Lubricant choices *(from left to right):* butter, cream, gel, and oil.

the client may report a burning sensation where the therapist is massaging. Several factors must be considered when choosing a lubricant.

Does It Nourish the Skin?

Ingredients such as cold-pressed vegetable, nut, and seed oils and plant essences are good for the skin, whereas ingredients such as mineral oil and isopropyl alcohol can clog pores and deplete skin nutrients. Mineral oil has a molecular weight of over 500, which does not permit it to be absorbed by the skin, and it is a petrochemical. Although stearyl and cetyl alcohol do not nourish the skin, they are safe and often used as emulsifiers and stiffening agents. Always read the ingredient list to ascertain its contents.

How Will the Skin React to It?

Certain skin types will be sensitive to some products and not to others. During the initial massage consultation, inquire about allergies to nuts or other products that are ingredients in massage lubricants. Keep a copy of all ingredient lists on hand, and allow the client to read the ingredient list for prior approval. Because lubricant sensitivity cannot always be predetermined, keep a hypoallergenic lubricant handy to use when the need arises. *Hypoallergenic* does not mean that the product will not cause allergic reactions, rather that the product underwent lengthy testing and the majority of the people in the study were unaffected. Scented lubricants increase the likelihood of allergic reactions. Many allergic reactions do not show up for 24 to 48 hours after the product is in contact with the skin, which means that most allergic reactions will not be apparent until a day or two after treatment.

How Will My Linens React to It?

Oils or products that have high oil content are more likely to stain linens. If the aforementioned products are used, massage linens such as bolster covers and bottom sheets are more likely to become oil stained and will require frequent replacing.

Avoid using oil-stained linens because they appear soiled and unsanitary. Even clean unstained sheets used in a massage practice where oil is the primary lubricant will emit a rancid odor over time.

How Much Does It Cost?

The cost factor will depend on your pocketbook and how much importance is placed on lubricant quality. Quality costs. If you subscribe to a business philosophy of *only the best for my clients,* then you will invest in a relatively more expensive lubricant. These additional costs are usually passed on to the client in higher fees.

Once a lubricant choice is made, allow the client to choose between unscented and scented. If the client is interested in a scented lubricant, then place a small amount on the back of his or her hand. Once approved, proceed with the massage. If not approved, select another scent or suggest unscented. If the client has allergies or other hypersensitivities, then an unscented hypoallergenic is recommended.

Never apply the lubricant directly on the client's skin. Place the proper amount in your own hands, warming it by rubbing the fingers and palms together. Apply lubricant only on the area you will be massaging, never on adjacent areas. If too much lubricant is accidentally used, wipe off the excess with the back of your hand.

The amount of lubricant you use will depend on:
- **Texture:** Texture refers to the feel of a lubricant and how it glides on the skin. Some lubricants are slippery and some are tacky.
- **Emolliency:** The more emollient the lubricant is, the less lubricant and reapplications are needed. An *emollient* is a substance that softens or moisturizes the skin.
- **Skin dryness:** Dry skin requires more lubricant and reapplication than nondry skin.
- **Body hair:** Areas with a plethora of body hair require more lubricant and reapplication than skin without hair. Additionally, use linear over circular movements because they are less likely to mat and tangle the hair.
- **Massage type and therapist intent:** In relaxation and wellness massage, the therapist primarily uses gliding strokes, and a reasonable amount of lubricant is needed. Specific massage, such as that used in sports and rehabilitation, requires the therapist to grasp superficial layers of skin and fascia. Only a small amount of lubricant is needed.

In general, excessive amounts of lubricant will reduce tissue manipulation, and inadequate amounts increase friction and will pull and irritate the skin. Experience will teach you how much to use in which circumstance. Less is better; adding more lubricant is easier than removing it.

TYPES OF LUBRICANTS

Cream

Massage cream is the best-selling massage lubricant and has been so since the early 1990s. Cream is more emollient than other lubricants and has a viscous quality, which gives it a staying power almost equal to that of massage oils and gels. Because it cannot be spilled as oils, gels, or lotions can, cream is less messy. Cream is not likely to stain clothing but is a relatively more expensive lubricant.

Butters

Having the similar consistency of massage cream, body butters are made from fruit, nuts, or seeds. The three most common butters are cocoa, jojoba, and Shea. These butters are naturally rich in vitamins A and E. They are extremely hydrating and moisturizing and have an excellent rapport with the skin. Butters are used for healing and soothing chapped or irritated skin. As butters are worked into the skin, body temperature will cause them to melt, so use sparingly. **Cocoa butter**, also known as theobroma oil, is obtained from cacao seed and is commonly found in stick form. Cocoa butter is recommended for therapists who are treating specific tissues. African **Shea butter**, extracted from the tree's fruit (called nuts), is mostly used as an ingredient in cream. **Jojoba** is almost a liquid wax and is taken from the desert shrub's seeds; it is chemically similar to the skin's oil (sebum). Allergic reactions to body butters are rare.

Oils and Gels

Used sparingly, oils and gels are excellent lubricants because they are relatively inexpensive. Cost depends on the source of the oil and the expense to the manufacturer to extract it. Some body treatments call for Ayurvedic oils, which are food-grade oils, oils you have in a kitchen. Because of their superior quality, nut and seed oils are preferred for massage. Additives such as vitamin E and essential oils can be used. Vitamin E, an antioxidant, also acts as a preservative, which is important because of oil's quick rancidity. Essential oils are used for a wide range of effects; essential oils and aromatherapy are addressed in the spa chapter (Chapter 24). Gels have a relatively longer shelf life, are hypoallergenic and unscented, and do not contain alcohol or mineral oil, so they are excellent for sensitive skin types.

Avoid mineral oil because it is a known *carcinogen* (cancer-causing agent). Mineral oil, or liquid petroleum, is not miscible in body oils and depletes skin nutrients. Mineral oil may clog the skin's pores. Most lotions and creams contain mineral oil because it is relatively inexpensive and has an infinite shelf life. Baby oil is primarily mineral oil.

One drawback of oil or gel as a lubricant is that an accidental spill spells disaster on walls or carpet. Clothing does not fare well after an encounter. If you use or plan to use oil or gel, address this factor with the client so he or she can plan accordingly, which usually involves the client bringing a change of old clothes to wear after the session. Caution needs to be taken because nut and seed allergies are common. Avoid using oils and gels on clients who have oily skin.

Some massage oil manufacturers sell a product to be added to the wash to help remove the appearance and smell of oil from linens. When using oils as your primary medium, this product would be an asset.

Some therapists mix their oil or gel with lotion in a 50/50 solution.

Lotion

Lotions are formulated to be used in two different settings: rehabilitation and spa. Therapists who treat specific injuries and conditions prefer *deep-tissue lotions* because these lotions offer the least amount of glide and the most control. Lotions are tackier than other lubricants, and they create a slight drag on the skin. *Hydrating lotions* are primarily used as finishing treatment in a three-step skin procedure (exfoliate, mineralize, and moisturize). Lotion will not leave the skin feeling greasy. However, lotion does not have the staying power of oil or cream and is quickly absorbed in the skin. Therefore you will use more lotion than oil or cream, but lotion is less expensive than cream.

Powder

Baby powder, talc, powdered chalk, or cornstarch is used when doing manual lymphatic drainage and massage during a pregnant woman's labor process. It affords little friction reduction but does leave a greasy residue. Be careful when applying powder because particles can enter nasal passages and cause the client or therapist to sneeze or cough.

Liniments

Liniments are alcoholic, oily, or soapy agents used as **analgesics** (agents that reduce pain) and to create the sensation of heat. All liniments are **rubefacient**, which means they redden the skin because the ingredients cause irritation. As reddening occurs, the skin's vessels dilate and increase local blood supply. Avoid using liniments or liniment-type lotions on a client's hands and feet, near mucous membranes, or before heat treatments.

Lubricant Dispenser

When choosing a lubricant dispenser, preventing cross-contamination is a primary concern. Either a single-use container or a pump dispenser works best. The downside to using a pump dispenser is that, if dropped, it may become damaged. The dispenser can be placed on the massage table between the client's knees for easy therapist access and to prevent it from being knocked off the table during massage. Placing the dispenser on the floor is not recommended because it requires the therapist to bend over or squat over when reapplying.

Holsters that suspend dispensers from straps are available; they allow dispensers to be worn around the therapist's waist or hips. When therapists are asked about the practicality of holsters, reviews are often mixed.

Storage and Shelf Life

Once purchased, store all massage lubricants (with the exception of powder) in a cool, dark location out of direct sunlight. In this condition, massage lubricants should last approximately 12 to 18 months. The product's shelf life can be extended up to an additional year with refrigeration or freezing; allow them to return to room temperature before use.

MASSAGE SUPPLIES

Massage supplies are items such as paper towels and drinking cups that are bought and used often. They are needed to provide a clean, sanitary, and comfortable massage environment. Some massage supplies are used for the massage itself; others are personal care items such as hair spray, contact lens solution, and cotton balls. Use the checklist (Figure 3-6) also provided on the *Evolve* website when shopping for supplies. Blank lines have been added to the checklist for items you wish to include in your massage office. Bottled water may be supplied either for personal use or for client use. Candy or mints may be needed if a client needs sugar, such as in a diabetic emergency.

> **evolve** *Log on to the Evolve website and access your student account. Print out the Massage Supply Checklist and use it when stocking your massage room with supplies.* ■

FURNISHING THE MASSAGE ROOM

The fixtures, furniture, and furnishings for the massage room require brief mention. These items help create the proper atmosphere where the massage takes place. These items include a mirror, clock, water dispenser, wastebasket, supply cabinet, chairs and stools, a place for your client's clothes and personal items, and wall hangings. Window treatments, light sources, and floor and wall treatment also deserve discussion. The massage room is an important element of the massage experience. It states how the therapist feels about his or her work.

Mirror

A mirror is essential for massage rooms. Clients use mirrors to groom themselves after a massage. Therapists use full-length mirrors to aid in client assessment. Mirrors also reflect light or room objects and can be used to make a space appear larger.

Clocks

Wall or desk clocks help to keep the therapist on a schedule, and they help regulate timed treatments such as ice packs or facial

---

MASSAGE SUPPLY CHECKLIST

☐ Lubricant

☐ Liquid soap

☐ Disposable gloves and finger cots

☐ Cleaning and disinfectant supplies

☐ Box of facial tissues

☐ Paper towels

☐ Toilet paper

☐ Cotton balls

☐ Disposable cups

☐ Hairspray

☐ Contact lens solution

☐ Waterless hand cleaner

☐ Bottled water

☐ Mints or candy

Facial Massage Supplies:

☐ Makeup remover

☐ Cleansing cream

☐ Toner/astringent

☐ Moisturizing cream

☐ Clay masque

☐ Other: _____

☐ Other: _____

_____

FIGURE 3-6 Massage supply checklist.

masques. The clock should be quiet and visible to the therapist rather than the client, for whom it may be a distraction.

Water Dispenser

Clean, pure drinking water is an important nutrient in maintaining health. Most people do not drink enough fluids. A conveniently located water dispenser makes getting the water that your body requires easy. Clients will want to take advantage of the water dispenser as well. Part of your massage can include offering clients water before and after the massage.

Wastebasket

A wastebasket is needed in the massage room for used paper towels, facial tissue, gloves, and other disposable items. Most state laws require the wastebasket to close with a lid. Lidded wastebaskets with foot pedals are preferred to those with lids that need to be lifted by hand for sanitation reasons.

Supply Cabinet

A supply cabinet is needed to stow massage linens, supplies, lubricant, and equipment. Hinged doors are preferred to open shelves if items need to be out of sight. Cabinets or closets fitted with louvered doors allow stowed items access to open air and allow music from hidden speakers to move through slats. Line shelves with laminate (e.g., Formica); it resists stains from lubricant dispensers and linens and is easy to clean and disinfect.

Chairs and Stools

A chair provides a place for the client to sit while removing trousers, stockings, shoes, and socks. Depending on available space and personal taste, the therapist may choose a simple straight-back chair, a plush and oversized chair, a chaise lounge, or an ottoman. Upholstery fabrics are available in a wide variety of colors and textures.

The therapist uses a stool to sit comfortably when performing head, neck, hands, or feet massage (see Figure 6-9). Use a stool that can be raised or lowered. Height adjustment mechanisms range from hydraulic to manual rotation. A hydraulic stool can be quietly adjusted while the therapist is sitting on the stool. The stools requiring manual rotation are often noisy and involve the therapist's standing to adjust or readjust the height. Some therapists use a large inflatable physioball as a stool.

Place for Client's Personal Items

Most therapists ask the client to remove some or all of his or her garments, glasses, and jewelry. A place can be provided for these items such as wall hooks, a coat tree, a freestanding locker, or a valet.

If the designated place for clients to prepare for the massage is a small table and chair, then provide a small dish or basket for smaller items such as keys, pocket change, wallet, eyeglasses, wristwatches, and jewelry. In this way, clients can

easily take their personal property with them if they move from one location to another.

Wall Hangings

Massage therapists use wall hangings in their massage rooms for many reasons.

- **Ambiance:** When choosing a wall hanging for ambiance, consider color and content. Warm or soft colors such as peach and beige are calming and tranquil. Bright, intense colors such as red and yellow stimulate the nervous system. In representational art, nature scenes depicting waterfalls, ocean waves, open meadows, or nature settings provide a relaxing environment. Visual art is music for your eyes. Keep it simple; if it is too busy, it may distract from the massage experience. Make a brief statement, not an exclamation. Solicit the aid of a trusted friend or family member if help is needed when choosing art. For example, save your prints of the American Civil War for your living room.
- **Inform and educate:** Anatomical and trigger point charts or acupuncture meridian charts are often used by therapists as wall hangings. These wall hangings provide quick reference for locating muscles, bony markings, trigger points, acupressure points, and other important areas of the body. They are also used for educating the client about musculoskeletal anatomy and mechanisms of pain and discomfort. Charts are used to create a clinical atmosphere. Many anatomical chart companies offer desktop flip charts that can be stored on a bookshelf and referred to as needed.
- **Professionalism:** Framed diplomas, certificates, and awards help portray the therapist as a professional who has attained success and community respect. These item help instill a sense of confidence in clients by demonstrating achievement, accomplishments, experience, and commitment. Many massage therapists prefer to hang their diplomas and awards in their offices and to keep the studio atmosphere artistic and relaxing; the studio space belongs to clients. Other suggestions are photos of the therapist receiving awards or giving lectures.

Window Treatments

Window treatments include blinds, shades, and draperies and are available a wide variety of styles and colors. Window treatments can be simple or serve as part of the overall décor. Fabric-covered blinds are more attractive than the vinyl and aluminum versions, but they are more expensive. All window treatments can be stained when touched by oily hands. Window coverings serve many important functions.

- **Decoration:** When choosing window treatments as decoration, the material (wood, textile, or metal), color, and shade of the walls and floor must be taken into consideration. For example, patterned draperies typically do not look good against patterned wallpaper. Ask someone who has talent or training in interior design if assistance is needed.
- **Reduce sound:** Vertical or horizontal blinds do little to reduce sound, whereas heavy fabric draperies absorb sound and reduce its travel. If the massage room is near

a busy or noisy area, then draperies can go a long way to cut down noise. Special batting can be purchased to add to the drapery material, which further reduces sound travel and echoing.

- **Block or filter light:** Massage therapists prefer window treatments that block light over those that filter light. Creating or increasing the lighting by turning on a lamp or opening a window blind is easier than decreasing daylight moving through light-filtering material.
- **Privacy:** For privacy, all windows that provide view into massage rooms should be covered by window treatments.

Flooring

Carpet is the best choice for flooring in a massage room. As an insulator, carpet provides warmth and sound absorption. Carpeted floors create a measure of client safety; oily feet create a liability risk on smooth flooring. If the massage room happens to have smooth flooring, carpet or a carpet remnant can then be cut to fit the room. A throw rug creates a tripping or slipping hazard.

Sound Proofing

Along with heavy draperies and carpet flooring, interior walls can be insulated, or sound-absorbing panels can be placed in the massage room. Textured wallpaper, hanging pictures, and other large decorations on the walls will minimize echoing sounds. Hollow-core doors can be replaced with solid-core doors to further reduce undesired sound.

> *"Where the spirit does not work with the hand, there is no art."*
> Leonardo da Vinci

MASSAGE ROOM ENVIRONMENT

The atmosphere of your massage room sets the tone for your client's experience. Ideally, you want a space that is quiet, private, serene, easy to heat or cool, and draft free. The room should be free of pet dander, as well as tobacco and cleaning solution odors. Supplies such as bolsters, blankets, lubricants, and pillows should be within the therapist's reach during the session but not where they can create an obstacle for the client. Convenient access to a restroom is desirable.

A dinner party metaphor is often used to explain the importance of atmosphere. When planning, preparing, and serving a meal for a special guest, adjustments are made to make the dining experience extraordinary. The table is set using clean, attractive linens. The host pulls out the fine china and crystal and polishes the silver flatware. A special flower arrangement is placed in the room. Soft music plays in the background, and the lights are dimmed. Give clients the same care and consideration by treating them as honored guests.

The importance of ambiance cannot be overstated. The Chinese symbol for space is the Japanese symbol for gates. Open the gates to relaxation and healing by creating a space

where these can occur. The atmosphere should begin when the client drives up to the office and should be maintained all the way to the massage room. Atmospheric considerations include lighting, music, temperature, and room color. Examples are listed here to stimulate the therapist's imagination and to help with goal setting.

MINI-LAB

If possible, receive massages from therapists who practice a variety of different styles. After the experience, write a summary on how you felt about the massage environment. Use this information when deciding décor. This mini-lab can be expanded to include the therapist's interviewing skills and the massage technique used.

Light

Lighting serves several purposes and requires differing amounts. First, enough lighting must be provided so clients can fill out paperwork, remove garments, safely maneuver around the room, get on and off the massage table, dress, and exit the office. Adequate lighting is needed for the therapist to assess skin condition before and during the massage. Decreased lighting is needed during the massage to assist in client relaxation.

Natural light, or sunlight, is the best light source. Room light from a window is easily adjusted through window treatments. Window glass can be tinted to reduce harsh sunlight.

During overcast days or after dusk, indirect lighting can be used. Indirect indicates that the light source is obscured from view by shades or baffles. This effect can be achieved with floor or table lamps, recessed ceiling lights in the room's corners, or a string of lights placed strategically in the room. To illuminate a dark area, use a nightlight behind a large object such as an oversized vase.

Many therapists enjoy candlelight in their massage rooms. Although candles are unbeatable for creating a relaxing ambiance, they are also a fire hazard. Regardless of how careful you are, candle wax spills, and soot deposits occur on shelves and walls. Decide if the benefits outweigh the risks.

Music

Music hath charms to soothe the savage breast, and although clients are not savages, they do respond to music. Music is art for the ears. Music for massage helps clients relax (if the music is soft and slow), and it helps therapists maintain a soothing rhythm when applying massage movements.

Keep an assortment of music selections on hand. Some therapists allow clients to bring their own music selections to the session. Although music, as with room décor, is a matter of taste, most therapists prefer a slow, even melody. Most classical selections are not appropriate because of the ebb and flow of crescendos and decrescendos.

Be cautious of New Age music because many selections contain jumpy melodies that are stimulating to the nervous system. Some music stores include a music category called

STEVEN HALPERN, PhD

Born: April 18, 1947.

"Mother Nature gave us eyelids. She didn't give us ear-lids or body-lids."

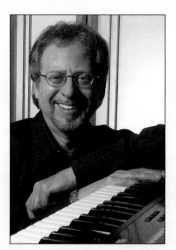

As the true pioneer in the field of relaxation music, Steven Halpern is far from being simply a gifted musician. His eternal thirst for knowledge has benefited the field of massage therapy, and any therapist who has used any of his music can attest to this undeniable fact. His extensive research has taken music to a scientific level and beyond.

Halpern's interest in music actually began when he was a toddler growing up in Long Island, New York. Surprisingly, his parents never played music in the home. In fact, Halpern often crawled down the hallway of his apartment building to the doors of neighbors who were playing music. This action allowed him to follow his heart and listen to music that he truly enjoyed at a very young age. A short while after starting in the school music program, he found himself becoming bored with just playing *little black dots written by dead white composers*. This boredom led to his involvement in jazz, which allows a great deal of improvisation.

During college in the late 1960s, Halpern's curiosity about music led to his revolutionary research on the effects of certain rhythms on the human body. At the time, it was practically a virgin field. Few schools would allow such research, but fortunately Halpern was introduced to the University of California at Sonoma, where he had access to biofeedback equipment and conducted investigations on the effects of music using subtle rhythms, gentle tones, and nontraditional harmonics. The result has been the hallmark of his approach to composition. "One of the most fundamental responses of the human organism is that it is easily rhythm entrained to an external rhythmic stimulus," he says. "In other words, if there is a steady beat, your heart and pulse will naturally synchronize to that rhythm." This concept explains why relaxing to music that has a beat faster than a resting heartbeat is impossible.

This theory instantly made Halpern's music popular with massage therapists and clients. After hearing this new type of music, people actually hired him to play live as they were receiving massages. Many massage professionals claimed that as a result of listening to his music, clients were actually relaxing before a hand was even placed on them. Thus therapists received much less resistance from clients, which, in turn, resulted in making therapists' work much easier.

Although music is important, Halpern reminds us not to forget about other forms of sound. Having a great deal of control over his or her environment, a therapist needs to be aware of the noises that are often taken for granted. Halpern says that he is amazed at how many therapists have a loud ticking clock or a noisy air conditioner. These factors should be addressed before music can even be considered. Many of us have conditioned ourselves to block out certain sounds. Halpern states, "Mother Nature gave us eyelids. She didn't give us ear-lids or body-lids." Whether we are consciously aware of it, a person's entire body is picking up and responding to all sounds.

Halpern notes that "while listening to true relaxation music, an altered state can be entered . . . whereas dancers say they become one with the music, a massage therapist can become one with the massage. This state allows therapists to consciously lose track of the exact strokes they are going to do next, yet they always seem to do exactly the right ones." He claims that some of the best massage professionals say that such music has helped them reach the zone in which the realm of massage lives and a wonderful healing energy can be tapped. He admits that this phenomenon has yet to be scientifically documented, but after hearing it from so many people, he believes that it must be true. Halpern invites all massage professionals to keep their awareness and hearts open to this idea because it can be of great service and benefit to their clients. "Music is much more powerful, and the effects of music are much more pronounced than most people realize," says Halpern. "In the past 25 or 30 years, people have forgotten how to listen in a lot of respects, but I now start to see people come back."

minimalism, which is suitable for massage. Nature sounds such as waves breaking on the shore, whale songs, and thunderstorms, combined with orchestral music, are good choices (as long as no surprising screeches or cackling birds are heard). Additionally, trickling water sounds may stimulate urination is some clients.

MINI-LAB

Lie on your massage table in the prone and the supine positions to get a client's perspective. Note what the major issues are: sights, sounds, smell, and so on. Do what you can to accentuate the positive and minimize the negative.

Room Temperature

A comfortable temperature for a massage room is approximately 75° F. Once room temperature is set, be prepared to make adjustments to address individual client needs. For example, clients who are warm-natured or those who are pregnant may request a fan blowing to keep them comfortable.

Clients may have difficulty relaxing if the room temperature is too cool. As the massage progresses, pulse rate, respiration rate, and blood pressure decrease as blood returns to the body's core. As a result, most clients become chilled during the massage, although they felt comfortable at its beginning. Address this issue before the massage begins because, as you may recall, warming a chilled client is more difficult than cooling a warm client. Blankets or an electric heating pad can help clients stay warm and comfortable. See the section on blankets for more information.

The therapist is unable to gauge room temperature by his or her own comfort. During the massage, the massage therapist's body temperature rises because of physical exertion. Wearing clothes made of natural fibers that fit loosely to allow air to evaporate perspiration helps keep the therapist comfortable. A small oscillating fan placed on the floor and directed at the therapist's feet could be helpful.

Color

The areas where color plays an important role are walls, flooring, window treatments, and linens. Choose colors that contrast well, such as tan walls and sage green linens or green walls and beige linens. Neutral colors work best because they do not excite the client's nervous system.

Colors used in the massage room are divided into two categories, warm and cool. Warm colors naturally bring a feeling of warmth but also stimulation; cool colors can make a room feel cool but also relaxing. Shade or hues of color have an impact and must be considered when making decisions regarding color.

Warm colors are reds, browns, yellows, and oranges; cool colors are blues, violets, and greens. White is the absence of color, and black is the combination of all colors. Either choose what you like or ask for assistance from an artistic friend or colleague.

evolve *After logging on to your Evolve student account, download and print out the massage room layouts for a massage practice. Using a new sheet of paper, draw your ideal massage room.* ∎

MINI-LAB

Using all the elements discussed in this chapter, design your massage room.

SAFETY GUIDELINES FOR THE TREATMENT FACILITY

The following are suggestions for providing a treatment facility that is safe and accessible for all clients.

- Comply with all state and municipal building fire and safety codes.
- Establish and maintain current liability insurance coverage. The original or copy of this policy must be kept on the premises at all times and made available for inspection.
- Maintain an operative fire extinguisher and heat or smoke detectors on the premises. Fire extinguishers must be located at eye level and in clear view (ratings specified by the city ordinance).
- Have a fire escape route posted in the office and clearly mark all building exits.
- Provide safe and unobstructed human passage in the public areas. Safe passage includes level flooring. Omit area rugs because they can be a slipping or tripping hazard.
- Choose only nonslip flooring, especially in bathrooms and wet areas.
- Bathrooms should be accessible to the physically challenged and should include a wheelchair-height lavatory with lever-style faucets. Grab bars should be located near the toilet for clients who need assistance transferring to and from the toilet seat.
- Lever-style door handles are required for physically challenged people.
- Have a designated handicapped-accessible parking space. Slopes, not steps, between the parking space and the building, should be available for use. The space should be marked with the international symbol for accessibility. Exterior ramps should be designed so that they drain easily and do not hold water.
- Public telephones should have an adjustable volume control.
- Maintain a list of all emergency telephone numbers by the telephone: the local fire station, police department, sheriff's department, local hospital, and ambulance.
- The street address should be outside the building in clear view, which will make locating your business easier for emergency assistance.
- Maintain all equipment used to perform massage services in safe condition, which includes checking and tightening your massage table hinges, knobs, and locks before each business day.

SUMMARY

Career success depends not only on knowledge, skills, and abilities but also on your capacity to use wisely the tools of the trade. Massage equipment or tools include the massage table, face rests, arm shelves, carrying cases, table carts, linens, bolsters, and massage lubricants. Equipment should be chosen with consideration to ergonomics, client comfort, longevity, and investment wisdom.

The massage table is your most important tool. When purchasing a stationary or a portable massage table, table manufacturers let you decide the specifications of features such as width, height, length, frame, padding, and fabric.

Massage linens include towels, sheets, blankets, pillowcases, bolster and face rest covers, and so on. Popular linen fabrics are flannel, cotton, cotton blends, and percale.

Massage media or lubricants include oils, gels, creams, butters, lotions, powders, and liniments. Good lubricants should nourish the skin. The therapist must consider client reactions and effect of fabrics when choosing a lubricant.

The massage room environment ties everything together. Considerations should be made for temperature, lighting, color, music, decorations, and client comfort.

Finally, the treatment facility must be safe for all who enter.

Using these recommendations can produce a great saving of time and money and improve the quality of the therapist's work.

CASE STUDY:

Lost Possessions

Tiffany owns and operates one of the oldest and most reputable massage therapy salons, Southern Comfort, in her hometown. She has two associate therapists, Juanita and Suzanne, who work with her. One of the salon's most frequent clients, Rebecca, the wife of the town's mayor, scheduled a massage with Juanita at 10 AM. Rebecca was feeling happy, sad, and tired. For the last few months, she had been planning her only daughter's wedding. The wedding was this last weekend, and Rebecca was ready to unwind.

That afternoon, Rebecca telephoned the salon to report that she left her wedding ring in the massage room. She described the ring to Tiffany as a very expensive platinum and diamond solitaire that was given to her by her husband on their 10-year wedding anniversary. After a brief conversation, a highly emotional Rebecca claimed that she does not remember putting it on her finger after the massage.

Tiffany searched the massage room and was unable to locate the ring. Rebecca returned to the salon and searched the massage room as well. She emptied her purse onto the massage table; both Rebecca and Tiffany looked for the ring. Tiffany looked at the appointment book and noticed that both therapists used the massage room after Rebecca's massage. Tiffany told Rebecca that she would ask both Suzanne and Juanita if a ring was found in the massage room and that she would call Rebecca if it were found.

If you were Tiffany, how would you approach Suzanne and Juanita about the missing ring?

If Rebecca sounded accusatory, how should Tiffany deal with the situation professionally?

If you were Rebecca, how would you react to Tiffany's plan of action? Is Tiffany doing enough to solve the problem?

---

evolve

Go to *Chapter Extras* on Evolve for additional illustrations and resources for this chapter. *Extras* for this chapter include:

1. Crossword puzzle (downloadable form)
2. Standard and adjustable face rest frames and cushions (illustration)
3. How To Set Table Height (video clip)
4. Massage chair (illustration)
5. Desktop model massage chair (illustration)
6. Case study (text)

MATCHING

Place the letter of the answer next to the term or phrase that best describes it.

A. Analgesics
B. Butters
C. Cream
D. Hypoallergenic

E. Indirect
F. Liniments
G. Loft
H. Memory

I. Mineral oil
J. Portable tables
K. Reduce friction
L. Rubefacients

_____ 1. Extracted from fruit, seeds, or nuts

_____ 2. Most popular massage lubricant

_____ 3. Synonym for foam thickness

_____ 4. The ability of foam to return to its original height after being disturbed

_____ 5. Alcoholic, oily, or soapy agents used to create a sensation of heat

_____ 6. Agents that reduce pain

_____ 7. Products that redden the skin and cause irritation

_____ 8. Accounts for 90% to 98% of all massage table sales

_____ 9. Product that underwent lengthy testing with the majority of persons experiencing no side affects

_____ 10. Primary reason to use a massage lubricant

_____ 11. Light source obscured from view by shades or baffles

_____ 12. Avoided when selecting a massage oil

INTERNET ACTIVITIES

Locate the website for massage table companies, such as http://www.oakworks.com and http://www.goldenratio.com. Read about table options. Write down criteria needed for you to determine which table options might be good for your practice.

Using these same websites, read about table accessories, writing down criteria needed when deciding on which table accessories might be good for your practice.

Visit http://www.cfsan.fda.gov/~dms/cos-224.html, and read the U.S. Food and Drug Administration's criteria for using the label *hypoallergenic* on products.

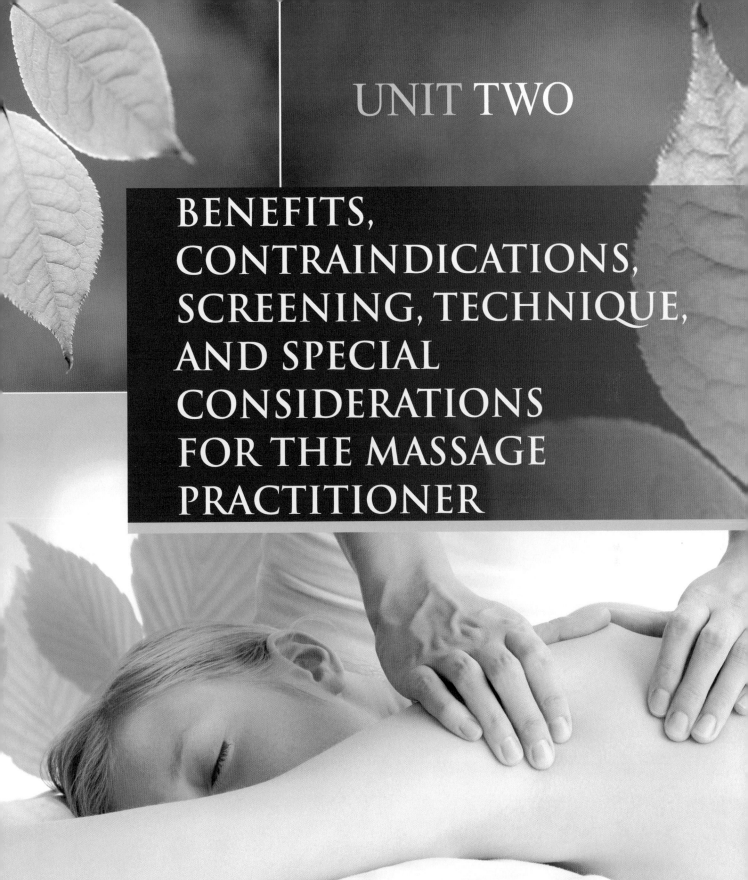

UNIT TWO

BENEFITS, CONTRAINDICATIONS, SCREENING, TECHNIQUE, AND SPECIAL CONSIDERATIONS FOR THE MASSAGE PRACTITIONER

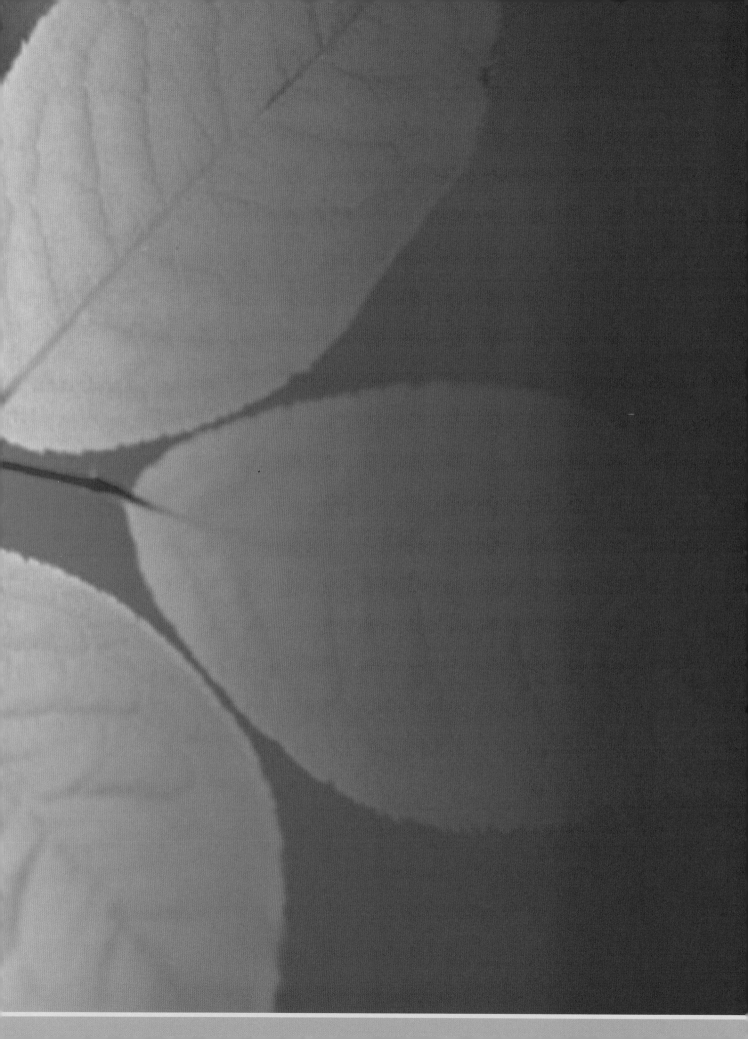

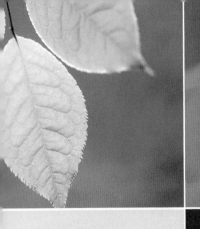

"The pessimist sees difficulty in every opportunity. The optimist sees the opportunity in every difficultly."
—Winston Churchill

Infection Control, Safety, Health, and Hygiene

STUDENT OBJECTIVES

After completing this chapter, the student should be able to:

- Define pathology, and give examples of pathogenic agents
- Discuss the role of feedback mechanisms and how they help maintain homeostasis
- Contrast and compare disorders with disease
- Contrast and compare the terms *signs* and *symptoms*
- Contrast and compare local and systemic diseases
- Contrast and compare the terms *acute*, *subacute*, and *chronic*
- Contrast and compare exacerbation with remission
- Contrast and compare malignant with benign
- Contrast and compare the terms *host* and *reservoir*
- State the types of diseases and disorders
- Discuss how infectious diseases can be transmitted
- Identify the host-pathogen relationship
- Name the recommended guidelines for sanitation, and explain how they control infection
- Outline the suggestions for providing an environment that meets high sanitation standards
- List the guidelines for providing a safe massage
- Discuss glove use in a massage practice, and determine when gloves might be necessary
- Demonstrate the recommended hand washing procedure
- Devise a plan to promote health and proper hygiene

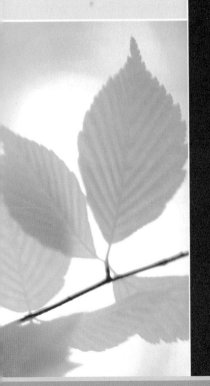

INTRODUCTION

Massage therapy is one of the safest, least intrusive, and most effective treatment modalities in the health care field today. However, the client is susceptible to injury. Contagious or communicable diseases may be transferred to clients by unclean hands and fingernails and by unsanitary equipment and supplies. A client may have a condition worsen by massage, which might have been prevented through proper screening. Precautions are needed to protect clients and include procedures such as routine hand washing and clinic modifications that minimize disease transmission and prevent accidents. Good hygiene and sanitation are the best ways to prevent the spread of disease. These standards are a part of professional massage conduct across the country.

Hippocrates, the father of Western medicine, declared that physicians should "do no harm." The therapist must adopt a policy of impeccable cleanliness before coming into contact with a client. This chapter examines procedures regarding infection control. These procedures will assist the therapist in providing an environment that is safe. Principles and activities that promote personal health and hygiene will assist in the overall success of the therapist's work.

DISEASE AWARENESS: INTRODUCTION TO PATHOLOGY

As health care professionals, massage therapists seek to improve the health and well-being of their clients through massage therapy. Regardless of the work setting or treatment style, the massage therapist will encounter clients who have diseases or medical conditions and who are under medical supervision. The therapist needs to be aware of disease and its agents so as to control its transmission. To build understanding, a fundamental overview of pathology is needed. **Pathology** is the study of biological and physical manifestation of disease. Disease occurs when a disruption of the body's homeostasis occurs.

Health and Homeostasis

Homeostasis is constancy of the body's internal environment. The body consists of cells, tissues, organs, systems, and their associated fluids. Homeostasis is a dynamic process. As internal conditions change, the body's equilibrium can adapt only over a narrow range. For example, blood glucose levels normally stay between 70 and 110 milligrams of glucose per 100 milliliters of blood. Blood glucose levels that stay outside this range, either above it or below it, may not be compatible with life.

Every body structure, from microscopic cells to complex organ systems, helps keep the internal environment within normal limits.

The body's homeostasis is constantly being challenged. Disturbances can come from the external environment, such as intense cold or lack of oxygen, or they can come from inside the body, such as water levels in the blood that are too low. Homeostasis can also be challenged by psychological stresses, such as demands from family or work. In most cases, the disturbance of homeostasis is temporary, and the body is able to restore it quickly. If the disruption is extreme, then homeostasis may not be restored. In the case of uncontrolled diabetes mellitus, blood glucose levels can be above 110 milligrams per 100 milliliters of blood because glucose is not entering the body cells that need it. If left uncontrolled long enough, then death might occur.

Homeostasis is maintained by the interplay of regulatory processes. The two major systems of the body that regulate homeostasis are the nervous system and the endocrine system. They can work together or independently to correct changes in homeostasis. The nervous system sends messages as nerve impulses to counteract imbalances. The endocrine system secretes chemical messengers called hormones into the bloodstream. Nerve impulses cause rapid changes, whereas hormones usually work slowly but no less effectively.

Role of Feedback Systems

The body regulates its internal environment through feedback systems. Feedback systems are cycles of events in which conditions in the body are constantly monitored, evaluated, modified, remonitored, reevaluated, remodified, and so forth. *Negative feedback systems* reverse a disruption in a controlled condition. For example, normal body temperature is 98.6° F. This is a controlled condition. When the external environment becomes very warm, body temperature can increase as well. This change is a disruption in the controlled condition; therefore, to remain in homeostasis, several mechanisms exist that cool the body and maintain homeostatic body temperature. These mechanisms include perspiring and bringing blood to the surface (the skin become flushed) so that excess heat can be lost. These mechanisms reverse the disruption in the controlled condition. Most of the feedback systems of the body are negative feedback systems.

Positive feedback systems strengthen or reinforce a change in a controlled condition. Positive feedback systems continue until they are interrupted by some mechanism outside of the system. An example of this mechanism is an immune system response when it is challenged by a disease-producing organism. White blood cells fight off the body's intruders. When a disease-producing organism enters, it stimulates the proliferation of white blood cells, which is a change in a controlled environment. The white blood cells secrete chemicals that stimulate the formation of more white blood cells. With more white blood cells, even more chemicals are secreted to stimulate the formation of even more white blood cells. This process represents continual strengthening or reinforcement of the change. The white blood cells will proliferate until large enough numbers are produced to create an army that destroys the invading organism. This positive feedback system will continue until the organism is contained and the need to form more white blood cells no longer exists.

Body in Disease

The body stays healthy as long as controlled conditions within the body are maintained by feedback systems. If, however, some aspect of the body loses its ability to contribute to homeostasis, equilibrium in other parts of the body, or the body as a whole, may be disturbed. If a moderate imbalance exists, then a disorder or disease may result. If the imbalance is severe enough, then death may occur.

A **disorder** is any functional abnormality. **Disease**, a more specific term, is any illness that is characterized by certain signs and symptoms. **Signs** are objective changes in the body that can be observed and measured. They include swelling, rashes, fever, high blood pressure, and paralysis, among others. **Symptoms** are subjective changes in the body of which only the person experiencing them is aware. These changes include headaches, nausea, and anxiety, among others. A **syndrome** is a group of signs and symptoms that occur to present a pattern that defines a particular disease or abnormality. Down syndrome is a genetic disorder in which the person has delayed mental development, short stature, round face, eyes that are Asian in appearance, and possibly heart abnormalities.

A **local disease** can affect only one area of the body. An example is a foot fungus. A **systemic disease** affects large parts of the body or the entire body. Periods of **exacerbation** (period of full-blown symptoms) and **remission** (period of partial or complete disappearance of symptoms) are often noted. An example of a systemic disease is lupus, an inflammatory disease of connective tissues, which are found everywhere in the body. **Acute diseases** have an abrupt onset of severe symptoms that run a brief course (less than 6 months) and then resolve or, in some cases, bring death. **Chronic diseases** develop slowly and last longer than 6 months. In some cases, chronic illness lasts a lifetime. **Subacute** is a term recently coined to describe a condition in which the client appears to be well with regard to an absence of measurable signs but is still experiencing symptoms.

Diagnosing is the science and skill of distinguishing diseases or disorders from one another. It is based on the signs and symptoms of the patient, physical examination, and specialized testing. Only trained health care providers can make diagnoses. Diagnosing clients is beyond the scope of practice for massage therapists.

Types of Diseases

To understand how to reduce the likelihood of disease transmission, disease itself must be examined. This section will explore types of diseases and delineate which ones are contagious and which ones are not contagious.

The types of diseases are autoimmune, cancerous, deficiency, degenerative, genetic, infectious, and metabolic. Disorders are also divided into two important categories: congenital and traumatic.

- **Autoimmune diseases** are part of a large group of diseases marked by an inappropriate or excessive response of the body's immune functions. The immune system fails to distinguish between the body's tissue and something that is foreign to the body, such as an invading organism. The immune system then attacks the tissue, which not only affects the targeted tissue but also depletes the immune system, allowing other invaders to infect the body. Examples of autoimmune diseases are rheumatoid arthritis, in which the synovial membranes of joints are attacked; systemic lupus erythematosus, in which the connective tissue of the body is attacked; and multiple sclerosis, in which the covering (myelin sheath) of nerves in the central nervous system is attacked. Autoimmune diseases are not contagious.

- **Cancerous diseases** are characterized by the uncontrollable growth of abnormal cells. The excess tissue that develops when body cells divide without control is called a *neoplasm* or *tumor*. Tumors can be either cancerous or harmless. A cancerous tumor is called **malignant** and will often **metastasize** or spread cancerous cells to other parts of the body. A **benign** tumor does not metastasize, but it may become life threatening if, as it grows, it puts pressure on vital areas, such as a tumor within the brain. Cancer is not contagious.

- **Deficiency diseases** are caused by a lack of an essential vitamin, mineral, or nutrient in the individual's diet, or they are caused by the individual's inability to digest and absorb a particular nutrient properly. This deficiency typically interferes with the body's growth, development, and metabolism. Types of deficiency diseases are scurvy caused by a deficiency of ascorbic acid or vitamin C, rickets caused by a deficiency of vitamin D, and beriberi caused by a deficiency of thiamine or vitamin B1. Pernicious anemia is due to inadequate absorption of vitamin B_{12} because of a lack of intrinsic factor from the stomach. Deficiency diseases are not contagious.

- **Degenerative diseases** refer to tissue breakdown caused by an overuse syndrome or one that may occur naturally as a result of the aging process. Examples of degenerative diseases are osteoporosis, Alzheimer's disease, and macular degeneration. Degenerative diseases are not contagious.

- **Genetic diseases** are caused by an abnormality in the genetic code. Genes are the cell's hereditary units. They are arranged in single file along chromosomes, which are located in the nucleus of the cell. Each gene codes for a single protein. All the genes on the chromosomes code for all the proteins in the body and are responsible for the physical makeup of each person. Genetic diseases can be passed from one generation to the next. Examples of genetic diseases are cystic fibrosis, sickle cell anemia, Turner's syndrome, muscular dystrophy, spina bifida, and hemophilia. Genetic diseases are not contagious.

- **Infectious diseases** are caused by biological agents such as viruses, bacteria, fungi, protozoa, or parasites. Also known as communicable diseases, infectious diseases are transmitted by **reservoirs,** or sources of infection, which can be living (e.g., person, animal) or inanimate (doorknob, locker room floor), either by direct or indirect contact. **Hosts** are the organisms in which the disease-causing agents or pathogens are residing. Examples of infectious disease are the common cold, strep throat, acquired immunodeficiency syndrome (AIDS), pneumonia, measles, scabies or lice infestation, hepatitis A and hepatitis B, most fungal infections, and tuberculosis. All infectious diseases are contagious, some more than others.

- **Metabolic diseases** are physiological dysfunctions that disrupt the body's metabolism. Examples are Cushing's disease, which is an overproduction of the hormone cortisol; diabetes, which is an underproduction of the hormone insulin or an insensitivity of body cells to insulin; cardiovascular conditions, such as high blood pressure; and kidney failure, which results from the kidney's inability to filter wastes out of the blood. Metabolic diseases are not contagious.
- **Congenital disorders** are present at birth. They may be caused by genetic abnormalities, or they may be caused by a maternal diet that is deficient in nutrients or by habits of the mother while the baby is in utero, such as use of recreational drugs, alcohol, or tobacco. Other causes of congenital abnormalities include in utero exposure of the baby to radiation, poisons, certain medications, disease-causing organisms such as Rubella, or oxygen deprivation of the baby before or during birth. Examples of congenital disorders include Down syndrome, cerebral palsy, and certain heart defects. Congenital disorders are not contagious.
- **Traumatic disorders** are injuries that can disrupt homeostasis. Examples of traumatic disorders are open wounds, bone fractures, contusions, and concussions. Traumatic disorders are not contagious.

TABLE TALK

A **disability** is the loss, absence, or impairment of physical or mental fitness. **Handicap** refers to a congenital or acquired mental or physical defect that interferes with normal functioning of the body system or the ability to be self-sufficient in modern society.

Agents of Disease

A **pathogen** is a biological agent capable of causing disease. Microorganisms, or microbes, are single-cell pathogens. One way to develop a disease is to be exposed to a pathogen. Effective exposure results in contamination. **Contamination** occurs when an infectious, or pathogenic, agent resides in or on an organism. Pathogens can be airborne or fluid-borne, or they can infect by direct contact.

Four basic pathogenic agents can cause disease in the body: (1) bacteria, (2) fungi, (3) protozoa, and (4) viruses (Table 4-1).

Bacteria

Most bacteria are not pathogenic and do not require living tissue for survival. Some bacteria are important for plant growth, such as nitrogen-fixing bacteria in the soil. Others are used for processing certain foods such as bread, cheese, yogurt, and wine. Helpful bacteria also occur as natural flora in the body (i.e., mouth, intestines) and aid digestive processes. Harmful bacteria are transmitted directly from person to person, from animal to person, or from a **fomite** (inanimate object). Bacteria may enter the body through ingestion and lead to diseases such as botulism and Salmonella. Improper food handling, such as chopping vegetables or fruits after handling raw meat or chopping on unclean surfaces, can contaminate food. Another frequent method in which a person may obtain bacteria is failure to wash hands after using the toilet and then touching the nose or mouth. Bacterial transmission can also occur by touching, or by coughing or sneezing on a person. Failure to adhere to proper hand washing procedures increases the chance of bacterial transmission. Some diseases that are caused by bacteria are boils, tuberculosis, strep throat, and tetanus.

Fungi

Fungal agents include molds and yeast. Warm, moist environments promote growth of these agents. Only a few varieties are pathogenic. When an individual has a fungal infection, it is typically superficial, tenacious, and difficult to eradicate. Generally, fungal spores are transmitted by a fomite. For example, athlete's foot fungus may be picked up off a locker room floor. Some fungal infections can infect the body internally, such as thrush, which is a yeast infection of the tissues of the mouth. In a person with severely impaired immune function, fungi can become systemic and may be life threatening. Fungi can be transmitted directly from person to person. *Candida albicans,* which normally grows in the mucous membranes of the mouth and vagina, can be found in the axilla and under the breast, and it can be transmitted to another person through touch. Other fungal infestations are ringworm and jock itch, which occur on the skin.

Protozoa

Protozoa are single-cell organisms and are considered the simplest form of animal life. Pathogenic protozoa can only survive in a living subject and are commonly transmitted through contact with feces, contaminated food and water, or an insect bite or sting. Protozoa are responsible for diseases such as trichomoniasis, amebic dysentery, African sleeping sickness, and malaria.

Viruses

Viruses are nonliving entities because they do not carry out independent metabolic activities. They can replicate themselves only within the cell of a living plant or animal. Viruses consist of a core of DNA or RNA surrounded by a protein coat. They attach to the plasma membrane of the host cell and inject their genetic material into the cell, where it travels to the nucleus. The viral genetic material then incorporates itself into the host cell's DNA. Because DNA is a blueprint or code for proteins, the cell reads the code and synthesizes

TABLE 4-1 Relationships Among the Organism or Pathogen, the Reservoir, and Resultant Infection or Disease

ORGANISM OR PATHOGEN	RESERVOIR	INFECTION OR DISEASE
Bacteria		
Escherichia coli	Colon, manure	Food poisoning, diarrhea, gastroenteritis
Staphylococcus	Skin, hair, nose	Cellulitis, pneumonia, impetigo, acne, boil
Streptococcus	Throat, skin, genitalia, perianal area	Strep throat, impetigo
Mycobacterium tuberculosis	Lungs	Tuberculosis
Neisseria gonorrhoeae	Genitalia, rectum, mouth, eye	Gonorrhea, pelvic inflammatory disease, eye infection
Rickettsia rickettsii	Tick	Rocky Mountain spotted fever
Borrelia burgdorferi	Tick	Lyme disease
Clostridium botulinum	Food (improperly handled)	Botulism
Salmonella enteritidis	Food (improperly handled)	Salmonella
Clostridium tetani	Fomite, insect	Tetanus
Helicobacter pylori	Duodenum, stomach, saliva	Ulcers
Escherichia coli	Digestive tract	Urinary tract infection
Chlamydia mycoplasma	Urinogenital tract, genital lesion	Chlamydia
Fungi		
Candida albicans	Mouth, skin, genitalia, colon	Thrush, dermatitis, vaginal infection
Trichophyton mentagrophytes, Epidermophyton floccosum	Fomite, skin	Athlete's foot, ringworm
Trichophyton or Epidermophyton floccosum	Fomite, skin, genitalia	Jock itch
Protozoa		
Plasmodium falciparum	Mosquito	Malaria
Trichomonas vaginalis	Urinogenital tract	Trichomoniasis
Trypanosome rhodesiense	Tsetse fly	African sleeping sickness
Entamoeba histolytica	Water, feces	Amebic dysentery
Viruses		
Human immunodeficiency virus	Body fluids	Acquired immunodeficiency syndrome
Influenza virus, types A, B, and C	Droplets, lung	Influenza
Measles virus	Droplets	Measles
Mump virus	Salivary gland, testicle	Mumps
Human papillomavirus	Skin	Wart
Rhabdovirus	Saliva, brain tissue	Rabies
Herpes simplex, type 2	Mucous membrane, genitalia, rectum, blisters	Herpes, genital

the corresponding protein. After the viral genetic material has become part of the host cell's DNA, the cell synthesizes viruses instead of its usual proteins. The cell will make viruses until the cell bursts from proliferation. Each virus will then travel and infect a new host cell. Viruses are difficult to treat because they easily mutate, or change, and because antibiotics are ineffective against them (antibiotics work only on living organisms). Viruses are usually transmitted from person to person, from insect to person, or animal to person. Viral diseases include the common cold, influenza, AIDS, measles, mumps, rabies, herpes simplex, viral hepatitis, and Ebola.

In addition to bacteria, fungi, protozoa, and viruses, parasites can also enter the body and cause disease. **Parasites** are organisms that live in or on a host organism and rely on that host for nourishment. Examples of parasites are tapeworms, hookworms, lice, and scabies.

Modes of Transmission

For infections to pass successfully from one infected agent or person to another, a mode of transmission is required. An important point to note is that modes of transmission are used for noninfectious, though no less serious, toxic agents (animal and insect venoms, asbestos, some carcinogens). By understanding the various modes of transmission, massage therapists and their clients can help protect themselves from disease.

Direct Physical Contact

Pathogens and toxic agents can enter a host through contact with mucous membranes and with intact or broken skin.

- **Mucous membranes:** This route includes the touching of an infected mucous membrane to an uninfected mucous membrane such as in the nose, mouth, and genitals and the exchange of bodily fluids and secretions by oral, genital, or rectal sexual activity. This route is how sexually transmitted diseases (STDs) are spread.

- **Intact skin:** This method of transmission includes contact with someone or something that is infected with agents or pathogens such as fleas, scabies, lice, ticks, and fungi. Other diseases can be transmitted by contact with toxins such as poison oak, poison ivy, and poison sumac.
- **Broken skin:** This type of transmission involves pathogen entry and toxin introduction through breaks in the skin. The skin can be broken because of an accident, surgery, an animal or insect bite or sting, skin eruptions from a prior infection, a hangnail, or a self-inflicted wound, such as that caused by intravenous drug use. Some parasites such as hookworms gain entry to the body through breaks in the skin. Rabies and malaria are two examples of diseases transmitted by bites or stings.

Indirect Physical Contact

Pathogens and other disease-producing substances can enter a host by ingestion or inhalation.

- **Ingestion:** This type of transmission includes the consumption of contaminated water, undercooked meats, or food that has not been properly stored or refrigerated. Another method of ingestion of pathogens is through unwashed hands. The oral-fecal route, for example, is the mode of transmission of hepatitis A.
- **Inhalation:** This mode of transmission includes infectious agents and toxins that are inhaled and then absorbed through the lining of the lungs. Although no direct contact takes place, contamination occurs after the person comes into contact with airborne droplets of fluid arising from the respiratory tract and salivary glands of the reservoir, primarily through coughing, sneezing, massaging, or talking within a 3-foot distance. Most respiratory diseases are spread by this method. Asbestos fibers, coal dust, textile fibers and tar, and particulates in cigarette smoke are toxic agents that are inhaled and can cause diseases such as emphysema and lung cancer.

Host-Pathogen Relationship

The ability of the pathogen to cause disease in a person depends on various factors that include (1) the portion or number of organisms that gain access, (2) the areas of the body that are attacked, (3) the pathogen's ability to spread and replicate itself, and (4) the pathogen's resistance to host defenses. Thus a weak host with a strong pathogen results in disease, whereas a strong host with a weak pathogen will overcome the introduction of disease.

The body's natural defense mechanisms against exposure to pathogens are (1) physical and chemical barriers, such as intact skin, the skin's surface acidity, mucus, cilia, digestive enzymes, perspiration, and vaginal secretions; (2) inflammation, which helps keep the infection contained; and (3) the body's immune response. In most instances, the first two defenses are successful in keeping pathogens from either entering the body or invading into deeper tissues. If the pathogens penetrate the physical and chemical barriers and if inflammation cannot keep it contained, then the immune response will go into action to destroy the pathogen. If chronic stress, malnutrition, radiation, some medications, or a preexisting illness (e.g., AIDS) suppresses the person's immune system, then the person is then increasingly susceptible to diseases caused by pathogens.

Some signs and symptoms that demonstrate the organism's attempt to overcome a pathogen are fever, mild nausea, altered metabolism, cardiovascular changes (e.g., increased heart rate), anemia, elevated white blood cell count, and a general feeling of low energy.

The disease process includes the course of infection, the pathogen's incubation stage, the period of exacerbation, and often a phase of remission. Remission may be spontaneous or the result of therapy or, in some cases, may represent the disease's cure.

> *"A musician must make music, an artist must paint, a poet must write, if he is to be ultimately at peace with himself."*
> Abraham Maslow

INFECTION CONTROL FOR MASSAGE THERAPISTS

In general, massage therapists are exposed to no more viruses and bacteria than the average person. However, given that the therapist is touching an unclothed person, a risk exists of transferring pathogens from client to therapist and from therapist to client. Additionally, an increased risk exists of transferring pathogens from one client to another. Massage therapists who are hospital based or work with individuals who are sick or injured are at an increased risk for contacting and spreading disease. Infection control through sanitation procedures will decrease this possibility.

Pathogens that the therapists are most likely to contact are fungi, yeast, bacteria, and viruses. Therapists may unknowingly spread infection from one part of the client's body to another during massage. For example, bacteria may be spread if boils are open. Viruses can spread through inhalation of infected droplets. A foot fungus on the client can be spread to other parts of the body by massage. Additionally, fungi, bacteria, and viruses can be spread through contact with linens, massage tools, and open containers of lubricant. These methods of transmission are why massage therapists need to learn, implement, and practice universal precautions.

In December 1991, the Occupational Safety and Health Administration (OSHA) supported and helped pass federal legislation that requires all health care providers to adhere to a plan that helps prevent the exposure to and spreading of bloodborne and fluidborne pathogens. Body fluids that can carry harmful microorganisms are mucus, sputum, respiratory droplets, semen, vaginal secretions, blood, saliva, breast milk, urine, and feces, as well as cerebrospinal, synovial, pleural, peritoneal, and pericardial fluids. From this legislation, the Centers for Disease Control and Prevention (CDC) established *universal precautions* to reduce the transmission of communicable disease. These precautions protect the client and the health care provider.

Universal precautions include mandatory hand washing, use of gloves, protective eyewear, masks for the nose and face, protective clothing, laundering linens and uniforms, cleaning or disinfecting equipment, and observing proper methods for disposing of used medical supplies and biological material. Universal precautions are required when performing invasive medical procedures or when handling body fluids. Invasive medical procedures involve puncturing or penetrating body tissues or entering a body cavity.

How involved do massage therapists have to become with these medical precautions? The answer to this question varies according to the therapist's practice. Although massage therapists are not involved with surgical procedures, they do occasionally enter a body cavity such as the mouth for temporomandibular joint (TMJ) massage (in areas of the country where it is legal to do so). A therapist who works in a medical clinic or hospital, where the population of sick people is great, has a greater exposure risk than the therapist who works in a private practice. In a clinical setting, the therapist may be required to perform rehabilitative therapy on patients who have pins, wires, stitches, staples, or open wounds near the treatment area, and thus an increased risk exists of the massage therapist's spreading contagion to the client.

Contact with body fluids seldom occurs in a private massage therapy practice; a small blemish may break, lesions or minute scabs on recently shaved legs may drain, a client may cough or sneeze and expel mucus, or a nauseated client may vomit. These and similar situations must be handled according to sanitary procedures, which involve the use of methods to eliminate the presence of pathogens; such procedures are outlined here.

A large part of infection control is to have a plan designed to prevent **cross-contamination** (the passing of microorganisms from one person to another). This prevention is best achieved by following guidelines of and procedure for sanitation. **Sanitation** involves the application of measures to promote a healthful, disease-free environment. Similar to universal precautions, sanitary procedures include laundering the massage linens after each use, disinfecting massage equipment and supplies, and following proper hand-washing procedures.

In some circumstances, state law or employers require the massage therapist to be immunized against diseases such as Rubella, rubeola, poliomyelitis, diphtheria, tuberculosis, and hepatitis B. Some employers of massage therapists, such as hospitals, may highly recommend vaccinations but not require them. However, if the massage therapist chooses not to get immunized, then he or she will be sent home in the event of an outbreak. The time spent away from work will vary with the disease in question. The following guidelines for sanitation will guide the massage therapist in ensuring the highest quality of health care possible.

Guidelines of Sanitation

- *Use a standard hand-washing procedure.* Wash and dry hands thoroughly before and after performing massage therapy. One example is provided later in this chapter.
- *Avoid wearing ornate jewelry while at work.* Wearing rings, bracelets, or wristwatches while performing massage therapy is not advised because removing microorganisms from small cracks and crevices found in ornate jewelry is difficult. Furthermore, jewelry or any sharp object can also potentially injure the client or break the protective barrier of gloves.
- *Keep fingernails clean, short, and without nail polish.* Long fingernails or cracked nail polish provide hiding places for microorganisms and is not in keeping with sanitary standards. Long fingernails can also injure the client or break the protective barrier of gloves. Artificial nails present a high risk for fungal infections for the therapist, which can be transmitted to the client.
- *Keep hair clean, and choose a hairstyle that keeps the hair out of the way, or secure the hair so that it does not touch the client.* Because of its porosity, hair is a source of harmful microorganisms.
- *Use clean linens for each massage, and launder all linens after use.* Clean linens will help reduce the likelihood of infection and demonstrate to the client the therapist's commitment to quality of care.
- *Adhere to a safe method of handling contaminated linens and massage tools.* In the event of body fluid seepage, remove the linens with gloved hands. Wash contaminated linens separately in hot water, using laundry detergent and ¼ cup of chlorine bleach. Another recipe is 2 ounces or ¼ cup of chlorine bleach to 20 ounces or 2½ cups of water. Dry linens using hot air. Once contaminated linens have been removed from the massage table, use paper towels to absorb the spill, and then clean the area with mild soap and water. Next, disinfect the table with a solution of water and chlorine bleach in a 10:1 solution. Discard the contaminated gloves and paper towels in a safe manner (determined by the local department of health). Finally, wash and dry your hands.

(4-2)

  - Implements used during the massage such as stones or T-bars that become contaminated should be immersed a 10% bleach solution or a 70% alcohol solution for 10 minutes.
  - These implements can be enclosed with plastic wrap before use. The plastic wrap can then be discarded after use.
- *Treat any substance that cannot be identified as unsafe.* Use the method previously described for handling contaminated linens when confronted with an unidentifiable substance.
- *Wear a clean uniform each day.* Do not wear massage uniforms, including a laboratory coat (if one is worn), for other purposes. The uniform should not fit too loosely because it will brush up against the client when the therapist leans

over the table. The sleeves should be short to allow for easy washing and use of forearms and elbows. Short sleeves are also more sanitary than long sleeves because they do not touch the client's skin. Avoid contact between contaminated linens and the uniform. If any exposure to the uniform occurs with contaminated fluids or droplets, wash the garment with a ¼ cup of chlorine bleach added to the detergent and wash water while laundering. Dry using hot air.

- *Use a pump dispenser or a clean single-use dish for massage lubricant.* Cross-contamination can occur if the lubricant becomes contaminated and reused. To prevent cross-contamination, use only closed dispenser-type containers. Use of open-jar containers poses a risk for cross-contamination because the therapist must remove the lubricant from the jar, place it on the client's skin, and reach back into the jar for additional lubricant. Unless a single-use container is used, the lubricant in the container is used for another massage. The therapist can use a clean spatula or tongue depressor to remove enough lubricant for single-client use and place it on a disposable palette or in a sanitary dish.

- *Use gloves when appropriate.* Disposable gloves are to be worn anytime the therapist has a cut or open wound on the hands, when handling contaminated linens, when disposing of trash, or when disinfecting massage equipment that contains body fluids. A finger cot may be used over a bandage to keep the edges smooth or instead of a glove if the area of broken skin is contained to one finger. Guidelines for protective glove use are found in the section entitled Glove Use. Another alternative to finger cots or gloves is a product that can be painted over a cut to seal.

- *Do not perform massage when ill or when experiencing coldlike symptoms.* These symptoms include sneezing, coughing, fever, or a runny nose. In these cases, canceling appointments or arranging for an associate to substitute is preferred over wearing a surgical mask to prevent the spread of airborne pathogenic microorganisms. In some states (e.g., Arkansas), working while ill is against the law for the massage therapist. If the therapist does sneeze or cough while performing massage, then he or she should wash them or use a waterless antimicrobial agent to disinfect the hands.

- *Avoid working under the influence of alcohol or recreational drugs.* Making good judgments regarding infection control is difficult while under the influence of mood-altering substances.

- *Avoid massaging clients who are ill.* This precaution will help prevent disease transmission.

> ### TABLE TALK
> Tree oil can be used as a disinfectant and antiseptic.

The following are additional suggestions for providing an environment that is sanitary.

- *Provide an operative toilet and lavatory with hot and cold running water in a private restroom setting.* Each restroom should be equipped with toilet tissue, a soap dispenser with soap or other hand-cleaning material, sanitary towels or other hand-drying device such as a wall-mounted electric hand dryer, and a waste receptacle. Massage establishments located in buildings housing multiple businesses under one roof, such as a shopping mall, or in hotels may substitute a centralized restroom. Facilities and fixtures should be kept clean, well lit, and adequately ventilated to remove offensive odors.

- *Maintain clean shower facilities and other related equipment.* These facilities and equipment include the whirlpool bath, sauna, steam cabinet, or steam room.

- *Remove all trash from the premises daily.* Trash left on premises may attract vermin or produce unpleasant odor. Make sure all trashcans are lined with a removable bag.

- *Exterminate all insects, termites, and rodents on the premises.* Vermin are a source of disease.

SAFETY GUIDELINES: FOR THE MASSAGE

The following guidelines will assist the therapist in providing a safe massage.

- Obtain and maintain training or certification in first aid and cardiopulmonary resuscitation (CPR).
- Keep a first-aid kit on the premises in a location known by all personnel.
- After each massage, wipe the client's feet to remove the lubricant. This precaution decreases the likelihood of the client's slipping and falling. The therapist may wish to spray witch hazel, isopropyl alcohol, or a natural product such as pure grain alcohol on the client's feet and wipe it off with a paper towel to remove the lubricant more effectively. However, do not use alcohol on client's feet if the skin is broken or if athlete's foot is present.
- Be able to identify endangerment sites and contraindications, and modify or postpone massage until safe to do so. Information regarding endangerment sites and contraindications are found in the following chapter.

Glove Use

When should a massage therapist use gloves? The following are several guidelines.

- When handling any form of blood, other body fluid or secretions, or any unidentifiable substance. This area includes removal of contaminated massage linens and cleaning of contaminated equipment.
- When removing trash.
- When the therapist has a break in the skin or a skin infection on one or both hands.
- When entering the oral cavity, such as for internal TMJ massage.
- When the client requests that the therapist wear gloves.
- When the therapist does not feel comfortable without them. In this case, discuss reasons for glove use with the client, and involve him or her in the decision. Get an airtight agreement before proceeding with the massage. Do not pretend that the client will not notice that you are wearing gloves.

If one or several of these conditions are present, then the therapist may decide that the risk factor is high enough to warrant double gloving or postponing the massage.

Make sure the gloves fit the therapist's hands. The therapist should be aware that glove use might reduce palpatory abilities until this new skill is acquired. Performing massage with gloved hands also increases friction, especially in areas of thick body hair, which may be uncomfortable for the client.

Before gloving, the therapist needs to wash his or her hands and dry them thoroughly. Put on the gloves discreetly and quietly. If a glove is torn or damaged during a procedure, then it must be removed, hands must be rewashed, and a new glove is put on immediately.

The two most popular gloves used in the health care industry are latex and vinyl. Each type has its assets and liabilities.

- Latex gloves are very thin and very strong and conform to the therapist's hands as though a second skin. They are available in a variety of sizes and are affordably priced. However, most massage lubricants are oil based and break down latex glove material. If latex gloves are used, then a water-based lubricant is needed. Additionally, many people have latex allergies or are sensitive to latex. Symptoms can include rashes, itching, or, more seriously, respiratory difficulties. If any of these symptoms occur,

then the massage therapist needs to remove the gloves immediately and seek medical attention.
- Vinyl gloves may be used with oil-based lubricants and are fine for clients with latex allergies. Vinyl gloves are thicker than latex gloves and greatly reduce tactile sensitivity until the therapist becomes skilled at palpating while using them. They do not have the stretch capability of latex; therefore they do not conform to the therapist's hands as readily as do latex gloves. Vinyl gloves are also more expensive than latex gloves.

 Care must be taken when removing and disposing of gloves to restrict possible contamination from the glove surface. One safe method of glove **(4-3)** removal is to peel the first glove from the cuff to fingers so that it is inside out (Figure 4-1, *A*). Then, the removed glove is placed into the palm of the other hand (Figure 4-1, *B*) so that when the second glove is peeled off, the first will be contained inside (Figure 4-1, *C*). The removed gloves need to be discarded in a closed container (Figure 4-1, *D*). Even after careful removal and discarding of the used gloves, the therapist should wash and dry his or her hands thoroughly.

---

evolve *After logging on to the Evolve website and accessing your student account, click on the segment involving proper glove removal and follow the steps outlined above.* ■

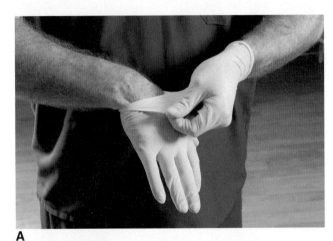

A

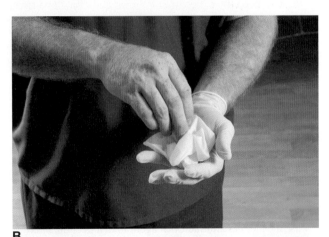

B

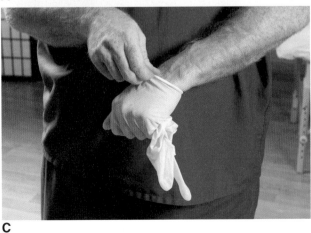

C

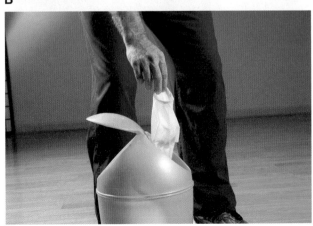

D

FIGURE 4-1 Proper removal of disposable gloves. **A**, Pulling off one glove. **B**, Putting the removed glove in the palm of the gloved hand. **C**, Removing the other glove with the first removed glove inside. **D**, Disposal of the used gloves.

Hand Washing

The number-one source of microorganism cross-contamination is by contact with human hands, and the best measure to prevent the spread of infection is proper hand washing. Hand washing removes and/or destroys pathogens from the forearms, hands, and nails. Other hand washing techniques include the use of special hand-cleaning solutions that are used without water. These high–alcohol-content gels are designed for field use in sporting events and on-site chair massage appointments where hand washing may not be convenient or even possible. The massage therapist needs to be sure to follow the directions listed on the container.

Massage therapists must wash their hands before and after each massage, as well as during the session if deemed

necessary. Remember that using gloves does not preclude hand washing. The hand washing procedure described here is recommended for health care professionals to ensure that appropriate steps have been taken to protect them and their clients.

(4-1)

Hand Washing Procedure

1. Approach the sink. Turn on the valves (Figure 4-2, *A*). Adjust the hot- and cold-water valves until the water is a comfortable temperature and the water is not splashing in the sink.
2. Wet hands, forearms, and elbows, keeping the hands lower than the elbows, which will prevent water, soil, and microorganisms from running up the arms and onto garments (Figure 4-2, *B*). Using a nailbrush or orange stick, clean underneath the fingernails (Figure 4-2, *C*).

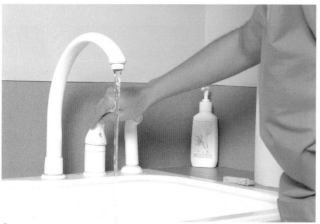

A

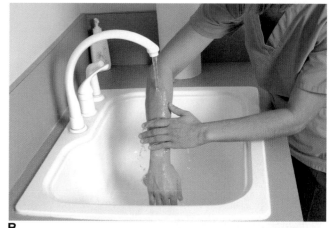

B

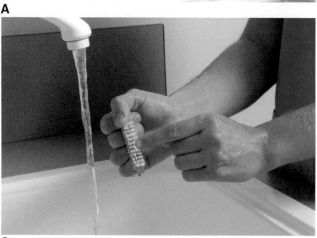

C

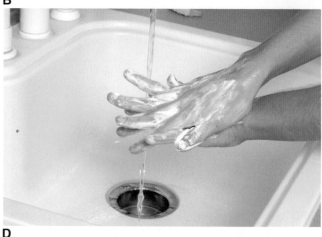

D

FIGURE 4-2 **A**, Turning on the water. **B**, Wetting hands, forearms, and elbows. **C**, Cleaning underneath fingernails, **D**, Soaping the hands. **E**, Rinsing, **F**, Drying the hands. **G**, Turning off the water.

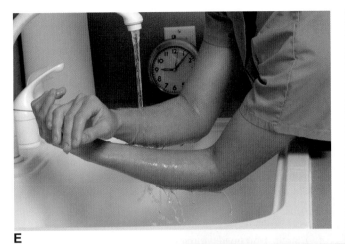

E

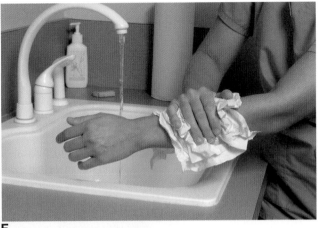

F

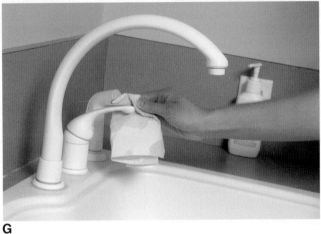

G

FIGURE 4-2 (*continued*)

A single-use fingernail brush or orange stick is preferred. Nails must be cleaned before hands.

3. Use soap; generate lather in your hands, and briskly rub the soap up the forearms using a firm, circular motion. When washing, include the areas between the fingers (Figure 4-2, *D*). Massage soapy hands, forearms, and elbows for at least 15 seconds. If the skin on the fingers, hands, forearms, or elbows is broken, or if accidental emission of and contact with body fluids such as blood, mother's milk, or semen occur, then increase the hand-washing time to 2 minutes.
   a. The friction created by rubbing hands together is essential to emulsify the oils on the skin and to lift microorganisms and dirt from the skin's surface. These unwanted impurities become suspended in the lather, which will be rinsed away.
   b. Liquid soap in a pump dispenser is preferred over bar soap because the soap does not become contaminated by direct contact and is therefore more sanitary. If bar soap is used, then rinse the bar before and after use. Liquid dishwashing soap or baby wash can be used as an alternative to liquid hand soap.
4. Rinse the hands and forearms thoroughly until all lather is removed (Figure 4-2, *E*). Allow the water to run from the fingers to the elbows. This rinsing technique ensures that the hands will be the most sanitary area. Do not skimp on this step. Leaving soap residue on the skin may result in chapped or dry skin.
5. Using clean paper towels, dry the hands and forearms well (Figure 4-2, *F*). Using the same paper towels, turn off the water valves (Figure 4-2, *G*). If washing hands before massage, then continue to use the same paper towels to open door handles until reaching the room in which the massage is performed.
6. Discard the paper towels (do not touch the wastebasket).

TABLE TALK

Instead of counting to 15 while generating lather during hand washing, many therapists mentally sing the Happy Birthday song twice.

evolve *Hand washing is an important aspect of the health care profession. Log on to the Evolve website and view the segment on proper hand washing. While you are there, watch the section on sanitation to review important guidelines for the massage therapist.* ■

HEALTH AND HYGIENE FOR MASSAGE THERAPISTS

As health care providers, we subscribe to habits that promote proper health and good hygiene. These habits help the therapist obtain and maintain the stamina needed to conduct a massage practice and demonstrate commitment to the profession and clientele by making the statement that he or she cares about health.

When attending massage school, the instructor often addresses the physical, mental, and emotional demands that are inherent in any service or health care profession. Internship is often seen as a trial run to determine how the student fares with a full schedule. Internship can feel as though training for an athletic event. Oddly, the definition of training is that the body is stressed and then adapts; it is restressed, it then readapts, and so on. The therapist must be prepared for the demand placed on his or her body during the course of a workday. If the therapist is prepared for this inevitability, then the likelihood of injury or an energy slump is reduced. Being a health care provider is also mentally and emotionally draining. Plan for this consequence with activities geared toward pleasure and fun.

Health is a condition of physical, mental, and social well-being and the absence of disease or other abnormal condition. René Dubos, often quoted in nursing education, says, "The states of health or disease are the expressions of the success or failure experienced by the organism in its efforts to respond adaptively to environmental challenges." In other words, health is a reflection of how well our bodies adapt to our environment. Good health helps our bodies adapt to changes. Regarding why dinosaurs vanished, the answer is often *because they could not adapt.* Additional information on activities to increase strength, flexibility, stamina, and hand-developing exercises can be found in Chapter 6.

Remember that we cannot give away what we do not already have. The best gift we can give to our clients is to give to ourselves first. *Charity begins at home* means that self-care is not being selfish but being self-nurturing in a way that allows us to pass along our gifts to others. The health tips described here can be used to achieve good health in our own lives so we can become better caregivers.

Health can be broken down into three primary elements: (1) nutrition, (2) exercise, and (3) relaxation. The suggestions here address all three health aspects. Each day, the therapist takes time to attend to health-promoting activities; you and your clients will reap the benefits.

- Exercise at least three times a week for 30 minutes for cardiovascular fitness.
- Lift weights three times a week (consult a fitness trainer for a personal program).
- Stretch or practice yoga to keep yourself flexible.
- Drink water daily—at least ½ ounce per 1 pound of body weight per day.

- Eat healthy, high-fiber foods, and maintain a balanced diet for your energy needs.
- Limit your intake of salt, sugar, caffeine, and alcohol.
- Avoid all forms of tobacco use.
- Start the day with morning meditation or quiet time to avoid a stressful day. Schedule stress breaks of at least 15 minutes to relax, especially on crowded days. Breathe slowly and deeply while allowing your body and mind to rest in a comfortable position.
- Remember to schedule regular massage therapy for yourself.
- Honor your emotions by expressing them appropriately. Keep a journal, talk with a counselor, or join a peer support group.
- Laugh. Surround yourself with positive, happy people. Go to a comedy club. Tell stories with old friends. Watch a Monty Python or a Marx Brothers movie. Avoid taking yourself too seriously.
- Stimulate yourself intellectually, spiritually, and emotionally on a regular basis. Go to art galleries, museums, worship services, and concerts. Read a book, write poetry, or see a foreign film. Talk about religion and politics with someone who has differing philosophies.

Hygiene is defined as the collective principles of health preservation. In states requiring licensure of massage therapists, good grooming and hygiene are required by law. Proper hygiene habits not only preserve health but also protect the public from the transmission of microorganisms. A list of tips has been compiled to aid you in practicing a hygiene regimen.

As you observe these hygiene tips, develop and maintain a respect for the diversity of different cultures found throughout the globe. What may be offensive to some is commonplace to others, and what is hygienic to some may be offensive to others. Each therapist must apply these tips to his or her own situation, common sense, and knowledge of local customs.

- Bathe or shower daily. Use an antiperspirant or deodorant if necessary.
- Wash your hair often.
- Brush your teeth at least twice a day, and floss daily to keep gums healthy. Regular brushing removes plaque and reduces the growth of bacteria. Because massage requires close contact with clients, you may elect to use a mouthwash or avoid food that can cause an offensive odor on workdays.
- Shave often or keep facial hair neat, trimmed, and well groomed.
- Keep fingernails clean, short, and neatly trimmed.
- If you perspire heavily while performing a massage, then wear sweatbands at the wrists and forehead to ensure that perspiration does not drip onto the client's skin.
- Avoid perfumes, colognes, or scented lotions. Respect the client's allergies and hypersensitivities.
- Wash your hands thoroughly after using the toilet and before and after each massage session.

SUMMARY

Pathology is the study of disease as it is exhibited biologically and physically. Many types of diseases exist: autoimmune, cancerous, deficiency, degenerative, genetic, infectious, and metabolic. Two significant disorders are congenital and traumatic. A biological agent that is capable of causing disease is known as a pathogen. Examples of pathogens are bacteria, fungi, protozoa, and viruses; they may be airborne or fluidborne or infect by direct contact. Exposure to a pathogen results in contamination. Once contaminated, the organism may or may not become infected, depending on the strength of the pathogen and the resistance of the host to the invading organism.

Once infection occurs, pathological conditions will develop that disrupt homeostasis shown by the presence of measurable symptoms that deviate from the body's normal functions. Identifying the path of infection allows transmission to be controlled.

To control infection in a massage practice, a therapist must be familiar with correct sanitary procedures, including hand washing, glove use, and disinfecting of equipment. Regardless of the work setting or treatment style, the massage therapist will encounter clients who have various pathological abnormalities, who are under medical supervision, and who are taking prescription medications. Information regarding these situations will assist the therapist in making treatment choices for their clients.

CASE STUDY:

More Than Just an Accident

Margaret was a recent graduate from the Gulf Coast School of Massage. She acquired her state license and began her practice at a well-established chiropractic clinic. Margaret massaged the physicians' patients before their spinal adjustments. The patients loved the massage, and the physicians loved that the patients reported improving more quickly with the addition of the massage before the spinal adjustments.

Mark was Margaret's next client. It was Mark's first massage at the clinic. He was a car sales associate uptown and was recently involved in a minor car accident. Mark's chiropractor gave clearance for him to begin receiving massages. Because Margaret was asked to address his back, neck, and shoulder only, Mark left on his trousers.

When Margaret reentered the massage room, Mark was lying prone with the sheet draped across his back and legs. Margaret lowered the sheet and observed a large portion of his back covered with red circles. The edges of the circles were slightly elevated, and she noticed a slight odor to his skin.

Should Margaret continue with the massage?

Should Margaret ask the client or his physician about the circles?

When should she make the inquiry?

Should she consult the physician before, after, or during the massage?

---

evolve

Go to *Chapter Extras* on Evolve for additional resources for this chapter. *Extras* for this chapter include:

1. Crossword puzzle (downloadable form)
2. Hand washing photo sequencing (photographs)
3. Case study (text)

MATCHING I

Place the letter of the answer next to the term or phrase that best describes it.

A. Acute
B. Chronic
C. Congenital
D. Diagnosing

E. Disease
F. Homeostasis
G. Local
H. Signs

I. Subacute
J. Symptoms
K. Syndrome
L. Systemic

_____ 1. Means present at birth

_____ 2. Constancy of the body's internal environment

_____ 3. Illness characterized by certain signs and symptoms

_____ 4. Objective changes in the body that can be observed and measured, such as swelling, rashes, fever, high blood pressure, and paralysis

_____ 5. Subjective changes in the body of which only the person experiencing them is aware, such as headaches, nausea, and anxiety

_____ 6. A group of signs and symptoms that present a pattern to define a particular disease or abnormality

_____ 7. Diseases affecting only one area of the body, such as foot fungus

_____ 8. Diseases affecting large parts of the body or the entire body

_____ 9. Diseases that have an abrupt onset of severe symptoms that run a brief course and then resolve or cause death

_____ 10. Diseases that develop slowly and last a lifetime or longer than 6 months

_____ 11. Describes a condition in which the person appears to be well with regard to absence of measurable signs but is still experiencing symptoms

_____ 12. Science and skill of distinguishing diseases or disorders from one another based on signs and symptoms of the patient, physical examination, and specialized testing

MATCHING II

Place the letter of the answer next to the term or phrase that best describes it.

A.	Autoimmune	F.	Degenerative	K.	Metastasize
B.	Benign	G.	Exacerbation	L.	Neoplasm
C.	Cancerous	H.	Genetic	M.	Oncology
D.	Communicable	I.	Infectious	N.	Remission
E.	Deficiency	J.	Malignant		

_____ 1. Diseases marked by inappropriate or excessive response of the body's immune system

_____ 2. Diseases characterized by uncontrollable growth of abnormal cells

_____ 3. Synonymous with the word *tumor*

_____ 4. Study of tumors

_____ 5. Cancerous tumors

_____ 6. Spreading of cancer cells

_____ 7. Tumors that do not metastasize

_____ 8. Diseases caused by a lack of essential vitamins, minerals, or nutrients in the individual's diet or caused by an inability to properly digest and absorb a particular nutrient

_____ 9. Associated with the disease process, periods of full-blown symptoms

_____ 10. Associated with the disease process, periods of partial or complete disappearance of symptoms

_____ 11. Diseases in which body tissues break down by overuse or as a result of the aging process

_____ 12. Diseases caused by an abnormal genetic code

_____ 13. Diseases caused by viruses, bacteria, fungi, protozoa, or parasites

_____ 14. Synonymous with the term *infectious*

MATCHING III

Place the letter of the answer next to the term or phrase that best describes it.

A. Centers for Disease Control and Prevention
B. Cross-contamination
C. Fomite
D. Fungi

E. Hand washing
F. Host
G. Hygiene
H. Parasites

I. Pathogen
J. Reservoir
K. Sanitation
L. Virus

_____ 1. Source of infection

_____ 2. Organism in which disease-causing agents or pathogens reside

_____ 3. Disease-causing agent

_____ 4. Entities such as molds and yeast

_____ 5. Nonliving entities that can replicate themselves only within the cell of a living plant or animal

_____ 6. Inanimate object

_____ 7. Organisms that live in or on a host organism and rely on the host for nourishment

_____ 8. Established universal precautions to reduce the transmission of communicable diseases

_____ 9. Passing of microorganisms from one person to another

_____ 10. Application of measures to promote a healthful, disease-free environment

_____ 11. Best habit of infection control

_____ 12. Principles of health preservation

INTERNET ACTIVITIES

Visit the website for the Center for Disease Control and Prevention (http://www.cdc.gov). Go to Diseases and Conditions, then to Risk Factors. Note how smoking and tobacco use predisposes someone to health problems.

While on the website for the Center for Disease Control and Prevention (http://www.cdc.gov), locate statistics on AIDS, noting the most common age of diagnosis and region of highest and lowest reported cases.

While on the website for the Center for Disease Control and Prevention (http://www.cdc.gov), locate its mission statement. Do you think the CDC fulfills its mission?

Bibliography

Applegate EJ: *The anatomy and physiology learning system,* ed 3, Philadelphia, 2006, Saunders.

Damjanov I: *Pathophysiology for the health-related professions,* ed 3, Philadelphia, 2006, Saunders.

Frazier MS, Drzymkowski JW: *Essentials of human diseases and conditions,* ed 3, Philadelphia, 2004, Saunders.

Gould BE: *Pathophysiology for the health professions,* ed 3, Philadelphia, 2006, Saunders.

Jacob S, Francone C: *Elements of anatomy and physiology,* Philadelphia, 1989, Saunders.

Larson E, Mayur T, Laughon BA: Influence of two hand washing frequencies on reduction in colonizing flora with three products used by health care personnel, *Am J Infect Control* 23:17, 1989.

Louisiana State Department of Social Services: *Uniform federal accessibility standards accessibility checklist,* Baton Rouge, La, 1995, United States Architectural and Transportation Barriers Compliance Board.

Ogg S: Personal communication, Lafayette, La, 1997, Lafayette General Hospital.

Pliszka M: *The truth about antibacterial soaps,* Twins Magazine, Jan/Fab 2006, pp 38-39

Salvo SG, Anderson SK: *Mosby's pathology for massage therapists,* St Louis, 2004, Mosby.

Thibodeau G, Patton K: *Anatomy and physiology,* ed 6, St Louis, 2006, Mosby.

Thibodeau G, Patton K: *Structure and function of the body,* ed 12, St Louis, 2004, Mosby.

Torres LS: *Basic medical techniques and patient care for radiologic technologies,* Philadelphia, 1993, JB Lippincott.

Tortora GJ: *Introduction to the human body: the essentials of anatomy and physiology,* ed 5, Hoboken, NJ, 2000, Wiley, John & Sons.

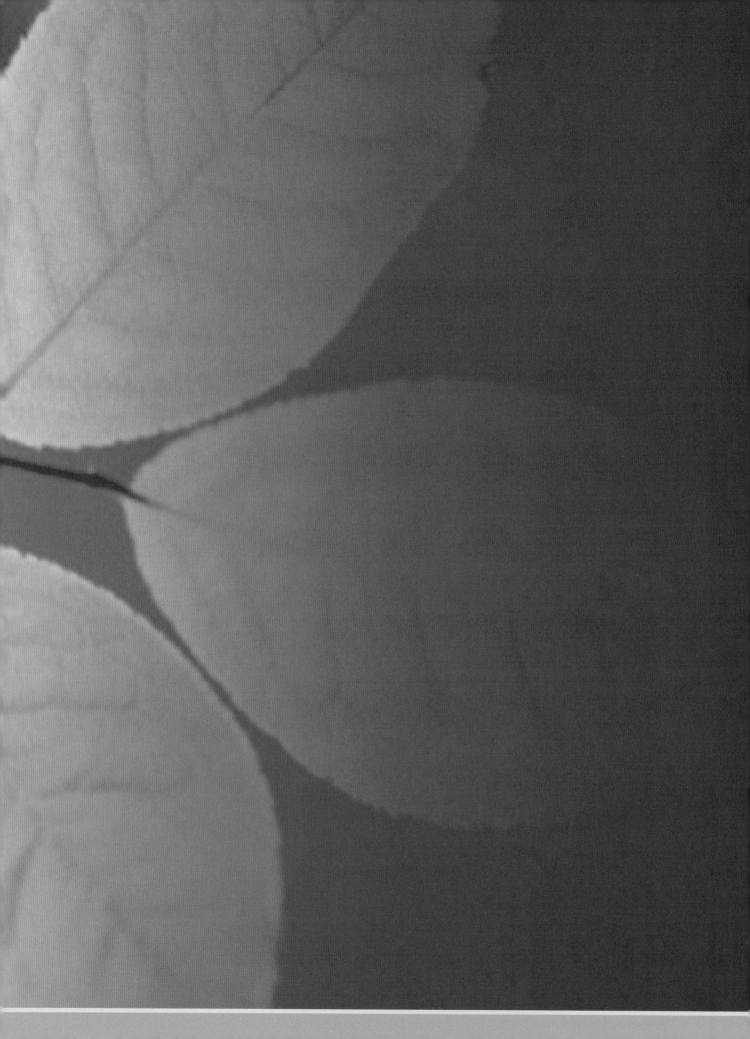

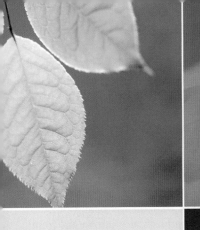

CHAPTER 5

"He who feels it knows it more."

—Bob Marley

Massage Physiology: Research, Effects, Indications, Contraindications, and Endangerment Sites

STUDENT OBJECTIVES

After completing this chapter, the student should be able to:

- Discuss the importance of skin as an organ system, especially with regard to touch and pressure
- Examine the scientific method and touch research
- Discuss the safety of massage
- Compare mechanical and reflexive responses of massage
- Discuss the effects of massage on various body systems and body tissues
- Using the gate theory, discuss how massage relieves pain
- Identify special populations that would benefit from massage therapy
- Identify guidelines for local and absolute contraindications of massage therapy
- Recognize and modify treatment over endangerment sites

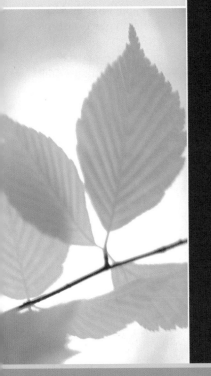

INTRODUCTION

Massage therapy has been found to be beneficial for a significant number of conditions such as reducing stress, reducing pain, decreasing depression, preventing premature birth, enhancing growth and development, increasing attentiveness, increasing neuromuscular function, and enhancing immune function. This chapter addresses the scientific method for which research is structured and how research is vital to the validity of our profession. First, however, we must pause to show reverence for the medium of touch, namely the skin. Next, specific individuals who conducted groundbreaking touch research are featured, as well as their research findings. Then, the effects of massage are detailed by body system and grouped by special populations.

A massage therapy session can simply provide a restful and refreshing interlude in an individual's busy life. Also, massage therapy has been an effective remedy for musculoskeletal conditions involving muscle tension. Massage therapy has recently gained a reputation for being beneficial in the treatment of other conditions. Interest has increased in the research of alternative and complementary therapies. This heightened interest has resulted in the establishment of the National Institutes of Health's Office of Alternative Medicine and improved funding for research of these therapies. Massage therapy was one of the first disciplines to receive funding from this agency. The Massage Therapy Foundation's mission includes supporting scientific research and developing the Massage Therapy Research Agenda, which can be found at *http://www.massagetherapyfoundation.org/or_methods.html.*

Awareness of research supporting the healing arts is essential for the massage therapist. In the course of practicing massage therapy, questions about conditions treated or techniques used may come to mind. Research assists in understanding persons to whom we deliver services and their needs and provides support for effective therapies.

Although massage is effective for many bodily ailments, a few conditions are evident for which massage is *contraindicated.* If massage therapy is to be administered safely, then the prudent professional will screen clients for these conditions.

Various anatomical landmarks are also evident for which caution is recommended or where downward pressure should be avoided. These topographical regions, known as *endangerment sites,* are regions in the body where nerves, blood vessels, and other fragile structures lie near the surface of the skin. Locations of the major endangerment sites are included in this chapter.

SKIN AND THE SIGNIFICANCE OF TOUCH

The sense of touch is the massage therapist's main avenue used to affect another human being and is the body's main method of gathering information about itself. In contrast, an artist uses the sense of vision, and a musician uses the sense of hearing to communicate with others. Touching can affect us physiologically, cognitively, psychologically, and emotionally.

Aristotle was the first to enumerate the five senses. Of all the senses, only touch involves the entire body. The other four senses reside in the head. Indeed, touch is not one sense but many. Touch can detect deep pressure or light stroking. It can differentiate between the weight of a feather and the skin's immersion in water.

The skin is temperature sensitive. It can distinguish between the warmth of wooden bleacher seats on a summer day and the cool shade found beneath the live oaks lining the still bayous of the South. It communicates intrusions, from the tickle of a kitten's fur to the intense pain of a nail piercing your shoe sole.

Touch is the most primitive of all sensations. Among the many studies that have been conducted, touch is the earliest sensory system to become functional in the human embryo. When the embryo is less than 6 weeks of age, measuring less than an inch long from crown to rump, light stroking of the upper lip or wings of the nose will cause bending of the neck and trunk away from the source of stimulation. At this stage of gestation, neither the eyes nor ears have developed.

The skin and the brain arise from ectoderm, the same cells that give rise to the entire nervous system, including the sense organs of smell, taste, hearing, and vision—all of which keep the organism informed about what is going on in its environment. Because of the ectoderm connection, the skin is considered exposed neural tissue and, in contrast, the brain is immersed skin. We can therefore regard the skin as a superficial nervous system.

Perhaps the fact that touch is such a primal sensation is precisely what makes it such a powerful therapeutic tool. Our first lessons about love and tenderness are learned through the medium of touch. Whether breast- or bottle-fed, our first meals were touch centered. Touch communicated some of our early experiences with pain. Quite often, this sense played a major role in the physical and emotional healing of those same wounds. Everyone, whether nurse or patient, massage therapist or client, parent or child, lover or friend, can look back on a time when touch played a personal role that was extremely important.

Touch is our first means of communication, and the skin is our main organ of sensation. We can see, hear, and think about something, but through touch the event becomes part of our personal experience. Touch can alter how we perceive the world. Touch can also stimulate us to action.

MINI-LAB

Write about a time in your life when touch was meaningful to you in a personal way.

"There are a number of very important irreversibles to be discovered in our universe. One of them is that every time you make an experiment you learn more; quite literally, you can not learn less."
Buckminster Fuller

SCIENTIFIC METHOD

Every massage effect featured in this chapter is in the context of a broad field of study called science. **Science** is a method of inquiry that attempts to prove or disprove hypotheses (calculated guesses) using a rational, logical method. The *scientific method* is a dynamic process, similar to problem solving in everyday life. With observations and vigorous tests called *experiments,* scientists address a hypothesis until a reasonable conclusion is reached. Scientists use an experiment to search for cause and effect. In other words, they design an experiment so that changes to one item cause something else to vary in a predictable way. These changing quantities are called *variables*. Variables are a key element of the scientific method.

Rigorous experiments that eliminate any influence or biases not being tested are called *controlled experiments*. If the results of observations and experiments are repeatable, then they may verify a hypothesis and eventually lead to enough confidence in the concept to call it a *theory*. Theories in which scientists have an unusually high level of confidence are sometimes called *laws*. Experiments may disprove a hypothesis, a result that often leads to the formation of a new hypothesis.

Two main types of research are discussed here: quantitative and qualitative. *Quantitative research* is a method that numerically measures variables using tight controls so the outcome can be attributed to a specific factor or set of factors while the scientist remains as objective as possible.

Several types of quantitative research exist: descriptive, correlational, quasiexperimental, and experimental. *Descriptive research* describes the variables (or factors) of interest (e.g., Does massage lower blood pressure?). *Correlational research* examines the relationship between two or more variables (e.g., Does a relationship exist between massage or acupuncture and reported reduction of intensity of low back pain?). *Quasiexperimental* and *experimental* research searches for the cause and effect between variables, differing in the amount of control exercised over the research project (e.g., Is massage or acupuncture more effective than other therapies in reducing low back pain?). Quasiexperimental research is much more likely to be used in behavioral research than experimental research because the more stringent control of experimental research is not possible. For instance, the subjects might be obtained in a convenient manner rather than randomly chosen (e.g., subjects or the sample will be clients who present to a specific massage therapy setting to have massage therapy for neck and upper back pain during a 3-month period.). The people who are being studied (the sample) in quantitative research are referred to as *subjects*.

Figure 5-1 summarizes some of the basic concepts of how new scientific principles are developed.

By necessity, quantitative research is reductive. Data, such as blood pressure, surveys, questionnaires, observations, or interviews, are collected and coded with numbers (for example, by using numerical scales, such as the Likert-type questionnaire, discussed later in this section). The data

1 . Stating the question: What are you trying to discover from your experiment? What do you hope to achieve?

2 . Research the topic: Investigate what past scientists have learned about your question. This information will help you carry out the experiment.

3 . State the hypothesis: After perusing past research, you should have some idea about what you think will happen in your experiment. State your hypothesis in a way that is measurable (quantitative).

4 . Test the hypothesis by conducting an experiment: With the hypothesis in mind, develop an experiment for testing whether it is true or false. This involves changing one variable and measuring the impact this change has on other variables. When you are conducting an experiment, it is best to measure the impact of only one variable.

Scientists usually run the experiment several times to verify that the results are consistent. Each time an experiment is performed, it is called a *run* or a *trial*.

5 . Analyze the results: The data collected during the experiment/s are organized and analyzed to summarize what the experiment has revealed.

6 . Draw a conclusion: The conclusion explains the meaning of the results. Did the experiment support or disprove the hypothesis? Does additional research need to be conducted?

7 . Communicate the findings: Publish an article or present the findings of the experiment at a professional meeting.

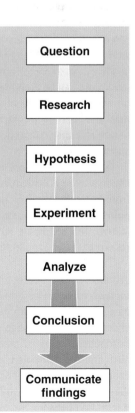

FIGURE 5-1 The scientific method.

analysis for all types of quantitative research involves numbers so that statistical analyses can be performed. Variables then are factors, ideas, or concepts that can be measured numerically. Statistics are used to describe the variables, examine the relationships between variables, or examine the differences between groups on measured variables, such as the subjects had a mean or average blood pressure of 120/80 mm Hg. Every step of the research is governed by rules and guidelines from how subjects are obtained and how many subjects are needed to which statistical tests are appropriate for the type of study and the level of measurement (nominal scale, ordinal scale, interval scale, or ratio scale). Nominal measurement names or puts the variables into exclusive and exhaustive categories such as gender (1 = male subjects; 2 = female subjects). The number has no meaning. Ordinal measurement provides a ranking of variables, and each number indicates rank order with uneven intervals and nothing more. An example using back pain is 0 = no pain, 1 = a little pain, and 2 = a lot of pain. Interval scale numbers indicate a continuum with equal distance between the scales and can be added and subtracted, but absolute zero does not exist. Fahrenheit temperature is commonly used to describe this measurement. Ratio measurement has the attributes of all the previous measures and has an absolute zero; a variable can have a complete absence of the factor being measured, such as heart rate. Therefore a heartbeat of 100 beats per minute is twice as fast as a heartbeat of 50. The methods used to set up the experimental design should be explained in the published article.

As a means of evaluating responses to massage therapy, clients might be asked to complete a Likert-type questionnaire about their satisfaction with the massage experience. The person completing the Likert-type questionnaire is forced to answer each question ranging from 1 (most negative) to 5 (most positive). An average can be obtained for each question, or a total score can be compiled and an average for the total questionnaire obtained. Another means of examining response to massage therapy might be to monitor physiological signs before and after the session such as heart rate, blood pressure, and respirations.

Qualitative research is an attempt to examine phenomena in a more holistic manner. The phenomena are examined from the subjects' (the people being examined) senses and points of view. The scientist does not attempt to remain objective. In fact, being subjective is desirable in qualitative research.

The types of qualitative research are phenomenological, grounded theory, ethnographic, and historical. *Phenomenological research* describes the experience as it is lived by the participants. For example, the subject describes the experience of having massage therapy at the onset of a migraine headache. *Grounded theory* is based on the meaning of reality and the symbols used as people interact; thus it often examines a process. (For example, words are symbols, but they often differ in meaning between people. The process of interaction between the massage therapist and the client with

the goal of decreasing pain might be studied.) *Ethnographic research* provides description of individual human societies such as groups of massage therapists, exploring their beliefs, values, attitudes, and behaviors. *Historical research* examines past events. One example is to review records of meetings held to achieve licensure of massage therapists in a state. Its purpose is to understand something that happened and is recorded in the past within a group. The people who are being studied (the sample) in qualitative research are referred to as *participants*.

Data are collected for qualitative research using observations in natural settings and open-ended interviews of participants and examining written material. Data analysis revolves around words or themes rather than numbers. At first glance, the qualitative research method seems to be less constrained by rules than quantitative research. Rigor in qualitative research involves maintaining integrity with the philosophical basis of the research. Data analysis and data collection occur simultaneously and require great skill in managing both at the same time. Analysis involves extensive review of the data and eventual identification of themes and patterns. Finally, the data are interpreted from the researcher's perspective.

As a means of evaluating clients' experiences with massage therapy, the clients might be asked to respond to the following question: What are your experiences with massage therapy? The responses to open-ended questions would be taped with the clients' permission and transcribed. The transcripts would then be examined extensively for themes or patterns. The researcher would then interpret the findings. Qualitative research can be more difficult to accomplish than quantitative research because of the lack of sequential steps. Qualitative research is usually interesting to read because the narrative reads more as a story.

Science is a dynamic process of getting closer and closer to the truth. Scientists drive the process of science, but our culture drives the kinds of questions we ask and how we attempt to answer them. As you study the concepts presented in this chapter, as well as the unit on anatomy and physiology, keep in mind that these concepts are not set in stone. Science is a set of rapidly changing ideas influenced by what our culture would like to know and understand.

FOUNDATIONAL TOUCH RESEARCH

Many physicians, nurses, biochemists, and psychologists have developed studies on the effects of touch. These studies address physical, intellectual, psychological, and emotional themes. Several studies discussed here are considered groundbreaking and fundamental. Following are brief summaries from research that focus on touch as a medium of communication. As you read these summaries and draw your own conclusions, apply the concepts you develop to your attitude about massage and to your role as a caregiver.

Rene Spitz and Wayne Dennis

Both Rene Spitz and Wayne Dennis studied children in orphanages in different parts of the world (e.g., Iran, Lebanon, United States). Rene A. Spitz, a Hungarian psychiatrist and pioneer in touch deprivation research, explored the development (or lack of development) of institutionalized children. In his 1945 study involving babies, Spitz followed the social development of babies who, for various reasons, were removed from their mothers early in life. Some children were placed with foster families, whereas others were raised in institutions such as orphanages and nursing homes. The nursing home lacked a family-like environment. More than a third of these children died. A large percentage were still living in institutions after 40 years. All survivors experienced some form of physical and mental delay. Spitz claimed that these individuals were depressed. This condition is now considered an attachment disorder.

In another study, Spitz observed young children in an orphanage who were fed and kept clean and were initially in good physical condition but who received no consistent affection from a sole caregiver. The long-standing absence of emotional warmth took an enormous toll on the children, primarily on their emotional development but also on their physical growth and development. These babies tended to wither away and die. Of 91 such babies he observed, 27 died in their first year of life, followed by seven more the second year. In other homes, up to 90% died in early infancy. Babies who did survive in institutions were classified as hopeless. Spitz concluded that providing only for a baby's physical needs is not sufficient for normal development. Tactile stimulation is essential to normal development and even to survival.

In the 1950s Dr. Wayne Dennis published his findings on what he called infant and child retardation. His research was based on his experience at an orphanage in Beirut, Lebanon. He found that the facility that contained the orphanage was more than adequate, but because of the orphanage's meager income, personnel was limited to one employee to 10 infants. The children were taken out of the cribs only for feedings, diaper changing, and a daily bath. The children remained in the crib until they began to pull up on the sides. From that point, they were placed in a playpen during the daylight hours with two other children. Opportunities for touch were very limited. A large number of these children died, even though they were receiving adequate nutrition and hygiene. The children who did survive were dwarfed or deformed.

The explanation Dennis gave for his findings of marasmus (wasting away) combined with the tragic death rates of the Lebanese orphanages were the result of touch deprivation and lack of physical stimulation and learning opportunities. The employees were so busy providing for their physical needs, they did not have time to hold and caress the infants. When aides were hired to rock and sing to these children, mortality rates dropped 70%.

---

evolve *Log on to the Evolve website to see a child affected with marasmus. This is the condition that infants in Lebanese orphanages had in Wayne Dennis's study. Locate similar studies that feature touch as an important element in human (and mammalian) growth and development. Use the Article Report Form located on the Evolve website to document your scientific studies.* ■

Harry Harlow

In 1958 Dr. Harry Harlow, another pioneer in touch research, conducted experiments at the University of Wisconsin that involved the isolation of monkeys during their early developmental stages. After a period, these touch-deprived monkeys exhibited evidence of emotional and social impairment. The lack of touch during their early developmental years had left them disturbed and socially inept. Most female monkeys refused mating, becoming hostile and aggressive when approached. The monkeys that did mate rejected or harmed their young. Harlow observed that during periods of isolation, the infant monkeys valued tactile stimulation more than they did nourishment. Harlow then created two artificial surrogate mothers. One was a bare wire sculpture of a monkey that housed a bottle of formula. The other was a fur-covered wire monkey that felt and smelled similar to other monkeys but offered no food. The infant monkeys preferred to cling to the mother who provided a semblance of physical contact without nourishment rather than to the wire models that provided food (Figure 5-2). Harlow's studies implied that babies who had been removed from their mothers suffered and displayed major dysfunction as they developed and when they themselves became mothers.

Bernard Grad

Dr. Bernard Grad, a Canadian biochemist, conducted his groundbreaking touch research on mice and barley seedlings in the early 1960s. In the first of his double-blind studies, 300 mice were selected and injured in the same manner. One third were allowed to heal without intervention, one third were held by medical students who did not profess to heal, and one third were held by a reknowned faith healer. After just 2 weeks, the mice held by the faith healer recovered remarkably faster than the mice in both of the other groups.

For the barley seed study, Grad soaked the seeds in a saline solution to get them off to a bad start. The seeds were then divided into three equal groups. The first group was watered with tap water. The second group was soaked using water held by disinterested students, and the last group was irrigated with water that was held by a renowned faith healer. The seeds that were watered by the healer held water, sprouted faster, grew taller, and contained more green chlorophyll than either of the other two groups.

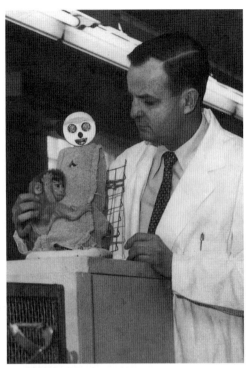

FIGURE 5-2 Harry Harlow 1906-1981.

Abraham Maslow

In the 1960s, Abraham Maslow, a renowned psychologist, placed the needs of human beings in a sequential order, from the most basic and concrete to the most ideal and abstract (Figure 5-3). He believed that these needs directed all human behavior, and as these basic needs are met, other needs of the hierarchy begin to emerge until the individual reaches what he terms self-actualization. Maslow called this progression the *Theory of Human Motivation*.

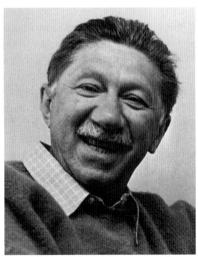

FIGURE 5-3 Abraham Maslow 1908-1970.

Maslow states that we have basic human needs, beginning from the concrete, biologic needs of food and water to abstract needs of self-actualization. Maslow characterized the self-actualized person as self-accepting, striving to help others, and engaging in activities that will help the person achieve the highest potential. His model was later redesigned, with the help of other psychologists, to a more comprehensive list of human needs (Box 5-1). An interesting point to note is that touching and skin contact are ranked very high on the list, just below the individual's need for a safe shelter. Many massage therapists attest to the fact that clients often receive massage to get their touch needs met.

Delores Krieger

In the 1970s Dr. Delores Krieger, a professor at New York University, became interested in touch healing through studies such as Grad's (Figure 5-4). Krieger was fascinated with the idea that intent was so important in healing touch. Using noninvasive techniques, Krieger wanted to apply

---

BOX 5-1

Hierarchy of Human Needs

1. Survival
2. Safety
3. Touching, skin contact
4. Attention
5. Mirroring and echoing
6. Guidance
7. Listening
8. Being real
9. Participating
10. Acceptance
    - Others are aware of, take seriously, and admire the *real you*
    - Freedom to be the *real you*
    - Tolerance of your feelings
    - Validation
    - Respect
    - Belonging and love
11. Opportunity to grieve losses and to grow
12. Support
13. Loyalty and trust
14. Accomplishment
    - Mastery, power, control
    - Creativity
    - Having a sense of completion
    - Making a contribution
15. Altering one's state of consciousness; transcending the ordinary
16. Sexuality
17. Enjoyment or fun
18. Freedom
19. Nurturing
20. Unconditional love, including connection with a Higher Power

Data from Glasser, 1985; Maslow, 1962; Miller, 1981; Weil, 1973.

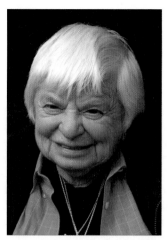

FIGURE 5-4 Delores Krieger.

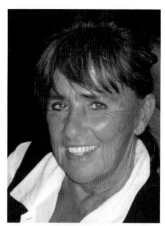

FIGURE 5-5 Tiffany Field.

the concepts of Grad's work in a way that might help her patients.

Through Krieger's research, a tangible relationship emerged between touching and healing. She was able to measure an increase in the hemoglobin content of the blood, which directly corresponded to levels of touching. Hemoglobin is the oxygen-carrying molecule in red blood cells. In Krieger's study, when a healthy person placed his or her hands on or near an ill person for 10 to 15 minutes with the intent to heal, this action was enough to cause the measurable increase.

MINI-LAB

Touching with Intent

1. Locate a partner.
2. Assign one person to be the giver and one person to be the receiver, and ask them to sit facing each other.
3. The receiver extends his or her hands, palms up. The giver places his or her hands on the receiver's hands, palms down. Both the giver and the receiver close their eyes.
4. The giver becomes unfocused, disinterested, and mentally distracted as the receiver stays open and passive for 2 minutes.
5. After that time, the giver becomes very aware, interested, and concerned about the receiver. This attitude is maintained for 2 minutes.
6. Reverse roles and repeat.
7. Share your experiences with each other. Did you notice any differences when the attitudes changed? Does intent really alter how touch is received? How can you use this information during a massage therapy session?

Tiffany Field

Dr. Tiffany Field, professor of pediatrics, psychology, and psychiatry at the University of Miami School of Medicine, began a research project to study the effects of massage on 40 premature babies (Figure 5-5). One half of the group was massaged three times a day for 15 minutes for 10 days.

The massaged infants gained 47% more weight than those who were not massaged. They spent less time in the hospital than the babies who were not massaged, even though both groups of babies had the same number of feedings and averaged the same intake per feeding. The massaged babies were also more active and alert and stayed approximately 6 fewer days in the hospital. The massaged babies were also more socially active and more responsive and had better coordination and motor skills than the babies who were not massaged (1986).

In 1992 Dr. Field formally established the Touch Research Institute (TRI) at the University of Miami School of Medicine through a start-up grant from Johnson & Johnson. The TRI is devoted solely to the study of touch and its application in both science and medicine. Research efforts actually began in 1982 and continue today. The TRI had researched the effects of massage therapy at all stages of life, from newborns to senior citizens. In these studies, the TRI had shown that touch therapy has many positive effects on health and well being.

HOW SAFE IS MASSAGE?

The most common form of massage, Swedish massage, is considered a very low risk for therapy, especially when the therapist tailors the session to the client's needs such as duration, pressure, and areas to avoid because of conditions such as thrombosis. To accomplish this task, most massage therapists acquire formal training. During their training, class hours are devoted to learning massage strokes, routines, how to screen clients for possible contraindications, and devising a treatment plan. Many hours are also spent learning anatomy, physiology, and pathology. Anatomical, physiological, and pathological knowledge is essential to understanding effects and contraindications and to locating endangerment sites. Ultimately, the therapist will conduct a client intake interview, perform a massage treatment based on a personalized treatment plan that addresses the client's needs.

However, how safe is massage? Can a client become injured?

To reiterate, massage is one of the safest modalities of complementary medicine and physical therapy. The probability that a well-trained, licensed therapist will harm a client is highly unlikely. In an article published in the *Journal of the American Medical Association,* liability claims against massage therapists were compiled and analyzed. The percentage of claims filed against massage therapists was less than one tenth of 1% (1990-1996). With regard to serious personal injury, the injured party always indicated that the form of massage used was too vigorous and aggressive, which led to injuries. These injuries include displacement of a ureteral stent, a hepatic hematoma after deep-tissue massage, and the deterioration in hearing among individuals who received deep-neck massage. In addition to the aforementioned cases, several reports of adverse reactions to shiatsu have been published, the most serious being a retinal artery embolism with partial loss of vision associated with work on the neck area. Documentation on this subject reported from Edzard Ernst in his published research entitled *The Safety of Massage Therapy* asserted that, despite these scattered reports, serious reactions to massage are extremely rare. Most claims were related to minor injures such as bruising and other soft-tissue damage. A significant portion of claims filed were related to sexual misconduct. Most massage schools are now teaching or are increasing hours devoted toward the therapeutic relationship, which includes the study of ethics and boundaries.

Because 500 hours represents the national average of training required in the states that mandate massage, the low rate of filed claims clearly indicates that these 500 hours are adequate to train a safe, competent massage therapist. Areas of specialization are available for additional training.

MECHANICAL AND REFLEXIVE RESPONSES TO MASSAGE

The body responds to pressure in one of two ways. One is a mechanical response, and the other is a reflexive response. A **mechanical response** occurs as a result of pressure, force, or range of motion. Tissues are pulled, lifted, rubbed, compressed, and manipulated. Examples of the mechanical responses to pressure are increased blood circulation, reduced swelling, and the reduced formation of scar tissue.

To create a **reflexive response** in the body, nerves are stimulated, which, in turn, activates a reflex arc. Examples of reflexive responses are decreased arousal of the sympathetic nervous system (i.e., general relaxation), triggering of stretch receptors (e.g., muscle spindles), increased diameter of blood vessels, and reduced blood pressure. Massage responses can be primarily mechanical or reflexive in nature, but both responses are closely related and often occur simultaneously.

EFFECTS OF MASSAGE

Both mechanical and reflexive responses are linked to massage techniques that deliver moderate to deep pressure, which stimulates pressure receptors. This type of massage is often referred to as *Swedish massage* or *therapeutic massage.* Some of the benefits outlined in this chapter are related to touch, but most are linked to Swedish massage. One study in particular implemented deep Swedish massage or deep-tissue massage. In this study, massage using light pressure generally produced adverse results. In fact, the study was criticized because it stated that massage did not have any effect on circulation. However, after closer examination, the fact that only light pressure was used for the experimental (massaged) group was discovered.

In a study conducted by Daniel Cherkin and colleagues, speculation was offered to explain why massage was effective in treating low back pain. As you would expect, effects on soft tissues were noted. Other factors attributed to massage effectiveness were the client spending 1 hour in a relaxed environment, receiving ongoing attention from the therapist, being touched in a therapeutic context, and increased body awareness during and after the massage. Education about exercise and other positive lifestyle changes was another benefit clients received as part of their massage.

Do the effects of massage last? Most benefits cease shortly after the massage treatments are terminated, but this is also true of other health-related treatments such as diet, exercise, and meditation. The key to long-term effects is the education clients receive concerning lifestyle habits and changes. These changes can be a healthy diet, frequent walks, and increased fluid intake. Clients are also taught other methods of self-care such as how to breathe for relaxation, a basic self-massage routine, or the stretching of muscle groups. Massage does have long-lasting effects on some specific injuries or pathological conditions. These effects include reducing scar tissue formation, decreasing edema, loosening lung phlegm, and relieving constipation. Chronic conditions often require ongoing massage treatments.

Massage therapy and the response it creates within the body can affect the cardiovascular system, lymphatic and immune systems, skin and related structures, nervous and endocrine systems, muscles, connective tissues, respiratory system, digestive system, and urinary system. Also noted are miscellaneous effects and indications for specific conditions and individuals.

This next lengthy section includes a listing of the documented effects of massage. Although every effort has been made to cite reliable sources, varying degrees of the quality of the research can be found (see the previous section on Scientific Method). Literature on massage therapy tends to lack the rigorous application of empirical research methods and is many times anecdotal in nature. The reference section at the end of this book has a complete list of works cited. If you have any concerns about a particular claim, then obtain the actual research and peruse the study.

Effects of Massage on the Cardiovascular System

- **Dilates blood vessels.** Superficial blood vessels become dilated resulting from reflex action.
- **Improves blood circulation.** Deep stroking improves blood circulation by mechanically assisting venous blood flow back to the heart. The increase of blood flow is comparable to that associated with exercise. The fact that local circulation during a massage increases up to three times more than circulation at rest has been documented.
- **Decreases blood pressure.** Blood pressure is decreased by blood vessel dilation. Both diastolic and systolic readings decline and last approximately 40 minutes after the massage.
- **Creates hyperemia.** Increased blood flow creates a hyperemic effect, which is visible on some skin types.
- **Stimulates release of acetylcholine and histamine.** These two substances are released as a result of vasomotor activity, thereby helping prolong vasodilation.
- **Replenishes nutritive materials.** Increased circulation aids in the delivery of products such as nutrients and oxygen to cells and tissues.
- **Promotes removal of waste products.** Increased circulation also aids in the removal of metabolic wastes. The notion is often said that massage *dilutes the poisons*.
- **Reduces ischemia.** Massage reduces ischemia. Ischemia is linked to pain and trigger-point formation.
- **Reduces heart and pulse rates.** Massage decreases heart rate through activation of the relaxation response.
- **Increases stroke volume.** Stroke volume is the amount of blood ejected from the left ventricle during each contraction. As the heart rate decreases, more time exists for the heart's lower chambers (ventricles) to fill with blood. The result is a larger volume of blood pushed through the heart, thereby increasing stroke volume.
- **Increases red blood cell (RBC) count.** The number of RBCs and their oxygen-carrying capacity are increased. This effect is due to (1) promoting the spleen's discharge of RBCs, (2) recruiting blood from engorged internal organs into general circulation, and (3) stimulating stagnant capillary beds and returning this blood into general circulation.
- **Increases oxygen saturation in blood.** When RBC count rises, oxygen saturation of the blood increases.
- **Increases white blood cell (WBC) count.** The presence of WBCs increases after massage. The body may perceive massage as a mild stressor (an event to which the body must adapt) and recruits additional WBCs. The increase in WBC count enables the body to protect itself more effectively against disease.
- **Enhances the adhesion of migrating WBCs.** The surfaces of WBCs become increasingly sticky after a massage, thereby increasing their adhesive quality and therefore their effectiveness.

- **Increases platelet count.** Massage has been found to increase the number of blood platelets.

Effects of Massage on the Lymphatic and the Immune Systems

- **Promotes lymph circulation.** Lymph circulation depends on pressure: from muscle contraction, pressure changes in the thorax and abdomen during breathing or applied pressure from a massage. Hence, massage promotes this circulation.
- **Reduces edema.** Massage reduces edema (swelling) by enhancing lymph circulation.
- **Decreases the circumference of an area affected with edema.** When an area swells, the diameter increases. When the swelling subsides, circumference decreases.
- **Decreases weight in patients with edema.** Fluid retention adds weight to an individual. When edema is addressed with massage, weight is consequently reduced.
- **Increases lymphocyte count.** Lymphocytes are types of WBCs. This effect indicates that massage supports immune functions.
- **Increases the number and function (or cytotoxicity) of natural killer cells, CD4 cells, and CD4/CD8 ratio.** All the aforementioned cells are types of WBCs. This increase further suggests that massage strengthens immune functions.

Effects of Massage on the Skin and Related Structures

- **Increases skin temperature.** Warming of the skin indicates a reduction of stress.
- **Improves skin condition.** As circulation increases, added nutrients are made available to the skin, thereby improving its condition, texture, and tone. Clinical observations have determined that massage also improves the appearance (i.e., color and texture) of the skin.
- **Stimulates oil glands.** Stimulation of the oil (sebaceous) glands causes an increase in oil (sebum) production. This stimulation improves the skin's condition and reduces skin dryness.
- **Improves skin conditions.** Unless a condition contraindicates massage, skin conditions may improve by decreasing

redness, reducing thickening or hardening of the skin, increasing healing of skin abrasions, and reducing itching.

Effects of Massage on the Nervous and the Endocrine Systems

- **Reduces stress.** Activating the relaxation response reduces stress.
- **Reduces anxiety.** Interestingly, a reduction in anxiety is noted in both the person who received the massage and the person who gave the massage.
- **Promotes relaxation.** General relaxation is promoted through activation of the relaxation response. Relaxation has a diminishing effect on pain.
- **Decreases beta wave activity.** Associated with relaxation, a decrease in beta brainwave activity occurred during and after the massage (confirmed by electroencephalogram [EEG]).
- **Increases delta wave activity.** Increases in delta brainwave activity, which occur during massage, are linked to sleep and to relaxation; both are promoted with massage (confirmed by EEG).
- **Increase in alpha waves.** An increase in alpha brainwaves during massage indicates relaxation (confirmed by EEG).
- **Increases dopamine levels.** Increased levels of dopamine are linked to decreased stress and reduced depression.
- **Increases serotonin levels.** Increased levels of serotonin suggest a reduction of both stress and depression. Theories suggest that serotonin inhibits pain signals, indicating that increased levels of serotonin also reduce pain.
- **Reduces cortisol levels.** Massage reduces cortisol levels by activating the relaxation response. Elevated levels of cortisol not only represent heightened stress but also inhibit immune functions.
- **Reduces norepinephrine levels.** Massage has been proved to reduce norepinephrine, a stress hormone.
- **Reduces epinephrine levels.** Epinephrine, another stress hormone, is reduced with massage.
- **Reduces feelings of depression.** Both chemical and electrophysiological changes from a negative to a positive mood were noted and may support the decrease in depression after massage therapy. Depression associated with chronic pain was also reduced.
- **Decreases pain.** Massage relieves local and referred pain, presumably by increasing circulation, thereby reducing ischemia. Massage also stimulates the release of endorphins (endogenous morphine), enkephalins, and other pain-reducing neurochemicals. General relaxation brought on by massage therapy also has a diminishing effect on pain. The pressure of a massage interferes with pain information entering the spinal cord by stimulating pressure receptors, further reducing pain. Massage interrupts the pain cycle (see Table Talk: Massage and the Pain Cycle) by relieving muscular spasms, increas-

ing circulation, and promoting rapid disposal of waste products (Figure 5-6). Massage also improves sleep patterns. During deep sleep, a substance called somatostatin is normally released. Without this substance, pain is experienced.

> ### TABLE TALK
>
> **Massage and the Pain Cycle**
>
> The pain cycle is initiated when painful stimuli result in reflex muscle contraction and localized muscle splinting or guarding. The localized muscle guarding restricts movement and decreases local circulation, which restricts the amount of oxygen available to the tissues and the removal of metabolic waste products. The subsequent swelling creates more pain. From this point, muscle splinting is intensified, and the cycle repeats itself. A more generalized secondary pain results that outlasts or exceeds the original discomfort. Massage interrupts the pain cycle on all levels.

- **Reduces analgesic use.** Because pain is reduced with massage, the need for excessive use of pain medication is also reduced.
- **Activates sensory receptors.** Depending on factors such as stroke choice, direction, speed, and pressure, massage can stimulate different sensory receptors, affecting massage outcome. For example, cross-fiber tapotement stimulates muscle spindles, which activates muscular contraction, whereas a slow passive stretch and deep effleurage activate Golgi tendon organs, thereby inhibiting contraction. Activation of pressure receptors reduces pain (see Table Talk: The Gate Theory).
- **Faster and more elaborate development of the hippocampal region of the brain.** As part of the limbic system, development of the hippocampal region is related to superior memory performance.

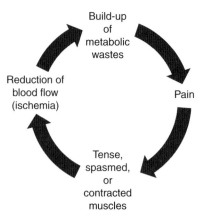

THE PAIN CYCLE

FIGURE 5-6 Massage interrupts the pain cycle.

The Gate Theory

In 1965 Ronald Wall and Patrick Melzack postulated the gate theory of pain relief, which explains why massage, ice, and heat are effective in the treatment of pain. The *gate theory* states that transmission of impulses into the spinal cord is *gated* (can be open or shut). Gating is affected by the degree of activity, or transmission, in sensory nerves. Multiple signals may be competing for the same gate—or entrance into the spinal cord. The one who hits the gate first wins. The gate then closes and prevents or inhibits other nerve impulses.

Nerve-transmission speed is affected by nerve diameter. Impulses traveling along larger nerve fibers are faster than those traveling along smaller nerves. Sensory nerves for pressure, temperature, and sharp acute pain lie close together in large concentrations near the body's surface. These sensory nerves are long and large in diameter and transmit impulses quickly, protecting the body from harm. Strong stimuli to these receptors generate a quick sensory input to the spinal cord. A reflex is generated to move the affected body part out of harm's way. Touching a needle or a hot pan elicits this type of immediate reflex response.

The sensory receptors for aching pain originate in the deeper tissues. These nerves are composed of short, thinner nerve fibers, which tend to transmit pain that has been present for some time (i.e., headache, dull pain) and requires no immediate protective action. These nerves transmit stimuli that are of lesser importance and lesser consequence to the body. The purpose of the deep, slower transmitting nerves is to make the conscious mind aware that a problem exists, which can be used to prevent overuse or dependence on an injured body part.

Suppose that a gymnast is having performance compromised by soreness in the right calf. This pain originates from the deeper, slower nerves. When a pressure stimulus such as massage is applied to the calf, the new sensory input travels along the faster, larger nerve network, entering the spinal cord first. The gate closes, excluding pain information from entering the cord. The body experiences the pressure of the massage stroke as an interruption of pain.

Massage therapists can use the gate mechanism when applying pressure, heat, and cold. All of these have the potential to interfere or interrupt pain signals.

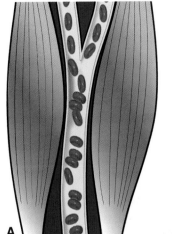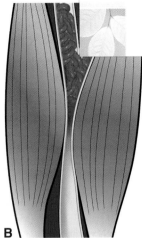

FIGURE 5-7 Muscle tensions relationship to blood flow. **A**, Blood flow within relaxed muscle. **B**, Blood flow within contracted, tense muscle.

Effects of Massage on Muscles

- **Relieves muscular tension.** Massage relieves muscular restrictions, tightness, stiffness, and spasms (Figure 5-7).
- **Relaxes muscles.** Muscles relax as massage reduces excitability in the sympathetic nervous system.
- **Reduces muscle soreness and fatigue.** Massage enhances blood circulation, thereby increasing the amount of oxygen and nutrients available to the muscles. Increased oxygen and nutrients reduce muscle fatigue and postexercise soreness. Massage promotes rapid disposal of waste products, further reducing muscle fatigue and soreness. Massage interrupts the pain cycle. A fatigued muscle recuperates 20% after 5 minutes of rest and 100% after 5 minutes of massage. A reduction in postexercise recovery time was indicated by a decline in pulse rate and an increase muscle work capacity.

- **Reduces trigger point formation.** Trigger point formation in both muscle and fascia is greatly reduced by massage.
- **Manually separates muscle fibers.** Compressive strokes and cross-fiber friction strokes separate muscle fibers, thereby reducing muscle spasms.
- **Increases range of motion.** When muscular tension is reduced, range of motion is improved. The freedom of the joints is dictated by the freedom of the muscles.
- **Improves performance (balance and posture).** Many postural distortions are removed when trigger points and muscle tension are reduced. Range of motion increases, gait becomes more efficient, the posture is more aligned and balanced, and performance is improved as the net result.
- **Lengthens muscles.** Massage mechanically stretches and broadens tissue, especially when combined with Swedish gymnastics (joint mobilization and stretches). These changes are detected by Golgi tendon organs, which inhibit contraction signals, further lengthening muscles. Massage retrains the tissue from a contracted state to an elongated state, thereby increasing resting length. This principle is one of the principles behind neuromuscular reeducation.
- **Increases flexibility.** By lengthening muscles and promoting relaxation, massage has also been shown to increase flexibility.
- **Tones weak muscles.** Muscle spindle activity is increased during massage strokes (e.g., tapotement, vibration). An increase in muscle spindle activity stimulates minute muscle contractions, thereby helping tone weak muscles. This effect is particularly beneficial in most cases of prolonged bed rest, flaccidity, and atrophy.
- **Reduces creatine kinase activity in the blood.** Creatine kinase is an enzyme that helps ensure that enough adenosine triphosphate (ATP) is available for muscle contraction. By reducing the activity of creatine kinase in the blood, massage indirectly helps decrease muscle spasm, which increases muscle relaxation.

- **Decreases electromyography (EMG) readings.** Decreased EMG readings signify a decrease in neuromuscular activity and reduction of neuromuscular complaints.

MINI-LAB

Sit in a chair with your feet flat on the floor. Moving only your head and neck, look over your left shoulder, and notice how far you can comfortably move. Do the same, looking to the right. With your right hand, grab the top of your right shoulder. As you apply pressure, slowly move the shoulder up and down 10 times. Maintain the pressure, and roll your shoulder back 10 times, then forward 10 times. Do this same movement with the left shoulder. Squeeze the back of your neck. Without releasing the pressure, turn your head (as if saying *no*), nod your head (as if saying *yes*), and move your nose in a circle clockwise and counterclockwise 10 times each. After the *squeeze and move* activity, look over your right and left shoulders again. Notice how much farther you can go. This increase is the result of self-administered massage.

Effects of Massage on Connective Tissues

- **Reduces keloid formation.** Massage applied to scar tissue helps reduce keloid formation in scar tissue beneath the site of massage application.
- **Reduces excessive scar formation.** Deep massage reduces excessive scar tissue formation, helping create an appropriate scar that is strong yet does not interfere with the muscle's ability to broaden as it contracts.
- **Decreases adhesion formation.** Deep, specifically applied massage helps decrease adhesions. This decrease, in turn, facilitates normal, pain-free motion of the affected muscles and joints.
- **Releases fascial restrictions.** Pressure and the heat it produces convert fascia from a gel state to a solid state (thixotropy), thereby reducing hyperplasia. Softening of the fascia surrounding muscles allows them to be stretched to their fullest resting length, thereby increasing joint range of motion and freeing the body of restricted movements.
- **Increases mineral retention in bone.** Massage increases the retention of nutrients such as sulfur and phosphorus in bones.
- **Promotes fracture healing.** When a bone is fractured, the body forms a network of new blood vessels at the break site. Massage increases circulation around the fracture, thereby promoting fracture healing. Increased circulation around a fracture leads to increased deposition of callus to the bone. Callus is formed between and around the broken ends of a fractured bone during healing and is ultimately replaced by compact bone.
- **Improves connective tissue healing.** Occurring only with deep-pressure massage, proliferation and activation of fibroblasts were noted. Fibroblasts generate a connective tissue matrix, which promotes tissue healing by increasing collagen production and increasing the tensile strength of healed tissue.

- **Reduces surface dimpling of cellulite.** Massage flattens out fat deposits located under the skin and makes the skin seem smoother. Cellulite (a type of fat) appears as groups of small dimples or depressions under the skin caused by an uneven separation of fat globules below the skin's surface, which are displaced by manual manipulation. Massage does not reduce the amount of cellulite below the skin; instead, it temporarily alters the shape and appearance of cellulite.

Effects of Massage on the Respiratory System

- **Reduces respiration rate.** Massage slows down breathing because of activation of the relaxation response.
- **Strengthens respiratory muscles.** The muscles of respiration have a greater capacity to contract, thereby helping improve pulmonary functions.
- **Decreases the sensation of dyspnea.** Dyspnea (short or difficult breathing) is lessened as a result of massage.
- **Decreases asthma attacks.** Through increased relaxation and improved pulmonary functions, a person with asthma experiences fewer attacks after massage.
- **Reduces laryngeal tension.** Laryngeal tension may occur from excessive public speaking or singing. Massage reduces the stress on the larynx and tension on the muscles of the throat.
- **Increases fluid discharge from the lungs.** The mechanical loosening and discharge of phlegm increase with rhythmic alternating pressures. Tapotement (cupping) and vibration on the rib cage are often used to enhance this effect. Phlegm loosening and discharge are further enhanced when combined with postural drainage (promoting fluid drainage of the respiratory tract through certain body positions) and when the client is encouraged to cough.
- **Improves pulmonary functions.** Relaxation plays a significant role in how massage improves pulmonary function, but massage also loosens tight respiratory muscles and fascia. The affected pulmonary functions are as follows:
  - **Increased vital capacity.** This measurement is the amount of air that can be expelled at the normal rate of exhalation after a maximum inhalation, representing the greatest possible breathing capacity.
  - **Increased forced vital capacity.** This measurement is the amount of air that can be forcibly expelled after a forced inhalation.
  - **Increased forced expiratory volume.** This measurement is the volume of air that can be forcibly expelled after a full exhalation.
  - **Increased forced expiratory flow.** This measurement is the volume of air that can be forcibly expelled after a full inhalation.
  - **Improved peak expiratory flow.** This measurement is the greatest rate of airflow that can be achieved during forced expiration beginning with the lungs fully inflated.

Effects of Massage on the Digestive System

- **Promotes evacuation of the colon.** By increasing peristaltic activity in the colon through massage, movement of bowel contents toward the anus for elimination is aided.
- **Relieves constipation.** Because evacuation of the colon is promoted, constipation is relieved.
- **Relieves colic and intestinal gas.** Increased peristaltic activity also helps relieve colic and the expulsion of intestinal gas.
- **Stimulates digestion.** Massage also promotes activation of the relaxation response, which stimulates digestion.

Effects of Massage on the Urinary System

- **Increases urine output.** Massage activates dormant capillary beds and recovers lymphatic fluids for filtration by the kidney, which, in turn, increases the frequency of urination and amount of urine produced. Massage is also relaxing and thus stimulates the parasympathetic nervous system, which promotes general homeostasis, thereby increasing urine output.
- **Promotes the excretion of nitrogen, inorganic phosphorus, and sodium chloride in urine.** Levels of these metabolic waste products are elevated in urine after massage.

Miscellaneous Effects of Massage

- **Reduces fatigue and increases vigor.** Many clients experienced a sense of renewed energy after massage.
- **Improves sleep patterns.** When clients who have had massage therapy went to sleep, they reported a deeper sleep and felt more rested after waking.
- **Reduces job-related and posttraumatic stress.** Massage reduces many types of stress, including job-related and posttraumatic stress.
- **Improves mood.** The mental health status and mood improved after massage.
- **Decreases feelings of anger.** Clients reported a decrease in aggression and feelings of anger with massage.
- **Improves body image.** Massage improved body image in clients who stated having a poor body image before the massage.
- **Improves self-esteem.** Individuals who received and who gave massages reported enhanced self-esteem.
- **Promotes communication and expression.** Individuals who received and gave massages reported an increase in the quantity and quality of their social interactions. They talked more freely and openly and enjoyed themselves more during these interactions. Massage can also assist the ease of emotional expression with relaxation.
- **Improves lifestyle habits.** After massage, clients reported improved lifestyle habits such as increased activities of daily living (ADL), fewer cups of coffee, fewer physical symptoms, fewer visits to the physician, and increased levels of exercising (e.g., walking).
- **Increases physical well-being.** Massage enhances well-being through stress reduction and subsequent relaxation.
- **Reduces touch aversion and touch sensitivity.** Victims of rape and spousal abuse reported a reduction in touch aversion after massage. Hypersensitivity to touch was reduced in other individuals.
- **Increases academic performance.** A decrease in math computation time and an increase in accuracy were noted in massage studies.
- **Increases mental alertness.** Massage increases mental alertness by relaxing the body and mind and by removing stress.
- **Satisfies emotional needs.** Clients reported using the therapeutic relationship to satisfy their emotional needs for attention, acceptance, caring, and nurturing touch.

"There's an alternative. There's always a third way, and it's not a combination of the other two ways. It's a different way."
David Carradine

INDICATIONS OF MASSAGE FOR SPECIFIC CONDITIONS AND SPECIAL POPULATIONS

Most individuals can benefit from massage therapy. This section focuses on specific conditions that have been documented to benefit from massage. For further reading, please see the bibliography at the end of the chapter.

- **Alzheimer's disease.** Massage decreased physical expressions of agitation (e.g., pacing, wandering) and improved sleep patterns.
- **Anemia.** An increase in RBCs and an increase in oxygen saturation in the blood suggest that massage is beneficial for individuals with anemia.
- **Asthma.** Studies indicate that massage improved pulmonary functions and reduced the occurrence of asthma attacks.
- **Attention deficit hyperactivity disorder (ADHD).** Individuals diagnosed with ADHD who receive massage were observed to be less fidgety and hyperactive and spent more time completing assigned tasks. Students themselves reported an improved short-term mood state.
- **Burn victims.** Burn victims who were massaged experienced a decrease in pain and itching and reduced anxiety before débridement. Massage also reduced feelings of depression and anger.
- **Cancer.** Edema, pain, fatigue, anxiety, nausea, and feelings of anger and depression were reduced when patients with cancer had routine massages. Massage also increased lymphocyte and natural killer cell counts.
- **Cerebral palsy (CP).** Massage promotes circulation of blood and lymph and relieves muscular tension in individuals with CP. Increases in flexibility were also reported.
- **Chronic fatigue syndrome (CFS).** Clients with CFS experience reduced feelings of depression and anxiety

JOHN F. BARNES, PT

Born: February 3, 1939.

"The master therapist is real, calm, nonjudgmental, intelligent, sensitive, strong yet flexible, supportive, compassionate, empathic, and joyful."

One of the major differences between *myofascial release* and many other forms of bodywork is that, at its best, it allows the therapist to bring more to the table. It is systematic, physiologically grounded, and intuitive without apology. The founder of myofascial release, John Barnes, is a physical therapist and teacher who values a wide range of modalities such as the work of Ida Rolf, Milton Trager, John Upledger, and Paul St. John.

Barnes's father died when he was 3 years of age, and he was raised by his mother. He remembers enjoying being alone in the forest and learning to be so quiet that the wildlife would venture out. He studied karate and, as a result, learned about the role of *Qi*. As a junior in high school, Barnes knew he wanted to be a physical therapist.

With warm eyes, a burly build, and a full beard, Barnes resembles the type to live in a log cabin and love nature—and he does. He as been called an old soul and does not scoff at the label. He does not believe in assembly-line quick fixes. How could he? He knows how insidious pain can be.

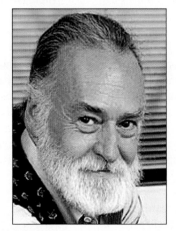

As a teen, Barnes was lifting weights and could not get out of a dead squat, so he turned a back flip and landed on his tailbone with an extra 300 pounds to boot. Not long afterward, his back locked up just as he was about to kiss a girl with whom he was infatuated. Nevertheless, he did not pay much attention to his condition. He had youth on his side and charged on, until a skiing accident left him in worse condition. Surgery made a big difference, but the pain left an indelible scar.

Robert Calvert of *Massage Magazine* quotes Barnes as saying, "I don't really mean this should happen, but in a way, every physician or therapist should be severely injured, and not just hurt for a week or two or a month, but a couple years. It's a whole different story when you are a prisoner in your own body. I felt broken, and I was broken. It was a horrible, horrible experience."

Yet another injury led Barnes to explore the advantage of alternative therapies that had been offered in his traditional physical therapist training. He began to blend experience with principles from different disciplines and

and fewer symptoms such as fatigue. CFS affects muscle strength; improved grip strength was also documented.
- **Constipation.** Elimination problems were relieved through massage.
- **Diabetes.** Blood glucose levels, anxiety, and depression were reduced with massage. An increase in dietary compliance was also reported.
- **Eating disorders.** Patients with anorexia nervosa and bulimia stated a reduction of depression and anxiety. These individuals stated that they experienced an improvement in eating habits and an increase in positive body image.
- **Edema.** Swelling resulting from edema was reduced with massage, as long as the swelling was not a result of inflammation or disease.
- **Fibromyalgia.** Not only were stress, anxiety, and feelings of depression reduced, but decreases in pain, stiffness, fatigue, and insomnia were also documented in individuals

with fibromyalgia. Massage was rated more effective than standard physical therapy or prescriptive drugs.
- **Headaches.** Most headaches (muscular, cluster, eye strain, mental fatigue, and sinus) were relieved with massage. People also reported a reduction in headache frequency and headache duration but not always in intensity. One study did report less analgesic use as a result of pain reduction.
- **High blood pressure.** Massage decreased blood pressure (both systolic and diastolic readings) and helped promote healthy lifestyle habits in patients with high blood pressure (hypertension).
- **Individuals infected with the human immunodeficiency virus (HIV).** The number of natural killer cells, CD4 cells, and CD4/CD8 cell ratio increased after 1 month of massage therapy. These cells are important because they have been shown to provide protection against acquired immunodeficiency syndrome and opportunistic

JOHN F. BARNES, PT (*continued*)

discovered how fascia and energy flow are connected. Basically, myofascial release is based on understanding the role of fascia, a web of interconnected tissue that travels the body without interruption. It surrounds individual cells, organs, and systems and then wraps it all up in one huge package, head to toe. This network also serves as the communication medium from cell to cell and organ to organ. Trauma, posture, or inflammation can change the consistency of the web, solidifying and shortening fibers and blocking the flow of messages that are necessary for homeostasis. This web, if pulled too tightly in one place, can leave other areas restricted, creating pressure on nerves, muscles, organs, and bones.

As a physical therapist, Barnes's style had always been focused, slow, and rhythmic. Sometimes his touch was light. Sometimes the tissue beneath his hands granted him deeper access. He did not know he was practicing *myofascial release,* per se, until he attended a physicians' course on connective tissue. Afterward, he began to see and treat the interrelationship of the whole body—including the mind or spirit—rather than the isolated sore neck, bum knee, or other body part. This shift in thinking not only enhanced the results of his work but also stirred up emotions that demanded his attention. As his work evolved, so did Barnes. (The goal of myofascial release is not necessarily to incite emotional response, but considering the pervasive nature of myofascial system and the complex nature of humans, many forms of bodywork are considered and

may eventually be proved to be therapeutic for emotional and physical trauma.)

Barnes started teaching other people his form of bodywork in the mid-1970s. His task begins by reawakening the therapist's ability to *feel* what is happening with the body. Then he teaches the techniques to evaluate and release restricted areas in a systematic way. In his opinion, a comprehensive program should also include exercise and flexibility programs, movement awareness facilitation techniques, instruction in body mechanics, mobilization and muscle energy techniques, nutritional advice, biofeedback, and psychological counseling.

Even with such a systematic and comprehensive approach, Barnes is realistic about results. Therapists do not *fix* clients; we can offer tools for change not only in the form of bodywork but also in *mindwork.* When we get right down to the nitty gritty, we cannot help our clients unless they are ready to help themselves. This thought is a humbling one, yet being proficient and humble is a good starting point.

Barnes's advice for beginning massage therapists is to continue learning advanced methods after graduating from the typical 500-hour program. Simply reading about a bodywork concept or simply being introduced to a modality is insufficient to practice it successfully and, in some cases, may lead to learning bad habits or faulty techniques. Barnes suggests learning as many forms of bodywork as possible to adapt to the wide range of client needs.

diseases. Massage also helped individuals infected with HIV to relax.
- **Hospitalized patients.** Massage increased relaxation, provided a sense of well-being, and produced a positive mood change for patients. Most (more than two thirds) attributed enhanced mobility, greater energy, increased participation in treatment, and faster recovery to massage therapy.
- **Hospice patients.** Hospice patients experienced reduced pain and had a decline in heart rate and blood pressure, indicating decreased stress and anxiety.
- **Infants.** Preterm, cocaine-exposed, HIV-exposed, and full-term infants experienced less colic, less repetitive crying, and improved feeding habits and gained more weight than infants in the same categories who were not massaged. Massage was found more effective than rocking for inducing infant sleep.
- **Injuries.** Massage speeds the healing of overuse injuries, sprains, and strains.

- **Insomnia.** Inducing relaxation alleviates insomnia.
- **Low back pain.** Addressing trigger points decreases low back pain. Medical costs were reduced by approximately 40% along with reduced analgesic use. Massage increased range of motion and promoted relaxation. Patients reported that massage made them feel cared for, happy, physically relaxed, less anxious, calm, and restful and gave them a feeling of closeness with the individuals who gave massages. Massage was rated more effective than standard physical therapy or prescriptive drugs.
- **Lung disease.** For clients with chronic obstructive pulmonary disease, massage strengthened respiratory muscles, reduced heart rate, increased oxygen saturation in blood, decreased shortness of breath, and improved pulmonary functions. Respiratory drainage is encouraged through cupping tapotement and vibration. Clients with cystic fibrosis further reported decreased anxiety and improved mood with massage treatments.

- **Multiple sclerosis (MS).** Individuals with MS who received massages experienced reduced anxiety and depression, improved self-esteem, and positive body image and implemented changes to their lifestyle that promoted health such as exercising and stretching.
- **Nerve entrapment.** Conditions of nerve entrapment, such as carpal tunnel syndrome, thoracic outlet syndrome, and sciatica, were relieved by release of the myofascial component.
- **Pervasive developmental disorder (PDD).** Massaged children with PDD or autism spent less time in solitary play and had an increase in attention to sounds and their social relatedness to their teachers. Behaviors such as touch aversion were reduced.
- **Poor circulation.** Massage improved blood circulation.
- **Pain (chronic).** Pain levels decreased, most often significantly. The depression and anxiety associated with individuals with chronic pain improved, as well as their quality of life.
- **Pregnancy and postpartum.** Massaged pregnant women reported fewer obstetrical and postpartum complications, reduced prematurity rates, shorter and less painful labors, improved psychological support, and fewer days in the hospital after labor and delivery. When nurses, midwives, or spouses massaged the pregnant or laboring women's perineal area, injury such as tearing during fetal delivery was reduced. Feelings of postpartum depression declined with massage. Depressed adolescent mothers reported less stress, anxiety, and depression.
- **Premenstrual syndrome (PMS).** Massage reduced swelling, pain, and anxiety and improved the mood of women experiencing PMS.
- **Psychiatric patients.** Child, adolescent, and adult psychiatric patients were observed to be better adapted to a group, and the medical staff reported better clinical progress with massage. A decrease in depression and anxiety was noted with reduced cortisol levels and norepinephrine blood levels and increased dopamine levels. In many individuals, a decreased self-destructive behavior was reported, and the mental health status improved in the people in the massaged group. A decrease in the episodes of dysfunctional behavior was found in patients with dementia.
- **Rheumatoid arthritis.** Massage reduced trigger point formation, provided relief from pain and anxiety, reduced morning stiffness and edema, and increased range of motion of the joints. Studies also revealed an increase tolerance of exercise and other educational approaches.
- **Stress and anxiety.** Stress and anxiety are reduced by activation of the relaxation response.
- **Temporomandibular joint (TMJ) dysfunction.** The muscular component of TMJ dysfunction was addressed with massage, and reduced pain and dysfunction was the result.

Once the benefits and indications of massage are known, an understanding of contraindications and endangerment sites becomes clear. For instance, by increasing lymph circulation, massage affects the tissue and fluids of the body; because massage increases the circulation of blood, thrombosis must be a contraindication.

> *"It's time again. Tear up the violets and plant something more difficult to grow."*
> James Schuyler

CONTRAINDICATIONS FOR MASSAGE THERAPY

During the assessment process, the therapist takes into consideration information obtained from the client. Some of this information comes through direct questioning, and some is obtained through observation and palpation (Table Talk box, this page). All information gathered culminates in a treatment plan that establishes goals and addresses modifications. In most instances, only slight adjustments are made, such as propping up a stiff shoulder so the client is comfortable lying on the table or using only light pressure over the abdomen because of a hernia. Some conditions warrant avoiding an area, such as the site of a recent burn or a client's feet because of a sebaceous cyst. Some conditions and symptoms may even preclude massage altogether. The presence of a disease or physical condition that makes treating a particular client in the usual manner impossible or undesirable is called a **contraindication.**

Ruling out the presence of any conditions in which massage may have harmful effects is the duty and obligation of the therapist.

> **TABLE TALK**
>
> If the client refuses to disclose his or her medical history, then the therapist has the right to refuse treatment.

The two categories of contraindications are *absolute* and *local.* Conditions in which massage is inappropriate, is not advised, and may be harmful to the client are known as **absolute contraindications.** Only rarely would a physician order massage under these conditions, but some exceptions occur, such as preeclampsia.

Many conditions or diseases are **local contraindications** in which massage can be administered while avoiding the infected area or the area in question.

> **evolve** *Identifying contraindications is a hallmark of a competent therapist. After logging on to the Evolve website, locate the comprehensive list of contraindications grouped by type. Use this list as a reference and study guide.* ■

Although massage is inappropriate in cases of absolute or local contraindications, the therapist may elect to use an energetic modality such as polarity that involves little or no physical contact. In other cases in which contraindications exist, advanced techniques such as lymphatic drainage may be appropriate. A well-trained, experienced therapist should possess the critical thinking skills involved in making these

---

BOX 5-2

Treatment Guidelines

Treat as a Local Contraindication If:

The condition is due to an injury that is less than 72 hours old (e.g., whiplash, ankle sprain).

Pressure causes unwarranted pain (e.g., corn, callus, bunion).

The area is inflamed (e.g., carpal tunnel syndrome, acute bursitis).

The area in question is confined to a small space that can be easily avoided (e.g., athlete's foot [foot or feet], irritable bowel syndrome [abdomen]).

The area presents an abnormal finding such as suspicious lumps, masses, or moles.

Treat as an Absolute Contraindication If:

If inflammation is widespread or if the condition is acute or exacerbated (e.g., rheumatoid arthritis, lupus).

If the condition is due to an infectious agent (e.g., fungi, virus) or disease (e.g., strep throat, pneumonia, scabies).

Until his or her physician can be consulted if the client's symptoms become more severe for any or no apparent reason (Parkinson's disease, scleroderma), which is revealed during the premassage assessment process. Make sure the client has signed a medical release form.

If condition represents a medical emergency (e.g., meningitis, appendicitis).

---

important decisions with the client. Record extensively in the client's records all discussions regarding his or her conditions and the type of treatment plan on which the two of you agree.

Much of the client intake and assessment involves screening clients for the appropriateness of massage. Some helpful guidelines follow, as shown in Box 5-2.

If a client has a condition or disease that is indicated for massage, then treat as a cautious indication and follow several basic guidelines, which include:

- Tailor the massage to client's vitality and stamina (e.g., slower, gentler massage; a massage of shorter duration; assisting the client on and off the table).
- Position the client for comfort (e.g., side lying position for pregnant clients, seated position for paraplegics, extra bolstering for clients with spinal abnormalities, semireclining for clients with emphysema).
- Obtain physician clearance before the initial treatment to acquire more information regarding client's health status (e.g., arteriosclerosis, cerebral palsy). Make sure the client has signed a medical release form.

Obtaining a pathology book written specifically for massage therapists that lists each one of these conditions is highly recommended, such as our companion text: *Mosby's Pathology for Massage Therapists,* by Salvo and Anderson. This and similar texts define each pathological condition and details how to proceed (or not proceed) with massage.

> *"It is the heart that understands*
> *and the hand that soothes."*
> Martha Rogers

ENDANGERMENT SITES

Endangerment sites are areas of the body that contain superficial, delicate structures that are relatively unprotected and are therefore prone to injury. These sites merit caution during treatment. In most instances, the therapist simply adjusts pressure or avoids pointed or sustained pressure. Endangerment sites include structures such as nerves, blood vessels, organs, and small or prominent bony projections. These areas may be treated during a massage session, and they often are, but cau-

tion must be exercised, working slowly, lightly, and carefully when in or around these sites. Exceptions to this rule would be energy work and techniques with which little or no pressure is used, such as therapeutic touch.

This section examines types of endangerment sites and why caution is warranted. In the next section, areas of the body where most endangerment sites exist are identified.

- **Nerves.** When nerves are compressed during massage, the client may experience numbness, tingling, burning, or shooting pain. That massage will damage the nerve is doubtful, but these sensations may alarm your client or make him or her feel uncomfortable. If the pressure is prolonged, then the client may experience a temporary loss of motor control.
- **Blood vessels.** Pressure applied to superficial blood vessels may cause a temporary reduction in blood flow and may possibly affect blood pressure. When massaging an area where a superficial artery is present, apply light pressure and feel for a pulse. If a pulse is felt, then avoid prolonged pressure on the specific pulse location (see Figure 19-15 and 19-16 for blood vessel locations). Caution areas for arteries also include the neighboring veins of the same name, with the exception of the aorta, the carotid artery, the great saphenous vein, and the jugular vein. Arteries and veins lie in proximity to each other, and caution of one vessel generally reflects caution of the other. Note that many of these endangerment sites are common pulse point locations (see Figure 19-10).
- **Bony structures.** Compression of certain small, fragile, or prominent bony areas may cause pain and bruising.
- **Organs and glands.** Pressure or striking movements such as tapotement to the kidney or eye area may cause bruising, sharp pain, nausea, or temporary dysfunction. Swollen lymph nodes are also endangerment sites.

The following specific locations of each type of endangerment site can be located on the endangerment site map (Figure 5-8). All endangerment sites are bilaterally symmetrical with the exception of those located on the midline of the body. Remember, you can and should work these areas, but be mindful of the following structures:

- **Abdomen.** The structures of which to be aware regarding pressure in the abdomen include the abdominal and

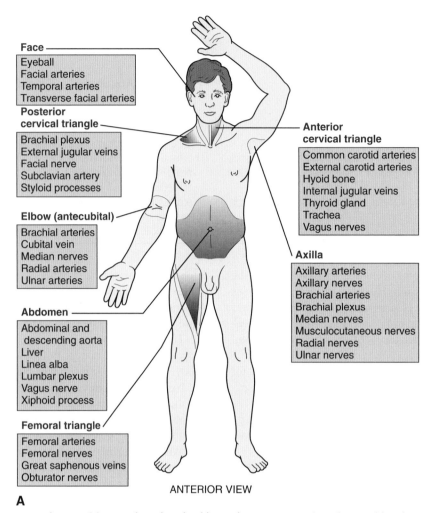

Face
- Eyeball
- Facial arteries
- Temporal arteries
- Transverse facial arteries

Posterior cervical triangle
- Brachial plexus
- External jugular veins
- Facial nerve
- Subclavian artery
- Styloid processes

Elbow (antecubital)
- Brachial arteries
- Cubital vein
- Median nerves
- Radial arteries
- Ulnar arteries

Abdomen
- Abdominal and descending aorta
- Liver
- Linea alba
- Lumbar plexus
- Vagus nerve
- Xiphoid process

Femoral triangle
- Femoral arteries
- Femoral nerves
- Great saphenous veins
- Obturator nerves

Anterior cervical triangle
- Common carotid arteries
- External carotid arteries
- Hyoid bone
- Internal jugular veins
- Thyroid gland
- Trachea
- Vagus nerves

Axilla
- Axillary arteries
- Axillary nerves
- Brachial arteries
- Brachial plexus
- Median nerves
- Musculocutaneous nerves
- Radial nerves
- Ulnar nerves

ANTERIOR VIEW

A

FIGURE 5-8 Endangerment site map. Massage therapists should exercise extreme caution when working these areas. **A**, Anterior view.
Continued

descending aorta, liver, linea alba (connective tissue band running down the abdominal wall, which can herniate), lumbar plexus, vagus nerve (deep pressure on psoas major may stimulate the vagus nerve and cause symptoms such as sweating and nausea), and xiphoid process (can fracture under heavy pressure).
- **Axilla.** The axilla contains several nerves and blood vessels that can become compressed during massage, such as the axillary and brachial arteries, as well as axillary, median, musculocutaneous, radial, and ulnar nerves, all branches of the brachial plexus.
- **Elbow.** The elbow is divided into a front (antecubital) and a back (cubital) area. Endangerment areas of the elbow include the brachial, radial, and ulnar arteries, as well as the median and the radial and ulnar nerves.
- **Face.** Avoid direct pressure on the eyeball, temporal artery (runs vertically anterior to the ear), facial arteries (alongside the upper and lower jaw), and transverse facial arteries (anterior to the ear).
- **Femoral triangle and medial thigh.** The borders of the femoral triangle are the muscles gracilis and sartorius and inguinal ligament (see Chapter 16). This area contains the

femoral arteries and nerves, great saphenous veins, and obturator nerves.
- **Low back.** Do not get carried away with the striking tapotement or the electrical massager on the low back. Two structures for which to watch out here are the floating ribs and kidneys (located retroperitoneally).
- **Popliteal.** Located behind the knee are the common peroneal and tibial nerves and the popliteal arteries.
- **Throat.** The throat region contains two triangular regions, the anterior and posterior cervical triangles.
  - *Anterior cervical triangle's* defining borders—the trachea, the base of the jaw (mandible), and muscle sternocleidomastoid—contains seven endangerment sites, which are the common carotid arteries, external carotid arteries, hyoid bone, internal jugular veins, thyroid gland, trachea, and vagus nerves.
  - *Posterior cervical triangle,* which uses the clavicle (collar bone) and the muscles sternocleidomastoid and trapezius, as its defining borders and presents the following endangerment sites: brachial plexus, external jugular veins, facial nerve, subclavian artery, and styloid processes of the temporal bone.

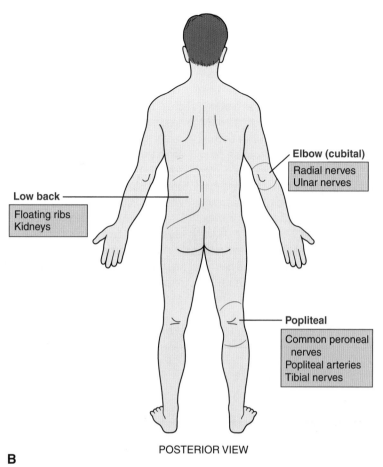

Elbow (cubital)
Radial nerves
Ulnar nerves

Low back
Floating ribs
Kidneys

Popliteal
Common peroneal
nerves
Popliteal arteries
Tibial nerves

B

POSTERIOR VIEW

FIGURE 5-8, **cont'd**. **B**, Posterior view.

SUMMARY

Massage has a powerful impact on the health and functioning of the body and has beneficial effects on virtually every body system. Nonetheless, massage is *not* the ultimate answer for all problems and ills. The massage therapist who has studied and learned the indications and contraindications inspires confidence in his or her clients by demonstrating a strong grasp of anatomy, physiology, and pathology. This learning includes the science of how massage provides pain relief through mechanisms such as the gate theory. No greater gift can be given to a client than the attention to and caution against contraindicated conditions and vascular, nervous, osseous, and other miscellaneous endangerment sites. In this way, the therapist also demonstrates an appreciation for his or her own abilities, an awareness of his or her own limitations, and an unflagging reputation for acting in the best interest of his or her clients.

CASE STUDY:

Dehydration

Judy made an appointment with her massage therapist, Becky, after canceling the last two massage appointments. Three months before, Judy had been laid off from her job of 11 years. This layoff came as a blow to her already lowered self-esteem resulting from a marital separation she did not want. Along with bouts of deep sadness and crying, Judy had also begun drinking vodka in the evening to cope with her loneliness. Many evenings, Judy went to bed without dinner because she was not hungry. She spent most of her time during the day tending to her home and yard. Returning to the workforce was not something for which Judy was ready. Luckily, she had a sizable amount in her savings account; thus money was not something about which she had to be worried.

When Judy got to Becky's office, she was anticipating the warm room, the relaxing music, and the smell of clean linens. Becky greeted her with a friendly smile and began asking Judy about her health since her last visit. Judy claimed that her health was fine; she had not been ill. She did tell Becky that she was under a lot of emotional turmoil over her recent separation from her husband.

Becky escorted Judy to the massage room and left while Judy prepared herself. When Becky reentered the room, she turned back the sheet to expose Judy's back. Judy was a petite woman, but she had apparently lost some weight. As the massage began, Becky noted that Judy's skin was mottled and cool and that, after it was compressed and lifted during a pétrissage, it remained elevated or *tented* for a few seconds before becoming smooth again. Becky paused her massage unconsciously, now uncomfortable with continuing; she suspected Judy was dehydrated.

If you were Becky, how would you approach Judy with regard to her physical condition?

If Judy were not receptive to your feedback, would you be satisfied that you had fulfilled your duty and proceed with the massage, allowing her to be responsible for her own health, or would you contact the emergency relative on her intake card to make sure he or she was aware of the situation?

If you were Judy, how might you react to the information that you are dehydrated?

---

evolve

Go to *Chapter Extras* on Evolve for additional illustrations and resources for this chapter. *Extras* for this chapter include:

1. Crossword puzzle (downloadable form)
2. Rene Spitz (illustration)
3. Bernard Grad (illustration)
4. Article report form (downloadable)
5. Vessel diameter and its effect on blood pressure (illustration)

MATCHING

Place the letter of the answer next to the term or phrase that best describes it.

A. Absolute
B. Contraindication
C. Decubitus ulcers, thrombophlebitis,
        ganglion cysts
D. Endangerment sites

E. Gate theory
F. Local
G. Mechanical
H. Osteoporosis, diabetes mellitus,
        hypertension

I. Pink eye, impetigo, ringworm
J. Reflexive
K. Science
L. Touch Research Institute

_____ 1. A method of inquiry that attempts to prove or disprove hypotheses using a rational, logical method

_____ 2. A program that was established in 1992 by Dr. Tiffany Field at the University of Miami School of Medicine

_____ 3. A physiological response caused by pressure, force, or range of motion

_____ 4. Examples of absolute contraindications

_____ 5. A physiological response caused by stimulated nerves

_____ 6. States that nerves compete for entrance into the spinal cord

_____ 7. The presence of a disease or physical condition that makes treating a particular client in the usual manner impossible or undesirable

_____ 8. Examples of caution indications

_____ 9. Contraindication in which massage is inappropriate, is not advised, and may be harmful to the client

_____ 10. Contraindications in which massage can be administered while avoiding the infected area or the area in question

_____ 11. Areas of the body that contain superficial delicate structures that are relatively unprotected and are therefore prone to injury

_____ 12. Examples of local contraindications

INTERNET ACTIVITIES

Visit the website for Touch Research Institute (http://www.miami.edu/touch-research). Locate two abstracts, and compose a summary of the research.

Using a search engine, locate information on the scientific method, or visit http://teacher.pas.rochester.edu/phy_labs/AppendixE/AppendixE.html. Write a one-page report on common steps used during research studies.

Visit http://www.researchmethods.com and locate types of research designs, outlining their strengths and weaknesses.

Bibliography

Ahles TA et al: Massage therapy for patients undergoing autologous bone marrow transplantation, *J Pain Symptom Manag* 18:157-163, Sep 1999.

Anderson KN, editor: *Mosby's medical, nursing, and allied health dictionary,* ed 6, St Louis, 2002, Mosby.

[Anonymous]: The mainstreaming of alternative medicine, *Consumer Reports* 65(5):17-25, 2000.

Applegate EJ: *The anatomy and physiology learning system,* ed 3, Philadelphia, 2006, Saunders.

Barr JS, Taslitz N: Influence of back massage on autonomic functions, *Phys Ther* 50(12):1679-1691, 1970.

Beeken JE et al: The effectiveness of neuromuscular release massage therapy in five individuals with chronic obstructive lung disease, *Clin Nurs Res* 7(3):309-325, 1998.

Bell AJ: Massage and the physiotherapist, *Physiother JCSP* 10(50):406-408, 1964.

Benjamin PJ: *Tappan's handbook of healing massage technique,* ed 4, Upper Saddle River, NJ, 2004, Prentice Hall.

Bernal GR: How to calm children through massage, *Childhood Educ* 74:1, 1997.

Bodian M: Use of massage following lid surgery, *Eye Ear Nose Throat Mon* 48(9):542-547, 1969.

Bonica JJ: The management of myofascial pain syndromes, *Phys Ther Rev* 39:6, 1959.

Burns N, Grove S: *Understanding nursing research*, ed 3, Philadelphia, 2004, Saunders.

Cady SH, Jones GR: Massage therapy as a workplace intervention for reduction of stress, *Percept Motor Skills* 84:157-158, 1997.

Cassileth BR, Vickers AJ: Massage therapy for symptom control: outcome study at a major cancer center, *J Pain Symptom Manag* 28:244, 2004.

Chang M, Wang S, Chen C: Effects of massage on pain and anxiety during labor: a randomized controlled trial in Taiwan, *J Adv Nurs* 39(1):68-74, 2002.

Cherkin DC et al: Randomized trial comparing traditional Chinese medical acupuncture, therapeutic massage, and self-care education for chronic low back pain, *Arch Intern Med* 161:1081-1088, 2001.

Coward DD: Lymphedema prevention and management knowledge in women treated for breast cancer, *Oncol Nurs Forum* 26(6):1047-1053, 1999.

Cuthbertson DP: Effects of massage on metabolism: a survey, *Glasgow Med J* 2:200-213, 1933.

Cyriax J: Treatment by manipulation, massage, and injection. In *Textbook of orthopedic medicine,* vol 2, ed 11, London, 1984, Bailliere-Tindall.

Deardorff J: Massage therapy rubs sufferers the right way, *Chicago Tribune*, June 5, 2005, p Q7.

De Domenico G, Wood E: *Beard's massage,* ed 4, Philadelphia, 1997, Saunders.

Denison B: Touch the pain away, *Hol Nurs Pract* 18(3):142-153, May/Jun 2004.

Dennis W, Pergrouhi N: Infant development under environmental handicap, *Psychol Monogr: Gen Appl* 71:1-13, 1957.

Dennis W: Causes of retardation among institutionalized children, *J Genet Psychol* 96(7):1-12, 1960.

Despard LL: *Textbook of massage and remedial gymnastics,* ed 3, New York, 1932, Oxford University Press.

Diego MA et al: HIV adolescents show improved immune function following massage therapy, *Int J Neuroscience* 106:35-45, 2001.

Eisenberg DM et al: Trends in alternative medicine use in the United States, 1990-1997: results of a follow-up national survey, *JAMA* 280(18):1569-1575, 1998.

Ernst E: Complementary therapies in palliative cancer care, *Cancer* 91(11):2181-2185, 2001.

Ernst E, Fialka V: The clinical effectiveness of massage therapy-a critical review, *Forsch Kimplementärmed* 1:226, 1994.

Ernst E: The safety of massage therapy, *Rheumatology* 42:1101-1106, 2003.

Evans P: The healing process at a cellular level: a review, *Physiotherapy* 66(8):256-259, 1980.

Fassbender HG: *Pathology of rheumatic diseases,* New York, 1975, Springer-Verlag.

Ferell-Torry AT, Glick OJ: The use of therapeutic massage as a nursing intervention to modify anxiety and the perception of cancer pain, *Cancer Nurs* 16(2):93-101, 1993.

Fiechtner J, Brodeur R: Manual and manipulation techniques for rheumatic disease, *Med Clin North Am* 86(1):91-103, Jan 2002.

Field T: Massage therapy, *Med Clin North Am* 86(1):163-171, Jan 2002.

Field T: *Massage therapy research,* ed 1, Oxford, 2006, Churchill Livingstone.

Field T: *Touch in early development,* Hillsdale, NJ, 1995, Lawrence Erlbaum Associates.

Field T: Chronic fatigue syndrome: massage therapy effects on depression and somatic symptoms in chronic fatigue, *J Chron Fatigue Syndr* 3:43-51, 1997.

Field T: Sexual abuse effects are lessened by massage therapy, *J Bodywork Movement Ther* 1:65-69, 1997.

Field T: Children with asthma have improved pulmonary functions after massage therapy, *J Pediatr* 132(5):854-858, 1998.

Field T, Bauer C, Nystrom J: Tactile/kinesthetic stimulation effects on preterm neonates, *Pediatrics* 77(5):654-658, 1986.

Field T, Hernandez-Reif M, Seligman S: Juvenile rheumatoid arthritis: benefits from massage therapy, *J Pediatr Psychol* 22:607-617, 1997.

Field T, Seligman S, Scafidi F: Alleviating posttraumatic stress in children following hurricane Andrew, *J Appl Dev Psychol* 17:37-50, 1996.

Field T et al: Massage reduces anxiety in child and adolescent psychiatric patients, *J Am Acad Child Adolesc Psychiatr* 31(1):125-131, 1992.

Field T et al: Massage and relaxation therapies' effects on depressed adolescent mothers, *Adolescence* 31(124):903-911, 1996.

Field T et al: Massage therapy for infants of depressed mothers, *Infant Behav Dev* 19(124):109-114, 1996.

Field T et al: Massage therapy reduces anxiety and enhances EEG pattern of alertness and math computations, *Int J Neurosci* 86:197-205, 1996.

Field T et al: Autistic children's attentiveness and responsivity improved after touch therapy, *J Autism Dev Disord* 27:333-338, 1997.

Field T et al: Burn injuries benefit from massage therapy, *J Burn Care Rehabil* 19:241-244, 1997.

Field T et al: Job stress reduction therapies, *Altern Ther Health Med* 3:54-56, 1997.

Field T et al: Labor pain is reduced by massage therapy, *J Psychosom Obstetr Gynecol* 18:286-291, 1997.

Field T et al: Massage therapy lowers glucose levels in children with diabetes mellitus, *Diabet Spectr* 10:237-239, 1997.

Field T et al: Adolescents with attention deficit hyperactivity disorder benefit from massage therapy, *Adolescence* 33(129):103-108, 1998.

Field T et al: Bulimic adolescents benefit from massage therapy, *Adolescence* 33(131):555-563, 1998.

Field T et al: Elder retired volunteers benefit from giving massage therapy to infants, *J Appl Gerontol* 17(2):229-239, 1998.

Field T et al: Pregnant women benefit from massage therapy, *J Psychosom Obstet Gynaecol* 19:31-38, 1999.

Field T et al: Massage therapy effects on depressed pregnant women, *J Psychosom Obstet Gynaecol* 25(2):115-123, Jun 2004.

Fraser J, Kerr JR: Psychophysiological effects of back massage on elderly institutionalized patients, *J Adv Nurs* 18:238-245, 1993.

Garner DM, Olmsted MP, Polivy J: *Anorexia nervosa: recent developments in research,* New York, 1983, Alan R Liss.

Gehlsen GM, Ganion LR, Helfst R: Fibroblast responses to variation in soft tissue mobilization pressure, *Med Sci Sports Exerc* 31(4):531-535, 1999.

Goldberg J, Seaborne D, Sullivan S: The effects of therapeutic massage on H-reflex amplitude in persons with a spinal cord injury, *Phys Ther* 74(8):728-737, 1994.

Grad B: The influence of an unorthodox method of treatment on wound healing in mice, *Int J Parapsychol* 3:5-24, Spring 1961.

Grafelman T: *Graf's anatomy and physiology guide for the massage therapist,* Aurora, Colo, 1998, DG Publishing.

Hammer WI: The use of transverse friction massage in the management of chronic bursitis of the hip or shoulder, *J Manipulative Physiol Ther* 16(2):107-111, 1993.

Harlow H, Harlow M: Learning to love, *Am Sci* 54:244-272, 1966.

Herandez-Reif M: Multiple sclerosis patients benefit from massage therapy, *J Bodywork Movement Ther* 2:168-174, 1998.

Herandez-Reif M et al: Migraine headaches are reduced by massage therapy, *Int J Neurosci* 96:1-11, 1998.

Hernandez-Reif M et al: Cystic fibrosis symptoms are reduced with massage therapy intervention, *J Pediatr Psychol* 24:183-199, 1999.

Hillard D: Massage for the seriously mentally ill, *J Psychosoc Nurs Ment Health Serv* 33(7):29-30, 1995.

Holland B, Pokorny M: Slow stroke back massage: its effect on patients in a rehabilitation setting, *Rehabil Nurs* 26(5):182-186, 2001.

Hovind H, Nielsen SL: Effect of massage on blood flow in skeletal muscle, *Scand J Rehabil Med* 6(2):74-77, 1974.

Hulme JH, Waterman V, Hillier F: The effect of foot massage on patients' perception of care following laparoscopic sterilization as day case patients, *J Adv Nurs* 30(2):460-468, 1999.

Hymel GM: *Research methods for massage and holistic therapies,* ed 1, St Louis, 2006, Mosby.

Ironson G et al: Massage therapy is associated with enhancement of the immune system's cytotoxic capacity, *Int J Neurosci* 84:205-218, 1996.

Jacob S, Francone C: *Elements of anatomy and physiology,* Philadelphia, 1989, Saunders.

Jacobs M: Massage for the relief of pain: anatomical and physiological considerations, *Phys Ther Rev* 40(2):93-98, 1960.

Jancin B: Massage effective in treating chronic low back pain, *Fam Pract News* 29:22, 1999.

Johanson R: Perineal massage for the prevention of perineal trauma in childbirth, *Lancet* 355(9200):250-251, 2000.

Jones NA, Field T: Massage and music therapies attenuate frontal EEG asymmetry in depressed adolescents, *Adolescence* 34(135):529-534, 1999.

Juhan D: *Job's body, a handbook for bodyworkers,* Barrington, NY, 1987, Station Hill Press.

Khilnani S et al: Massage therapy improves mood and behavior of students with attention-deficit/hyperactivity disorder, *Adolescence* 38(162):623-638, Winter 2003.

Kim EJ, Buschmann MT: The effect of expressive physical touch on patients with dementia, *Int J Nurs Stud* 36(3):235-243, 1999.

Kresge CA: Massage and sports. In *Sports medicine, fitness, training, injuries,* Baltimore, 1987, Urban and Schwarzenberg.

Krieger D: Therapeutic touch: the imprimatur of nursing, *Am J Nurs* 75(5):784-787, 1975.

Krusen FH: *Physical medicine,* Philadelphia, 1941, Saunders.

Leivadi S, Hernandez-Reif M, Field T: Massage therapy and relaxation effects on university dance students, *J Dance Sci* 3:108-112, 1999.

Lindrea KB, Stainton MC: A case study of infant massage outcomes, *MCN Am J Matern Child Nurs* 25(2):95-99, 2000.

Little L, Porche DJ: Manual lymph drainage, *J Assoc Nurses AIDS Care* 9(1):78-81, 1998.

Lucia SP, Richard JF: Effects of massage on blood platelet production, *Proc Soc Exp Biol Med* 31:87, 1933.

Lundeberg T: Long-term results of vibratory stimulation as a pain relieving measure for chronic pain, *Pain* 20:13-23, 1984.

Lundeberg T et al: Vibratory stimulation compared to placebo in alleviation of pain, *Scand J Rehabil Med* 19:153-158, 1987.

Lundeberg T et al: Effect of vibratory stimulation on experimental and clinical pain, *Scand J Rehabil Med* 19:153-158, 1988.

MacGregor HE: Can massage cure? As a healing aid, hands-on therapy gains credibility at leading medical centers, *Los Angeles Times,* November 22, 2004, p F1.

Mannoia V J: *What is science? An introduction to the structure and methodology of science,* Washington, DC, 1980, University Press.

McKechnie A et al: Anxiety states: a preliminary report on the value of connective tissue massage, *J Psychosom Res* 27:125-129, 1983.

Meek S: Effects of slow stroke back massage on relaxation in hospice clients, *Image J Nurs Sch* 25(1):17-21, 1993.

Melzack R, Wall PD: Pain mechanisms: a new theory, *Science* 150(699):971-979, 1965.

Menard MB: An introduction to research methods for massage therapists, *Massage Ther J* 33(3):113-118, 1994.

Mennell JB: *Physical treatment,* ed 5, Philadelphia, 1945, Blakiston.

Merck manual, ed 17, Whitehouse Station, NJ, 1998, Merck and Company.

Mitchell JK: *Massage and exercise in system of physiological therapeutics,* Philadelphia, 1984, Blakiston.

Mock HE: Massage in surgical cases. In *AMA handbook of physical medicine,* Chicago, 1945, Council of Physical Medicine.

Modi N, Glover J: *Massage therapy for preterm infants.* Research paper presented at the Touch Research Symposium, April 1995.

Montagu A: *Touching: the human significance of the skin,* ed 2, New York, 1978, Harper and Row.

Morelli M, Seaborne DE, Sullivan J: Changes in H-reflex amplitude during massage of triceps surae in healthy subjects, *J Orthop Sports Phys Ther* 12:55-59, 1990.

Morelli M, Seaborne DE, Sullivan J: H-reflex modulation during manual muscle massage of human triceps surae, *Arch Phys Med Rehabil* 72:915-919, 1991.

Moyer CA, Rounds J, Hannum JW: A meta-analysis of massage therapy research, *Psychol Bull* 130(1):3-18, Jan 2004.

Mueller B, Spine-health.com: Massage therapy for lower back, 2002. Available at: *http://www.spine-health.com/topics/conserv/massage/massage1.html*

Myers TW: *Anatomy trains: myofascial meridians for manual and movement therapists,* New York, 2001, Churchill Livingstone.

Nixon N et al: Expanding the nursing repertory: the effective of massage in postoperative pain, *Aust J Adv Nurs* 14:21-26, 1997.

Nordschow M, Bierman W: Influence of manual massage on muscle relaxation: effects on trunk flexion, *Phys Ther* 42:653-657, 1962.

Ottoson D, Ekblom AT, Hansson P: Vibratory stimulation for the relief of pain of dental origin, *Pain* 10:37-45, 1981.

Pemberton R: Physiology of massage. In *American Medical Association handbook of physical therapy,* ed 3, Chicago, 1939, Council of Physical Therapy.

Premkumar K: *Pathology A to Z, a handbook for massage therapists,* Baltimore, 1999, Lippincott Williams & Wilkins.

Preyde M: Effectiveness of massage therapy for subacute low-back pain: a randomized controlled trial, *CMAJ* 162(13):1815-1820, 2000.

Prudden B: *Pain erasure,* New York, 1980, Random House, Ballantine Books.

Puustjarvi K, Pontinen PJ: The effects of massage in patients with chronic tension headaches, *Acupunct Electrother Res* 15(2):159-162, 1990.

Quinn C, Chandler C, Moraska A: Massage therapy and frequency of chronic tension headaches, *Am J Publ Health* 92(10):1657-1662, Oct 2002.

Reed B, Held JM: Effects of sequential connective tissue massage on autonomic nervous system of middle-aged elderly adults, *Phys Ther* 68(8):1231-1234, 1988.

Rich GJ: *Massage therapy: the evidence for practice,* St Louis, 2002, Mosby.

Richards A: Hands on help, *Nurs Times* 94(32):69-72, 1998.

Rodenburg JB et al: Warm-up, stretching, and massage diminish harmful effects of eccentric exercise, *Int J Sports Med* 15:414-419, 1994.

Rogeness GA, Javors MA, Pliszka SR: Neurochemistry and child and adolescent psychiatry, *J Am Acad Child Adolesc Psychiatry* 31(5):765-781, 1992.

Rowe M, Alfred D: The effectiveness of slow-stroke massage in diffusing agitated behaviors in individuals with Alzheimer's disease, *J Gerontol Nurs* 25(6):22-34, 1999.

St. John P: *St. John neuromuscular therapy seminars, manual I,* Largo, Fla, 1995, Author.

Salvo SG, Anderson SK: *Mosby's pathology for massage therapists,* St Louis, 2004, Mosby.

Samples P: Does sports massage have a role in sports medicine? *Physician Sportsmed* 15(3):177-183, 1987.

Sansone P, Schmitt L: Providing tender touch massage to elderly nursing home residents: a demonstration project, *Geriatr Nurs* 21(6):303-308, 2000.

Schachner L et al: Atopic dermatitis symptoms decrease in children following massage therapy, *Pediatr Dermatol* 15:390-395, 1998.

Schanberg S: Genetic basis for touch effects. In Field T, editor: *Touch in early development,* Hillsdale, NJ, 1984, Lawrence Erlbaum Associates.

Scull CW: Massage: physiological basis, *Arch Phys Med* 26:159-167, 1945.

Sherman K et al: A survey of training and practice patterns of massage therapists in two US states, *BMC Complem Altern Med* 5:13, 2005.

Sims S: Slow stroke back massage for cancer patients, *Nurs Times* 82:47, 1986.

Smith L et al: The effects of athletic massage on delayed onset muscle soreness, creatine kinase, and neutrophil count: a preliminary report, *J Orthop Sports Phys Ther* 19(2):93-99, 1994.

Smith M et al: Benefits of massage therapy for hospitalized patients: a descriptive and qualitative evaluation, *Altern Ther* 5(4):64-71, Jul 1999.

Smith MC et al: Massage therapy and hospitalized patients, *J Nurse Midwifery* 44(3):217-230, 1999.

Spitz R: Hospitalism: an inquiry into the genesis of psychiatric conditions of early childhood, *Psychoanal Study Child* 2:53-74, 1945.

Stewart K: Massage for children with cerebral palsy promotes tactile stimulation, *Nurse Times* 96(1):51, 2000.

Sullivan SJ: Does massage decrease laryngeal tension in a subject with complete tetraplegia? *Percept Mot Skills* 84:169-170, 1997.

Sullivan SJ et al: Effects of massage on alpha motoneuron excitability, *Phys Ther* 71(8):555-560, 1991.

Sunshine W et al: Fibromyalgia benefits from massage therapy and transcutaneous electrical stimulation, *J Clin Rheumatol* 2:18-22, 1997.

Thibodeau G, Patton K: *Anatomy and physiology,* ed 6, St Louis, 2006, Mosby.

Thibodeau G, Patton K: *Structure and function of the body,* ed 12, St Louis, 2004, Mosby.

Tortora GJ: *Introduction to the human body: the essentials of anatomy and physiology,* ed 5, Hoboken, NJ, 2000, John Wiley and Sons.

Tortora GJ, Grabowksi SR: *Principles of anatomy and physiology,* ed 11 New York, 2005, John Wiley and Sons.

Travell J: Referred pain from skeletal muscles, *N Y State J Med* 55:2, 1955.

Travell JG, Simons D: *Myofascial pain and dysfunction, the trigger point manual,* Baltimore, 1992, Lippincott Williams & Wilkins.

Trombley J, Thomas B, Mosher-Ashley P: Massage therapy for elder residents: examining the power of touch of pain, anxiety, and strength building, *Nursing Homes* 52(10):92-96, Oct 2003.

Trotter J: Hepatic hematoma after deep tissue massage, *N Engl J Med* 341:2019-2020, 1999.

Van Der Riet P: Effects of therapeutic massage on pre-operative anxiety in a rural hospital: part 1 and part 2, *Aust J Rural Health* 1(4):248-257, 1993.

Venes D, Thomas CL, Taber CW, eds: *Taber's cyclopedic medical dictionary,* ed 20, Philadelphia, 2005, FA Davis.

Vickers A, Zollman C: Massage therapies, *BMJ* 319:7219, 1999.

Voss DE, Ionta MK, Myers BJ: *Proprioceptive neuromuscular facilitation,* Philadelphia, 1985, Harper and Row.

Wakim KG: *Manipulation, traction and massage,* New York, 1976, Robert E Krieger.

Wakim KG et al: The effects of massage on the circulation in normal and paralyzed extremities, *Arch Phys Med* 30:135-144, 1949.

Walach H, Guthlin C, Konig M: Efficacy of massage therapy in chronic pain: a pragmatic randomized trial, *J Altern Compl Med* 9(6):837-846, 2003.

Wheeden Q et al: Massage effects on cocaine-exposed pre-term neonates, *J Dev Behav Pediat* 14(5):318-322, 1993.

Weeks VD, Travell J: Postural vertigo due to trigger areas in the sternocleidomastoid muscle, *J Pediatr* 47(162):315-327, 1955.

Weinrich SP, Weinrich MC: Massage and pain in cancer, *Appl Nurs Res* 3(4):140-145, 1990.

Williams RE: *The road to radiant health,* College Place, Wash, 1977, Color Press.

Zeitlin D et al: Immunological effects of massage therapy during academic stress, *Psychosom Med* 62:83-84, 2000.

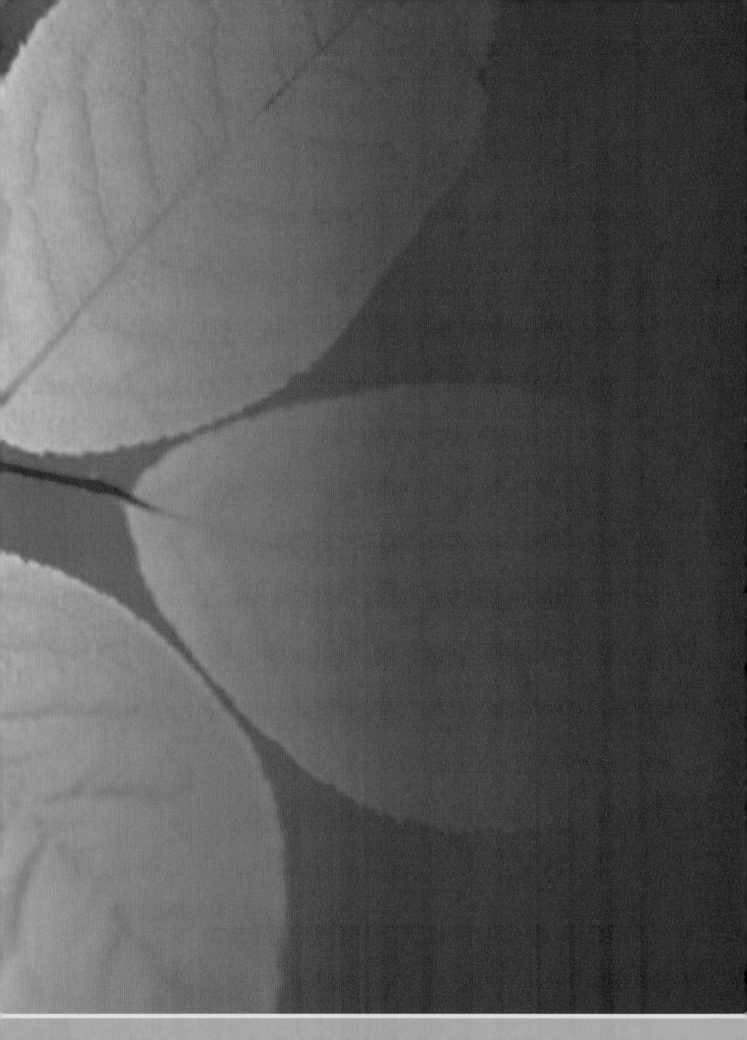

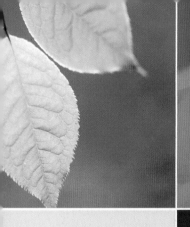

CHAPTER 6

*"Hands are the heart's
landscape."*
—Pope John Paul II

The Science of Body and Table Mechanics

STUDENT OBJECTIVES
After completing this chapter, the student should be able to:

- Discuss ways to reduce the risk of repetitive motion injuries
- Implement the concepts of health that relate to the practice of body mechanics
- Identify basic foot stances
- Explain guidelines for proper body mechanics
- Use appropriate positioning equipment and bolstering devices and position the client in the prone, supine, side-lying, and seated positions
- Properly drape the client with sheets and towels
- Maintain appropriate draping while the client rolls over
- Assist the client on and off the massage table while maintaining the appropriate drape

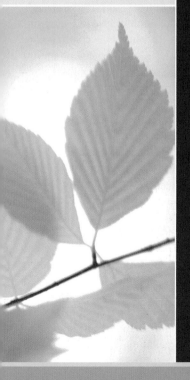

INTRODUCTION

To ensure a successful long-term career in massage, the therapist must maintain his or her own physical condition and avoid pitfalls associated with repetitive motion injuries. To accomplish this task, we examine some of the causes of repetitive motion injuries and two important aspects of massage therapy: body mechanics and table mechanics.

Body mechanics includes the principles of strength, stamina, breathing, stability, balance, and groundedness and centeredness. It also encompasses the practice of foot stances, body postures, and leverage techniques to enhance treatment effectiveness and reduce the risk of injury. **Table mechanics** addresses the practical issues of setting the table height and positioning, bolstering, and draping your client in a manner that is professional, ethical, and efficient. Assisting the client on and off the table is also addressed as it involves both body and table mechanics.

REPETITIVE MOTION INJURIES

The number-one reason that massage therapists decide to leave the industry is not professional burnout or missed employment opportunities; it is because of injuries resulting from repetitive motions and cumulative trauma to the wrist and fingers. Our bodies were designed to be in motion. We begin to have problems when we stop moving or start moving the same joints repetitively. Even with the use of proper body mechanics, body tissues react negatively when the same motion is repeated excessively. Because this type of injury can shorten your career, let us examine repetitive motion injuries in detail.

Repetitive motion injuries, also known as repetitive strain injuries (RSIs), are basically self-inflicted injuries related to poor biomechanics, including general posture, sporting movements, and work habits. A repetitive or constant motion, combined with compressive forces or joint hyperextension, causes injury to soft tissues. The resulting injury is usually cumulative in nature, having built up from self-abuse over an extended period. This injury type encompasses a broad spectrum of injuries. The most common types of repetitive motion injuries are carpal tunnel syndrome, thoracic outlet syndrome, tennis elbow, and rotator cuff strain. The symptoms and damage are progressive, unless the inefficient biomechanics or repetitive strain is altered. The general symptoms of RSI are related to the inflammation response: pain, redness, heat, swelling, limited range of motion. Initial symptoms are usually limited to the soft tissues. The progression of injury typically goes from muscle soreness; to increased tonus; to the formation of trigger points; and, in some cases, to nerve entrapment. Chronic RSIs may result in neuropathy, subluxation, deterioration, or trauma to the joints that includes bursitis and arthritis and even stress fractures of involved bones.

The muscles of the anterior forearm quickly become large and tight because of repeated finger flexing. Over time, the flexor retinaculum begins to compress against the tendons and nerves supplying the hand. You may begin to feel a numbness or weakness in the forearm, wrist, or hand. The digits most likely involved are the middle and ring fingers and the thumb. Compression damage and nerve entrapment may occur because of excessive trigger point work with the tips of the fingers and thumb or with the tip of the elbow. If you begin to have symptoms, then massage the entire arm, pectoralis major and minor, and the neck musculature.

To prevent these injuries from occurring, not only frequent massage of the anterior forearm muscles is recommended, but also strengthening of the posterior forearm muscles. A 3-pound barbell can be used to strengthen these muscles.

For our clients, improper work habits are probably the leading cause of these types of injuries, and most are preventable. A little education is all that is required to help alleviate this problem. Initially, the client has to be made aware of the potential damage being done to his or her body, as well as the warning signs and symptoms and the consequences of the damage. The client can then implement a new work habit. This again involves education of proper body mechanics such as lifting and keyboarding. The only way to break an old bad habit is to replace it with a new good one. The worst thing about repetitive motion injuries is that they take time to occur. By the time they are symptomatic, we are already in the habit of doing an activity improperly.

An example of a job-related RSI is the office worker who holds the telephone to his or her ear with the shoulder to free the hands to do other things. Years of this behavior, especially if he or she favors one shoulder, may lead to headaches, muscular tension, and eventually degenerative disk disease or herniation. This consequence may sound like an exaggeration, but it is not. How can the seemingly innocuous act of holding the telephone to the ear with the shoulder lead to degenerative disk disease? It simply happens through the mechanisms of muscular imbalance and postural distortion.

Muscular imbalances are common in the body. They occur when the strength of one muscle or muscle group is greater than that of the opposing muscle or muscles. Quadriceps muscle imbalances are a common cause of hamstring tears in sprinters and hurdlers. So what does this example have to do with the telephone? Holding the telephone by using the right side of the head, neck, and shoulders contracts muscles such as the right trapezius, right scalenes, and right levator scapulae. This daily activity occurring over a period of several years develops these muscles; they become stronger, enlarged, and tighter. With this type of muscular imbalance, postural distortions come into play. The stronger right neck muscles begin to compress the cervical vertebrae. The weaker muscles on the left have less pressure across the cervical joints. Over time, the action of right lateral flexion and rotation actually disrupts the integrity of the disks between the vertebrae. If the disk migrates (bulges) toward the left because of the increased vertebral compression on the right, then the disk may press against the left nerve root, causing an impingement or pinched nerve. The pattern often appears as neck pain on one side of the body and arm numbness or pain on the opposite side. Preventive measures are simple enough: an earphone with wraparound microphone or a speakerphone.

As you can surmise, these types of injuries will not only affect your work as a therapist, but clients will present these types of injuries to you. Pain is the great equalizer. It eventually gets everyone's attention; therefore pay attention to your body, or your client's body, when it is speaking to you.

The best ways for you to reduce the likelihood of RSI affecting you are to:

- Use a variety of strokes.
- Avoid wrist hyperextension.
- Rest your hands by spacing appointments.
- Adjust table height.
- Avoid sustained pressure (more than 1 minute).
- Keep your body physically fit through a fitness program.
- Use proper body mechanics.
- Receive massage.
- Prepare for the massage with movement (next section).

PREPARING FOR THE MASSAGE

 (6-9) The following exercises are designed to assist the therapist in preparing shoulders, wrists, and hands for the physical exertion involved in massage therapy.

- **Warm-up:** Begin by rubbing your palms and fingers together, creating friction and warmth; then vigorously rub the backs of your hands and arms. Shake your hands and fingers at the wrists, and then drop your hands to your sides and roll your shoulders forward for 10 repetitions (Figure 6-1, *A*). Reverse the direction, and rotate your shoulders backward. Perform this movement sequence 10 times. This quick warm-up is effective for preparing the hands right before a massage or before other hand-developing exercises. Remember to breathe as you move.

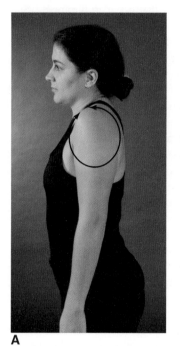
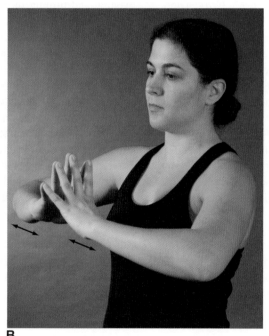
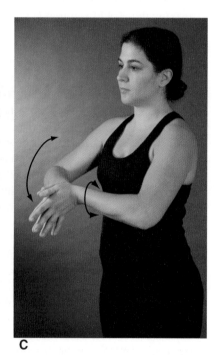

A **B** **C**

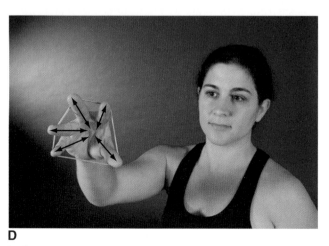
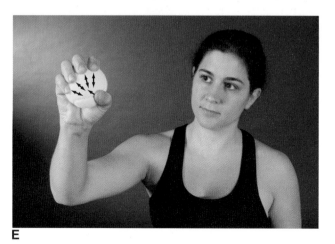

D **E**

FIGURE 6-1 **A**, Therapist rolling shoulders. **B**, Therapist applying and releasing pressure while maintaining contact. **C**, Therapist performing hand swishing. **D**, Therapist using fingers to stretch a rubber band. **E**, Therapist squeezing a ball.

- **Finger stretch:** Press your finger pads together as you keep your wrists apart approximately 6 to 8 inches. Spread fingers apart. Release this pressure while maintaining contact (Figure 6-1, *B*). Repeat the press-and-release sequence 10 times.
- **Wrist circles:** Begin with your arms at your sides. Flex the elbows 90 degrees while lifting your hands in front of you to chest level. With your fingers relaxed and extended, circle wrists in one direction for 10 revolutions, and then reverse the direction for 10 revolutions. Repeat wrist circles in both directions, but this time, close your hands into a fist. Perform 10 revolutions in both directions.
- **Hand swishing:** Press your palms and fingers together at chest level with fingertips pointing up to your chin. Quickly rotate your forearms until fingers are now pointing downward toward the toes and then reverse back to the starting position. This motion should be playful, quick, and vigorous (Figure 6-1, *C*). NOTE: The elbows and shoulders remain fixed while the wrists rotate together.
- **Rubber band stretch:** Place a thick rubber band around the outside of the fingers at the level of the nail. Stretch the rubber band as you move the fingers apart (Figure 6-1, *D*). Repeat 10 times. Switch hands, and repeat the sequence.
- **Ball squeeze:** Place a tennis ball or racquetball in the palm of your hand, and wrap your fingers around it. Squeeze the ball as hard as you can for 5 seconds (Figure 6-1, *E*). Repeat 10 times. Switch hands, and repeat the sequence.
- **Reach and pull:** Start with your open palms at your sides. Pull your hands up to chest, height, closing the palms into fists. Without stopping, continue the upward thrust of your hands over your head, stretching your fingertips out and inhaling simultaneously. Reverse the direction, bringing your arms back down. Close your hands as you pass your chest, and reopen them as they reach your sides, exhaling forcefully. Keep your pace slow and your movements graceful. Repeat the sequence five times. Stop immediately if you become lightheaded.

evolve *Log on to your student account using the Evolve website and retrieve images related to this section on Preparing for the Massage (therapist rubbing hands together, therapist shaking hands vigorously, therapist circling wrists with fingers extended, therapist circling wrists while making a fist, and therapist reaching and pulling). Create two other activites and share them with your classmates.* ■

BODY MECHANICS

Body mechanics is the proper use of postural techniques to deliver massage therapy with the utmost efficiency and least amount of trauma to the therapist. Also known as *bio-*

mechanics, proper body mechanics influences the execution of the massage, decreases fatigue and discomfort during and after the massage, and helps prevent repetitive motion injuries. The key to a long healthy career as a massage therapist is the ability to provide treatment without incurring injury. Proper body mechanics is as critical to a successful practice as are anatomical knowledge, manual skills, and business acumen. Few occupations use upper-body strength at the force or frequency as massage. Incorrect working posture and poorly executed hand techniques can increase stress on the joints, creating RSIs.

Bonnie Prudden, in her book, *Pain Erasure: The Bonnie Prudden Way* (1980), classifies occupations into five categories, according to the degree of physical activity required to perform the job. These categories are (1) *sitting,* (2) *standing,* (3) *walking,* (4) *active,* and (5) *strenuous* occupations. She lists massage therapy in the strenuous category because of the expenditure of physical energy and the use of torque (twisting and turning motions that occur in the torso). She also states that strenuous occupations often result in back pain (Box 6-1). As stated in the prior section, an important part of body mechanics lies in taking steps to prepare our bodies for the massage. Engaging in a fitness program can help us do just that.

An important point to note is that most members of Western cultures focus on strength and stamina as the primary goal of a fitness regimen. Eastern cultures focus on building balance and the ability to become grounded and centered as the foundations of health; strength and stamina come with discipline. Both viewpoints have merit. The concepts discussed here combine several key principles of both Eastern and Western cultures. All fitness activities help you explore the body's landscapes and increase vigor. Anyone with health problems should consult a physician before initiating any fitness program; but generally, if a person is healthy enough to do massage, then he or she is healthy enough to exercise.

The elements of body mechanics and the kata in martial arts are similar in nature. To help us better understand these systems of movement, the ancient practices of kendo and aikido need to be examined. Students of these martial arts are required to follow four basic principles: (1) *eyes first* (for focus and attention), (2) *footwork next* (foot position for weight transference), (3) *courage third* (assessing timing, space, your opponent, and how you are going to initiate your movements), and (4) *strength last* (body moves into action, or weight effort). Notably, strength and weight effort come last in the list. If we apply these principles to massage therapy, then focus, foot stance, and assessment come before the massage strokes.

MINI-LAB

Using a full-length mirror in your massage room, occasionally observe your body mechanics during a massage. Adjust your stance when needed.

BOX 6-1

Occupations and Related Pain Hazards (Occupations Classified by Kind or Degree of Physical Activity Required)

Sitting	Standing	Walking	Active	Strenuous
Accountant	Bank teller	Detective	Carpenter	Athlete
Administrator	Barber	Flight attendant	Carpet layer	Construction worker
Anesthetist	Bartender	Floorwalker	Dairy worker	Dancer
Architect	Beautician	Librarian	Electrician	Diver
Artist	Blacksmith	Nurse	Farmer	Heavy equipment operator
Astronaut	Butcher	Orderly	Fireman	Linesman
Author	Cafeteria server	Postal carrier	Forester	Longshoreman
Bookkeeper	Clerk	Real estate agent	Maintenance	Martial arts instructor
Broadcaster	Cook	Restaurant wait staff	Mason	Massage therapist
Bus driver	Dental hygienist	Service station attendant	Mechanic	Miner
Cab driver	Dentist	Train conductor	Painter	Steel worker
Chauffeur	Physician	Usher	Photographer	Wood worker
Computer programmer	Electrologist	Watchman	Plumber	
Crane operator	Elevator operator		Police officer	
Dispatcher	File clerk		Sailor	
Draftsman	Hairdresser		Ski instructor	
Editor	Machinist		Soldier	
Educator	Sales clerk		Sports coach	
Electronics repairer	Sculptor		Tree remover	
Engineer	Surgeon			
Executive	Teacher			
Glass blower	Veterinarian			
Jeweler				
Keypunch operator				
Lawyer				
Pilot				
Psychiatrist				
School bus driver				
Secretary				
Student				
Telephone operator				
Truck driver				
Weaver				

Sitting

Sitting occupations often put trigger points in the upper and lower back. Because the body is constantly bent, the groin may be involved. If excessive weight impairs circulation, then the legs and buttocks, which are constantly compressed against chairs, become involved.

Standing

Occupations requiring long hours of standing in one place contribute to the risk of low back pain. The upper back is also in danger, as are the arms and the shoulders and neck. Swelling may also occur in the feet and ankles.

Walking

Occupations requiring ordinary walking are not at risk. However, when the walking includes carrying (postal carrier or restaurant server staff), the back is in danger.

Active

Active occupations all entail danger. For example, carpenters damage their elbows and experience tennis elbow, the plumber working with pipe threaders and large wrenches puts trigger points in the chest muscles, the mason strains the back, and the ski instructor damages the legs and lower back.

Strenuous

Strenuous occupations often result in back pain, and the injuries often involve torque, such as the ladder that gets away, the barrel that rolls the wrong way, or anything that pulls the torso with a twisting motion.

Modified from Prudden B: *Pain erasure: the Bonnie Prudden way,* New York, 1980, Ballantine Books.

PAUL ST. JOHN, LMT

Born: July 27, 1945.

*"Where all the growth is in this profession and in life is the line of most resistance.
Oftentimes we resist so much of what life wants to teach us and why we're here."*

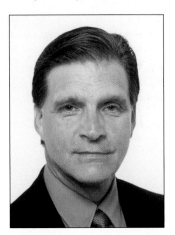

The St. John method of neuromuscular therapy is a comprehensive program of soft-tissue manipulation techniques that balance the central nervous system with the structure and form of the musculoskeletal system. On a more basic level, it is the study of how form affects function. The St. John method can free the body to move, stand, and simply *be* the way it was created to be from a structural and biochemical model.

Unlike some therapies that relax individuals and relieve minor pain, deep neuromuscular work zeroes in on both the problem and the effect. According to St. John, the five principles of neuromuscular therapy are (1) biomechanics, (2) postural distortion, (3) trigger points, (4) nerve entrapment–nerve compression, and (5) ischemia, all of which upset homeostasis.

Much of the charisma and commitment of Paul St. John, the man behind the method, was captured by Robert Calvert in an interview for *Massage Magazine*. St. John was 3 years of age when his father, an illegal alien, was deported. Young St. John was a street kid and an average student who later discovered a learning disability. Playing high school football, he suffered a broken back, his first injury. This injury led him to take a U.S. Army recruiter's aptitude test. After doing exceptionally well, however, St. John still was not quite ready to join. Instead, his mother's battle with cancer motivated him into a career in radiology. While practicing radiology, he was drafted into military service during the Vietnam War. When his aircraft was shot down, two Chinese physicians accomplished in minutes what the hospital, which managed his earlier leg injury in high school, had not been able to do in weeks.

After he returned home, his family hounded him to get a job. He hitchhiked to Florida and worked as a garbage collector until his third injury. With debilitating pain and mounting health bills, he experienced no improvement. A friend in chiropractic care then introduced St. John to the work of Dr. Raymond Nimmo, who was responsible for a technique known as *receptor tonus*. St. John studied this technique and soon began helping friends cope with pain. He then began massage therapy school and is now a teacher and therapist who never wants to lose touch with clients.

His own encounters with pain and other persons living with pain fuel his desire to do even more. He considers himself a perpetual student.

Today, St. John is changing the quality of lives with his methods, giving hope to people who have not found relief through conventional means. "Medicine has unconsciously become totally function oriented," explains St. John. "It ignores form, but if you have someone with a collapsed diaphragmatic posture, then peristaltic action and nutrient absorption is affected. The stomach collapses and loses tone. The medical community might suggest a laxative. You've got to treat the cause and not the effect. America spent over $4 billion for analgesics, medicines to suppress symptoms, this past year [1997]."

St. John shares the results of one of his latest cases. "A young woman who was about to have surgery to correct her scoliosis spent some time at my clinic. Doctors were going to put a rod in her back. We corrected her curvature 27%, and we have the x-rays to prove it."

St. John goes on to share other relationships between structure and disease. "Parkinson's patients almost all have a distortion in their cranium. In many stroke victims a forward-head posture of 6 to 8 inches is seen. This traps the arteries. Patients with cardiac problems usually have a slumping shoulder posture. An abdominal posture affects the diaphragm, aorta, vena cava, and esophagus. That's why so many of these people develop hiatal hernias.

"Neuromuscular therapy is the best value for the money. If your carburetor needs fixing, you get it fixed, right? But we let our bodies stay broken down."

After treatment, St. John's clients ask, "Why hasn't my doctor done this? It makes so much sense!" Nonetheless, skeptics abound. A man with a bad knee who had practically been dragged to the clinic told St. John, "I know what's wrong with my knee. I'm 72 years old." St. John then pointed to the patient's good knee and said, "Oh yeah, so how old is that knee?"

"He had a belief," explains St. John, "a belief in permanence creating a state of mind called *inertia*. So I created doubt by asking him about his good knee. Doubt is energy in itself. Once I created doubt in the permanence of his condition, it opened the door for me to point out

PAUL ST. JOHN, LMT (*continued*)

that his right shoulder and pelvis were inferior, the knee was twisted and compressed, the left shoulder and pelvis were elevated."

St. John has many success stories, but because of his commitment to his work, he has little time to recount them all. He has patients waiting. The interview is over with these words of advice for the beginning therapist: "Take personal responsibility. Specialize in a certain area if you really want to make a living. Techniques that work best conform to the laws of the universe. One third medicine is intellectual; two thirds is art."

In an earlier interview, St. John offers direction for anyone seeking success. "People who accomplish great things are ordinary people who have great dreams. It's not that they are more gifted and God has smiled upon them. People who become great have great work ethics and they put a lot of sweat equity into it. They aren't lucky people, you know; they work hard, and they're committed."

PRINCIPLES OF BODY MECHANICS

In Chapter 4, the concept of health is examined in the context of nutrition, exercise, and relaxation. However, this chapter explores some concepts related to these three areas of health, which are vital to the principles and practice of massage therapy. These principles are (1) strength, (2) stamina, (3) breathing, (4) stability, (5) balance, and (6) groundedness and centeredness.

Strength

Massage requires physical strength. If you do not possess adequate strength through exercise and proper diet, then you not only fatigue faster, but are also increasingly prone to injury. You may be asked to assist your client on and off the table or lift and move a client who is elderly or physically challenged. The best activities to add muscle strength to your body are floor exercises (e.g., sit-ups, push-ups) and weight or resistance training. Muscles become stronger when they are challenged. Because massage involves the entire body, all major muscle groups should be addressed during strength training.

Stamina

Most massage sessions last at least 1 hour. The therapist must possess enough stamina and endurance for all clients all day long, which usually means including some cardiovascular training in the fitness program. Thirty minutes three times a week is the minimum time to spend to enhance health and influence stamina. Between sessions, you might want to try the 60-second energy snack shown in Box 6-2. It contains no calories, and it is loaded with energy. Additional complex carbohydrates added to a balanced diet are the best fuel food for keeping your energy level high. Make sure you get plenty of rest. Good body mechanics suffers when a therapist is tired. Fatigue can also be reduced by proper breathing technique.

Breathing

Proper breathing will help the therapist relax, pace massage movements, and fuel muscles. Proper breathing technique enhances our mental and physical health, thereby positively affecting the quality of massage. According to William Barry, author and instructor, correct breathing is often referred to as

---

BOX 6-2

60-Second Energy Snack

1. Slap the palms of your outstretched hands together, and rub them rapidly for 5 seconds (out of earshot of clients).
2. Hold your warmed palms over your cheeks and eyes for 5 seconds.
3. Make your hands into claws, and apply vigorous tapping tapotement to the scalp for 5 seconds.
4. Apply loose-fist tapotement up and down each arm for 10 seconds.
5. Gently grasp the hyoid bone, and mobilize it from side to side to stimulate the thyroid gland.
6. With your right hand, cup your palm around the back of your neck and squeeze firmly approximately 10 times.
7. Repeat Step 6 with the left hand while nodding the head at the same time.
8. Repeat Step 6 with the left hand while shaking the head at the same time.
9. With the right hand, reach across the midline of your body, grasp the top of your left trapezius, and squeeze firmly approximately 10 times.
10. Repeat Step 9 to the right trapezius with the left hand.
11. Perform three sets of shoulder rolls forward and three backward.
12. Pincer-grip the thumb web of each hand, and hold for 3 seconds (omit this step if you are pregnant).
13. Shake the hands out.
14. Stomp the feet several times.

You are now energized and ready to go!

the *foundation of massage.* Try combining volitional breathing and massage therapy. As you massage, strokes requiring the therapist to reach are accompanied by expiration, and return strokes are accompanied by inspiration. Some deep-breathing modifications such as sighing and yawning may be indicators that the body needs more oxygen. If yawning occurs, then take a few slow deep breaths. Deep breathing is also a great way to release tension. Encourage your clients to sigh or yawn before, during, and after the massage. Placing your tongue on the roof of your mouth encourages nasal breathing.

Aikido masters often use breathing to guide the students to shrink their focus to a space approximately the size of a quarter, 2 inches below and behind the navel. This ancient center of gravity is called the **dantien** (Chinese term). This space is a topographic *and* meditative point of reference known for thousands of years in many cultures as the center of physical and spiritual balance. A simple way to experience the power of this energetic center is to allow your breath to move into and out of the **hara**, a Japanese term used to describe the lower abdomen (Figure 6-2). On expiration, the therapist should contract the muscles of the pelvic floor to lower the center of gravity and splint the lower back muscles to help maintain a straight back. Additionally, this form of abdominal breathing helps lower the center of gravity and contributes to stability.

Stability

Effective body mechanics requires the therapist to move from a stable base, with the feet forming the foundation for all movement. The lower portion of the body is capable of providing approximately two-and-a-half times more power and greater stability than the upper body, just as walking is easier than doing push-ups. Proper body mechanics transmits force from the therapist to the client by using lower body stability. The upper body becomes a flexible conduit while the therapist remains free of injury. With both feet firmly planted, force is transmitted from a stable base shared by both feet and legs (Figure 6-3).

The greater the number of points of contact, the more stable the object becomes. Compare the relative stability of a pogo stick, ironing board, tripod, and chair. The tripod and chair are stable, but the pogo stick is not. Techniques requiring the therapist to stand with most or all of his or her weight on one leg constitute poor body mechanics. Precise articulations from the upper extremity are not possible while continually leaning on the client. Furthermore, the center of gravity is much higher, further reducing stability. The therapist needs a

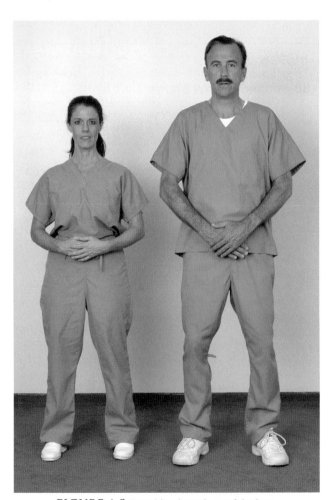
FIGURE 6-2 Breathing in and out of the hara.

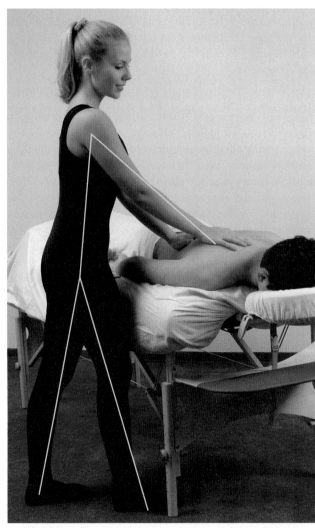
FIGURE 6-3 Both feet flat on the floor provide a stable base.

stable base of support. In fact, when the therapist works from a stable body stance, he or she is more responsive to the client. Stability is the prerequisite to balance.

Balance

Proper body mechanics is a direct result of balanced posture that respects the laws of gravity. Gravity is the mutual attraction of two objects toward each other, such as your body and the earth. When you are balanced, energy expended during the massage is reduced. The center of gravity, the point at which the body is balanced, is generally between the fourth and fifth lumbar vertebrae on the front of the spine, or an inch or two below and behind your navel (dantien). The principle of balance can be expanded to an emotional and spiritual awareness or energetic experience of ourselves in relation to our surroundings. Exercises that encourage balance include yoga and martial art disciplines such as tai chi, qi gong, and aikido, which can also be used for meditation or grounding.

MINI-LAB

Choose a partner. Have him or her stand with feet 24 inches apart. Ask your partner to concentrate on his or her head. After a moment, gently and gradually begin pushing against his or her shoulder. Question your partner about how his or her body responds to the change. Next, ask your partner to concentrate on an area between the fourth and fifth lumbar vertebrae on the front of the spine or approximately 1 to 2 inches below and behind your navel. After allowing time for concentration, give another gentle push. Have your partner report on the difference he or she felt during each push. Which area of concentration felt more stable? Switch roles and allow your partner to gently push you. Compare experiences, noting similarities or differences. The area that felt more stable is the area from which you initiate your massage movements.

Groundedness and Centeredness

Embedded in the art of massage are two concepts, groundedness and centeredness, which refer to the *mental, emotional,* and *physical* states of consciousness. The connection between the body and the mind is fundamental; the two are difficult, if not impossible, to separate. The best way to illustrate this intimate relationship between mind and body is to consider what happens to the body when you are under mental or emotional stress. The body responds by mirroring that state of mind; headaches and insomnia are common. Conversely, when people are physically ill or in chronic pain, they are affected mentally and emotionally, which is often expressed by their attitude. Mundane tasks become difficult, and we either show our emotions too easily or not at all. Thus taking time to prepare our minds helps us become more compassionate and sensitive therapists.

The martial art aikido is helpful for guiding the massage therapist into useful application of movement principles. When teaching the concept of centeredness to students of

aikido, masters often tell the students to place their weight underside and allow themselves to feel light on top. As mentioned earlier, abdominal breathing from the hara helps ground the therapist.

When you are grounded, you may feel the presence of God, nature, or your higher power, in addition to the company of your client. You become part of a larger whole and recognize that you are just a vessel for healing and positive change. The therapist might imagine that all tensions are draining from his or her body, and he or she connects to the ubiquitous energy and power that bring peace and serenity (Box 6-3). Using the vessel as a psychological and spiritual reference point, the stress, tension, and excess energy that are released by the client during a massage are not absorbed by the therapist but are channeled to the grounding source itself. Being both grounded and centered makes a difference in how you deliver the massage; it will help you stay focused on the task at hand. By clearing your mind and experiencing the moment, your body mechanics will be greatly enhanced.

FOOT STANCES RELATED TO BODY MECHANICS

We do not just massage with our hands; our whole bodies play a role in how massage is delivered. The placement of the feet influences the type and direction of the massage stroke, while providing a stable base. Remember, the lower extremities have two-and-a-half times more available strength than the upper extremities; thus using the body's natural strength to deliver massage makes sense. Foot placement, the source of a stable base, has a profound effect on body mechanics and body alignment.

The therapist typically uses one of two foot stances when delivering massage strokes: the *bow* and *warrior stances.* Both bow and warrior stances provide a secure foundation and balanced body posture. The foot stance used most often depends on the style of massage you perform and the type of strokes used. When a bow or warrior stance is used, each foot makes contact with the earth at three points (Figure 6-4; see

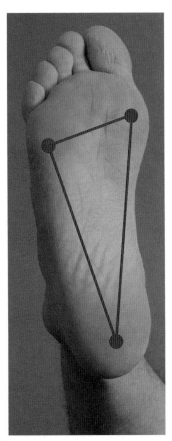

FIGURE 6-4 The foot forms a base of support with three points of contact.

Chapter 14 for more information). Both feet represent six points of contact. This double-tripod structure provides a stable foundation for movement. While moving from both the bow and the warrior stances, let it be initiated from a stable base (feet planted firmly on the floor) up to the center of balance (dantien) and then through the arms and hands (see Figure 6-3).

Bow Stance

(6-10) Also known as the *archer stance* or *lunge position,* the **bow stance** is often used when applying any stroke in which the therapist proceeds from one point to the next along the client's body (i.e., effleurage) while the therapist faces the head or foot of the table. The therapist's feet are placed on the floor in a 30- to 50-degree angle, one pointing straight forward *(leading foot)* and the other pointing toward the side *(trailing foot).* The leading foot points in the direction of movement (Figure 6-5, *A*). Distance between the two feet will vary.

When applying massage along a limb or trunk, keep knees flexed while shifting weight between the leading and the trailing feet; if not, then balance may be lost. Avoid movements that bring the knee beyond the placement of the leading foot. For longer strokes, place the trailing foot behind the leading foot, and then step forward with the leading foot (Figure 6-5, *B* and *C*).

With the bow stance, you will shift your body weight forward then back to return to an original position, without

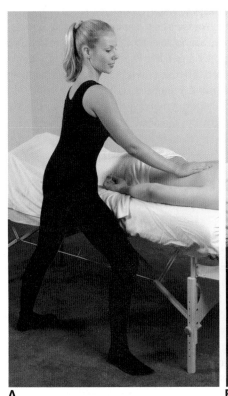

A

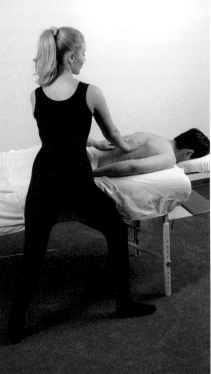

B

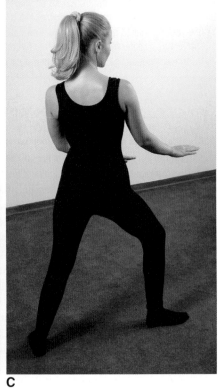

C

FIGURE 6-5 **A**, Therapist in bow stance from side angle. **B**, Therapist in bow stance from back angle. **C**, Therapist in bow stance from back angle without table and client.

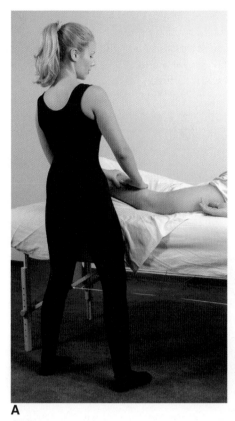 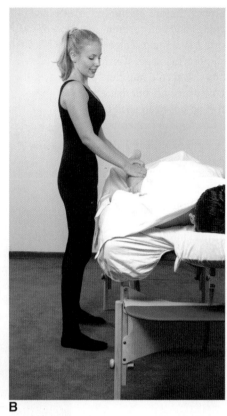 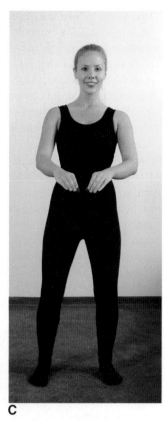

A   **B**   **C**

FIGURE 6-6 **A**, Therapist in warrior stance from, back angle. **B**, Therapist for side angle. **C**, Therapist from front angle without table and client.

bending over or losing contact with the client and while maintaining a constant flow. Keep the upper and lower torso in as straight a line as possible, using rotational movements when needed. Bend at the hips and not the waist while proceeding with a stroke. When possible, get behind your hands while working in the bow stance.

 Warrior Stance

(6-10) Also known as the *horse stance,* the **warrior stance** is used to perform massage strokes that traverse relatively short distances, such as pétrissage and most friction strokes, and while reaching over to the far side of the client's body. The therapist faces the opposite side of the table while both feet are placed on the floor a little more than hip distance apart with toes pointing forward (Figure 6-6). The actual distance between both feet depends on therapist's height and hip size. Shorter people have a lower center of gravity; their feet tend to be closer together. Taller people have a higher center of gravity; their feet tend to be farther apart.

If you are having difficulty maintaining balance, then readjust your foot distance until movement in the stance feels effortless. Once the proper foot distance is located, soften your knees by allowing them to flex slightly. Keep your hips pointed forward and your back straight. Your shoulders should be relaxed while your hands and arms are moving, transferring the load through the torso to the legs and feet.

As long as both feet are on the floor, lean forward with your thighs resting against the table. Shift your weight from one foot to the other as your hands move across the client's skin. This stance works particularly well for a two-handed alternating pétrissage. If a lifting or lowering action is required to apply a massage stroke, then raise or lower your body by bending your knees and keeping your back straight.

evolve *Log on to the Evolve website for self-care suggestions for the therapist. Write down at least three more ways to reduce and relieve tension between sessions.* ■

 GUIDELINES FOR PROPER BODY MECHANICS

(6-11) 1. **Check table height.** If working on a table that belongs to someone else or if someone else has borrowed your table, then check the table height before beginning the massage to make sure table height is appropriate for you. Proper table height allows you to use your weight rather than your strength to increase pressure.

2. **Wear comfortable attire.** Wear sensible supportive shoes with low or no heels and good arch supports. In addition, clothing should be comfortable, should allow the therapist freedom of movement, and should appear professional. Cotton clothes are best because they absorb the body's perspiration, which helps keep you cool.

3. **Warm up before massage.** Warm up before giving a massage, especially on cold mornings and before strenuous routines such as active assisted stretching, Trager, body mobilization techniques, and sports massage. Warm muscles are less susceptible to injury than cold muscles. Stretching can be done as part of the warm-up, but make sure that some other form of warm-up has been used to increase the heart rate and blood flow before stretching. See prior section entitled Preparing for the Massage for some movement suggestions.

4. **Use a variety of strokes.** Most massage routines incorporate an assortment of strokes. Changing from effleurage to pétrissage to tapotement to friction requires the therapist to change the position of both hands and feet, thus reducing fatigue and repetitive motion injuries. As the therapist, you must also listen to your own body. If the right forearm is becoming fatigued, then use the left arm more; if compressive movements are irritating wrist and knuckle joints, then change to a lifting move such as pétrissage.

5. **Get behind your work.** Position yourself, as much as possible, directly behind your work. Both arms and legs should face the direction in the area you are working or in which pressure is applied. When pushing a heavy object, you would not stand beside it; you would stand directly behind.

6. **Check in with low back, hips, knees, and feet.** Keep your back straight by tilting your pelvis backward (posterior tilt), which flattens out the low back and reduces an exaggerated lumbar curve. Use the penny-pinching technique (see the Mini-Lab for instructions). Hips should be level and knees slightly bent. Keep your feet planted firmly on the ground while standing. Shift weight from one foot to another to reflect what your hands are doing. Freda Whalen, a massage therapist and teacher, tells students to suck it (pull in abdomen), tuck it (posterior tilt of pelvis), and drop it (lower shoulders and flex knees).

7. **Position shoulders, arms, wrists, and fingers.** Place your shoulders comfortably on top of your rib cage, relaxed and dropped. Do not hunch over or round the shoulders while working, and try to keep them over the hips, when possible. Avoid raising your shoulders toward your ears. Keep your upper arms close to your upper body whenever possible. When your upper arms are far away from your body, they tend to fatigue more quickly.

8. **Keep the wrists as straight as possible** (Figure 6-7). At times, flexing and extending the wrist will be necessary, but remember that the greater the pressure, the straighter the wrist should be. Hyperextending the wrist while applying pressure can produce overuse injuries such as tendonitis and carpal tunnel syndrome. When not being used, keep wrists and fingers relaxed.

9. **Do not let the digits become hyperextended while applying direct pressure**. Use braced finger and thumb techniques to avoid joint hyperextension (Figure 6-8).

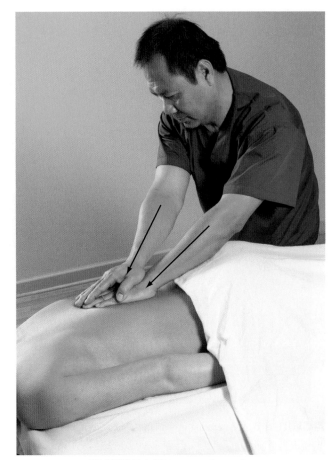

FIGURE 6-7 Proper wrist angle.

10. **Lean or sit.** Lean, sit, or brace yourself against the table when needed; do not push or force movement. Most Swedish moves require that the therapist be in motion, but some modalities require the therapist to lean on the client, brace him or herself against the table, or sit on the table for a short time. When leaning into the client, make sure both feet are on the floor and you are not overly contracting your arm and shoulder muscles to produce downward force. Avoid staying on your feet for long periods. A stool can be used while performing foot, neck, or facial routines (Figure 6-9). Keep both feet flat on the floor with the back straight while seated. This position maintains a stable base and reduces strain on the upper body.

11. **Align your spine.** Keep your spine in correct alignment by maintaining your head over your neck and shoulders. Move the body as a unit. Avoid a forward head posture. When working on a muscle or group of muscles, keep your eyes forward, your neck straight, and your head erect. If you spend a great amount of time looking down, then your neck may become stiff. If you must observe your work, then lower yourself to the level of your hands by kneeling down on the floor or sitting on a stool. Look up, out the window, or at the corners of the ceiling occasionally to stretch the anterior neck musculature. Another way to reduce the strain

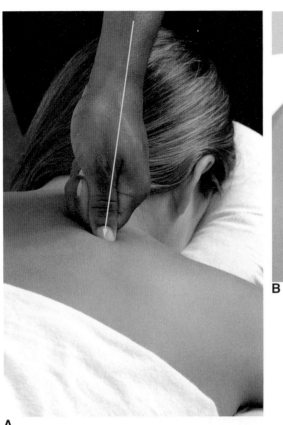

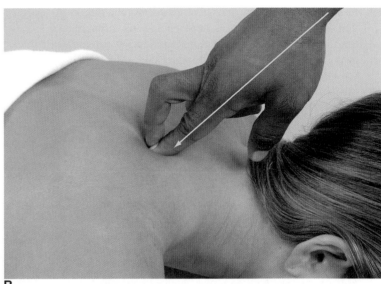

B

A

FIGURE 6-8 **A**, Braced thumb technique. **B**, Braced finger technique.

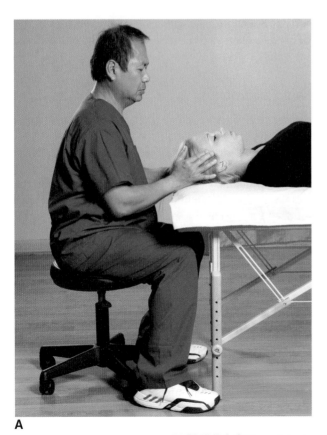

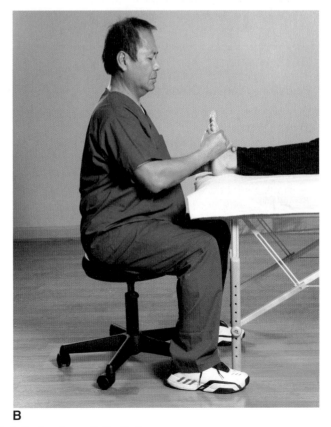

A

B

FIGURE 6-9 Therapist using stool. **A**, For head area. **B**, For foot area.

on your neck is to turn your head away from the direction of the massage stroke. Experiment with different head and neck positions for different massage strokes to discover which positions are more comfortable for you (Box 6-4).

12. **Stretch.** Take stretch breaks while walking from one side of the table to the other. Use this time to shake out your arms, stretch your neck, and relax. Between massage sessions, spend a few minutes doing exercises to strengthen and stretch the muscles of the hands.

13. **Breathe.** During the massage, use deep, full abdominal breathing. This action will aid in self-relaxation and helps keep a steady pace with your massage strokes. Apply the pressure stroke while exhaling and the return stroke while inhaling. While you breathe, be aware of facial expression; keep your jaw unlocked and your forehead relaxed.

14. **Move smoothly.** Find your *own* rhythm and then move *with* it. For example, pétrissage can be done more efficiently in the warrior stance, with a side-to-side rocking motion. The rocking motion itself can be learned from an instructor, but the rate or rhythm is an internal component that originates between the therapist and client. Keep your movements smooth and flowing. What is jerky and rough for you is jerky and rough for your client, too.

15. **Lift correctly.** If you have to lift during the massage, then keep the heaviest part of the client's body close to your body. Use your legs, not your back, when lifting. Know your own limits. Do not try to lift a body part that is too heavy. Ask for assistance.

BOX 6-4

Body Mechanics Quick Check

The following is a list of questions for determining correct body mechanics during the massage:

1. Is your massage table the correct height for you?
2. Are you warming up before your first massage of the day and stretching between massage sessions?
3. Are your knees slightly bent?
4. Are your feet firmly planted on the ground?
5. Are you shifting your weight as you move, working with your whole body?
6. Are your wrists straight?
7. Are your thumbs and fingers supported while applying direct pressure?
8. Is your back straight and your pelvis posteriorly tilted?
9. Is your head centered over your neck and shoulders?
10. Are you using a variety of strokes in your massage? Are you positioning yourself behind your strokes?
11. Is a stool nearby to be used during facial and foot massages?
12. Is your face relaxed and your jaw unlocked during the massage?
13. Are you using proper lifting techniques?

   If you answered *no* to one or more of these questions, then you may be at risk for stress, strain, and injury resulting from poor body mechanics.

MINI-LAB

To experience a posterior-tilted pelvis, try the penny-pinching technique. While standing, imagine that you have a penny between your buttocks. To keep the penny from falling to the ground, contract your gluteal muscles, and *pinch* the penny. This simple exercise straightens your back muscles, pulls in your abdominal muscles, and tilts your pelvis backward.

MINI-LAB

Stand in front of a full-length mirror. Place one foot 18 inches in front of the other, and place your hands on your hips. Lunge forward, shifting your weight from the back leg to the front leg. As you move forward and backward, keep your shoulders and hips level. Look in the mirror to check your progress. Maintaining a good posture while you are in motion promotes good working posture while performing massage therapy.

"Close your hand—do you feel absence or presence"?
Brenda Hefty

TABLE MECHANICS

The science of table mechanics involves a variety of practical considerations concerning the placement of the client on the table during treatment. These considerations include (1) client positioning (prone, supine, side-lying, or seated), (2) positioning equipment (bolsters, cushions, and pillows), and (3) draping (towels or sheets).

Client Positioning

Once you have interviewed your client and directed him or her to the massage table, you must determine how to position the client while he or she receives the massage. Client positioning promotes client comfort and relaxation through proper body alignment, and it addresses medical and health issues because some conditions may require the client to be positioned on the table a specific way. Considerations for specific medical conditions are addressed in the pathology section of each anatomy and physiology chapter, as well as the adaptive massage chapter.

Ask yourself in what position would you like the client to lie: prone, supine, side-lying, or seated position? How do you position the client's joints during the massage (e.g., head and neck, knees, and ankles)? Does the client have any health condition or physical limitations that would require an adjustment to the table or additional bolstering?

The last question addresses the client who has a condition that time on the table might make worse. For example, some clients may have sinus problems that limit time spent in the prone position. A swollen ankle may need additional support and elevation. A client with severe lordosis may need a cushion under his or her abdomen while in the supine position.

Regardless of which positions you and the client decide, a good question to ask your client is, "How can you become even more comfortable?" This process allows you to fine-tune the client's position and address his or her comfort needs.

Positioning Equipment

(6-1) To provide greater client comfort and proper body mechanics in the prone, supine, or side-lying position, use positioning equipment and bolstering devices. Cushions support the client's individual joints, which, in turn, help relax the muscles. The most commonly bolstered areas are the *face and head, neck, ankles, and knees.* Special placement of bolsters for clients in the side-lying position is discussed in the draping section of this chapter. In the absence of commercially manufactured bolsters, a rolled-up towel, blanket, or pillow may be used.

Many therapists store bolsters under the table, on a low shelf, or on the floor. The therapist may bend down to get these bolsters, replacing them in the storage areas before the client rolls over and before the client gets up when the massage is finished. Typically, three bolsters are used per session. If you see six clients per day, then you will be bending and reaching for bolsters frequently in the course of a workday. Avoid bending over because this action alone may cause low back strain. Instead, squat down to get bolsters, stand the bolsters on their end in a convenient corner, or place them on a shelf at chest level for easy frequent access.

Position the seam running lengthwise on the bolster away from the client's body, which prevents any uncomfortable sensations or compression marks left on the client's skin. Always drape the bolster or pillow with a protective covering such as a towel, pillowcase, or specially designed bolster cover. These covers are washed after each client use. The bolster may also be placed between the bottom sheet and the table surface. Remove the bolster before your client gets off the massage table to dress.

Prone Position

(6-2) In the **prone** position, the person is in a horizontal position while lying face downward. The most commonly supported areas when the client is in the prone position are anterior ankles and the head-neck complex. If possible, use a face rest or specially designed prone pillow, which allows your client to keep his or her neck straight while lying face down. The best way to adjust a face rest for maximal client comfort is to have the client lie prone on the table; making sure all cams are unlocked, have the client lie comfortably and pull the face rest up while you lock the cams. Some tables possess a wide slit for the face, allowing the client to lie prone without a face rest. If a face rest is not available, then one or two standard-size pillows may be used, placing them either horizontally or diagonally under the forehead and shoulders.

Large-breasted women may need additional pillow support under the breasts or lengthwise along the sternum.

A vinyl-covered 3- or 6-inch diameter bolster under the anterior ankles allows the hips, legs, and ankles to relax fully during the massage. Try both sizes to see which one works best for each client. If the client complains of his or her low back feeling strained by lying prone, then a pillow or soft cushion placed under the abdomen or pelvis reduces the anterior curve, which may reduce the strained feeling. For added shoulder and arm relaxation, an arm shelf or linen-draped stool placed under the face rest can be used for a forearm rest (Figure 6-10, *B*).

Supine Position

(6-3) In the **supine** position, the person is lying horizontally on the back. When the client is in the supine position, the most commonly supported areas are the posterior cervical region and the posterior knees. Use of a knee bolster helps relax the low back. This client position is also the best for addressing the abdomen, with the knees flexed and while in the supine position.

A soft cloth-covered cervical pillow is best placed under the cervical region, not the occipital region (Figure 6-11). A rolled-up bath-size towel can be used as a cervical pillow; fold both long sides toward the middle, leaving a 1-inch space down the middle before rolling the towel (Figure 6-12). If you are working on a narrow table and have a large client, then consider providing a side extension accessory, giving additional width to the table and support for your client's arms (Figure 6-13). While you are massaging the client's feet in the supine position, place a pillow, cushion, or rolled towel under the feet to elevate them, which provides easier access to the feet and facilitates proper body mechanics for you. This added foot support also assists dependent drainage in cases of lymphedema. You may sit on the massage table or on a stool while massaging the client's feet. Avoid permitting the client to raise his or her own feet simultaneously because his or her low back may be strained. Instead, ask him or her to place one foot on the pillow at a time or lift the client's feet for him or her onto the pillow.

If needed, the therapist can use a semireclining position for pregnant clients, clients with respiratory problems, or any client who is more comfortable in this position. The semireclining position has the client's upper body elevated approximately 30 degrees. See Figure 20-11 in this text.

Side-Lying Position

(6-4) The side-lying or lateral recumbent position is preferred for pregnant clients, some older adults, and for persons with various other conditions. The client may lie in either a right lateral or a left lateral recumbent position. Ask the client to lie on the side on which he or she feels most comfortable, but you may dictate the direction. The client will spend most of the treatment time on the first side because much of the body can be accessed from this position.

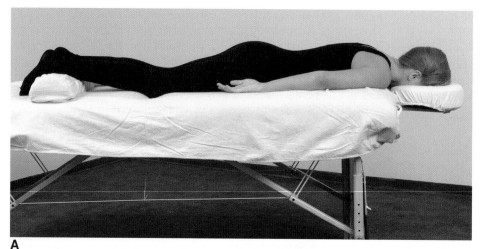

A

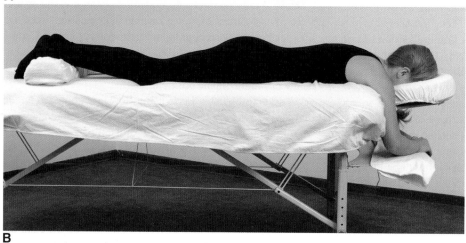

B

FIGURE 6-10 **A**, Prone client with bolsters and face rest. **B**, With the addition of arm shelf.

Ask the side-lying client to slide back so his or her backside is near the edge of the table (approximately 4 inches). This position will not only make it easier for the therapist to work the client's back, but it also provides additional table space in front of the client for pillows to be placed. Use three or four pillows; place the first pillow underneath his or her head. The next pillow should be placed under the upper arm (the side of the body not against the table), supporting his or her arm and shoulder. The last is positioned under the upper knee and ankle; this pillow helps relax the hip and low back. If the hip, knee, and ankle are not all in

the same horizontal plane, then add another pillow until the proper alignment is achieved. Proper alignment is imperative; if the ankle is unsupported, then the hip outwardly rotates. This rotation may cause tightening of the outward rotator musculature and may aggravate sciatic conditions. Two additional smaller pillows may be added under the wrist of the lower arm and under the lower ankle (side of the body touching the table). Figure 6-14 demonstrates proper pillow positioning for the side-lying position.

Because the back, parts of the legs, and feet are approached from a side position, the therapist adjusts his or her

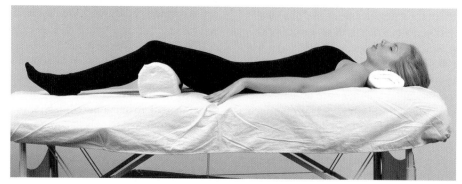

FIGURE 6-11 Supine client with bolsters.

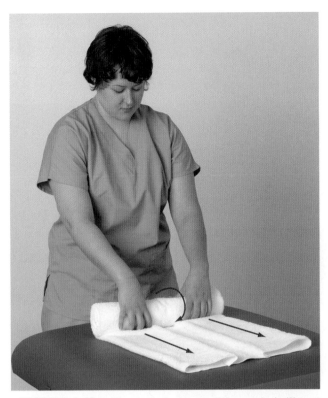

FIGURE 6-12 Rolling up bath-size towel for cervical pillow.

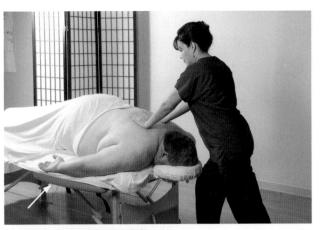

FIGURE 6-13 Table widening accessory.

body position for the best leverage, which may include using a stool, squatting, or kneeling down on the floor.

Roll the client over and complete the massage on the second side-lying position; treatment time spent should be considerably shorter than with other areas. Before your client changes positions, or before he or she gets up from the massage table after the session, remove all pillows and bolsters to reduce obstacles that may impede a smooth recumbent-to-upright transition. See the section Draping Your Client for the Massage Session for more information on draping the side-lying client.

MINI-LAB

Acquire approximately six pillows of various sizes, a massage table, and a partner. Ask your partner to lie on the massage table in the supine position, and use the pillows to create a variety of comfortable positions. Once all possibilities are explored, remove the pillows from the massage table and ask your partner to turn over and lie on his or her side. Use the pillows again to position your partner's arms, legs, and so on. Repeat the activity in the prone position. This method will help you discover new and creative ways to work with pillows as positioning equipment.

Seated Position

(6-5) The seated position is a massage given while the client is seated. The client may be sitting in an ordinary chair or a specially designed massage chair. Devices are also available that sit or clip onto a tabletop that accommodate the client who is leaning forward.

When an ordinary chair is used, the client may lean forward and rest his or her head on a cushion placed on the top of a nearby table (Figure 6-15). The seated position may be preferable in one of the following situations:
- The client prefers a seated massage.
- A massage table is not available.
- Adequate physical space is not available to set up a massage table or to use proper body mechanics during the massage.
- The client has a condition (e.g., handicap, pain, mobility problem, medical condition) that makes getting on or off a massage table difficult.
- The client is in a wheelchair. NOTE: Transferring to a massage table or chair may not be feasible for the client. Work with him or her in the wheelchair. Simply roll the chair up to the side of the massage table so that the client's legs are underneath. Lock the wheels in position, lean the client forward on a cushion, and proceed with the massage. See Chapter 10 for more details.
- The client has reservations about removing clothing for the massage.
- If you have decided that the seated position is best for serving your client, then refer to Chapter 27 for specific details on how to position your client for comfort and accessibility.

How to Begin?

Prone? Supine? How do you decide? What are the pros and cons of beginning prone or supine? Some therapists prefer to start their clients prone and end the massage with their clients supine, or vice versa, whereas other therapists let the clients decide. The following sections detail the possibilities.

Beginning Prone, Ending Supine

Most clients complain of back-related pain. Beginning the client in the prone position allows you to massage this essential area first. Ending supine allows your client's sinuses to drain; otherwise, the client may leave your office with a stuffy head from lying prone last. Beginning prone also allows the genital region of the body to be underneath the client's body (a physically and emotionally vulnerable

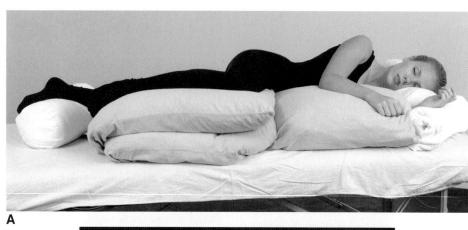

A

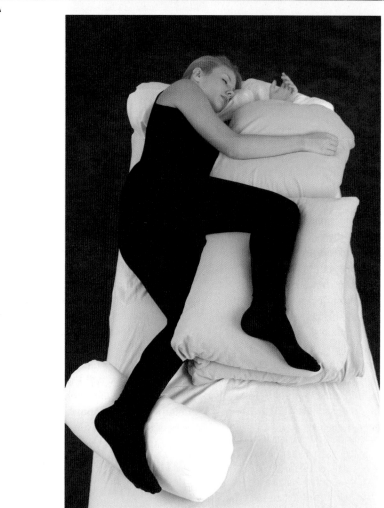

B

FIGURE 6-14 **A**, Side-lying client with pillows. **B**, Side-lying client seen from above.

area) and allows time for trust between the client and therapist to develop. Even with the best face rest, the client's neck may become stiff while lying prone. Beginning prone and ending supine allows the neck to be worked during the last half of the session to reduce or eliminate any neck stiffness that may have occurred from lying prone. Many therapists wrap their clients up in the bottom sheet as a human cocoon. Ending supine allows this type of treatment conclusion.

Beginning Supine, Ending Prone
Clients often enjoy conversing with their therapists but also enjoy silence during the massage. When you begin the massage with the client in the supine position, eye contact between client and therapist is easy. Conversation may flow effortlessly from the client. The client who rolls onto his or her abdomen often signals a time of quiet rest. Ending prone also allows the back to be worked last, which is often a primary area of complaint.

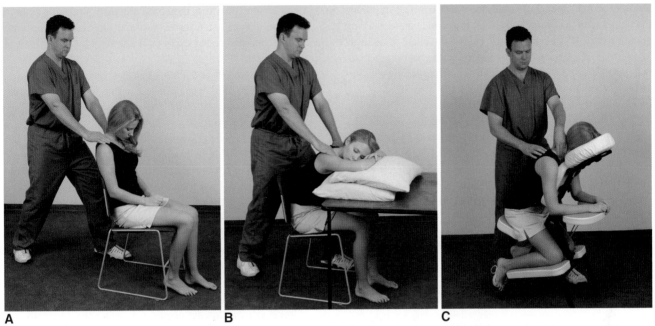

FIGURE 6-15 **A** and **B**, Client receiving seated massage in chair. **C**, Client receiving seated massage in special massage chair.

After these considerations, weigh the pros and cons, and decide which position sequence you or your client prefers. No matter how you begin, you may decide to finish the massage with the client in the side-lying position, allowing him or her to rest before getting up off the table. The side-lying position also facilitates stretching of the client's back, especially if you ask him or her to pull both knees to the chest into a fetal position.

Draping Your Client for the Massage Session

Draping is essentially covering the body with cloth. The purpose of using a drape during massage therapy is to (1) provide a professional atmosphere, (2) support the client's need for emotional privacy (modesty), (3) offer warmth, and (4) provide access to individual parts of the client's body. Covering up the body with cloth allows the client to be undressed while receiving the massage.

The primary comfort consideration is warmth. As the massage progresses, the client becomes relaxed and shifts into a parasympathetic state. When this shift occurs, a drop in basal body temperature and blood pressure occurs. The client may become chilled and have difficulty relaxing. Always ask the client if he or she is comfortably warm at least twice during the session—once before you start the massage and again halfway through. If the client indicates that he or she is chilled, then additional draping may be added by placing a blanket across the top sheet. On the flip side of the issue, your client may become too warm as a result of pregnancy or being peri- or postmenopausal. If this discomfort occurs, then expose more body surface area, provided the following areas remain draped: the genital region on both men and women, the gluteal cleft, and in some regions breast area on female clients.

The drape not only constitutes the therapist's professional and ethical boundaries, but it also represents the client's modesty boundary. With regard to modesty of either the therapist or the client, three basic rules apply. The *first rule* is the state or local laws regarding draping. This rule is your minimal draping standard, and you cannot drape with less than the law requires without endangering your license. The *second rule* is to honor the client's individual request for draping. As long as it does not conflict with your state laws, you may add extra draping or remove superfluous draping. The *third rule* is that the massage therapist also has to be comfortable with the level of draping. For example, a female client may schedule a massage from a therapist in a state that has no massage therapy legislation. The female client may be perfectly comfortable with no top drape, but the therapist may be uncomfortable with this situation. In this case, the therapist discusses the situation with the client. The resolution may range from the massage performed with a top drape or the client locating a different therapist. When in doubt, always go for more drape than for less. This precaution is respectful to the client's privacy and a way to protect therapists from misunderstandings. For more information regarding draping and ethics, see Chapter 2.

Expose only the body areas being massaged. For example, if you are massaging the back, then both legs should be draped. If you are working on the posterior aspect of the left leg, then the back *and* the right leg should be draped.

Lifting, fluffing, or moving the sheet in such a way as to make the fabric leave the client's body is improper. The sudden feeling of air space may violate the client's feelings of warmth, security, relaxation, and privacy, thus detracting from the massage experience. Avoid lifting the sheet off the client's body for the process of turning over. When an anchoring method of turning (described in the sheet and towel draping sections of this chapter) is used, the client can feel the drape in contact with his or her body at all times and can feel secure about privacy. If you accidentally expose the client, look away and redrape the exposed area. Generally, the best thing to do is to acknowledge your error with a simple pardoning of yourself while remaining composed. A look of horror on your face only makes the uncomfortable situation worse.

The two main types of drapes are sheets and towels. Become proficient at using *both* types of drapes because you may find yourself in a situation requiring the use of the one you do not normally use. Be patient with yourself while learning draping techniques; time and practice are required. Proper draping is considered an art in itself. A challenge for most new therapists is turning the client over while keeping the draping securely in place. In turning the client, most accidental exposures occur.

MINI-LAB

One way to practice draping is to put on a pair of bright undergarments over your regular attire. Lay on a table with the drape over you. Have a classmate practice turning you over while *not* exposing your bright undergarments.

Towel Draping

(6-6) Towels are often used as draping materials. They are thicker, heavier, and more opaque than sheets; they are also smaller and easier to use when accessing treatment areas such as the abdomen. Typically, one towel is used for draping male clients, and two towels are used to drape female clients; however, provide more drape if a client requests it. A flat or fitted sheet is used as a table cover beneath the client, with one or more towels draped over the client.

When using towel draping, fold the towel back or under to reveal the area to be massaged. In most circumstances, the towel stays where it is folded, but it may be secured by tucking underneath the body. Avoid using towels when a client is in a side-lying position; they typically do not provide enough coverage. Never use a towel to drape the face rest because the terry material leaves pits on a client's face as a result of compression.

Towel draping male clients – Instruct the client to undress, lie on the table, and drape himself with one towel across the pelvis. After you reenter the room, grasp the bottom corner of the towel closest to you with your lower hand and the top corner of the towel (opposite side of the table) with your upper hand. Pull these corners apart until slight traction is felt. While maintaining traction and keeping the center of the towel over the pelvis, rotate the towel 90 degrees, with the top hand pulling the far corner of the towel across the midline of the clients body to the hip nearest the therapist. At the same time, with the same speed, move the lower hand away until the corner held is on the opposite side of the client's body. The towel is now draped down the legs (Figure 6-16). The towel will be turned back to its original position before the client is turned over.

Towel draping female clients – Instruct the client to undress, lie on the table, and drape herself crossways with the two towels—one across her torso and the other across her pelvis. The two towels should be parallel to each other but perpendicular to the client's body, as an equal sign (=). After you reenter the room, use the technique detailed previously to rotate the bottom towel 90 degrees. When towel rotation is complete, the bottom towel will be parallel to the body, creating a T where it meets the top towel (Figure 6-17). The towels will be returned to the equal-sign formation before the client is turned over.

Accessing the abdominal area on female clients – Towel draping is convenient for accessing the abdomen in the supine position. The top towel is pulled down until the top edge is at the level of the clavicles. The bottom corners of the top towel are lifted with both hands and the towel is fanfolded on itself across the breasts to act as a bikini top. Care must be taken to keep the female breasts covered while the abdomen is being exposed (Figure 6-18, *A*). To redrape the client's abdomen, simply anchor the top edge of the towel with one hand at the

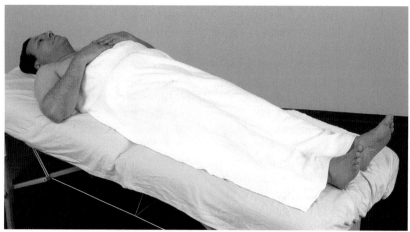

FIGURE 6-16 Client on table with towel draped down legs.

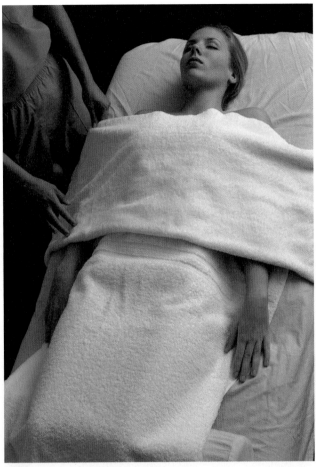

FIGURE 6-17 Supine female client with two towels draped across chest and hips.

sternum and pull the center of the towel down toward the lower towel, unfolding the fanfolds as you go (Figure 6-18, *B*). Make sure the knees are flexed when working the abdomen.

Turning the client prone to supine – NOTE: This discussion assumes that the therapist is using two towels. Modify the instructions for a single towel.

When turning the client from prone to supine, the direction of rotation should be *toward the therapist*. This direction prevents undraping the client accidentally. First, remove all positioning equipment from the table before turning the client over. Instruct the client to scoot down until his or her head is resting on the table and off the face rest, guiding the towels down with him or her for proper coverage. Rotate the lower towel back to the equal sign position if the towel placement is still in the T formation.

Reach across the table and grasp the top corner of the top towel with your upper hand and the lower corner of the top towel and upper corner of the bottom towel with your lower hand. Anchor the towel edges nearest you by leaning on them, thus securing them to the table (Figure 6-19). Instruct the client to turn to face you, and continue turning until he or she is all the way over onto the back (180 degrees). Use verbal instructions and hand gestures such as tapping the table to direct the client as to which way to turn. Return

the bottom towel to the T formation before proceeding with the massage. Place bolsters under the client's neck and behind the knees.

Turning the client supine to prone – NOTE: This discussion assumes the therapist is using one towel on a male client. If needed, then modify the instructions for two towels.

When turning the client from supine to prone, the direction of rotation should be *away from the therapist*. This direction prevents undraping the client accidentally. First, remove all positioning equipment from the table and rotate the towel until it is perpendicular to the body. Anchor the towel against the table with your body. Instruct the client to turn to face away from you, and continue all the way over until he or she is on the abdomen (Figure 6-20). Use verbal instructions and hand gestures such as tapping the table to direct the client as to which way to turn. The client may scoot up and make use of the face rest. Rotate the towel 90 degrees until the towel is parallel to the client's body, draping him or her from the waist to the ankles. Place a bolster under the ankles.

Sheet Draping

(6-7) Two sheets are required for each client: one sheet draped over the client and one sheet covering the massage table. Clients and therapists may prefer using sheets because they are already familiar with this arrangement; it is how beds are made. Twin-size sheet sets are preferred (fitted sheet for the table drape and flat sheet for the client drape), but a double-size flat sheet folded in half may be used as the table drape. Arrange the top flat sheet neatly on the bottom sheet, folding down the top corner edge to reveal the bottom sheet. This arrangement gives the draped massage table an inviting appearance. As you undrape specific areas of the body for massage, tuck the ends of the fabric underneath the client's body. Untuck the sheet, and redrape when moving to a different area for massage.

Accessing the abdominal area on female clients – The easiest method of accessing the abdominal area requires the use of a towel or pillowcase. A towel is draped on top of the sheet, across the breasts, and perpendicular to the body. The top center edge of the towel is held at the level of the clavicles with one hand. The other hand pulls the sheet out from under the towel without moving the towel from its location. Once the sheet is clear of the towel, the sheet is folded back to expose the abdomen, with the towel acting as a bikini top (see Figure 6-18, *A*). Make sure the knees are flexed when working the abdomen.

Turning the client prone to supine – When turning the client from prone to supine, the direction of rotation should be *toward the therapist* (Figure 6-21). This direction prevents undraping the client accidentally. Remove all positioning equipment from the table. Uncover the feet because they may become entangled in the sheet while the client is turning over. Instruct the client to scoot down until his or her head is resting on the table and not on the face rest. Grasp and slightly elevate the sheet along the opposite edge of the table, while anchoring the sheet with your thighs on the side of the table closest to you. The therapist's hands are holding the sheet at

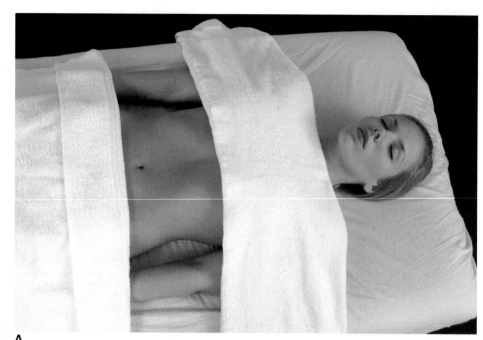

FIGURE 6-18 **A**, Supine female client with towel draping, abdomen exposed. **B**, Therapist holding top of towel while unfolding fanfolds with the other hand.

A

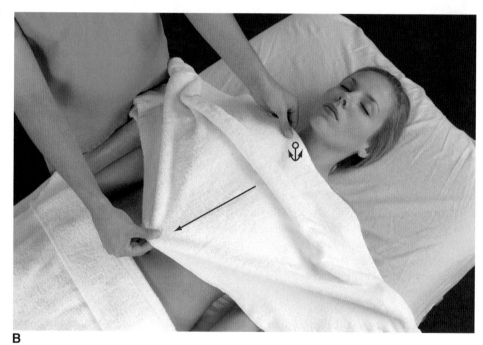

B

the level of the client's shoulder and pelvis. Instruct the client to turn and face you and to continue turning until he or she is all the way onto the back (180 degrees). In some instances, a helpful technique is to pull a little extra top sheet material toward the therapist before beginning to turn the client. Reinforce your instructions by the use of hand gestures such as tapping the table to direct the client as to which way to turn.

Turning the client supine to prone – When turning the client from supine to prone, the direction of rotation should be *away from the therapist* (Figure 6-22). This direction prevents undraping the client accidentally. Remove all positioning equipment from the table, and uncover the feet to prevent

getting entangled in the sheet while the client is turning over. Slightly elevate and hold the sheet along the opposite edge of the table while anchoring the edge of the top sheet on the side of the table closest to you. Instruct the client to turn away from you and continue all the way over until he or she is on the abdomen. Ask the client to center him or herself on the table and to move up and make use of the face rest. Place a bolster under the ankles. Reinforce your instructions by the use of hand gestures such as tapping the table to direct the client as to which way to turn.

Side-lying using sheet draping – Drape the side-lying client with a sheet. Proceed with the massage as usual, exposing

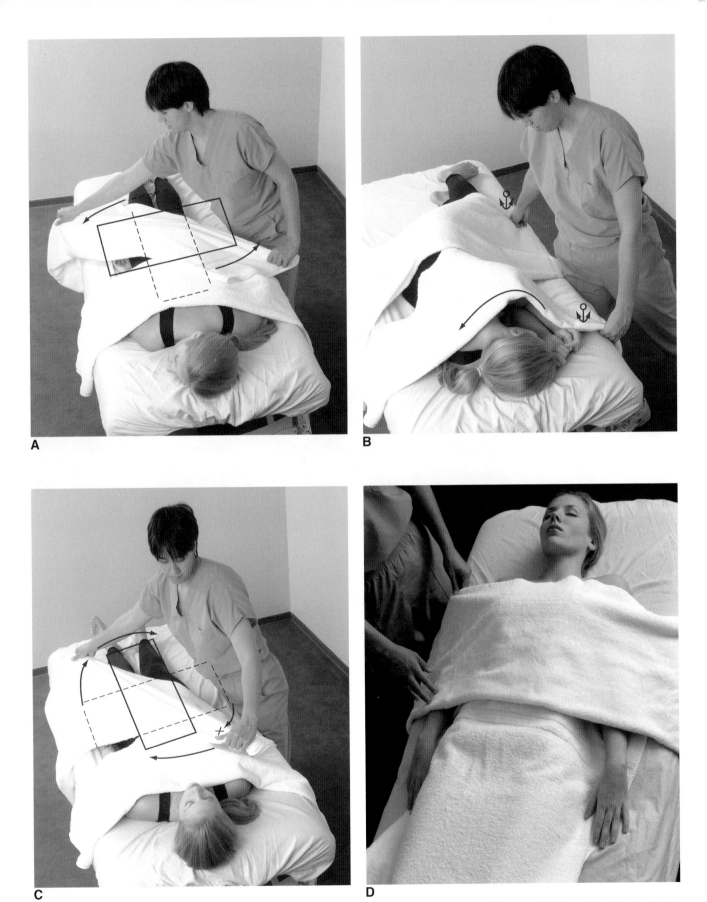

FIGURE 6-19 **A**, Therapist rotating lower towel back parallel on prone female client. **B**, Client rolling over while therapist maintains, holds, and anchors towel. **C**, Therapist rotating lower towel back to T formation. **D**, Supine client draped with towels in a T formation.

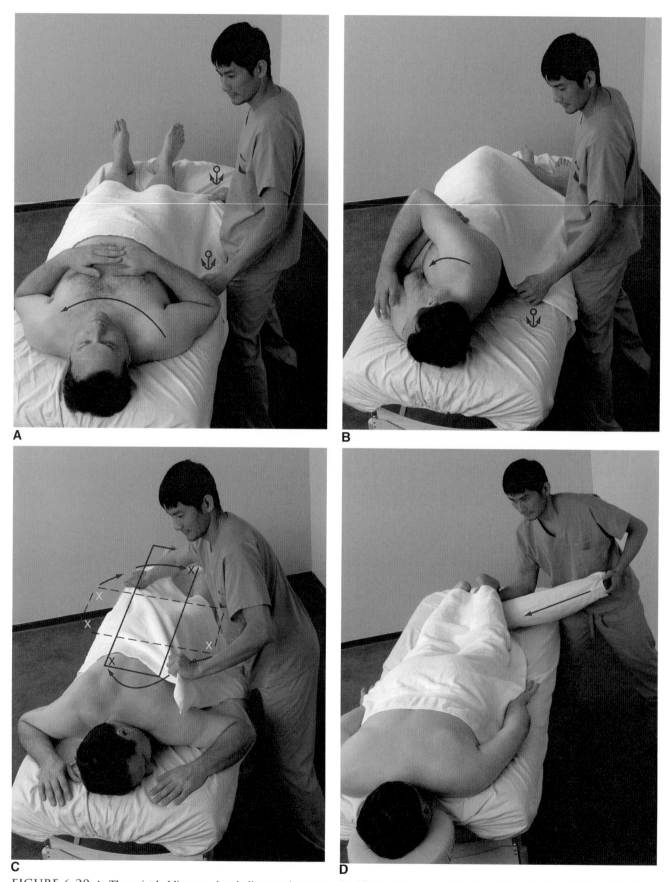

FIGURE 6-20 **A**, Therapist holding towel and client ready to turn. **B**, Client rolling over while therapist maintains, holds, and anchors towel. **C**, Therapist rotating towel 90 degrees. **D**, Client draped with towel down legs and therapist placing a bolster under the ankles.

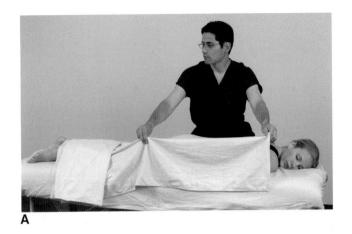

A

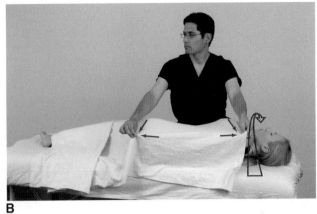

B

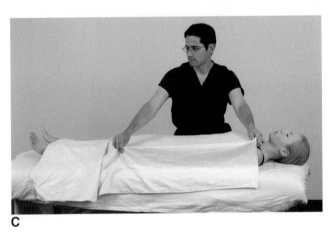

C

FIGURE 6-21 **A**, Prone female client with feet uncovered, ready to turn while therapist lifts and holds sheet in place. **B**, Client in mid-turn while therapist holds sheet in place. **C**, Client now in supine position.

one area at a time. When the back and neck are uncovered, use a towel folded in half lengthwise, draping it over the client's side to secure the sheet drape (Figure 6-23, *A*). The arm is worked from the front while the client is draped from the chest down (Figure 6-23, *B*). For the bottom leg, drape as you would if the client were lying prone or supine (Figure 6-23, *C*). For the top leg, undrape and tuck the sheet back around under the leg (Figure 6-23, *D*). The back can be worked while the therapist is seated in a stool or chair (Figure 6-23, *E*).

Turning the client from supine to side-lying or from side-lying to opposite side – Remove all positioning equipment from the table, except the head pillow. With the client in the supine position, grasp the sheet along the opposite edge of the table while anchoring the sheet with your thighs on the side of the table closest to you (Figure 6-24). Ask the client to turn and lay on the side that feels most comfortable. The client will roll 90 degrees or a quarter turn either toward or away from you. Use the bolstering recommendations located in the Positioning Equipment section earlier in this chapter. Remember to place all cushions *under* the drape, which may take some practice. The massage time is usually shorter on the second side than it is on the first side because the back and neck were already addressed.

ASSISTING A CLIENT ON AND OFF THE MASSAGE TABLE

From time to time, a client may need assistance getting on the table or sitting up and getting off the massage table once the massage is complete. Geriatric clients may use a low, stationary stool when getting on the table. The therapist may offer his or her forearm as a brace maneuvering on or off the table.

Assistance is most often requested by clients when getting *off* the table. A variety of methods assists the client getting off the table while keeping the client comfortably draped and protecting the therapist's back against injury. This method assumes the therapist is using sheets as the drape; however, towels may be substituted.

Remove all positioning equipment used during the massage, and explain the procedure to the client. The client needs to be in the supine position; thus you may have to ask him or her to roll over. Follow these steps:

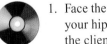

1. Face the client while standing with the side of your hip or thigh against the massage table at the client's waist level (Figure 6-25, *A*).

(6-8) 2. Place your closest arm under the client's closest arm, and grasp under and behind his or her shoulder.

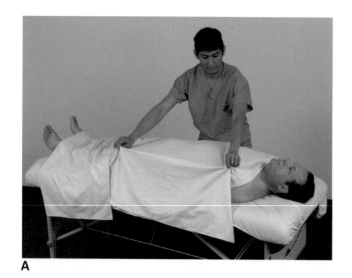

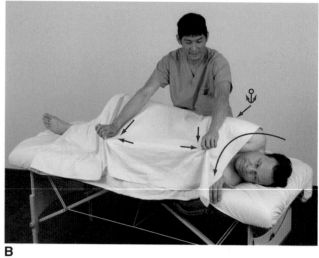

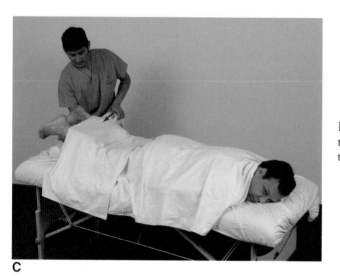

FIGURE 6-22 **A**, Supine male client with feet uncovered, ready to turn while therapist lifts and holds sheet in place. **B**, Client in mid-turn while therapist holds sheet. **C**, Client now in prone position.

Ask the client to reach under your arm and grasp your closest arm or shoulder (Figure 6-25, *B*).

3. Slide your other arm under the client's back until you are supporting the opposite shoulder from behind. Grasp the edge of the top drape while supporting the shoulder with your arm (Figure 6-25, *C*).

4. With the client assisting, raise him or her to a seated position. Use your legs, not your back, to assist in lifting.

5. Pull the sheet loosely about the client's neck and shoulders while continuing to secure the top edge of the drape (Figure 6-25, *D*).

6. Reach over the client's knees, and cup your palm around and over the side of his or her opposite knee (Figure 6-25, *E*).

7. While supporting the client's back with your upper arm, pull his or her knees toward you in a swivel so that the client's lower legs dangle off the table edge (Figure 6-25, *F*).

8. Maintaining your upper arm around the client's shoulders, use your other arm to support the client into a standing position (Figure 6-25, *G*). Do not let go of the top edge of the drape until your client has it securely in his or her hand and drapes him or herself appropriately.

MINI-LAB

To generate bioenergy, begin by rubbing your hands together vigorously for 1 minute. Separate them approximately 5 inches, and be receptive to a light sensation between your hands. It may feel like the attraction or resistance of two magnets. Experiment by moving your hands very slightly closer together and then farther apart. Let your right hand move in a small circle while your left hand is still. Reverse. Imagine a ball of energy between your hands. Move your hands back and forth, and imagine the ball becoming malleable. Breathe in and out slowly as your hands move. Imagine the ball growing as you separate your hands and compressing as you move your hands together. Finally, separate your hands as far as possible, and turn the palms outward, allowing the ball of energy to dissipate.

evolve *How to assist a client off the table is featured on the Evolve website that accompanies this text. Log on and access your student account, then locate the course materials and click on Chapter 6. Click on "How to Assist a Client Off the Table."* ■

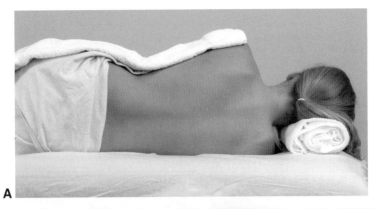

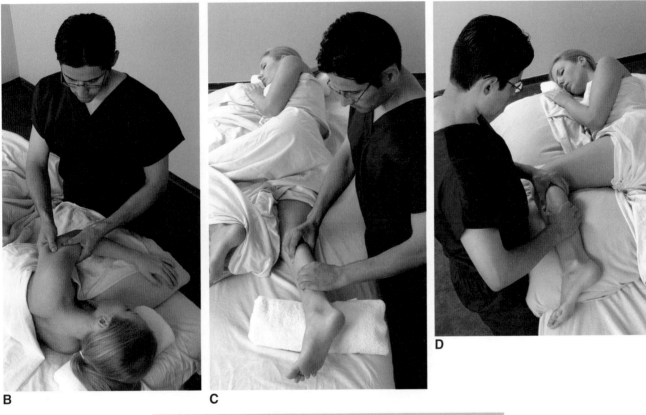

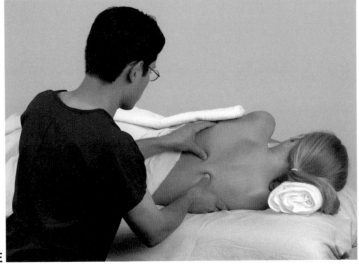

FIGURE 6-23 **A**, Side-lying female client with back exposed while towel holds sheet in place. **B**, Therapist massaging client's arm. **C**, Therapist massaging client's lower leg. **D**, Therapist massaging client's upper leg. **E**, Therapist massaging client's back.

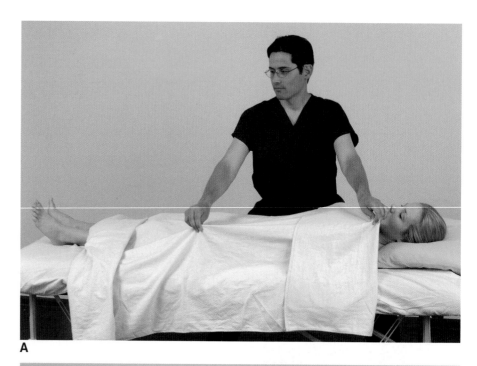

A

FIGURE 6-24 **A**, Supine female client with head pillow, ready to turn while therapist holds sheet in place. **B**, Side-lying client rolling over. **C**, Client on other side with bolsters and pillows in place.

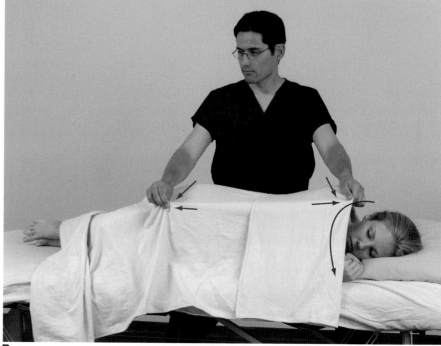

B

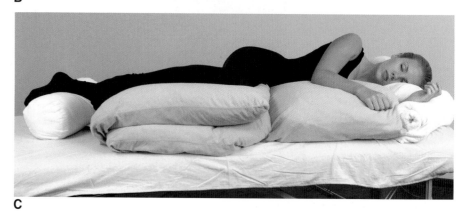

C

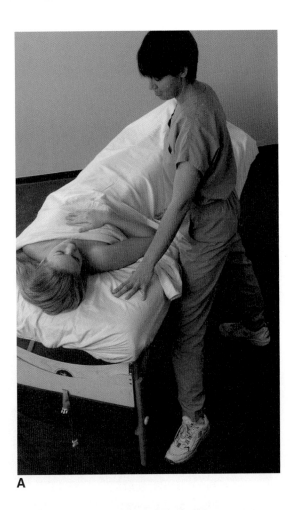

A

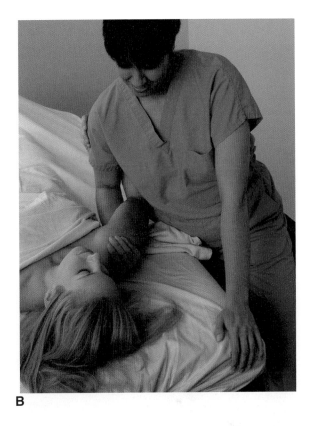

B

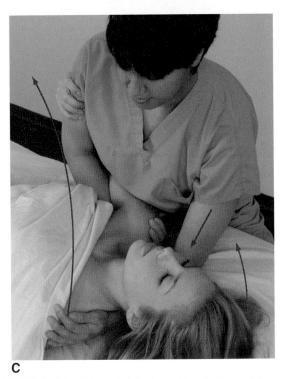

C

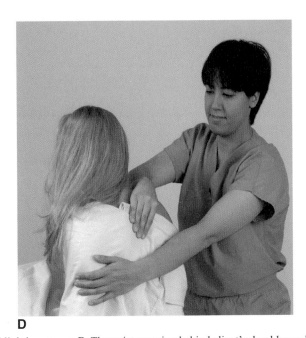

D

FIGURE 6-25 **A**, Therapist's body position before assisting client, highlighting stance. **B**, Therapist grasping behind client's shoulder and client grasping behind therapist's shoulder. **C**, Therapist sliding other hand under client to opposite shoulder. **D**, Therapist adjusting and securing drape once client is in seated position.

Continued

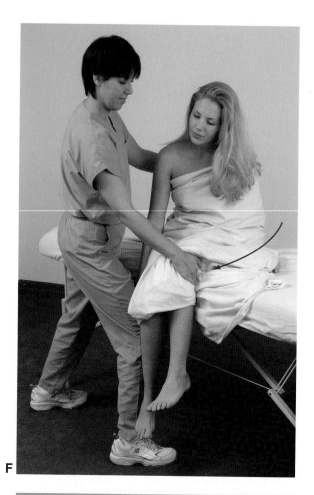

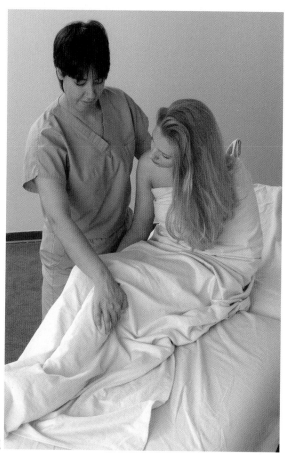

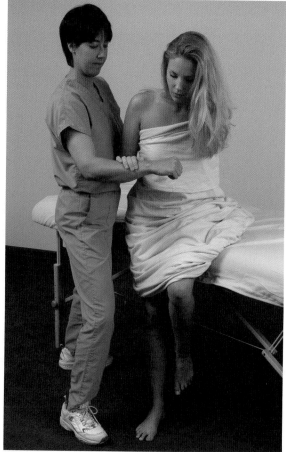

FIGURE 6-25, **cont'd E**, Therapist reaching over both client's knees. **F**, Therapist rotating client until feet dangle off table edge. **G**, Therapist maintains drape while client gets off table, using therapist's other arm as support.

SUMMARY

As a precursor to giving the massage, we have explored two subjects that must be taken into consideration regarding both the client and the therapist. One topic is *body mechanics,* which refers to personal health care and the proper use of postural techniques to deliver massage therapy with the utmost efficiency and with minimum trauma to the therapist. Body mechanics reduce the physical toll taken on the therapist's body both on a daily basis and cumulatively over a long career. Specifically, body mechanics includes the use of foot stances, body postures, and leverage techniques based on the principle elements of strength, stamina, proper breathing, stability, balance, and being grounded or centered. Each of these elements is essential to the success of the massage. Use self-care techniques to prevent or treat minor aches and pains that arise from working too hard or too long. The other main topic is the study of *table mechanics,* which is composed of setting the table height, positioning, bolstering, and draping the client. Proper table mechanics ensures that every step has been taken to provide a physically secure and emotionally comfortable space for the client in a way that is time and energy efficient to the therapist.

CASE STUDY:

Head Lice

Contessa had been working at a very chic midtown salon doing massages on their upscale clientele for approximately 4 years. One of her regulars was Julia, wife of a prominent local attorney and stay-at-home mom to three kids. Julia, who also receives other salon services, came in faithfully every week for a 90-minute massage. Contessa usually spent the first hour massaging Julia's back while Julia was prone and then turned her supine for the last 30 minutes. Julia usually napped when she was face down, but she liked to spend the last 30 minutes chatting. As they were talking about kids and parenting, Julia suddenly exclaimed, "Oh! I almost forgot, please save the last 5 minutes or so for a scalp massage. My oldest daughter, Jill, came home with head lice, and ever since then, I can't stop thinking about it, and the very thought makes my head itch. I think Jill got them when she went to spend the night with one of the girls in her dance class." As Contessa began

to comply with Julia's request for a scalp massage, she realized that visible nits, the egg sacs for the lice, were attached to some of Julia's own hair shafts. Contessa finished the massage without saying anything. She knew that she should tell Julia, but she was afraid of ruining the relaxation effect of the massage, afraid of Julia's reaction, and afraid of losing her as a client.

If you were Contessa, how might you have approached Julia with the news?

Should Contessa share the information with the other employees at the salon, especially Julia's hairdresser?

What steps does Contessa need to take as far as sanitizing her table, linens, and face rest?

If you were Julia, how might you have received the news that you were infested with head lice?

evolve

Go to *Chapter Extras* on Evolve for additional illustrations and resources for this chapter. *Extras* for this chapter include:

1. Crossword puzzle (downloadable form)
2. Therapist doing wrist extension curls for the prevention of repetitive motion injuries (illustration)
3. Warming up activities (video clip)
4. Positioning equipment (video clip)
5. Bioenergy (illustration)
6. Case study (text)

MATCHING

Place the letter of the answer next to the term or phrase that best describes it.

A. Body mechanics	E. Dantien	I. Strenuous
B. Bow stance	F. Prone	J. Supine
C. Breathing	G. Repetitive motion injuries	K. Warmth
D. Draping	H. Side-lying position	L. Warrior stance

_____ 1. Postural techniques used to deliver massage therapy with the utmost efficiency and with minimal trauma to the therapist

_____ 2. According to Bonnie Prudden, how the profession of massage therapy is classified

_____ 3. The position of a client when lying on his or her abdomen

_____ 4. Covering the body with a cloth for professionalism, client's emotional privacy, and warmth, while accessing the client's body for massage

_____ 5. According to William Barry, the foundation of massage

_____ 6. The center of gravity located 1 to 2 inches below and behind the navel

_____ 7. The foot stance most often used when applying effleurage or any stroke in which the therapist proceeds from one point to the next along the client's body, one foot pointing in the direction of movement

_____ 8. The foot stance used to perform massage strokes that traverse relatively short distances, both feet placed on the floor with toes pointing forward at a little more than hip distance apart

_____ 9. Injuries related to inefficient biomechanics—a constant motion, combined with compressive forces, causing injury to soft tissues

_____ 10. Position preferred for pregnant women, some older adults, and persons with various other conditions

_____ 11. In the art of draping, the primary comfort consideration

_____ 12. The position of a client when lying on his or her back

INTERNET ACTIVITIES

Visit the website http://www.saveyourhands.com and read the section Prevention Tips.

Visit the Centers for Disease Control and Prevention website at http://www.cdc.gov. Using the search feature, look up information on carpal tunnel syndrome. Write a brief report, applying this information to massage therapy.

Visit http://www.massagetoday.com and click on All About Massage Therapy. Choose a particular massage modality, and write a short report, highlighting the modalities, goals or objectives.

Bibliography

Barry W: Massage body mechanics, *Massage Magazine,* vol 60, 1996.

Barry W: Personal communication, Houston, Texas, 2006.

Beck MF: *Theory and practice of therapeutic massage,* ed 4, Albany, NY, 2005, Thomson Delmar Learning.

Coughlin P: *Principles and practice of manual therapeutics,* New York, 2002, Churchill Livingstone.

Fritz S: *Fundamentals of therapeutic massage,* ed 3, St Louis, 2003, Mosby.

Frye B: *Body mechanics for manual therapists: a functional approach to self-care.* ed 2, Stanwood, Wash, 2004, Fryetag Publishing.

Grafelman T: *Graf's anatomy and physiology guide for the massage therapist,* Aurora, Colo, 1998, DG Publishing.

Greene L: *Prevention tips.* Available at: *http://www.saveyourhands.com.*

Prudden B: *Pain erasure,* New York, 1980, M Evans and Co.

Torres LS: *Basic medical techniques and patient care for radiologic technologies,* Philadelphia, 1993, JB Lippincott.

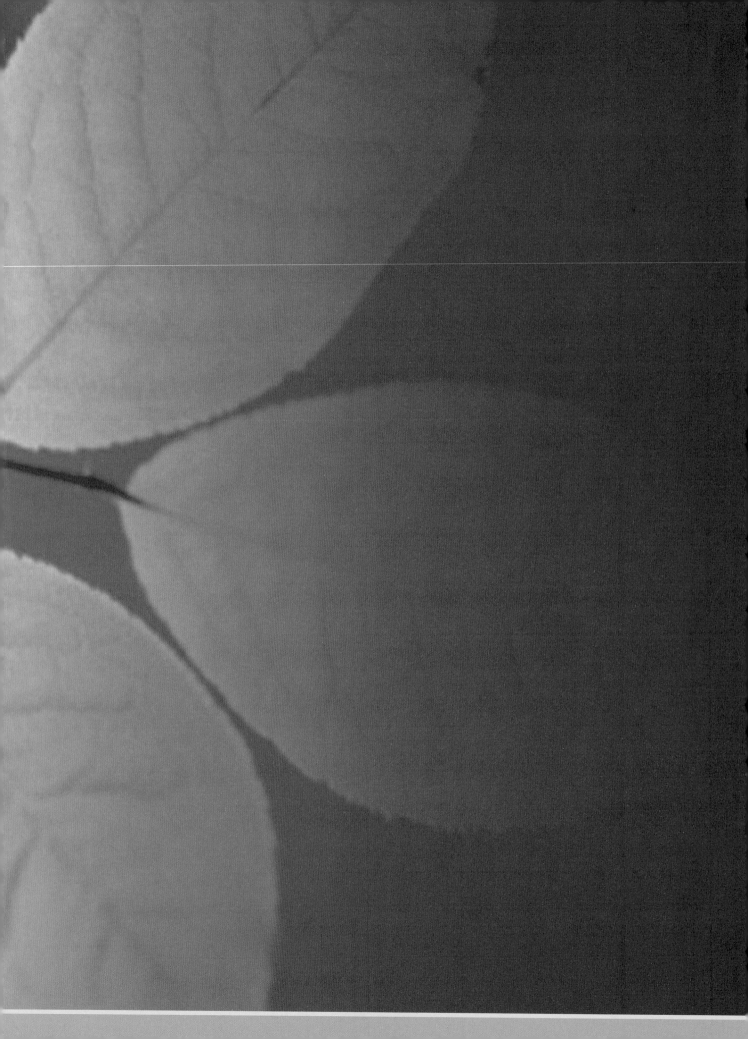

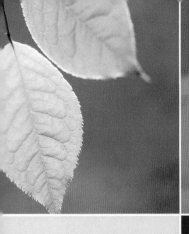

CHAPTER 7

"It is not the same to talk of bulls as to be in the bullring."
—Spanish proverb

Swedish Massage Movements and Swedish Gymnastics

STUDENT OBJECTIVES

After completing this chapter, the student should be able to:

- Describe and implement the following basic elements used in applying Swedish massage strokes: intention, touch, pressure, depth, direction, excursion, speed, rhythm, continuity, duration, and sequence
- Describe and perform the five basic Swedish massage strokes and their variations: effleurage, pétrissage, friction, tapotement, and vibration
- Perform Swedish gymnastics (stretches and joint mobilizations) on articulated body segments

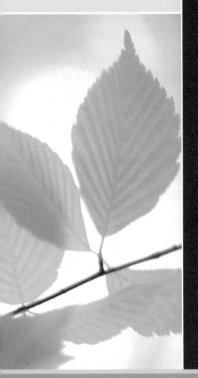

INTRODUCTION

(7-1)   Massage has been around for millennia, probably since early man hit his head on the roof of the cave and instinctively began to rub it to reduce the pain. Massage in Asian countries developed according to Eastern philosophy, spirituality, theories of energy movement, and clinical practice. Massage in Western society was originally based on early religious and medical ideas and has evolved under the influence of modern medicine, biology, and sports models. This chapter concentrates primarily on a Western style of massage, Swedish massage.

Swedish massage is the systematic and scientific manipulation of the soft tissues of the body for the purpose of establishing or maintaining good health. One writer defined massage as organized, intentional touch. Massage is used for a variety of reasons: to bring a client to a deeper level of relaxation, to rehabilitate, to prevent an injury, or to slow the progression of an illness.

The era of modern massage began to develop in the early nineteenth century, when a wide variety of practitioners were advocating massage and developing their own systems. The most important of these writers was Pehr Henrik Ling (1776-1839), a Swedish physiologist and gymnastics instructor. Because of his nationality, Ling's system became commonly known as *Swedish massage,* and he became known as both the father of Swedish massage *and* physical therapy.

The most widely used system of massage therapy in North America is the Swedish system. The five basic massage strokes or movements are (1) effleurage, (2) pétrissage, (3) friction, (4) tapotement, and (5) vibration. Dutch physician Johann Mezger promoted Swedish massage using the Western medical model and is given credit for introducing and popularizing the use of French terminology into the profession (see Chapter 1).

Swedish gymnastics, part of the Ling system, is also discussed in this chapter. The primary movements used in Swedish gymnastics, which include stretches and joint mobilizations, can be performed actively and passively. Furthermore, the therapist can assist or resist active movements.

Understanding the effects of these movements on the body is essential to the *scientific application* of massage. *Masterful application* requires the addition of one basic ingredient—practice, practice, and more practice. Recall any distinguished musical composer or performer; a musician practices scales before advancing to symphonies.

A master of massage, as with a martial arts master or professional dancer, no longer has to think about the moves; he or she has totally integrated science and art—the physical, emotional, intellectual, and spiritual aspects of movement—into his or her own body. The massage therapist uses the whole being when practicing the craft. This technique includes using all of the sensory facilities, spatial awareness, and client receptiveness for meticulous execution of massage strokes. Your skills of massage will evolve and mature as you evolve and mature as a therapist.

The massage session is not a rigid progression. Rather, it is a dynamic process, and the massage routine is simply a road map to help you learn your way around. As we discuss a massage routine, keep in mind that room, and even a need, exists for creativity. You can invent massage strokes. For instance, you can massage the palm of the hand and the sole of the foot at the same time. You might try massaging around the scapula and up the neck simultaneously, thereby creating a unique massage stroke. Your session will indeed be unique as long as you keep the client as the central focus of the massage.

"It's not the age; it's the mileage."
Harrison Ford as Indiana Jones in *Raiders of the Lost Ark*

ELEMENTS IN APPLICATION OF STROKES

During your study of massage therapy, you quickly discover that applying massage movements is much more than placing your hands on the body and manipulating skin, muscle, and fascia. Skillful application of massage strokes is a blend of the hand movements themselves and your body mechanics, as well as pressure and depth, direction, excursion, rhythm and continuity, speed, duration, and sequence. These elements affect not only the body's response to massage therapy but also the intensity of the response.

A client seeks massage therapy services for many reasons, but what a client may yearn for are the three Ts—touch, talk, and time. In our advanced, technological society, many people feel distant and out of touch. The time your client spends on your table or chair has many benefits that cannot be scientifically measured. Massage is an art *and* a science.

As you begin your study of massage, your initial struggle is just to remember the names and order of the strokes. As you practice, your strokes integrate the qualities listed in this chapter, and they will vary within a session and from client to client. Let us examine these concepts to deepen your understanding, and then use them as you evaluate your own progress and digest the critiques of others.

Intention

Intention is a consciously sought goal or a desired end. All other elements in the application of massage are dependent on intention. Our intention during a massage can alter the result of the session. If you approach the massage with personal or therapeutic agendas, then you may not be able to listen to what the body is telling you. This approach is similar to having a one-sided conversation with someone; when you do all the talking, all you hear is yourself! Sometimes in massage therapy our desire to help interferes with our actual ability to observe what the client needs to happen. It helps to be willing to approach the massage table as a tabula rasa, or blank slate, willing to listen and feel.

In massage, touch is not a monologue but rather a dialogue. The client's body leads you in a certain direction, and you follow. Your hands, in turn, communicate with the client's tissue, and it responds accordingly. Spoken communication and the tissue response you feel in the client's skin give you the information you need to create therapeutic impact. Your hands become sensitive miniature microphones sensing restrictions in the tissue. With this information, you can verify or discard your original therapeutic assessment and offer the client the fullness of your therapeutic abilities.

Then, if we combine the approaches of the two preceding paragraphs, we can create a session that is client focused and experience led. In this time of being both full and empty, the massage therapist can bring awareness to the clients and initiate the dialogue that can effect positive change.

Touch

Touch is the medium of massage and a powerful therapeutic tool. In this context, touch is not casual but full of meaning and intention. In some methods, touch is a modality in and of itself (e.g., in therapeutic touch, healing touch). Touching the client on the head, feet, or back is one of the best ways to begin and end the massage session (Figure 7-1). In many instances, a moment of quietness accompanies the initial contact with your client, giving him or her the opportunity to become accustomed to you without distracting conversation.

Pressure and Depth

Pressure is the application of force applied to a surface (the client's body). Usually the therapist uses his or her own hands, elbows, or forearms when applying pressure; however, hand-held tools can be used. Pressure may also be applied with the knees or feet when integrating the use of Eastern techniques.

Achieved through the application of pressure, *depth* is the distance traveled into the body's tissues. The therapist can control the amount of pressure exerted on the tissues, but the client often influences depth during treatment. A tense, contracted muscle prevents the therapist from going deep into the tissues (guarding). A relaxed muscle will yield and allow the therapist to push deep into the tissues. Hence the depth achieved is a combination of the calculated depth and the muscle receptivity or resistance.

Initially the pressure should be light to moderate, gradually adding more pressure until the desired effect is achieved. More pressure may be applied simply by changing your body position to put more (or less) of your own body weight into the stroke or by lowering (or raising) your massage table. Avoid applying pressure past the client's pain threshold. Pressure tolerance is best known by asking the client. The amount of applied pressure is ultimately determined by the intention of the massage and client tolerance. Pressure to

MINI-LAB

The following exercise is designed to increase your level of sensitivity as a massage therapist and to strengthen your proprioception. Select a partner, and decide which of you is the giver and which is the receiver. Sit facing each other, and raise your hands just below shoulder level. Gently flex your fingers; allow your fingertips to touch your partner's fingertips. Both the giver and the receiver then close their eyes.

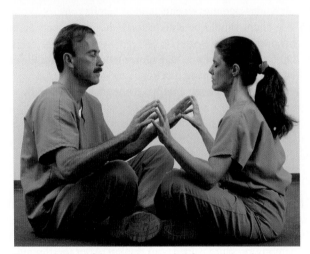

Demonstration of the position needed for push hands.

The designated giver slowly begins to move his or her hands in space, allowing the receiver to follow his or her hands while remaining connected by fingertips. This movement may feel awkward at first, but as the receiver expands his or her awareness, it begins to feel as though the two are dancing. After a minute of practice, switch roles.

After the exercise, ask yourself the following questions. How confident were you as the giver? How did you feel as the receiver? When you were the giver, did your receiver relax and follow you, or did he or she tense up? Sometimes people have a tendency to follow by anticipating the moves instead of experiencing the moves. The more sensitive the receiver becomes, the easier it is to follow the giver. How can this type of sensitivity apply to massage therapy?

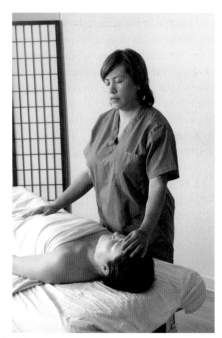

FIGURE 7-1 Therapist touching supine client in a quiet, focused manner.

affect lymph flow is different from pressure to reduce the hypersensitivity of a trigger point. After tissue release has occurred or the desired results have been accomplished, gradually release the pressure.

The amount of pressure that the therapist uses depends on the following:

- Purpose or intent of the massage stroke
- Condition of the tissue before the application of a massage stroke
- Massage stroke the therapist is using
- Area on the body where the pressure is being applied
- Response of the client (i.e., reaching the client's pain threshold) during the application of pressure

If too much pressure is used, then the client guards by tensing the muscle, decreasing the stroke's effectiveness so that little depth is achieved. Too much pressure irritates tissues, causing soreness and/or bruising. Avoid heavy pressure on delicate or thin-tissued areas such as the face, dorsum of the hand, and anterior throat. Thick muscular areas such as the back, legs, or hips can withstand greater pressure. Sufficient pressure is needed to create positive tissue changes, as evidenced by hyperemia, softening of tight bands, and deactivation of trigger points. Most documented massage benefits come with activation of deep pressure receptors. With appropriate training, practice, and common sense, you can make good pressure judgments.

As pressure is being applied, observe the client's facial expressions, changes in breathing patterns, or any other messages of discomfort. Distorted facial features or an alteration in the client's breathing (e.g., shallow breathing, holding the breath) often indicates pressure that is too great. The client may lift a limb or lift the head up off the table to indicate discomfort. In many instances, the therapist simply increases the surface area contacting the client's skin without reducing pressure. For example, if you are using a fingertip to apply pressure, then change to the palm of your hand.

Keep your pressure consistent as your hands move over the client's skin, releasing pressure while maintaining contact. The use of even pressure and anticipated motion helps build trust with your client. It is easier for relaxation to take place when the client feels safe. If each long movement feels like a roller-coaster ride, then the client will always be braced for the next unpredictable push.

Direction

The direction in a massage can vary from down and forward (effleurage), to inward and up (pétrissage), to downward, and back and forth (friction). Direction of pressure can make the difference when locating a trigger point. When looking at a trigger point map, locate a desired point on the body. Place your thumb on the spot, and without removing your thumb, move the direction of pressure as if looking at a compass. Move up, or north, toward the right, or east, down, or south, and to the left, or west. To locate the trigger point, you may have to navigate southwest, northeast, and so on. Continue exploring the tissue beneath the skin until the tender spot is located.

When working a tender area, apply the direction of pressure against the bone, using the bone as if it were a backboard.

Excursion

Excursion is the distance traversed during the length of one massage stroke, typically effleurage. Once the therapist has applied the desired pressure and direction of a stroke, the next consideration is how far across the skin the movement should go. The therapist decides if the massage movement will cover the length of the muscle, then the area of tissue restriction, or a topographical region such as the lower leg or the lateral border of the scapula.

Excursion has a relationship with body stance and foot placement. Longer strokes are best achieved while standing in the bow stance; shorter strokes are done in the warrior stance. Proper foot stance is vital to ensure a smooth continuum of the excursion without a change in pressure or a break in flow.

Speed

Speed refers to the change of your hand position over time or how rapidly (or slowly) a massage movement is being executed. The therapist determines the stroke speed, but the following general rules apply:

- Rapid massage movements tend to be stimulatory.
- Slow massage movements tend to be relaxing.
- The client should be able to track the movements across his or her skin.
- Quick delivery of massage movements may alarm the client, causing a tensing reaction.
- Fast massage movements have a tendency to fatigue the client.
- The therapist cannot palpate and assess tissues if the hand speed is too fast or too slow.

Rhythm and Continuity

The repetition or regularity of massage movements is its *rhythm*. Massage therapy is delivered using both strong (forte) and soft (piano) elements. A distinct connection exists among pressure, speed, and rhythm. Alter the rhythm of the massage to fit the intent of the session; a slower technique is ideal for stress reduction, whereas a faster tempo is more stimulatory and is ideal for pre-event sports massage.

The concept of *continuity* in massage refers to the uninterrupted flow of strokes and to the unbroken transition from one stroke to the next. Relaxing is more difficult for the client when the massage lacks smooth rhythm and fluid continuity. During the massage, the therapist should keep his or her hands relaxed and flexible, which allows them to be lifted, without losing contact, around the bony regions and contours of the body. Rhythm and continuity come not only from what the hands are doing but also from what the rest of the therapist's body is doing (e.g., foot placement, distance between the client and the therapist) and the height of the table.

Duration

Duration refers to the length of time spent on an area, which may be difficult to determine. Working an area too long is setting the stage for disaster. The desire to help may be overwhelming because you really want to help and, well, more massage is better, right? Wrong. More massage, especially deep pressure massage, often creates a mild inflammatory response. Learn to work effectively by using a variety of strokes, and use ice packs after treatment if you suspect the client may become sore. Massage soreness is similar to exercise soreness or even overexposure to the sun. You really do not know you have overdone it until later and often not until the next day.

Sequence

A sequence is the arrangement and order of massage strokes. The therapist combines massage strokes in a series of movements based on the client's plan of care. Typically, effleurage is applied initially to evaluate and warm up the tissues. Pétrissage often follows effleurage to work on tissues more deeply. Friction is used to address specific areas. Vibration and percussion may be used when the therapist deems them necessary. A series of ending effleurages often flushes out the area. Using a sequence also helps prevent repetitive motion injury to the therapist.

Routine

The union of these aforementioned elements results in a routine. In the classroom and under the supervision of a caring and experienced instructor, you will learn several routines. Learning a routine from a book is difficult, at best. By its very nature, routines are dynamic. Each time you begin a massage, your routine will change. As you evolve as a therapist, your routine will change. With each postgraduate seminar you attend, your routine will change. With each massage you receive, your routine will change. Stay in tune with the client during the routine. A conscientious therapist continually listens to the client and the client's body, modifying his or her original protocol as needed.

> ### TABLE TALK
>
> Client empathy is one of the reasons that receiving massages from other therapists is so important for you, as the therapist. By getting back in touch with what a client experiences, you will be a more attentive and sensitive therapist.

CLASSIFICATION OF SWEDISH MASSAGE MOVEMENTS

The five basic Swedish massage strokes have been categorized into groups according to their application. These groups are *effleurage, pétrissage, friction, tapotement,* and *vibration.* Each of these strokes is described, technically discussed, and photographically represented. Also included are stroke variations. Sometimes the description of these moves may seem as though they are describing a kitten; you have a better chance of understanding them through sight and touch. Hence learning these strokes takes more than a book. Rely on your experienced instructor or instructors to demonstrate properly each move, to model technique as you go, and to guide your practice. Use the self-assessment guide to help you evaluate your progress (Box 7-1).

Hybrid strokes exist in Swedish massage, as they do in most systems. Some pétrissage variations such as ocean waves combine lifting and squeezing followed by a downward compression often seen in effleurage strokes. Pincement tapotement is a hybrid of pétrissage and tapotement because it has elements of both. The classifications presented here are based on tradition, research, observation, and experience (Table 7-1). Feel free to reinterpret the definitions and regroup the variations.

Effleurage (Gliding Strokes)

Description

(7-2) The most commonly employed Swedish stroke is effleurage (ef-flur-ahzh). The term comes from the French word *effleurer,* which means to flow or glide. **Effleurage** is the application of unbroken gliding movements that are repeated and follow the contour of the client's body. These movements may be linear or circular. This stroke may be applied with the therapist's hands (palm, knuckles, fingertips) or forearm; the pressure may be either superficial (gentle) or deep. Variations are *one handed, two handed, alternate hand,* and *nerve stroke.*

Effleurage is used to introduce touch and for applying lubricant. It is excellent for assessing and exploring surface and underlying tissues. It is also the stroke used to begin and

> ## BOX 7-1
>
> ### Massage Therapist's Self-Assessment Guide
>
> - Are the movements smooth and easy for you to perform? Are the movements jarring, rough, or abrupt?
> - Are your transitions smooth?
> - Is your own body as fluid, easy, and open as the movement qualities you want to give to the client?
> - Do you leave time for the client to respond?
> - Do you know how far a stroke needs to go? Are your excursions long enough, or are they too long?
> - Is the depth sufficient without invasion or intrusion?
> - Do you know when to stop so as not to overwork part of the body?
> - Do you use your body well (positioning, stance, leverage, and wrist angle)? Are your body mechanics complementing your massage movements?
> - Are you working within an appropriate amount of time?
> - Is the session feeling whole and integrated?
> - Does your client feel honored and invited?

TABLE 7-1 Massage Strokes and their Variations

MASSAGE STROKE	VARIATIONS
Effleurage *(gliding)*	One handed *(raking, ironing, circular)*
	Two handed *(heart, circular)*
	Alternate hand *(raking, circular)*
	Nerve stroke
Pétrissage *(kneading)*	One handed
	Two handed *(praying hands, ocean waves)*
	Alternate hand
	Fulling
	Skin rolling
Friction	Superficial warming *(sawing)*
	Rolling
	Wringing
	Cross-fiber
	Chucking
	Circular
Tapotement *(percussion)*	Tapping *(pulsing, raindrops)*
	Pincement
	Hacking *(quacking)*
	Cupping
	Pounding *(rapping)*
	Clapping
	Diffused
Vibration *(shaking)*	Fine
	Jostling
	Rocking

end a massage because it is so proficient at moving blood and lymph. Effleurage can be used to prepare tissue for deeper massage and to flush out the tissue after using other strokes. In many instances, effleurage is the only stroke needed to eliminate discomfort in a painful area. Effleurage can be used on virtually every type of body surface, making it the preferred transition stroke to use between other strokes.

Technique
The hand placement used in most effleurage variations is shaped as the letter L (Figure 7-2). Effleurage is, in effect, a *pushing* of the tissue both downward and away from the therapist and is delivered using a *lean-and-drag* technique. When working on the extremities, apply pressure **centripetally**, or toward the heart (or center). This action promotes venous blood flow. Once the excursion is complete, drag your hands back using no added pressure and only the weight of your hands. Remember to maintain contact during each repetition. Additionally, a deeper effleurage is more effectively delivered by going more slowly.

When working the extremities, work the area most proximally first, proceeding distally. For example, the posterior thigh is massaged from the knee to the hip first and then the calf from the ankle to the knee. If a stroke has several phases or progressions up the leg or arm, then apply more pressure when gliding from distal to proximal. When applying

effleurage on the back, centripetal application does not apply because the heart is centrally located.

Avoid hyperextension of the wrist by keeping the angle between 100 and 180 degrees. This action reduces repetitive motion injuries such as carpal tunnel syndrome. The therapist's hands, arms, shoulders, back, and legs should all be aligned along the path of movement to reduce injuries and increase the ease of stroke application (Figure 7-3).

The hands should be relaxed and the movement even. Mold your hands to the contours of the client's body. Gradually increase the pressure with each repetition. Reduce pressure over bony areas. Effleurage is often repeated six

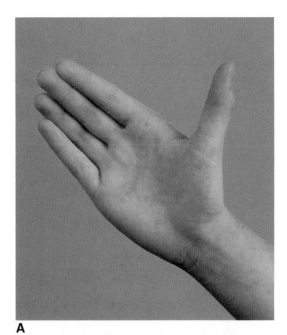

A

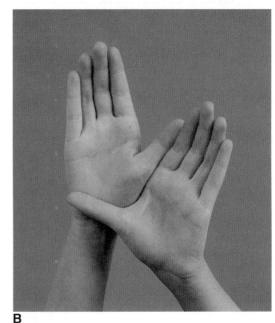

B

FIGURE 7-2 Hand(s) in L formation used in effleurage. **A,** One hand. **B,** Two hands joined.

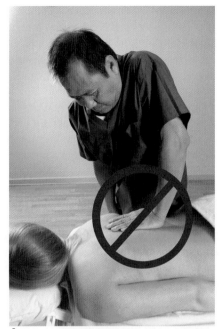

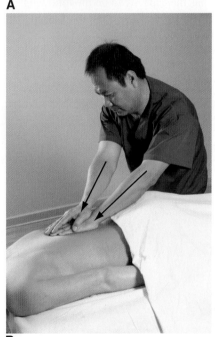

FIGURE 7-3 Incorrect **(A)** and correct **(B)** wrist alignment.

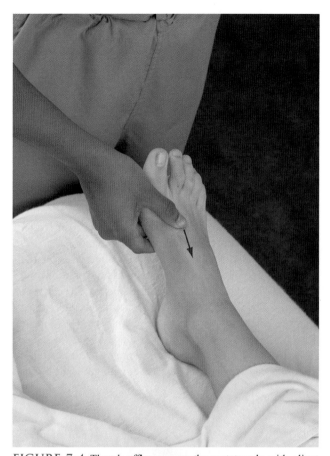

FIGURE 7-4 Thumb effleurage up the metatarsals with client supine.

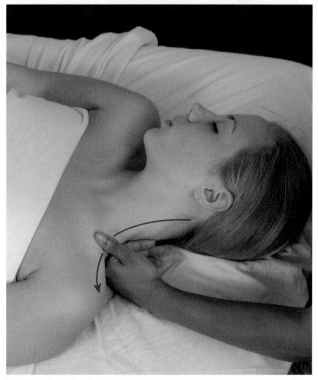

FIGURE 7-5 Fist effleurage down upper trapezius with client supine.

times on an area or until the desired effect is achieved (e.g., hyperemia, release of taut bands of tissue). Remember to apply pressure in only one direction, or you may induce friction.

Variations

One-handed effleurage – This variation implies that one hand or one thumb is used to apply gliding pressure and is used for small areas such as in between the metacarpals or metatarsals (Figure 7-4) or in the neck and shoulder area (Figure 7-5). The hands may be stacked to help increase pressure. Fingertips moving together or apart in one direction is called *raking*. A deep one-handed effleurage is often referred to as *ironing effleurage* and is often done with the forearm (Figure 7-6), fist, or palm of hand. The deeper the glide, the slower the move should be. *Circular* one-handed effleurage can be performed around the shoulder, hip, and knee and also on the abdomen (Figure 7-7).

Two-handed effleurage – Two-handed effleurage is executed using both hands gliding on the skin simultaneously. The hands may glide together or move apart. This variation works well up or down the back in a heart shape or *heart effleurage* (Figure 7-8), up the leg (Figure 7-9), or up the arm (Figure 7-10). Two hands may be used to perform the *circular two-handed effleurage* (Figure 7-11). A variation of two-handed effleurage is to alternate your hands.

Alternate-hand effleurage – To perform alternate-hand effleurage, glide one hand or thumb across the skin, lifting it up as the other hand or thumb follows behind in succession (Figure 7-12). Done properly, the sequence resembles a paddlewheel (Figure 7-13). The index and middle finger forming the letter V may be placed on either side of the spine. This variation, known as *alternate finger raking,* is used to move from one side of the table to the other without losing contact with the client (Figure 7-14). *Alternate-hand circular effleurage* can be performed as one hand circles a region and the other hand moves behind the first hand in a half circle or a crescent shape (Figure 7-15). Because of the full- and half-circle sequence, this variation is also known as *sun-moon.* Move both hands in the same direction in all variations of effleurage (opposing directions is used in pétrissage).

Nerve stroke – Considered a light effleurage, nerve stroke is feather-light finger tracing over the skin. This finishing stroke is typically done at the end of massaging a body segment and at the completion of the massage. Avoid pressure that is too light because it may be perceived as ticklish or produce goose bumps. The stroke may be applied to bare skin or clothed clients (sports or seated massage) or through the massage drape. The direction of nerve strokes is always down the body, superior to inferior or proximal to distal because downward movements are more relaxing (Figure 7-16). Many therapists regard nerve stroke as *icing on the cake*.

Benefits

Effleurage has the capacity to do the following:

- Warms bodily tissues, thereby making them more extensible

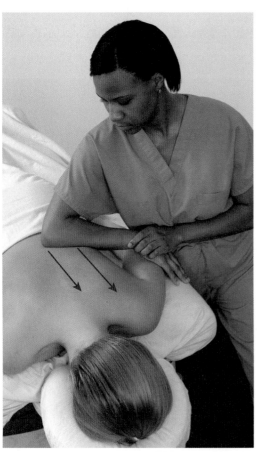

FIGURE 7-6 Forearm iron effleurage on the back with client prone.

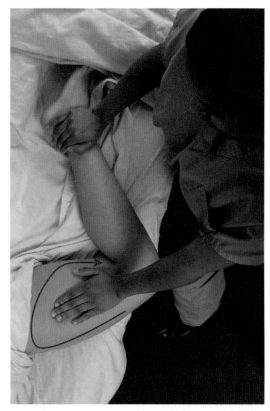

FIGURE 7-7 Palmar circular effleurage on a prone client's iliotibial band with knee flexed and hip outwardly rotated.

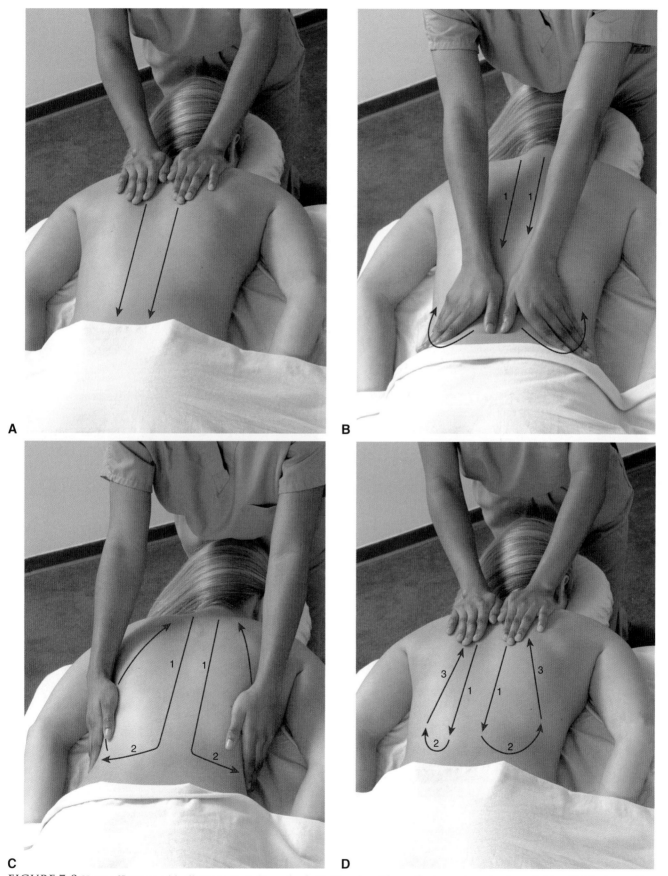

FIGURE 7-8 Heart effleurage with client prone. **A**, Down back. **B**, Stopping at base of spine and moving toward sides. **C**, Moving up the sides of the back. **D**, Back to original position.

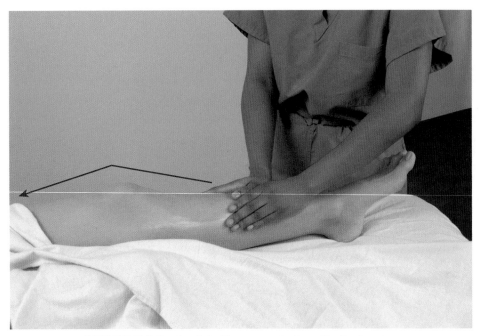

FIGURE 7-9 Two-handed effleurage up the leg with client supine.

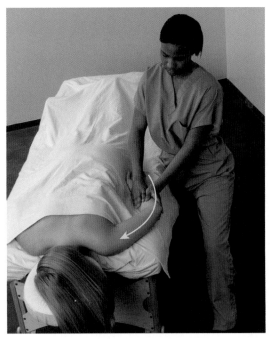

FIGURE 7-10 Two-handed effleurage up arm with client prone.

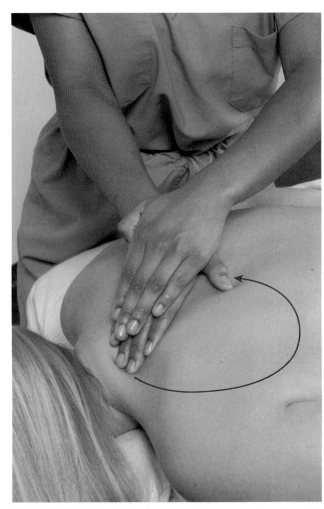

FIGURE 7-11 Two-handed circular effleurage on shoulder with client prone.

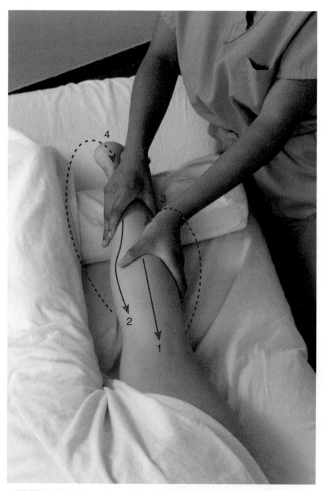

FIGURE 7-12 Alternate hand effleurage on prone client's leg.

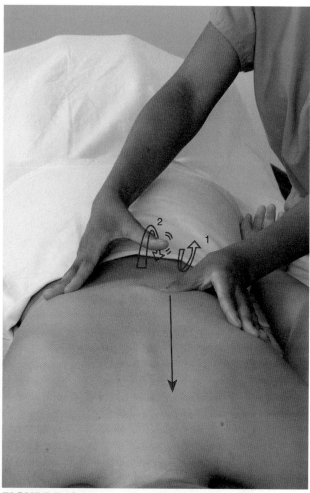

FIGURE 7-13 Alternate hand (thumb) effleurage up one side of the paraspinals.

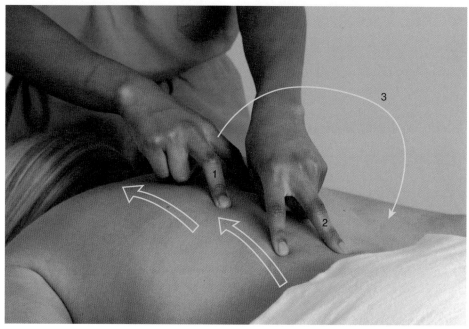

FIGURE 7-14 Raking up the paraspinals.

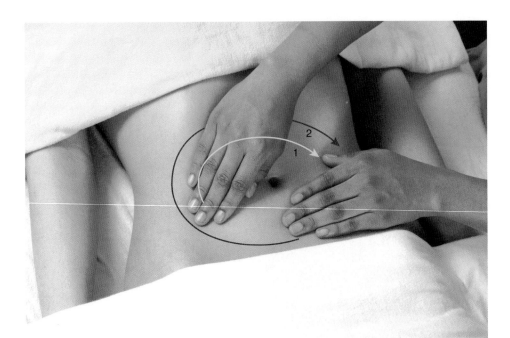

A

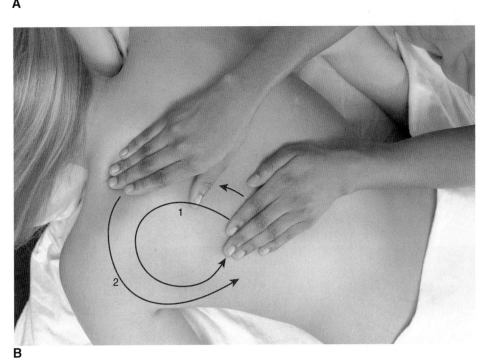

B

FIGURE 7-15 **A**, Alternate hand circular effleurage on abdomen with client supine. **B**, Alternate hand circle effleurage on shoulder.

- Relaxes the client and prepares an area for deeper strokes
- Soothes an area after deep work
- Addresses places too painful for deep, specific work
- Calms the nervous system when done slowly
- Stimulates the nervous system when done quickly
- Aids in the moving of wastes out of congested areas (also known as flushing)
- Creates length in a muscle, if applied with fiber direction

- Increases blood and lymph circulation
- Soothes tired, achy muscles
- Relieves insomnia

evolve Log on to your student account from the Evolve website and view the basic strokes demonstration and their variations from this chapter. Use this as you practice at home. ■

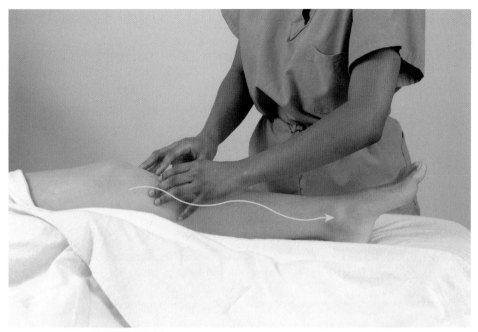

FIGURE 7-16 Nerve stroke down the leg while client is supine.

Pétrissage (Kneading Strokes)

Description
(7-3) The term *pétrissage* (peh-tre-sahzh) comes from the Frenchword *petrir*, meaning to mash or to knead. In a Swedish massage routine, pétrissage typically follows effleurage strokes. The application of **pétrissage** consists of a cycle of rhythmic lifting, squeezing, and releasing of tissue, working parallel to the muscle fibers. Pétrissage is the stroke of choice to *milk* the tissue of metabolic wastes and draw new blood and oxygen into the tissues. This technique also stretches and broadens tissues. Repeating effleurage strokes after pétrissage is important to flush stirred-up wastes from an area, thereby moving them toward the circulatory system. Pétrissage strokes can also be followed with friction, then with effleurage strokes. Several variations of pétrissage are *one handed, two handed, alternate hand, fulling,* and *skin rolling.*

Technique
Grasp the skin or muscle with the hand in a C formation (Figure 7-17). Lift up the skin and the underlying muscle tissue and firmly knead, wring, or squeeze. This movement should raise the muscle from its usual position, away from the bone. As you relax the grasp, repeat the first move with the opposite hand (Figure 7-18). Repeat the lifting, compressing, and releasing using one or both hands simultaneously or alternately. Work in one area using several repetitions before proceeding to another area. Imagine that the palm of your hand is a suction cup and that you are *slurping* up tissue. The focus is on lifting the tissue and moving it horizontally then vertically.

In general, pressure should be applied in a rhythmic circular pattern in at least two directions to achieve alternate compression and relaxation of the muscle. When working large muscular areas such as the back, use as much of the hands as possible. Use enough pressure to engage the muscle but not so much that you cause pain. If your client has a lot of body hair, then small, circular moves may mat and pull the hair. As an alternative, use the back-and-forth pattern (as with ocean waves, described later), or perform the pétrissage movement on top of the drape. Do not lose contact with the skin while switching hands.

Variations
One-handed pétrissage – As much as the entire hand or as little as the pads of the fingers and thumb can be used to lift the tissue (Figure 7-19). This variation is well suited for smaller muscular areas such as the arms, top of the trapezius (Figure 7-20), or the arms and legs of a child.

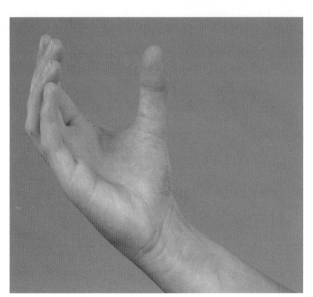

FIGURE 7-17 Hands in a C formation often used in pétrissage.

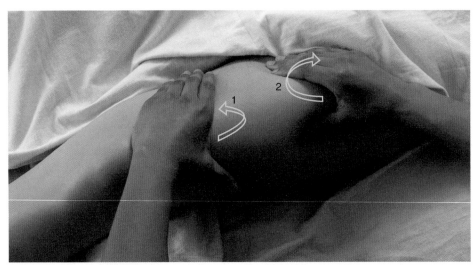

FIGURE 7-18 Alternate hand pétrissage on quadriceps.

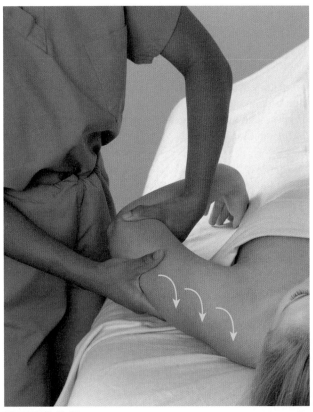

FIGURE 7-19 One-handed pétrissage of triceps with inwardly rotated shoulder and flexed elbow on supine client.

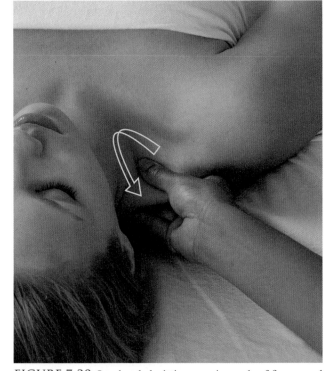

FIGURE 7-20 One-handed pétrissage using pads of fingers and thumb on upper trapezius with client supine.

Two-handed pétrissage – The technique for two-handed pétrissage is the same as for one-handed pétrissage, except both hands are lifting, compressing, and releasing the tissue simultaneously. Two hands are often used to address larger muscular areas such as the back and thighs. One variation uses the heels of both hands on the sides of the heel or a muscle belly, lifting it up before releasing it. To help maintain proper position, the fingers are interlaced in a praying hands position (Figure 7-21). Another variation of two-handed pétrissage adds compression to the stroke, covering both the top and sides of an area (Figure 7-22). Use a back-and-forth movement while the hands oppose each other, lifting the sides and pressing down while on top. Because the hands are moving across the body in waves, this variation is called ocean waves. This variation is typically applied across a large muscular area or horizontally down the back (Figure 7-23). Another variation of two-handed pétrissage is to alternate your hands.

Alternate-hand pétrissage – Lift the skin and the underlying tissue with one hand and compress. Next, lighten the grip

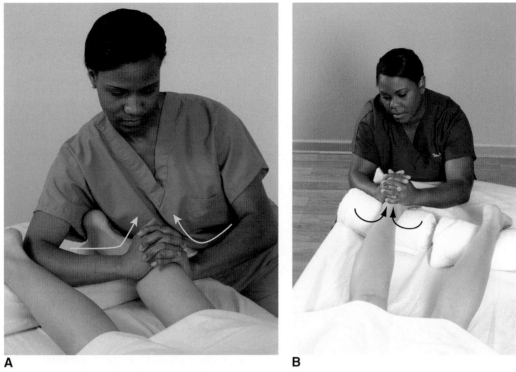

A   **B**

FIGURE 7-21 **A**, Praying hands two-handed pétrissage on prone client's calf **B**, Praying hands two-handed pétrissage on prone client's heel.

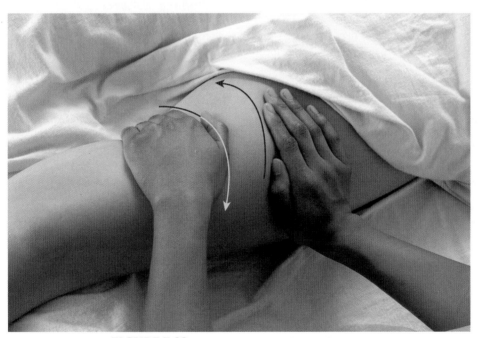

FIGURE 7-22 Ocean waves across the anterior thigh.

enough to allow the muscle tissue to be released while still remaining in contact with the skin (Figure 7-24). Repeat the first move with the opposite hand. Duplicate the sequence, alternating both hands (see Figure 7-18).

Fulling pétrissage – Grasp the tissue with both hands; lift it up and away from the bone while spreading it out laterally (Figure 7-25). It should feel as though you are kneading the muscles around the bone. Repeat the movements until the

tissues feel warm and elastic. Fulling pétrissage is effective for broadening muscles and their related tissues and mimics the movement of a muscle when it contracts. Because of this effect, fulling pétrissage is often referred to as *broadening*.

Skin rolling – Skin rolling involves lifting and compressing the skin and superficial fascia. Skin rolling is a technique essential to *Bindegewebsmassage* (connective tissue massage) and myofascial release. Because no downward force

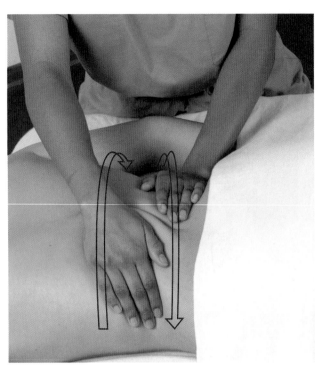

FIGURE 7-23 Ocean waves across the low back.

is used, skin rolling is one of the few massage techniques that may be applied over bony areas. It may be initially uncomfortable for the client; therefore move gently and respect the client's pain threshold. Some areas are vascular and sensitive; therefore overworking an area may leave the client bruised and sore.

Remove any excess lubricant. Hot packs may be used to prepare the skin and fascia. Grasp and lift the skin between the fingers and thumbs, compressing the tissue. Roll the skin

as though you were rolling a pencil, using your fingers to scoop up the skin as you move across the area (Figure 7-26). Continue the rolling technique until the designated area has been treated. Tissue may be lifted using the sides of two hands (Figure 7-27). The skin may also be lifted between the thumb web of one hand and the fingers of the other hand (Figure 7-28). Because the superficial fascia lies in several planes, lift and roll the skin in several directions. If the skin is not lifting, then do not force the tissue into this position. You should address the area two or three times in a session, allowing time between each application.

Benefits
Pétrissage affects a client physiologically by doing the following:
- Increasing blood flow
- Working out metabolic wastes
- Reducing local swelling
- Relieving general fatigue
- Improving cellular nutrition
- Mechanically relaxing and lengthening the muscle
- Addressing tension *under* the surface
- Reducing muscle soreness and stiffness
- Stimulating the nervous system
- Softening superficial fascia
- Producing analgesia by stimulating the release of pain-relieving substances such as endorphins (during skin rolling)

Friction

(7-4)

Description
The term *friction* comes from the Latin word *frictio,* meaning to rub. Friction typically follows pétrissage in the sequential order of massage strokes. **Friction**

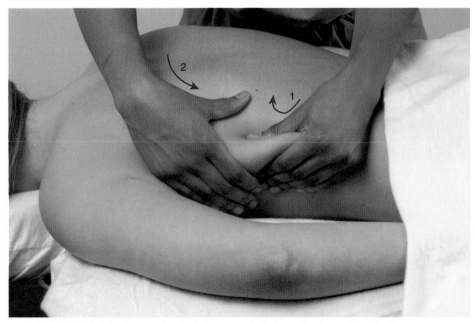

FIGURE 7-24 Alternate hand pétrissage on latissimus dorsi muscle with client prone.

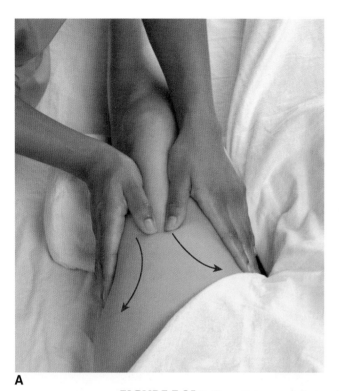

A

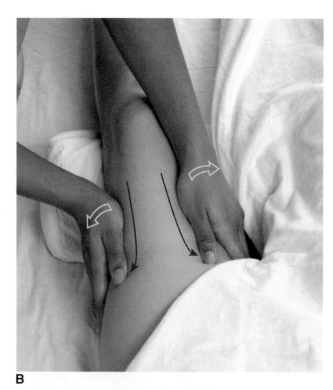

B

FIGURE 7-25 Fulling pétrissage on the quadriceps. **A**, Top of thigh. **B**, Down sides of thigh.

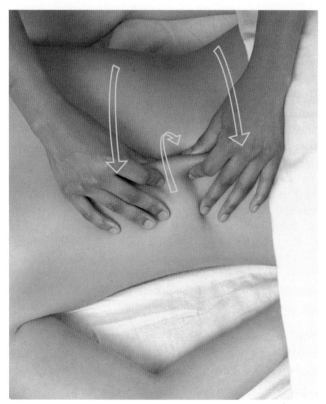

FIGURE 7-26 Skin rolling pétrissage on the back.

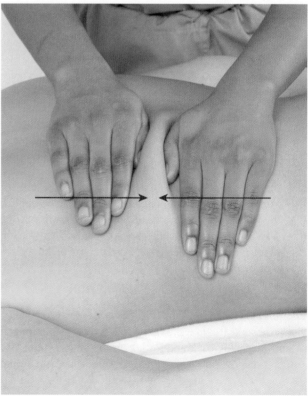

FIGURE 7-27 Skin lifted between two hands while they lie flat over client's back.

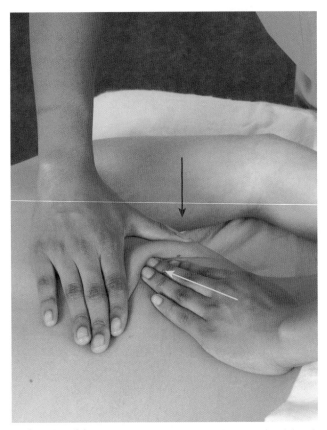

FIGURE 7-28 Skin lifted between fingers of one hand and thumb web of the other.

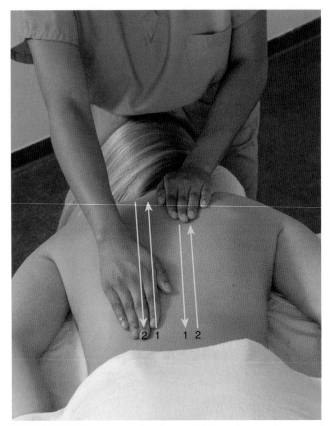

FIGURE 7-29 Alternate hand superficial friction on the back of prone client.

massage is performed by rubbing one surface over another. Because this stroke increases circulation, it is often used for areas that have little or no blood supply, such as ligaments and tendons. Varieties of friction range from general techniques such as *superficial warming, rolling,* and *wringing* to deep, specific techniques such as *cross-fiber, chucking,* and *circular.* General friction is used to address large areas such as the back or the arm. Deep friction is well suited for tender areas, trigger points, and areas that lack muscle bulk such as the ankle, the sides of the head, or the suboccipital region. Friction may be applied with the palm of one or two hands, or specific work may be done with the tips of the thumb, fingers, or elbow. The variation depends on the intent of the massage and the size of the surface area to be treated.

Technique

Friction may be applied superficially or deeply. For superficial or general friction, the therapist's hands, palms, finger, or knuckles slide back and forth over the client's skin. Use lighter pressure for these varieties. For deep, penetrating friction, the therapist's hands do not slide over the skin but move the skin (and the superficial fascia) across tissue layers beneath the skin. Friction may be circular, pressing down and around an area, or linear reciprocating movements may be used. Deep frictioning techniques are typically done dry, using little or no lubricant.

Variations

Superficial warming friction – Also known as a *heat rub,* superficial warming friction generates heat by creating resistance to motion. Place both hands palm down on the client's skin. The fingers of each hand should be together firmly. Move the hands briskly and simultaneously in opposite directions, one hand moving toward you and the other moving away from you (Figure 7-29). The hands should pass each other in midstroke and continue to alternate as pistons. Begin to pick up speed to build resistance and create heat. The muscles of the shoulder and upper arm are used to propel the hands, reducing the stress on the therapist's hands. The fingertips, knuckles, or ulnar surface of one or both hands may be used if the surface area treated is small (Figure 7-30). The latter variation is called *sawing* (Figure 7-31). Superficial warming friction may also be done with a towel, rubbing it quickly on the client's skin. This is called *towel friction.*

Rolling friction – Rolling is best suited for the extremities. Compress the tissue firmly with open palms and extended fingers of both hands. Roll the skin, muscle, and surrounding tissues around the bone, moving both hands in opposite directions. As you roll the tissue around an extremity, use back-and-forth movements (Figure 7-32) while you compress the tissue and slide your hands from distal to proximal. The client may assist by holding the limb still.

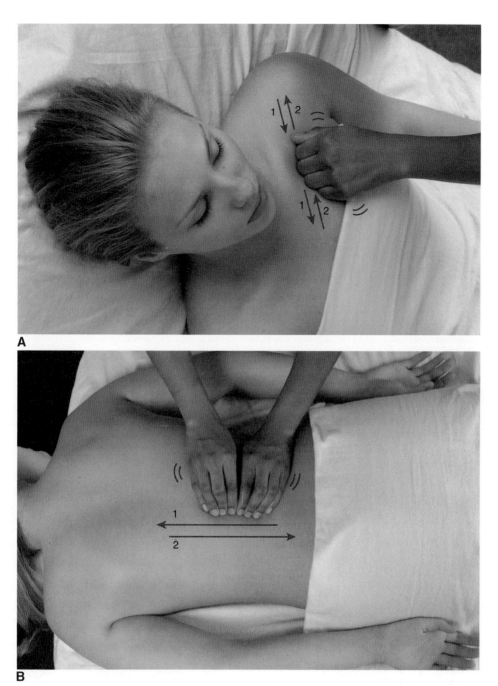

FIGURE 7-30 **A**, Superficial warming friction using knuckles of one hand on pectoralis major below clavicle with client supine. **B**, Superficial warming friction using fingertips up and down the paraspinals.

Wringing friction – While compressing the lubricated tissue on all sides with the palmar surfaces of the hands and fingers, move the hands in opposing directions. Slide the hands toward the trunk of the body during the movement (distal to proximal). Wringing friction is performed vigorously, as though you were wringing water out of a cloth (Figure 7-33). This movement is best suited for arms, legs, and fingers. To wring the fingers and other small body areas, modify your technique; compress the tissue using only the fingers rather than your entire hand.

Cross-fiber friction – Also known as *deep transverse friction,* cross-fiber friction is a precise and penetrating form of friction popularized by Dr. James Cyriax of London (see page 171), who called it the most rehabilitative massage stroke. The direction of movement should be across and perpendicular to the pattern of muscle fibers. Success of this method depends on the therapist's ability to identify contracted or injured tissue by palpation and then apply the technique. The therapist must have a good knowledge of muscular fiber patterns.

One or more fingers are placed on the skin at the exact site of a pain or injury. Applying firm, consistent pressure in one or both directions, move the fingers in a back-and-forth motion (Figure 7-34). The fingers and skin must

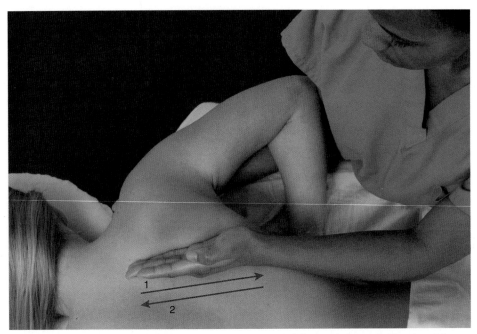

FIGURE 7-31 Sawing superficial friction using the ulnar sides of the hands on medial border of the scapula.

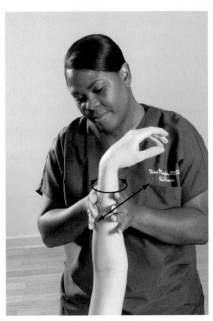

FIGURE 7-32 Rolling friction on extended arm with client supine.

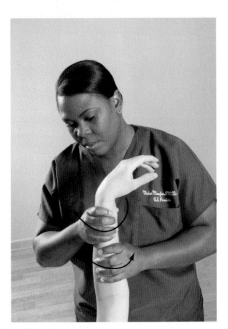

FIGURE 7-33 Wringing friction on extended arm with client supine.

move as one unit, or a blister may form. Apply moderate to heavy pressure, according to the client's tolerance, for up to 15 seconds. Repeat if needed. Being a rehabilitative stroke, cross-fiber friction is remarkably effective in treating most muscular, tendinous, or ligamentous injuries, especially when adhesions and fibrosis are involved (Figure 7-35).

Chucking friction – Chucking friction, or *parallel friction,* refers to deep friction applied in the same direction as muscular, tendonous, or ligamentous fibers. The therapist uses his or her thumb or fingers to rub back and forth, moving the superficial tissue over the underlying structure.

Chucking is usually performed using one hand while the other hand is supporting the limb that is being massaged (Figure 7-36). This movement is often applied between bony areas (e.g., metacarpals, metatarsals, forearms, legs).

Circular friction – Circular friction uses small, circular movements that glide superficial tissue layer over underlying tissue layer in several different directions using the fingers or palm of hand (Figure 7-37). This movement is particularly useful around joints and on bony areas (Figure 7-38). Palmar friction is also great to use before skin rolling and myofascial release and must be applied using quick, circular movements.

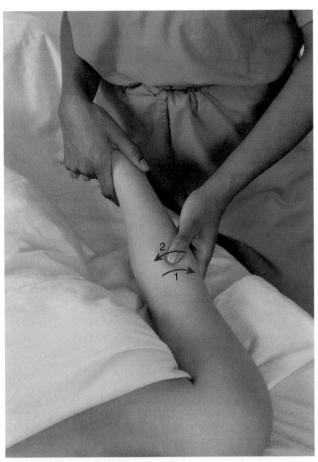

FIGURE 7-34 One thumb cross-fiber technique on the forearm musculature.

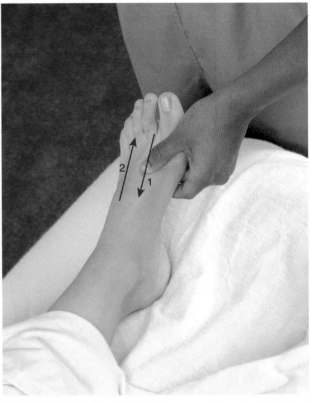

FIGURE 7-36 Chucking friction on metatarsals with client supine.

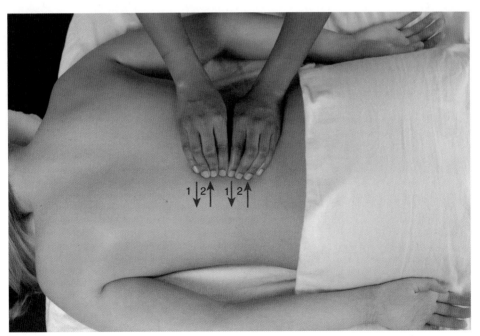

FIGURE 7-35 Cross-fiber friction of the paraspinals using the tips of several fingers.

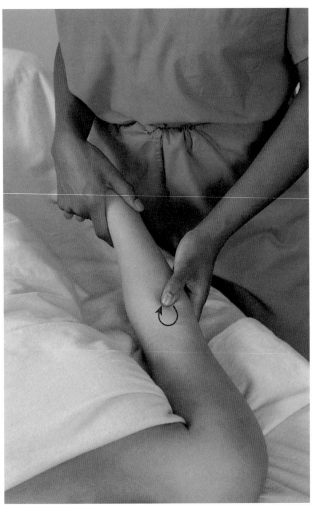

FIGURE 7-37 Circular friction on the forearm musculature.

Benefits

Friction can benefit the client through the following:

- Generating heat
- Dilating the capillaries
- Increasing circulation
- Promoting venous blood flow
- Loosening stiffness in joints
- Relaxing muscles
- Improving the glandular action of the skin
- Promoting proper scar formation by reorganizing collagen, creating a more biofunctional pattern (This result is accomplished by stressing the scar formation at the injury site, using mild, controlled pressure in a specific direction. Stress, in this instance, is defined as response to a demand placed on it.)
- Breaking down and freeing adhesions
- Softening hyperplasia
- Mimicking muscle broadening and stretching that occurs in normal muscle movement
- Reducing trigger and tender point formation
- Reducing trigger and tender point activity

MINI-LAB

To illustrate how cross-fiber friction can have an effect on scar tissue repatterning, perform the following activity. Place 50 toothpicks in a haphazard formation under a thick towel. Lay your hand, palm down, on the towel and begin moving your hand using a back and forth motion. Continue moving your hand for several minutes and notice what happens to the toothpick arrangement. Do they remain haphazard, or do they line up straight? How does this exercise relate to applying cross-fiber friction on restricted fascia or a scar? Write down your conclusion and share it with your class.

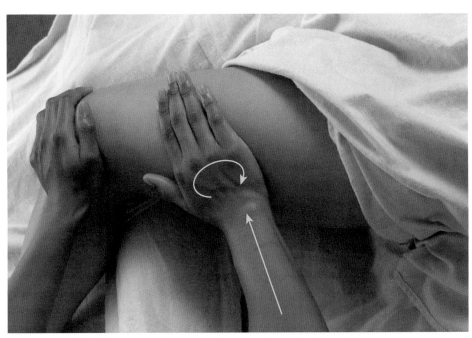

FIGURE 7-38 Palmar circular friction on the iliotibial band.

Tapotement (Percussive Strokes)

Description

(7-5)   **Tapotement** involves repetitive staccato striking movements of the hands, moving either simultaneously or alternately. This stroke may be delivered with the ulnar surface of the hand, tips of the fingers, open palm, cupped palm, or back, knuckles, or ulnar surface of a loosely closed fist. Performed skillfully, tapotement has a pleasant, stimulating effect. The word *tapotement* (tap-ot-mon) is a French derivation of an Old French term, *taper*, that means a light blow, which, in turn, was derived from the Anglo-Saxon term *ta-eppa,* meaning to tap, in the sense of draining fluid from a cavity. At first, this word origin may seem strange, but interestingly enough, the mechanical impact of the tapotement techniques is still used by respiratory therapists and nurses to loosen phlegm congestion in the lungs. The synonym *percussion* comes from *percussio,* which means a striking.

The technique variations are *tapping, pincement, hacking, cupping, pounding,* and *clapping.* The style of the percussion depends on the location where it is employed and the desired effect. Muscular areas such as legs and hips may absorb more force in the delivery, and thin-tissued or delicate areas such as the face require a smaller, lighter tap. Most therapists use tapotement to finish an area or end the massage, along with nerve stroking. Avoid the application of tapotement immediately after exercise because this stroke can activate muscle spindles, causing cramping. Heavy tapotement over the kidneys in the low back area is not advised because they are not adequately protected by bodily tissues. You may want to warn the client about the loud noise that often accompanies some tapotement varieties (e.g., quacking, cupping, clapping).

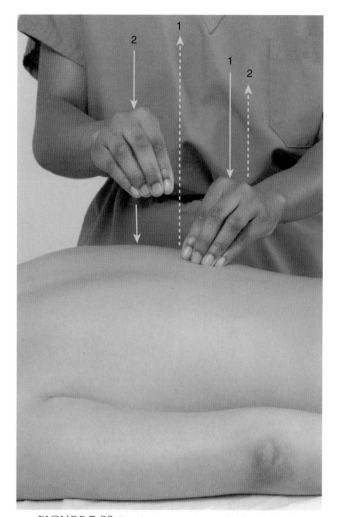

FIGURE 7-39 Tapping tapotement applied to the back.

Technique

The percussion may be applied directly to the skin or through the drape. When applying tapotement, begin with light pressure and moderate strike speed, gradually increase speed, and finally diminish speed and depth. The stroke is delivered rhythmically, allowing your hands to spring back after contact. This sudden bounce-back reduces the impact. The client should feel the onset and removal of pressure. Keep your wrists loose and your fingers relaxed while making skin contact. Proper percussive techniques should be learned under the supervision of a qualified instructor because percussion delivered with too much force can bruise a client. Different variations require the therapist to use different parts of his or her hands.

Variations

Tapping – Using your fingertips of one or both hands, strike the body's surface. Modifying the time and speed of the tap produces several varieties of tapping tapotement. Rapid but consistent delivery of pressure and speed produced *tapping tapotement* (Figure 7-39). A hard version of tapping punctuation tapotement is excellent for the soles of the feet. *Pulsing tapotement* is performed using one hand, with an alternate deep and light tap. The deep tap is comparable to a full note, and the light tap is comparable to a half note. The sound produced by the soft and hard tap reverberates as the sound or feel of a beating heart (*lubb-dubb, lubb-dubb*). Commonly used on the face or scalp, *raindrops tapotement* feels similar to light rain—each fingertip of the hand strikes the skin lightly at a different time (Figure 7-40).

Pincement – Pincement, or *plucking,* tapotement lifts the skin much the same way as the skin rolling technique mentioned previously. The skin is grasped using a quickly delivered striking motion, lifted, and released while the fingers of the opposite hand follow suit (Figure 7-41). This action is classified as a tapotement but resembles pétrissage because of its distinct lifting effect.

Hacking – Using the ulnar edge of one hand or both hands alternately, strike the surface of the client's skin. The hands should be held loosely with the finger slightly spread. On contact, the momentum of the stroke causes each finger to contact the one above it. This action produces a slight vibratory action coupled with the percussive action. Hacking *along* muscle fibers, with the fingers parallel, produces relaxation in the muscle (Figure 7-42).

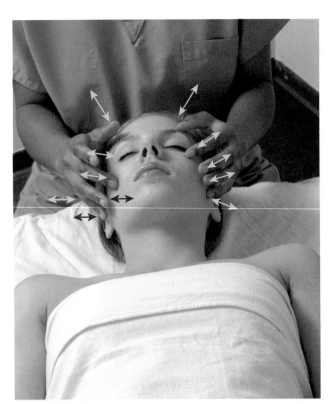

FIGURE 7-40 Raindrops tapotement on the face of supine client.

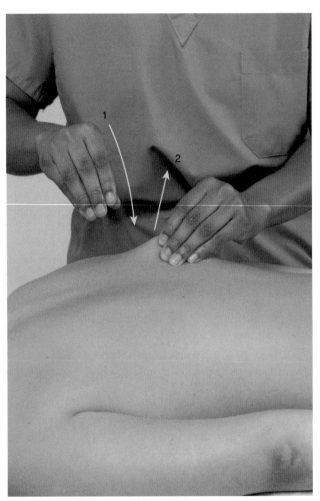

FIGURE 7-41 Pincement tapotement on the back.

Hacking applied *across* large muscles, with the fingers perpendicular (across the grain), stimulates muscle spindles. Minute contractions of the muscle are the result. A variation of hacking, *quacking* places the palms of both hands together. The skin is struck using only the sides of the third, fourth, and fifth finger. It is best if the fingers are slightly apart before the strike. The air moving out of the hands during the strike makes a quacking sound (Figure 7-43).

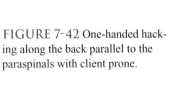

FIGURE 7-42 One-handed hacking along the back parallel to the paraspinals with client prone.

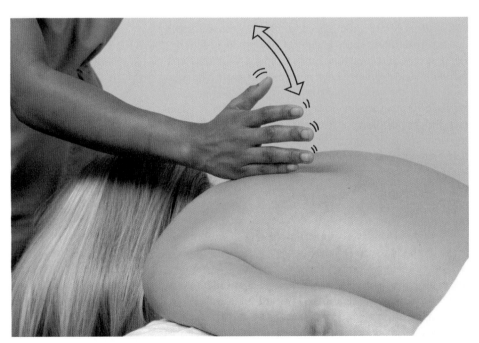

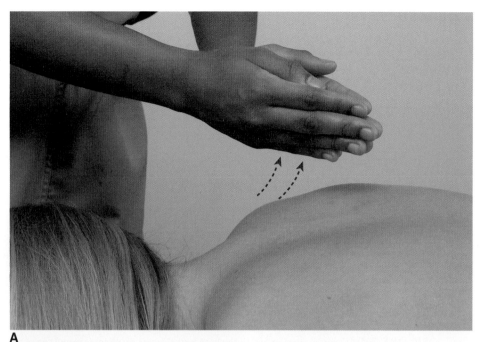

A

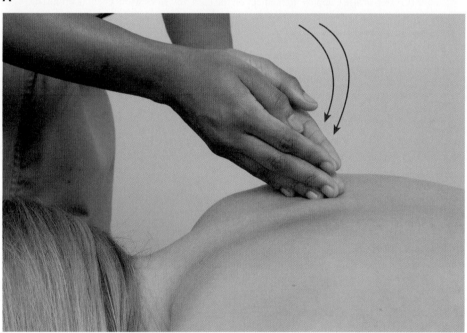

B

FIGURE 7-43 Quacking tapotement on the rhomboids with client prone. **A**, Hands lifted. **B**, Hands in contact with skin.

evolve To see alternate hands hacking perpendicular to the hamstrings on a prone client, log on to the Evolve website and go to the course materials for Chapter 7. ■

Cupping – Curve the palmar surface of the hand into a cup, as if holding water. Strike the client's skin with the edges of a cupped hand, making a muffled horse-hoof sound (Figure 7-44). A vacuum is created when lifting the palm from the skin's surface—hence the hollow sound of suction. Cupping is the stroke of choice for loosening mucus and phlegm in the chest cavity. Additionally, the stroke is vigorous and may induce coughing. Therapists using this type of stroke therapeutically should interrupt the technique to allow for coughing and have plenty of tissues on hand for the client. An often helpful approach is to orient the client with the head lower than the chest by using pillow bolsters under the abdomen and chest to induce positional drainage. Make sure you end this section with several soothing strokes. This type of tapotement may not be considered a pleasant experience; therefore make sure that you thoroughly explain the procedure before treatment. Chapter 20 has more information about postural drainage.

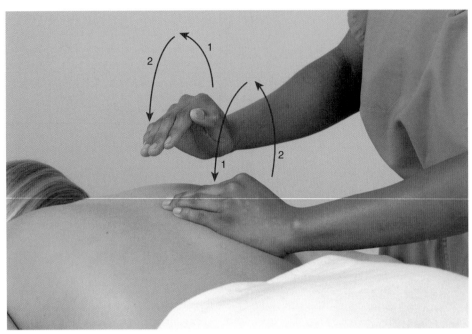

FIGURE 7-44 Cupping tapotement on the back and sides while client is prone.

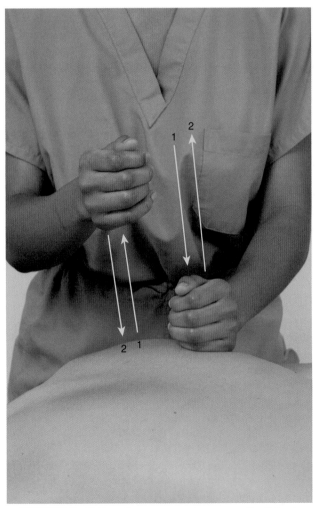

FIGURE 7-45 Pounding tapotement on prone client's back.

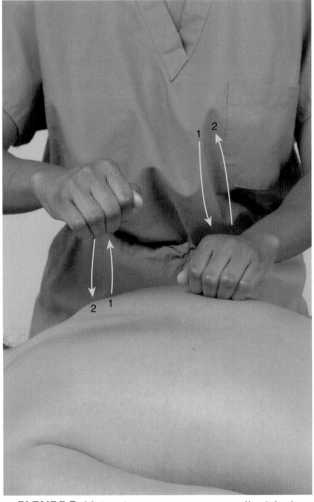

FIGURE 7-46 Rapping tapotement on prone client's back.

evolve *Log on to the Evolve website to view a demonstration of a therapist using postural drainage positioning. In addition, Chapter 20 has more information about postural drainage.* ■

Pounding – Pounding tapotement is performed with the sides of one or both loose fists, contacting the skin alternately. These blows are delivered rhythmically using moderate pressure (Figure 7-45). Pounding tapotement, or *loose fist beating,* is used on large, muscular areas such as the posterior legs and the hips. The loose fists may be placed knuckle down, striking the skin's surface as though the therapist is knocking on a door (Figure 7-46). This variation is called *rapping.*

Clapping – Clapping, or *slapping,* tapotement is performed with the palmar surface of the hands and fingers, striking the skin with alternate strokes (Figure 7-47). The fingers are held together. A loud smacking sound is heard if done correctly. A light upward slapping may be done on the sides of the face. Although this stroke is often invigorating, clapping tapotement is not recommended for use on clients who are known to be survivors of abuse because it may trigger painful memories of past episodes of abuse.

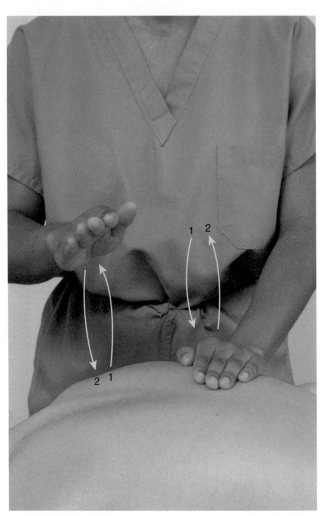

FIGURE 7-47 Slapping tapotement on prone client's back.

Diffused – Lay the palmar surface of one hand on the client's skin. Use a loosely clenched fist to strike the dorsal surface of your relaxed open hand to diffuse the force (Figure 7-48). Diffused tapotement is commonly used over the abdominal region. Drag the open hand across the skin as you move across the skin's surface.

Benefits

The massage therapist may use tapotement to do the following:
- Stimulate nerve endings initially, becoming more sedative if continued
- Aid in decongesting the lungs by loosening and mobilizing phlegm in the respiratory tract
- Tone flaccid muscles
- Increase local blood flow
- Access deeper structures such as hip rotators
- Create an ultrasound effect manually
- Relieve pain (perhaps as a result of the gate theory)
- Desensitize a hypersensitive area after a few minutes of tapotement stimulation

Vibration

Description

(7-6) The term **vibration** comes from a Latin term that means *a shaker.* Vibration is rapid shaking, quivering, trembling, or rocking movements applied with the fingertips, full hand, or an appliance. Done properly, you will be able to observe the tissue moving near the area of contact. As in tapotement, the client should feel the onset and removal of pressure. However, vibration differs from tapotement in that the hands do not break contact with the client's skin. Performing vibration correctly requires coordination and practice. The three categories of vibration are *fine, coarse,* and *rocking.* Vibration is the most physically demanding massage stroke (Box 7-2). Many therapists use an electrical device to apply vibration. A discussion on the use of such appliances is included in this section.

Technique

Each variety of vibration requires a slightly different delivery. Fine vibration uses the fingertips or hands to tremble the skin. When applying coarse vibration, the therapist grasps the muscle or limb with one or both hands and shakes or pulls it vigorously. Rocking involves pushing the client's body with one hand or tossing the body back and forth on the table between two hands. The therapist will notice that each body has its own type of movement pattern, depending on the size of the body, density of the tissues, and health of the joints. Avoid imposing an unnatural rhythm on the body.

Variations

Fine vibration – Place the fingertips of one or both hands on the skin and begin a trembling movement by rapidly contracting and relaxing the arm, keeping the fingers and wrist stiff. Fingers should be moving side to side or up and down

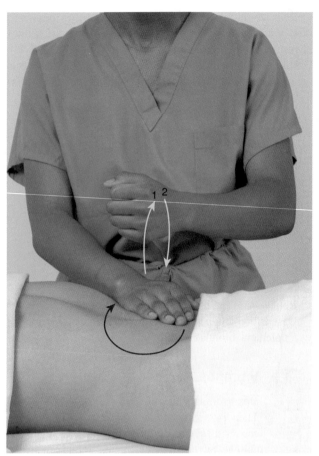

FIGURE 7-48 Diffused tapotement on supine client's abdomen.

while maintaining contact with the skin (Figure 7-49). This type of vibration is especially useful over the abdomen to increase peristalsis, stimulating digestion and elimination. The therapist's hand may remain in one location or glide down or around an area, such as the back, legs, or arms, while applying the quivering movement (Figure 7-50).

Another way to apply fine vibration is to compress and lift the tissue into your hands (Figure 7-51). Done properly, the stroke feels as though you are slurping up the tissue in your hands. Once this action is done, begin trembling the hand that is in direct contact with the tissue.

BOX 7-2

Ultrasound

Ultrasound is acoustic mechanical vibration of high frequency that produces thermal and nonthermal effects. Therapeutic ultrasound is unique because it falls within the acoustic spectrum and not within the electromagnetic spectrum. Physical and physiotherapists use an ultrasound machine to project microwaves beyond human hearing. Although ultrasound therapy is outside the scope of massage therapy, sonic (sound) energy can be transmitted into the body during tapotement delivery. Therapeutic ultrasound is known for its thermal effects, but its acoustic pressure changes are the most important. Therapeutic ultrasound is referred to as *micromassage*. It is also interesting that lower frequencies of sound penetrate farther into the tissue than higher frequencies.

Jostling – Jostling, or *coarse vibration,* can be used on a muscle belly, joint, or limb. When applying this technique to muscle, grasp the muscle belly or bellies and shake vigorously, but rhythmically, back and forth (Figure 7-52). This action may feel similar to rolling friction. Shortening the muscle by moving the attachments closer together creates slack in the muscle before applying vibration. Example: When jostling the hamstrings on a prone client, make sure the knee is flexed. If applied to a limb, then use one or both hands to grab the limb securely. The most proximal joint (e.g., shoulder or hip) is preferred. Add a small degree of traction by leaning back, shaking the limb (Figure 7-53). As in fine vibration, you can slide your hands down the limb, supporting it from behind, thumping it on the table (Figure 7-54). Coarse vibration can loosen up muscles surrounding a joint and is the principle stroke used in the Trager technique.

Rocking – Rocking vibration requires a pitch-and-catch motion. Push, or *pitch,* the body with one or both hands, then retrieving, or *catching,* it as the body swings back toward you (Figure 7-55). Pitch and catch the body until it begins to move easily or fluidly. You can also pitch and catch the body using one hand on each side of the body (Figure 7-56). A wonderful bodily sensation for the client, rocking is often physically taxing to the therapist, who should closely monitor his or her own personal exertion for setting the duration of the stroke. Not unlike pushing someone on a swing, timing of this stroke is everything. Some bodies have a quicker rattle,

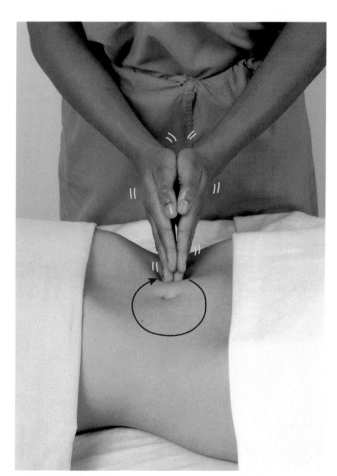

FIGURE 7-49 Fine vibration on abdomen with client supine.

JAMES HENRY CYRIAX, MD, MRCP

Born: 1904; died: June 17, 1985. Physician. Father of orthopedic medicine.

"He could often be seen walking backwards along Lambeth Palace Road round to the bus stop on Westminster Bridge so as to keep an eye on the oncoming buses."

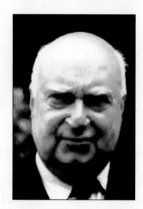

James Cyriax was born in London to Edgar and Annyuta (Kellgren) Cyriax, both of whom studied medicine. His mother's family used exercise and manipulation in the treatment of musculoskeletal disorders, something that was not a common practice at the time and that became very influential in Cyriax's medical career.

Young James was educated at University College School (Gonville) and Caius College (Cambridge) before finally graduating from St. Thomas's Hospital Medical School (London). Soon after passing his qualifying medical examinations, Cyriax became affiliated with St. Thomas's Hospital in the department of orthopedic surgery. He is generally given credit for coining the term *orthopedic medicine* and was probably one of Great Britain's most noted orthopedic practitioners. In 1938 Cyriax transformed the massage department at St. Thomas's into the first department of orthopedic medicine. His new department did much to help transform the art of manipulation into a science that was practiced by trained medical physicians and physical therapists.

Especially important among Cyriax's contributions was his system of soft-tissue diagnosis. According to his book *Textbook of Orthopedic Medicine* (1982 edition), Cyriax had a four-step process for determining problems of soft tissues: (1) active motion (to assess the patient's range of motion, strength, and willingness to move the affected area); (2) passive motion (to assess the degree of motion available and the direction of limitation, the use of palpable sensation at the end of passive motion that Cyriax called *end-feel,* and the determination of resistance felt by the practitioner during the end-feel testing); (3) resisted contractions (to determine the reaction of the muscle, tendon, and bony attachments to contraction); and (4) palpation (to confirm involvement of the structures suggested by the preceding three steps in the diagnostic procedure; Hayes et al, 1994).

In an effort to determine the exact location of a soft-tissue lesion, Cyriax's work is extremely important (although not without numerous critics) in that it helps therapists identify the tissues causing the pain and, consequently, select the best methods of treatment to diminish the pain. In general, Cyriax advocated the use of manipulation, deep friction massage (without the use of creams or oils), and the injection of selected drugs in the treatment of soft-tissue lesions. Even though Cyriax's ideas were (and remain) controversial, he provided the first systematic diagnostic approach to determine the cause of a patient's soft-tissue disorder.

An important point to note is that Cyriax was a firm believer in deep-tissue massage (deep transverse friction), either alone or in conjunction with passive or active movements, for the treatment of muscular, ligamentous, and tendinous lesions. In his book *Textbook of Orthopedic Medicine* (1982 edition), he wrote, "Deep transverse friction restores mobility to muscle in the same way a manipulation frees a joint. Indeed, the action of deep transverse friction may be summed up as affording a mobilization that passive stretching or active exercises cannot achieve."

According to Cyriax's obituary in the *British Medical Journal* (July 1, 1985), he was apparently *persona non grata* within the British medical establishment because of his nontraditional views and consequently was never elected a fellow of the British Royal College of Physicians. His work continues to be scrutinized, as an examination of the various journals within the physical medicine profession attest. He was an individual who brought out the extremes in individuals, with both his supporters and critics being adamant about their views. Regardless, Cyriax was instrumental in advancing the concepts of manipulation and massage in the medical profession, making incalculable contributions to those professions.

A key indicator of the importance of James H. Cyriax's contributions is the fact that his book *Textbook of Orthopedic Medicine* is presently in its ninth edition.

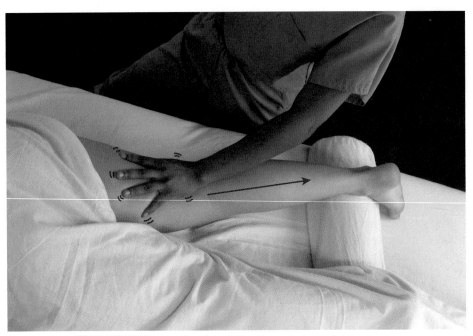

FIGURE 7-50 Fine vibration sliding down the leg with client prone.

whereas others have a slow, full rock. Support the client's own movement pattern, whether it is a rattle or a rock. The gentle rocking in a mother's womb or in a parent's arms is probably the first motion your body experiences. Even as adults, we find comfort in this sensation.

Use of mechanical vibration – Place a towel on the client's skin for a more comfortable delivery of mechanical vibration.

If a corded unit is used, then the cord must be long enough to reach the area of treatment from an electrical outlet. Make sure the cord does not touch the client. If the cord is long enough, then drape it over your shoulder while holding the appliance. Never leave the appliance on the floor or the cord stretched out; someone may trip over it. Check the cord often for wear, and replace it immediately if it is frayed.

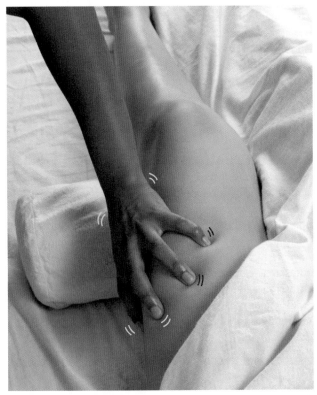

FIGURE 7-51 Fine vibration slurping up the tissue on the quadriceps with client supine.

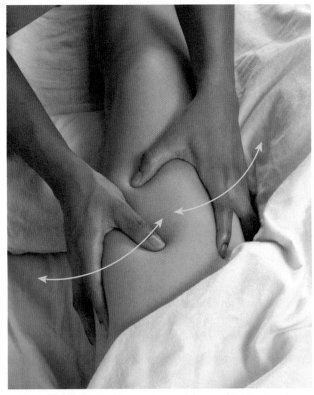

FIGURE 7-52 Jostling on the quadriceps with client supine.

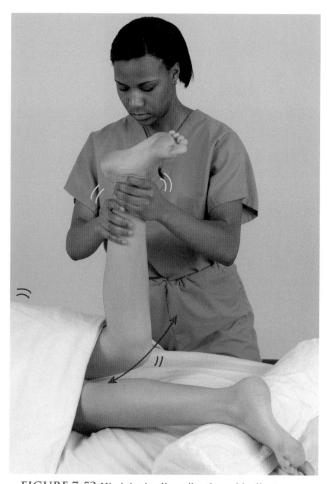

FIGURE 7-53 Hip joint jostling vibration with client prone.

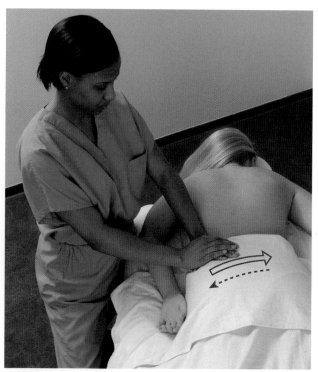

FIGURE 7-55 Rocking vibration using hand-over-hand with client prone.

The use of handheld vibrators or electric vibrators that strap to the back of your hand should be kept to a minimum. Prolonged use of these appliances has a harmful effect on the nervous system of the therapist. Vibration applied on one area for more than a few minutes will create an unpleasant numbing sensation. After prolonged mechanical vibration, a rash may appear, indicating tissue irritation. Prolonged vibration can also break down collagen. In many instances, massage therapists who frequently use handheld electric vibrators experience nerve damage of the hand. In some cases, nerve damage was so severe that opening a jar lid was difficult and painful.

Benefits
Used during a massage, vibration does the following:
* Enhances general relaxation
* Increases circulation
* Stimulates muscle spindles, thereby creating minute muscle contractions
* Relieves pain
* Relieves upper respiratory tract congestion, including sinus congestion
* Stimulates peristalsis of the large intestine
* Moves gas in the lower gastrointestinal tract
* Stimulates synovial fluid production in joints when applied with traction
* Accesses deeper structures such as hip rotators
* Reduces trigger and tender point activity

"Often the hands will solve a mystery that the intellect has struggled with in vain."
C. G. Jung

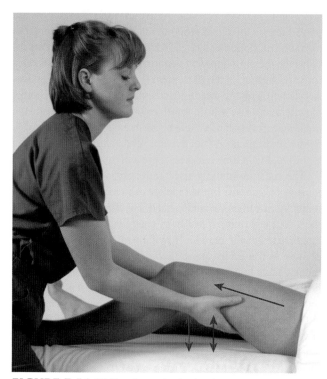

FIGURE 7-54 Sliding down the back of the leg while coarsely vibrating with client supine.

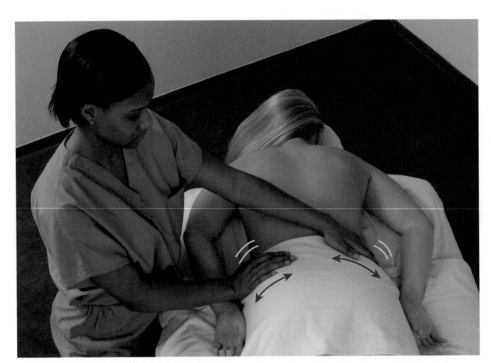

FIGURE 7-56 Rocking vibration with two hands on either side of the hips with client prone.

MINI-LAB

To demonstrate the ability to relax the body during vibration, perform the following activity. With a partner, decide who will be the giver and who will be the receiver. Stand approximately 18 to 24 inches apart. The giver grasps the receiver's wrist and pulls, using moderate force. Note the response of the receiver's body. Let go and again grasp the receiver's wrist. Pull, using moderate force, only this time rock or shake the arm as you do so. Note the response of the receiver's body. Ask the receiver to share his or her experience with both techniques. Perform the exercise again, reversing roles. Is tensing up and resisting the forward movement more difficult while your body is being rocked? Might the rocking movement also be providing a distracting element, interfering with the body's tendency to stiffen?

SWEDISH GYMNASTICS

During the massage, the therapist takes special care to address the client's needs with massage strokes, applying pressure up to the client's tolerance on tender areas. To further assist the client in restoring healthy tissue and pain-free movements, the therapist may use another method of the Swedish system called **Swedish gymnastics.** These movements are used to reduce pain, restore mobility, and maintain health. These movements of joints (range of motion) and muscles (stretching) provide a variety of treatment options, add a kinesthetic element to the session, and can easily be applied before, during, or after the massage. If the latter two are used, then you may need to wipe off any excess lubricant. Ideally, the therapist uses Swedish gymnastics to mobilize and stretch articulated segments of the client's body. Also referred to as *therapeutic exercise,* much of Swedish gymnastics can be used by the client at home to extend the benefits received during the massage.

Description

(7-7)

The movements used in Swedish gymnastics can be classified into two primary categories, (1) *passive* and (2) *active.* **Passive movements** are applied by the therapist while the client remains relaxed (or passive). **Active movements** involve the therapist describing or demonstrating the movement while the client actively performs the movement. Active stretching has two variations: (1) *active assisted* and (2) *active resisted.* **Active-assisted movements** are performed by the client while the therapist assists throughout the range of motion or stretch. **Active-resisted movements** involve the therapist applying gentle resistance while the client is actively engaged in the movement (Figure 7-57). When active-assisted or active-resisted movements are performed at home, the client may use a wall, towel, or other object to provide the assistance or resistance. Active movements are vital to health. Passive movements do not dynamically engage the muscle and therefore do not tone muscles or prevent muscle atrophy.

The most commonly used movements are *stretches* and *joint mobilizations.* In the practice of massage, stretching and joint mobilizations go hand in hand. The therapist may mobilize the joint, performing a stretch by changing the joint position to lengthen a specific muscle. How far a muscle can be stretched or how well a joint can be mobilized depends on numerous factors, including the client's flexibility, genetic limitations, the health of the involved joint, fascial restrictions, muscle tension, muscle guarding, past injuries, and past surgeries. *Flexibility* is the ability of muscles and other soft tissues to lengthen and shorten through the range of motion for which they are intended. Although these factors may reduce a person's ability to move, we can use massage therapy and Swedish gymnastics to increase flexibility, reduce pain, and restore function.

Joint mobilizations involve moving a joint through its normal range of motion. **Stretching** involves a single muscle (and its synergist) being drawn out to its fullest length. Be familiar with the type of joint with which you are working and the movements possible at that joint and the muscles causing the movement. The information found in Chapters 13, 14, 15, and 16 will prove invaluable. Furthermore, use proper body mechanics when applying stretching or joint mobilizations because they are physically demanding on the therapist, particularly when the client is large. Avoid stretching or mobilization if swelling is present around the area.

The purpose of this section is to give the beginning massage therapist a basic understanding of both stretching and joint mobilizations and to foster a desire for further learning. Books and workshops are available to assist the student in this task. Additionally, massage therapists should check their state's definition of scope of practice for the inclusion or exclusion of Swedish gymnastics (stretching modalities and joint mobilizations).

Technique

Use caution if any abnormality is present, such as a surgical replacement, pins or wires, and any conditions in which movement must be limited or avoided, such as edema, inflammation, osteoporosis, rheumatoid or osteoarthritis, dislocations, scoliosis, spondylolisthesis, spondylosis, and hypermobility. The body must be warmed up before applying stretches or joint mobilizations. If the movements are performed before the massage, then the therapist may use rocking vibration or superficial warming friction over the treatment area. If the client performs the movements at home, then light activity should be done before the stretches or mobilizations. The principle is simple; similar to clay, warm tissues are pliable and can move and stretch without tearing. Cold tissues tend to be rigid and less malleable, making them more susceptible to injury.

Avoid fast, bouncy, or *ballistic* movements because they can cause the muscle to contract, thereby limiting the effec-

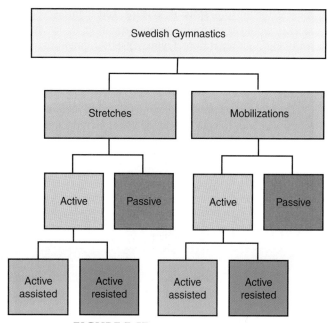

FIGURE 7-57 Swedish gymnastics.

tiveness of the movement. A succession of ballistic movements can cause irritation or even tear the muscle, fascia, tendons, and ligaments (Box 7-3). The lengthening and sweeping motions should be gentle and not induce pain. Avoid overextending or overtreating; use a *static* stretch. The client should try to relax and inhale at the beginning of the movement and exhale during the stretch or mobilization. Take the joint through three range-of-motion exercises or a muscle through three stretch repetitions. **Range of motion** is movement around a joint or set of joints. Hold the stretched

BOX 7-3

Stretch Reflexes

The two types of reflexes associated with stretching are the *myotatic stretch reflex* and *inverse stretch reflex.* Each reflex is associated with a corresponding sensory nerve initiating the reflex. Both reflexes are safeguards activated by extremes in movement. The myotatic stretch reflex is initiated when a muscle is pulled suddenly, initiating contraction. The receptor detecting the abrupt stretch, the *muscle spindle,* is located within the muscle belly. An impulse is sent to the spinal cord, thereby triggering a motor response of contraction. This reaction is designed to protect the joint from further movement in that direction and the muscle from overstretching by causing the muscle to contract. The force of the muscle contraction is somewhat related to the force and speed of the stretch that triggers it.

The *Golgi tendon organs* mediate the second stretch reflex, the inverse stretch reflex. These receptors measure changes in distance or degree of tensile force between the fibers of the muscle-tendon junction. When Golgi tendon organs are stimulated by slow, low-force stretches, they inhibit regular muscle contraction, thereby relaxing the entire muscle and allowing maximal stretching.

In summary, myotatic stretch reflex stimulates muscle spindles, which initiates muscle contraction; inverse stretch reflex stimulates Golgi tendon organs, which inhibits muscle contraction.

muscle for up to 5 seconds, release, and then take up the slack and hold again for the second repetition. Repeat for the third and final repetition. Try to sense movement drag and end-feel (see Chapter 26). These feelings offer vital feedback as to the condition of the tissues and the limitations of motion.

The techniques presented in the following section are basic passive movements. A brief description of the movement is presented with pictorial representation. Both mobilization and stretches are addressed in the prone and supine positions. Practice these Swedish movements with an instructor or an experienced therapist.

Neck

(7-8) Movements of the neck include flexion, extension, lateral flexion, and rotation. These movements, performed while the client is in the supine position, include *neck circles, neck lateral flexion, neck lateral flexion with rotation,* and *neck forward flexion* (Table 7-2). Apply these movements using gentle to moderate pressure.

Wrist and Hand

(7-9) The four movements of the wrist are abduction, adduction, flexion, and extension. Do not apply excessive pressure while moving the wrist and

TABLE 7-2 **Neck Gymnastics**

MOVEMENT	FIGURE NUMBER	STRETCH OR MOBILIZATION	PRONE OR SUPINE	DESCRIPTION
Neck circles	7-58	Mobilization	Supine	Place one hand on the client's forehead, rocking the client's head back and forth while your other hand intermittently pulls the tissue in lamina groove on the opposite side up and toward you.
Neck lateral flexion	7-59	Stretch	Supine	With one hand, pull the client's head toward the near shoulder while your hand stabilizes the client's far shoulder.
Neck lateral flexion with rotation	7-60	Stretch	Supine	With one hand, hold and pull the client's head (rotated toward the near shoulder) toward the near shoulder while your other hand stabilizes the client's far shoulder. Repeat with client's head rotated toward far shoulders.
Neck forward flexion	7-61	Stretch	Supine	With one or both hands, hold the client's shoulders while your criss-crossed forearms support the client's posterior head and neck as the head is lifted toward the chest.

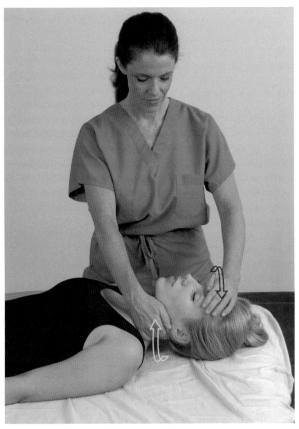

FIGURE 7-58 Neck circles.

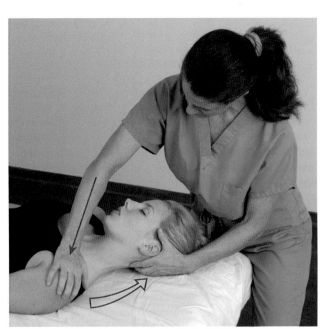

FIGURE 7-59 Neck lateral flexion.

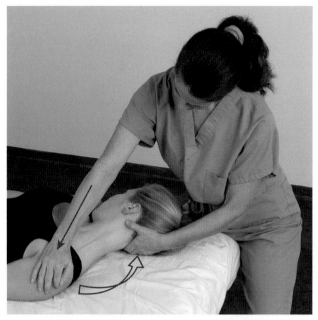

FIGURE 7-60 Neck lateral flexion with rotation.

hand. Swedish gymnastics used for this area, which can be done while the client is lying prone or supine, are *flip wrist, interlace fingers during movements, metacarpal scissors, circumduct fingers,* and *pull fingers* (Table 7-3).

 (7-10) ### Shoulder and Elbow
The movements of the shoulder are flexion, extension, adduction, abduction, rotation, and circumduction. The elbow permits flexion, extension, and rotation. Most of the basic gymnastic movements are best applied while the client is supine but can be adapted for the prone client. The basic movements are *pull arm down side, pull abducted arm, push adducted arm, pull arm overhead, big shoulder circles,* and *little shoulder circles* (Table 7-4).

 (7-11) ### Chest
The Swedish gymnastics movements for the chest area use simple pulling and compressing of the ribcage while the client is supine. Hence these

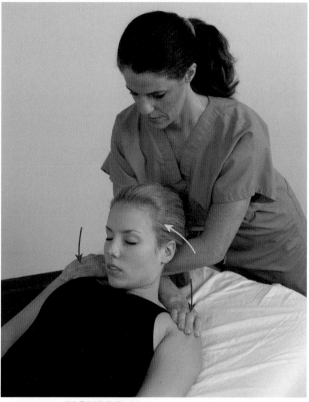

FIGURE 7-61 Neck forward flexion.

movements are called *lift ribcage* and *compress ribcage* (Table 7-5).

 (7-12) ### Back
The Swedish gymnastics movement for the spine uses a lengthening and twisting motion on the supine-lying client and is called *spinal twist* (Table 7-6). The upper or lower portion of the spine may be isolated with a simple modification.

 (7-13) ### Hip and Knee
Some hip movements are adduction, abduction, and circumduction. Both the hip and knee can flex and extend, as well as medially and laterally

TABLE 7-3 Wrist and Hand Gymnastics

MOVEMENT	FIGURE NUMBER	STRETCH OR MOBILIZATION	PRONE OR SUPINE	DESCRIPTION
Flip wrist	7-62	Mobilization	Prone or supine	Use your fingers below the client's wrist to flip it while your thumbs stabilize the top of the client's wrist.
Interlace fingers during movements	7-63	Mobilization	Prone or supine	Interlace your fingers with the client's fingers while moving the wrist into flexion, extension, abduction, and adduction as your other hand stabilizes the client's flexed arm above the wrist.
Metacarpal scissors	7-64	Mobilization	Prone or supine	While holding the client's metacarpals, alternately move them up and down.
Circumduct fingers	7-65	Mobilization	Prone or supine	With one hand, hold the client's hand while your other hand circumducts each finger and thumb with mild traction.
Pull fingers	7-66	Stretch	Prone or supine	With one hand, hold the client's hand while your other hand pulls each of the client's fingers and thumb.

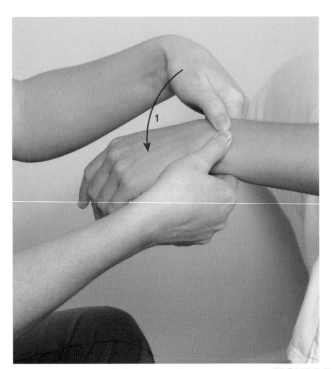 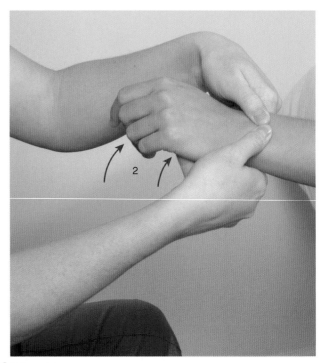

FIGURE 7-62 Flip wrist.

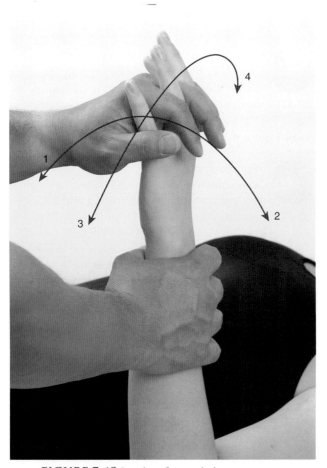

FIGURE 7-63 Interlace fingers during movements.

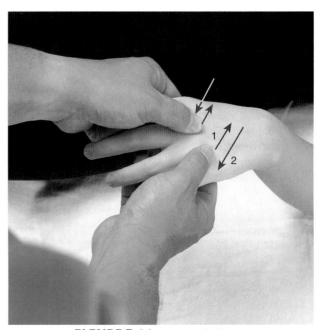

FIGURE 7-64 Metacarpal scissors.

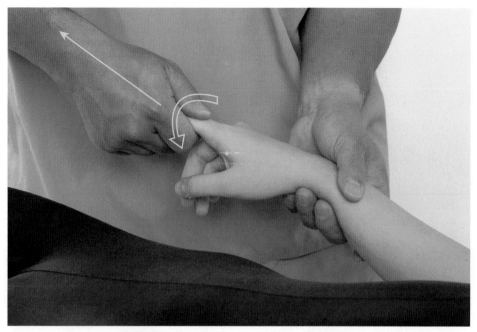

FIGURE 7-65 Circumduct fingers with traction.

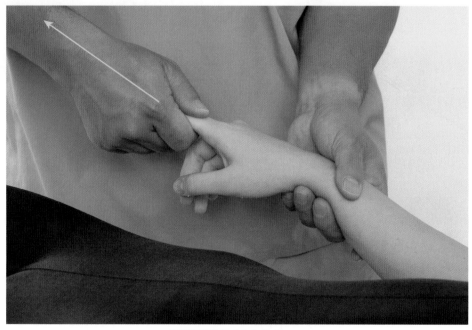

FIGURE 7-66 Pull fingers.

TABLE 7-4 **Shoulder and Elbow Gymnastics**

MOVEMENT	FIGURE NUMBER	STRETCH OR MOBILIZATION	PRONE OR SUPINE	DESCRIPTION
Pull arm down side	7-67	Stretch	Prone or supine	While standing tableside, grasp the client's wrist and pull firmly down toward the toes several times.
Pull abducted arm	7-68	Stretch	Prone or supine	While standing several feet away from the table's side, grasp the client's wrist and pull the arm straight out to the side firmly several times.
Push adducted arm	7-69	Stretch	Supine	Push the client's shoulder and arm horizontally across the table.
Pull arm overhead	7-70	Stretch	Supine	While standing at the head of the table, grasp the client's wrist and pull firmly several times.
Big shoulder circles	7-71	Mobilization	Supine	Beginning with the client's arm at his or her side, pull arm up over the client's head then down to side by bending the elbow while maintaining traction during the movement.
Little shoulder circles	7-72	Mobilization	Prone or supine	Grasp above and below the client's shoulder, moving it in a circular direction.

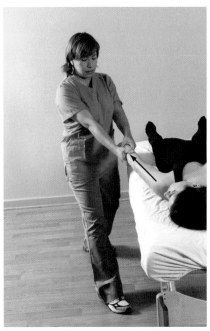

FIGURE 7-67 Pull arm down side.

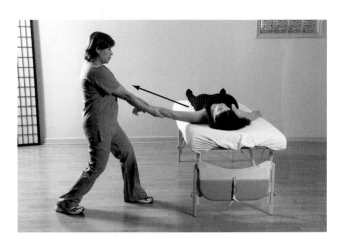

FIGURE 7-68 Pull abducted arm.

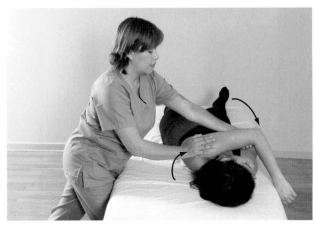

FIGURE 7-69 Push adducted arm.

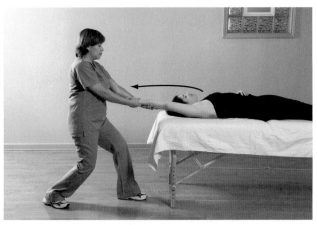

FIGURE 7-70 Pull arm overhead.

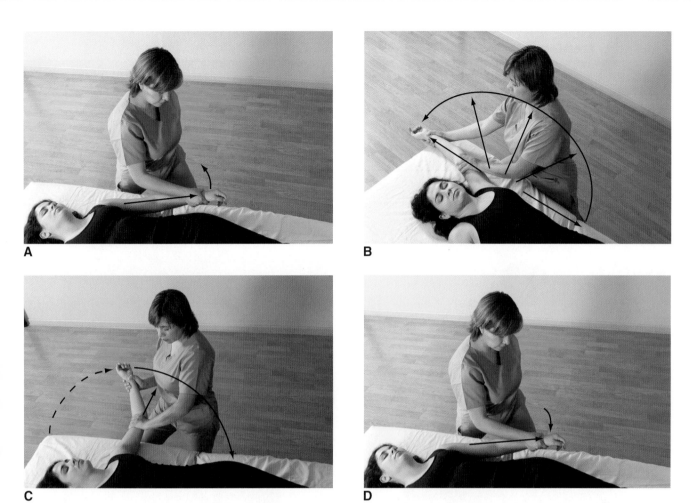

FIGURE 7-71 Big shoulder circles.

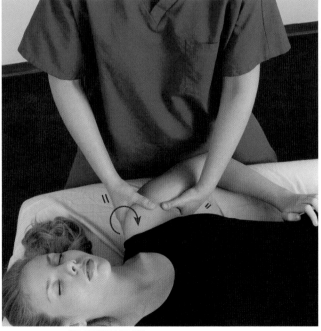

FIGURE 7-72 Little shoulder circles.

TABLE 7-5 **Chest Gymnastics**

MOVEMENT	FIGURE NUMBER	STRETCH OR MOBILIZATION	PRONE OR SUPINE	DESCRIPTION
Lift ribcage	7-73	Stretch	Supine	While reaching across table, grasp the back of the client's ribcage, pulling up and toward you. Release and repeat.
Compress ribcage	7-74	Mobilization	Supine	Using one or two hands, gently compress the client's ribcage down several times. Release after each compression.

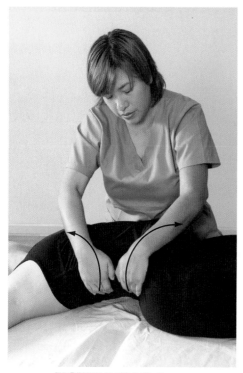

FIGURE 7-73 Lift ribcage.

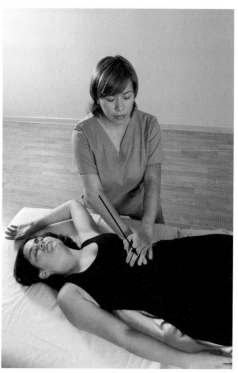

FIGURE 7-74 Compress ribcage.

rotate. Most Swedish gymnastics can be applied while the client is prone or supine. These basic movements are the *leg pull, leg rock, hip clock stretch, hip circles, groin stretch, hip rotations, heel to hip,* and *hip hyperextension* (Table 7-7).

Ankle and Foot
The ankle and foot movements, which include dorsiflexion, plantar flexion, inversion, and ever-
(7-14) sion, can be applied while the client is prone or supine. These gymnastics movements are *plantar flex ankle, dorsiflex ankle, leg rotations* (using the foot to mobilize the hip), *metatarsal scissors, circumduct toes,* and *pull toes* (Table 7-8).

Benefits

Benefits of Swedish gymnastics include the following:
- Promotes relaxation
- Decreases pain
- Increases circulation
- Relieves muscle soreness
- Aids in rehabilitation
- Increases and maintains flexibility and range of motion
- Reduces muscle guarding
- Resets the muscular tone around a joint, thereby increasing joint mobility
- Stimulates synovial fluid production
- Increases kinesthetic awareness
- Improves body alignment and posture
- Assists the therapist in assessing tissues

TABLE 7-6 **Back Gymnastics**

MOVEMENT	FIGURE NUMBER	STRETCH OR MOBILIZATION	PRONE OR SUPINE	DESCRIPTION
Spinal twist	7-75, A	Stretch	Supine	With the client's near leg bent and the foot placed on the lateral side of the far knee, push the bent knee away from you while pulling the far shoulder toward you.
	7-75, B			Anchor far shoulder while you pull bent far knee toward you and down.
	7-75, C			Anchor near shoulder while you push bent near knee away from you.

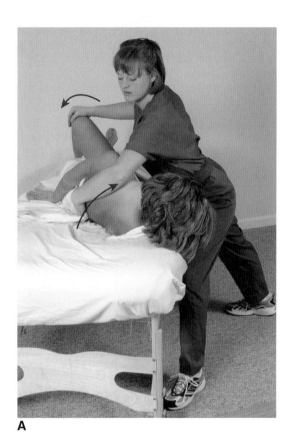

A

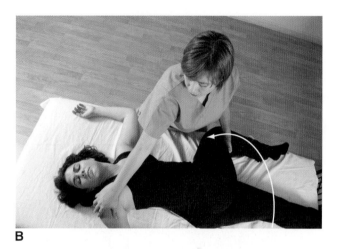

B

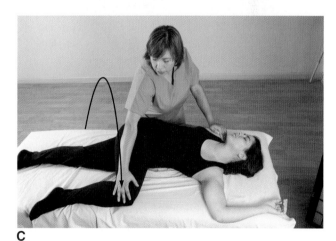

C

FIGURE 7-75 Spinal twist.

TABLE 7-7 **Hip and Knee Gymnastics**

MOVEMENT	FIGURE NUMBER	STRETCH OR MOBILIZATION	PRONE OR SUPINE	DESCRIPTION
Leg pull	7-76	Stretch	Prone or supine	While standing at the foot of the table, grasp the client's ankle and pull firmly several times.
Leg rock	7-77	Mobilization	Supine	While standing tableside, place your hands above and below the client's knee and rock back and forth.
Hip clock stretch	7-78	Stretch	Supine	Flex the client's hip and knee while supporting both the knee and heel; imagining that the client's lower leg is the hour hand of a clock, push and stretch the hip in a 10 o'clock, 12 o'clock, and 2 o'clock stretch.
Hip circles	7-79	Mobilization	Supine	Move the client's flexed hip and knee in a circular direction. Reverse direction
Groin stretch	7-80	Stretch	Prone or supine	Place the client's flexed far leg on the table with the foot by the straight near knee; stretch by gently compressing the near knee.
Hip rotations	7-81	Mobilization	Prone or supine	Picking up the client's near leg above and below the knee, rotate the hip by pushing the leg in, to the side, and out several times. Reverse direction.
Heel to hip	7-82	Stretch	Prone	Flex the client's near knee, bringing the heel toward the hip.
Hip hyperextension	7-83	Stretch	Prone	Pick up and hyperextend the client's near hip while the knee is flexed. The lifting hand should be placed above the near knee.

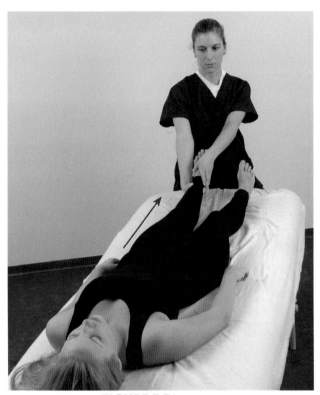

FIGURE 7-76 Leg pull.

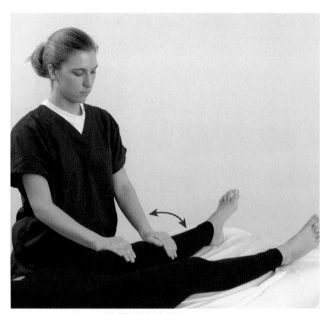

FIGURE 7-77 Leg rock.

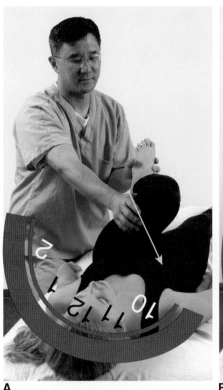

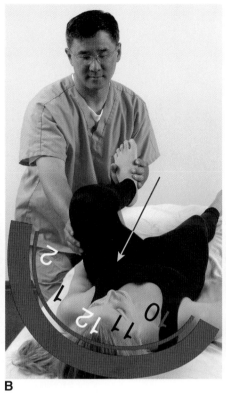

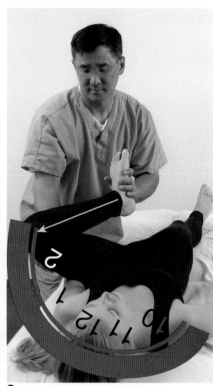

A   B   C

FIGURE 7-78 Hip clock stretch.

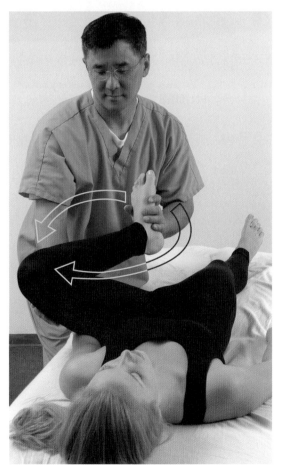

FIGURE 7-79 Hip circles.

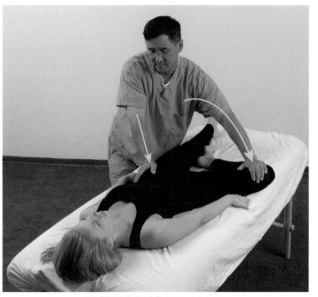

FIGURE 7-80 Groin stretch.

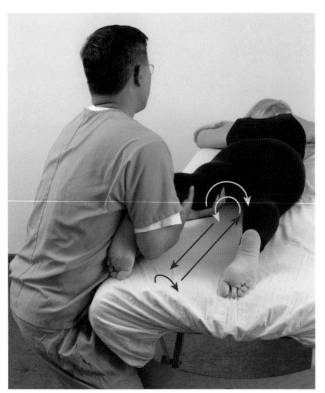

FIGURE 7-81 Hip rotations.

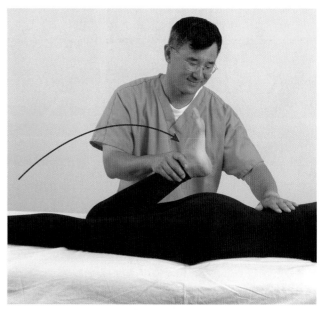

FIGURE 7-82 Heel to hip.

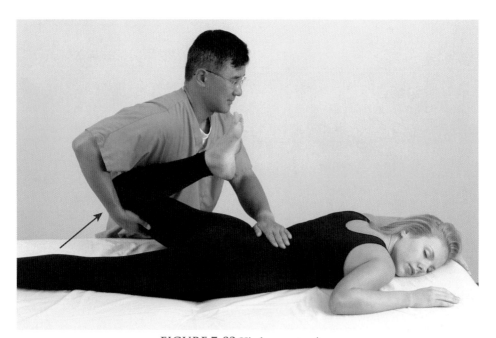

FIGURE 7-83 Hip hyperextension.

TABLE 7-8 **Ankle and Foot Gymnastics**

MOVEMENT	FIGURE NUMBER	STRETCH OR MOBILIZATION	PRONE OR SUPINE	DESCRIPTION
Plantar flex ankle	7-84	Stretch	Prone or supine	While holding the client's heel with one hand, push down on the top of the foot with the other hand.
Dorsiflex ankle	7-85	Stretch	Prone or supine	Hold the client's heel with one hand while pushing the ball of the foot toward the knee with the other hand.
Leg rotations	7-86	Mobilization	Supine	Rotate the hip by circumducting the toes as you hold the client's heel as though a handle. Reverse direction.
Metatarsal scissors	7-87	Mobilization	Prone or supine	While holding the client's metatarsals, move them up and down.
Circumduct toes	7-88	Mobilization	Prone or supine	Support the client's foot with one hand while the other hand circumducts each toe with mild traction.
Pull toes	7-89	Stretch	Prone or supine	With one hand, hold the client's foot while your other hand pulls each of the client's toes.

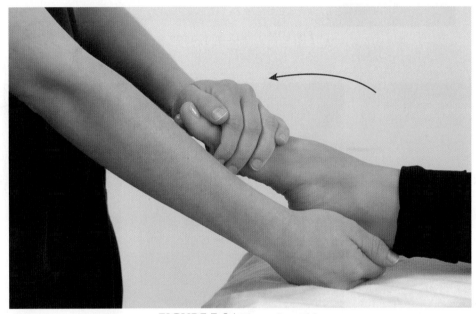

FIGURE 7-84 Plantar flex ankle.

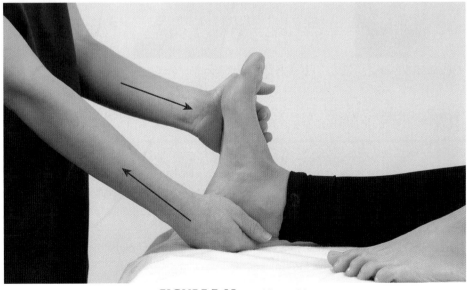

FIGURE 7-85 Dorsiflex ankle.

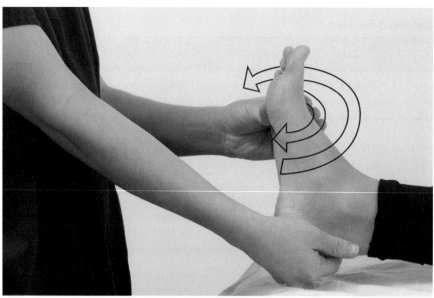

FIGURE 7-86 Leg rotations.

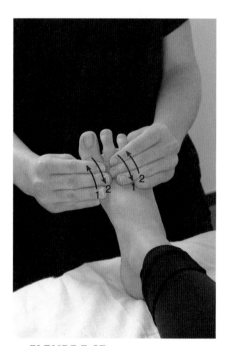

FIGURE 7-87 Metatarsal scissors.

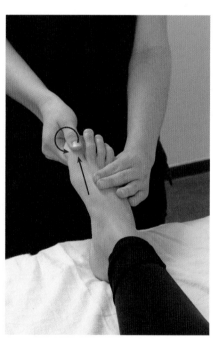

FIGURE 7-88 Circumduct toes.

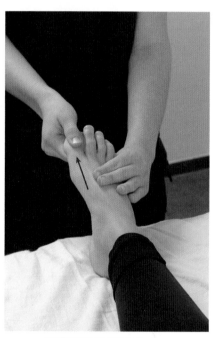

FIGURE 7-89 Pull toes.

SUMMARY

Massage may be used to relax the body or to rehabilitate an injury. Swedish massage is the grandparent of most Western forms of massage therapy. It uses the following five main strokes: effleurage, pétrissage, friction, tapotement, and vibration. Execution of these strokes can be measured by several qualities, including intention, touch, depth, pressure, direction, excursion, speed, rhythm, continuity, duration, and sequence.

Swedish gymnastics, performed on articulated body segments, includes stretches and joint mobilizations and can be performed actively and passively. Active movements can be assisted or resisted.

CASE STUDY:

Client Gifts

Chastity, a massage therapist, had a marriage that was coming to an end. She worked in a contract labor setting for another massage therapist, Jill. To minimize expenses, Chastity was looking for a cheaper apartment. Chastity had had a difficult time with the separation, and the stress was evident to many of her clients. One client, Bill, had questioned her until she had finally divulged her dilemma. That night, Bill talked the problem over with his wife, Marjorie, and then offered to let Chastity stay at their camp on the river, rent free, until she got back on her feet financially. Chastity was so excited to finally get a break. When Jill came in to close the books for the day, Chastity was bubbling over and proceeded to tell her boss about her new living arrangements. Jill was quiet for a moment and then said, "Chastity, we need to talk."

Jill's view was that accepting free rent from a client, especially one of the opposite gender, was an unethical decision. "What will you do if he just shows up and lets himself in unexpectedly?" Jill asked. "What if he asks for legitimate favors? Aren't you going to feel somewhat indebted?"

Jill tried to get Chastity to understand her point of view, but Chastity just became sullen and eventually hostile. "I thought you'd be happy for me," cried Chastity, barely able to hold back the tears.

Despite the fact that Chastity had been a loyal and productive employee for several years, Jill told her that she had to make a choice—find another living arrangement or find a new job.

If you were Chastity, how would you analyze the situation ethically? How would you approach Jill for further dialogue on the subject? What would your decision be in regard to the situation?

If you were Jill, what would you do to put yourself in Chastity's place?

What, if any, compromise would you be willing to make?

If Chastity chooses to stay, what kind of dialogue might prevent further similar occurrences?

If Chastity chooses to leave, what kind of references would you give to a prospective employer?

---

evolve

Go to *Chapter Extras* on Evolve for additional illustrations and resources for this chapter. *Extras* for this chapter include:

1. Crossword puzzle (downloadable form)
2. Effleurage (video clip)
3. Pétrissage (video clip)
4. Friction (video clip)
5. Vibration (video clip)
6. Tapotement (video clip)
7. Mechanical vibration (illustration)
8. Case study (text)

MATCHING

Place the letter of the answer next to the term or phrase that best describes it.

A. Active-assisted movements
B. Active movements
C. Active-resisted movements
D. Continuity
E. Cross-fiber friction
F. Effleurage

G. Friction
H. Joint mobilization
I. Nerve stroke
J. Passive movements
K. Pétrissage

L. Rhythm
M. Stretching
N. Swedish gymnastics
O. Tapotement
P. Vibration

_____ 1. Movements that are described or demonstrated by the therapist while the client actively performs the movements

_____ 2. The repetition or regularity of massage movements

_____ 3. The uninterrupted flow of massage strokes; unbroken transition from one stroke to the next

_____ 4. Gliding movements that are repeated and follow the contour of the client's body

_____ 5. Considered a light effleurage, the massage stroke that consists of feather-light finger tracing over the skin

_____ 6. Massage stroke that consists of rhythmic lifting, squeezing, and releasing of the tissue

_____ 7. Massage stroke performed by rubbing one surface over another

_____ 8. A precise and penetrating form of friction, popularized by Dr. James Cyriax of London, in which the direction of movement is across and perpendicular to the tissue fibers

_____ 9. Repetitive staccato striking movements of the therapist hands on the client's skin

_____ 10. Rapid shaking, quivering, trembling, or rocking massage movements applied with the fingertips, a full hand, or an appliance

_____ 11. Part of the Swedish system that consists of active and passive stretches and joint mobilizations to reduce pain, restore mobility, and maintain health

_____ 12. Movements applied by therapist while client remains relaxed (or passive)

_____ 13. Active movements performed by client with therapist assisting

_____ 14. Therapist applies gentle resistance while client is actively engaged in a movement

_____ 15. Moving a joint through its normal range of motion

_____ 16. Drawing out a single muscle (and its synergist) to its fullest length

INTERNET ACTIVITIES

Visit http://www.thebodyworker.com and click on Psychology. Scroll down the article until you see the featured word Intention. After reading, write a short paragraph on the subject.

Visit http://www.massagetherapyfoundation.org and click on Students. Locate the Student Case Report, and, after reading, discuss the report with a classmate.

Visit http://www.thebodyworker.com and click on Self Care. Scroll down the article until you see the featured phrase Self Care Tips. Jot down a few suggested tips. Use the suggestions in the text and the ones on your list to create a poster board to display in class.

Bibliography

Anderson B: *Stretching,* Bolinas, Calif, 1980, Shelter Publications.

Beck MF: *Theory and practice of therapeutic massage,* ed 4, Albany, NY, 2005, Thomson Delmar Learning.

Benjamin PF, Tappan: *Tappan's handbook of healing massage technique,* ed 4, Upper Saddle River, NJ, 2004, Prentice Hall.

Chaitow L: *Modern neuromuscular techniques,* ed 2, New York, 2003, Churchill Livingstone.

Coughlin P: *Principles and practice of manual therapeutics,* New York, 2002, Churchill Livingstone.

Drez D: *Therapeutic modalities for sports injuries,* St Louis, 1989, Mosby.

Hayes KW et al: An examination of Cyriax's passive motion tests with patients having osteoarthritis of the knee, *Phys Ther* 74(8):697-708, 1994.

Juhan D: *Job's body, a handbook for bodyworkers,* ed 3, Barrington, NY, 2003, Station Hill Press.

Kendall FP, McCreary EK, Provance PG: *Muscles: testing and function,* Baltimore, 1993, Lippincott Williams & Wilkins.

Krieger D: Therapeutic touch: the imprimatur of nursing, *AJN* 75(5):784-787, 1975.

Mackey B: Massage therapy and reflexology awareness, *Nurs Clin North Am* 36(1):159-170, 2001.

Mattes A: *Active isolated stretching,* self-published by Aaron Mattes, 2000.

Mennell JB: *Physical treatment,* ed 5, Philadelphia, 1945, Blakiston.

Moore KL: *Clinically oriented anatomy,* ed 5, Baltimore, 2005, Lippincott Williams & Wilkins.

Platzer W: *Color atlas and textbook of human anatomy: locomotor system,* vol 1, ed 3, New York, 1984, Thieme.

Prudden B: *Pain erasure,* New York, 1980, M Evans.

Reed B, Held JM: Effects of sequential connective tissue massage on autonomic nervous system of middle-aged and elderly adults, *Phys Ther* 68(8):1231-1234, 1988.

St. John P: *St. John neuromuscular therapy seminars: manual I,* Largo, Fla, 1995, self-published.

Thompson C: Oil on troubled waters? *Nurs Times* 97(15):74-77, 2001.

Travell JG, Simons D: *Myofascial pain and dysfunction, the trigger point manual,* Baltimore, 1992, Lippincott Williams & Wilkins.

Venes D, Thomas CL, Taber CW: *Taber's cyclopedic medical dictionary,* ed 20, Philadelphia, 2005, FA Davis.

Voss DE, Ionta MK, Myers BJ: *Proprioceptive neuromuscular facilitation,* Philadelphia, 1985, Harper and Row.

Williams RE: *The road to radiant health,* College Place, Wash, 1977, Color Press.

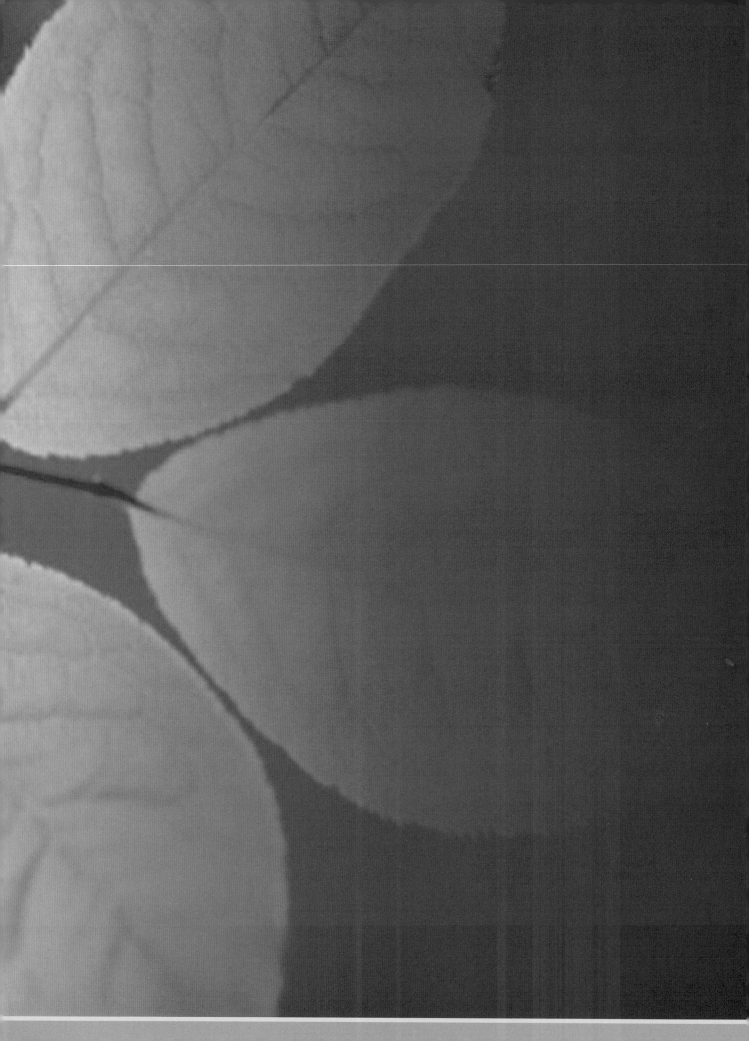

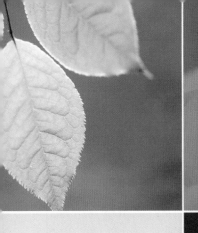

CHAPTER **8**

Assessment and Planning

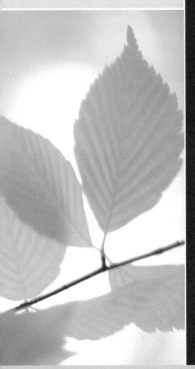

STUDENT OBJECTIVES

After completing this chapter, the student should be able to:

- State the value of assessment and planning
- List reasons for collecting and documenting client information
- Develop a client intake form
- Design an informed consent document
- Contrast and compare a client's right of refusal and a therapist's right of refusal
- Contrast and compare SOAP and APIE notes
- Conduct a client interview, using the interview skills and assessment domains discussed in the chapter
- Using data collected on the PPALM form, formulate a plan of care
- Define *subjective* and *objective* data
- State how data collection enhances the client-practitioner relationship
- List the minimum paperwork needed for a new client's initial session
- Discuss items to be included in the plan of care
- Use progress reporting to network with other health care professionals
- Outline important guidelines of the Health Insurance Portability and Accountability Act

INTRODUCTION

This chapter will examine the process of collecting client information, performing client assessment, and developing a plan of care. Because this process includes dialogue via an interview, it enhances feelings of connection and trust between the client and the therapist, forming the foundation of a positive, committed, and cooperative therapeutic relationship.

An effective therapist listens carefully to the client, identifying his or her needs, desires, and expectations, and then customizes the plan of care based on client intake and assessment. This process is documented, which reflects the quality of care for the client.

Experience is the best teacher. By palpating, questioning, listening, and treating, the massage therapist develops a sense of what is familiar, which, in turn, breeds knowledge, enhances skill, and promotes confidence. With practice, a client's intake, assessment, and plan of care will flow effortlessly.

 ## IMPORTANCE OF ASSESSMENT AND PLANNING

(8-1) For the massage to have a satisfying outcome for the client, the therapist needs a map. Each client possesses his or her own unique map, and the therapist's responsibility is to read the map and then follow it to the desired end—a satisfied client. Without this map, or treatment plan, the therapist cannot predict where he or she is going and may end up with an unsatisfied client, one who is not likely to return.

To draw this map, the therapist must collect information, conduct assessments, and then devise and execute a plan. This chapter focuses on these tasks.

An overall approach of assessment and planning is required to address client expectations and to prioritize needs. The systematic approach outlined in this chapter uses a diagram to arrange the information gathered in the assessment process and then to develop a treatment plan. The treatment plan serves as an organizational framework for the massage. The diagram itself is known as the **client web.** It encompasses all of the steps that the therapist takes in client assessment. **Assessment** is the process involved in appraising a client's condition based on subjective reporting and objective findings. The client's goals and objectives for the session will determine the length and depth of the assessment. Five assessment domains are featured, assisting the therapist in data collection.

From these steps, the therapist and the client develop a treatment plan. **Planning** is the therapist's strategy used to help the client achieve his or her goals, established once the assessment data are analyzed. The treatment plan is completed before the massage begins.

All information relevant to the assessment and client's plan of care is documented.

REASONS FOR COLLECTING AND DOCUMENTING CLIENT INFORMATION

Documentation is the process of providing written information regarding client care. A massage therapist needs to collect and document client information for many reasons. A primary reason is to create a holistic picture of the client's health, both past and present. This picture is the basis for planning the session, also known as *plan of care* or *treatment plan*. The **treatment plan** outlines steps the therapist will follow to provide a tailor-made session for each client, thereby improving professional services.

Second, documentation is a vital tool for communicating with other health care providers regarding how to serve the client's best interest, as well as how the client responded previously to the massage. The written word is the communication of choice in all professional arenas. Guidelines for sharing this information between your office and another health care provider are outlined in the Health Insurance Portability and Accountability Act (HIPAA) section presented later in this chapter.

Next, systematically collecting and documenting client information sharpen the therapist's critical thinking skills. Through written record, the therapist can confirm his or her educated assessments, choice of modalities, decisions to avoid or focus on an area, and pressure judgments. Alterations are made based on client response.

Another reason for assessment and documentation is that client records are legal evidence, which serves to protect the therapist by establishing professional accountability. Written communication decreases liability risks by verifying the information your client has shared with you and supports the treatment that the client received. Adequate and accurate documentation also helps in supporting payment reimbursement, improving the quality of client care, and demonstrating to the public that the therapist followed accepted standards of care mandated by law, the profession, and the health care facility. In the legal world, if an action is not documented, it was not done.

Furthermore, many state licensing boards are mandating systematic collection and ongoing documentation, which may be used in peer review, licensing determinations, and other legal proceedings.

Finally, relying on memory is poor record keeping. Written records serve to jog memory and to outline particular details for review; the more detailed and specific client notes are, the more accurate the assessment and planning will be. Given that written information is recorded on paper, or documented, the therapist can reread them when needed.

At this time, SOAP notes are the standard documentation method in the medical and paramedical fields.

Minimum paperwork consists of a health history or an intake form, a consent form, and a plan of care. However, observational test forms, policies and procedures, and therapy protocols are recommended for professional practice. Additional paperwork such as progress reports will be needed if you plan to assist the client with insurance or other forms of reimbursement or when following prescriptive directives.

Prescriptive directives: A prescription is a written order by a physician or other qualified health care provider to a person properly authorized to dispense or perform the order. The order is usually for medication, therapy, or a therapeutic device. If a therapist accepts a prescription for therapy, the prescription must then specify massage therapy, not physical or occupational therapy.

The prescription may instruct the therapist to *evaluate and treat* at the discretion of the therapist, or it may state a specific modality such as soft-tissue mobilization or massage. The prescription may also state how the massage is to be *taken* or *administered*. Massage is *taken* in increments known as sessions, with a specific time frame such as 60 minutes *(strength)*. The prescription may also specify frequency,

---

TABLE TALK

Prescription Versus Referral Form

Massage therapists have direct access to the public, meaning that no prescription or referral is needed to receive treatment. However, most insurance companies require documentation of referral or prescription when insurance is billed for massage services. In these cases, a medical physician, chiropractic physician, physician assistant, or nurse practitioner must complete one of two forms: (1) prescription and (2) referral.

A *prescription,* which literally means *take thou this,* is a written order by a physician or nurse practitioner authorizing massage therapy treatment. These orders are usually written on the physician's own personalized prescription pad. Parts of a prescription include the following:

- Date of the order
- Client's name
- Diagnosis and diagnosis code
- Treatment order
- Frequency of treatments
- Duration of treatments
- Referring health care provider's name, signature, and contact information

A *referral form* is generally produced by the provider (you) and given to and filled out by a health care provider authorizing massage therapy treatment. These forms may be personalized with the massage therapist's logo, name, address, telephone number, fax number, and other contact information. The form should have room for the patient's name, diagnosis, treatment choices (preferably with check boxes), and blank spaces for frequency and duration. At the bottom is a space for signature and office address stamp. These referral forms can be given one at a time to a specific patient who is seeking your services, and the patient can bring it to his or her physician for completion, or the therapist can drop a tablet of these forms off at the office of physicians who support massage therapy for their patients. Keep in mind that it does not matter on whose form the order is written. Just as you have your choice of pharmacy for medication, you also have your choice of therapist for massage. As with prescriptions, you cannot treat an order for physical therapy with massage therapy.

---

such as once a week, and duration, such as 6 weeks *(dosage).* If you have any problem understanding the order, call the physician's nurse or assistant to verify the order. At the end of the prescriptive period, the client returns to the referring health care provider for follow-up and evaluation. The original prescription becomes a permanent part of the client's file. The client may request a copy, and some insurance companies may require a copy as well, but the therapist retains the original.

OWNERSHIP AND RETENTION OF CLIENT RECORDS

Client records are considered the property of the owners of the facility where they were created. For example, a therapist in private practice owns his or her clients' records; client records acquired in a spa or clinic are the facility's property.

As a protection in the event of litigation, records should be kept until the applicable stature of limitations period has elapsed, which is generally 4 years after the last date of client service. This procedure is also the recommendation of the National Certification Board for Therapeutic Massage and Bodyworkers (NCBTMB), but requirements may vary from state to state.

Massage client records are not protected under the law because they are subject to subpoena by a court of law. However, treat client records with the same care for confidentially that a physician's office would use.

SUBJECTIVE VERSUS OBJECTIVE DATA

During the assessment process, the massage therapist collects subjective and objective information and combines these findings to formulate a plan of care.

Subjective Data
Subjective data are any information learned from the client or the client's family and friends; this information includes most written information obtained on the intake form and information gathered during conversation. The information is referred to as *subjective* because the client cannot present the information without personal bias—it is his or her perception or point of view. Of special note are the client's chief concern or complaint and his or her explanations of various symptoms. Important symptoms such as headaches, fatigue or depression, loss of sensation or the sensation of pins and needles, and painful or stiff joints are helpful to know because this information will affect the session. Listening is the primary skill used when gathering subjective information.

Objective Data
Objective data are measurable and quantitative and obtained by the therapist through **empirical** means (measurable and verifiable via the senses). Objective findings include the size and shape of a mole, whether the right shoulder is higher than the left shoulder, or whether the left knee is more swollen

(larger) than the right knee and by how much. The data may be a comparison of range of motion in one hip joint to the other. The main skills used for gathering objective information are observation and palpation, even though all senses participate in the process.

MINI-LAB

Without the use of sight, work in pairs and use palpation to find and note the differences among bone, muscle, tendons, lymph nodes, veins, arteries, and hair. This activity will help sharpen your palpatory skills.

Palpation, or palpatory assessment, is done through touching with purpose and intent and is an essential skill; massage therapists *see* with their fingers. Assessing tissues through touch includes locating muscle origin and insertion via tendons and bony markings, noting differences between muscle tension and tone, locating muscle spasms and trigger points, and locating fascial restrictions.

Palpation can detect temperature differences. Decreased circulation and interference with neurological health are two frequent causes of cool hands and feet. Temperature is commonly increased with fever and infection, inflammation, and tissue irritation. The therapist uses descriptive terms such as hot, swollen, or ropey, to record palpatory findings.

Comparing Subjective and Objective Data

To understand the difference between objective and subjective information, look at the following example. If a client comes into a massage therapist's office and enters his or her height and weight on the intake form, this information is subjective. If the therapist uses a tape measure and a scale to determine the client's height and weight, the information is objective.

> *"The body tells the story. It is, in fact, a living autobiography."*
> Elaine Mayland

DOCUMENTING FORMATS: SOAP NOTES VERSUS APIE NOTES

Client information must be organized. The two most popular formats are the SOAP note and the APIE note. The notation form used will depend on which system is in place where the therapist is employed or, if self-employed, the therapist's preference. All client records contain a baseline of information that is standard care for each client. Both formats have their strengths and weaknesses, but SOAP notes are the most widely used. Whatever format you decide, documentation of a client's complaint, condition, and treatment plan must be consistent, concise, and comprehensive.

SOAP stands for subjective, objective, assessment (or diagnosis), and plan.

In the initial SOAP note, the *S* is the *subjective* section that contains the client's experience of his or her condition, including symptoms, when and how the condition started, what makes it better or worse, and what has been done about it until now, as well as the results. In future sessions, the *S* section will state the client's updated, current experience of his or her condition, including impressions or responses to the previous session.

The *O* is the *objective* section that contains the therapist's visual and palpatory findings, as well as the results of any examinations or tests.

If you are working under prescriptive directives or billing insurance, all subjective and objective data must directly correspond to the physician's diagnosis.

The *A* is the *assessment* section that states the physician's diagnosis. In future sessions, the *A* section will contain therapist notes of what was done for that session.

The *P* is the *plan* portion that contains the treatment plan as directed by the physician, including the type, duration, and expected outcome or results. In future sessions, the *P* section will outline modalities and techniques used for future sessions and any suggested stretching or exercise.

One criticism of this format is that it lacks flexibility and usually focuses on only one problem. In addition, no consistency exists as to what *A* or *P* means or what information is placed in the *A* or the *P* sections of the format. For example, *A* might mean assessment, activity, or even analysis; *P* might mean procedure (past or present tense) or planning (future tense). For this reason, always include a legend.

Another variation of the SOAP note is the SOAPIER note. This abbreviation stands for subjective, objective, assessment (or diagnosis), plan, implementation, evaluation, and review.

The second most widely used format is the APIE format. APIE stands for assessment, plan of care, implementation, and evaluation. This format is becoming increasing popular because it encompasses a broader spectrum of client care than SOAP notes.

The *A*, or *assessment,* section contains subjective data and objective data, as well as the physician's diagnosis. Assessment addresses pretreatment conclusions.

The *P,* or *plan* (treatment plan), portion states what should be done today and in the near future. This section is written before the massage.

The *I,* or *implementation,* section contains the modalities applied during that day's session. This section is written after the massage.

Finally, the *E,* or *evaluation,* section is the therapist's determination of treatment outcome to date. Evaluation addresses posttreatment conclusions.

Let us compare formats in Boxes 8-1 and 8-2.

> *"The question is not what you look at, but what you see."*
> Henry David Thoreau

BOX 8-1

SOAP Note Format

SOAP Note

Client Name: _Rebecca Johnson_   Date: _5/15/07_

S: Pain in right shoulder, 8 on 10 pt pain scale; Client states difficulty brushing and washing hair, difficulty tucking in shirt and hooking bra straps (difficulty raising arm above chest height)

O: Elevated right shoulder, TP's in infraspinatus, supraspinatus, and rhomboids

A: Adhesive capsulitis

P: Deep pressure massage to right upper back, neck, and shoulders, ice for 20 minutes post massage, self-massage, area at home twice a day for 3 minutes

Therapist's signature: _Jane Smith_

Legend: S=Subjective   O=Objective   A=Assessment   P=Plan

BOX 8-2

APIE Note Format

APIE Note

Client Name: Rebecca Johnson   Date: 5/15/07

A: 8 on 10pt pain scale in right shoulder, which is elevated. Client states discomfort in right shoulder and difficulty brushing and washing hair, difficulty tucking in shirt and hooking bra strap (difficulty raising arm above chest height). TP's in infraspinatus, supraspinatus, and rhomboids - adhesive capsulitis

P: Deep pressure massage to right upper back, neck, and shoulders, ice for 20 minutes post massage, self-massage area at home twice a day for 3 minutes

I: Completed a 30 minute focused treatment session addressing increased tonus and TP's in R rotator cuff, trapezius, levator scapulae, rhomboids, biceps, and pecs

E: Continue same treatment protocol 3 times a week for 3 weeks and re-evaluate

Therapist's signature: _Jane Smith_

Legend: A=Assessment   P=Plan of care   I=Implementation   E=Evaluation

NEW CLIENT: INITIAL SESSION

From the moment a client enters the massage therapist's office until the time he or she leaves, the massage experience is literally and figuratively in the massage therapist's hands. Client experience depends on the therapist's communication skills, critical thinking skills, and hands-on skills. During the client's initial session, time is spent gathering client information, obtaining consent for therapy, performing assessments, and devising a plan of care.

As stated earlier, the primary reason for collecting and documenting client information is to create a holistic picture of the client's health. In this way, the therapist will create a session that is based on this particular client's needs and expectations by following a plan of care. The fact that some therapists are successful and some are not is not happenstance. Massage therapists who develop a large clientele are masters at finding and meeting, or exceeding, client's expectations.

Each step will be addressed here, from the client intake form, to the consent document, to the interview. Then, the plan of care is discussed and finalized.

Preparing the Client Intake Form

The therapist should create a basic intake form for new clients to complete. Information on the client intake constitutes the first part of a client record. To keep from overlooking and forgetting vital information, a well-designed client intake form is essential and should encompass a variety of entries, such as the client's personal and contact information, as well as health and medical histories (Figure 8-1). Please note that third-party payers, such as insurance companies, may have their own particular forms for use if you are a part of their provider network. Questions the therapist should ask while designing an intake form are as follows:
- Readability. Is the type large enough?
- Organization. Is it organized logically?
- Brief. Is it confined to a single page?
- Convenient. Can the client check off or circle quickly items that apply?
- Necessary. Is the information requested relevant and important for the therapist to know?

---

evolve *It behooves a therapist to look at many different intake forms before designing the one for their practice. Access your student account from the Evolve website that accompanies this text to view, download, and print out several variations of client intake forms.* ■

General biographical information is a standard part of all information forms and includes:
- Client's name and address
- Preferred contact telephone numbers (home, office, or cell, but lets the client dictate which is preferred)

- Date of birth
- Date at which the information is being recorded

Other facts to include:
- A person to contact in an emergency
- The name and telephone number of regular physician or health care provider
- The referring person

Conditions or situations that have relevance to a massage therapist and may need to be included in a checklist format:
- Allergies
- Arthritis
- Blood clots
- Easily bruised
- Cancer
- Diabetes
- Heart condition
- Infection
- Inflammation
- Kidney disorder
- Medical supervision
- Pregnancy
- Previous motor vehicle accidents or trauma
- Ruptured or bulging disk
- Seizures
- Stroke
- Surgeries (including cosmetic surgeries)
- Varicose veins or thrombophlebitis

Presenting the Intake Form

After greeting the client, escort him or her to a quiet area with adequate lighting for reading and writing. The client is given a writing utensil and the health intake form on a clipboard to complete. If a health care provider requested massage services, important forms such as prescriptions or a referral forms are then obtained from the client at this time.

While the client is filling out the form, the massage therapist should be available for questions. If the client is unable or unwilling to fill out the form, the therapist my obtain data by asking questions and writing down the client's responses on the intake form. Some therapists prefer to write down the information instead of asking the client to do so. For one thing, they can read their own handwriting. It also provides the perfect opportunity to ask any questions to clarify information immediately. The therapist signature is needed, indicating that he or she assisted in completing the form.

MINI-LAB

Collect a variety of intake forms from other professionals, including massage therapists, physicians (medical, chiropractic, dental, etc.), hospitals, physical therapists, and counselors. Use these forms to create your own *health intake form.* Ask your teacher or a massage therapist to critique your form for flow and relevance. Redesign the form until it is complete and precise.

SOFT TISSUE THERAPEUTICS
JANE SMITH and ASSOCIATES
Client Intake Form

Name:_____

Address:_____

Telephone (_____)_____ Telephone (_____)_____

Date of birth:_____ Occupation:_____

Emergency contact:_____ Telephone (_____)_____

Previous massage experience:_____

Are you under medical supervision?_____

Regular physician:_____ Telephone (_____)_____

Referring by:_____

Check all that apply:

☐ allergies   ☐ heart condition   ☐ previous MVA/trauma
☐ arthritis   ☐ infection   ☐ ruptured/bulging disk
☐ blood clots   ☐ inflammation   ☐ seizures
☐ bruise easily   ☐ kidney disorder   ☐ stroke
☐ cancer   ☐ medications affecting blood clotting   ☐ surgery
☐ diabetes   ☐ pregnancy   ☐ varicose veins/thrombophlebitis

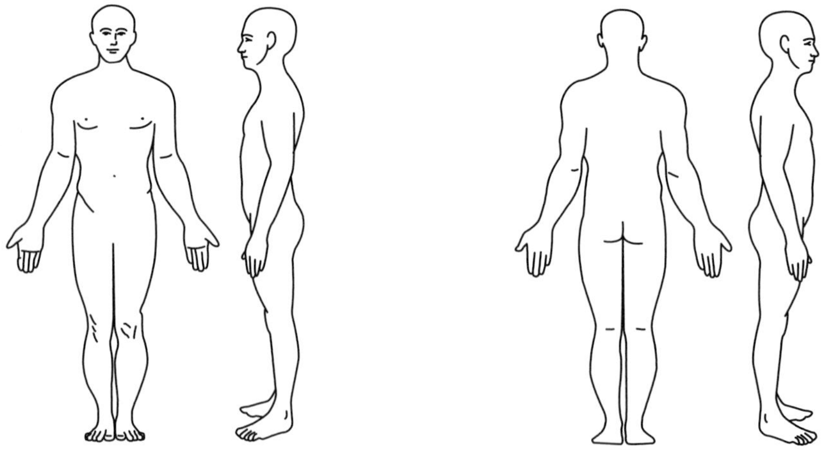

Identify your painful areas on these drawings using an X

Please briefly explain all checked items:_____
_____
_____

Signature:_____ Date:_____

FIGURE 8-1 Sample client intake form.

Informed Consent

Informed consent is a client's authorization for professional services based on information that the massage therapist provides. Essentially, informed consent is permission for treatment and is a common principle in all health care fields. The consent may be on a separate document or combined on the health intake form. Ideally, the contents of the document are discussed with the client during the interview so he or she has a chance to ask questions and receive answers before signing. If the therapy is provided to a minor, then a parent or guardian needs to sign the consent. If the client signs the consent without reading, then part of the therapist's responsibility is to read or review its contents with the client.

The informed consent document should contain the following:

- *Therapist's credentials:* This information includes the massage school the therapist attended, the year he or she graduated, any postgraduate training and certifications held, any college diplomas he or she has, and professional affiliations. If the massage therapist works in an office in which several therapists share client intake forms and consent documents, then this information needs to be verbalized to the client. Sharing therapist qualifications with a client helps establish a foundation of trust in the emerging therapeutic relationship. For appointments away from the office, create a presentation binder with copies of certificates, diplomas, and licenses, as well as a résumé or short autobiography.
- *Description of modalities:* This information will depend on the therapist's education, skills, and abilities and will vary among therapists.
- *Expectations and potential benefits:* Outline the positive effects of a particular modality, why it is used, or how it can influence the client's symptoms.
- *Potential risks and possible undesirable side effects:* One potential risk of massage is a blood clot that may become dislodged. Some potential massage side effects may include soreness, bruising, and mild inflammatory response. The therapist can suggest using ice and increasing water intake to reduce these side effects. Such suggestions are to be documented in the treatment plan section of the PPALM form. Unless both benefits and risks are listed, the consent is not a valid, legally sound document.
- *Statement of scope of practice:* Assure the client that the therapist does not diagnose medical conditions or prescribe and that services are not a substitute for medical treatment.
- *Right of refusal:* The right of refusal by the *client* means that he or she has the right to terminate the session at anytime or for any reason. The right of refusal by the *therapist* means that, when a contraindication is suggested or presented, the therapist has a right, responsibility, and even an obligation to refuse to treat the client or the local area involved until the client obtains written or verbal permission to proceed from a qualified health practitioner. We also have the right to refuse a client who makes us feel unsafe or who makes continued sexual advances once warned.
- *Professional and ethical responsibility:* Provide the client with written information on how to report professional misconduct to national, state, or other regulatory boards or agencies. The informed consent document should include a request that any changes in the client's health be passed on to the therapist.
- *Information use:* Include information on how the client's records will be used and stored, as well as the circumstances for its disclosure (see HIPAA guidelines).
- *Office policies:* Include established business procedures and policies of your practice. Time spent on these issues can go a long way in establishing boundaries and avoiding conflicts with regard to the therapeutic relationships, including dual relationships, fee schedules and payment policies, returned checks, and missed appointments.

MINI-LAB

Pair up with another student. Decide who will be the therapist and who will be the client. Ask the client to complete an intake form. Afterward, the therapist looks over the form, examines it for correctness, fills in any omitted information, and makes certain that the form has been signed and dated. Next, discuss the information on the consent document, and answer any questions to the best of your ability. Reverse roles and repeat.

The following are samples of items to include in the consent. Any or all can be used.
- The therapist's credentials are _____
OR
- The therapist has told me of his or her credentials.
- The information attained on the intake form is true to the best of my knowledge.
- I freely give my permission to receive massage therapy treatments.
- I understand that massage is contraindicated for some medical conditions and that obtaining a physician's clearance, release, or prescription may be necessary before beginning treatment.
- The primary modalities used will be [list modalities]. Secondary modalities will be [list modalities].
- Using these modalities, the client can expect [list goals]. These are the potential benefits of massage.
- Potential undesirable effects of massage are [list undesirable effects].
- I agree to inform the therapist of any experience of pain during initial and subsequent sessions.
- I understand that I have the right to refuse any treatment or ask that it be modified in regard to pressure or modality.
- I understand that I will be draped during treatment in accordance with state laws and that I may request additional draping if desired.
- During future sessions, I agree to update the therapist on changes in my health status and medical history and

understand that no liability on the therapist's part shall exist if I should neglect to do so.

- I understand that massage therapy should not be construed as a substitute for medical examination, diagnosis, and treatment and that I should see a medical physician, chiropractic physician, or other health care specialist to address concerns that are outside the scope of a massage therapist's practice.
- I have been asked to report any professional misconduct to [list agencies or other resources].
- I understand that information obtained from me will be used only to provide a safe professional treatment and will be stored in a locked file cabinet. If any outside agency requests this information, it will be released only after written permission is obtained from me or through a court order.
- Client signature _____
- Therapist signature _____
- Date of signatures _____

THE INTERVIEW

The person conducting the client interview is the attending therapist. The purpose of the interview is twofold. First, the interview gives the therapist greater insight into the client's overall health and any conditions he or she may have. The therapist can ask for specific information and necessary details. This information will help the therapist screen for contraindications or realize the need for adaptive measures during treatment, such as the use of pillows or the side-lying position.

Second, the interview gives the therapist a chance to gather details needed to provide a better service. These details include the primary purpose of the session and personal likes and dislikes. This information goes a long way in establishing a positive working relationship that often results in client satisfaction and continued patronage. Collaboration with the client is needed to design a plan of care that suits his or her needs and wishes. The interview and resultant plan

MILTON TRAGER

April 20, 1908 – January 20, 1997

"Not until we experience it is it more than just words. After we experience it, there is no need for words."

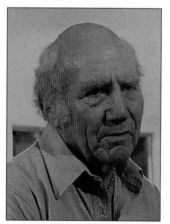

It is the roaring '20s in sunny Miami. However, for a high school dropout who lied about his age to get the $0.65-an-hour job at the post office, it is all work. He barely has time to breathe—until today. Today the posted health tip instructs him to do so and to sign his name indicating that he had done so.

Milton Trager slowly inhaled, then exhaled. He had no idea that he possessed a talent that would develop—without outside influence—into a revolutionary method of bodywork. That one deep breath put Trager in touch with his body for the very first time. "It was the beginning of me," he recalls. Soon he started working out at the beach, doing acrobatics, developing his muscles, and listening to the waves as he swayed to their ebb and flow. Fascinated by the movements of boxers in the ring, he took up the sport. One day he offered to *turn the table* and massage his trainer. His trainer was stunned at his ability. From there he went home to massage his father, who had severe sciatic pain. After four treatments, the pain was gone, never to return.

At 19, Trager helped a child walk who had not walked in 4 years. The proverbial 90-pound weakling had grown

into a strong, agile young man whose acrobatic antics along his mail route captured the attention of the Hollywood studios. However, his unique mode of hands-on therapy went virtually unnoticed.

He enlisted with the Navy medical corps. After his release, he decided it was time to get the credentials that would make physicians take notice of his work. However, the only medical school that would accept a 42-year-old person was in Guadalajara, so he headed south with his wife and embarked on the arduous task of earning a medical degree in a completely Spanish-speaking environment.

Establishing a medical practice was difficult for someone with his background, but the Tragers finally settled in Honolulu. Sadly, the medical community remained deaf and blind to his work. However, Trager did not need the medical community's blessing to know what he was doing was right. His method of holding, listening to, rocking, and freeing the body continued to evolve.

By chance, a well-known psychologist experienced Trager's methods and convinced Trager to demonstrate at Esalen, a workshop and meeting place for developing human potential. Jack Liskin, Trager's biographer, writes:

of care is an essential step in developing the therapeutic relationship.

The interview is also an opportunity for the client to ask questions. Unfortunately, we are living in a *blame* society, and a legal aspect exists. For the protection of the therapist, the completion of a client intake, informed consent, and explanation of treatment and products used in the treatment is essential.

Tips for Documenting

(8-4)
- The therapist's name and signature, along with the date of the session, should always be on the form.
- Maintain confidentiality.
- Use blue ink color. Currently, blue is the preferred ink color for documentation of client records because it differentiates an original from a facsimile or a photocopy. However, more important, the color ink should be consistent from initial treatment until release. Changing from

blue to black then back to blue may cause a record to be thrown out of a court proceeding because it might appear as though the other color were added as an afterthought instead of as part of the original treatment documentation.
- Correct errors with a single line and initials, avoiding correction fluid and tape.
- Use precise and correct medical terminology. Be careful of intangible words such as *energy* or *energy work*. For a medical record or a chart that will be read by someone working for an insurance company, using words that describe exact anatomy, physiological response, or specific technique is best.
- If a client misses an appointment, document this event with an entry on his or her client record indicating *no show* or *canceled, no reschedule*.
- Be careful with abbreviations and use of symbols. Remember, one reason to document is that this information may be shared with others. *SOB* might offend someone, even though it often means *shortness of breath*.

MILTON TRAGER (*continued*)

"And so it was that an aging and unusual doctor with an unusual talent, unattached to any movement, New Age or conventional, came face-to-face with the California counterculture." (From Liskin J: *Moving medicine: the life and work of Milton Trager, M.D.*, Barrytown, NY, 1996, Station Hill Press.)

The Trager Approach uses nonintrusive movements to lull the body into a better, more mobile, lighter state of being by releasing deep-seated physical and mental patterns.

Essential to Trager work is a state that has been termed *hook-up,* which means that the practitioner becomes so totally focused that he or she achieves a hypersensitivity to body cues. "It's as though the practitioner's mind and body communicates, without using words. And what is being said to the receiver is, though you may have hidden them from your consciousness, you hold the keys to unlock patterns that are holding you physically and mentally hostage. I'm just here to give your body the cues to gently remind you of your own potential—nothing more."

A Trager session does not end with table work. Mentastics reinforces the results. *Mentastics* is Trager's term for mental gymnastics, the gentle, mindful movement exercises that help the body recall positive physical or mental changes that occurred on the table and reinforce these changes.

Though Trager never cared for explaining his work, people who experienced, practiced, and witnessed its results have filled in the gaps.

"The practitioner uses the vast sensory capacities of the skin and deeper tissue to transmit messages. Using wavelike, moving rhythms that are at the core of all forms and matter of life, it communicates its messages thousands of times during a session to break habitual patterns," writes Liskin in *Moving Medicine, The Life and Work of Milton Trager, M.D.*

Trager never cared to be referred to as a genius, guru, or healer, claiming instead to have a talent. However, his talent touched lives and changed minds about what was possible.

For instance, Betty Fuller, a frequent seminar leader at Esalen, was prepared to live the rest of her days in chronic pain. When Trager reached out to examine her, she practically shrieked, "No one touches my neck." Nonetheless, Trager persisted in his gentle but unyielding manner. Soon she was pain free and became Trager's first instructor. In Trager she saw the same deep reverence for the mind's ability to heal the body that she had experienced as a student of Moshe Feldenkrais. Trager turned to Fuller to protect his name and his work, and in April of 1980 the Trager Institute was founded (from *Massage Magazine,* May/June 1997). Today practitioners all around the world are using the Trager Approach and Mentastics Movement Education techniques to ease headaches, back pain, and the debilitating effects of Parkinson's disease, cerebral palsy, polio, and multiple sclerosis.

- Write legibly. Documentation that cannot be read is worthless.
- Use sentence fragments to highlight the information gained from the client, as well as objective assessments, but be sure the fragment makes sense to the reader.
- Use direct quotes when applicable.
- Keep in mind the scope of practice. You can make observations of a client, but you cannot diagnose a condition. For example, *anxiety* is a medical diagnosis. You can, however, report when the client says, "I feel stressed out."

How much time is needed during the interview? – The reasons for the client's visit will determine how much time is spent during the interview and planning phase. The generally healthy client with no specific complaints does not require a lengthy interview (i.e., a 4-minute average). In contrast, a client coming to receive massage for a recent injury or painful symptom may need a lengthier discussion and a focused evaluation of posture, gait, or range of motion.

Keep in mind that a client may not want to spend more than a total of 10 minutes filling out a health questionnaire and being interviewed. The trick is to be thorough and fast. The client usually wants to spend most of the appointment time receiving massage. In fact, the client may choose to arrive 5 to 10 minutes before the scheduled appointment to complete the intake form.

Setting – The location of the interview sets its tone. The goal is to establish a productive climate for the exchange of information. This goal is achieved by an atmosphere of warmth, safety, and comfort. Focus on the physical comfort of the room by addressing details such as lighting, temperature, and seating of relatively close proximity. Prominently display all certificates and diplomas in the area where the interview takes place so as to add a sense of professionalism. Professional attire demonstrates to the client that the therapist is serious about his or her role as therapist.

Attend to aesthetic details of the interview such as paper quality, attractive layout of printed material, fine-writing pen, and choice of aromatherapy to make the experience more enjoyable for the client. Ask yourself if the setting reflects who you are in a unique and memorable way. A therapist who is empathic and genuinely concerned for the client can do a lot to warm even the most clinical (such as a hospital) or busy (such as a salon) environments.

 Interviewing skills – Some behaviors exhibited during an interview express care and concern, and some do not. Some questions are appropriate

(8-3) information-gathering instruments, and some are not. Following is a list of skills that can be developed to increase the success in obtaining client information during the interview while setting the stage for an enjoyable experience for both the client and therapist (Figure 8-2).

- *Sit facing the client at his or her eye level*. This arrangement helps create an atmosphere of interaction and rapport, instilling a sense of trust and goodwill.
- *Begin with a brief orientation*. If you did not discuss this information with the client previously, tell him or her why the interview is needed and how long the interview should take.
- *Consider the background or education of the client*. Use words that the client understands. Anatomical names and medical terminology may be inappropriate for clients who do not have the background or training in these areas.
- *Do not lose control of the interview.* Loss of control can occur when the client strays to other topics.
- *Use open- and closed-ended questions*. *Open-ended questions* offer little restriction when answering and allow the client to reflect and to clarify his or her own thoughts and feelings, thus producing more accurate subjective information. *Closed-ended questions* are more direct and require a *yes* or *no* response, helping to keep the client focused on the interview. Examples of closed-ended questions are "Are you thirsty?" or "Would you like a blanket to help keep you warm?" Examples of open-ended questions are "How can I help you be more comfortable?" "What brings you to the clinic?" "Tell me about it," or "Anything else?"
- *Listen carefully, asking reflective questions if needed*. Reflective questions restate the answer that the client gives to determine whether the therapist heard it correctly. Types and examples are:
  - To learn more about a patient's viewpoint, ask, "Can you tell me more about that?"
  - To clarify a muddled point, ask, "I'm not sure I understand. Would you explain further?"
  - To clarify a vague point, ask, "Would you give me an example of that?"
  - If a patient does not understand or know how to answer a question, say, "I'll repeat the question for you. The question was [restate the question]." Then pause.
- *Use silence*. Silence has many benefits; it gives the client time to talk, think, and gain insights, allowing the therapist to acquire a greater understanding of his or her client. Use this technique judiciously to avoid giving the feeling of disinterest or judgment.

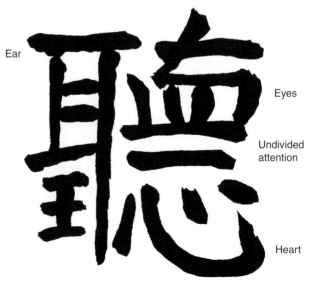

Ear
Eyes
Undivided attention
Heart

FIGURE 8-2 Chinese character depicting communication.

- *Signal your interests*. This signal is conveyed by maintaining eye contact and by occasional nodding or using appropriate facial expressions that coincide with the tone of the message. Neutral phrases or sounds, such as *really, uh-huh, hmm, I see,* and *okay* show interest and encourage communication. Even though documentation is taking place, balance note taking with maintaining eye contact with the client. Avoid glancing at the clock or ruffling through papers as though you are in a hurry.
- *Avoid the following:*
  - Agreeing or disagreeing with a client
  - Indicating that a client's response is *right, wrong, good, poor,* or *interesting*
  - Suggesting an answer or interpreting a question for a client
  - Giving your own opinions

TABLE TALK

Necessary Versus Palliative Care

Necessary and appropriate care relates to the client regaining function and the ability to perform his or her activities of daily living. **Palliative care**, also called *comfort care*, is care that is directed toward reducing or relieving the intensity of uncomfortable symptoms but that cannot effect a cure. In some cases, palliative care represents pain management.

Conducting the Interview

(8-2) This section features a special format for compiling and analyzing information using assessment sion domains to establish an appropriate plan of care. During the interview, the therapist views the client intake form and asks the client questions about five specific areas; answers to these questions create the map used for treatment plan. These area are **p**urpose, **p**ain and discomfort, **a**llergies and skin conditions, **l**ifestyle and vocation, and **m**edical history (PPALM). All information gathered during the interview will be documented. This next section breaks down the interview process into specific tasks.

Reviewing the intake and consent forms – The first step is to review the information the client has written on the initial intake and consent forms. Make sure that these forms are complete, dated, and signed.

Direct questioning – If lines are blank, ask the client for the information requested, and write it on the form. Next, begin to highlight health and individual issues that will affect the massage session. The PPALM system with its assessment domains is used during the interview and the planning process.

The five *assessment domains* (purpose, pain, allergies and skin conditions, lifestyle and vocation, and medical history) encompass observable and palpable data, as well as information from direct client inquiry; thus it includes both subjective and objective information (Figure 8-3). These assessment domains help prevent errors of omission. Each domain will be discussed in the interview, documenting relevant information to provide a picture of the client in the present tense.

Each assessment domain is discussed with the client, with the therapist documenting information on a sheet of paper, most often on the backside of the client intake form. Even though some information requested is listed on the client intake form (i.e., medical), the therapist will return to the information, even if the comment is, "So, Mrs. Brown, I see that you do not have any health conditions that would affect your massage today," pausing for her remark. Asking the client for this information directly not only builds rapport but also provides the opportunity to learn more about the client.

The therapist can place this information vertically (Figure 8-4, *A*) down the page or use a webbing diagram. The idea is to put the information down in a way that helps the therapist *see* how to serve that particular client best. Additional extensions of the client web can be made to create related pockets of information (e.g., medications). If nothing has been found to report in a particular domain, place a symbol such as ∅ instead of leaving it blank to indicate that the domain was addressed with the client. The length of time and depth of the interview are determined by the session's purpose, which is the first question the client answers.

TABLE TALK

How an individual collects and processes information comes into play when choosing a documentation method. Left brain–dominant individuals might prefer linear documentation, whereas right brain–dominant individuals might choose circular or web documentation methods.

The assessment domains:
- **P**urpose of session
- **P**ain and discomfort
- **A**llergies and skin conditions
- **L**ifestyle and vocation
- **M**edical and health information

Note that these assessment domains go *hand-in-hand* with a massage practice, as does the acronym PPALM (referred to as P-PALM, a two-syllable word). Given that massage therapists have a broad practice spectrum ranging from

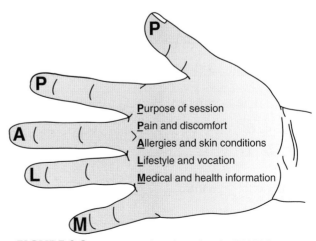

FIGURE 8-3 Assessment domains using the PPALM system.

Client Name: _Rebecca Johnson_

PPALM

P—Relief of pain in R shoulder

P—R shoulder, 8-10 pt scale, elevated, TP's in infraspinatus, rhomboids

A—None

L—Inactive since pain began, difficulty raising arm above chest height (brushing and washing hair)

M—Surgery on left knee in college, no residual effect, keloid scar

Treatment Plan –

- 30 minutes deep massage to right upper back, neck, and shoulders
- Target rotator cuff, rhomboids, levator scapulae, trapezius, pecs, and biceps
- Ice 20 minutes post massage
- Time permitting, 5 minutes on old scar
- Self-massage right shoulder at home 2X a day for 3 min

Therapist signature: _Jane Smith_   Date: _5/15/07_

Client signature: _Rebecca Johnson_

| Legend: | P=Purpose | P=Pain | A=Allergies and skin conditions | L=Lifestyle | M=Medical history |

FIGURE 8-4 Sample of linear diagramming for PPALM notation.

wellness to rehabilitation, information within each assessment domain varies from general and nonspecific to detailed and precise.

 Let us examine the assessment domains closely. ***Purpose of session:*** The first thing to document is the client's reason for wanting massage or his **(8-2)** or her chief concern today. Be clear about what motivated today's visit. What must happen for the client to be satisfied? Are his or her expectations reasonable? If you do not understand the client's goals, you will not meet his or her expectations and probably will not get another chance. Write this information down. Remember that the length and depth of the interview are determined by the session's purpose.

Pain and discomfort: This assessment domain concerns the subjective reporting of the client's pain. Guidelines are often used in which pain can be assessed. To help remember these guidelines, use the acronym OPPQRST (Figure 8-5), which stands for:
- **O**nset: When did it start?
- **P**rovocative: What makes it worse?
- **P**alliative: What makes it better?
- **Q**uality: How would you describe the pain?
- **R**adiation: Does the pain radiate?
- **S**ite: Where does it hurt?
- **T**iming: When did the pain start, and how often does it hurt?

When asking a client to describe the quality of the pain, a 1- to 10-point pain scale can be used, with 10 being the worst (Figure 8-6). Qualitative descriptors such as *mild*, *moderate*, and *severe* can be used. Other descriptors may be sharp, dull, or tingling. This information should be recorded for each session to develop a graph or trend of improvement or exacerbation.

When appropriate, assessment tests and measures can be done, including palpation, postural analysis, range of motion (measure of movement around a joint or set of joints), and gait. Although strength and other tests of muscle, tendon, and ligament integrity are within our scope of practice, these skills are usually learned through advanced training in areas such as clinical and sports massage, neuromuscular

massage, and myofascial release. See Chapter 26 for more information on these and other types of advanced objective assessments.

Allergies and skin conditions: This domain includes questions, observations, and palpations regarding:
- Skin disorders and diseases (e.g., rashes, boils, acne, impetigo)
- Skin temperature
- Skin color
- Bruises or varicosities visible on skin
- Sensitiveness to smell, such as cleaning products or aromatherapy
- Allergies to any ingredient in massage lubricant (e.g., nuts) or any plant from which an essential oil may be derived

Lifestyle and vocation: Factors that contribute to this domain are:
- Occupation
- Leisure
- Stress level
- Nutrition
- Regular exercise

Include assessment questions that ask how the client is using his or her muscles daily. Investigate his or her frequent activities at work and home, such as sitting, standing, chasing small children, and carrying heavy books. Assess general soft-tissue health by asking about regular exercise or sports activity.

Habits such as diet, fluid intake, sleep habits, and use of tobacco and alcohol affect tissue health. Questions about these issues help the client begin to make connections between how he or she feels and his or her lifestyle choices. Here, you will gain information concerning muscle health, potential areas of muscle stress, and expected tissue response and recovery time after your massage.

When asked, "How's your stress level?" a client may indicate a high level of stress. If so, your treatment plan might include some stress-reduction massage, which may mean suggesting that the client schedule a longer massage in the future.

O	**P**	**P**	**Q**	**R**	**S**	**T**
Onset	**Provocative**	**Palliative**	**Quality**	**Radiation**	**Site**	**Timing**
Ask the client:	Ask the client:	Ask the client:	Ask the client:	Ask the client:	Ask the client:	Ask the client:
• When did it start?	• What makes it worse?	• What makes it better?	• How would you describe the pain?	• Does the pain radiate?	• Where does it hurt?	• How often does it hurt?

FIGURE 8-5 Pain assessment using OPPQRST.

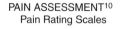

PAIN ASSESSMENT[10]
Pain Rating Scales

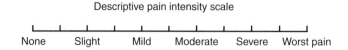

Descriptive pain intensity scale

None   Slight   Mild   Moderate   Severe   Worst pain

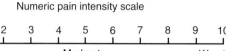

Numeric pain intensity scale

0   1   2   3   4   5   6   7   8   9   10

No pain   Moderate   Worst pain
                            pain

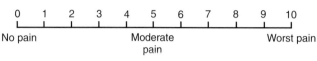

A

PEDIATRIC PAIN ASSESSMENT
Wong-Baker Faces Pain Scale

Brief word instructions: Point to each face using the words to describe the pain intensity. Ask the child to choose face that best describes his or her pain and record the appropriate number.
From Hockenberry MJ: Wong's nursing care of infants and children, ed 7, St. Louis, 2003, Mosby. Reprinted by permission

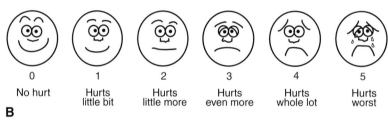

| 0 | 1 | 2 | 3 | 4 | 5 |
| No hurt | Hurts little bit | Hurts little more | Hurts even more | Hurts whole lot | Hurts worst |

B

FIGURE 8-6 **A**, 10-pt pain scale. **B**, The Wong-Baker Faces Pain Rating Scale.

___Medical and health information:___ Using the medical information from the client intake form, paraphrase any medical conditions to the client. This information will help determine contraindications for massage. Ask the client to explain in detail about any unfamiliar conditions or medications or herbal supplement. Pay particular attention to the medication types listed in Box 8-3. Keep in mind that certain medications can cause symptoms. Acquiring and referring to a pathology text with massage applications can be useful. Other information to include:

- Specific medical events such as surgeries (purpose)
- Accidents and injuries
- Medications, including over-the-counter and herbal supplements (purpose)

---

evolve *Log on to the Evolve website that accompanies this text and read the case study. Write responses to the questions regarding the study and share them with your instructor.* ■

"Pay attention to your patient's allergies or you will have to pay attention to his lawyer."
Rebecca Swanson, MD

Ruling Out Contraindications

(8-5) As the therapist is collecting information on the client intake form and during the interview process, he or she is also screening each client for the inappropriateness of massage, or contraindications. A **contraindication** is the presence of a disease or physical condition that makes treating a particular client in the usual manner impossible or undesirable. Conditions are stated as contraindications based on how massage affects physiological factors that are interfaced with the alteration in the client's physical status perhaps due to a disease process. If a local or absolute contraindication is determined through assessment, then it influences how massage will be applied, or it may rule out massage therapy entirely. Box 8-4 lists some helpful guidelines that were presented in Chapter 5 (Box 8-4).

Next, let us examine how this information will be used to develop the plan of care.

FORMULATING THE PLAN OF CARE

(8-6) During the planning process, the therapist uses the intake information to outline the parameters and set the course of action for the massage session. It represents the approach the therapist will use to address a client's massage

BOX 8-3

Medications That May Affect Massage Therapy

During the client intake and assessment, the therapist queries the client regarding medications that are injected, ingested, or administered via a skin patch. The following information will help guide the therapist in making proper modifications to the massage treatment with regard to a client on prescribed or over-the-counter medications.

Nonsteroidal antiinflammatory drugs (NSAIDs): Massage techniques such as deep effleurage; deep pétrissage; ischemic compression; and deep, specific frictions (e.g., cross-fiber, linear, circular) need to be carefully monitored or avoided because application of these techniques may result in bruising. This group of drugs includes many over-the-counter preparations. When asking about medication use, be sure to ask specifically about over-the-counter drugs because many clients do not consider these preparations as medications.

Examples: acetaminophen (Tylenol), acetylsalicylic acid (aspirin), Aleve, celecoxid (Celebrex), clinoril, diclofenac (Voltaren), ibuprofen (Motrin, Advil, Nuprin), indocin, naprosyn, naproxen (Anaprox), nuprin, paclitaxel (Taxol), relafen, vinblastine (Velban, Velsar), vincristine (Oncovin, Vincasar).

Muscle relaxers: Same as for *narcotic analgesics*.

Examples: cyclobenzaprine, dantrolene, diazepam (Valium), Equagesic, Flexeril, Lioresal, Norgesic Forte, Parafon Forte, Soma, Succinyl-choline.

Narcotic analgesics: Caution is merited because these medications depress sensory information entering the nervous system. The therapist relies on client feedback to help gauge pressure and force of techniques that include joint mobilizations and stretching. When tissue does not respond by tightening, the sensory feedback loop is reduced or lost, and the client may be injured as a result of excessive pressure or aggressively applied movements.

Examples: Buprenex, codeine, Darvocet, Darvon, Demerol, Dilaudid, Dolophine, Duragesic, hydrocodone, Lorcet, Lortab, morphine, Nubain, OxyContin, Percocet, Percodan, pethidine, Roxanol, Stadol, Talwin, Tylox, Vicodin.

Corticosteroids: Taking these medications, especially over a period of 30 days, results in loss of integrity of various body tissues. Muscles may atrophy, and connective tissues of the skin, ligaments, joints, bones, and tendons may weaken. Massage that stresses these structures, such as joint mobilizations, ribcage compressions, stretching, heavy percussion, skin rolling, wringing, deep friction (cross-fiber, chucking, and circular), should be monitored or avoided. This precaution is particularly true for women who have or are at risk for osteoporosis (i.e., postmenopausal women or older adults).

Examples: cortisone (Cortone), hydrocortisone (Cortef), prednisone (Deltasone, Orasone), prednisolone (Prelone, Pediapred, Orapred), triamcinolone (Aristocort, Kenalog), methyl prednisolone (Medrol), dexamethasone (Decadron), betamethasone (Celestone).

Antidepressants and antipsychotics: Same as for *narcotic analgesics*.

Examples: aripiprazole (Abilify), clozapine (Clozaril), Olanzapine (Zyprexa), risperidone (Risperdal), sertindole (Serlect; sertindole is not on the U.S. market as of this writing), quetiapine (Seroquel), ziprasidone (Geodon), alprazolam (Xanax), diazepam (Valium), lorazepam (Ativan), ketazolam (Loftran; ketazolam is not available in United States), chlordiazepoxide (Librium), clonazepam (Klonopin), estazolam (Prosom), flurazepam (Dalmane), oxazepam (Serax), temazepam (Restoril), triazolam (Halcion), estazolam (Prosom), flurazepam (Dalmane), midazolam (Versed), oxazepam (Serax), temazepam (Restoril), triazolam (Halcion).

Anticoagulants and platelet inhibitors: Massage techniques such as deep effleurage; deep pétrissage; ischemic compression; and deep, specific frictions need to be carefully monitored or avoided. These specific techniques often produce a mild inflammatory response that usually resolves within 48 hours. Performing these techniques when a client is taking these medications may result in bruising and excessive soreness.

Examples: acetylsalicylic acid (Aspirin), dipyridamole (Persantin), heparin, streptokinase, warfarin (Coumadin), clopidogrel (Plavix).

Transdermal patches: Do not massage within a 4-inch radius of the patch. Massage near the skin patch has the ability to alter the absorption rate of the medication. Additionally, asking a client to remove a transdermal patch is typically outside the massage therapist's scope of practice. These patches are often used to administer nitroglycerine, birth control, antinausea medication, and medication used to stop smoking or to reduce pain (lidocaine).

Injected medications: Avoid the area of injection for at least 10 days after last injection. Massage over a recent injection site increases the absorption rate of the medication. Avoid heat application over the injection site for at least 10 days. Avoid ice over the site for at least 3 days.

BOX 8-4

Treatment Guidelines

Treat as a <u>Local</u> Contraindication If:

The condition is due to an injury that is less than 72 hours old (e.g., whiplash, ankle sprain).

Pressure causes unwarranted pain (e.g., corn, callous, bunion).

The area is inflamed (e.g., carpal tunnel syndrome, acute bursitis).

The area in question is confined to a small space that can be easily avoided (e.g., athlete's foot [foot or feet], irritable bowel syndrome [abdomen]).

The area presents an abnormal finding such as suspicious lumps, masses, or moles.

Treat as an <u>Absolute</u> Contraindication If:

Widespread inflammation exists or the condition is acute or exacerbated (e.g., rheumatoid arthritis, lupus).

The condition is due to an infectious agent (e.g., fungi, virus) or disease (e.g., strep throat, pneumonia, scabies).

Until his or her physician can be consulted if the client's symptoms become more severe for any or no apparent reason (Parkinson's disease, scleroderma), which is revealed during the premassage assessment process. Make sure the client has signed a medical release form.

Condition represents a medical emergency (e.g., meningitis, appendicitis).

therapy needs. The plan is based on all the information the massage therapist has gathered—the client's intake form, the interview, and other assessments such as palpation. After integrating all this information, the massage therapist uses his or her critical thinking skills, knowledge of anatomy and physiology, massage therapy skills, and understanding of the effectiveness of techniques to determine what will work best for the client. The plan also takes into account the client's financial and time restraints. With practice, the planning process will flow naturally.

Take care not to encroach on the professional boundaries of other practitioners involved in the client's care. If a physical therapist has assigned activities for the client such as exercise, then adding more or different activities might be inappropriate. Similarly, avoid commenting negatively on the assignments from other practitioners. If client permission is given, network directly with the client's health care provider to discuss any concerns regarding the client.

A good plan of care includes:
- **Techniques** and **areas** to include or avoid
- **Recommendations**: Unless state law restricts you, recommendations for self-care are part of your professional activities. Self-care supports soft-tissue healing, promotes active care, and reduces unnecessary or inappropriate provider dependency. Suggest an activity that would fit easily into the day and that would tie into something the client does daily. For example, suggest gentle movements of the neck under a warm shower stream. These activities are to be performed between scheduled appointments. Other examples are:
  - Stretches
  - Self-massage with or without tennis balls
  - Stress-reduction techniques such as meditation, guided imagery, breathing exercises, and strolling outdoors
  - Sleeping with proper support
  - Nutrition such as increasing intake of fiber and water
  - Ergonomics such as computer monitor height or getting a telephone headset
  - Regular exercise
  - Salt and soda bath (1 cup each; soak for 20 minutes)
  - Ice and heat
- Duration, frequency, and length of treatments
- **Reassessment:** These are methods used to measure improvement of the client (e.g., decrease in pain and increase in range of motion)
- **Referrals:** Refer the client to a chiropractor, a nutritionist, a personal trainer, biofeedback technician, yoga or tai chi instructor, or any other appropriate services to benefit the client and help him or her achieve the desired goals.

The plan of care may also include:
- Whether the client needed assistance
- Use of support or bolstering devices that are out of the ordinary
- Use of any adjunctive therapies such as aromatherapy or hydrotherapy
- Suggested reading material such as books found in local bookstores and libraries

After discussing the proposed plan of care with the client, make any appropriate revisions. Once the plan is complete, ask the client to sign and date the document. This signed document represents a give-and-take dialogue that must exist in a therapeutic relationship.

Subsequent Sessions

Following the initial session, prepare for future sessions by briefly reviewing your PPALM notes for that client. This review will assure the client of your attention to his or her care and provide for client safety as you review any health concerns, noting any lack of progress that may necessitate modification of the original treatment plan.

You may need to update the record regarding progress toward the client's goal as indicated by the session's purpose. This update includes how long relief was experienced, which areas are feeling better, which areas still need attention, and whether the client experienced any adverse effects such as soreness or bruising. Also include any changes (better or worse) in the frequency, intensity, or duration of pain.

Be careful to keep the client's specific desired results and goals clearly in mind. Given the variability of client response, the therapist often has difficulty knowing how often and how many massages may be needed to achieve the client's desired results or goals. In general, the initial period consists of frequent sessions, tapering off as symptoms subside.

Ideally, you hope to see a decrease in the frequency and severity of the client's symptoms, most notably pain, and an increase in flexibility and range of motion. Be sure to include self-care activities such as using ice packs, stretching, and performing self-massage so that the client takes responsibility for maintaining therapeutic progress. A session's goals need to be realistic within the confines of the time allowed for the session. Short- and long-term goals can be determined following the first session, after the therapist's palpatory assessment and evaluation of the client's response to therapy. Short-term goals are increments of progress toward a larger goal. Short-term goals generally focus on a client's immediate problem; long-term goals focus on restoration of normal or enhanced function.

> *"The body never lies."*
> Martha Graham

---

evolve Try your hand at creating treatment plans by viewing the client interviews located in the course materials for this text in Chapter 8. Share them with your instructor for additional suggestions on how best to proceed with a particular client. ■

NETWORKING WITH OTHER MEMBERS OF A HEALTH CARE TEAM

A client assembles a team of health care providers, usually with the assistance of his or her primary care provider, such as a physician. Members are selected according the client's needs, as well as the professional skill and expertise of the health care providers. For this approach to work, team members must converse with one another and share information. Written documentation in the form of progress and narrative reports are the primary tools used to communicate your initial and subsequent assessment and to summarize client progress. Before the transfer of client information, the therapist must obtain the client's consent through written release.

Release Form

Because of its confidential nature, a signed release form must be obtained from the client. The release form gives the therapist authorization to release certain information to specific parties. The form should have the client's name, the institution and address maintaining the client records, and the institution and address of the receiving institution. Ask the client to sign and date the release form, and obtain a signature from a witness. The release of information should have an expiration period. If the client is a juvenile, then a parent or guardian must sign. An example of a medical release form is presented in Figure 8-7.

Only the information requested should be released. Carefully review the signed release form to ensure that the correct records are sent.

If a client is unwilling to release his or her information, then do not release the client's records. Exceptions include legally required disclosures, such as those ordered by subpoena, as well as those dictated by statute to protect public health or welfare or those considered necessary to protect the welfare of a client or third party.

MINI-LAB

Using a medical dictionary such as *Dorland's Illustrated Medical Dictionary* or a reference book such as Travell and Simons' *Myofascial Pain and Dysfunction,* find and define words that might be used to describe a knot or ropiness, tonus or tension, thickening or swelling, tenderness or discomfort, and numbness. Use these appropriately in the objective portion of your treatment record.

Progress Report

Progress reports are addendums to previous client records such as the intake form and the PPALM assessment and planning form; progress reports summarize client progress over an extended period. The therapist should consider a progress

---

RELEASE OF MEDICAL INFORMATION

I authorize: Name of person or institution: _____
                                          (Provider of information)
              Street address: _____

              City, state, ZIP code: _____
To release client information to: _____

              Name of person or institution: _____
                                          (Recipient of information)
              Street address: _____

              City, state, ZIP code: _____
              Attention: _____

Client's name: _____   Date: _____

Signature of client or legal guardian: _____

Complete address: _____

Relationship, if not the client: _____   Client's date of birth: _____

The authorization will automatically expire one year from the date of signature, unless specified otherwise.

FIGURE 8-7 Medical release form.

report at times of reassessment, which are usually 30 days in an acute case but may be longer in chronic cases.

Progress reports may be formal and sent on letterhead to the referring professional as a mechanism to keep him or her up to date on the progress made in massage therapy, as well as thanking him or her for the referral. The report itself includes:

- Initial or most recent client assessment
- Summary of client progress
- Current treatment plan

Present all information chronologically. If the therapist is recommending continuing client care, then the progress report would include:

- Goals for future sessions
- Plan of care used to accomplish these goals

Also include a statement acknowledging that the client will be referred back to the health care provider for evaluation at the close of the prescriptive period. The following is a sample of a progress report (Box 8-5).

Narrative Report

One type of progress report is called a **narrative report** because it can be lengthy, covering many sessions and prescriptive periods. A well-organized vignette captures the client's condition and how the therapist addressed the condition. The format of a narrative report tells a story, and although it can be expanded to include more information, recording a more concise summary of the session is sometimes necessary. The goal of narrative report writing is to provide a more detailed history of the client's condition, treatment, and treatment response.

In most cases, the initial assessments and latest assessments are used as the measures to show improvement. The application of massage therapy and the client's responses are discussed in detail; to resolve symptoms, to continue progress, or to maintain progress currently achieved, you may present justification for continuing therapy, if appropriate.

Use a classic letter format such as the following one shown (Box 8-6). Factors that can increase the ease and speed of reading are lists with bullets for multiple items of the same type and check-off style forms. A letter that is well organized and easy to read increases the likelihood that the receiver will review the report. By using standard forms, you will save time in report writing.

Begin with an opening statement to introduce the client and his or her complaint. The report may also contain the plan of care suggested by the physician's diagnosis on which you and the client have agreed. Also include a statement acknowledging that the client will be referred back to the health care provider for evaluation at the close of the prescriptive period. Information to include in the report is:

- All initial assessments
- All current assessments
- Modalities used and locations applied
- Summary of progress, including goals achieved
- Status of client
- Suggestions for future plan of care

BOX 8-5

Thank your for referring Mrs. Margaret Hebert to my office. Our initial appointment was on October 16, 2006.

Initial Assessments:
Constant, severe neck pain (8 on 10-pt pain scale)
Shoulder pain, moderately severe on the right (6 on a 10-pt scale) and on the left (7 on a 10-pt scale)
Unable to look over her shoulders; difficulty driving
Unable to lift her arms above her shoulders; difficulty dressing and grooming
Generalized neck and shoulder tension
Daily headaches that increase in intensity in the posterior region of the head and that interfere with work, sleep, and daily activities
A 1½ to 2–inch forward head posture
Internally rotated shoulders
High right shoulder
High left iliac crest
Acutely tender and severely hypertonic muscles: posterior cervicals, anterior cervicals, scalenes, anterior and posterior rotator cuff, paraspinals, trapezius, triceps, and coracobrachialis

Summary of Client Progress:
Intermittent mild to moderate neck pain (4 on 10-pt pain scale)
Shoulder pain mild on the right (4 on a 10-pt pain scale)
Full cervical lateral rotation; increased lateral flexion with no pain
Ability to lift arms carefully above her shoulders as needed
Decreased neck and shoulder tension
Occasional headaches, which are decreased by 50% following the first week
Mild to moderate hypertonic muscles: scalenes, paraspinals, trapezius, subscapularis, serratus anterior, and pectoralis minor

Current Plan of Care:
Eight 30-minute sessions, one per week
Additional self-care activities
Maintenance plan of massage once a month for 6 months also recommended

I will report back to you by December 18, 2006. Please contact me if you have any questions or comments.

TABLE TALK

Narrative Versus Progress Reports

- Narrative reports summarize entire personal injury case from beginning to end.
- Progress reports summarize improvement month by month.

- Narratives are written for attorneys and reviewed by insurers and are several pages in length, a fee is usually charged.
- Progress reports are written for referring health care providers, are a few paragraphs in length, and are complimentary.

Either of these reports may be required for insurance authorization in managed care systems.

BOX 8-6

LETTERHEAD

Date
Person requesting narrative report
Address
Claim #:
Re: [Client's name]

Mrs. Margaret Hebert was first seen on October 16, 2005, as a referral from Dr. Feelgood with a diagnosis of tension headache. The initial prescription included massage to neck and shoulders for 30 minutes, twice a week, for 8 weeks. The client is being referred back to Dr. Feelgood for follow-up evaluation. Mrs. Hebert describes the onset of headaches following a front-end motor vehicle accident on October 15, 2005, in which she remembers gripping the wheel and being thrown forward and backward. She states she was wearing a seatbelt. She does not remember hitting any structure in the car. Mrs. Hebert initially exhibited the following complaints:

- Constant, severe neck pain (8 on 10-pt pain scale)
- Shoulder pain, moderately severe on the right (6 on a 10-pt scale) and on the left (7 on a 10-pt scale)
- Unable to look over her shoulders; difficulty driving
- Unable to lift her arms above her shoulders; difficulty dressing and grooming
- Generalized neck and shoulder tension
- Daily headaches that increase in intensity in the posterior region of the head and that interfere with work, sleep, and daily activities

Evaluation of Mrs. Hebert revealed postural distortions that traditionally exacerbate cervical discomfort, notably:

- A 1½ to 2–inch forward head posture
- Internally rotated shoulders
- High right shoulder
- High left iliac crest

Range of motion is significantly decreased bilaterally in lateral flexion and rotation R . L. Palpatory findings revealed acutely tender and severely hypertonic muscles in the following areas: posterior cervicals, anterior cervicals, scalenes, anterior and posterior rotator cuff, paraspinals, trapezius, triceps, and coracobrachialis

Significant involvement of the fascial system and superior soft tissues that contributes to boggy, congested tissue and to extreme tension in the cranial fascia

Initial treatment consisted of a myofascial release over the neck and shoulder area to begin restoring elasticity and circulation to the superior tissues. Massage techniques were used to warm and prepare the area. Sustained pressure was used to address isolated tender areas. Massage was then used to flush the area. Stretching of the involved muscles was performed to lengthen taut bands of tissue. Ice was applied to the entire upper back, neck, and shoulder area to reduce inflammation. Progression in therapy depth was based on positive tissue response and client comfort.

Presently, Mrs. Hebert reports the following:

- Intermittent, mild to moderate neck pain (4 on 10-pt pain scale)
- Shoulder pain, mild on the right (4 on a 10-pt scale)
- Full cervical lateral rotation; increased lateral flexion with no pain
- Ability to lift arms carefully above her shoulders as needed
- Decreased neck and shoulder tension
- Occasional headaches, which are decreased by 50% after the first week

Current palpatory findings reveal mild to moderate hypertonic muscles in the following areas: scalenes; paraspinals, trapezius, subscapularis, serratus anterior and pectoralis minor.

Mrs. Hebert has residual postural distortions contributing to cervical discomfort; patient exhibits a forward head posture of 1 inch.

Based on Mrs. Hebert's positive response to therapy, I believe continued therapy would contribute to resolution of her residual symptoms. My therapy plan would focus on continued release and depth progression, adding self-care activities for long-term maintenance of progress to date. Eight sessions tapering in frequency based on Mrs. Hebert's resolution to date may bring her to at least 75% of her preinjury state. A maintenance plan of massage once a month for 6 months is also recommended.

Health Insurance Portability and Accountability Act of 1996 (HIPAA)

HIPAA (Public Law 104-191) was signed by President Clinton on August 21, 1996, and became effective in 2001 by the U.S. Department of Health and Human Services. HIPAA was designed to improve the productivity of the American health care system. This piece of legislation has four main purposes:

1. Protect and enhance the rights of consumers by providing them with access to their health information and controlling the inappropriate use of that information

2. Improve the quality of health care in the United States by restoring trust in the health care system among consumers, health care professionals, and the multitude of organizations and individuals committed to the delivery of care

3. Improve the efficiency and effectiveness of health care delivery by creating a national framework for health privacy protection that builds on efforts by states, health systems, individual organizations, and individuals

4. Promote administrative efficiency through standards regarding electronic transactions

Just because a massage therapist does not need to be HIPAA compliant does not mean that the rules do not extend when conducting business with agencies that must be compliant. In fact, the massage therapist is required to meet all the same standards for securing privacy as other covered entities (agencies that must be HIPAA compliant). This issue is regarded as a *chain of trust*.

HIPAA Guidelines for Massage Therapists
- Obtain a signed informed consent from each client.
- Always obtain a signed written consent form or medical release form from the client before any information about your client is disclosed to a third party (see sample).
- Do not disclose any information regarding clients to individuals in your office.
- Protect electronic client files by assigning passwords to anyone who has access to them. Computers that are connected electronically to the Internet must be fitted with a firewall to protect information from hackers.
- Obtain client authorization before dispensing any marketing material such as newsletters, facsimile referrals, greeting cards, or e-mail.
- Place confidentiality notices on all facsimiles and e-mails (Box 8-7).
- Store client files in a locked fireproof cabinet and restrict access.
- Create a client information sheet outlining how you intend to use the information obtained from the client, how

this information will be maintained and stored, and under what circumstances this information will be disclosed, as well as how the therapist will obtain permission for such incidences, how copies can be obtained by the client of his or her files, how long these files will be kept once the client is released, and how these records will be destroyed. Give a copy of this document to each client. Go over each item with the client, asking him or her to sign and date a separate statement that he or she received the *Notice of Privacy Policies*.
- Keep the appointment book and all client files out of view.
- When talking on the telephone, do not use the caller's name if others who might overhear are in the room.
- If you have a computer in your office, make sure the screen is out of view or shows a screen saver when clients or unauthorized individuals are nearby.

TABLE TALK

Self-Report Forms

During initial and subsequent sessions, the therapist can periodically use *self-report forms* to evaluate client progress and symptom resolution at the beginning of any session. The self-report form describes the client's perception of his or her symptoms; the client answers questions or indicates on a body map the area of discomfort. The form contains simple pictures of a body (front and back) for the client to mark or circle areas in which discomfort exists.

BOX 8-7

HIPAA Confidentiality Notice

The document inside this electronic transmission contains confidential information belonging to the sender that is legally privileged. This information is intended only for the use of the individual or entity named above. The authorized recipient of this information is prohibited from disclosing this information to any other party and is required to destroy the information after its stated need has been fulfilled, unless otherwise required by law. If you are not the intended recipient, you are hereby notified that any disclosure, copying, distribution, or action taken in reliance on the contents of these documents is strictly prohibited. If you received this electronic transmission in error, please notify the sender immediately to arrange for the return of this information.

SUMMARY

One of the most valuable skills a therapist can use is to be an effective listener and communicator. Most of the subjective data on a client will be gathered by a written health intake form and premassage interview. A well-written intake form contains the client's personal information, health and medical history, and an informed consent to agree to massage therapy treatment. The consultation also assesses client pain levels.

Objective data will be gathered through therapist observation and palpation of the soft tissues for condition and anomalies. These observations are made during the premassage interview, the assessment, and during the massage treatment itself.

By assessing and understanding the client's current health status and chief concerns, you can devise a treatment plan and determine the appropriate massage therapy techniques.

The cooperative nature of the process is shown by the formation, evaluation, and modification of therapy goals.

CASE STUDY:

If It Itches, Scratch It

George is a dedicated massage therapist working for two chiropractors in a midsize clinic. He performs 15-minute, area-specific massages that are insurance reimbursed. He has been working on Ann Marie for neck and back strains caused by an on-the-job accident. In the third week of her treatment, George makes a discovery. After finishing massaging her back, he asks her to turn over so he can begin the neck work. George notices that Ann Marie is scratching at her chest periodically. He notices a red rash outline visible above the top of the drape.

"How long have you had that rash?" asks George, "I hadn't noticed it before."

"Oh, it's not a rash," replies Ann Marie, "my doctor says it's scabies."

George immediately recoils from her. "That's highly contagious, Ann Marie. Are you taking anything for it?"

"Oh, he gave me some cream to rub on it," says Ann Marie, "but I stopped using it because it went away. But now it's back. I'm just waiting for it to go away again."

"It's not going to go away by itself!" explodes George, irritated that he and his other clients had been exposed to a possible infestation. "It's a parasite, a microscopic bug that bores into your skin and lays its eggs there. That cream has to be used to kill not only the adults but also the hatching egg larvae to stop the cycle. You've not only hurt yourself, but you've also exposed me and my other patients to this. I'm sorry, but I can't work on you anymore until you're clear and I have a release from your medical doctor."

Did George overreact to Ann Marie's news? What are other ways might George have handled the situation, including possible consequences of each possibility?

Should George inform the physicians and staff, given that Ann Marie also has contact with their treatment tables?

What steps should George take to decontaminate his linens, table, and accessories?

How do you think Ann Marie feels?

evolve

Go to *Chapter Extras* on Evolve for additional illustrations and resources for this chapter. *Extras* for this chapter include:

1. Medical release form (downloadable)
2. PPALM form (downloadable)
3. Client web PPALM form sample (downloadable)
4. Client web PPALM form (downloadable)
5. Sample consent form (downloadable)
6. Sample physician referral form (downloadable)
7. Crossword puzzle (downloadable form)
8. Sample intake form (downloadable)
9. APIE form (downloadable)
10. SOAP form (downloadable)
11. Client interviews (video clips)

MATCHING

Place the letter of the answer next to the term or phrase that best describes it.

A. Assessment
B. Client web
C. Documentation
D. Empirical

E. Informed consent
F. Narrative report
G. Objective
H. Palpation

I. Planning
J. Progress report
K. Range of motion
L. Subjective

_____ 1. The process of providing written information regarding client care

_____ 2. The measure of movement around a joint or set of joints

_____ 3. A diagram used to arrange information gathered in the assessment process

_____ 4. A summarization of client progress spanning through numerous sessions and prescriptive periods

_____ 5. The process involved in appraising a client's condition based on subjective reporting and objective findings

_____ 6. Client's authorization for professional services based on information provided by the therapist

_____ 7. A summarization of client progress over an extended period, usually 30 days or the length of a prescriptive period, whichever comes first

_____ 8. The strategy used to help the client achieve his or her goals, as established by analyzed assessment data

_____ 9. Information learned from the client or the client's family and friends

_____ 10. Data that are measurable and quantitative

_____ 11. Term denoting information that is verifiable through the senses

_____ 12. Assessment through touching with purpose and intent

INTERNET ACTIVITIES

Visit the American Health Information Management Association at http://www.myphr.com/ and click on Starting a Personal Health Record and then Step-by-Step Guide to Creating a PHR. After reading, list the 7 recommended steps and share this information with your teachers and classmates.

Visit http://www.privacyrights.org/index.htm and choose Medical Records. Locate and click on HIPAA Basics: Medical Privacy in the Electronic Age. After reading 1-6, write an essay on how this important document might relate to massage therapists.

Visit http://www.medicalassistant.net/soap_example.htm and scroll down to the five examples of SOAP notes listed on the webpage. Note the abbreviation key toward the bottom of the page. After reading, write three examples of SOAP notes for massage clients and allow your instructor to critique them.

Bibliography

Abdenour J: *TN magazine: the professional magazine with the personal touch,* Mountvale, NJ, 1999, Medical Economics Company.

American Health Information Management Association: Time for a HIPAA tuneup? 2006.

American Massage Therapy Association: Code of ethics, Evanston, Ill, 1994, The Association.

Boltn R: *People skills,* New York, 1979, Simon & Schuster.

Burley-Allen M: *Listening: the forgotten skill,* New York, 1995, John Wiley & Sons.

Chaitow L: *Palpation skills: assessment and diagnosis through touch,* New York, 1998, Churchill Livingstone.

Charting made incredibly easy, Springhouse, Pa, 1998, Springhouse Corporation.

D'Ambrogio KJ, Roth GB: *Positional release therapy—assessment & treatment of musculoskeletal dysfunction,* St Louis, 1997, Mosby.

Davis NM: *Medical abbreviations: 7000 conveniences at the expense of communications and safety,* ed 5, Huntington Valley, Pa, 1990, Neil M Davis Associates.

Dilks T: Personal communication, Lake Charles, La, 2005.

Dimond B: *The legal aspects of complementary therapy practice: a guide for health care professionals,* New York, 1998, Churchill Livingstone.

Dolan DW: *Objective structural findings in massage therapy: key to insurance reimbursement & specially physician referrals.* Jacksonville, Fla, 1995, Advanced Therapeutics America.

e-university: Documentation, 2005. Available at: *http://www.childbirths .com/euniversity/documentation.htm*

Expert 10—minute physical examination, St Louis, 1997, Mosby.

Health Privacy Project: Welcome to Health Privacy 101, 2006. Available at: *http://www.healthprivacy.org*

Ignatiavicius DD, Bayne MV: *Medical-surgical nursing: a nursing process approach,* ed 2, Philadelphia, 1995, Saunders.

Jusdon K, Hicks S: *Law and ethics for medical careers,* ed 3, New York, 2003, Glencoe McGraw-Hill.

Lowe WW: *Functional assessment in massage therapy,* Corvallis, Ore, 1995, Pacific Orthopedic Massage.

Loving J: *Massage therapy: theory and practice,* Stanford, Conn, 1998, Appleton & Lange.

Mackey B: Massage therapy and reflexology awareness, *Nurs Clin North Am* 36(1):159-169, March 2001.

McKay M, Davis M, Fanning P: *Messages: the communication skills book,* ed 2, Oakland, Calif, 1995, New Harbinger Publications–Mosby.

National Association for Nurse Massage Therapists: *Standards of practice,* June 1, 2006.

National Certification Board of Massage Therapy: *Code of ethics,* McLean, Va, June 1, 2006.

Natural Wellness. *Ethics: therapeutic relationships.* Self-published manual, 2004.

Reese-Berryman N: *Muscle and sensory testing,* ed 2, Philadelphia, 2005, Saunders.

Rubino J: *Been there done that,* Charlottesville, Va, 1997, Upline Press.

Salvo SG, Anderson SK: *Mosby's pathology for massage therapists,* St Louis, 2004, Elsevier Mosby.

Rose MK: The art of the chart: documenting massage therapy with CARE notes, *Massage and Bodywork,* 2003.

Shealy NC: *Alternative medicine–the complete family guide,* Versailles, Ky, 1996, Rand McNally.

St. John P: *St. John neuromuscular therapy seminars manual I,* Largo, Fla, 1995, self-published.

Sohen-Moe C: Taking care of business: the ultimate client interview, *Mass Ther J* 133-136, Fall 1996.

Starlanyl D, Copeland ME: *Fibromyalgia and chronic myofascial pain—a survival manual,* ed 2, Oakland, Calif, 2001, New Harbinger Publications.

Strong J et al: *Pain: a textbook for therapists,* New York, 2002, Churchill Livingstone.

Successful business handbook, Evergreen, Colo, 2001, Associated Bodywork & Massage Professionals

Thibodeau G, Patton K: *Anatomy and physiology,* ed 6, St Louis, 2006, Mosby.

Thompson DL: *Hands heal essentials,* Baltimore, 2005, Lippincott Williams & Wilkins.

Torres LS: *Basic medical techniques and patient care for radiologic technologies,* Philadelphia, 1993, JB Lippincott.

U.S. Department of Health and Human Services: Guidance on compliance with HIPAA transactions and code sets, 2006. Available at: *http://aspe.hhs.gov/admnsimp/HIPAACP.pdf*

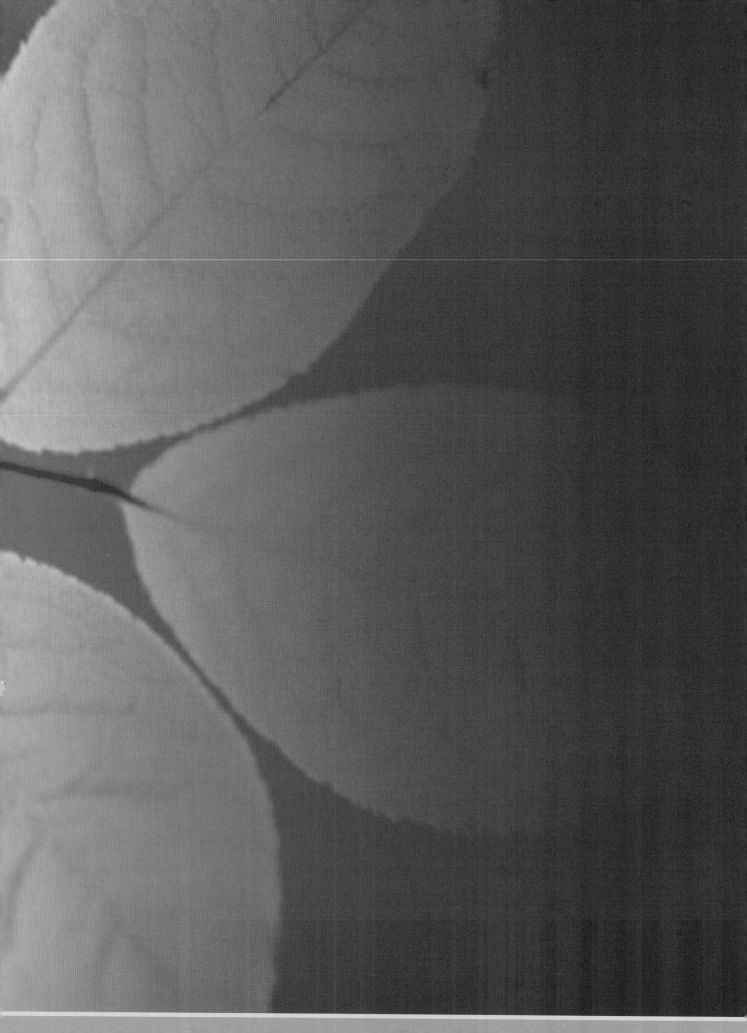

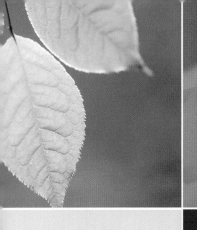

CHAPTER 9

Pregnancy and Infant Massage

Susan G. Salvo, BEd, LMT, NTS, CI, NCTMB
Maria Mathias, MS
Wayne Mathias, BS

"You are entirely engrossed in your own body and the life it holds. As if you were in the grip of a powerful force; as if a wave had lifted you above and beyond everyone else. In this way there is always a part of a pregnant woman that is unreachable and is reserved for the future—her baby."
—Sophia Loren

STUDENT OBJECTIVES

After completing this chapter, the student should be able to:

- Differentiate between a normal pregnancy and one that is high risk
- Address issues of client comfort when having a pregnant woman as a client
- Properly screen a pregnant client for precautions and contraindications
- Provide a massage that is safe for all expectant mothers who have a normal, healthy pregnancy
- Support the pregnant client using modified supine and semireclining positions
- Modify the massage treatment for a normal pregnancy
- Implement treatment modifications for second and third trimesters
- Offer massage suggestions for the father to help his pregnant wife during her pregnancy and the birth of their child
- Offer health-related suggestions to the pregnant client
- Distinguish major differences between infant massage and adult massage
- List the benefits of infant massage for parents and babies
- Explain why the parent rather than a therapist should massage the baby
- Name the infant state that is preferred for infant massage
- List infant cues that indicate a readiness or willingness to be massaged
- List infant cues indicating that the baby is becoming intolerant to massage
- Describe ways to handle crying babies in classroom settings

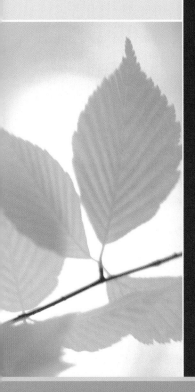

INTRODUCTION

All mothers share the miracles of conception, gestation, and birth. Within 9 short months, a new life comes forth; lives of the parents, the grandparents, and the baby's siblings are altered forever.

A pregnant woman's body progresses through tremendous changes during the childbirth experience—pregnancy, birth, and postpartum. Many of these changes are physically taxing and uncomfortable. Her uterus expands to 20 times its previous size, breasts more than double their size, her pelvis widens and the ligaments slacken, blood volume increases 50%, and her breathing rate increases so that approximately 20% more oxygen is taken in. These changes represent a partial list. As her body grows, the expectant mother often yearns for pampering and self-nurturing. The stress that often accompanies this period can complicate the pregnancy, as well as the delivery. Much of this stress can be relieved with massage.

"Pregnant women are becoming more aware of what massage can offer them. I haven't met a pregnant woman who didn't like massage. They savor the moment, because they know that at the end of nine months, moments of free time and quiet are few and far between," says Sallie Mowles, LMT, who specializes in prenatal massage at Urban Oasis in Chicago. Furthermore, many women are postponing childbirth until they have achieved other goals, such as careers and higher education. Because of this choice, women in their late 30s and 40s are becoming pregnant and may experience the physical stress of pregnancy to a higher degree than younger women. Massage is a way to reduce many of the discomforts associated with pregnancy. Please note that *this chapter is not intended to instruct students or therapists on how to apply massage techniques on pregnant clients who have pregnancy-related complications or who are considered high risk.* These special clients require therapists with special skills and postgraduate training. This chapter will discuss comfort issues and treatment modifications to provide women with normally progressing pregnancies with safe massage during this special time.

HOW NORMAL PREGNANCY PROGRESSES

Joining of an egg with a sperm (fertilization) takes place at any time up to approximately 24 hours after ovulation. The fertilized egg, or zygote, travels through the fallopian tube to implant in the uterus. This event begins the gestational process, or **pregnancy**, and involves the sequence of events including implantation, continues to embryonic and fetal growth, and ends in birth. Normal pregnancy is divided into three trimesters.

First Trimester (14 Weeks from the First Day of the Last Period)

Baby: The baby develops from a zygote to a 3-inch-long embryo. The baby has a body with arms, legs, nails, and ears, and the heartbeat can be heard at day 26.

Mother: The mother's uterus grows. Structural changes are minimal, but the hormone relaxin begins to affect joints at week 10. She may have frequent headaches and feel tired, dizzy, and nauseated, with or without vomiting, all probably because of hormonal changes. Her blood volume and heart rate and metabolism increase. She may experience frequent urination. Hormones raise the body temperature to create an incubation effect.

Second Trimester (14 to 28 Weeks)

Baby: The baby grows to 11 inches in length and 1½ pounds in weight. Fingerprints, eyebrows, and eyelashes form. At 16 weeks, the baby becomes sensitive to light. At 24 weeks, the baby's hearing is now well developed. At 29 weeks the baby's eyes can open and look toward a light source.

Mother: The mother begins to *show,* and her body changes to accommodate her growing baby. Her ribs may move up and out, her pelvis expands, and resultant back pain may occur. Her center of gravity changes to adapt to extra weight in front. Her diaphragm elevates at its rib attachments, and her breathing is mostly costal as abdominal breathing becomes difficult. The linea alba begins to separate as the rectus abdominis moves out of the way to accommodate the baby. Muscle cramping may occur. The skin begins to stretch. Breasts are often tender and swollen. She should feel the baby move by the end of the second trimester.

Third Trimester (28 to 40 Weeks)

Baby: The baby grows from 14 or 16 inches and from 2½ or 3 pounds at the start to 20 inches in length and 5 to 9 pounds in weight. Lungs develop by week 34. The baby's eyes track movement, and sleep patterns develop.

Mother: The mother may experience shortness of breath and difficulty breathing as uterus ascends into ribcage. Moving and walking become more and more difficult. She may develop hemorrhoids, varicose veins, heartburn, hiatal hernias, trouble sleeping, edema in ankles and legs, and carpal tunnel syndrome.

After a gestation period of approximately 40 weeks (10 lunar months), the uterus begins a complex process called **labor**. The three stages of labor are:

1. Dilation: The time from the onset of labor to complete cervical dilation (10 cm or 4 inches). Rupture of the amniotic sac occurs during this stage.
2. Expulsion: The time from complete cervical dilation to delivery.
3. Placental stage: The time after delivery until the placenta or *afterbirth* is expelled by powerful uterine contractions. These contractions also constrict torn blood vessels that occur during delivery to prevent hemorrhage.

The secretion and ejection of milk by the mammary glands is called *lactation.* During late pregnancy and the first few days after birth, the mammary glands secrete fluid called *colostrum* (first milk). True milk appears approximately the fourth day postpartum. It contains more lactose and fat than colostrum, but both contain antibodies that protect the infant from disease during the first few months of life.

BENEFITS OF PREGNANCY MASSAGE

Healthy pregnant women with a low-risk pregnancy can receive massage and all the benefits that come with it. In addition to the fact that massages during pregnancy feel good, many benefits exist for the expectant mother and her baby. Studies conducted by Dr. Tiffany Field and her colleagues at the University of Miami School of Medicine have credited prenatal massage with most of the following:

- Relieves fatigue
- Reduces headaches
- Reduces muscular discomforts such as spasms, leg cramps, and stiffness
- Keeps skin supple to help prevent stretch marks
- Assists muscles in preparation for labor and delivery
- Helps control blood pressure
- Relieves pain associated with pressure on the sciatic nerve
- Strengthens the immune system
- Improves lymphatic and blood circulation, the latter of which increases tissue oxygenation
- Reduces insomnia
- Reduces stress, anxiety, and depression
- Enhances self-image
- Helps prepare the perineum for fetal delivery (see Table Talk)
- Helps relax mother between contractions during labor
- Reduces postpartum stress and depression

TABLE TALK

Perineal massage increases tissue elasticity and decreases the likelihood of tearing the perineum during fetal delivery (stage 2 labor). Because the perineum is located in the genital region, the massage therapist is not permitted to administer perineal treatments. Perineal massage can be self-administered or administered by her husband or birth coach. Perineal massage is most beneficial during the last 6 weeks of pregnancy and during the first and second stage of labor.

The announcement of pregnancy is not a joyous occasion for all women. Some women are shocked, stunned, or confused, whereas others are elated. Some women may be struggling with new responsibilities facing them as parents, how the new family member will affect the relationship between them and their husbands, and how the new baby will affect family finances, including concerns about baby's health or resentments about discomforts surrounding their pregnancies. All of these inner stresses are normal and understandable.

The therapist can provide much-needed compassion to support the transformation the expectant mother is undertaking. Pregnancy is often a time for reflection and introspection. Frequently, unresolved childhood issues come to the forefront. Active listening and massage will help her better cope with the stress surrounding her pregnancy; caring, nurturing touch brings comfort and solace during this time.

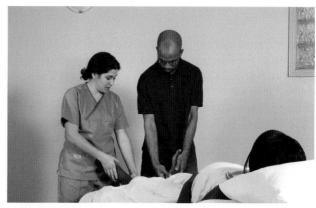

FIGURE 9-1 The husband can help reduce pregnancy discomforts through massage.

Along with the benefits for the expectant mother, benefits for the baby may exist. A recent study cited the negative effects of maternal stress on the developing fetus. Findings indicate stressed pregnant women produce fetal heart rates that stay higher longer. This response has also been linked to retarded fetal development and higher risks of heart disease and diabetes later in the baby's life.

Massage benefits can extend to the expectant mother's relationship with her co-parent. Offer the husband the opportunity to attend massage sessions with his pregnant wife. Teach him massage strokes he can do at home to bring her much-needed relief (Figure 9-1). This activity will also facilitate the bond between father and baby as he lightly massages his wife's belly. Invite him to make loving statements to both his wife and the new life within her. In this way, family bonding is enhanced and nurtured through touch. Family bonding helps strengthen the shared love and responsibility of this new life, which belong to both parents.

"There are some people who just can't seem to concentrate. They can't hold on to their part of the conversation. Their attention wanders; their eyes always seem to have a slightly glazed-over look. Sometimes snapping a finger in their face brings them back, but only for a short time, for their brains have been programmed to respond to stimuli that no one else notices. These people are called mothers."
Beverly Slapin

DISCOMFORTS OF PREGNANCY

Regardless of individual circumstances, a pregnant woman's body is challenged, changed, and stressed in many ways. The sweet burden of motherhood begins long before the baby is born. Throughout her pregnancy, an expectant mother watches her body change and experiences new aches and pains with each passing month.

Each woman's physical condition before pregnancy will have some bearing on the scope and variety of the discomforts that she experiences. Understanding the causes of the discomforts of pregnancy is the first step toward helping to alleviate them.

Anemia

During pregnancy, blood volume increases 30% to 50%. This increase causes a functional decrease in the number of red blood cells and a subsequent anemia because blood is more dilute. Other causes of anemia are folic acid or vitamin B_{12} deficiency, blood loss, or disease such as sickle cell disease. Depending on the cause, her physician may prescribe iron supplements. Anemia also contributes to fatigue.

Backaches

Backaches are a common complaint during pregnancy, especially during the fifth through the ninth month. During pregnancy, the ovaries and the placenta produce large amounts of relaxin. The purpose of relaxin is to increase the flexibility of the pelvis, to help cervical dilation, and to ease delivery of the baby. By week 10, the hormone relaxin is in sufficient amount to produce ligament laxity, which may affect joint stability (mainly the sacroiliac [SI] and hip joints and the pubic symphysis).

As the uterus protrudes in the front of her body, the mother leans backward to compensate. This changes her center of gravity, rotates her pelvis forward, and places even more stress on the SI joints, lumbar spine, and the abdominal muscles. Stress is also placed on weight-bearing joints. Other muscles stressed in this postural shifting are pectoralis major, quadratus lumborum, the entire pelvic floor, iliopsoas, and the paraspinals. Additional contributing factors are fetal positioning and referred pain from overstretched uterine ligaments.

The main paired ligaments that help support a growing uterus, as well as the increased weight in the abdomen during pregnancy, are:

- Broad ligaments that extend from the sides of the uterus to the sides of the pelvis
- Round ligaments that extend from the uterus and attach to the lower region of the pelvis

Overstretching of the broad ligaments (see Figure 23-7) may create sciatic-like pain (low back and buttock) in the pregnant woman. This pain is most often felt during and after the sixth month of pregnancy. True sciatica involves compression of the sciatic nerve, which is a different condition.

Round ligament pain is felt diagonally on one side from the superior uterus to the groin. The sensation is often felt as a pulling or sharp pain on either side of the lower abdomen. Common causes of round ligament pain are quickly standing from a sitting position or suddenly turning while standing, sitting, lying down, or coughing.

Breast Tenderness

The vascular supply increases to breasts, and they become enlarged and tender by the eighth week. Stretch marks may appear, as well as chloasma around the areola because they are preparing for their job of nourishment once the baby has arrived.

Charley Horse (Leg Cramps)

The extra weight and the heavy uterus pressing on the blood vessels are the cause of most leg cramps during pregnancy. The mother's physician may prescribe a multimineral supplement to reduce cramping in case the cause is a mineral imbalance. Charley horses are especially noticeable at night.

Edema

Interstitial fluid volume increases 40% in the third trimester, causing edema. Because the growing uterus puts pressure on blood vessels in the lower extremity, lower legs and feet are most edematous. Edema is more prevalent at the end of the day than it is at other times and is worse during the summer months than it is during other seasons. Temporary carpal tunnel syndrome may develop as edema compresses the contents of the carpal tunnel.

Elimination Problems

Frequently, a pregnant woman experiences frequent urination, which intensifies as the uterus enlarges and bladder capacity decreases. Progesterone causes decreased peristaltic activity and decreased muscle tone of the colon, which causes constipation. This event is compounded by the fact that her organs must move aside, and the growing baby compresses the sigmoid colon. Constipation may become severe if the pregnant client is taking iron supplements. Straining and the pressure exerted on the pelvic floor commonly result in hemorrhoids.

Fatigue

Being pregnant puts a strain on the body (eating, breathing, eliminating for two) and requires a great deal of energy. Pregnancy-induced anemia and hormonal changes cause the pregnant woman to feel sluggish. Getting a full night's rest is difficult if frequent urination is a problem. Nausea certainly costs the expectant mother energy, and feelings of depression or anxiety can be draining. Even though fatigue is felt throughout pregnancy, most pregnant women experience an energy boost in the second trimester.

Gastrointestinal Complaints (Indigestion, Heartburn, and Gastroesophageal Reflux Disease)

The burning sensation associated with indigestion and gastroesophageal reflux disease (GERD) often extends from the bottom of the breastbone to the lower throat. During pregnancy the placenta produces progesterone, which relaxes the smooth muscles of the uterus; it also relaxes the valve between the esophagus and the stomach, allowing gastric acids to seep back up the esophagus. Progesterone also slows down motility, making digestion sluggish. As the pregnancy progresses, the uterus expands and crowds the abdominal cavity, slowing elimination and pushing up the stomach acids.

Many women start getting indigestion and GERD in the second half of pregnancy. Intestinal gas is often experienced in the last trimester.

Headaches

Pregnancy hormones, postural changes and compensation, sinus congestion, stress, dehydration, and increased neck and shoulder muscle tension contribute to the headaches of pregnancy. Discontinuing caffeine intake also can cause headaches. For most women, pregnancy headaches diminish or disappear during the second trimester, when hormones stabilize and the body grows accustomed to its altered chemistry.

Nausea (Morning Sickness)

Approximately 75% of pregnant women have nausea and sometimes vomiting during their first trimester. Nausea can begin as early as 10 days after fertilization occurs and normally fades by the end of the third month. Some women feel queasy off and on throughout pregnancy. Common causes of pregnancy-related nausea are elevated human chorionic gonadotrophin, elevated adrenocortical hormone levels, and altered carbohydrate metabolism. If nausea is excessive, she may be dehydrated, with resulting acidosis. Ask her to consult with her physician because this condition usually requires hospitalization.

Respiratory Conditions (Shortness of Breath, Allergies, Sinus, and Nasal Congestion)

Approximately 30% of pregnant women have congestion without any other cold symptoms while they are pregnant. Congestion usually starts in the third month of pregnancy and can last until the baby is born. Elevated and sustained levels of estrogen and progesterone cause an increase in blood flow to nasal mucosa, which results in swelling and increased mucus production. Furthermore, blood volume increases along with the vascularity of the nasal mucosa; both lead to swollen nasal membranes.

Pregnancy can also make allergies worse or cause sensitivity to allergens and other irritants. As the uterus grows, the lower ribs flare out, the diaphragm elevates, and her thoracoabdominal organs must move aside as well. This change often causes shortness of breath. Accessory respiratory muscles (scalenes, sternocleidomastoid, and pectoralis minor) are often used for breathing.

Stretch Marks

As the scales show weight gain in the later stages of pregnancy, stretch marks may appear on the abdomen, buttocks, thighs, hips, or breasts. At least one half of all pregnant women get stretch marks, although they are less common among women with dark skin. Stretch marks start out pink, reddish brown, or very dark brown, depending on the color of your skin, and later fade though never totally disappear.

Vascular Problems

The scales will show weight gain; varicose veins are not uncommon. As the uterus grows, pressure is exerted on large abdominal veins, which, in turn, increase pressure in leg veins. Blood volume increases during pregnancy, which adds to the burden on the venous system. Progesterone relaxes smooth muscles, dilates peripheral blood vessels, and contributes further to varicose veins and even hemorrhoids (varicose veins in the rectum). Many women first develop varicose veins or find that they get worse during pregnancy.

INTAKE PROCESS

When a client schedules an appointment and announces that she is expecting, ask how far along she is in her pregnancy. If she is still in her first trimester (12 weeks or less), schedule her massage after week 12. Given that the primary concern is for the mother and baby's health and well-being, and because most miscarriages occur during this time, postponing massage is best.

Make sure the pregnant client's physician is aware that she is receiving massage by asking her to obtain a statement from her physician. This document should state that your client's pregnancy is normal. If it is not, state the complication. Make sure the document contains the physician's name, office location and telephone number, and consent to massage treatments. The document must be signed and dated by the physician. Place it in your client's file.

Along with a customary intake form, inquire about the following during the premassage interview featured in Chapter 8:
- Current and previous pregnancies
- Due date
- Breast soreness
- Nausea or vomiting
- Incompetent cervix or other uterine abnormalities
- Placenta previa or placenta abruptio
- Reduction of fetal movement within last 24 hours
- Swelling in arms, hands, legs, or feet
- Circulation problems in legs
- Have been or are currently inactive or placed on bed rest by physician
- Vaginal bleeding or discharge within last 24 hours
- Over 36 years of age
- Anything you care to mention that will help you receive a safe massage today

The goal of the intake and interview for a pregnant massage client is to rule out any high-risk factors and conditions that would contraindicate massage, as well as to guide the therapist in how to prepare an appropriate plan of care.

Even when the aforementioned statement is obtained, her pregnancy can change course quickly. Conduct a premassage interview each visit. If complications arise, then avoid massage until she is cleared again for massage.

CONTRAINDICATIONS AND HIGH-RISK FACTORS

Concerns of Miscarriage

The first trimester marks the least change in the woman's body, but the most development takes place in the embryo. Because of this crucial time, massage is best postponed until the woman begins her fourth month or second trimester of pregnancy. The first trimester also marks the time that many women experience pregnancy-related ailments such as nausea, vomiting, fatigue, hypersensitivities to taste and smell, and mood swings. Hence the second and third trimesters are wonderful times to begin prenatal massage.

TABLE TALK

The first trimester is an excellent time to recommend Kegels (pubococcygeus exercise). Kegels are a regimen of isometric exercises involving voluntary contractions of the muscles of her pelvic diaphragm and perineum in an effort to increase tone of the pelvic floor. Laxity and weakness of the pelvic floor muscles, often a result of childbirth, may predispose certain women to looseness of the vaginal wall and to urinary incontinence. The technique involves the familiar muscular squeezing action that is required to stop the flow of urine while voiding. Instruct the pregnant client in how to duplicate the squeezing, pulling-up action. Hold the contraction for 6 to 10 seconds, allowing the muscles to relax between contractions. Perform four to six repetitions of the contraction in a series, and repeat the series three to four times each day.

High-Risk Pregnancy

Along with customary contraindications discussed earlier in this text, avoid massage (unless directed by her physician) if the expectant mother's pregnancy is considered *high risk*. **High-risk pregnancies** are ones that put the mother, the developing fetus, or both at higher-than-normal risk for complications during or after the pregnancy and birth. Some factors are:
- Abnormalities or infections of the urogenital tract
- Complications caused by pregnancy itself, which can turn a normal pregnancy into a high-risk pregnancy, such as gestational diabetes or preeclampsia
- History of miscarriage
- History of preterm labor or delivery
- Hypertension
- Maternal age (younger than 15 and older than 35 years)
- More than five previous pregnancies
- Prepregnant weight is less than 100 pounds or the woman is obese
- Twins, triplets, or higher order multiples
- Vaginal bleeding or discharge
- When prenatal tests indicate fetal abnormalities
- When women with chronic illnesses become pregnant

Additional Contraindications

Avoid massage in the following situations, even if the pregnancy is considered normal or low risk:
- Physician disapproves of massage during pregnancy.
- Severe, persistent, or unexplained pain is present anywhere in the body.
- Nausea, vomiting, or diarrhea occurs.
- Back pain is accompanied by bleeding or other discharge, abdominal cramping, or persistent uterine contraction, which is often an indicator of preterm labor.

Massaging a Pregnant Woman's Legs

Lower extremity is locally contraindicated if the client:
- Has extremely poor circulation in the legs (with or without pain)
- Is inactive
- Is on bed rest, as directed by her physician
- Has severe or pitting edema

TREATMENT GUIDELINES

Several factors help make a pregnancy massage an enjoyable experience for both the mother and the therapist (Box 9-1). Following are numerous recommendations and suggestions.

Duration and Frequency

Massage can be performed for any duration from 10 minutes to 1 hour. Recommendations are to massage once a week during the second trimester and twice a week, or more, during the third trimester.

Table Height

Because getting on and off the massage table may be difficult for the client as her pregnancy progresses, the therapist might shorten the legs to lower the table when appropriate. A lower table height is preferred when massaging in the side-lying position.

Draping

Therapists should use a sheet for adequate coverage. Additionally, a thick bath-size towel may be needed to help secure placement of the sheet drape when it may slide off the client (Figure 9-2).

BOX 9-1

Supplies for Pregnancy Massage

Four to five firm standard-size bed pillows
One to two firm king-size pillows (for knee and ankle support in the side-lying position)
Pillowcases to fit the pillows
Small, round cervical pillows or bath-size towels to be rolled up

---

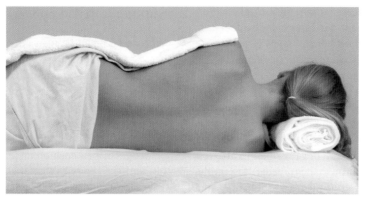

FIGURE 9-2 Using a towel to secure the sheet drape.

Table Width

Massage tables are often narrow. A standard table width is intended to help the therapist establish and maintain proper body mechanics. However, when performing a side-lying massage, the tabletop may be too narrow to accommodate the pregnant client with pillows in place. Either place a thick pad on the floor and perform the massage on the floor, or widen your tabletop with table accessories designed to do so (see Figure 3-3).

Avoid Prone Position

Tables and support systems intended to place the pregnant women in the prone position have questionable safety, and the advisability of their use is uncertain. Intraabdominal pressure is exerted during low back massage, and added strain is exerted on the supporting ligaments and muscles when in a face-down position. Prone positioning is contraindicated during pregnancy. This position is not a client preference; providing a safe and knowledgeable pregnancy massage is the responsibility of the therapist.

Client in Pain While on the Table

If a client experiences back, side, or abdominal pain while repositioning or getting off the massage table, then assist her in lying down until the pain subsides. She can try moving again more slowly afterward. This type of pain is usually related to stressing of uterine ligaments.

Modality Restrictions

- Avoid connective tissue and myofascial release techniques because of the presence of the hormone relaxin.
- Avoid heating blankets and hot packs because she is often overheated.
- Avoid techniques that require pulling on the lower extremities because pain caused by separation of the pubic symphysis can occur.
- Avoid direct and sustained pressure between the anklebone and heel. This area in reflexology is related to the uterus and vagina.
- Avoid scented lotions and all aromatherapy because many pregnant women have an aversion to strong odors (Boxes 9-2 and 9-3).

Abdominal Massage

Avoid deep abdominal massage during the entire pregnancy and for 3 months following childbirth. If the client has breast soreness (or is nursing), make modifications to her position while prone (refer to the section Large Breasts or Breast Implants in Chapter 10). Obtain permission. Use the entire

---

BOX 9-2

Essential Oil Recommendations for Pregnant Clients Past Their First Trimester for Home Use

Lavender
Rosewood
Rose
Frankincense

Make sure they are used in dilutions appropriate for a child (diluted by one half).

BOX 9-3

Essential Oils and Scents to Avoid During Pregnancy and Breast Feeding

Angelica	Davana	Peppermint
Anise	Fennel	Pimenta racemosa
Basil	Geranium	Rockrose
Birch	Ginger	Rosemary
Bitter almond	Hyssop	Sage
Camphor	Jasmine	Savory
Cedarwood	Juniper	Star anise
Chamomile	Laurel	Tarragon
Cinnamon	Marjoram	Thyme
Citronella	Myrrh	Valerian
Clary sage	Nutmeg	Wintergreen
Clove bud and leaf	Oregano	Yarrow
Coriander	Pennyroyal	Ylang-ylang
Cornmint		

hand, and apply light circular effleurage in a clockwise or horizontal direction. Allow your hand to gradually decrease in weight, as you slowly lift it off her abdomen as a whisper. Do not use tapotement or pointed, forceful, or deep pressure on the pregnant client's abdomen.

Massaging the Medial Thigh

The clot-dissolving properties of the blood decrease during pregnancy. A pregnant client is at an increased risk for blood clots. Blood clotting is more likely in veins than in arteries because blood moves slowly through them. Veins most likely to be at risk for blood clotting are the iliac, femoral, and great saphenous, all of which are located in or near the medial thigh region. Massage on these veins can loosen a clot or clot fragment. It can become lodged in the heart or lungs as they travel in the bloodstream. Use only gentle pressure in the medial thigh region, and restrict your techniques to the use of an open, flat hand.

> **TABLE TALK**
>
> Suggest that the client use light, gently self-applied abdominal massage while singing or speaking to her baby. She can use single or double (figure 8) circles. Recommend that she use a natural, highly emollient cream to increase the elasticity of her skin.

Comfort Issues

Treatment guidelines would not be complete without mentioning issues of client comfort. The following are tried and true suggestions to increase the comfort and pleasure of the massage experience for the pregnant client.

- The room should be well ventilated. Use an osculating fan to circulate the air. Remember to avoid heating packs and heating blankets. Pregnant women's hormones raise body temperature and create an incubation effect.
- Suggest that she use the restroom before and perhaps during the massage. Pregnant women tend to urinate frequently because of pressure on the urinary bladder by the growing fetus.
- Avoid water sounds in the massage music (e.g., rain, waterfalls, bubbling brooks). This sound may intensify the already frequent urge to urinate.
- Offer her a glass of pure water before, after, and perhaps during the massage, especially if she is nursing.
- Have lemon drops, peppermints, or ginger candy nearby. Candy may relieve nausea.
- Be responsive to the pregnant woman's mood, both in conversation and body language. Be willing to make adjustments in techniques, pressure, or her position on the table.
- Given that she may be dealing with emotions, as well as physical discomforts, have tissue handy!

PREGNANT CLIENT POSITIONING

Following are recommended safe positions for the pregnant client during the massage. Experiment with pillow positioning until optimal comfort and support are achieved.

Supine: Left Tilt

When a pregnant woman is lying supine, gravity will force her uterus to lie against her spine, thereby compressing the abdominal aorta and inferior vena cava. Pressure on these important vessels may cause a condition known as *supine hypotensive syndrome* (reduction of blood and oxygen to the fetus and mother's lower extremities).

To prevent this condition, place a small pillow, rolled towel, or wedge-shaped cushion under her right pelvis and trunk to tilt her lower body to the left 15 to 20 degrees (Figure 9-3). This elevation toward the left will move the uterus off the spine, maintaining normal blood circulation.

Supine: Semireclining

Support an expectant mother's head, shoulders, and back at a 45-degree angle when lying supine as stated above. Tilt her body to the left by placing a pillow or cushion under her right flank. A thick pillow can also be placed under the lower arms and behind the knees for additional comfort (Figure 9-4).

Side Lying

Ask the client to lie on the side on which she feels most comfortable. The client will spend most of the treatment time on this side, given that much of the body can be accessed from this position. Request that the client slide back so her backside is near the edge of the table. This position not only makes the therapist's work easier but also provides additional table space in front of the client for placement of pillows.

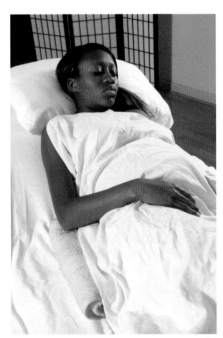

FIGURE 9-3 Pregnant client lying supine with a wedge under her right flank, tilting her to the left.

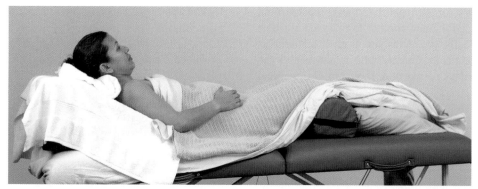

FIGURE 9-4 Pregnant client in semireclining position with additional pillow supports.

Use three or four pillows. Place the first pillow underneath her head. The next pillow should be placed under the upper arm (the side of the body not against the table) for support of her arm and shoulder. The last pillow props the knee and ankle and should lie in a horizontal plane with the hip on the same side. If the hip, knee, and ankle are not on the same plane, then use another pillow until the proper height is achieved. Three additional smaller pillows may be added under the wrist of the lower arm, under the lower ankle (side of the body touching the table), and under the abdomen (Figure 9-5).

Because the back, parts of the legs, and feet are approached from a side position, the therapist adjusts his or her body position for the best leverage. This adjustment may include using a stool, squatting, or kneeling on the floor.

Seated

Draping for a pregnancy-seated massage requires the client to bring a large short-sleeved shirt that buttons down the front. Disrobing for the massage involves her removing her shirt and brassiere and putting on the large shirt backwards. Be sure she does not attempt to button it. The unbuttoned shirt will provide the therapist with access to her back, neck, shoulders, forearms, and hands while the client

remains relaxed and comfortable during the massage. A hospital gown will do the trick as well.

Position a chair with its back against a table, and place a thick pillow on the tabletop. Have your pregnant client sit on the chair and lie against the pillow on the table by leaning forward.

MASSAGE DURING LABOR

Massage is a wonderful tool that helps the pregnant woman cope with the demands of labor. Realistically, most massage therapists cannot be on call day or night waiting for a message that the client is in labor. Additionally, labor may take many hours, or the massage therapist may be faced with false labor. All trips to the hospital or birthing center require that the therapist cancel and reschedule previously scheduled sessions. Massage for the pregnant client in labor will not be addressed for these reasons. Special considerations are needed when massaging during this special event. Please refer to one of the excellent references at the end of the chapter for more information.

MASSAGE POSTPARTUM

Once the baby is born, the mother's body begins its journey back to a prepregnant state. Some texts refer to this time as the *fourth* trimester. Postpartum massage can help the mother by reducing tension and soreness in muscles and enhancing relaxation. Vaginal bleeding (lochia) for the first 2 weeks postpartum for a vaginal birth and up to 6 weeks after a cesarean section (C-section) is normal and not a contraindication.

Back pain is not uncommon if the client was given an epidural. In fact, the new mother may experience pain and discomfort in and around the area where the epidural was administered. Avoid the area of the injection and a 1-inch area around the epidural for 72 hours.

Normal Vaginal Births

If the mother experienced a normal vaginal birth, no restrictions for prone and supine positions are necessary. The uterus will return to normal size relatively quickly with massage

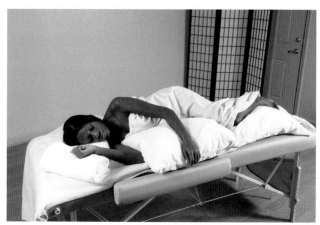

FIGURE 9-5 Client in side-lying position with pillows properly placed. Note the table widening device.

done every 4 hours for 10 days to 2 weeks postpartum. Teach and encourage the new mother to massage her own abdomen. Additionally, the rectus abdominis heals and returns to normal relatively quickly with massage and can begin as early as 3 days postpartum. Draw muscles together toward the midline and manually vibrate them. Knead the two sides of the rectus abdominis as they are moved toward the midline.

C-Section

Working on a client who underwent a C-section can be challenging. She may experience back and abdominal pain from the C-section. Feeling achy all over is not uncommon, resulting from inactivity while recuperating from a surgery. Next, add the stress from caring for a newborn while recovering from surgery. Finally, she may find that standing upright after surgery compounds back pain. Massage, once it is physician approved, will go a long way in relieving back discomfort.

Get written permission from her physician. Once obtained, use side-lying and supine positions for up to 8 weeks postsurgery. If an abdominal mesh was implanted, avoid the abdomen for 3 months and any deep abdominal (i.e., psoas) work indefinitely.

Massage and Nursing Mothers

Nursing mothers often feel tension in the back, neck, shoulders, and arms. Much of this tension stems from holding the baby during feedings. Nursed babies eat more frequently than babies who are not nursed; this variable may affect how much rest the mother can get. She may also sleep during feedings in some uncomfortable sleeping positions.

Offer the nursing client water before and after the massage because her fluid needs increase during this time. She may elect to wear her nursing bra during the massage because she may leak milk. Her breasts may be sore and tender, and she may feel more comfortable in a side-lying position during the massage. The therapist may even skip massage in the prone position. Be accommodating to all session adjustments that may add comfort. If mother's milk accidentally spills on the linens, treat them as contaminated.

INTRODUCTION TO INFANT MASSAGE

Infant massage in the postpartum period is a natural transition of the baby being massaged in utero to being massaged in the outside world. A mother who has just experienced massage during her pregnancy can understand the many benefits of massage for her new baby. Massage can accommodate the ongoing love from one world to the next, as well as provide an opportunity for the father's early involvement in nurturing the baby.

> **evolve** *Log on to your student account for* Massage Therapy Principles and Practice, 3e, *and locate the course materials for Chapter 9. Read the "History and Development of Infant Massage" for a better understanding of infant massage.* ■

Benefits of Infant Massage for Infants

Infant massage may:
- Help foster parent-infant bonding as a result of intimate interaction time between parent and baby.
- Relieve discomfort from teething, congestion, gas, and colic.
- Promote digestion by activating the relaxation response.
- Stimulate the nervous system through the stimulation of the skin while speeding myelination of the nerves and enhancing neurological development.
- Increase blood flow, ensuring that oxygen and nutrients reach the infant's cells and tissues.
- Slow and deepen respiration rate.
- Improve muscle tone through activation of sensory and motor neurons.
- Encourage midline orientation and sensory awareness after tactile stimulation.
- Increase vocalization, thereby assisting in speech and language development.
- Promote deeper and longer sleep for the baby.

Benefits of Infant Massage for Parents

Infant massage can:
- Assist parents in acquiring self-confidence and self-esteem in their parenting roles.
- Enhance and reinforce parental skills and validate the parental role.
- Help ease the stress of a working parent by reinstating the connection with the infant.
- Offer parents time to relax by providing focused time and attention with their infant.
- Help increase the parent's ability to relax the child in times of stress.
- Help release the pituitary hormone prolactin in both mothers and fathers. In women, prolactin is involved in milk production and may help foster maternal feelings. In men, the belief is that prolactin stimulates the desire to protect and nurture the infant.
- Enhance communication between the parent and infant.
- Provide a special time for intimacy between fathers and their children.
- Help parents learn to read infant behavior, making parenting easier.

> *"A baby is born with a need to be loved—and never outgrows it."*
> Frank A. Clark

Importance of Bonding

Bonding is a reciprocal relationship that goes from the caregiver to the infant and from the infant to the caregiver. According to Drs. Marshall Klaus and John Kennell, bonding is a "solid connection between the parent and child that nourishes the infant on a core level, the process that attaches the infant to reality." Bonding occurs when certain elements are in place soon after the baby's birth. These elements include skin-to-skin contact, odor or scent, high-pitched voice, prolonged eye contact, warmth, and the reestablishment of biorhythmic activity that existed between the mother and the baby in utero. Infant massage is especially suitable as a vehicle for all of the necessary elements for parent-infant bonding, a process that builds trust and intimacy, calls forth the innate protective and nurturing instincts in parents, and sets the tone for long-term quality of the parent-child relationship.

evolve *Log on to the Evolve website to read a short story about the process of bonding and attachment.* ■

Infant Massage Is *Different* from Adult Massage

Perhaps the easiest way to describe infant massage is to begin with how it differs from adult massage. Much of what we assume to be true of massage for adults is perhaps not only untrue but also just the reverse for babies.

For instance, if an adult is stressed and overwhelmed, then the assumption is that getting a massage will be beneficial. Most adults are quite capable of letting go, surrendering to gravity and sinking into the massage table. Babies are not programmed to do so. In fact, they are in the process of being imprinted by each touch and image as they engage in the world. A stressed baby is usually ready to disengage. Stress for a baby means lower tolerance and limited resources to cope with more stimulation such as massage. Massage is one more thing with which to deal and usually is not what is needed at that time.

Unlike adults, babies often participate in massage in a social way, with their eyes wide open and body in motion, rather than being a passive recipient. Remember, the parents are sharing in a bonding process by loving and touching baby with their hands and heart. A nurturing two-way relationship is going on, which is different from the professional boundaries and comparatively distant touch of a massage therapist. This nurturing is part of a process of attachment that occurs for months and is nature's way of ensuring that the family falls in love with the baby.

Infant massage is not a 1-hour appointment, and it never lasts 1 hour. At its best, massage is, for parent and baby, a timeless dimension of hanging out, being attentive, and performing a creative partnered dance orchestrated by a parent, who is really hearing and seeing the baby and offering thoughtful and spontaneous nurturing.

Comparing Infant Massage with Adult Massage
- Babies are going through a period of attachment and bonding with the parent who is massaging them; adults are not.
- Babies may not have good thermal regulation and may need to stay partially dressed for warmth; adults can ask for a blanket.
- Babies will get massaged in various locations, such as the floor, parent's bed, couch, or even on a parent's body; adults get massaged on a massage table.
- The mother or father massages babies; a therapist massages adults.
- Babies need to be massaged with a cold-pressed, edible oil because they often put their hands in their mouths; adults are safe with a wider range of lubricants.
- Baby massage may be done in 5, 15, 30 minutes, or more, depending on the baby's tolerance and parent's state; adults receive a 1-hour massage and wish it were longer.
- Babies should receive massage 30 to 45 minutes after feeding, which is a good idea for adults too but not as necessary.
- Babies are too sensitive for scented massage lubricants and prefer the smell of their parents; adults often prefer scented lubricants.
- Babies prefer the parent's voice or quiet; adults generally prefer music or quiet.
- Babies cannot walk away if the massage is really bad; adults can.
- Older babies and toddlers play during the massage; adults lie there.
- Babies may fall asleep during massage, signaling that the massage is over, which is not necessarily so for adults, who may continue to get massaged as they snore.
- Babies who get overstimulated during massage will cry; adults who get overstimulated will either fall asleep or talk.

GETTING STARTED

The infant massage instructor begins by informally interviewing the parent to learn what he or she is hoping to achieve during the session (Figure 9-6). Perhaps the parent is looking for a way to calm the baby or a way to relieve the pain of gas and colic. Next, find out what the baby already seems to like or dislike. Perhaps the baby enjoys having his or her head stroked and may be ticklish or have sensitive feet. Use and affirm the parent's wisdom as you initiate touch and massage in their family. This insight may include the parent's opinion as to what position the child will prefer while being massaged. Supine, prone, side lying, sitting upright, and standing are possibilities, with the addition of support, which depends on the baby's age and stage of development.

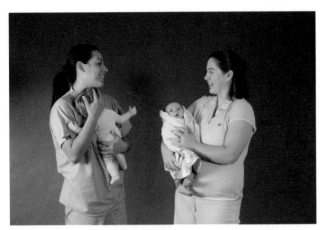

FIGURE 9-6 Infant massage instructor talking to parent. Note the instructor holding a doll.

After the initial interview, wash your hands before teaching, even though you are not touching the baby. Families are concerned about germs, and rightfully so, given that some babies are prone to illness. This gesture is a sign of professionalism and respect to the family. If you are sick, cancel the teaching session until you are well.

> ### TABLE TALK
>
> Do not massage the baby for 30 minutes after bottle feeding. However, because breast milk is predigested, the baby can be massaged shortly after eating.

INFANT BEHAVIOR AS A GUIDE

Teaching the family to recognize and use the baby's behavioral states will assist the family in finding the best time to massage the baby. For example, a state such as *deep sleep* is an obvious statement to postpone the massage until later.

Perhaps equally important is being attentive to a baby's rapid transitioning from one state to another, such as moving from crying to sleep (a baby's state of consciousness can shift in an instant). The parents have to be willing to adapt to the baby's new behavioral state. Additionally, some babies become disoriented when their position is changed or as their behavioral state begins to shift. Both instructor and parent should watch the baby closely and be prepared to shift with the baby's change in behavior, even if these changes occur during the course of the massage.

Infants exhibit predictable behavioral states that cycle in times of both sleeping and wakefulness. Being aware of these behavioral states can help parents choose the best time to massage their baby. These states are:

- Deep sleep
- Light sleep
- Drowsiness
- Quiet alert
- Active alert
- Crying

While coaching parents to massage the baby, teach them these behavior states and encourage them to observe their babies and note in which behavioral state the baby may be. The most appropriate behavioral state for infant massage is the quiet alert state in which the motor activity, facial expression, and breathing are relaxed while baby's eyes are open and appear bright, interested, observant, and quietly alert. Although the baby's natural tendency is to follow a cycle, states can be activated by external stimuli such as noise, activity, or of course massage. One moment, the massage can be nurturing, and the next moment, it can become the stressor.

RESPONDING TO CRYING

While facilitating infant massage with parents and their babies, the instructor will witness a variety of cries triggered by a wide range of distresses. Be willing to stop wherever you are in the session. The baby must be allowed to set the course of the massage.

If a parent is uncomfortable or hesitant about responding to the baby while crying, avoid encouraging him or her to comfort the baby. A parent's intuition with his or her baby should always be respected, even if your own instinct is the opposite. With more experience, the parent will gain a greater skill in really listening to the baby.

Asking parents if they know what the baby seems to be saying is appropriate. Sometimes parents may know, and other times they may not. However, by supporting the spontaneous expression of the crying infant with intuitive listening, and by maintaining a welcoming presence for the expression, we open the door to a baby's emerging into the world around him. We do not encourage parents to simply let their baby cry or to do something to stop the crying but to attend to the baby's cries by trying to discern what type of cry it is, thereby learning to understand the baby.

Cries of pain or overstimulation need to be carefully studied and considered because your teaching will vary, depending on the type of cry it is. In public, start listening whenever you are around a baby who is crying; automatically tune in to the sound and ask yourself, "What kind of cry is this? What is this cry expressing?" Of course, "I'm hungry" cries, "Change my diaper" cries, and "I've got gas" cries can occur. However, release cries that simply say, "Hear my grief" and "Hear my rage!" can also occur. This kind of crying is emotional crying, sometimes called *talk crying*. You may witness very young babies looking right into their parent's eyes and expressing their feelings of frustration, anger, or grief. The release cry is a way for the baby to communicate the release of stress, and optimally the parent will respond by listening and acknowledging. If you have ever cried because you are stressed out, then you know the crying is different than that of a specific emotion. Additionally, the cry can be one of fatigue for some babies who have a hard time dropping into sleep.

*"When I was born I was so surprised that
I did not talk for a year and a half."*
Gracie Allen

MINI-LAB

To learn about crying, start listening to it. Listen to babies' cries everywhere. What do you hear? Listen to the tone, the pitch, and how it fluctuates back and forth from stronger to softer. Do you hear emotion in the crying? If so, what emotion do you hear? How does the cry affect you internally?

TYPICAL STROKES FOR MASSAGING BABIES

When individualizing touch and massage for an infant, strokes are created and refined as a session progresses. However, already having at least a handful of tried and true strokes ready for use throughout the session is a good idea. Some strokes are easily adaptable for use over much of the body. These strokes include, but are not limited to, touch-holds, thumb-over-thumb stroking, thumb spreading, and full-hand stroking.

When applying these strokes, focus on the mechanics of the touch relative to pressure, pacing, rhythm, direction, and so forth while observing whether the parent is connecting to the baby with the touch and whether the baby is tolerating it. Additionally, note that, depending on the age and development of the baby (e.g., 4 months, 8 months), the comfort positioning of the infant can appear very different. Following are some strokes that can be adapted.

Touch-Holds

Warmly holding an area of the body lets the baby know you are starting (or ending) the massage on that body part.

Swedish Milking

Using your full palms, massage with long fluid strokes toward the heart.

Thumb-Over-Thumb

In this technique, rhythmic stroking occurs with thumb-over-thumb in the motion of windshield wipers.

Thumb Spreading

Starting with thumbs together, spread laterally to the sides. This stroke is less stimulating than thumb-over-thumb stroking.

Rather than applying strokes as a routine, try to view the application of touch as a continuum from calming touch to stimulating touch. For instance, when introducing touch to a newborn's arm, the most calming touch would be a touch-hold, warmly holding the arm with no movement. If this touch is acceptable to the baby, try holding the arm with one hand and pressing lightly with the other. This touch can still be calming though more stimulating than a touch-hold. Then increase the stimulation by holding with one hand (calming and organizing) and stroking with the other hand (stimulating). Finally, if the baby is still tolerating the touch, then stroke with both hands. As always with infants, all of these movements should be done very slowly and with parent and instructor constantly observing the baby to make sure the touch and massage is being tolerated.

Infant Cues: Reading the Baby

Another key to individualizing massage is recognizing infant behavioral cues. According to Dr. Kathryn Barnard, certain facial expressions and gestures imply specific needs and feelings. We can generally group these cues as indicators of an infant's need or openness for engagement or for disengagement. Babies can only accommodate so much stimulation before they need a break. They want to interact (engage) for a while; then they need to take a break (disengage) before they are ready to interact again. Taking these breaks helps the infant regroup and be available for more interaction. Attentiveness to these cues translates into a deep level of empathy and ultimately the ability to attend to a baby's needs.

Clinically, more than 108 known infant behavioral cues exist that parents can learn to recognize so that in each moment the massage approach can be adapted to fit the baby. Engagement cues are similar to magnets for parental attention: baby smiling, cooing, bright eyes, making eye contact, reaching toward parent, and so forth. These cues are potent signals that the baby is ready to interact.

Compared with the number of engagement cues that tell us that the infant is ready to interact with the parent, perhaps a tenfold number of disengagement cues exist that appeal for the parent to stop what is happening. Some cues are obvious and send an alarm to a parent, such as crying, gaze aversion, arching, splayed fingers and toes, or leg kicking. One cue by itself, such as a sneeze, may suggest only a slight stress. However, when the sneeze is accompanied by other cues such as arching and pushing away, this increasing cluster of signals should be viewed as a growing announcement that the direction of the massage needs to change before the infant becomes overstimulated. Whatever is happening with touch and massage in that moment is no longer working for the baby. A word of wisdom is to watch, listen, and then act.

If these behavioral cues are missed and the massage is continued, the baby will become increasingly stressed. What to do next? Have the parents stop the massage and give the baby a comfort break. Try to reduce the stimulation in the room; maybe turn off the CD player if one is playing, lower your own voice, reposition the baby, or adjust the lights or temperature. Sometimes a baby may need to be held or fed. However, if the baby continues to get fussier, then the massage needs to stop. In this case, other educational strategies can be done for the remainder of the session, such as teaching the parent about benefits and cues or asking a questions such as, "How is it going for you as a parent?"

If you are able to proceed with the massage after the comfort break, the parent should offer the massage more slowly so the touch is in accord with the baby. Slow is good in infant massage. Actually, slow for infant massage is slower than what we normally consider as slow. Slow movement is less stimulating than fast movement and encourages both baby and parent to be aware and present. Similarly, firm but gentle touch is more grounding and less stimulating than light touch, as is using a full hand rather than fingertips. Less is more. If you can succeed in helping a parent tune into the baby, to go slowly,

and to watch closely for and respond to behavioral cues, then he or she will not require a lot of strokes or information.

MINI-LAB

Without judgment, observe parent-infant interaction and notice how the parents calm their baby. Do they use movement, voice, touch, or visual engagement? What else do you observe?

Using a Doll to Teach Parents to Massage Their Babies

A good doll for teaching infant massage is one with flexible limbs and a weighted body that can be positioned to match the positions of a baby. Infant massage instructors use dolls

VIMALA SCHNEIDER McCLURE

Born: June 7, 1952

"Do all the good you can in all the ways you can, for all the people you can for long as ever you can."
P. R. Sarkar

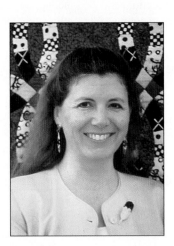

Vimala Schneider McClure, the pioneer of infant massage in the United States, always had the feeling that she was put on earth to fulfill a specific purpose. At age 21, the starry-eyed humanitarian sold everything she had and took off for India. "I was terrified," she confided, "but my sense of purpose was so strong it was worth putting myself in harm's way."

In India, McClure studied with yogi master P. R. Sarkar until a bout with malaria cut her trip short and landed her in a New York hospital for a couple of weeks.

McClure had recurrences for years afterward, and her health has never been perfect. McClure is a diethylstilbestrol (a drug given to prevent miscarriages now proved to have adverse effects) daughter. As a child, she had open-heart surgery. She had 11 operations and has lost "every expendable organ." Today, she experiences severe fibromyalgia.

Somewhat recovered from the malaria, McClure returned to India and worked in an orphanage. There, she learned the art of infant massage from an assistant. Out of necessity, the nun who ran the orphanage spent much of her time begging for money for its support; thus McClure

was left to care for the children along with two Indian girls. "They couldn't speak my language, and I couldn't speak theirs," she remembers. In the evenings, when the courtyard cooled off to 90° F, she learned traditional Indian baby massage.

"They've done it in India for 10,000 years or more," she explains. Mothers massage their infants and pass along the skill to their daughters. "I began to see how relaxed these children were…how different [they were] from American children. They were easier with each other and less aggressive. Boys and girls alike walk around with their arms around each other. Then it began to click. I began to see massage as something that could change lives. A good analogy is that we're like a cup, and the more love that goes into that cup, until it is overflowing, the more you can give. If your cup didn't get filled as a child, then you're always looking for someone to fill it up."

McClure points out that every mammal species licks its young, which is not just for cleaning. It is a bonding process that stimulates the whole system. Without this stage, mothers kill their offspring, or offspring are to demonstrate positioning, massage strokes, and interpersonal dynamics such as talking. If the baby is changing positions, then the instructor will mirror the same positioning with his or her doll to facilitate a seamless flow from one stroke to the next.

Given that parents are often sleep deprived and overwhelmed with new parenting responsibilities, teach slowly to avoid adding to their stress. Actually, parents cannot learn and process a lot of new skills and strokes; therefore in each session, give them just the few massage movements that they are able to take in and their baby can tolerate (Figure 9-7). Parents can practice between sessions and keep building on their skills each week, and the baby's tolerance increases over time. In this way the massage is effective both for parents and baby.

Parents want to know that they are doing the strokes correctly. Teach them that they need to look to the baby for confirmation rather than to the instructor, and attune to the baby for affirmation rather than zeroing in on the mechanics via the instructor. A baby is a person; connect to this person to determine what works best.

Parents are taught to ask permission before they begin a massage with their baby. Initially, this action may be just a show of thoughtfulness from the parent to a baby who as yet has no answers, but as the baby grows, asking permission to massage becomes an authentic sign of respect. If the baby indicates *no,* then the massage is postponed, regardless of how much the mother or father was looking forward to it.

Babies cannot tell the parents what they like; thus the parents (along with the instructor) need to discover what works for their baby. Infants cannot tolerate massage as long as adults can; thus parents need to be prepared to be finished when baby is finished. This time can be perhaps 5 minutes, 15 minutes, or 30 minutes. The length of time varies with each child and each session, as well as with the time constraint

VIMALA SCHNEIDER McCLURE (*continued*)

affected down the road in the same way that abused children may perpetuate abuse.

McClure returned to the United States in 1976 and became pregnant with her first of two children. In addition to everything about massage and yoga she had learned in India, she asked friends to teach her some Swedish massage techniques to develop a routine for her newborn. In her book *Infant Massage: A Handbook for Loving Parents,* she writes: "This joyful blend provided my son with a wonderful balance of outgoing and incoming energy, of tension release, and stimulation. Additionally, it seemed to relieve the painful gas he had been experiencing that first month."

McClure began to keep copious notes. Eventually, she invited mothers over to show them what she was doing. During these sessions, she distributed a small hand-made flyer.

One of McClure's tiny flyers fell into the right hands, and she was invited to speak at a childbirth education conference. There, she met the owner of a baby products company who asked, "Have you ever thought about writing a book? Write one, and I'll publish it."

McClure had already done so, and *Infant Massage: A Handbook for Loving Parents* became, and still is, the definitive work on infant massage. Pressed by others to begin an organization, she founded the International Association of Infant Massage, which is a worldwide operation now, but she receives no money for her pioneering training except for royalties from the book. "I was zero percent motivated by money at the time. I didn't think about how much profit I could make. I didn't think of my work as a business venture. At this point in my life, I'm not so sure how smart that was," she confesses.

For the beginning massage therapist, McClure's advice is to start with a different mindset regarding infant massage because what happens between parent and child is different from what happens during a therapeutic massage. McClure says, "It's the act of bonding and impacting a lifetime. That's why I trained instructors to teach parents rather than training massage therapists to massage infants. As an instructor, you have to allow parents to develop their own style. Even if they don't apply strokes in an expert manner, the message comes through. You have to empower parents and not allow them to turn over their power to the instructor as the expert."

McClure considers the rearing of her two children her main mission in life. Asked how she would respond if her daughter said she was off to some third-world country to find her purpose, McClure admits, "I'd try to talk her out of it. I'm too much a mom. But if it was something she positively had to do, I'd give her my blessing." She continues to write and to help parents develop closer, more meaningful relationships with their children. Her other works include *The Tao of Motherhood, A Woman's Guide to Tantric Yoga*, and her current book, *The Path of Parenting: Twelve Principles to Guide Your Journey.*

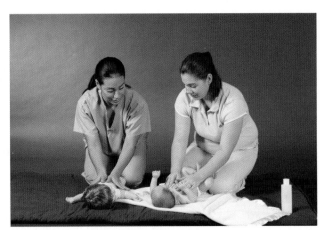

FIGURE 9-7 Teaching a parent infant massage.

of the parent. Babies also do not do as well as adults with unconscious touch from their parents. You know how a massage feels when a therapist is hurrying or not paying attention. The same feeling goes for the infant. If the parent is acting hurried or having difficulty focusing, then the massage will not feel good to the baby.

Given that the parent is the one who is massaging the baby, success is attributed to parental competence rather than to the skills of either a massage therapist or an infant massage instructor. Parental success will ensure the continuity of infant massage in the family, thereby sustaining or deepening the attachment and the quality of the family's life.

Students are often amazed to hear that massage is not always so great for a baby. It can be, but we have to discover the ingredients to make massage wonderful for the baby and the parent in that moment. Remember that *less is more*. Infant massage is not about the volume of strokes or even the amount of coverage of the baby's body; it is about sharing a moment of time and going deeper into it together.

Organizing Your Environment for Infant Massage

Warmth
The environment should be warm and without drafts. Oil will wick heat off the baby's body; therefore the room temperature should be approximately 5° to 10° warmer than usual. Babies are calmer in warmer temperatures than they are in colder temperatures. Some babies do not have good thermal regulation. If they do tend to get chilled, keep areas that are not being massaged covered with a blanket. Additionally, keeping them partially dressed or partially covered may work, especially for newborn or very young babies.

Lighting
Natural light or low light is best. Babies can become overstimulated with fluorescent lighting, much as adults do.

Where to Do the Massage at Home
Massage can be given on the floor, bed, couch, recliner, or wherever the parent spends time with the baby.

Noise
Keep the environment free from distractions such as ringing telephones, television, or radio noise. However, some households are active with other children; thus you may need to be accommodating with this rule.

Positioning
Parents need back support without having to lean over too far to look at the baby during the massage. Parental positioning is as crucial as that of the baby.

The baby's positioning will vary from baby to baby and will be adjusted to appropriately fit the developmental age of the baby. The position initially used in the massage will change as the massage progresses and as the baby grows and develops.

Lubricant
The most preferred types of oil to use are grape seed, safflower, and olive. Avoid mineral oils because they clog the skin's pores and are not digestible. Also avoid scents; they may cause an allergic reaction in a sensitive baby.

Music
Soft background music can assist the parent in creating the rhythm for the massage, as well as promote the relaxation response. The favorite music for the baby is the parent's voice singing a lullaby or just talking or humming.

Who Massages the Baby?

Infant massage belongs, first of all, to the parents. Both the mother and the father should learn, if possible. Grandparents can massage the baby if the parents approve. Infant massage can be fun to do with their grandchild and can enhance their bonding. Other family members can also join the massage team; provided the parents are comfortable with this, it is safe for the baby, it does not threaten the parent-child relationship, and parents are acting as the gatekeeper. Unfortunately, both physical and sexual abuse runs in some family systems. Family members need to be informed of the same learning of infant cues, asking permission throughout the session, observing the baby, and stopping when the infant is done. As child advocates, infant massage instructors need to watch family dynamics closely and make it safe for the baby.

ADAPTING TO THE GROWING CHILD

For the crawler, the idea of *massaging what comes up* is often a surprise for massage therapists. One minute, the parent is massaging a leg, and the next minute, the child has turned over and the parent continues on the back. This adaptation seems different than to what most of us are accustomed. The session is simply not static and passive anymore. Parents follow the baby's lead.

Toddlers have even more mobility than infants, and parents learn to massage on the run. To help engage the toddler with the massage, some parents will play, sing, and accompany their strokes with rhymes.

It is never too late for parents to learn to massage their children. Families have been taught to massage their children who are at varying ages and developmental stages, from birth through the teen years, with all enjoying the connection with one another. Parents report a feeling of increased closeness to their children.

Creating magical moments for your family requires only your presence. This dimension is always in place, waiting for you to step into it and to transform what you are doing into a *happening,* a scene of compassion, insight, and lifelong memories for both the child and the parents.

BECOMING AN INFANT MASSAGE INSTRUCTOR

Much can be learned about infant massage from books. However, no shortcut can substitute for the practical experience that prepares you to teach parents how to massage their babies. Postgraduate continuing education in the form of infant massage instructor certification training is a 4-day immersion into infant massage, complete with observation of the trainer teaching a group of families and student practicum teaching with families during the course.

To discover the best instructor trainer, ask how long the teacher has been training instructors and whether the trainer consistently teaches families. It is your responsibility to ensure the best training possible. Ultimately, you will get the most from a trainer who is active on more than a casual basis and knows the work from years of experience with families. Such a trainer can bring freshness and liveliness to the learning environment and can share meaningful stories that provide insight into the many questions that students have.

Following the basic instructor certification training for the well baby, extra training courses are available for working with families with children who have special needs or who are biologically or environmentally at risk. More can

always be learned, and a variety of avenues can be taken to help you grow as an infant massage instructor. Supervision by an experienced instructor trainer, review of your videotaped sessions, and private preceptorships are available to assist in the infant massage instructor's development.

PRECAUTIONS AND CONTRAINDICATIONS FOR INFANT MASSAGE

Special Precautions of Infant Massage for the Well Baby

- Jaundice: Red blood cells are not breaking down properly, and these cells can be spread with massage.
- Reflux: Wait at least 30 minutes after feeding. The baby needs to be elevated 45 to 90 degrees during the massage and held upright for 10 to 15 minutes after the massage. Another suggestion is to avoid massaging up the back.
- Nausea, vomiting, and diarrhea: These signs indicate illness or detoxification. Massage is not recommended.
- The instructor should not assume that discomfort of gas or colic is simply that; it can indicate an internal medical condition. If relief is not apparent soon, then parents should consult with their physician.

Contraindications for Babies Who Are at Risk or Have Special Needs

Precautions exist for the baby who is premature, both in the nursery and following discharge. Further continuing education is needed for an instructor to gain proficiency in this branch of infant massage. This precaution also exists for working with families with babies with special needs or with medical or neuromotor conditions. These challenging conditions need to be considered to design a safe and suitable massage plan for the family.

SUMMARY

This chapter has provided you with a brief overview of the world of pregnancy and infant massage. Both of these areas require a deep connection with pregnant women and their families and with a field in which you never stop learning; each situation will teach you something new. Massage does make a difference, a huge difference in many cases, and changes the lives not only of parents and babies but of the therapist and instructors as well.

CASE STUDY:

Up in Smoke

Susan was a mother of four children and a wife of a loving husband. For their fifteenth wedding anniversary, Susan's husband bought her a massage with her therapist, Delilah. He had been laid off of work recently and saved up to give this anniversary gift to his wife. She had been stressed as a result of a recent diagnosis of a chronic illness. He would stay home with the children while she relaxed.

Susan was diagnosed with chronic obstructive pulmonary disease, specifically chronic bronchitis. She had smoked for 20 years, which had taken its toll on her lungs. Susan's physician instructed her to avoid cigarette smoke. She was currently on a drug regimen to quit smoking, and it was successful.

When Susan arrived for her appointment, she was ready for tranquil moments. The receptionist greeted her and asked her to have a seat and that Delilah would be with her shortly.

When Delilah called Susan to the massage room, she was anticipating the smell of clean linens, soothing music, and an inviting atmosphere. To her surprise, an overwhelming stench of cigarette smoke was in the room and on Delilah's clothes. Delilah greeted her with a welcoming smile and asked Susan about her health since her last visit. Susan informed her of the recent diagnosis. She told Delilah about the avoidance of cigarette smoke. Delilah, who was a cigarette smoker, thought nothing of this news

because she did not smoke in the building.

Approximately 10 minutes into the massage, Susan started to feel nauseated and began to cough. Delilah asked her if she would like a glass of water. Susan nodded. Delilah left the room. When Delilah returned, Susan was still coughing and nearly dressed. Susan drank the water and told Delilah that she could not continue with the massage, stating that she had a headache and felt queasy. Delilah believed that Susan was upset as well.

How should Delilah respond to Susan's sudden illness?

Should Delilah address the belief that Susan seemed upset? If so, how might she do this?

If Delilah were told the truth, how might she respond to the criticism?

Once told, should Delilah assume responsibility and refund the charges?

Given that this session was a gift, how should Delilah involve the gift giver?

Should Susan be referred to a nonsmoking therapist for future sessions?

How should Susan tell Delilah about the offensive odor?

Susan does not want to change therapists because she loves Delilah's work; therefore how might she address the situation for future sessions?

How might Susan tell her husband that the massage was an awful experience?

---

evolve

Go to *Chapter Extras* on Evolve for additional illustrations and resources for this chapter. *Extras* for this chapter include:

1. Sample infant massage routine (text)
2. Crossword puzzle (downloadable form)
3. Case study (text)
4. Pregnancy and infant massage (video clip)

MATCHING

Place the letter of the answer next to the term or phrase that best describes it.

A. Bonding
B. Broad
C. Doll
D. First
E. Fourth
F. High risk

G. Incubation
H. Morning sickness
I. Parents
J. Permission
K. Postponement

L. Progesterone
M. Prone
N. Quiet alert
O. Round
P. Second

_____   1.   The question parents must ask before they begin massaging their baby

_____   2.   According to the chapter, the persons to whom infant massage belong

_____   3.   In the first trimester, the effect created by hormones that raise body temperature

_____   4.   The trimester during which the mother begins to *show*

_____   5.   The ligaments in which overstretching creates sciatic-like pain in pregnant women

_____   6.   The ligaments that may create a pulling or sharp pain on either side of the lower abdomen

_____   7.   The hormone that relaxes the smooth muscle of the uterus and the valve between the esophagus and the stomach and that slows down gastrointestinal tract motility

_____   8.   The condition that approximately 75% of pregnant women experience during their first trimester

_____   9.   The trimester that marks the least change in the woman's body but the most development in the embryo

_____   10. The month that the pregnant woman should have entered to safely begin pregnancy massage

_____   11. The term given to pregnancies that put the mother, the developing fetus, or both at higher-than-normal risk for complications to develop during or after the pregnancy and birth

_____   12. The position that is contraindicated during pregnancy

_____   13. The term that is used to describe the solid connection between the parent and the child that nourishes the baby on a core level

_____   14. The preferred behavioral state for the baby to receive massage

_____   15. The item that an infant massage instructor uses to model both strokes and relational dynamics

_____   16. The event that should happen with massage if the baby becomes overstimulated

INTERNET ACTIVITIES

Visit http://www.infantmassageinstitute.com and click on Why Infant Massage? Write a short paragraph on the subject.

Visit http://www.marchofdimes.com and click on Pregnancy and Newborn. Locate the section on Special Topics and click on Birth Defects and Genetics. Choose a condition and prepare a short report.

Visit http://www.americanpregnancy.org and click on Pregnancy Complications. Choose a complication, and, after reading, discuss with the class how massage can affect a pregnant client with this particular condition.

Bibliography

Applegate EJ: *The anatomy and physiology learning system,* ed 3, Philadelphia, 2006, Saunders.

Artal R, Friedman MJ, McNitt-Gray JL: Orthopedic problems in pregnancy, *Phys Sports Med* 18:93-105, 1990.

Avery MD, Van Arsdale L: Perineal massage: effect on the incidence of episiotomy and laceration in a nulliparous population, *J Nurse Midwifery* 32(3):181-184, 1987.

Bernard K: *Keys to caregiving. Nursing child assessment satellite training (NCAST) manual,* ed 2, Seattle, 1995, University of Washington School of Nursing.

Eisenberg A, Murkoff HE, Hathaway SE: *What to expect when you're expecting,* New York, 1991, Workman Publishing.

Engelmann GJ: Massage and expression or external manipulation in the obstetric practice of primitive people, *Massage Ther J* 33(3):34-40, 92-110, 1994.

Evans M: Complementary therapies: reflex zone therapy for mothers, *Nurs Times* 86(4):29-31, 1990.

Gorsuch R, Key M: Abnormalities of pregnancy as a function of anxiety and life stress, *Psychosom Med* 36:353, 1974.

Grafstrom AV: A short review of mechano-therapy in connection with obstetrics, *New York Med J* 64:746-748, 1896.

Guthrie RA: Lumbar inhibitory pressure for lumbar myalgia during contractions of the gravid uterus at term, *J Am Osteopath Med Assoc* 80:264-266, 1980.

Heller S: *The vital touch,* New York, 1997, Henry Holt and Company.

Hiniker PK, Moreno LA: *Developmentally supportive care, theory and application,* Norwell, Mass, 1994, Children's Medical Ventures.

Inkeles G: *Massage and peaceful pregnancy,* New York, 1983, Putnam Publishing Group.

Klaus MH, Kennell JH, Klaus PH: *Bonding: building the foundations of secure attachment and independence,* San Francisco, 1983, Addison-Wesley.

Knaster M: Researching massage as real therapy: an interview with Dr. Tiffany Field, *Massage Ther J* 33(3):45-53, Summer 1994.

Leboyer F: *Loving hands: the traditional art of baby massage,* New York, 1997, Newmarket Press.

Leigh S: Aromatherapy: making good scents, *Mothering* 59:77-79, 1991.

Mathias M, Mathias W: *Infant touch and massage instructor manual,* Albuquerque, NM, 2002, Self-published manuscript.

Milinare C: *Birth,* New York, 1990, Random House.

Napolitano R: Loving pregnancy massage: a manual for practitioners and educators, *Natural Wellness,* Pine Bush, NY, 2000.

Osborne-Sheets C: Massage and the pregnant pelvis, *Mass Ther J* 37(2):88-96, 1998.

Osborne-Sheets C: *Pre- and perinatal massage therapy*, San Diego, 1998, Body Therapy Associates.

Ostgaard HC et al: Prevalence of back pain in pregnancy, *Spine* 17(1):53-55, 1992.

Parvati J: Hygieia: a woman's herbal, *Freestyle Collective,* Moab, 1991, Freestone Publishing Co.

Rich P: *Practical aromatherapy,* Bath, UK, 1994, Parragon Book Service.

Salvo S: *Massage therapy: principles and practice,* ed 1, Philadelphia, 1999, Saunders.

Salvo SG, Anderson SK: *Mosby's pathology for massage therapists,* St Louis, 2004, Mosby.

Schrag K: Maintenance of pelvic floor integrity during childbirth, *J Nurse Midwifery* 24(6):26-30, 1979.

Schneider McClure V: *Infant massage: a handbook for loving parents,* New York, 2000, Bantam Books.

Stillerman E: *Mother massage: a handbook for relieving for relieving the discomforts of pregnancy,* New York, 2006, Dell Publishing.

Thibodeau G, Patton K: *Anatomy and physiology,* ed 6, St Louis, 2006, Mosby.

Turner Bernhardt R: Massage therapist as doula, *Massage Ther J* 33(3):46-48, 1994.

Waters B: *Massage during pregnancy,* ed 3, 2003, Bluewaters Press.

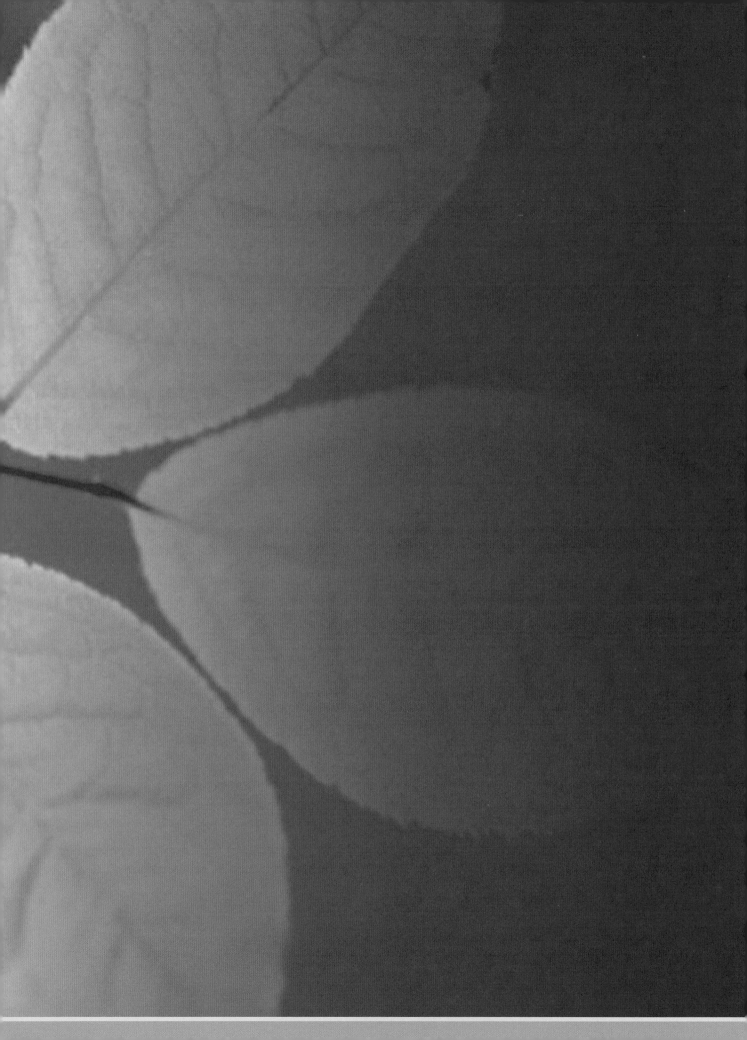

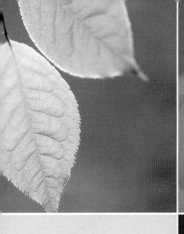

CHAPTER 10

"It is only with the heart that one can see rightly. What is essential is invisible to the eye."
—Antoine de Saint-Exupéry

Adaptive Massage

STUDENT OBJECTIVES

After completing this chapter, the student should be able to:

- Modify the client's position to accomodate his or her special needs
- Adjust massage techniques to suit the client's various conditions
- Identify important considerations when working with chronically or terminally ill clients
- State the guidelines to follow when working with clients who have cancer
- Apply modifications required when working with clients who are HIV positive or who have AIDS
- Define physical changes noted in most geriatric clients
- Explain modification that may be needed when working with large clients
- Accommodate clients who have visual, auditory, or speech impairments
- Adjust massage to accommodate someone who is physically challenged or in a wheelchair
- Discuss emotional releases, and describe ways they can be handled appropriately

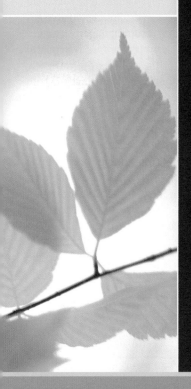

INTRODUCTION

The standard massage routine is designed to suit the needs of the average client, who may represent the majority of your clientele. However, you will encounter individuals who have unique situations that include physical, emotional, and health-related challenges. You will need to accommodate these individuals and modify or adapt massage therapy to fit their special needs. Client needs may range from relatively simple ones such as bolstering for breast implants or spinal abnormalities; to communication modifications for persons with speech, vision, or hearing impairments; to moderate needs such as working around central venous catheters, colostomy bags, and pacemakers; to emotional needs for persons who have been sexually abused or have chemical dependencies; and to clients living with chronic or terminal illnesses such as cancer and acquired immunodeficiency syndrome (AIDS).

The most important way to assist individuals who need adaptive massage is to view them as people first and their special needs only as a secondary consideration. Generally, the best approach is to regard all injuries and conditions with the attitudes of gentleness, kindness, and acceptance. Many clients who have special needs may be touch deprived, and massage can go a long way to provide safe touch and meet psychosocial and physiological needs. Adopting this attitude sets the stage for a therapeutic relationship that can be fulfilling to both of you.

When adapting your massage for special populations, keep in mind that the massage strokes themselves may not change. The alterations come in how you modify the pressure, speed, duration, and frequency of the massage, as well as how you position your client on the massage table and how you follow other safety precautions. Adaptations to consider include the following:

- Amputations
- Implanted devices
- Colostomy or ileostomy
- Chronic or terminal illnesses
- Cancer
- Clients who are human immunodeficiency virus (HIV) positive or who are living with AIDS
- Geriatric clients
- Pediatric clients
- Large clients
- Hearing-impaired clients
- Speech difficulties
- Visually impaired clients
- Eye conditions or users of contact lens
- Spinal abnormalities
- Clients in wheelchairs
- Substance abuse and drug addiction issues
- Sexual abuse

The client may make you aware of his or her special need when he or she calls to get information about your services or to set up an appointment. If so, spend a few minutes looking up the condition in this textbook, a pathology book written for massage therapists, or a medical dictionary before the scheduled appointment. The best way to obtain information about a special need is to ask the client directly during the premassage interview. Each situation will be different, and you must be willing to be open minded, patient, tolerant, and flexible. Each client will teach you, if you are willing to listen and learn. Although each client will have different needs in the delivery of the massage, the therapist's boundaries should always be consistent. See Chapter 2 for an in-depth discussion of personal and professional boundaries and confidentiality issues for the massage therapist.

The following sections can help you make the necessary accommodations.

AMPUTATIONS

If your client has an amputation, obtain consent to massage the stump during the informed consent interview. Inquire about the actual surgical procedure; most clients know about their particular situation. For instance, if a midhumeral amputation has a smooth stump with no protruding bone, then knowing if the triceps or biceps was used to wrap the stump end would help. This knowledge helps you locate trigger points. While massaging the stump, ask the client if it is sensitive or numb. Use light tapotement, towel friction, or mechanical vibration to desensitize any hypersensitive areas. Many practitioners of energy work such as polarity and Reiki treat the energy field of the missing limb as though it were still present.

Approximately 70% of all people with amputations experience *phantom limb sensation* (feeling pain and other sensations in all or part of an amputated limb). The onset of pain occurs generally within the first week but may occur several months or years after the amputation. One possible explanation of this phenomenon is that a *neuroma* (tumor found in nervous tissue) forms on the severed nerve ends of the amputated limb. Another theory states that abnormal sensory input along afferent nerves in the amputated area enters the higher centers of the brain, resulting in pain. Another postulation is that nerves in the central nervous system still send out signals to the length of the missing limb. Clearly phantom limb sensation is complex and does involve both the peripheral and the central nervous systems. However, the calming effects of massage generally have a positive outcome on phantom limb pain regardless of the cause.

Amputations may not be obvious because of prosthetic appliances. Some clients may not want to remove prosthetic devices because of the time factors, whereas others are glad to be free of them for a while. Look out for chafing or friction wounds where the prosthetic limb fits to the stump. Avoid any inflamed areas, broken skin, or open wounds. Clients with leg amputations may walk using leg prosthetics and at other times may be on crutches or in wheelchairs (see the section Clients in Wheelchairs).

---

evolve *Log on to the course materials featured on the Evolve website for Chapter 10 to view drawings of an amputated limb and images of various prosthetic devises.* ■

IMPLANTED DEVICES

Central Venous Catheter

A central venous catheter, or central line, is a flexible tube that is inserted and sewn into a large vein (usually the right subclavian vein in the upper chest) and left in place for an extended period. This type of catheter is used to keep a vein open for dialysis, blood withdrawal, chemotherapy, and frequent administration of medications, which must be taken regularly or cannot be taken orally. The three common types of central venous catheters are Hickman catheters, Quinton catheters, and Groshong catheters. Another style of central venous catheter inserted under the skin of the chest wall, a port-a-cath, does not have an external opening.

The use of these catheters makes lying prone comfortably either difficult or impossible for the client. The massage therapist should use bolsters, pillows, or modifications such as a side-lying position for the client's comfort. Sometimes a small towel or washcloth over the area is all that is needed. The catheter is usually sutured to fascia and muscle. During the massage, the therapist should take precautions to avoid dislodging the catheter by exerting tension or excessive movement on nearby skin tissues. No traction should be performed in the area where the devices are located so as to avoid damaging the devices or surrounding tissues. Massage lubricant should not come into contact with the catheter dressing or sutures. If a catheter is placed in the arm, then the area below the catheter should not be massaged because these tissues may be sensitive. Massage work above the catheter in these extremities should be gentle.

Implantable Cardioverter Defibrillator

Implantable cardioverter defibrillator (ICD) is a device that is used to treat abnormal heart rates. It can detect heart rhythms that are too slow or too fast. When necessary, an ICD delivers an electrical shock to restore normal heart rate and rhythm. Similar to a pacemaker, the defibrillator is implanted under the skin near the clavicle. It is attached to one or more leads positioned in the right ventricle and right atrium. The electrical shock is painful to the client. The massage therapist may feel the shock if he or she is touching the patient when the device discharges. The feeling may resemble a tingling sensation, if felt at all, and is generally not harmful to the massage therapist. Massage is contraindicated once the device delivers a shock. The client should be referred for immediate medical attention. Other modifications are listed under Pacemaker.

Pacemaker

An artificial pacemaker is a device that is surgically implanted. It sends out small electrical currents to stimulate the heart to contract. Newer models are activity-adjusted pacemakers that automatically speed up the heartbeat during exercise. The artificial pacemaker is implanted under the skin, similar to an ICD, with wires going directly to the sinoatrial (SA) node or the atrioventricular (AV) node. Given that the site is usually sensitive, local massage is contraindicated.

The primary concern is to be sure the incision from the surgery has completely healed. While the client is prone, a soft pillow placed under the chest should be offered; this will provide added comfort for the client during the massage.

The leads (wires) going from the pacemaker to the heart often travel up and over the clavicle and down into the chest cavity. For this reason, the massage therapist should avoid vigorous massage on the pectoral region and movement of the arm over the head when mobilizing the shoulder joint because the lead connections may be disturbed.

Stent

A stent is a small, expandable, lattice-shaped metal tube or hollow perforated tube. The main purpose of a stent is to create an increase in vessel or duct diameter. Although the most popular use of stents is linked to the coronary arteries, they are widely used in several other structures, such as peripheral arteries and veins, bile ducts, esophagus, trachea or large bronchi, ureters, and urethra. Some stents are drug eluting; these medications potentially reduce the chance that the vessel will become blocked again.

During the premassage interview, ask the client to point out the location of the stent. If located superficially, then local massage is contraindicated. If within a deep vessel or duct, then err on the side of caution, and use only light pressure over or near the site.

BREAST IMPLANTS OR LARGE BREASTS

When massaging a woman with breast implants or large breasts, several options are available to make her more comfortable while she is lying prone. You may offer the client a rolled-up towel or cylindrical pillow placed under, above, or between her breasts, whichever is most comfortable. Many clients prefer a supportive device both above *and* below the breasts (Figure 10-1, *A*). Use a face rest that can be adjusted above the level of the table (Figure 10-1, *B*). Several massage table manufacturers now carry tables fitted with recessed channels that allow the client to lie prone comfortably (Figure 10-2).

In the supine position, accessing muscles in the chest area of full-figured women is sometimes difficult. If massage is needed in the pectoral region, the serratus anterior, or in the walls of the axilla, then you may ask the client to use the back side of her hand to cup the breast tissue and retract it medially (Figure 10-3). This technique establishes a safe physical boundary between client and therapist. You may decide to work on this area in a side-lying position with the client holding her top arm above the elbow with her bottom hand (Figure 10-4). These modifications are also useful to a postpartum or nursing mother.

COLOSTOMY OR ILEOSTOMY

A *colostomy* is an incision in the colon to create an opening that is affixed to the exterior abdominal wall. A bag is attached outside the body to collect fecal material that passes

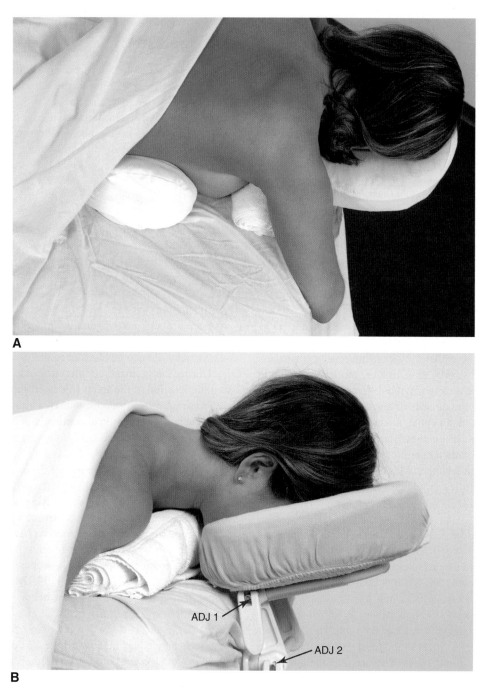

A

B

ADJ 1

ADJ 2

FIGURE 10-1 **A**, Prone large-breasted woman with cylindrical pillows above and below breast. **B**, Face rest adjusted properly, above the level of the table.

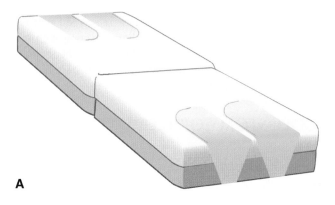

A

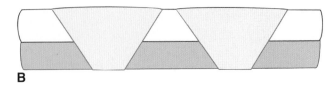

B

FIGURE 10-2 Breast comfort system in table padding. **A**, Superior/lateral view. **B**, Cross section.

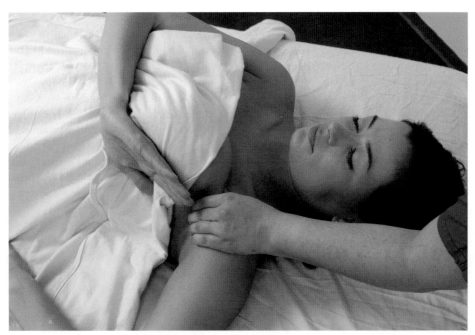

FIGURE 10-3 Woman retracting her breast tissue using the back of her hand.

through the opening. Colostomies are sometimes permanent; sometimes they are a temporary bypass method used in conjunction with other surgeries.

An ileostomy is similar to a colostomy except the *ileostomy* connects the small intestine (i.e., ileum) to the external abdominal wall. For both procedures, the end of the intestine is pulled through an opening made in the abdominal wall. The intestine is then folded outward onto itself and attached to the abdomen with stitches. This apparatus is called a *stoma*. Clients who have lower colostomies can regulate their bowels. The bowel

material of upper colostomies and ileostomies will be too loose to afford the client the ability to control bowel movements.

When clients who have a colostomy or ileostomy make an appointment for a massage, the massage therapist should recommend they not eat 2 hours before they arrive. This 2-hour delay will decrease bowel motility. Because of the anterior abdominal opening, these clients may not be able to receive massage in the prone position. Side-lying position can accommodate these special individuals. An extra pad may be placed under the massage linens in the event of bag spillage.

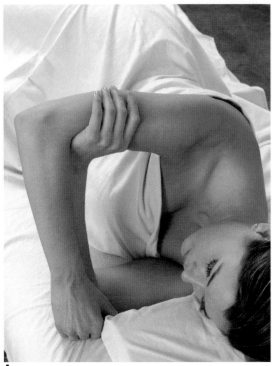

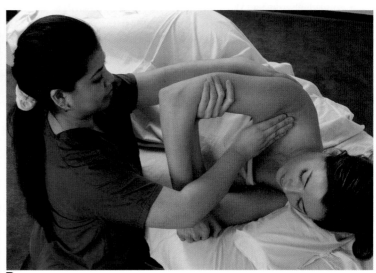

FIGURE 10-4 **A**, Side-lying large-breasted woman holding her upper arm away from her body. **B**, Therapist applying massage therapy.

The massage therapist can suggest to a client to empty his or her bag before the massage begins. A bag can burst or become unclipped during the session, spilling its contents. Should this event occur, the massage therapist needs to remain calm and reassure the client that accidents such as this do happen. The massage therapist should ask the client if he or she would prefer to clean him or herself up or if assistance is desired. If the client has a spinal injury, then he or she may require assistance. Disposable gloves and towels or washcloths should be available.

Lubricant should not be applied on or near the bag opening. Oily substances interfere with the ability of the adhesive or cement that anchors the bag to the skin.

> **evolve** To learn more about a colostomy, log on to your student account from the Evolve website and look at both the drawing of a colostomy and the photo of a stoma. ■

CHRONIC OR TERMINAL ILLNESSES

A *chronic illness* is a condition of the body for which no cure is known, such as multiple sclerosis, chronic fatigue syndrome, fibromyalgia, Parkinson's disease, lupus, and rheumatoid arthritis. A *terminal illness* is a condition in which the client is expected to die within a time frame, usually 6 months. With either illness, a gradual decline in health is expected; thus not getting any worse is considered an improvement. The long-term goal of the sessions is to add life to the client's years rather than years to the client's life. With improving the quality of life, suffering is reduced and personal comfort is increased.

People who are chronically or terminally ill will experience good days and bad days and have varying degrees of tolerance for and responsiveness to touch. Most therapists assert that working with clients who are ill requires intuition and awareness. Every session will be different, even if it is with the same client seen every week. Each client will be in a different stage of his or her illness. Some clients cry, some feel angry, some act mean, some feel happy, some feel bothered by their caregivers and just want to complain. Exercise empathy with every client, supporting his or her feelings with a compassionate, nonjudgmental attitude.

Once medical clearance is obtained, administer the massage more slowly, gently, more frequently, and for shorter periods than you would with a healthy client. The pressure is firm but broad (this technique helps bring a soothing touch and feeling of connection while preventing injury or discomfort). Respect what the client says regarding pressure and comfort by making immediate modifications. In most instances, deep pressure is not appropriate. Add some gentle Swedish gymnastics (stretching and joint mobilization) to the session if the client is feeling up to it. The purpose of these movements is to provide some mild form of exercise by moving the limbs that might be weak. Constantly monitor these clients during treatment because massage therapy can be tiring for them.

If working with hospice or doing a house call, the client may then prefer to be massaged in his or her bed. Even a gentle hand and foot massage is a welcomed experience. If you are giving the massage in the hospital, then check with the physician or nurse about additional information needed to serve the client most effectively. Work carefully around tubes, catheters, needles, monitors, and other medical equipment.

The intent is to ease pain. The attitude is one of deep respect, which requires the therapist to listen, both verbally and nonverbally, to what the client is telling you. This professional and respectful attitude will help create a respite, as well as a refuge.

End-of-Life Massage

Massage can be used at the end of life to reduce suffering and increase feelings of comfort. When massaging someone who is near the end of life, addressing your own feelings about death and dying would be helpful. You might attend workshops that are part of a local hospice program and read books on the subject. Several authors who have written books on the subject are Elisabeth Kübler-Ross, Stephen Levine, and Bernie Siegel. These resources may be helpful in working with people near the end of their life as they and their support people face grief issues.

Another goal of massage for individuals who are ill is to decrease the feeling of isolation and loneliness. Touch is an important method of relating when communicating verbally is difficult or impossible. Focused, gentle, and calm touch is often effective as a means of reassuring and calming someone who is confused or afraid.

Before you decide to work with a client who is dying or terminally ill, make a personal commitment to stay with him or her until death because abandonment is difficult to face at this time. Additionally, take care of yourself while caring for the ill. Find something, an outlet for the energy you spend around sickness, sadness, fear, and grieving. Know that you will probably become attached to the client, cry when death comes, mourn the loss, grieve with his or her family, and grow from this experience.

> *"Writing a novel is like driving a car at night. You can see only as far as your headlights, but you can make the whole trip that way."*
> E. L. Doctorow

Cancer

Cancerous diseases are characterized by the uncontrollable growth of abnormal cells. The excess tissue that develops when body cells divide without control is called a *neoplasm* or *tumor*. The study of tumors is called *oncology*. Tumors can be either cancerous or harmless. A cancerous tumor is called *malignant* and will often *metastasize,* or spread, cancerous cells to other parts of the body. Regardless of where a cancer may spread, however, it is always named for the place it begins. For instance, melanoma that spreads to the liver is still called melanoma, not liver cancer.

A *benign* tumor does not metastasize, but it may become life threatening if, as it grows, it puts pressure on vital areas, such as areas within the brain.

Many types of cancers have been identified, and they are named for the type of tissue from which they are derived. *Carcinomas* arise from epithelial tissue. *Melanomas* grow from melanocytes—skin cells that produce the pigment melanin. *Sarcomas* develop from muscle cells or connective tissue. *Leukemia* is characterized by rapid growth of abnormal white blood cells. *Lymphoma* is a cancer of lymphatic tissue.

Causes of cancer include carcinogens, oncogenes, and oncoviruses. *Carcinogens* are chemical agents or radiation that causes permanent structural changes in the genetic material of the cell. Examples of carcinogens include cigarette tar, radon gas, and ultraviolet radiation in sunlight. *Oncogenes* are cancer-causing genes. When these genes are inappropriately activated, they transform a normal cell into a cancerous cell. The way in which oncogenes become activated is unclear. *Oncoviruses* cause cancer by stimulating cells to divide abnormally. For example, the human papillomavirus (HPV) causes cervical cancer in women.

Some cancers, such as leukemia, do not form tumors. Instead, these cancer cells involve the blood and blood-forming organs and circulate through other tissues, where they grow.

You likely know someone who has or has had cancer. It is the leading cause of death in individuals 35 to 64 years of age and the second leading cause of death in individuals 65 and older (the first being heart disease in this age category). The American Cancer Society advocates massage to comfort and help improve the quality of life for patients with cancer, although not to specifically treat cancer. Cancer may be a reason to begin, continue, or increase the frequency of massage treatments. Besides the benefits of relaxation, improved sleep, pain reduction, and increased blood flow, massage also bolsters immune functions, reduces or prevents lymphedema, decreases nausea, and improves the quality and survival of skin during radiation therapy (perhaps as a result of the high-quality moisturizers in massage lubricants). Massage also reduces fatigue, which affects 72% to 95% of all patients with cancer.

In the recent past, cancer was viewed as a contraindication for massage. This incorrect perception prevented people living with cancer from receiving treatments. The prevailing thought was that massage therapy increased the circulation of blood and lymph. Given that most malignancies spread via these routes, it must increase the chance of spreading the cancer throughout the client's body. No medical evidence supports this claim.

Currently, new and accurate information is available for massage therapists who want to work with patients with cancer. Because cancer and cancer treatments affect the entire body, leaving the person in a fragile condition, the massage therapist absolutely must be informed.

Here are a few important guidelines to help massage therapists when working with patients with cancer. For more detailed information, see Chapter 12 in *Mosby's Pathology for Massage Therapists*.

• Obtain medical clearance for massage from the client's health care provider.

• Use a side-lying position and/or special propping to increase client comfort if he or she is unable to lie prone because of central lines on the upper chest wall, radiation burns, or surgical wounds.
• Avoid massage over or near intravenous insertion sites, catheters, surgical wounds over known cancer sites, radiation burns, or known tumors sites.
• Adjust the treatment to the client's stamina. Suggest that the client receive massage on high-energy days and times. Massage received on low-energy days and times may actually feel depleting to the client.
• Massage may be contraindicated if the client's cancer has spread to the bones. If medical clearance has been obtained for massage, traction and joint mobilizations may be contraindicated or only cautiously used.
• If the client is experiencing nausea as a result of cancer treatments, then avoid pressure and speed that rocks the client. These activities include joint mobilizations, stretches, and jostling.

"Humility is not thinking less of yourself,
but thinking of yourself less."
Alcoholics Anonymous saying

Clients Who Are HIV Positive or Living with AIDS

AIDS is a fatal disease caused by HIV, affecting T lymphocytes of the immune system. It is diagnosed through antibody testing, a decline in specific (CD4) cells, and presenting diseases, including *Candida albicans* infection, *Pneumocystis carinii* pneumonia, Kaposi's sarcoma, persistent swelling of lymph nodes (lymphadenopathy), and chronic diarrhea.

Transmission occurs through contact with contaminated body fluids (blood, semen, vaginal secretions, and mother's milk) and by transplacental route. More directly, the virus is spread through sexual contact with an infected person, by sharing needles or syringes with someone who is infected, or less commonly through transfusions of infected blood or blood clotting factors. Nearly one million Americans are infected with HIV, most of them through sexual transmission, and an estimated 15 million cases of other sexually transmitted diseases (STDs) occur each year in the United States.

The average time between infection with the virus and symptom development and diagnosis is 8 to 10 years, but the incubation time is much shorter. Generally, symptoms of primary infection include enlarged lymph nodes, weight loss, fatigue, night sweats, and fever. Even a person who is HIV positive does not necessary have AIDS; scientists estimate that approximately one half of the people who are HIV positive will develop AIDS within 10 years after becoming infected.

In the United States, the Centers for Disease Control and Prevention (CDC) estimates that between 800,000 and 900,000 people are living with HIV or AIDS. Through December 2000, a total of 774,467 cases of AIDS had been reported to the CDC. Approximately 60 million people have been infected with HIV since the start of the global epidemic. At the end of 2001, an estimated 40 million people were living with HIV infection or AIDS. The United Nations AIDS program estimates five million new HIV infections occurred in 2001. An estimated three million adults and children died of HIV/AIDS in 2001.

HIV infection is often accompanied by psychological suffering such as depression, stress, and anxiety, which may increase HIV symptoms. Stress further suppresses the immune system.

No known cases have been reported of a massage therapist contracting HIV from a client while performing massage. Only one instance occurred of patients being infected by an HIV-infected health care worker. This case involved HIV transmission from an infected dentist to six patients.

If a person believes that he or she has been exposed to HIV, then this person should contact his or her health care provider and/or local HIV/AIDS foundation for testing, information, and free counseling.

Precautions
Sanitation and cleanliness are important for the client and the massage therapist. Because the immune system of the client with HIV is not fully functional, he or she is more susceptible to contacting infections through simple exposure. The massage therapist is a greater health hazard to the HIV infected client than he or she is to the massage therapist. Care needs to be taken so that any infectious disorders of the client are not spread to the therapist, and vice versa. Chapter 4 has information on *universal precautions*.

Keep in mind that a massage therapist may not be permitted to ask clients if they have HIV/AIDS if this information has not been released on the intake form. Contact the state board in which you practice to determine what information is within your rights to ask either verbally or on your intake forms.

Intact healthy skin is an excellent barrier against HIV and other viruses and bacteria. If a massage therapist has an open wound on the hands, then it needs to be covered or massages should not be performed until the wound has completely healed. Lubricants used in massage generally break down latex gloves. Use a water-based lubricant with latex gloves or use vinyl gloves. Wear gloves for tasks such as cleaning up blood or other body fluids.

Guidelines
- Tailor the massage to the client's vitality; ask about his or her vitality before each massage. A gentle massage of shorter duration may be indicated if the client is feeling

debilitated. However, many people living with AIDS can typically tolerate even a vigorous massage.
- Avoid open lesions, as you would with any client.
- Disinfect or carefully discard objects containing blood or body fluid.
- Inquire about areas that need to be avoided, including the most recent site of blood work.
- If the HIV-infected client has Kaposi's sarcoma, deep-pressure massage is contraindicated because it can cause internal bleeding.
- Limit joint mobilizations and stretching if the client is bedridden because inactivity affects bone integrity. This circumstance depends on the individual client. Joint mobilizations are beneficial for persons who are bedridden so as to maintain range of motion.
- Clean any contaminated linens by washing them separately in hot water with detergent and a quarter cup of chlorine bleach (Table 10-1). Dry linens with hot air. Some therapists treat all sheets as *hot* (i.e., a possible exposure hazard).
- Immerse all implements used during massage in either a 10% bleach solution or a 70% alcohol solution for 10 minutes.
- If you know or suspect that you have come into contact with body fluids, immediately wash the area of contact with hand soap for 2 minutes.
- Treat any unidentifiable substance on your massage table as infectious. In such cases, use latex gloves and the aforementioned bleach solution when cleaning the table.
- If massage is given in the hospital, check with the client's health care provider about information that serves the client. Work carefully around tubes, catheters, needles, monitors, and other medical equipment. Under these circumstances, a massage lasting less than an hour can bring comfort to an HIV-infected client.

MINI-LAB

AIDS is a socially and emotionally charged issue today. Discuss your thoughts and feelings about this subject with your classmates. Begin by stating how you define the problem, how it affects you as a massage therapist, and what precautions you will take in your practice.

Should massage therapists be routinely tested for HIV? Examine the legal, ethical, and medical ramifications, as well as personal and professional risk factors. What if you, as a massage therapist, discover that you are HIV positive? Should this discovery restrict you from performing or receiving a massage?

TABLE 10-1 Caring for Equipment

EQUIPMENT	CLEANING BLOOD	CLEANING OTHER BODY FLUIDS/SECRETIONS
Tables and accessories	1 part bleach to 10 parts water 7 parts alcohol to 10 parts water	Spray on bleach solution
Linens	¼ cup bleach + detergent + hot water wash + high dry cycle	Detergent + hot water wash + high dry cycle

When in doubt about any disinfectants that can be used in your practice, contact the local health department or state board of health.

"If there is one door in the castle you have been told not to go through, you must. Otherwise you'll just be rearranging furniture in rooms you've already been."
Anne Lamott

GERIATRIC CLIENTS

Geriatric, or senescent, clients represent the fastest-growing populations in the massage industry. **Geriatric** refers to someone who is 70 years of age or older. However, just as there are no typical 30 year olds, there are no typical 70 year olds. An elderly person can be quite active and independent, living without assistance with his or her activities of daily living. Some older adults require assistance with accomplishing various daily activities and may live at home or in an assisted living facility. Others can be frail and cannot function without skilled help. Most of the persons in this latter group are found in long-term care facilities, and the rest are often at home with family or caregivers.

TABLE TALK

35,000,000 American are over 65 years of age.
In 1900 the average American lived to be 46 years of age.
In 2000 the average American lived to be 76 years of age.
By 2025 Americans over age 65 will outnumber adolescents by more than 2 to 1.

In general, health and physical condition decline with age, but this varies from person to person. As we age, the following changes occur to the body:

- Nerve and reflex reaction time is reduced, thus more time is typically needed to perform tasks such as the intake and premassage interviews.
- Because of the effect of the nervous system, a loss or increased sensitivity to pain may occur.
- In most instances, a loss in hearing and vision, especially near-sighted vision, occurs that must be taken into consideration.
- A decrease in strength, muscle tone, and flexibility is often noted.
- Bones are not as strong as they once were. Joints begin to wear down, and mobility decreases.
- The skin appears pale and wrinkled and becomes thin, loose, and frail. Age spots may appear on the skin as a result of blood leaking from damaged and weak capillaries. Liver spots may be seen on the skin of older people, especially those who have been excessively exposed to the sun.
- Fat deposits decrease.
- In the case of inactivity, circulation may not be efficient. Atherosclerosis is fairly common among older adults.
- An increase in incontinence may result from loss of muscle tone in the urinary and gastrointestinal tracts.
- Common conditions and illnesses include strokes, diabetes, hypertension, Alzheimer's disease, Parkinson's disease, depression, cancer, arthritis, osteoarthritis, osteoporosis, constipation, poor circulation, and peripheral vascular disease.

Not all health problems are obvious; therefore conduct a through intake, taking extra time each visit to ascertain the client's current health status. Establish rapport by acclimating him or her to surroundings, helping create a sense of safety and security. Use a soft, clear voice, facing the client when speaking. When explaining procedures, tell him or her which parts of the body you will be massaging using simple, nonanatomical terms. Be sure your client understands what is being said, and allow time for asking and answering questions.

Provide adaptations to ensure the client's comfort and safety. The most comfortable positions are supine and side lying. Because elderly people may tire easily, a 30-minute session is often best. Deitrich W. Miesler, founder of Day-Break Geriatric Massage Institute, recommends a 5-minute introduction of unhurried effleurage, deep breathing, and gentle rocking, then 20 minutes of focused work on the feet, legs, shoulder, or neck (client determined), and then 5 minutes of closure work. Guard against chilling by using blankets over the client's body and, if appropriate, an external heat source such as a portable heating unit.

When massaging an elderly person, deep work should be avoided unless ordered by his or her physician. Because of decreased reaction time, possible insensitivity to pain, and thinning of the blood vessels and skin, damaging the skin or causing bruising is relatively easy; this can be prevented by reducing both treatment time and pressure. Avoid extreme neck mobilizations, which may harm the client because of loss of bone integrity. Instead, add some gentle Swedish gymnastics (stretching and joint mobilization) to arms and legs. The purpose of this approach is to provide some mild form of exercise by moving the limbs.

Many elderly people experience a sudden drop in blood pressure when they move from a recumbent position to an upright position. The clinical term for this drop is *orthostatic hypotension*. The massage therapist should assist the geriatric client into a sitting posture on the table (see Chapter 6), allowing time for the client to adjust to the change in position. You may choose to spend this time massaging the neck and shoulder region while he or she is seated on the massage table. Help the client to his or her feet if needed; otherwise, he or she may become dizzy while transferring off the table, lose balance, and fall.

Many elderly clients live or feel alone because their spouses have passed away or because family members are busy tending to their own families. If your client is living with family or friends or residing in a nursing home, then knock on the door of his or her room before entering, make sure you put objects back in their places if disturbed, and be patient if he or she needs extra time to dress. This extra time may provide an opportunity for elderly clients to talk and share their thoughts with you. Depression may also affect the elderly client. Be attentive and sensitive to the client's emotional needs. Many massage therapists offer discounts to elderly clients because most are living on fixed incomes.

TIFFANY FIELD, PhD

"The best pioneers are the ones actually out there doing massage. They get devotees just from having put their hands on them. That's what keeps the field alive and moving."

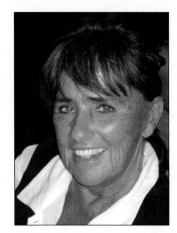

Tiffany Field has always been a woman on the move. As the daughter of an insurance executive and teacher, she lived in 12 different places when she was growing up, but now she has found her home—and her life's calling—on the beach in Hollywood, Florida.

She is not a massage therapist, and she has not developed any particular massage modality; however, her work has dramatically affected the credibility of the profession. Tiffany Field is a professor of pediatrics, psychology, and psychiatry, and she is the director of the University of Miami School of Medicine's Touch Research Institute (TRI). TRI was established in 1992 and is the only center in the world devoted solely to the study of touch and its applications in science and medicine.

According to a recent article in *Massage Therapy Journal,* by Mirka Knaster, Field holds a doctorate in developmental psychology and has 25 years of research experience, with numerous publishing credits, awards, and research grants. She has written for 50 professional journals and retains membership in more than a dozen professional organizations.

TRI evolved after her team's research findings supported touch as a factor that increased birthweight in premature infants. Premature infants who received massage gained weight faster and left the hospital earlier than infants who did not receive massage. With 470,000 premature births in the United States each year, up to $7.05 billion in annual savings might be realized.

The potential for Field's research and the cost-cutting measures earned her the grant money to explore touch therapy further. Currently, her group is studying the effects of massage on all ages, from cocaine-exposed newborns to arthritic geriatric patients. *Massage Therapy Reduces Anxiety and Enhances EEG Pattern of Alertness and Math Computations* is one of the most recent studies being conducted.

Some of the work being examined at TRI is particularly groundbreaking. Although breast cancer is still considered by many authors as a contraindication for massage, an ongoing breast cancer study shows an increase in natural killer cells (cells that kill cancer cells and other pathological microorganisms) after massage. In a society that values scientific proof, such findings might eventually make massage therapy a component of mainstream medicine.

Field has a hectic schedule that involves a great deal of travel for fund raising, overseeing projects, and writing grant proposals. To unwind, she swims daily; practices yoga, ballet, and tai chi when she has spare time; and, of course, gets a massage whenever she can.

For over a decade, Field has probably been one of the most instrumental individuals in helping increase respect for massage therapy and advises new massage therapists to "join a group practice to learn the ropes of operating a business."

PEDIATRIC CLIENTS

Children, or **pediatric,** clients are defined as people between 3 and 18 years of age. Anxious parents often accompany them because most pediatric massage addresses specific tissue problems from injury or illness, resulting in pain to the young client. During the premassage interview, explain the procedure to both the parents and the child, but informed consent must be obtained from the parents or legal guardians. In some states, a parent must also supervise while the massage is in progress. If the child is between the ages of 16 and 18, parental permission is recommended but not required. Keeping the parent in the room while massaging a child of the opposite sex would be prudent. This precaution is especially true, for example, when working in a sensitive area such as a pulled adductor injury in a young athlete.

Use special caution when working with adolescent boys. The reflexive sexual erection response is often sensitive; peripheral stimulation (i.e., massage) on the thighs and belly can trigger this reflex. Keeping the top drape bunched up in the groin area would be helpful to disguise any physical response to the massage. Stopping the massage for a brief period and stepping out of the room (perhaps for the reason of getting a drink of water) often reduces the neurological response.

In younger children, the massage session may last only 30 to 45 minutes because of the child's smaller stature, short attention span, short neural reflex, and increased metabolism. Use the extra time to establish a rapport with the client.

LARGE CLIENTS

When massaging the client who is large (i.e., obese or the somatotype known as an *endomorph*) or who has generous amounts of fragile subcutaneous tissue, two areas require special consideration. The first consideration is psychological and requires approaching the client with an attitude that is compassionate, caring, and nonjudgmental because large clients typically have a history of verbal abuse from society in general and health care providers in particular. Never badger a client about his or her weight or blame excessive size or weight on lack of morality or self-control. No one has a body that is perfect in all aspects. Make the accommodations necessary for his or her comfort, and proceed with the session.

The second consideration is physiological in which pressure must be applied carefully to areas that contain high quantities of adipose tissue, thus reducing possible tissue damage. Adipose tissue is extremely vascular, with each pound of tissue containing approximately 1 mile of capillaries, the most fragile of vessels, making adipose tissue extremely susceptible to bruising. Avoid deep stroking of adipose tissue because it can damage and break these vessels. The client may have large amounts of soft subcutaneous adipose tissue and yet may still have tense back and shoulder muscles that have become overdeveloped to support the extra weight. The back, neck, shoulders, hips, and sometimes legs of many larger clients may require extra massage work.

Palpation must be used to discern the difference between muscle and adipose tissue. If muscle fiber cannot be felt with gentle pressure, then avoid working deeply into the tissue. You can ask the client to contract a specific muscle or muscle group to help you decipher the difference. If the tissue does not respond with an increase in tone, then the tissue is probably adipose tissue, and deep work should be avoided. Sometimes gently retracting adipose tissue to access muscle tissue underneath is possible. Clients who have had recent weight loss may have areas that tend to hang in folds until the skin tightens. These areas should never be worked deeply or pinched; folds can be moved to the side while working on adjacent muscle and may be flattened out against the area to be worked so that the therapist can work through it while remaining attentive to pressure.

Inquire about the client's activity level. Just because someone is large does not necessarily mean that he or she is sedentary. For clients who are inactive, watch for signs of edema.

Another area of consideration when working with larger clients is the therapist's body mechanics and efficiency. Either lowering the table height before the client's visit or having a small platform on which to stand to gain height and leverage may help. Most table manufacturers offer electric lift or hydraulic tables that can be raised or lowered easily to a comfortable height.

Use a sheet or an extra-large towel as a top drape to provide adequate coverage. A client who is obese or excessively large may feel awkward or unsafe getting on and off the massage table. Have a footstool available, and be willing to offer assistance. If you have an electric or hydraulic lift massage table, then set it in the lowest position while the client is

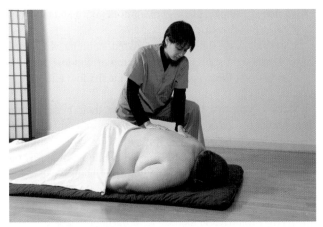

FIGURE 10-5 Massaging large client on floor.

getting on and off. If the client does not feel comfortable on your massage table, then he or she may need to receive the massage on the floor (Figure 10-5). Provide a comfortable floor mat for such an instance.

HEARING-IMPAIRED CLIENTS

An important point to remember is that hearing-impaired clients communicate perfectly well; they just receive and interpret sounds differently than those of us whose hearing is intact. Be aware that even a small hearing impairment can hamper a person's ability to understand what you say.

Allow more time for the premassage interview. When initiating conversation with a client with hearing impairment, get his or her attention before you begin to speak. Eye contact is considered a sign of attention. Tapping a person lightly on the shoulder or arm or waving a hand in the person's direction to gain his or her attention is perfectly acceptable. This approach is especially important when the client is lying face down in the face cradle and cannot see the therapist. Find out immediately if your client is a lip-reader, and use the information in the next paragraph during the interview process. Rephrase any sentence that the client with hearing impairment does not understand; do not just repeat the same words over and over in the same sequence. Allow time for him or her to respond. If you have a regular client who is hearing impaired, attending a class on sign language to be used during the interview process may be a good investment. If he or she has a sign language interpreter, then do not direct your conversation to the interpreter; make eye contact and talk directly with the person with the hearing impairment.

The following ideas help the therapist communicate better with a client who reads lips.

- Face the client and maintain eye contact through the conversation.
- Enunciate clearly and normally, but do not exaggerate your lip movements.
- Use facial expressions and body language to clarify your message. Do not be embarrassed to be expressive.
- Stand close and do not let any object obstruct the person's view of you.

- Do not eat, smoke, chew gum, or hold your hands in front of your mouth while you talk.
- Stand in a well-lighted place. Avoid standing with your back to a light source such as a lamp or window because this position throws your face into a shadow and makes seeing lip movements difficult.

Many people try to compensate for their hearing loss through the use of hearing aids. Do not assume that a hearing aid corrects hearing loss; it may just improve it slightly. If your client is wearing a hearing aid while he or she is on the massage table, then avoid moving your hands close to the client's ears. Proximity to the hearing aid generates feedback, producing an uncomfortable squeak in the wearer's ear. Some clients may remove the aid before or during the session.

Remember that clients who lost their hearing early in life may often have speech difficulties. When the cause of the speech difficulty is hearing loss, the client may pronounce words incorrectly. Many people make the mistake of assuming that someone with a speech problem is mentally handicapped. Remember that the client is only hearing impaired, not unintelligent. Talking very slowly or using exaggerated lip movements only serves to frustrate the client. Give him or her the dignity you would afford any hearing adult in normal conversation.

Many medical establishments use a flash card system for communicating with clients with hearing or speech impairment. The system consists of a single-card listing a set of simple questions. The answer area of the card has a *yes* and *no* block. The client responds by pointing to the appropriate answer. This principle can be used to create a pain tolerance level flash card for massage clients.

SPEECH DIFFICULTIES

If your client has difficulty articulating speech, or enunciating words, then ask him or her to repeat anything that is unclear or that you do not understand. Repeating what you heard to the client and giving him or her an opportunity to give you clarification or further instructions would be helpful.

During the premassage interview, inquire about any accommodations that can be made on his or her behalf. Be direct and inquire about the speech difficulty. The impairment may be the result of a physical abnormality such as cleft palate, aphasia (abnormal neurological condition causing difficult speech and verbal comprehension) resulting from a stroke or head injury, a regional dialect or accent, dementia resulting from drug use or illness, or inadequate pronunciation caused by deafness (see the section Hearing-Impaired Clients). If a client speaks a foreign language that you do not understand, then ask him or her about the possibility of bringing a support person to act as an interpreter.

VISUALLY-IMPAIRED CLIENTS

Visual impairment can range from mild to severe. Blindness is defined as central visual acuity (sharpness) of less than 1/10 (or 20/200 on the Snellen test). Other conditions are amblyopia (one eye is weak), scotoma (blind or partially blind area of the retina), and strabismus (crossed eyes, either inward or outward). Massage helps people with visual impairment because of their need for tactile stimulation; touch is one of the most important ways they define their world. Riesin (1996) found that visually-impaired cats and monkeys who received regular massage (tactile stimulation) did not experience mood swings whereas if massage was reduced, these animals became either hypo- or hyperemotional.

During the initial consultation, allow extra time to give and receive information. The best source of information comes from the client him or herself. Ask your client to explain his or her impairment and what assistance, if any, is needed. Do not feel offended if he or she declines your offer to help; the same is true for any client who is physically challenged.

Keep your facilities as barrier free as possible; the floor in your office, hallway, bathroom, and massage room should be free from clutter. Announce your presence when you step into the room, speaking in a normal tone of voice. Begin by addressing the client by name, and then state your name. When transferring a client with visual impairment from one area to another, stand just in front or to his or her left. The client may choose to touch your right elbow and follow you. Be a gentle guide, and give useful, meaningful directions. Describing the surroundings, using the face of a clock as a reference, may be helpful. Instead of saying, "There is a table in front of you," say, "There is a table at two o'clock." Go into detail about what you are going to do and what you would like him or her to do. Never begin a massage on a client with visual impairment until he or she knows that you are in the room, and maintain physical contact throughout the massage as much as possible.

If your client has a service dog, do not feed, pet, or interact with the dog without permission from the client. This kind of interaction distracts the dog, making its important task difficult.

MINI-LAB

Gather a blindfold (scarf or king-size pillowcase) and a dollar bill. Locate a partner. You are the *explorer*. Take a few dollars and stick them in your pocket. Your partner is the *attendant*. Ask your partner to blindfold you.

The attendant guides the blindfolded explorer, on foot and in silence, to a nearby store to make a refreshment purchase. After you walk back blindfolded, remove the blindfold and reverse roles. You are now the attendant, and your partner is the explorer. Return to your starting point by a different route.

Share your experiences with each other. This activity is designed to experience being without sight. You may notice a heightened sense of awareness in your other senses, such as hearing and skin sensations.

If a store is not a convenient destination, allow the students to walk a few blocks from the school and back. This activity can be done with earplugs and blindfolds.

Eye Conditions or Contact Lens Wearers

If the client is uncomfortable lying prone while using the face rest, show the client how to adjust the cushion to reduce eye compression while lying prone. Be sure to place the face rest cushion in its original position after the massage. If the client is still uncomfortable after the adjustment, then massage in the side-lying position. While the client is supine, avoid massage that is near or directly over the eyes.

If the client is wearing contact lenses, suggest that they be removed before the massage. Have contact lens solution available for lens storage after removal. If contact lens users do not remove them, then follow the guidelines in the earlier paragraph for both the prone and the supine positions.

> **evolve** *To view how to move the face cushion, log on to the Evolve website and click on course materials for Chapter 10.* ▪

Spinal Abnormalities: Kyphosis, Lordosis, and Scoliosis

When massaging a client who has spinal abnormalities, positioning or table mechanics provides a way in which the client can relax in a recumbent position. A client who has a spinal condition called *kyphosis,* or humpback condition, may be uncomfortable lying in the prone position. Place a cushion or supportive device under the clavicles, and offer a standard-size pillow or a face rest for his or her head when your client is in the prone position. If possible, adjust the face rest higher than the table height. In this way, your client can further relax and enjoy the massage.

Lordosis, or swayback, is common in clients who are overweight or who have flaccid abdominal muscles. A pillow under the anterior superior iliac spine while the client is in the prone position may relieve low back discomfort. Additionally, a bolster under the ankles and using pillows to correct externally rotated femurs may help release the hips. A 6- to 8-inch bolster behind the knees while the client is lying supine may also relieve pain associated with lordosis.

Scoliosis is a lateral spinal distortion that occurs mostly in women and girls (60% to 80%). Because the abnormal curve is in the thoracic region, the ribs and hips have distorted positions. Different degrees of spinal distortion exist; therefore offer your client with scoliosis several pillows, and suggest that the client position them until he or she feels supported and comfortable. More information on spinal abnormalities can be found in Chapter 13. You may elect to forgo massaging in the prone position.

> ## TABLE TALK
>
> Handicaps are about barriers. Disabilities are about conditions.

Clients in Wheelchairs

The first consideration when working with a client in a wheelchair is how he or she will enter your massage establishment. Most municipalities require businesses to be barrier free, but if yours is not, then schedule a home visit and perform the massage off site. Ask the client the reason for his or her wheelchair use. Spinal cord injuries must be treated differently than other conditions because of the loss of sensory input. Clients with amputations may have special needs that must be addressed (see the section Amputations).

When you speak to a client who is in a wheelchair, sit down in a chair or a stool or kneel down on the floor to be able to speak to him or her at eye level. Inquire about particular limitations. Avoid making assumptions; just because your client is in a wheelchair does not necessarily mean that he or she is paralyzed. People use wheelchairs for many reasons. The client may be experiencing any of the following:

- Amputation
- Depression
- Inability to walk long distances
- Obesity or inactivity
- Para-, hemi-, or quadriplegia
- Recovery from surgery
- Short-term injury (e.g., broken leg or foot)
- Spinal cord injury

For any long-term disease or trauma, loss of muscle function (motor paralysis) or loss of sensation (sensory paralysis) is often noted. The massage for clients in wheelchairs is tailored to the type of paralysis and the needs of the client. Of primary concern is that the client generally has large areas of numbness from the severed nerves. When working legs or arms that have no feeling, the therapist must use a pressure that is light, just enough to increase circulation, but not enough to cause any discomfort that cannot be discerned by the client. An important point to remember is that being paralyzed does not always mean that the client cannot detect pressure and vibration. Sometimes only motor nerves have been damaged, leaving the client immobile but with feeling. Other clients who have had sensory nerve or total spinal cord separation may be paralyzed and sensory impaired but may be able to feel vibrations in other parts of their bodies that still detect sensations.

Depending on time factors, reasons for impairment, and ability of the client to undress and transfer to and from the chair, some clients may elect to be massaged in the wheelchair. In most instances, this circumstance simply involves positioning the wheelchair at the side of the massage table and placing some pillows onto which the client can lean. If a table is unavailable, then place a cushion in the client's lap and have him or her lean onto it (Figure 10-6). A desktop model massage chair may be used. Occasionally, the height of the table may have to be adjusted to accommodate the wheelchair. Make sure that the wheelchair wheels are locked in place with the brakes before starting this type of seated massage. Clients with greater mobility usually elect to use the table.

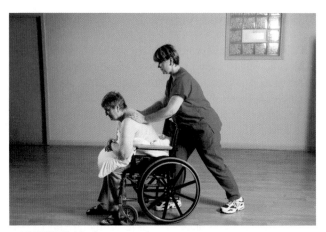

FIGURE 10-6 Client holding pillow in lap during massage.

During the massage, ask the client directly for valuable feedback regarding pressure, body warmth, and how he or she feels with regard to positioning. Modify your massage techniques and body mechanics as needed. Trigger points may be located in the shoulders and chest area from moving about in the chair. Generally speaking, the longer the client has been inactive, the weaker the bones become. Limit all range-of-motion exercises, especially on the neck, spinal column, and hip joints. Avoid using electrical vibrators. Assist the client on and off the table.

Observe wheelchair etiquette. Never push a wheelchair without permission from the person in the chair. When moving the client from the chair to the table, he or she can give you the best instructions on how to proceed. The person in the wheelchair usually has learned how to transfer, or move, him or herself in and out of the chair. Never assume that these clients are helpless; many of them have been trained to right themselves even after falling out of the chair.

"When you can't tell the difference between your own pleasure and your pain, then you're an addict."
Margaret Atwood

SUBSTANCE ABUSE AND DRUG ADDICTION ISSUES

Addictive or compulsive disorders develop when the individual starts using a mood-altering chemical as a temporary chemical escape from unpleasant emotions. Some of these uncomfortable feelings are pain, inadequacy, sadness, loneliness, anger, and fear. The behavior continues to escalate until the consequences of the addiction exceed the pain of the uncomfortable emotions that led to the substance, trapping the person in a cycle of pain and escape. Examples of chemical dependency disorders range from nicotine and caffeine addiction to alcohol and narcotic abuse.

Massage therapy may be part of the recovery process for clients with addictions because it is effective for relieving stress during periods of chemical withdrawals. Deep work should be avoided during the early stages of withdrawal because it may

intensify the release of toxins into the system, which may already be overburdened during the detoxification process. During episodes of **recidivism** (relapse into a previous condition such as substance abuse), massage can be used for its psychological and physiological benefits.

Although massage can assist the recovering addict through relaxation and increased body awareness, education and support are probably the best tools for overcoming this disorder. Most massage therapists are not licensed to provide counseling services, but they can offer these special clients acceptance and moral support as a part of their recovery. If the client is participating in a recovery program, then encourage him or her to continue. If not, then recommend a program that deals with the client's particular addiction issues, or refer him or her to a professional counselor.

SEXUAL ABUSE

You will likely meet clients who are survivors of sexual abuse. Abuse crosses all population barriers, with both perpetrators and survivors being men or women (boys or girls), straight or gay, old or young, poor or wealthy. The majority of these incidents tend to be perpetrated by family members, extended family members, friends of family members, or friends of the survivor (e.g., date rape). Many survivors require special consideration during massage therapy, and in some cases massage may even be contraindicated. This decision is generally up to the client, but he or she may need an extended period to build rapport with the therapist before any massage work actually begins. In any case, treatment can best be provided by a massage therapist who has an understanding of the dynamics of abuse and the steps for making massage therapy emotionally and physically safe.

One of the reasons that sexual abuse is so traumatic is that sex is such a powerful experience. It has the potential of being the ultimate expression of intimacy or one of the worst bodily assaults possible. Many survivors become people of extremes, often developing compulsive eating habits. These survivors may overeat to the point of obesity, cocooning themselves from others emotionally and physically by hiding inside excess body weight. Other survivors may relate to their bodies as the source of self-esteem and become compulsive about exercise and diet. Some survivors become anorexic or bulimic. To anesthetize the pain of the abuse, many survivors develop alcohol, nicotine, caffeine, and narcotic dependencies. Depression or chemical addictions often get most survivors of sexual abuse involved in counseling. As the survivor begins to peel back different layers of various issues, he or she discovers incidences of abuse underneath, or he or she may have always been aware of the abuse.

The extreme behaviors may also involve sexual inappropriateness. Many survivors may fear or encourage sexual interactions; they may have difficulty understanding appropriate sexual boundaries. For a victim of sexual abuse, part of the healing process is to be in contact with positive role models. As massage therapists, we must be aware of our own issues surrounding sexuality and possess good boundaries so we can role model this behavior. If you are not clear about your own boundary issues, or if you experience feelings of sexual attraction toward a particular client, then refer him or her to another therapist.

If a client confides in you that he or she has an abusive history, take extra precautions to ensure a nurturing, safe, and healing environment. Some suggestions are to close window blinds, turn off the telephone, and reduce noises that may trigger a startled response. *Ask the client if he or she knows what his or her triggers are.* Common triggers are perfume, certain body positions, touch in a particular area, lighting, a specific color, and certain kinds of music. Allow the client to set the boundaries from one massage to the next, and reassure the client that he or she has control of the session. Examples of boundaries are draping issues, areas on which to work, speed and depth of massage, and length of time an area is to be worked. In many instances, massage itself may act as a trigger mechanism for old abuse issues.

Occasionally, a client's physical body may *remember* a past traumatic event while receiving a massage. These repressed memories come to the conscious mind by a mechanism called **state-dependent memory,** which is triggered by duplicating the original position of a client, location or amount of pressure, body movements, emotions, and nervous system activation at the time the experience occurred. When your body assumes a particular position, or when a certain set of circumstances occurs, it may recall the experience (for example, when climbing on a bicycle for the first time in 20 years).

Some survivors of abuse coped with the original trauma by *leaving the body* so as not to feel, or to believe that the abuse was happening to someone else. This coping mechanism is called **disassociation.** Clients may relive abuse memories during a massage and repeat the disassociation. Signs of disassociation are the client becoming unresponsive, a distant look in the eyes, shaking, disorientation, loss of clarity between the present and the past, and a shift in breathing pattern.

Changing the coping mechanism by reminding the client to remain aware of his or her body is not your responsibility, nor is removing a coping skill. Learning to cope differently takes time, and we must honor the ways in which the client has learned to survive. We must also honor his or her need for emotional release. Do not continue massage if you have just retriggered the client because further disassociative touch can be traumatizing.

> *"All feelings, both positive and unpleasant, come out of the same faucet. To turn down the faucet on pain is to slow the flow of pleasant feelings as well."*
> Gay and Kathlyn Hendricks

Emotional Release During Treatment

Occasionally, survivors of abuse release physical or emotional tension during a massage session. These releases can exhibit themselves as a deep sigh, a stream of tears, laughter, shaking, uncontrollable muscle twitching, or in rare cases a thrashing temper tantrum. These emotional expressions may be an indication of pain, deep sadness, anger, or even rage. The causes of these releases may be suppressed emotions that are locked in the muscles and released through massage therapy. Muscle twitching may be a physical manifestation of body memories that were trauma induced during the time of the abuse and may occur at any time, not just during a massage. Some clients let down their defenses and release emotions during massage because of the high level of safety they experience with their therapists.

If the client is in counseling, his or her emotions are typically closer to the surface, and he or she is more likely to experience emotional releases. The most common form of emotional release is tears or crying. Chances are that the tears are not about physical pain. Here are some tips on handling your client's tears. If the client is aware that he or she is likely to experience a release during the session, then orient him or her by explaining the following process in advance:

- Approach the emotional expression with the attitude of total acceptance. Do not interfere with probing questions.
- Discontinue the massage, and make touch contact in an area that is neutral to the abuse (e.g., shoulders, arms, feet; Figure 10-7). This action should be determined before the massage begins. Most clients prefer to stop the massage because their bodies have another job now—crying. Avoid leaving the massage room unless instructed to do so by the client. Leaving the room may be interpreted as abandonment. Help provide a safe place for your client to experience and release these emotions without explanation or judgment.
- Do not be quick to offer facial tissues. Drying someone's tears or offering the tissue too fast can be taken as disapproval of crying and of the feelings beneath it.

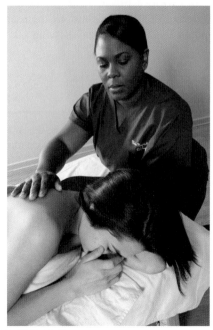

FIGURE 10-7 Therapist comforting crying client.

- When appropriate, remind your client that the tears, shaking, or fear is all right and that he or she is in a safe place. Ask the client if he or she would like to take a short break, offer them a comfort measure (e.g., stroking the client's hair, opening a window for fresh air), or end the massage session. However, avoid offering too many choices all at once; keep it simple.
- Regardless of which option the client chooses, be calm and accepting of the response, and never encourage or repress the response.
- Get in touch with your own feelings about others who express emotions. You must be willing to witness another person's pain without interrupting him or her. We may feel either empathic or uncomfortable with the client's tears, but we need to give the client the time and place to experience the emotion without interruption.
- We are not counselors, but we can support the client emotionally. You can be supportive with comments such as, "It's all right to cry; in fact it's good to cry," or "Tears are part of the natural cleansing process of the body."
- In most instances, continuing the massage is best, which allows the body to integrate the information. Clients may ask that the massage continue but to a less emotionally charged area such as the hands or feet.

Responding To Your Client After the Emotional Release

- If the client asks for an explanation of what happened, mirror back to him or her what you observed. Do not offer your personal interpretation or analysis; perhaps offer your understanding of state-dependent memory.
- Disassociation typically leaves the client in an emotional void. Many clients will be self-conscious. They may want to leave before they are ready to go back to the *real world*. Provide a safe, private space for them to integrate the experience, whether with you, by themselves, or on the telephone with their counselor. Avoid asking the client to leave while he or she is in a raw, open, wounded, or disassociated state.
- When appropriate, refer the client to a qualified mental health counselor.
- If you are truly uncomfortable with the client's emotional release, then be honest with yourself. Support the client through the experience as best you can while he or she is on the table. Later, share your feelings of apprehension with a counselor, preceptor, fellow therapist, or a peer support group. Process your feelings, and find out if you can get past your apprehension.

If you choose not to work with survivors of sexual abuse, discuss your limitations with your client during the consultation. Discussing how uncomfortable you are while he or she is on the massage table or immediately after the emotional release when he or she may feel vulnerable is inappropriate. Simply communicate only that you cannot provide the care the client needs. Make sure that you take ownership of the limitation or boundary, then refer the client to a massage therapist who is trained and comfortable in dealing with these issues.

Working with survivors of sexual abuse requires special skills and much empathy. If you are planning on working specifically with survivors, then familiarize yourself with these issues through reading (e.g., *The Courage to Heal and Allies in Healing,* by Ellen Bass and Laura Davis), attending seminars, or taking an introductory class at a university. Another resource is a support group called *Survivors of Incest Anonymous*. Although many support programs are available, no substitute exists for a qualified psychotherapist who specializes in sexual trauma. Obtain recommendations for psychotherapists in your area, and refer clients to them when appropriate.

As is true with all of your clients, always remember that confidentiality is a sacred trust. Everyone has painful psychological issues at some point in life. Protect the anonymity of your clients. Divulging personal information is their right alone.

SUMMARY

Massage is an adaptable medium; the sessions are diverse, with endless variations. By applying specific combinations of these variations, we can reach out to assist individuals with special needs who fall outside the average treatment session, including those with physical, emotional, and health challenges. These needs can be met by using adaptive massage techniques and basic client management to ensure client safety and eliminate restrictive barriers.

Client respect is the primary focus of adaptive massage. Regardless of whether you understand the client's condition, respect for him or her is essential before a therapeutic relationship can be established. The patients themselves are almost always the most valuable source of information. Once respect and communication have been firmly established, adaptive massage techniques can be used to heal and enrich the lives of your special clients. Working in this type of practice requires commitment, patience, discipline, and flexibility. It can also be one of the most gratifying areas of the profession.

CASE STUDY:

Seize the Day

Moxie is a middle-age African-American woman who recently had her second child. While in her early 20s, she began having anxiety attacks with occasional mild seizures. Her physician prescribed appropriate medication to control seizure activity. While she was pregnant, she discontinued the medication as directed by her obstetrician. Her physician told her to remain off the medication until she stopped nursing because the medication is excreted in her milk.

Many of Moxie's pregnancy-related discomforts were alleviated with massage. Her loving husband frequently bought her massage gift certificates to a local therapist, Chantell. Moxie received a massage at least twice a month. She had a standing appointment with Chantell, 2:00 PM every other Tuesday. A neighbor cared for Moxie's 2-month-old infant so she could get away and relax. The demands of a new infant on top of caring for a 2-year-old child and a new home were beginning to take a toll on Moxie. She tried hard to get the nourishment her body needed, but it was not easy.

Moxie was on time for her 2:00 appointment. She entered the massage room and began to prepare herself for the session. She felt unusually tired and thought, "Timing for this massage is perfect! I really need a break." She pulled the sheet over as she lay down on her back and closed her eyes.

Chantell entered the room and asked Moxie a few health-related questions. Moxie replied in single syllables. After approximately 5 minutes,

Chantell asked Moxie to comment on the pressure. Moxie did not answer. Chantell asked again. She looked down at Moxie and saw that her eyes were moving rapidly under her closed lids. Because Chantell had done an in-depth client intake, she knew about Moxie's history of seizures. Not ever seeing one in the past, Chantell assumed that Moxie was experiencing a seizure.

Chantell immediately discontinued the massage, anchored her leg to the tableside nearest her, and waited for the seizure to pass. While in school, Chantell was taught to place pillows around the massage table, but doing that meant she had to leave Moxie's side. What if Moxie fell onto the floor while Chantell was gathering pillows? Only two pillows were in the massage room; two pillows are not enough. Where should they be placed on the floor? The reality of the situation was very different than she expected.

If you were Chantell, how would you handle the seizure incident?

Once the seizure has passed, how would Chantell explain the incident to Moxie?

If you were Moxie, how might you feel coming out of the seizure?

If Moxie's seizure had been physical, how might Chantell respond?

If Chantell had called emergency services and an ambulance had been dispatched, what would happen if Moxie did not want to be treated once they arrived?

evolve

Go to *Chapter Extras* on Evolve for additional illustrations and resources for this chapter. *Extras* for this chapter include:

1. Central venous catheter (illustration)
2. Implantable cardioverter defibrillator (illustration)
3. Pacemaker (illustration)
4. Stent (illustration)
5. Manual communication skills for massage therapists (illustration series)
6. American Sign Language (ASL) (illustration series)
7. Positioning for clients lying prone who have kyphosis (photo)
8. Positioning for clients lying prone who have lordosis (photo)
9. Therapist using a desktopper (photo)
10. Mother supervising pediatric massage (photo)
11. Kaposi's sarcoma (photo)
12. Case study (text)
13. Crossword puzzle (downloadable form)

MATCHING

Place the letter of the answer next to the term or phrase that best describes it.

A. Central venous catheter   D. Geriatric   F. Phantom limb sensations
B. Colostomy   E. Pediatric   G. Recidivism
C. Disassociation

_____   1.   Feeling pain and other sensations in all or part of an amputated limb

_____   2.   A flexible tube sewn into a large vein to keep it open for dialysis, blood withdrawal, chemotherapy, or frequent administration of medications

_____   3.   An incision in the colon to create an opening between the bowel and the abdominal wall, with a bag attached outside the body to gather fecal material

_____   4.   Term to refer to someone who is age 70 or older

_____   5.   Term to refer to someone between 3 and 18 years of age

_____   6.   A coping mechanism in which the client *leaves the body* or believes his or her own past abuse has happened to someone else

_____   7.   A relapse into a previous condition

INTERNET ACTIVITIES

Visit the website for the National Hospice and Palliative Care Organization (NHPCO) at http://www.nhpco.org. List three of the most frequently asked questions about hospice care. Include answers to the questions.

Visit http://www.cancer.org and click on *Find Resources for Healthy Living.* List a few ways to prevent some common forms of cancer.

Visit the Centers for Disease Control and Prevention website at http://www.cdc.gov and research the states with the highest rate of AIDS/HIV. Hint: Click on *Diseases and Conditions,* then click on *HIV/AIDS,* then click on *Surveillance,* and then on *Basic Statistics.* Is your state or a neighboring state in the top 10?

Bibliography

Applegate EJ: *The anatomy and physiology learning system,* ed 3, Philadelphia, 2006, Saunders.

Barstow C: *Tending body and spirit: massage and counseling with elders,* Boulder, Colo, 1985, Cedar Barstow.

Bass E, Davis L: *The courage to heal,* Philadelphia, 1994, Harper-Collins Publishers.

Curties D: *Massage therapy and cancer,* Moncton, New Brunswick, Canada, 1999, Curties-Overzet.

Falconer J: Being of service, *Massage Bodywork: Nurture Body, Mind, Spirit Magazine* Feb/Mar 2002, pp 132-137.

Fritz S: *Fundamentals of therapeutic massage,* ed 3, St Louis, 2003, Mosby.

Gould BE: *Pathophysiology for the health professions,* ed 3, Philadelphia, 2006, Saunders.

Ignatiavicius DD, Varner Bayne M: *Medical-surgical nursing: a nursing process approach,* ed 2, Philadelphia, 1995, Saunders.

MacDonald G: Easing the chemotherapy experience with massage, *Massage Mag* 84:85-91, 2000.

MacDonald G: *Medicine hands: massage therapy for people with cancer,* Tallahassee, Fla, 1999, Findhorn Press.

Mathias M: Personal communication, 2006.

McConnellogue K: The courage to touch: massage and cancer, *Massage Bodywork: Nurture Body, Mind, Spirit Magazine* Dec/Jan 2000, pp 12-20.

McKay M, Davis M, Fanning P: *Messages: the communication skills book,* Oakland, Calif, 1987, New Harbinger.

Meek S: Effects of slow stroke back massage on relaxation in hospice clients, *Image J Nurs Sch* 25(1):17-21, 1993.

Miesler, Dietrich W. *Readings in geriatrics: topics for bodyworkers,* ed 3, Sunrise, Fla, 2001, Massage Review Publications.

Nelson D: *From the heart through the hands: the power of touch in caregiving,* Findhorn, Scotland, 2001, Findhorn Press.

Nelson D, Allen B: *Therapeutic massage in facility care: benefits, effects, and implementation,* Sunrise, Fla, 1996, Massage Review Publications.

Rich GJ: *Massage therapy: the evidence for practice,* St Louis, 2002, Mosby.

Rounseville C: Phantom limb pain: the ghost that haunts the amputee, *Orthop Nurs* 11(2):67-71, 1992.

Salvo SG, Anderson SK: *Mosby's pathology for massage therapists,* St Louis, 2004, Elsevier Mosby.

Scott D et al: The antiemetic effect of clinical relaxation: report of an exploratory pilot study, *J Psychosoc Oncol* 1(1):71-83, 1983.

Thibodeau G, Patton K: *Anatomy and physiology,* ed 6, St Louis, 2006, Mosby.

Thibodeau G, Patton K: *Structure and function of the body,* ed 12, St Louis, 2004, Mosby.

Tortora GJ: *Introduction to the human body: the essentials of anatomy and physiology,* ed 5, Hoboken, NJ, 2000, Wiley, John & Sons.

Tortora GJ, Grabowksi SR: *Principles of anatomy and physiology,* ed 11 New York, 2005, John Wiley & Sons.

Weidner N: Personal communication, 2002.

Williams D: Touching cancer patients, *Massage Mag* 84:74-79, 2000.

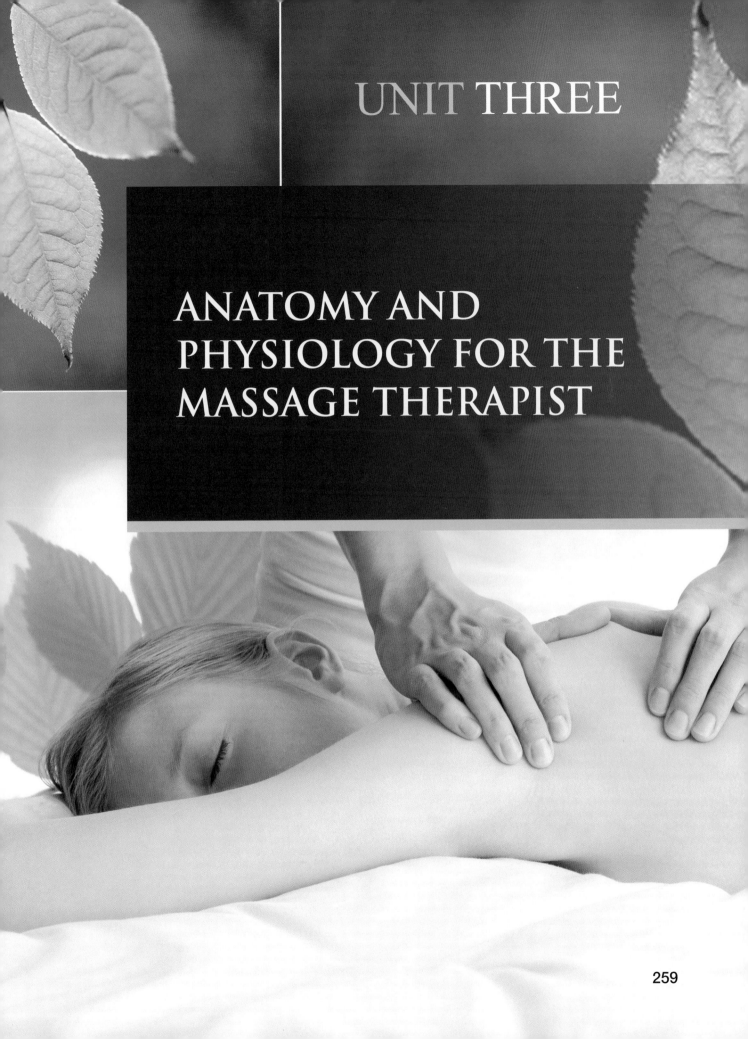

UNIT THREE

ANATOMY AND PHYSIOLOGY FOR THE MASSAGE THERAPIST

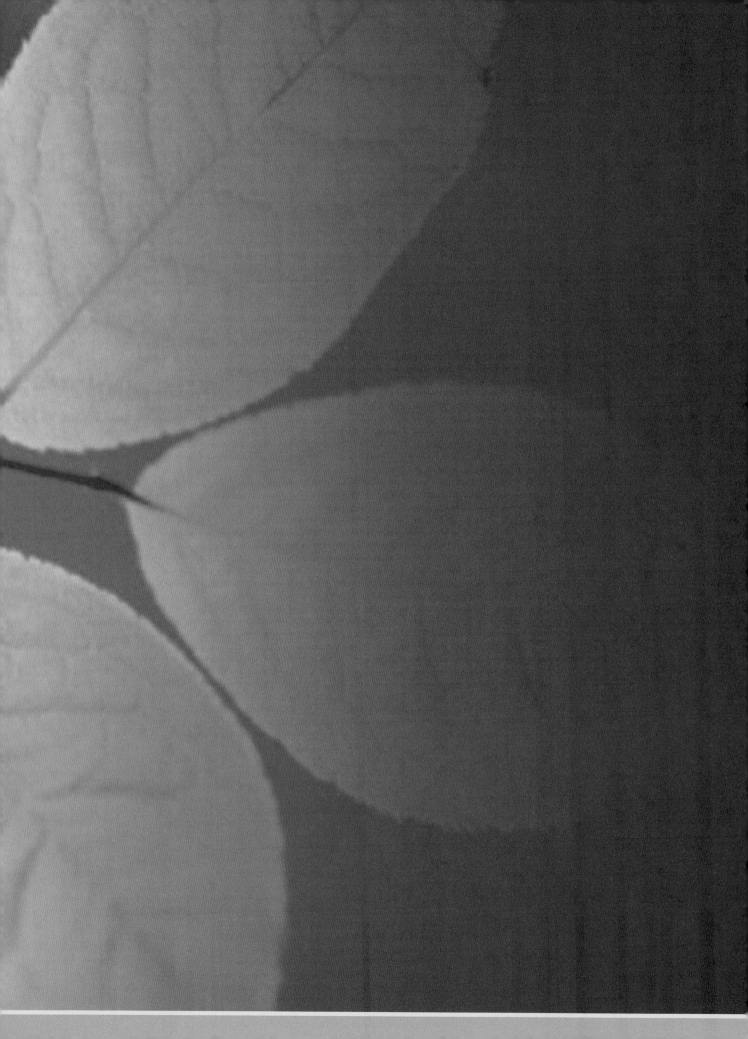

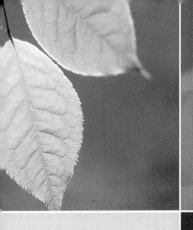

"The capacity to blunder slightly is the real marvel of DNA. Without this special attribute, we would still be anaerobic bacteria and there would be no muse."
—Lewis Thomas

Introduction to the Human Body: Cells, Tissues, and the Body Compass

STUDENT OBJECTIVES

After completing this chapter, the student should be able to:

- Define *anatomy*, *physiology*, *homeostasis*, and *metabolism*
- Place the levels of organization in a hierarchy from least to most complex
- Identify the parts of a cell, and discuss their functions
- Describe passive and active cell processes, and give examples of each
- Discuss the tissue types, and give examples of each
- Discuss fascia's property of thixotropy and how this property is used in massage therapy
- Outline the types of membranes, and state their secretions
- State the 10 main body systems detailing both anatomical structures and their functions
- Describe or stand in the Western anatomical position
- Indicate the planes of the body
- Differentiate among the main body cavities, their subdivisions, and the organs contained within them
- Identify the abdominopelvic quadrants
- State the terms used to describe anatomical directions; use them to express the location of body structures
- Identify the body's regions

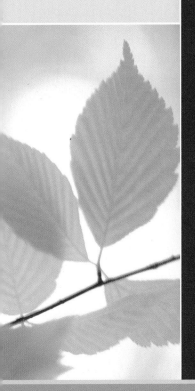

INTRODUCTION

You are about to embark on an unforgettable journey—a new path of self-discovery—into your own interiors. To begin, you have to learn a language and definitions, much of which is Latin and Greek. Basic anatomical terminology is crucial to your understanding of the anatomy and physiology that follows; to be an effective and skillful massage therapist, you must have a comprehensive knowledge of this material.

A clear visual picture of the many arrangements of cells and tissues will help you feel what is beneath your hands. As massage therapists, you will be manipulating and comparing numerous types of tissues. You will be compressing and stretching fascia (connective tissue), kneading the gluteus maximus (muscle tissue), chucking metacarpals (connective tissue), and gliding across the epidermis (epithelial and nervous tissues). All of these terms will be reinforced many times during your studies. This step is only the beginning—a first step on a memorable journey.

Anatomy and physiology are inseparable. Structure is determined by its function, and function is carried out through its structure. Another way of looking at this concept is that *form follows function.* For example, consider the form (or structure) of the lungs, a pair of thin-tissue organs. Lung tissue is suited for gas exchange. What organ (structure), with its thick, muscular walls, is suited for pumping fluids (function)? The heart, of course!

Our bodies are all physiological masterpieces. As you read this text, your heart is pumping blood, your lungs are moving air, your pupils are adjusting to reading conditions, and your nerves are monitoring both the internal and the external environments. These processes occur within us at every moment. During your study of anatomy and physiology, many wonders will be revealed. The philosopher Plato once noted that the "acquiring of knowledge is just a form of recollection." Learning anatomy and physiology is simply becoming aware of who you are already.

This chapter is designed to serve as a reference as you continue your studies in anatomy and physiology. Here, you will learn about cells, tissues, and their membranes. You will also be introduced to organ systems. The terms used to navigate your way around the body are presented. The reference used in directional terminology, structural landmarks, and body cavities is known as the *body compass.*

PREFACE TO ANATOMY AND PHYSIOLOGY

The two ways to approach the study of the human body are regionally and systemically. The *regional approach* is typically used in medical schools, especially in laboratory classes. In the cadaver laboratory, the student learns all the structures (i.e., skin, nerves, blood vessels, bones, muscles) within a body region such as the arm, leg, and chest. The *systemic approach* is needed during classroom lecture and explores one body system at a time (i.e., endocrine, respiratory, urinary). This approach is used in most of the chapters

in this unit. However, the regional approach is used in chapters covering skeletal and muscular nomenclature. A laboratory class format is the best way to approach the information presented in these two chapters. Both approaches are valid, and although we can look at each system individually or by region, an important point to remember is that the body functions as an interrelated whole and that all the systems balance and support one another.

Nearly everyone has some understanding of basic anatomy and physiology, if not from prior education classes, then from practical experience of one's own body. As we begin our study, getting a good definition of anatomical terms based on the medical model is important so that everyone speaks a common language.

Anatomy is the study of the structures of the human body and their positional relationship to one another (the head bone is connected to the neck bone and so on). The study of anatomy can be approached in many ways. *Gross anatomy* is the study of larger body structures such as bones, muscle, nerves, blood vessels, organs, and glands. *Microscopic anatomy* is the study of the smaller structures of the body, such as cells and tissues, which make up the larger structures and can best be seen through a microscope. *Applied anatomy* studies body structures and their morphological properties as it relates to the diagnosis and treatment of disease. *Comparative anatomy* studies the structures of all life forms to indicate a progression from the simplest to the most highly specialized. *Surface anatomy* studies the structural relationships of the body's surface and how they relate to internal structures.

Physiology is the study of how the body and its individual parts function in normal body processes. These processes are both physical and chemical. As with anatomy, different ways can be used to approach the study of physiology. *Comparative physiology* studies similarities and differences of vital processes. *Developmental physiology* studies embryonic development. *Pathophysiology,* or pathology, studies the physical and chemical processes involved in disease (discussed in Chapter 4).

To understand the relationship between anatomy and physiology better, a theater metaphor may be helpful. The stage, props, and cast of characters are the structures of the play (anatomy). How the characters relate to one another and the plot of the play is its function (physiology).

Within the study of physiology is an important concept called homeostasis. **Homeostasis** is constancy of the body's internal environment. It represents a relatively stable condition of the body's internal environment within a limited range. Even when the outside conditions change, the body's internal environment is relatively constant. Every body structure, from microscopic cells to complex organ systems, helps keep the internal environment within normal limits. Homeostasis is maintained by adjusting the metabolism of the body.

Metabolism is the total of all the physical and chemical processes that occur in an organism (i.e., those that are considered to be signs of life) and results in growth, generation of energy, elimination of wastes, and other bodily functions as they relate to the distribution of nutrients in the blood after digestion. Metabolism takes place in two steps: (1) *anabolism,* the constructive phase, in which smaller molecules (e.g., amino acids) are converted to larger molecules (e.g., proteins), and (2) *catabolism,* the destructive phase, in which larger molecules (e.g., glycogen) are converted to smaller molecules (e.g., pyruvic acid). Exercise, elevated body temperature, hormonal activity, and digestion can increase the metabolic rate, which is the rate determined when a person is at complete rest, physically and mentally. The metabolic rate is customarily expressed in calories as the heat liberated in the course of metabolism.

INTRODUCTION TO TERMINOLOGY

Anatomy, physiology, and pathology have their own language. Most sciences of the body were born in eighteenth century universities in which Greek and Latin were the languages used during lectures and in books. Hence most prefixes, suffixes, and word roots are based on Greek or Latin.

All medical terms possess one or more parts: a prefix, a root, and a suffix. Once you have become familiar with medical terminology, looking at a new term and ascertaining its meaning is relatively easy.

A *root* is the main part of a word, or its foundation. Some words combine two roots, such as *cardi-,* Greek for *heart,* and *vascular,* Latin for *vessel.* Most often, a vowel is used to combine the roots to aid in pronunciation. When combining

---

BOX 11-1

Commonly Used Plural Endings

Singular	Plural
-a; scapula	-ae; scapulae
-en; foramen	-ina; foramina
-is; testis	-es; testes
-is; iris	-ides; irides
-nx; larynx	-ges; larynges
-on; mitochondrion	-a; mitochondria
-um; bacterium	-a; bacteria
-us; nucleus	-i; nuclei
-x; thorax	-ces; thoraces
-y; cavity	-ies; cavities

---

the two aforementioned roots, the new term is *cardiovascular.* The most common combining vowel is the letter *o.*

A *prefix* is a syllable or syllables placed before a root to alter its meaning. For example, *pre-* is a prefix that means *before* or *front.* Add *pre-* before the root *cancerous* and it becomes *precancerous,* denoting a stage of tumor growth that is likely to develop, but has not yet developed, into cancer.

A *suffix* is a syllable or syllables placed after a root to alter its meaning (Box 11-1). For example, *-ectomy* is a suffix that means *to cut out,* usually in surgery. Add *-ectomy* behind

---

Biological Prefixes and Suffixes

PREFIX	MEANING	EXAMPLE
a-, an-	Lacking, without, not	Asymptomatic, anaerobic
ab-	Away from, absent, decrease	Abduct
ad-	Toward, near to, increase	Adduct
ante-	Front, before, toward	Anterior
anti-	Against, opposed	Antifungal
auto-	Self	Autoimmune
bi-, di-	Twice, double, two	Biceps, diencephalon
bio-	Life	Biology
cephal-	Head	Cephalitis
circum-	Around	Circumduction
contra-	Opposite, against	Contraindication
cryo-	Extreme cold	Cryotherapy
cyto-	Cell	Cytoplasm
de-	Separate, away from, down	Decapitate
dia-	Through	Diaphragm
dis-	Apart, away	Dislocation
dors-	Back	Dorsiflexion
dys-	Difficult, bad, labored	Dysfunction
ecto-, exo-, ex-	On the outer side	Ectoderm, exocrine, excise
endo-	Within, inside	Endometrium
epi-	Upon, over, in addition to	Epicondyle
eu-	Good, well, normal	Euphoria
extend-	Straighten	Extension

Continued

Biological Prefixes and Suffixes—cont'd

PREFIX—cont'd	MEANING—cont'd	EXAMPLE—cont'd
flex-	Bend	Flexibility
glu-, gly-	Sugar, sweet	Glucose, glycosuria
histo-	Tissue	Histology, homolateral
homeo-, homo-	Like, same	Homeopathy
hydro-	Water or hydrogen	Hydromassage
hyper-	Over, above, excessive	Hyperextension
hypo-	Under, below, deficient	Hypodermic
hyster-	Uterus, womb	Hysterectomy
infra-	Under, below, beneath	Infraspinatus
inter-	Between, together, midst	Intercostals
intra-	Within	Intravenous
meso-	Middle	Mesentery
meta-	Beyond, after, change	Metacarpals
mono-	One, single	Mononuclear
multi-	Many	Multifidus
narco-	Sleep, numbness, stupor	Narcolepsy
necro-	Death	Necrosis
ophthalmo-	Eye	Ophthalmologist
ot-	Ear	Otitis
para-	Alongside, beside	Parasympathetic
patho-	Disease	Pathophysiology
ped-	Foot	Pedicure
peri-	Around, about	Periosteum
post-	Rear, after, behind	Posterior
pre-, pro-	Before, front	Prenatal, protuberance
quad-	Four	Quadriceps
re-	Again, back	Realign
recto-	Straight	Rectum
retro-	Backward	Retroperitoneal
sub-	Under, beneath, below	Subscapular
super-, supra-	Above, over	Superficial, supraspinatus
syn-, sym-	Together, with, joined	Synarthrotic, symbiotic
therm-	Heat	Thermotherapy
thixis-	To touch	Thixotropy
trans-	Across, over, beyond, through	Transverse
tri-	Three	Triceps
uni-	One	Unilateral

SUFFIX	MEANING	EXAMPLE
-algia	Pain	Fibromyalgia
-ate	Use, action	Articulate
-cyte	Cell	Hemocyte
-ectomy	Excision or to cut out	Tonsillectomy
-emia	Blood condition	Hyperemia
-gen	Produce	Carcinogen
-gram	To record	Electrocardiogram
-ia, osis, ism	State or condition	Anemia, cyanosis, embolism
-iatry	Healing	Psychiatry
-itis	Inflammation	Arthritis
-oid	Shaped	Rhomboid
-ology	Study of	Urology
-oma	Tumor	Neuroma
-osis	Condition	Lordosis
-otomy	Incision or to cut into	Colostomy
-scopy	To view or examine	Orthoscopy
-stasis	Control, stopping	Homeostasis
-trophy	Nourish, grow, develop	Hypertrophy
-tropy	Turning	Thixotropy

the word *appendix,* and the new term is *appendectomy,* or surgical removal of the appendix.

The more you are exposed to medical terminology, the more familiar you will become with prefixes, suffixes, and roots. Learn to pronounce these terms while in class; echoing what the teacher says reinforces the pronunciation in your mind. Along with correct pronunciation, correct spelling is crucial. When in doubt, use a medical dictionary. Guessing is not advised because it might totally change the meaning of the word. Several medical terms sound similar but are spelled differently, such as ileum (a section of the small intestine) and ilium (a section of the pelvis).

Learning medical terms can be daunting at first, but with time and practice, it will reap many rewards, including better marks on tests featuring medical terms. You will soon discover that medical terminology makes sense and is easy to understand, once you are familiar with the prefixes, suffixes, and roots.

LEVELS OF ORGANIZATION: CELL TO ORGANISM

The human body can be considered as a universe, made up of very small parts organized to function as a unit. These parts follow a hierarchy based on their levels of complexity. The levels are chemical, cellular, tissue, organ, organ system, and organism levels. The *chemical level* encompasses the biochemistry of our body (e.g., water, hormones, deoxyribonucleic acid [DNA], oxygen, iron, compounds). The *cellular level* deals primarily with cells. Cells are composed of chemicals from the chemical level and can perform all the functions vital to life. The *tissue level* is composed of groups of cells possessing their own unique properties that perform specific function. The *organ level* is composed of two or more specialized groups of tissue that carry on specific functions (e.g., stomach, liver, brain). Related organs with complementary functions arrange themselves into organ systems that can perform certain necessary tasks, such as respiration and digestion. The *organism level* is the highest level of organization, representing living entities composed of several organ systems. All organ systems provide functions that promote life. The total of all structures and functions is a living individual (Table 11-1).

evolve *Log on to the Evolve website to view an illustration of the levels of organization.* ■

Think of these levels as the building materials of a house. The cells are similar to the individual parts such as nails, studs, tiles, bricks, and mortar. These materials are put together to make walls, floors, and ceilings, which correspond to the tissues of the body. Then put tissues together, and you get a room, which is similar to an organ. Several rooms may function as an organ system; the bedrooms might constitute one organ system; the bathrooms and kitchen constitute another. These systems are all linked together into one house, which is akin to the organism level. To understand the body, the smallest components are examined first, and then we proceed up to the organism level. Let us take a look at our cellular level.

MINI-LAB

In small groups or as a class, discuss the concept of being *alive*. Use a board or overhead projector to list all the ideas that accumulate. As you will discover, the concept of being alive is a very complex set of ideas.

CELL

In the late 1600s, Robert Hooke was examining plant tissue samples through a primitive microscope. He identified structures that reminded him of the long rows of cell rooms in a monastery. He named these cubelike biological structures *cells*. The **cell** is the fundamental unit of all living organisms and is the simplest form of life that can exist as a self-sustaining unit. Cells are the building blocks of the human body (Figure 11-1).

Scientists estimate that between 75 and 100 trillion active, living cells are in the body. Cells consist of four elements: (1) carbon, (2) oxygen, (3) hydrogen, and (4) nitrogen, plus trace elements, such as iron, sodium, and potassium, among others. These trace elements are extremely important for cellular functions: Calcium is needed for blood clotting (among other things); iron is necessary to make hemoglobin, which carries oxygen in the blood; and iodine is needed to make thyroid hormones, which control metabolism. Besides the four primary elements, water makes up approximately 60% to 80% of all cells.

TABLE 11-1 Levels of Organization

LEVEL	DESCRIPTION	EXAMPLES
Chemical	Biochemistry of our bodies	Atoms, molecules, compounds, water, hormones, DNA, oxygen, iron
Cellular	Basic unit of life	Bone cell, muscle cell, nerve cell
Tissue	Groups of cells that share a similar structure and function	Epithelial, connective, muscular, nervous
Organ	Complex structures of two or more tissue types performing a specific function	Heart, kidney, brain, lung
Organ system	Related organs with complementary functions that perform certain tasks	Circulatory, urinary, nervous, respiratory
Organism	Living entities composed of several organ systems; most complex level	*Homo sapiens*, fish, frog, butterfly

DNA, Deoxyribonucleic acid.

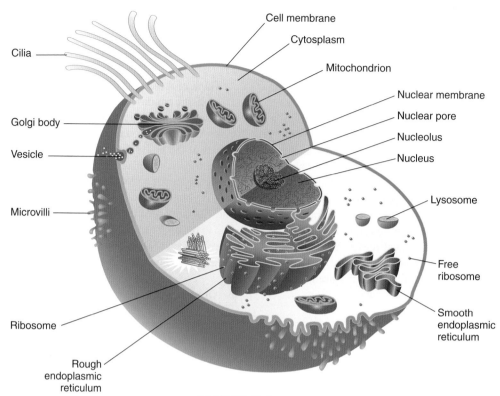

FIGURE 11-1 A cell.

The cell contains three basic parts: (1) cell membrane, (2) cytoplasm, and (3) organelles. Organelles include the nucleus, mitochondria, ribosomes, endoplasmic reticulum, Golgi body, and lysosomes (Table 11-2). The specialized nature of body tissues reflects the specialized function of their cellular makeup.

Cell Membrane

The **cell (plasma) membrane** separates the cytoplasm from the surrounding external environment. The membrane creates a *semipermeable* (some materials can freely pass, and others cannot) boundary that governs exchange of nutrients and waste materials. This membrane also responds to stimuli. Movement of molecules takes place by active and passive processes, which are discussed in the next section. The cell mem-

brane often contains projections such as *microvilli, cilia,* or *flagellum,* which help protect the cell and aid in its mobility.

Cytoplasm

Consisting primarily of water, **cytoplasm** (cytosol) is the gel-like intracellular fluid within the cell membrane. Floating in cytoplasm are cellular structures called *organelles,* which provide special functions. Functions of cytoplasm are to provide cellular nutrition and to support the organelles.

Organelles

Within the cell are **organelles** (little organs), which are necessary for metabolism. Each organelle possesses a distinct structure and function within the cell. Some organelles

TABLE 11-2 Cell Structures and Functions

PARTS OF CELL	ACTION
Cell membrane	Governs exchange of nutrients and waste materials
Cytoplasm	Provides cellular nutrition and supports organelles
Organelle:	
Nucleus	Control center of the cell; directs nearly all metabolic activities
	Contains DNA and RNA
Ribosomes	Synthesizes protein
Endoplasmic reticulum	Synthesizes proteins and lipids; assists in the transportation of these materials
Golgi body	Packing and shipping plant of the cell; alters proteins and lipids, packs and stores them till needed
Mitochondria	Power plant of the cell, responsible for cellular respiration; provides most of the cell's ATP
Lysosomes	Engulfs and digests bacteria, cellular debris, and other organelles

ATP, Adenosine triphosphate; *DNA,* deoxyribonucleic acid; *RNA,* ribonucleic acid.

function in reproduction, some store materials, and some metabolize nutrients. Types of organelles are the *nucleus, ribosomes, endoplasmic reticulum, Golgi body, mitochondria,* and *lysosomes.*

Nucleus

The **nucleus,** the largest and most obvious organelle in the cytoplasm, is the control center of the cell, directing nearly all metabolic activities. All cells have at least one nucleus at some time in their existence. Red blood cells lose their nuclei (anucleate) as they mature, and skeletal muscle cells possess many nuclei (multinucleate). The shape of the nucleus is usually spherical, and it is enclosed in a porous double-layer nuclear membrane. Each nucleus contains clusters of proteins, ribonucleic acid (RNA), and DNA, which make up chromosomes (our genetic code). Humans possess 23 pairs of chromosomes, although abnormalities can exist.

The DNA is similar in every cell of the body, but depending on the specific cell type, some genes may be turned on or off. This property is why a liver cell is different from a muscle cell and a muscle cell is different from a fat cell.

The *nucleolus* produces ribosomes, which move out of the nucleus to positions on the rough endoplasmic reticulum, where they are critical in protein synthesis.

Ribosomes

Ribosomes are small granules of RNA and protein in the cytoplasm. Their function is to synthesize protein for use within the cell and to produce other proteins that are exported outside the cell. Ribosomes may bind to rough endoplasmic reticulum or may float free in the cytoplasm. When the latter occurs, they are called *free ribosomes.*

Endoplasmic Reticulum

A complex network of membranous channels within the cytoplasm is **endoplasmic reticulum.** These structures often extend from the cell membrane to the nuclear membrane and may extend to certain organelles. The endoplasmic reticulum functions in the synthesis of protein and lipids and assists in the transportation of these materials from one part of the cell to another. Endoplasmic reticula are classified as *rough* or *granular* (ribosomes are attached to the surface) or as *smooth* or *agranular* (ribosomes are absent).

Golgi Body

The **Golgi body** is a series of four to six horizontal membranous sacs. Referred to as the *packing and shipping plant* of the cell, the Golgi body, associated with altering proteins and lipids, packs and stores them until needed. Once this process is complete, they are wrapped in a piece of the Golgi body's membrane, or vesicle, and jettisoned to the desired area, often out of the cell.

Mitochondria

An oval organelle, the **mitochondrion,** is considered the cell's *power plant* because it is a site for cellular respiration and provides most of a cell's adenosine triphosphate (ATP), which is the body's energy molecule. Mitochondria consist of an inner and outer membrane; the outer shell is smooth, and the inner, convoluted membrane contains many projections called *cristae.* These inner chambers increase the surface area to increase mitochondrion's metabolic properties.

Lysosomes

Membrane-bound organelles containing digestive enzymes are the **lysosomes.** Lysosomes can engulf pathogens, cellular debris, and other organelles and digest them, after which any reusable matter is returned to the cytoplasm for reuse. The lysosome can also cause self-digestion of the cell when the reduction of cells in an organ is needed, such as reduction in the size of the uterus after childbirth. Lysosomes also release their digestive enzymes at injury sites to help dispose of cellular debris.

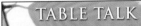

TABLE TALK

The death of cells in tissues or organs caused by disease or injury is called *necrosis.*

PASSIVE AND ACTIVE CELL PROCESSES

To survive, a cell must be able to carry on a variety of functions. In a majority of these processes, substances are exchanged across the cell membrane, which allows for the assimilation of oxygen, nutrients, and water; the elimination of pathogens; and the excretion of waste products. These processes can be classified as passive or active processes. Passive processes occur naturally by means of gradients of temperature, pressure, or concentration. The gradient or difference in levels of temperature, pressure, or concentration is the factor that drives the exchange of particles or fluid through the cell's membrane. Involving no active expending of energy by the cells, passive cell processes include diffusion, filtration, and osmosis.

Active processes are those that require an expenditure of energy (using ATP) by the cell itself to transport the products across the membrane. Active processes include active transport and endocytosis.

Passive Processes

Diffusion

Diffusion is the movement of molecules, or other particles, from an area of high concentration to an area of low concentration. This passive process continues until the distribution of particulates is equal in all areas (Figure 11-2).

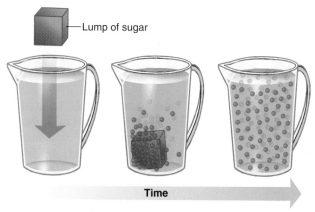

FIGURE 11-2 Diffusion in a liquid.

Log on to your student account from the Evolve website to view an image of diffusion through a membrane. List examples of when this cell process occurs in the human body. ■

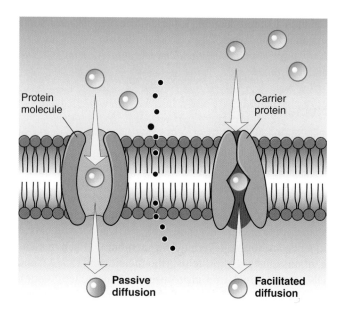

FIGURE 11-3 Passive and facilitated diffusion.

Diffusion can be easily demonstrated by filling a long baking pan with cool water and setting it somewhere where no vibration or movement can disturb the pan. Open a packet of colored soft drink mix (e.g., Kool-Aid), and gently sprinkle the powder in one corner of the pan. Even though no true currents are in the pan, the colored powder diffuses across the pan. When kinetic energy, or speed, of the particles is increased (e.g., by raising the temperature), the rate of the diffusion process also increases. The greater the energy is, and the higher the gradient is, the faster the rate of diffusion will be. Try the Kool-Aid experiment with a pan of hot water or by gently shaking the pan, and see how the rate of the diffusion process increases.

Facilitated diffusion is a special type of diffusion that uses a carrier protein to facilitate the diffusion process (Figure 11-3). Carrier proteins are contained in the cell membrane. Sometimes molecules in solution are too large to cross the cell membrane. When the solution outside the cell membrane has a high concentration of large molecules, the carrier proteins in the cell membrane assist the large molecules in crossing the membrane. The number of available carrier proteins limits facilitated diffusion. Many of the nutrients in our digestive tract enter our bloodstream through diffusion or facilitated diffusion.

Filtration

Filtration is the movement of particles across the cellular membrane because of pressure. A pressure gradient across a cell membrane is the force that drives the filtration process. The air filter on your furnace or central air conditioning unit is a good example. The vacuum created by the suction of the fan lowers the pressure behind the filter. The atmospheric pressure in the room is then greater than that behind the filter. The air flows through the pores of the filter, which is selective and traps the larger particles of dust, pet hair, and smoke. An example of filtration is the kidney's filtering of wastes out of the body across a special membrane.

Osmosis

Similar to diffusion, **osmosis** is the movement of a pure solvent such as water from an area of low concentration (most dilute) to an area of high concentration (least dilute). This action continues until the two concentrations equalize (Figure 11-4). In osmosis, water moves instead of particles to create equilibrium.

Unlike filtration, osmotic movement does not depend on pressure but rather on the concentration of dissolved elements that lie in the solutions on each side of a cell membrane or vessel wall. When the solutions contain particles that are too large to cross the membrane, diffusion cannot occur. Even though a cell membrane does not permit the particles to pass through its walls, the solvent fluid is still able to permeate the membrane. When your fingers are wrinkled from being in water too long, it is because water has been moved by osmosis from your body toward the particles in the water in which your hands have been.

Active Processes

Active Transport

Active transport moves important atoms and molecules such as ions against the concentration gradient from low levels to high levels to maintain such vital processes as nerve conduction (Figure 11-5). The mechanisms of active transport are both chemical and physical. The chemical part of the mechanism involves the breakdown of ATP to produce the energy needed for the transport. Scientists estimate that at least 40% of the ATP in the human body is used solely for active transport.

Ions are attracted to a protein molecule, or carrier protein, which is part of the cellular membrane. The outside wall of the carrier protein opens, as would a clamshell, and the ion is drawn inside and binds to it. The binding causes the chemical breakdown of ATP, which again transforms the shape of the carrier protein. The clamshell closes, and then the opposite side of the carrier protein opens again to release the ion to the inside

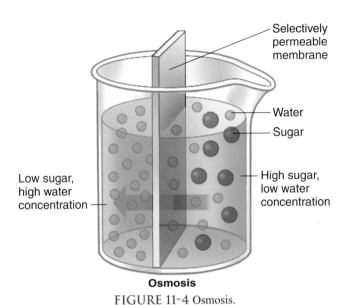

FIGURE 11-4 Osmosis.

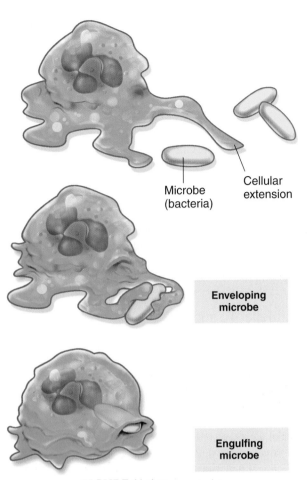

FIGURE 11-6 Phagocytosis.

of the cell membrane. This process is similar to an air lock in that only one door can be opened at a time and represents the physical component of the active transport mechanism.

Endocytosis

Endocytosis is a process that moves large particles across the cell membrane into the cell. The two main types of endocytosis are phagocytosis and pinocytosis, both of which are vital to the immune defense systems of the body.

Phagocytosis, or *cell eating,* is the process by which specialized cells ingest harmful microorganisms and cellular debris, break them down, and expel the harmless remains back into the body (Figure 11-6). Phagocytosis is chiefly characteristic of leukocytes found in the blood. The process includes five steps. Once the leukocyte locates the microbe through chemical attraction and targeted for destruction, it forms extensions to surround it. Next, it engulfs the microbe.

Third, a membranous sac is formed around the microbe as it becomes internalized. Fourth, lysosomal enzymes destroy the phagocytosed material. Finally, the digested microbial products are released.

Pinocytosis, or *cell drinking,* is almost identical to phagocytosis except that the targeted object is liquid (Figure 11-7).

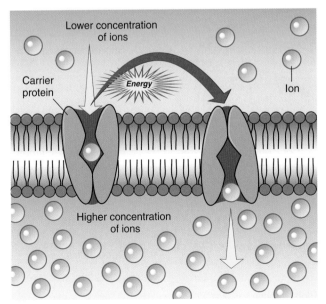

FIGURE 11-5 Active transport.

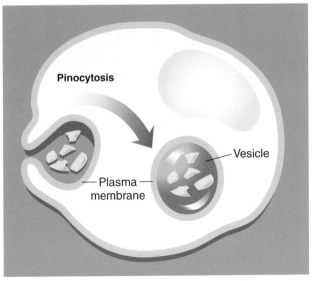

FIGURE 11-7 Pinocytosis.

In this process, the cell develops a saccular indention, drawing the molecule inside and then enclosing it. Pinocytic cells are more common than phagocytic cells.

BODY TISSUES

Tissues are defined as groups of similar cells that act together to perform a specific function. The study of tissues is known as *histology*. Only four major types of tissues are in the human body: (1) epithelial, (2) connective, (3) muscle, and (4) nervous (Figure 11-8).

Tissues organize themselves into organs. *Organs* are defined as groups of two or more tissue types that act together to perform a specific common function and have a consistently recognizable shape. To understand better the structure and functions of our body's organs, studying first the tissues that comprise the organs would be beneficial.

Epithelial Tissue

Epithelial tissue, or epithelium, lines or covers internal and external (skin) organs of the body; lines blood vessels and body cavities; and lines the digestive, respiratory, urinary, and reproductive tracts (Figure 11-9). The functions of this tissue include protection, absorption, filtration, secretion, excretion, and diffusion. Epithelial tissue is closely packed, typically avascular, and receives nutrition by diffusion from blood vessels in underlying connective tissues. Epithelium reproduces and regenerates quickly.

Connective Tissue

Connective tissue is the most abundant and ubiquitous tissue of the body. This tissue serves a wide variety of functions. Some connective tissue types serve as nutrient transport systems (housing nearly 25% of all body fluids), some defend the body against disease such as inflammatory processes, some possess clotting mechanisms, and others act as a supportive framework and provide protection for vital organs (Figure 11-10).

Connective tissue is highly vascularized, providing nutrition and oxygen to itself and nearby tissues (i.e., skin, muscle), with the exception of cartilage.

All connective tissue is composed of connective tissue cells scattered in a matrix. The matrix itself is a gelatinous liquid that is primarily composed of ground substance and protein. The ground substance is mostly water with some suspended solids such as carbohydrates, giving it viscosity. Within the ground substance are precursor cells called *fibroblasts,* which give rise to various connective tissue cells needed for metabolism and tissue healing (e.g., chondroblast, collagenoblast, osteoblast). The second component of matrix is long protein strands of collagen.

The arrangement of the fibers and the ratio of collagen to ground substance is the primary factor for determining the different types of connective tissues. Blood and lymph are dilute and have high amounts of ground substance. Bone has a very high ratio of collagen arranged to trap the mineral salts that give it density and firmness. The ligaments and fascia have a ratio of collagen to ground substance that is somewhere in the middle, giving it both durability and elasticity.

The five different classifications of connective tissue, some of which contain more than one type of tissue, are (1) liquid connective tissue (blood), (2) bone or osseous tissue, (3) cartilaginous tissue, (4) loose connective tissue, and (5) dense connective tissue (Table 11-3).

Liquid Connective Tissue
Also known as *vascular tissue,* **liquid connective tissue** consists of blood, lymph, and interstitial fluid. Blood contains three formed elements, two of which are cells (erythrocytes

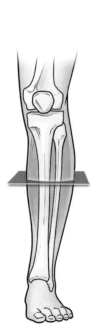
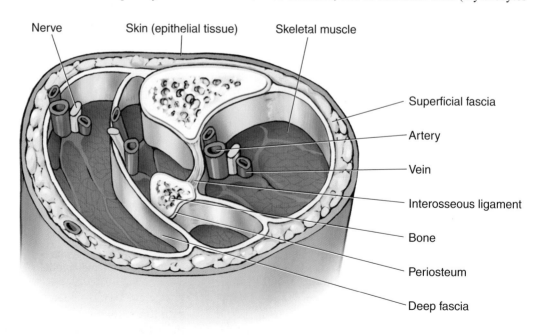

Nerve	Skin (epithelial tissue)	Skeletal muscle

Superficial fascia

Artery

Vein

Interosseous ligament

Bone

Periosteum

Deep fascia

FIGURE 11-8 Cross section of limb denoting tissue types.

Epithelial Tissue

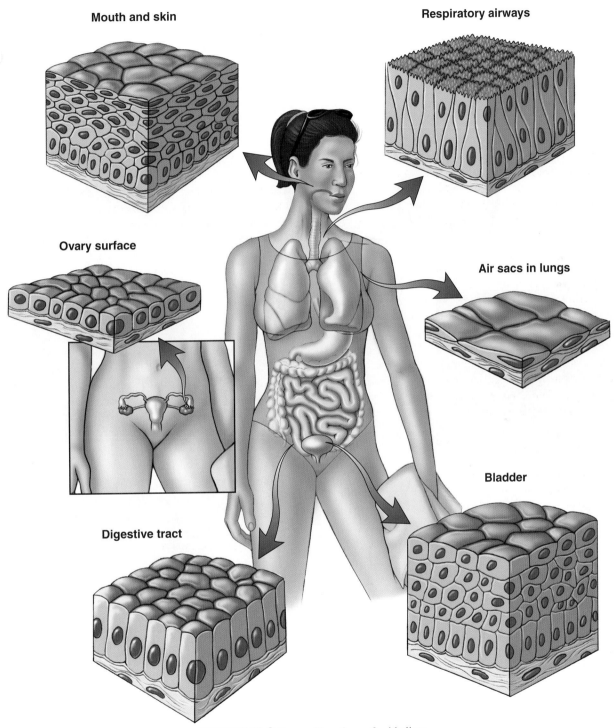

FIGURE 11-9 Types of locations of epithelium.

and leukocytes) and one of which is cell fragments (platelets). The fluid medium in which these elements are suspended is *plasma.* Lymph and interstitial fluid are the same substance, differing only in where they are located. Lymph resides in the lymphovascular system, and interstitial fluid bathes cells and tissues. Hence both lymph and interstitial fluid are chemically similar to blood plasma.

Bone

The hardest, most dense, and only slightly elastic connective tissue, **bone**, or *osseous tissue,* consists of compact bone, spongy bone, collagenous fibers (for strength), and mineral salts (for hardness). Bones are permeated by many blood vessels and nerves and are enclosed in membranous periosteum. Long bones contain yellow marrow in longitudinal

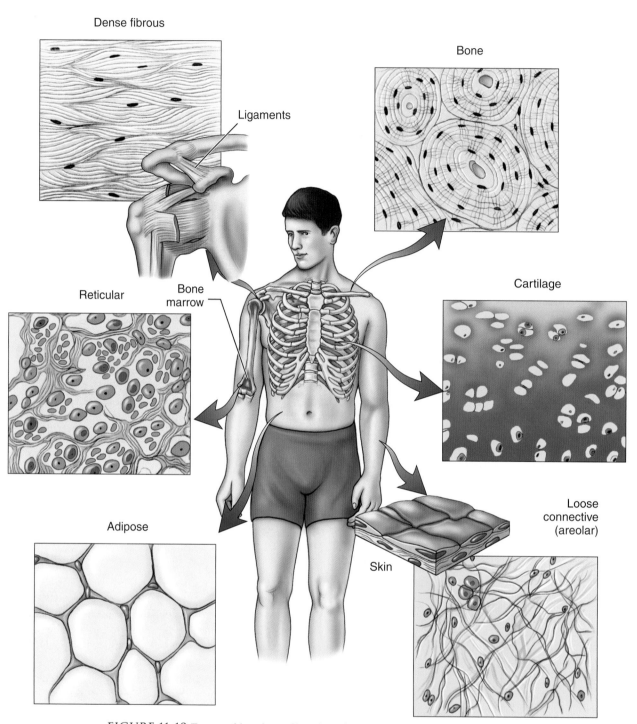

Connective Tissue

Dense fibrous

Ligaments

Bone

Reticular

Bone marrow

Cartilage

Adipose

Skin

Loose connective (areolar)

FIGURE 11-10 Types and locations of location of connective tissues (not all are shown).

cavities and red marrow in their articular ends. Blood cells are produced in active red marrow.

Cartilaginous Tissue

Cartilage is an avascular, tough, protective tissue capable of withstanding repeated stress and is found chiefly in the thorax, joints, and certain rigid tubes of the body (e.g., trachea, larynx, nose, ears). Temporary cartilage, such as that comprising

most of the fetal skeleton at an early stage, is later replaced by bone. Permanent cartilage remains unossified, except in certain diseases and, sometimes, in advanced age. Cartilaginous tissue can be divided into three subcategories: (1) hyaline cartilage, (2) fibrocartilage, and (3) elastic cartilage.

Hyaline cartilage (gristle) is an elastic, rubbery, smooth type of cartilage composed of cells in a translucent, pearly-blue matrix. The most common type of cartilage, hyaline

TABLE 11-3 **Connective Tissue Types**

TYPE	PROPERTIES AND EXAMPLES
Liquid Connective Tissue	
Blood	Fluid medium (plasma) containing erythrocytes, leukocytes, and platelets suspended in it
Lymph	Fluid of the lymphovascular system
Interstitial	Fluid bathing cells and tissues
Osseous Connective Tissue	
Bone	Consists of compact tissue, a spongy cancellous tissue, collagenous fibers, and mineral salts
Cartilage	
Hyaline	Most common type; elastic, rubbery, and smooth; covers ends of bones and part of the larynx and nose; forms the C-shaped rings of the trachea
Elastic	Soft and pliable, giving shape to the external nose and ears and the epiglottis and auditory tubes
Fibrocartilage	Greatest tensile strength of all cartilage types; found in intervertebral disks, meniscus of the knee, and between the pubic bones
Loose Connective Tissue	
Areolar	Most widely distributed; forms the superficial fascia
Adipose	Specialized for fat storage; insulates the body against heat loss; provides fuel reserves for energy; provides cushion around structures
Reticular	Forms the framework for bones and organs
Dense Connective Tissue	
Dense regular	Offers great strength and can resist pulling forces in one direction such as ligaments, tendons, retinacula, and aponeuroses
Dense irregular	Resists pulling forces in several different directions such as deep fascia, deep epidermis, periosteum

thinly covers the articulating ends of bones, connects the ribs to the sternum, and supports the nose, the trachea, and part of the larynx. The early fetal skeleton is mostly this cartilage type.

Fibrocartilage has the greatest tensile strength of all three cartilage types; it consists of a dense matrix of white collagenous fibers. Fibrocartilaginous disks are found between the vertebrae, in the knee joint, and between the pubic bones.

Elastic cartilage (yellow) is the softest and most pliable of all three kinds of cartilage, consisting of elastic fibers in a flexible fibrous matrix. It gives shape to the external nose and ears and internal structures such as the epiglottis, part of the larynx, and the auditory tubes.

Loose Connective Tissue

Loose connective tissue is regarded as the packing material of the body. It attaches the skin to underlying structures in a basement membrane, serves to wrap and support the body cells, fills in the spaces between structures (e.g., organs, muscles), and helps keep them in their proper places. The three types of loose connective tissue are (1) areolar, (2) adipose, and (3) reticular tissues.

Areolar connective tissue is one of the most widely distributed and possesses little tensile strength. Along with adipose tissue, areolar connective tissue forms the subcutaneous layer of the skin (superficial fascia). This layer of tissue also attaches the skin to its underlying tissues and structures.

Adipose tissue, or fatty tissue, is specialized for fat storage. This connective tissue, which includes yellow bone marrow, also insulates the body against heat loss, provides fuel reserves for energy, and provides a cushion around certain structures (e.g., heart, kidneys, some joints).

Reticular connective tissue forms the supportive framework of bones and of certain organs such as the liver and spleen.

Dense Connective Tissue

A fibrous connective tissue, **dense connective tissue,** consists of compact, strong, inelastic bundles of parallel collagenous fibers that have a glistening white color. The two types of dense connective tissue are (1) dense regular and (2) dense irregular.

Dense regular (organized) connective tissue offers great strength and can resist pulling forces, generally in two directions; examples are ligaments, tendons, retinacula, and aponeuroses. **Dense irregular (unorganized) connective tissue** resists pulling forces in several different directions; examples of dense irregular connective tissue are deep fascial membranes, dermis of the skin, periosteum, and the capsules of organs.

Muscle Tissue

Extremely elastic, **muscle tissue** is exceedingly vascular and has the unique ability to shorten (contract) and elongate (stretch) to produce movement. The three types of

One type of connective tissue, fascia, deserves more discussion because it relates directly to a massage therapist's work. The two types of fascia are (1) *superficial fascia,* which is immediately under the skin, and (2) *deep fascia,* which surrounds muscles, holding them together and separating them into functioning groups. The main difference is location. Some therapists view fascia as a single, but complex, body membrane.

The ground substance in fascia possesses two physical states: (1) a relatively thin fluid (sol state) and (2) a thicker, more gelatinous fluid (gel state). Fascia in its sol state has a fluid quality, is more pliant and elastic, and offers less-restricted movements. Fascia in the gel state is tougher, more inflexible, and can restrict the body's movements.

Fascia viscoelastic state can be altered to some degree because it possesses a property called thixotropism. This term refers to fascia's ability to change the ground substance in the matrix from one state to the other. The word *thixotropy* comes from the Greek root words meaning *to touch* and *turning.* Through touch and/or friction, fascia can *change* or *turn* the state of its ground substance in the matrix from a gel state to a sol state, or vice versa.

When the body is not in efficient posture, as in forward head posture, the spine no longer adequately supports the head in space. The muscles and fascia become the supportive tissue, adapting to the situation by becoming firmer. The fascia in the neck can turn from liquid (sol) to solid (gel) to help hold the head in this physically stressful position. The stiffness that the client feels is often fascia in a gel state. This restricted fascia must be addressed during the massage.

As we apply pressure and heat, either by friction or local and general application, thixotropy occurs, converting the gel state to the sol state. The fascia loosens, melts, and becomes more flexible and elastic. This softening of the fascia that surrounds the muscles allows the muscles to be manipulated to their fullest resting length, increase joint range of motion, and free the body from restrictions of movement. Thixotropism also occurs when the body is warmed by physical work, exercise, and stretching.

muscle tissue in the body are (1) smooth muscle, (2) cardiac muscle, and (3) skeletal muscle and are commonly referred to by their features or characteristics. Skeletal muscles are studied in detail in Chapters 15 and 16. More information on cardiac muscle can be found in Chapter 20; smooth muscle receives additional coverage in Chapter 22 (Table 11-4).

Smooth muscle (involuntary-visceral) forms the walls of hollow organs and tubes such as the stomach, bladder, uterus, and blood vessels. Consuming little energy, these cells are adapted for long, sustained contractions (Figure 11-11). The muscle cells are spindle shaped (pointed at both ends), and each contains one oval-shaped nucleus.

Skeletal muscle (voluntary-striated) fibers are cigar-shaped and are multinucleated; many nuclei are located near the periphery of the cell. Each skeletal muscle fiber contains bands of red and white material, which causes it to appear striped or striated under a microscope (Figure 11-12). Muscle contraction occurs when an electrochemical impulse crosses the myoneural junction and causes the thin filaments within the muscle fibers to shorten.

Cardiac muscle (involuntary striated) is located in the heart wall and is Y or H shaped (Figure 11-13). These shapes allow the cells to fit together similar to clasped fingers and help create the spherical shape of the heart. Between each cardiac muscle cell is a structure known as the *intercalated disk.* These disks assist in the transmission of a nervous stimulus from a cardiac muscle cell to another cardiac muscle cell.

Nervous Tissue

Nervous tissue consists of oddly shaped cells called *neurons,* which can detect and transmit electrical signals by converting stimuli into nerve impulses. Located in the

TABLE 11-4 **Muscle Histological Table**

	HISTOLOGICAL CHARACTERISTICS		
	SMOOTH	CARDIAC	SKELETAL
Synonyms	Visceral	Heart	Voluntary
Striations	No	Yes	Yes
Number of nuclei	Mononucleate	Mononucleate (can be multinucleate)	Multinucleate
Location of nuclei	Centrally located	Centrally located	Peripherally located
Shape of nuclei	Oval shaped	Oval shaped	Small, elongated
Shape of fibers	Spindle shaped	Y- or H-shaped	Cylindrical
Voluntary or involuntary	Involuntary	Involuntary	Voluntary
Distinguishing characteristics	Shape of fibers	Intercalated disks	Striations
Fatigue rate: rapid, slow, or none	Slow	None	Rapid
Discussion	Forms the walls of hollow organs and tubes (e.g., stomach, bladder, blood vessel); controls the transport of materials, moving them along or restricting their flow	Located in the myocardium; possesses intercalated disks, which operate like an electrical synapse	Attaches to bones or related structures; is the *flesh* of the body; must be stimulated by a nerve impulse to contract

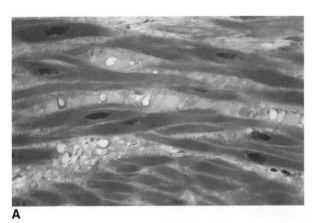

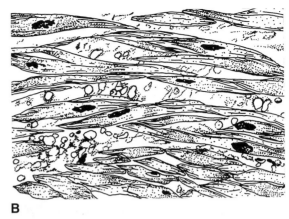

FIGURE 11-11 Smooth muscle. **A**, Pictomicrograph. **B**, Line drawing of the pictomicrograph.

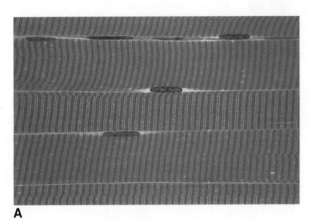

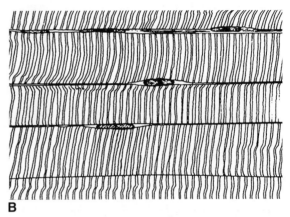

FIGURE 11-12 Skeletal muscle. **A**, Pictomicrograph. **B**, Line drawing of the pictomicrograph.

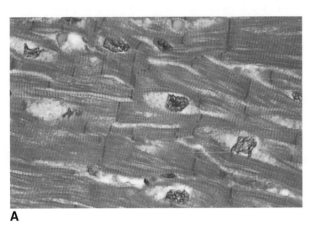

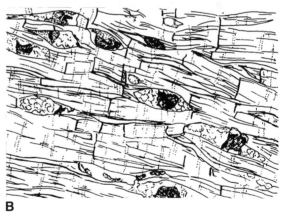

FIGURE 11-13 Cardiac muscle. **A**, Pictomicrograph. **B**, Line drawing of the pictomicrograph.

brain, spinal cord, and peripheral nerves, nervous tissue possesses characteristics of excitability and conductibility. Neurons detect changes both inside and outside the body, interpret the perceived information to provide a response (e.g., muscular contractions or glandular secretions), and are involved in higher mental functioning and emotional responsiveness.

The three principal parts of a neuron are (1) the cell body, which contains the nucleus and other standard cell machinery; (2) the dendrites, which transmit impulses to the cell body; and (3) the axon, which transmits impulses away from the cell body (Figure 11-14).

> *"When health is absent . . .*
> *Wisdom cannot reveal itself*
> *Art cannot become manifest*
> *Strength cannot be exerted*
> *Wealth is useless and*
> *Reason is powerless . . . "*
> Herophilies, 300 BC

DEANE JUHAN, MA

Born: April 18, 1945.

"The principle is elegantly simple. We learn to love by being loved, we learn gentleness by being gentle, we learn to be graceful by experiencing the feeling of grace."

Deane Juhan is a bodyworker, one of the first Trager-trained instructors, an anatomy teacher and lecturer for the Trager Institute, and author of *Job's Body: A Handbook for Bodyworkers.* As the title suggests, the book offers an answer to the age-old question of *why* regarding the Old Testament book of Job . . . but that is just for starters. The book explores "the various ways through which intuitive and informed touch can positively affect a wide variety of symptoms and help to change people's lives for the better." The book was 9 years in the making, which is surprising, considering the manner in which Juhan's words easily flow during casual conversation.

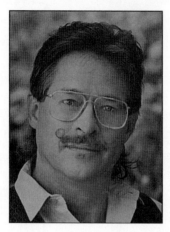

(Copyright © Karen Zurlinden Photography.)

Born to a woman who had *poor taste in men* and a soldier who did not hang around to become a father, Juhan was later adopted, growing up as an only child in Glenwood Springs, Colorado. His father worked for the state and never drew a large salary, but his parents were wise about using resources and were determined that their only child's education would receive top priority in their lives.

Juhan describes himself as an underachiever in high school. The University of Colorado introduced him to a whole new way of living, and he admits to being caught up in the novelty of its hip, liberal atmosphere until his junior year, when "his rudder finally bit the water," he says. At this point in his life, he became interested in the aspects of art, science, and civilization.

Juhan learned about Esalen, a workshop and meeting place for developing human potential in Big Sur, California, while working on his dissertation in literature. He actually managed to sneak in and start doing massage. He was so good at it. Juhan's first experience in anatomy was developing slides and lectures for *Structural Integration for Rolfing* lectures, but when he witnessed Milton Trager, he was hooked and abandoned all other methods to learn the Trager Approach.

"It was love at first sight," says Juhan. "I was attracted to his quality of being. It was his rich avuncular benevolence without all the preliminary folderol that made me want to learn to do what he did, so I threw myself into it and gave it my all."

Learning the approach did not come easy though for this hard-pushing 6-footer. His strength had always been,

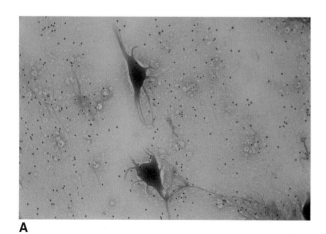

A

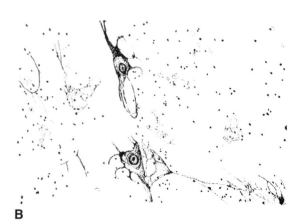

B

FIGURE 11-14 Nervous tissue. **A**, Pictomicrograph. **B**, Line drawing of the pictomicrograph.

DEANE JUHAN, MA (*continued*)

well, his strength. Nonetheless, Juhan broke down and cried when he saw his first Trager demonstration. Then, as he clumsily applied himself to unlearning everything he ever thought he knew about bodywork, Trager reduced his ego to ashes, hollering at him during training, slapping his hand away and taking over, always admonishing him to work lighter and softer and to quit trying so hard to get the job done.

Juhan points out that Trager's use of inducing a transcendental meditation state during a session, which has been called *hook-up,* is one of the things that sets Trager apart and makes the work so effective. During this hook-up, messages are communicated that have nothing to do with verbal and nonverbal interaction as we know it, and this exchange is the key to long-term change.

For the bodywork session, the goal is to connect with the client's sensory information, process what the practitioner helps the client discover or rediscover, then help the client *wake up* to the possibility for long-term change through movement. The practitioner lays down new patterns by repeating a movement message again and again. The feeling finally becomes etched on the client's awareness, creating an experience of length, relaxation, and pain-free movement.

Before this task can be achieved, however, the bodyworker needs to understand how the body works and what this *preverbal* language is all about. Juhan also argues for bodywork to "redress some of the underdevelopment and dysfunction we find associated with various pathological conditions." Most important, he wants to change the way we think about our bodies.

In short, Juhan asserts, we have stopped "listening to the only reliable source of self-regulation and preservation we have available. It is the direct result of century-long programming that has debased our subjective awareness." When we are in pain or simply feeling bad, instead of confronting what is at the root of our problem, we seek help outside the wisdom of our own bodies. We run to the physician, shrink, psychic, minister, and self-help section of the nearest bookstore. Nothing is wrong with any of these resources, of course, but Juhan reminds us that the only thing we truly know about the world is the way the body responds to it, and no one can know how our bodies are responding to stimuli the way we each individually can. In short, we are, to a very great degree, responsible for our own well-being.

Juhan writes in *Job's Body: A Handbook for Bodyworkers:* "For Job this was revelation—the perception that God was in his very flesh, in the throbbing of his heart, in the singing of his nerves, in the coiling of his muscles, to be touched and felt more intimately than an embrace."

As a beginning massage therapist, you are probably not seeking a revelation so much as you are a direction. You can probably guess that Juhan's advice is to look within. Choose the modality that will, according to Juhan, "flower in your psyche or experience. Look for what turns you on, look for what you love, not what the market says is hot."

BODY MEMBRANES

Membranes are thin, soft, pliable sheets of tissue that cover the body, line tubes or body cavities, cover organs, and separate one part of a cavity from another. Two important major types of membranes exist: epithelial and connective. *Epithelial membranes* are composed of epithelium and an underlying layer of connective tissue. Three types of epithelial membranes are (1) cutaneous, (2) mucous, and (3) serous. *Connective tissue membranes* are composed exclusively of various types of connective tissue. One type of connective tissue membrane exists in the body: synovial (Figure 11-15). Another type of membrane, meninges, surrounds the brain and spinal cord. However, since it does not secrete its related fluid, it is not included for discussion.

Cutaneous Membranes

Both tough and supple, **cutaneous membranes** cover the entire surface of the body. The skin is the largest organ of the body by weight and is composed of five layers of cells. The skin helps cool the body when the temperature rises by radiating the heat of increased blood flow in expanded blood vessels and by providing a surface for the evaporation of sweat. When the temperature drops, the blood vessels constrict and the production of sweat diminishes.

Mucous Membranes

Membranes that line openings to the outside of the body are called **mucous membranes** (mucosae). Essentially, skin continues into various parts of the body such as in the lining

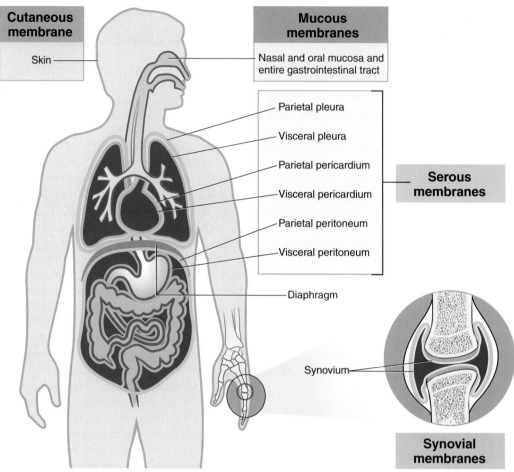

FIGURE 11-15 Types and locations of membranes.

of the vagina, the bladder, the lungs, the intestines, the nose, and the mouth. This type of membrane secretes the mucus that lubricates and protects associated structures. The mucosa of the digestive tract also aids in the processes of digestion and absorption.

Serous Membranes

Serous membranes line closed body cavities that do not open to the outside of the body. These membranes consist of two layers, (1) a *parietal layer,* which lines the wall of body cavities, often adhering to it, and (2) a *visceral layer,* which provides a peripheral covering to organs in closed body cavities. Examples of serous membranes are the pericardium, the pleura, peritoneum, and mesenteries. Serous membranes secrete a thin, serous fluid between the parietal and visceral layers. This fluid lubricates organs and reduces friction between the organs.

Synovial Membranes

Lining the joint cavities of freely moving joints (e.g., shoulder, hip, knee) are the **synovial membranes** or synovium. These membranes secrete synovial fluid, a viscous liquid that provides nutrition and lubrication to the joint so it can

move freely without undue friction. This fluid can also be contained in bursa sacs, located around the joint cavity, between tendons and bones, where friction is present, and in synovial sheaths surrounding a tendon of a muscle.

BODY SYSTEM OVERVIEW

Ten body systems make up the organism discussed in this section; all are interrelated and interdependent (Table 11-5).

"Think with the whole body."
Taisen Deshimaru

BODY COMPASS

Every good travel map has a compass drawing to indicate north, south, east, and west. The map also has some distance reference such as a scale of miles per a specific measure. Any map without these items is of little or no use. Imagine trying to read a map if you cannot understand the definitions of the words *south, 5 miles, 1 block,* or *by the lake.* Think of the anatomical drawings as your map, and consider this section of the book your body compass. You will learn new terms that constitute directions to help you find your way

TABLE 11-5   **Body Systems, Related Anatomy, and Physiology**

BODY SYSTEM	ANATOMY	PHYSIOLOGY
Circulatory system	Heart Blood and blood vessels Lymph Lymph vessels and glands	Transports and distributes gases, nutrients, antibodies, waste materials, and hormones; protects the body from disease; prevents hemorrhage by clotting mechanisms
Skeletal system	Bones Cartilage Ligaments Joints	Supports the body through a bony framework; protects the body's vital organs; gives leverage through muscle attachment; houses the mechanism of blood cell formation; stores fats and minerals
Integumentary system	Skin Hair Nails Oil glands Sweat glands	Protects the organism; absorbs substances such as fats, fat-soluble vitamins, oxygen, carbon dioxide, steroids, resins of certain plants, organic solvents, and salts of heavy metals; receives stimuli; regulates body temperature; eliminates wastes; converts ultraviolet rays to vitamin D
Respiratory system	Nose and nasal cavity Pharynx Larynx Trachea Bronchi and bronchioles Alveoli Lungs Diaphragm	Exchanges gases; detects smell; produces speech; regulates body pH
Reproductive system	Gonads (ovaries in females and testes in males) Ducts (Fallopian tubes in women and spermatic duct in men) Gametes (ova in women and spermatozoa in men) Uterus and vagina in women Penis, prostate, and urethra in men	Produces offspring and propagates the species
Muscular system	Skeletal muscles and related fascia Tendons	Creates movement; produces heat; maintains posture
Endocrine system	Pituitary Pineal Thyroid Parathyroids Thymus Adrenals Pancreas Gonads Hormones	Produces and secretes hormones; regulates body activities; maintains the body during times of stress; contributes to the reproductive process
Nervous system	Brain Spinal cord Meninges Cerebrospinal fluid Cranial nerves Spinal nerves	Receives sensory input; interprets and integrates all stimuli; initiates motor output; houses mental processes and emotional responses
Urinary system	Special sense organs Kidneys Ureters and urethra Urinary bladder and urine	Eliminates metabolical wastes; regulates blood pH and its chemical composition; regulates blood volume and fluid balance; monitors and helps maintain blood pressure; maintains homeostasis
Digestive system	Teeth Tongue Alimentary canal (tube from mouth to anus) Accessory glands (liver, gallbladder, pancreas, salivary)	Facilitates ingestion, digestion, absorption, and defecation

around the body. These terms include names for planes of the body, locations that are relative to the body planes, regional and directional terms for different aspects of the body, and the body cavities.

Anatomical Position

In Western medicine, to avoid confusion, all parts of the body are described in relation to other body parts using a standard body position called the **anatomical position** (Figure 11-16). In this position, the body is erect and facing forward, the arms are at the sides, the palms are facing forward with the thumbs to the side, and feet are about hip distance apart with toes pointing forward.

Planes of Reference

We live in a three-dimensional structure; our height, depth, and width help describe volume in space. Thinking of ourselves as flat is easy; mirrors and photographs give us the illusion that we are two dimensional, but we have sculpted fullness, curves, and angles. Because the body is three dimensional, we can refer to three planes or sections that lie at right angles to one another.

The **midsagittal** or **median plane** runs longitudinally (vertically) down the body, anterior to posterior, dividing the body into right and left sections. When a plane passes through the body parallel to the median plane, we have the **sagittal plane**. The **frontal** or **coronal plane** passes through the body side-to-side to create anterior and posterior sections. The **transverse** or **horizontal plane** passes through the body and creates superior and inferior sections (Figure 11-17).

Body Cavities

The body contains organs and other structures in closed spaces called *cavities;* the two main cavities are the dorsal and the ventral (Figure 11-18). The **dorsal cavity,** located on the back or posterior aspect of the body, is further divided into the cranial cavity (containing the brain) and the spinal or vertebral cavity (containing the spinal cord). The larger **ventral cavity,** located anteriorly to the dorsal cavity, is further divided by the diaphragm into the thoracic cavity and abdominopelvic cavity. The thoracic cavity contains the right and left pleural cavities (lungs) and the mediastinum (containing the pericardium, heart, great vessels such as aorta and vena cava, esophagus, and trachea).

The abdominopelvic cavity is further divided into the abdominal cavity and the pelvic cavity. The abdominal cavity contains the digestive system and its accessory organs. The pelvic cavity contains the organs of the reproductive and urinary systems and the rectum of the digestive system.

Abdominopelvic Quadrants

Anatomists divide the abdominopelvic region into four quadrants to help describe organ, pathological condition, or pain location. An imaginary line is drawn both horizontally and vertically through the umbilicus. This line divides the region into a *right* and *left upper quadrant* and a *right* and *left lower quadrant* (Figure 11-19). The right upper quadrant contains structures such as the duodenum, the hepatic flexure of the colon, the liver, and the right kidney and right adrenal gland. The left upper quadrant contains structures such as the left kidney and left adrenal gland, the majority of the pancreas, the spleen, the splenic flexure of the colon, and the stomach. The right lower quadrant contains the appendix, the cecum, the right ovary and fallopian tube (women), the majority of the right spermatic duct (men), and the right ureter. The left lower quadrant contains the sigmoid colon, cecum, the left ovary and fallopian tube (women), the majority of the left spermatic duct (men), and the left ureter. The midline contains the urinary bladder and the urethra. Review structures of each quadrant once they have been learned in subsequent chapters.

Directional References

This section defines the following terms used as directional references (Figure 11-20).

Anterior or **ventral**: pertaining to the front side of a structure. *The navel is anterior to the vertebral column.*

Posterior or **dorsal**: pertaining to the back of a structure. *The vertebral column is posterior to the lungs.*

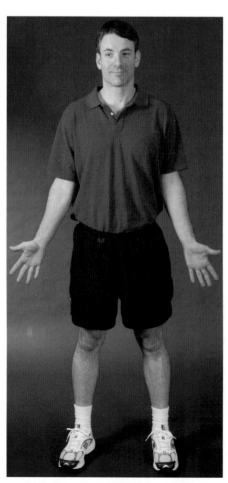

FIGURE 11-16 Anatomical position.

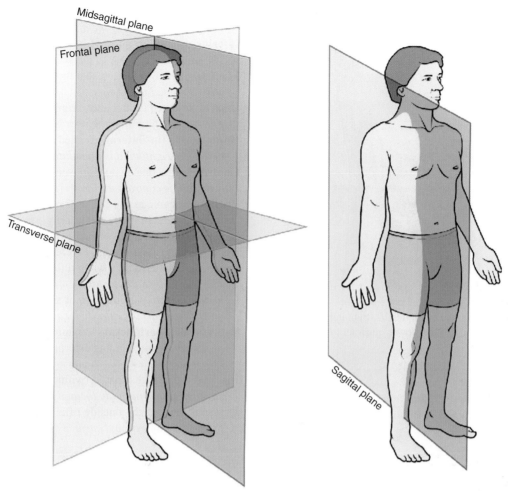

FIGURE 11-17 Planes of the body.

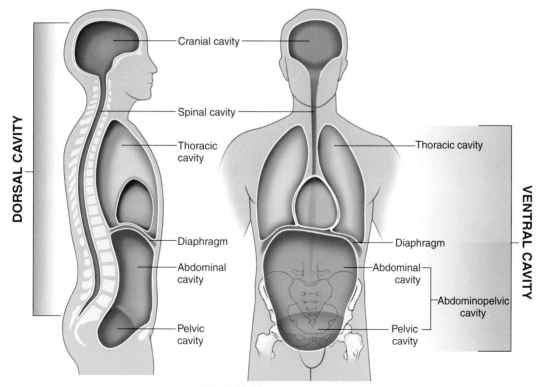

FIGURE 11-18 Major body cavities.

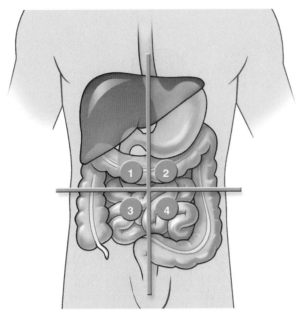

FIGURE 11-19 Abdominal quadrants; *1*, Right upper quadrant. *2*, Left upper quadrant. *3*, Right lower quadrant. *4*, Left lower quadrant.

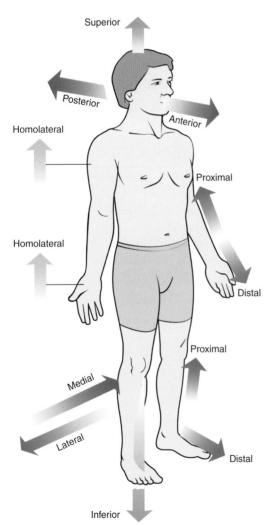

FIGURE 11-20 Directional terminology.

Superior or **cranial**: situated above or toward the head end. *The jaw is superior to the navel.*

Inferior or **caudal**: situated below or toward the tail end. *The sacrum is inferior to the skull.*

Medial: oriented toward or near the midline of the body. *The nose is medial to the ears.*

Lateral: oriented farther away from the midline of the body. *The ribs are lateral to the vertebral column.*

Homolateral (ipsilateral): related to the same side of the body. *The right hand is homolateral to the right elbow.*

Contralateral: related to opposite sides of the body. *The right foot is contralateral to the left foot.*

Proximal: nearer to the point of reference, usually toward the trunk of the body (used only when referencing the extremities). *The hip is proximal to the knee.*

Distal: farther from the point of reference, usually away from the midline (used only when referencing the extremities). *The foot is distal to the hip.*

Central or **deep**: pertaining to or situated at a center of the body. *The heart is centrally located.*

Superficial or **peripheral**: pertaining to the outside surface, periphery, or surrounding external area of a structure. *The skin is superficial to the bones.*

Internal: nearest the inside (within) of a body cavity. *The stomach is an internally located organ.*

External: nearest the outside of a body cavity. *The skin is located on the external surface of the body.*

Regional Terms

This section identifies regions associated with body areas such as the head and neck, upper and lower extremities, and anterior and posterior torso (Figure 11-21).

Head and Neck
   Buccal: cheek area
   Cervical: neck area
   Cephalic: head end
   Cranial (skull): head end
   Facial: face area
   Frontal: forehead
   Mandibular: lower jaw
   Mental: chin area
   Nasal: nose region
   Nuchal: posterior neck
   Occipital: posterior and inferior surfaces of the head
   Oral: mouth region
   Orbital (ophthalmic): eye area
   Otic (auricular): ear area

Upper Extremity
   Acromial: top of shoulder
   Antebrachial: forearm; between wrist and elbow
   Antecubital: space in front of elbow or at the bend of the elbow
   Axillary: armpit region
   Brachial: upper arm; between the shoulder and the elbow

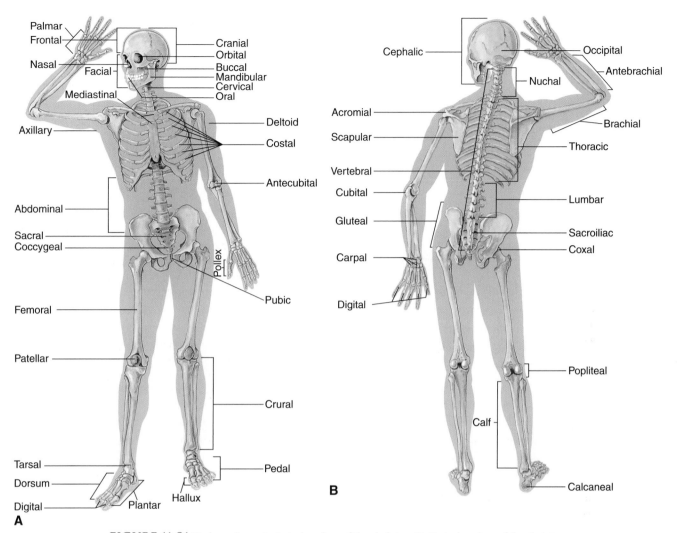

FIGURE 11-21 Body regions. **A**, Anterior view of the skeleton. **B**, Posterior view of the skeleton.

Carpal: wrist area

Cubital: elbow

Deltoid: curve of the shoulder and upper arm formed by the deltoid muscle

Digital (phalangeal): fingers and/or toes

Palmar (volar): anterior surface of the hand

Pollex: thumb

Anterior Torso

Abdominal (celiac): anterior trunk; between the thorax and the pelvis

Costal: ribs

Groin (inguinal): area where the thigh meets the abdomen

Mediastinal: portion of the thoracic cavity occupying the area between the lungs

Pectoral (mammary): upper anterior thorax

Pelvic: inferior region of the abdominopelvic cavity

Perineal: region between the pubis and coccyx; inferior pelvic cavity

Pubic: region of the pubic symphysis or the genital area

Thoracic: between the neck and the respiratory diaphragm

Umbilical: mid-abdomen or navel (scar left from the umbilical cord)

Posterior Torso

Coccygeal: bottom of the spine; upper region of the gluteal cleft

Gluteal (buttock): curve of the buttocks formed by the gluteal muscles

Lumbar: low back; between the ribs and the hips

Sacral: sacrum of the spinal column

Sacroiliac: between the sacrum and the pelvic bone

Scapular: the shoulder blade area

Vertebral: vertebrae of the spinal column

TABLE TALK

In anatomy, the upper leg is called the *thigh* and the lower leg is called the *leg*.

Lower Extremity

Calcaneal: heel

Calf (sural): posterior leg

Coxal: hip region

Crural: leg

Digital (phalangeal): fingers and/or toes

Dorsum: top of foot

Femoral: femur or the thigh area; between the hip and the knee

Hallux: great toe

Patellar: kneecap

Pedal: foot or feet

Plantar (volar): bottom surface or sole of the foot

Popliteal: posterior aspect of the knee

Tarsal: ankle

> **evolve** *Log on to the Evolve website and choose the "drag and drop" activity under course materials for Chapter 11.* ■

SUMMARY

An introduction to the human body includes a study of the basic structural building blocks of the body, their functions, and the directional references based on the Western medical model.

The first of these building blocks is the cell, the simplest form of life that can exist as an independent self-sustaining unit. Each cell is made up of a combination of a cell membrane, cytoplasm, and organelles. Cells function through the exchange of fluids, nutrients, chemicals, and ions, which is carried out by passive and active cell processes. Examples of passive processes are simple and facilitated diffusion, osmosis, and filtration. Active processes include active transport and endocytosis.

Cells organize to form tissues. The four divisions of body tissues are epithelial, connective, muscle, and nervous. Some tissues present themselves as membranes that protect organs or separate body cavities. The three types of bodily membranes are mucous, serous, and synovial.

Tissues organize to form organs, which are classified according to organ systems. The 10 organ systems of the body are the circulatory, skeletal, integumentary, respiratory, reproductive, muscular, endocrine, nervous, urinary, and digestive.

To negotiate these body systems, learning the language of the body itself is necessary. Our map consists of anatomical directions and planes of references, body cavities, and regional body landmarks.

evolve

Go to *Chapter Extras* on Evolve for additional illustrations and resources for this chapter. *Extras* for this chapter include:

1. Diagram of body systems (illustration)
2. Body system activity (worksheet)
3. Prefix and suffix game (online game)
4. Crossword puzzle (downloadable form)
5. Muscle tissue activity (worksheet)

MATCHING I

Place the letter of the answer next to the term or phrase that best describes it.

A. Anatomy	E. Filtration	I. Nucleus
B. Cell	F. Homeostasis	J. Phagocytosis
C. Cytoplasm	G. Lysosome	K. Physiology
D. Diffusion	H. Mitochondria	L. Semipermeable

_____   1.   Study of human body structures and their positional relationships

_____   2.   Study of how the body functions in normal body processes

_____   3.   Constancy of the body's internal environment

_____   4.   Fundamental unit of all living organisms

_____   5.   Property of the cell membrane in which some materials can freely pass and others cannot

_____   6.   Gel-like fluid within the cell membrane

_____   7.   Cell's control center, directing nearly all metabolic activities

_____   8.   Cell's power plant and site for cellular respiration

_____   9.   Membrane-bound organelle containing digestive enzymes

_____   10.   Movement of molecules from an area of high to low concentration

_____   11.   Movement of particles across cellular membranes caused by pressure

_____   12.   Process of ingesting, breaking down, and expelling harmful microorganisms and cellular debris

MATCHING II

Place the letter of the answer next to the term or phrase that best describes it.

A. Adipose
B. Connective
C. Cutaneous
D. Epithelium

E. Fibrocartilage
F. Hyaline
G. Mucous
H. Muscular

I. Nervous
J. Serous
K. Synovial
L. Thixotropism

_____ 1. Tissue type that lines or covers internal and external organs; blood vessels; body cavities; and digestive, respiratory, urinary, and reproductive tracts

_____ 2. Tissue type that serves in nutrient transport, defense, blood clotting, or organ protection

_____ 3. Cartilage that covers articulating end of bones, connects ribs to the sternum, and supports the nose, the trachea, and part of the larynx

_____ 4. Cartilage found between the vertebrae, in the knee joint, and between the pubic bones

_____ 5. Specialized for fat storage

_____ 6. Ability of fascia to change from one state to the other

_____ 7. Tissue type that produces movement

_____ 8. Tissue type that detects and transmits electrical signals by converting stimuli into impulses

_____ 9. Tough, supple membrane that covers the surface of the body

_____ 10. Lines open body cavities

_____ 11. Lines closed body cavities

_____ 12. Lines cavities of freely moving joints

MATCHING III

Place the letter of the answer next to the term or phrase that best describes it.

A. Anterior   E. Inferior   I. Peripheral
B. Contralateral   F. Lateral   J. Proximal
C. Distal   G. Medial   K. Superficial
D. Homolateral   H. Posterior   L. Superior

_____   1.   Synonymous with superficial

_____   2.   Pertaining to the front

_____   3.   Pertaining to the back

_____   4.   Situated above or toward the head

_____   5.   Situated below or toward the tail

_____   6.   Oriented toward the midline

_____   7.   Oriented farther from the midline

_____   8.   Related to the same side of the body

_____   9.   Related to opposite sides of the body

_____   10. Nearer to the point of reference, usually toward the trunk

_____   11. Farther from the point of reference

_____   12. Pertaining to the outside surface or periphery

MATCHING IV

Place the letter of the answer next to the term or phrase that best describes it.

A. Antebrachial   E. Buccal   I. Nuchal
B. Antecubital   F. Cervical   J. Orbital
C. Axillary   G. Cubital   K. Otic
D. Brachial   H. Mental   L. Pollex

_____ 1. Cheek

_____ 2. Neck area

_____ 3. Chin

_____ 4. Posterior neck

_____ 5. Eye

_____ 6. Ear

_____ 7. Forearm

_____ 8. Front of elbow

_____ 9. Armpit

_____ 10. Upper arm

_____ 11. Elbow

_____ 12. Thumb

MATCHING V

Place the letter of the answer next to the term or phrase that best describes it.

A. Calcaneal   E. Dorsum   I. Plantar
B. Costal   F. Hallux   J. Popliteal
C. Coxal   G. Lumbar   K. Sacroiliac
D. Crural   H. Mediastinal   L. Sural

_____   1.   Ribs

_____   2.   Portion of the thoracic cavity occupying the area between the lungs

_____   3.   Between the ribs and the hips

_____   4.   Between the sacrum and the pelvic bone

_____   5.   Heel

_____   6.   Calf area

_____   7.   Hip region

_____   8.   Leg

_____   9.   Top of foot

_____   10.   Great toe

_____   11.   Bottom surface or sole of foot

_____   12.   Posterior aspect of the knee

INTERNET ACTIVITIES

Go to http://www.madsci.org/~lynn/VH/planes.html and click on Transverse Animations. Identify as many structures as you can as the animation takes you through the transverse cross sections of the body.

Go to http://library.thinkquest.org/C004535/introduction.html and click on Cell Anatomy. Print out a picture of one of the cellular organelles found in the cytoplasm and be prepared to explain the purpose of the organelle.

Visit http://science.nhmccd.edu/biol/ap1int.htm#bonejoint and scroll down to Skin, Skeleton and Joints. Click on "Regional Body Terminology" to test your knowledge of body regions.

Bibliography

Abrahams P, Marks S, Hutchings R: *McMinn's color atlas of human anatomy,* St Louis, 2003, Mosby.

Applegate EJ: *The anatomy and physiology learning system,* ed 3, Philadelphia, 2006, Saunders.

Beers, MH, Berkow R: *The Merck manual of diagnosis and therapy,* Whitehouse Station, NJ, 2006, Merck Research Laboratories.

Como D, editor: *Mosby's medical, nursing, and allied health dictionary,* ed 6, St Louis, 2002, Mosby.

Crawley J, Van De Graaff KM: *A photographic atlas for anatomy and physiology,* Englewood, Colo, 2002, Morton.

Ferri FF: *2003 Ferri's clinical advisor, instant diagnosis and treatment,* St Louis, 2003, Mosby.

Gould BE: *Pathophysiology for the health-related professionals,* ed 3, Philadelphia, 2006, Saunders.

Goldberg S: *Clinical anatomy made ridiculously simple,* Miami, 2004, Medmaster.

Grafelman T: *Graf's anatomy and physiology guide for the massage therapist,* Aurora, Colo, 1998, DG Publishing.

Guyton A: *Human physiology and mechanisms of disease,* ed 6, Philadelphia, 1996, Saunders.

Gray HT, Pickering P, Howden R: *Gray's anatomy,* ed 29, Philadelphia, 1974, Running Press.

Haubrich WS: *Medical meanings: a glossary of word origins,* New York, 1984, Harcourt Brace Jovanovich.

Jacob S, Francone C: *Elements of anatomy and physiology,* Philadelphia, 1989, Saunders.

Juhan D: *Job's body: a handbook for bodyworkers,* ed 3, Barrington, NY, 2003, Station Hill Press.

Kalat JW: *Biological psychology,* ed 8, Belmont, Calif, 2003, Wadsworth.

Kapit W, Elson LM: *The anatomy coloring book,* ed 3, New York, 2002, Benjamin Cummings.

Kapit W, Macey R, Meisami E: *The physiology coloring book,* ed 2, New York, 1999, HarperCollins.

Lauderstein D: *Putting the soul back in the body: a manual of imaginative anatomy for massage therapists,* Chicago, 1985, self-published manual.

Marieb EN: *Essentials of human anatomy and physiology,* ed 8, New York, 2005, Benjamin Cummings.

Martini FH, Bartholomew EF: *Essentials of anatomy and physiology,* ed 3, New York, 2003, Benjamin/Cummings.

Merck manual, ed 17, Whitehouse Station, NJ, 1998, Merck and Company.

Moore KL: *Clinically oriented anatomy,* ed 5, Baltimore, 2005, Lippincott Williams & Wilkins.

Myers TW: *Anatomy trains: myofascial meridians for manual and movement therapists,* New York, 2001, Churchill Livingstone.

Netter FH: *Atlas of human anatomy,* ed 3, Teterboro, NJ, 2003, Icon Learning Systems.

Premkumar K: *The massage connection: anatomy and physiology,* ed 2, Philadelphia, 2004, Lippincott Williams & Wilkins.

Salvo SG, Anderson SK: *Mosby's pathology for massage therapists,* St Louis, 2004, Elsevier Mosby.

Thibodeau G, Patton K: *Anatomy and physiology,* ed 6, St Louis, 2006, Mosby.

Thibodeau G, Patton K: *Structure and function of the body,* ed 12, St Louis, 2004, Mosby.

Tortora GJ: *Introduction to the human body: the essentials of anatomy and physiology,* ed 5, Hoboken, NJ, 2000, Wiley, John & Sons.

Tortora GJ, Grabowksi SR: *Principles of anatomy and physiology,* ed 11 New York, 2005, John Wiley & Sons.

Venes D, Thomas CL, Taber CW: *Taber's cyclopedic medical dictionary,* ed 20, Philadelphia, 2005, FA Davis.

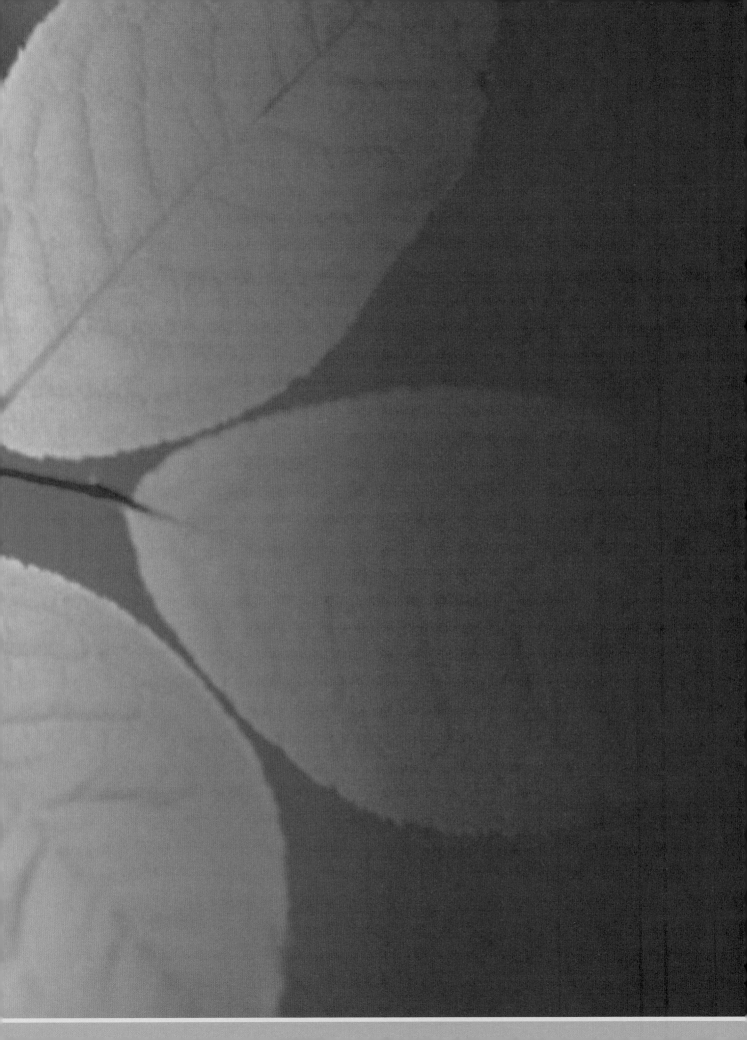

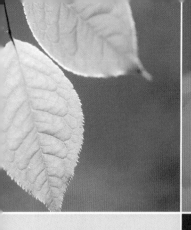

CHAPTER **12**

Integumentary System

*"The skin is no more
separate from the brain
than the surface of a lake
is separate from its depths.
They are two different
locations in a continuous
medium. To touch the
surface is to stir the depths."*
—Deane Juhan

STUDENT OBJECTIVES

After completing this chapter, the student should be able to:

- List the anatomical structures of the skin
- Describe the skin's physiological properties
- Define the regions of the skin, and give characteristics of each
- Name the epidermal cell types
- State the epidermal layers
- Explain epidermal growth
- Explain dermal growth and repair
- Outline the skin's glands, discussing each one
- Contrast and compare sudoriferous and sebaceous glands
- Differentiate between eccrine and apocrine sweat glands
- Name the main parts of a nail
- Define several factors that contribute to skin color
- Name types of pathological skin conditions, giving characteristics and massage considerations of each
- Contrast and compare common moles and melanomas

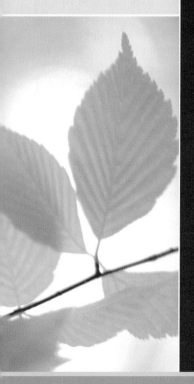

INTRODUCTION

Integument is another term used when referring to the skin. The integumentary system is the organ system that includes skin and its appendages, or derivatives, including hair, nails, and related glands. A relatively flat organ, the skin, by weight, is the largest organ of the body and houses the tactile system. Sensory receptors receive perceptual stimuli (e.g., heat, cold, movement, touch, pressure, pain). In fact, more than one half million sensory receptors from the skin are found entering the spinal cord.

The skin is classified as a membrane, a cutaneous membrane. Similar to a cell, this membrane defines our parameters. Housed within its layers are various tissues that carry out special functions such as waste elimination and temperature regulation. The skin forms natural openings such as the mouth, external ear canal, nose, urethra, vagina, and anus. These passageways to the digestive, respiratory, urinary, and reproductive systems can be classified as extensions of the external environment. No other body system is more easily exposed to infections, disease, pollution, or injury than the skin, yet no other body system is as strong and resilient.

The appearance of the skin reflects our physiology. At a glance, something about a person's nutrition, hygiene habits, circulation, age, immunity, parents (genetics), and environmental factors can be noted by the condition of the skin. Healthy skin is soft, flexible, moist, acidic, and blemish free. People spend millions each year on products from companies that promise to give users a more youthful appearance. Millions are also spent on surgical and nonsurgical procedures to darken the skin, remove wrinkles, lighten freckles, minimize scars, smooth out cellulite, remove unwanted hair, restore lost hair, and treat acne.

Not only does it reveal vital physiological data (e.g., circulation, fever), the skin also mirrors our emotional self. Through muscular expression and neurological impulses, the skin has the power to reflect an ever-changing stream of emotions. How people feel about themselves and others is reflected on the surface of the skin.

TABLE TALK

The skin covers an area of approximately 22 square feet (ft²) and weighs approximately 9 pounds (lb), making up 7% of body weight. A piece of skin the size of a quarter contains more than 3 million cells, 100 sweat glands, 50 nerve endings, and 3 ft of blood vessels. The skin is thinnest over the eyelids and thickest on the soles of the feet. The fingertips have approximately 700 touch receptors on 2 square millimeters (mm²) of surface area.

ANATOMY

Areas of discussion in this chapter include:
- Hair
- Nails
- Oil glands
- Skin
- Sweat glands

PHYSIOLOGY

- **Protection.** One of the primary functions of the skin is protecting the organism by acting as a physical, biological, and chemical barrier. The skin's physical barrier is essential for protecting underlying tissues from abrasion. The skin also provides limited protection from ultraviolet (UV) radiation through pigmentation. As a biological barrier, intact skin is an effective barrier against many pathogens (e.g., bacteria, viruses). Secretions provided by the skin's glands inhibit growth of these pathogens by providing an acid mantle, providing a chemical barrier.
- **Absorption.** The skin has limited properties of absorption. Substances that can be absorbed by the skin are fat-soluble substances (oxygen, carbon dioxide), fat-soluble vitamins (A, D, E, and K), steroids, resins of certain plants (poison ivy and poison oak), organic solvents (paint thinner, which can cause brain and kidney damage), and salts of heavy metals (lead, mercury, and nickel). The use of medicated transdermal patches is based on the absorption properties of the skin.
- **Sensation.** The skin is considered an extension of the nervous system. It receives stimuli such as pressure, pain, and temperature from the external environment and brings this information to the central nervous system. The most fundamental of all the senses is touch.
- **Body temperature regulation.** An increase in blood circulation to the skin's surface creates a property of temperature regulation. As the blood moves to the skin's surface and blood vessels dilate, heat is discharged into the atmosphere (Figure 12-1). In this way, our bodies radiate to release internal heat. Heat can also be dissipated through the evaporation of perspiration produced by specialized glands called *sudoriferous glands*. A limited amount of heat conservation is provided by the skin through shivering.
- **Waste elimination.** The skin functions as a mini-excretory system, eliminating wastes through perspiration. Sweat, a waste product, is a mixture of 98% water and 2% solids (e.g., salt ions, lactic acid, and other metabolical wastes). By contrast, urine is 96% water and 4% solids.
- **Vitamin D synthesis.** Located in the skin are precursor molecules that are converted by the UV rays in sunlight to vitamin D (with the help of liver and kidney enzymes). Vitamin D is important because it stimulates the absorption of calcium and phosphorus from food. Little UV light is required for this synthesis to occur; thus prolonged sunbathing is actually unnecessary.
- **Immunity.** Specialized cells, called Langerhans cells, are found in the skin that play an important role in immunity by attaching to and destroying pathogens. Additionally, these cells function along with helper T cells to trigger useful immunological reactions.

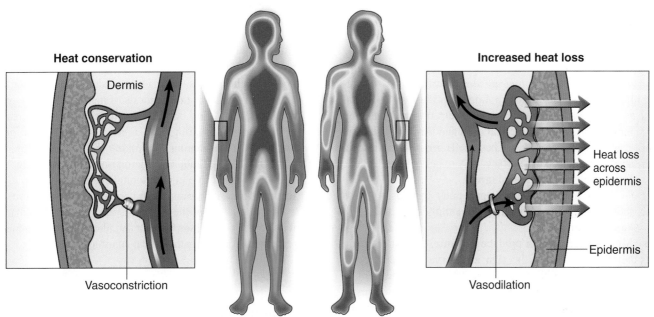

Heat conservation

Dermis

Vasoconstriction

Increased heat loss

Heat loss across epidermis

Epidermis

Vasodilation

FIGURE 12-1 Heat can be dissipated through the skin when superficial blood vessels dilate.

Terms and Their Meanings Related to the Skin

Term	Meaning
acne vulgaris	*Gr.* point; common or ordinary common acne
bruise	*O.Fr.* to break
corium	*L.* leather, skin
cutaneous	*L.* skin
cuticle	*L.* little skin
decubitus	*L.* lying down
dermis	*Gr.* skin
eczema	*L.* to boil out
epidermis	*Gr.* upon or over skin
follicle	*L.* sac, small
boil	*AS.* sore
granulosum	*L.* grain, small
integument	*L.* a covering
Krause	German anatomist (1833-1910)
lacrimal	*L.* tear
lucidum	*L.* clear
Meissner	German histologist (1829-1905)
melano	*Gr.* black
Pacini	Italian anatomist (1812-1883)
palpate	*L.* stroke or touch
psoriasis	*Gr.* itching
Ruffini	Italian anatomist (1864-1929)
scleroderma	*Gr.* hard, skin
seborrhea	*L.* tallow, to flow
sebum	*L.* grease, tallow
stratum	*L.* a layer, cover, or spread
sudoriferous	*L.* sweat, to carry or bear
wart	*L.* wart

Fr., French; *Gr.*, Greek; *L.*, Latin.

REGIONS OF THE SKIN

The skin is divided into two distinct regions: (1) epidermis and (2) dermis. The epidermis consists of four or five layers containing unique cells. The dermis is located under the epidermis and contains the blood vessels, many nerve receptors, hair follicles, and skin glands. A dermal-epidermal junction helps glue these two regions together. Underneath the skin is a layer of tissue known as the *subcutaneous layer.* The following sections examine these layers.

Epidermis

The **epidermis** is derived from ectoderm, the same embryonic cell layer that gives us the brain, spinal cord, and special senses. Contained in its layers are melanocytes, which contribute to the color of the skin, hair, and eye iris and absorption of UV light. The epidermis also contains pores; these openings allow passage for hair and specialized glands.

Composed solely of epithelial tissue, the epidermis is relatively avascular. Therefore all oxygen and nutrients must reach the epidermal cells by diffusion of tissue fluids from the underlying dermis. The cells of the epidermis are formed in the deepest epidermal layer, where they multiply and eventually push themselves up toward the surface, similar to a seedling or a budding tooth. As they move farther away from their source of nutrition, these cells become starved and eventually die. The superficial epidermal cells are constantly being sloughed off in an endless renewal process. The entire life cycle of skin cells from birth to death is 21 to 27 days.

Cell Types

The epidermis contains several types of epidermal cells. They are *keratinocytes, melanocytes,* and *Langerhans cells.*

- **Keratinocytes** are cells that are filled with an extremely tough, fibrous protein called *keratin,* which provides protection by waterproofing the skin's surface (it is insoluble in water). Its waterproofing properties serve a dual purpose: keeping water in and water out. They make up more than 90% of epidermal cells and form the principal structures of outer skin. These cells are dead and begin shedding at the skin's surface, only to be replaced by cells from the deeper epidermal layers.

  Where the skin enters open body cavities, such as the mouth and nose, the mucosa simply lacks the skin's keratinization.

- **Melanocytes,** which produce **melanin** or skin pigment, contribute color to the skin and serve to decrease the amount of UV light that can penetrate into the deeper layers of the skin. These cells are also found in hair and eye's iris. Both the melanocyte-producing hormone from the pituitary and genetics determine the amount of melanin produced in an individual.

  UV light stimulates the formation of this pigment and causes darkening of the melanin granules. Melanin serves as a protective shield for the skin from the damaging effects of sunlight and is activated by sunbathing (tanning). Freckles and moles are present when melanin is concentrated in one area.

  Albinism is a genetic condition in which the individual cannot produce melanin. An albino's hair and skin appear white or pale, and the iris of the eye appears pink or red because of the easy visibility of blood vessels.

Vitiligo is the partial or total loss of skin pigmentation, which occurs in patches. This may be as the result of a deep burn or scar that damages the melanocytes in a given area of the body. The skin in this area remains white and will not tan.

Certain hormones such as those secreted during pregnancy can stimulate the synthesis of melanin, which can produce a dark line between the navel and pubic area or give the childbearing woman *chloasma,* or a *mask of pregnancy,* by darkening the skin of the face and throat.

- **Langerhans cells,** another epidermal cell type, are thought to play a limited role in immunological reactions that affect the skin. They originate in bone marrow but migrate to the deep layers of the epidermis in early life. Together with helper T cells (see Chapter 19), they trigger immune reactions in certain pathological conditions.

---

evolve *Use your student account from the Evolve website to view images of various skin pigmentations such as a freckled face, an albino child, vitiligo, and chloasma.* ■

Epidermal Layers

Four epidermal layers, or *strata,* are typically found. However, in areas where friction is greatest (i.e., namely the soles of the feet and palms of the hands) an extra layer of skin is evident. From deepest to most superficial, these layers are the *stratum germinativum, stratum spinosum, stratum granulosum, stratum lucidum,* and *stratum corneum* (Figure 12-2).

- **Stratum germinativum:** This layer is the deepest layer of the epidermis. The stratum germinativum, or stratum

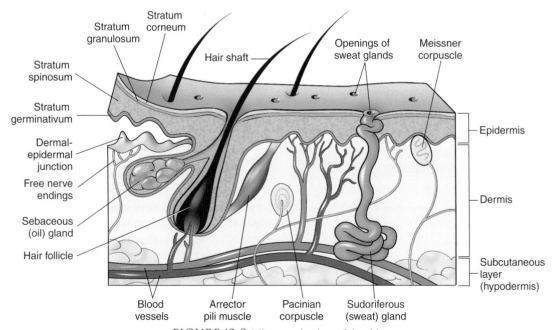

FIGURE 12-2 Microscopic view of the skin.

basale, undergoes continuous cell division and generates all other layers. This layer also contains Merkel disks, which are nerve endings responding to superficial pressure.

- **Stratum spinosum:** The stratum spinosum, or *prickly layer,* is a bonding and transitional layer between the stratum granulosum and the stratum germinativum, possessing cells of both these layers.
- **Stratum granulosum:** A layer of cells containing an accumulation of keratin granules distinguishes the stratum granulosum under a microscope. This layer is three to five cells deep, depending on the thickness of the skin. This layer also marks the beginning of change before the drying of the tissue.
- **Stratum lucidum:** In the thick skin of the hands and the feet, a translucent layer is found between the stratum corneum and the stratum granulosum. Similar to the stratum corneum, the stratum lucidum contains cells that are keratinized. In thin skin, the stratum lucidum is absent.
- **Stratum corneum:** This layer is the outermost layer of the skin. By the time these epithelial cells reach the surface, they are no longer living cells. These cells have become completely keratinized, ready to be sloughed off.

Epidermal Growth

As the surface cells of the stratum corneum are lost, replacement of keratinocytes by cell division is occurring in the stratum germinativum. New cells must be formed at approximately the same rate that old keratinized cells flake off to maintain a constant thickness of the epidermis. Cells push upward from the stratum germinativum into each consecutive layer, die, become keratinized, and eventually *desquamate* (fall away), as did their predecessors. Current research suggests that the surface of the epidermis is renewed approximately every 35 days.

Dermal-Epidermal Junction

Between the epidermis and the dermis is a specialized area where cells of the two regions meet. This basement membrane is called the dermal-epidermal junction and is easily identifiable with an electron microscope.

The dermal-epidermal junction not only cements the epidermis to the dermis but also provides support for the epidermis. Additionally, this junction serves as a partial barrier to the passage of some cells and large molecules.

Dermis

Also known as the corium, or *hide,* the **dermis** is the true skin. Leather products are the treated dermis of an animal. The dermis possesses a network of nerves and nerve endings that receive sensory information such as pain, pressure, touch, and temperature (Table 12-1). Application of massage techniques stimulates these sensory receptors. Located at various levels of the dermis are muscles, hair follicles, sweat and oil glands, and numerous blood vessels that help supply the epidermis with nutrients. This rich vascular network plays a critical role in regulating body temperature. The dermis is generally thicker on the posterior aspect than it is on the anterior aspect of the body and is thicker in men than it is in women; this difference may be the result of presence of certain hormones. More specifically, dermis is thickest on the palms of the hands and soles of the feet and quite thin over the eyelids.

Collagen, the main component of connective tissue, is an insoluble, fibrous protein that constitutes approximately 70% of the dermis and offers supports to the nerves, blood vessels, hair follicles, and glands. Within the collagen fibers are pliable fibers called *elastin,* which gives the skin its elasticity and resilience. As we age, fat is lost under the skin, which results in sags and wrinkles.

The loss of elasticity can be accelerated by excessive exposure to UV rays; perhaps one of the best ways to prevent

---

TABLE 12-1 **Sensory Receptors of the Skin**

NAME	DESCRIPTION
Meissner corpuscles	Mediate sensations of discriminative touch such as light versus deep pressure, as well as low-frequency vibration. Most numerous in hairless areas such as nipples, fingertips, and lips.
Pacinian corpuscles	Located in the deeper dermal layers, primarily in the hands and feet and in many joint capsules; they respond quickly to crude and deep pressure, vibration, and stretch and perceive proprioceptive information about joint position. Pacinian corpuscles adapt quickly to stimuli.
Merkel disks	Located in the epidermis; they respond to light and discriminative touch.
Hair root plexus	Also called hair follicle receptors, they detect hair movement and resemble a web of receptors wrapping around hair follicles.
Krause's end bulbs	Widely distributed in mucous membranes, more so than in the skin. Because of this feature, they are sometimes called *mucocutaneous corpuscles*. They are involved in discriminatory touch and low-frequency vibration. Some references indicate that these receptors are secondary thermoreceptors, detecting temperatures below 65° F, and are often called *cold receptors*.
Ruffini end organs	Located in the dermis and stimulated by deep or continuous pressure; they adapt slowly and permit us to stay in contact with grasped objects. Some references indicate that these receptors are secondary thermoreceptors, detecting temperatures ranging form 85° to 120° F, and are often called *heat receptors*.

premature wrinkling is to protect the skin from exposure to the sun. Avoiding the process of aging is impossible, but good nutrition, plenty of fluids, and daily skin care can retard the process.

Dermal Growth and Repair

The dermis does not continually shed and regenerate itself as do the cells of the epidermis. However, when the dermis is injured, fibroblasts in the dermis quickly reproduce and begin forming a dense collection of new connective tissue called a *scar*.

Deeper sections of the dermis are characterized by dense bundles of white collagenous fibers that arrange themselves in patterns. These patterns differ from one body area to another. The resultant pattern formation is called *Langer's cleavage lines* (Figure 12-3). If surgical incisions are made parallel to the Langer's lines, the resultant scar will then have less of a tendency to gape open, which often leads to a less noticeable scar. Conversely, incisions that go across Langer's lines tend to pull the edges apart and may retard healing.

If elastic fibers in the dermis are overstretched, such as the skin over the abdomen during later stages of pregnancy, these fibers may then weaken and tear. The result is a tiny linear scar commonly referred to as a *stretch mark*.

Subcutaneous Layer

Also known as *superficial fascia* or *hypodermis,* the **subcutaneous layer** is not a true region of skin but rather a loose layer rich in fat and areolar connective tissue. This layer contains nerve receptors called *Krause end bulbs* and *Ruffini end organs.* Also found in the subcutaneous layer is a band of adipose tissue called the *panniculus adiposus.* The thickness of the panniculus adiposus varies with age, gender, and health. Infants and children have a uniform fat layer under the skin. Women have an extra thickness of adipose over the breasts, hips, and inner thighs. Men have an accumulation of fat on the nape of the neck, deltoid and triceps muscles, and abdominal region of the body.

SKIN COLOR

Skin color variations are the result of the following factors:
- Melanin
- Amount of oxygen present in the capillaries of the dermis, which can give the skin a rosy cast to a blue or purple cast of cyanosis (excessive amounts of deoxygenated blood)
- Presence of the pigment bilirubin in the blood, which can produce the yellowish appearance of jaundice
- Presence of the pigment carotene in the skin, which produces the yellowish appearance of Asians

SKIN APPENDAGES

The appendages of the skin include the hair, nails, and glands.

Hair and Related Structures

Hair is made up of keratin filaments arising from a specialized follicle in the dermis. Its function is primarily protection. *Hair follicles* are the pouchlike structures in the skin from which hair grows. The hair shaft is what is seen and felt on the skin's surface. Hair covers almost the entire body. Only a few areas of skin are hairless, notably the palms of the hands and the soles of the feet. Hair is also absent from lips, nipples, and some areas of the genitalia. Heavier concentrations of hair are found in the axillae, scalp, on external genitalia, and above eyes and eyelids. Because of male hormones, men typically have extra hair growth on their face and chest.

Hair protects the scalp from injury and UV radiation. Eyebrows and eyelashes guard the eyes from foreign particles; hair in the nostrils and external ear canal protects the nose and ears, respectively. Hairs also function in light touch

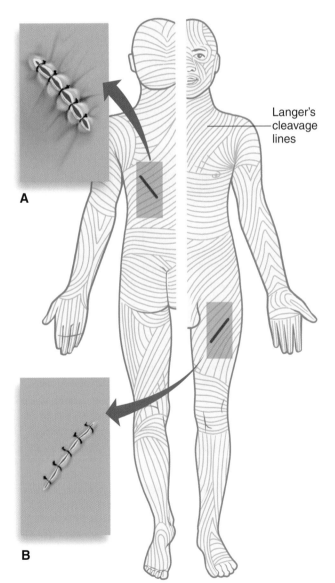

Langer's cleavage lines

A

B

FIGURE 12-3 Langer's cleavage line map, comparing incisions with Langer's lines perpendicular to cleavage lines (**A**) and parallel to cleavage lines (**B**).

ASHLEY MONTAGU, PhD

Born: June 28, 1905; died: November 16, 1999.

"To be kind, to be, to do, and to depart gracefully."

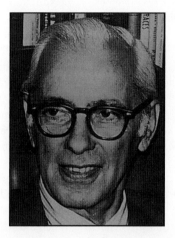

Born in London, Ashley Montagu studied at the University of London and the University of Florence before coming to the United States in 1927. He earned his doctorate from Columbia University in 1937. That same year, he published his first book, *Coming into Being Among the Aborigines.* Between 1937 and 1988, he authored more than 50 books, most of which are in their second or third editions.

Montagu's long and distinguished academic career included positions at some of the most respected schools in the country. He was a professor of anatomy at Hahnemann Medical College and Hospital, Philadelphia, from 1938 to 1949; chairman of the Department of Anthropology at Rutgers University from 1940 to 1955; and a lecturer at Princeton University from 1978 to 1983. During this period, Montagu also held many other concurrent positions in education, professional associations, the United Nations, and the media.

Montagu realized that touch is an enormously important experience for every human being, not only from birth but also from the moment that life begins in the womb. As a professor of anatomy and anthropology, he was inspired to begin researching the effects of touch and nurturing after reading an article on the effects of thyroid surgery on two groups of rodents. The first group, with a 75% survival rate, was cared for by a female physician who caressed each rodent at feeding time. In the second group, the animals all died rapidly. They were cared for by a male laboratory attendant who threw food into the cages and roughly clanged the door. The article noted this difference in treatment but attached no significance to it; however, Montagu did. After he shared this study with a class that he was teaching, a student from a farming area told Montagu that everyone knows that newborn animals must be licked by their mother or they soon die. Notions such as these were the clues that led Montagu to begin his research on effective nurturing. As a scientist, Montagu scientifically solved the mysteries concerning the attributes that make up what we understand to be love. In his own words, "It [love] is the communication to another, by demonstrative acts, of your profound involvement in their welfare."

Montagu's works have emphasized that a healthy mental state results from effective nurturing. Of his own findings, he says, "the most surprising of all things was that doctors had rarely understood this."

Most of Montagu's written work deals in some way with the human condition. His book *Touching: The Human Significance of the Skin* is a must-read resource for all massage therapists. He is also well known for *The Elephant Man* and *Man's Most Dangerous Myth: The Fallacy of Race,* now in its sixth edition.

Montagu's awards included the following:
- Distinguished Achievement Award from American Anthropological Association (1987)
- Darwin Award from the American Association of Physical Anthropologists (1994)
- American Humanist of the Year Award (1995)

Montagu received more than a dozen major awards and two honorary doctorate degrees during his long and prolific career. When asked once what he would like future massage therapists to remember, he said, "To understand that what they are doing is very important indeed. That by caressing another human being's body, in which you are trained to do, I hope, by communicating this involvement in their welfare, what you are doing is what human beings should always be doing, all the days of their lives—caressing other people."

because touch receptors that are associated with them are activated whenever the hairs move.

Hair has a variety of sizes and shapes. Hair is short and stiff in the eyebrow and flexible and long on the top, sides, and back of the head. A round shaft of hair produces straight hair. When the hair shaft is oval, the person usually has wavy hair. If the hair shaft is flat and ribbon-like, then the hair is curly or kinky. In fine hair, no medulla (inner core) is present in the hair follicle. Genetics determine most of our hair characteristics, from hair color to texture.

All shades of hair come from one or a combination of the three colors of melanin: brown, yellow, and black. Red hair is a combination of brown and yellow pigment. White hair often is the result of air in the hair follicle itself. Gray hair occurs when the amount of melanin deposited in the hair decreases or is absent. Aging, emotional distress, certain chemical treatments (chemotherapy), radiation, excessive vitamin A, and certain fungal diseases can cause both graying and hair loss.

Hair follicles can sometimes become irritated during a massage, which may be caused by the following:
- An allergic reaction to the lubricant
- Pulling of the hair
- Insufficient use of lubricant on the skin, causing undue friction

Arrector Pili

Arrector pili are the muscles of the hair. These tiny muscles contract when you are cold or experiencing emotions such as fright or anxiety. The hair is pulled upright, dimpling the skin surface with goose bumps. If an animal is cold, this action creates an insulating layer of air in the fur. Because most humans do not have fur, this effect is relatively useless. If an animal is frightened, this added volume allows the animal to appear larger and possibly deter an enemy.

TABLE TALK

Changes in Skin Caused by the Aging Process

Moisture: Skin becomes dryer and flakier.
Pigment: Skin color is paler in color.
Thickness: Wrinkling occurs especially on face and arms. The skin takes on a parchmentlike appearance, especially over bony protuberances, on the back of the hands, feet, arms, and legs.
Texture: Not only does wrinkling occur, but the skin also feels rougher and may possess lines and creases.
Turgor: When pinched, the skin may tent (poor turgor), especially if the client is dehydrated.

Skin Glands

The glands of the skin include sebaceous glands, sudoriferous glands, and ceruminous glands.

Sebaceous (Oil) Glands

Sebaceous glands, also known as *oil glands,* secrete *sebum,* rich in chemicals such as triglycerides, waxes, fatty acids, and cholesterol, which are mildly antibacterial and antifungal, lubricating both the hair and the epidermis. Although almost always associated with hair follicles, some specialized sebaceous glands open directly on the skin's surface in such areas as the glans penis, lips, and eyelids.

Overproduction of sebum, caused by hormones or disease, can make the skin appear oily; underproduction of sebum caused by nutritional factors and UV radiation makes the skin appear dry. Massage therapists can use massage to stimulate the production of sebum, which adds additional natural oils to the skin. The best massage movement for sebaceous gland stimulation is friction.

Sudoriferous (Sweat) Glands

Sudoriferous glands, or *sweat glands,* secrete sweat, or perspiration. They are regulated by the sympathetic nervous system and can be stimulated in response to excess heat or emotional arousal. The skin's surface possesses approximately 2 million sweat glands. Mammary glands, which are modified sudoriferous glands, are often regarded as part of the integumentary system.

The primary functions of sudoriferous glands are to regulate body temperature and to eliminate waste products. As perspiration evaporates, it carries large amounts of body heat away from the skin surface. The most rapid process of heat dissipation is evaporation of perspiration.

Approximately 1 pint of fluid and impurities is lost in each 8-hour period when a person is visibly sweating. When sweat production is high, replacement of lost minerals is essential. When the sweating is low, most of the sodium chloride present in the perspiration is reabsorbed in the skin. In this case, mineral depletion is minimal.

Sweat glands can be classified into two groups, (1) eccrine and (2) apocrine (Figure 12-4).
- *Eccrine sweat glands* are the most numerous, widespread, and important sweat glands. Eccrine glands function throughout life to produce the watery fluid called sweat, which is rich in salts, ammonia, uric acid, urea, and other wastes. They do not exist on the lips, the ear canal, the glans penis, and nail beds.
- *Apocrine sweat glands* are located in the deep subcutaneous layer in the axillary region, the areola of the breast, and the pigmented skin around the anus. They are much larger than eccrine glands and join hair follicles. They enlarge and begin to function at puberty, producing a more viscous and colored secretion than eccrine glands. In women, apocrine gland secretion show cyclical changes linked to the menstrual cycle. Odor produced by these glands is mainly the result of decomposition of the apocrine sweat by skin bacteria.

Ceruminous Glands

Ceruminous glands are a special variety of modified apocrine glands that release its secretion of the surface of the external ear canal. They secrete a waxy cerumen instead of watery sweat.

Nails

Nails are heavily keratinized, nonliving tissue that forms the thin hard plates found on the distal surfaces of the fingers and toes. The two main functions of the nails are (1) protection of the ends of the fingers and (2) use as a tool for tasks such as digging, scratching, and manipulation of objects.

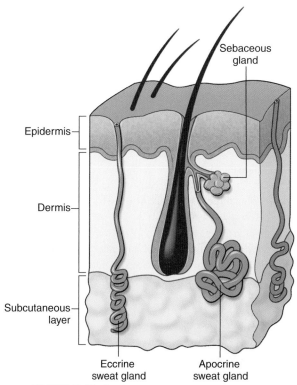

FIGURE 12-4 Eccrine and apocrine skin glands.

Nails are typically transparent but appear pinkish because of blood vessels present in the dermis below. If the blood contains an insufficient amount of oxygen, the nails appear bluish purple, or *cyanotic*. Nail changes, such as ridges and white spots, may occur as a result of poor nutrition or disease.

The **nail body** is the main and most visible part of the nail. Other nail structures are the nail bed, nail root, lateral nail folds, cuticle, lunula, and the free edge of the nail. Nail production takes place in the **nail root.** Nail growth occurs at approximately 1 mm per week. The **nail bed** is the skin beneath the nail; it appears through the clear nail, often as a series of longitudinal ridges. The *lateral nail*

folds are the edges of the nail where they meet the skin at the sides of the nail. This area is where hangnails occur. The **cuticle,** or *eponychium,* is the tough ridge of skin that grows out over the nail from its base. Also located here is the *lunula,* which is the whitish half-moon shape at the nail base. The most distal portion of the nail is the **free nail edge,** which is what is trimmed as a result of nail growth (Figure 12-5).

MINI-LAB

Spray the back of your hand with tap water. Blow on the damp surface, and describe the sensation as the water evaporates. Speculate how evaporation of water (sweat) from the skin surface can regulate the temperature of the body. Repeat the experiment with alcohol, which evaporates at a lower temperature than water, and compare the results.

NERVOUS SYSTEM'S ROLE IN TOUCH

The brain detects the sensation of touch in the parietal lobe of the cerebral cortex. The postcentral gyrus, an elevated area of brain tissue located in the parietal lobe, is where the axons that detect touch terminate. Keep in mind that the right postcentral gyrus represents the left side of the body and vice versa. An interesting fact is just how much gray matter is dedicated to each surface area (Figure 12-6). The hands, face, lips, jaw, and tongue take up approximately 80% of this neural space. The more space devoted to an area in the postcentral gyrus, the more sensory touch receptors are found in the corresponding part of the body. The more sensory receptors that are located in that part of the body, the more sensitive is the body part.

The skin functions as a large conductor of information such as heat, cold, pressure, pain, movement, and touch. The sense of touch is actually a complex composition of specialized receptors found in the skin. Touch and pressure

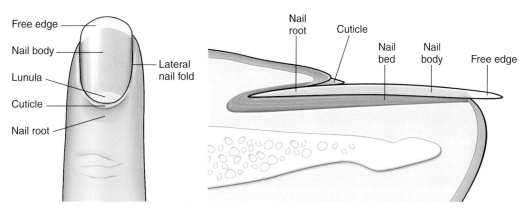

FIGURE 12-5 A cross section of a nail.

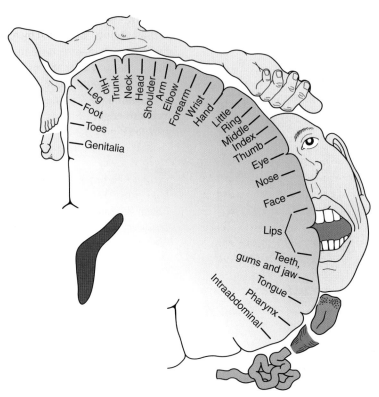

FIGURE 12-6 Illustration of the *homunculus*, meaning little man, in the postcentral gyrus

is an amalgamation of many sensations and is the least understood of all the senses. Touch provides sensory input and physical information about our surroundings. This sense also warns the body of damage, such as the cooking pot is hot or your finger is in the way as you cut an orange with a sharp knife. Following is a list of all the currently known receptors and their functions. Please note that *discriminative touch* means touch that is subtle and can be easily located in the skin. Conversely, *crude touch* is more easily identified but is more difficult to locate on the skin than discriminative touch.

- **Meissner corpuscle:** Also called a *tactile corpuscle,* this receptor mediates sensations of discriminative touch such as light versus deep pressure, as well as low-frequency vibration. Meissner corpuscles are most numerous in hairless areas such as nipples, fingertips, and lips.
- **Ruffini's corpuscle:** Located in the dermis, Ruffini's corpuscles alert us when the skin comes into contact with deep or continuous pressure. They adapt slowly and permit us to stay in contact with grasped objects. The ability to clutch a pencil or pen in your hand for long periods and still be able to feel it depends on these receptors. Some references indicate that these corpuscles are secondary thermoreceptors, detecting temperatures ranging from 85° to 120° F, and are often called *heat receptors.*
- **Pacinian corpuscle:** Located in the deeper dermal layers, primarily in the hands and feet and in many joint capsules, these receptors respond quickly to crude and deep pressure, vibration, and stretch and perceive proprioceptive information about joint position. Pacinian corpuscles

adapt quickly to stimuli; thus, for this reason, they respond only when the stimuli is first applied. In cross section, the shape of a Pacinian corpuscle resembles an onion slice.

- **Krause end bulb:** These receptors are found widely distributed in mucous membranes, more so than in the skin. Because of this arrangement, they are sometimes *mucocutaneous corpuscles.* They are involved in discriminatory touch and low-frequency vibration. Some references indicate that these receptors are secondary thermoreceptors, detecting temperatures below 65° F, and are often called *cold receptors.*
- **Merkel disk:** Located in the epidermis, these receptors respond to light touch and discriminative touch.
- **Hair root plexus:** Also called *hair follicle receptors,* these structures are light-touch receptors that detect hair movement and resemble a web of receptors wrapping around hair follicles. They may alert us to goose bumps or inform us of a small breeze or intrusive insect.

MINI-LAB

Take the bottom of a clear glass and press it into the heel of your hand. Describe the color changes and possible explanation for these changes. What would happen to the skin cells if the pressure were prolonged? How does this experiment reflect what happens to the skin when clients are bedridden? How can massage, with its circulatory effects, aid in preventing decubitus ulcers (bedsores)?

Using the Evolve website, access chapter-related activity "drag and drop" to review structures of the skin. Use it as review or a study guide for upcoming tests. ■

MOLE CHANGES

Observing any changes and reporting these changes to the client are added services in massage therapy. Because our profession uses the skin as the primary organ of contact, we have the unique opportunity to notice any changes in the skin's surface. These changes are noted both visually and tactilely.

Mole changes may occur often with people who are exposed to natural and artificial UV light. Mole changes may also be associated with friction or irritation from clothing (particularly bra straps), elastic waistbands, eyeglasses, or hard hats. Changes in moles should be noted and discussed with the client. A referral may be made to a physician for diagnosis and possible treatment.

Common moles and melanoma do not appear similar. Using the ABCDEF method of mole assessment listed here, you will be able to detect changing moles as they occur. Point these moles out to your clients, and ask them to continue checking their moles at home. A mirror can be used for hard-to-see places on the body. If moles have any of the abnormal characteristics listed here, then consult with a physician immediately.

- *Asymmetry.* Asymmetry means that if a line were drawn down the middle, it would not create two equal halves. Common moles are symmetrical and round. Malignant moles are asymmetrical.
- *Border.* The edges or borders of early malignant melanoma are uneven, often containing scalloped or notched edges.
- *Color.* Different shades of brown or black are often the first sign of a problem. Common moles are evenly shaded

brown. Black moles are darker than surrounding moles and should be checked by a physician.

- *Diameter.* Common moles are usually less than one-quarter inch in diameter (6 mm), the size of a pencil eraser. Early melanomas tend to be larger than common moles.
- *Elevated.* Common moles are smooth, and malignant moles are elevated.
- *Fast growing.* Common moles do not grow fast, if at all. Malignant moles change their size rapidly, indicating metastasis.

In addition to these criteria, look for a sore that does not heal properly, which may indicate skin cancer. Ask your client to check with his or her physician. The preceding boxed feature lists the massage effects of the skin and related structures.

PATHOLOGICAL CONDITIONS OF THE SKIN

Acne

Acne is a bacterial infection of the hair follicles and associated sebaceous glands (i.e., pilosebaceous units). Acne causes inflammation and pus formation. It usually begins at puberty and may continue throughout adolescence. Whiteheads are accumulations of dead bacteria, cell debris, and dead white blood cells. Blackheads are accumulations of dried sebum and bacteria in the gland and its duct. The black appearance is due to oxidation of the sebum. Acne is most commonly found on the face but can also appear on the chest, neck, shoulders, and back. Drainage of acne pustules (i.e., extracting) is beyond the scope of practice for most massage therapists. Check with your state board for more information. *Local contraindication of infected area.*

Athlete's Foot

Athlete's foot is a contagious superficial fungal infection of the foot characterized by discoloration of the skin and a ridge of red tissue. The skin may also break, bleed, or ooze clear fluid. The infected foot often has an unpleasant odor. *Local contraindication of infected area.*

Boils

A boil or an abscess is caused by the staphylococcal bacteria in the dermis or hair follicle. It is characterized by pain, redness, and swelling. Necrosis forms a core of dead tissue that may extrude. *Local contraindication of affected area. Avoid swollen lymph nodes.*

Bruise

A bruise is an injury that does not break the skin. It is caused by mechanical trauma such as a blow and is characterized by swelling, discoloration, and pain. The color of a bruise is

---

BOX 12-1

Effects of Massage on the Skin and Related Structures

Increases skin temperature. Warming of the skin indicates a reduction of stress.

Improves skin condition. As circulation increases, added nutrients are made available to the skin, thereby improving its condition, texture, and tone. Clinical observations have determined that massage also improves the appearance (i.e., color, texture) of the skin.

Stimulates oil glands. Stimulation of the oil (sebaceous) glands causes an increase in oil (sebum) production, which improves the skin's condition and reduces skin dryness.

Improves pathological skin conditions. Unless a condition contraindicates massage, pathological skin conditions may improve by decreasing redness, reducing thickening and hardening of the skin, increasing healing of skin abrasions, and reducing itching.

caused by blood from ruptured vessels that have leaked into the interstitial spaces. *Local contraindication until bruise turns yellowish. Massaging around the bruise while it is bluish-purple is fine*.

Burns

When heat, radiation, electricity, or chemical agents damage the skin, cells perish. The damage that results is called a *burn*. A formula is used for estimating the amount of body surface covered by burns. This formula is called the *Rule of Nines*, and it assigns 9% (or multiples of 9) to specific body areas. This formula is modified for infants and children because of the different body proportions. Burns can be classified into three categories, depending on the depth of damage to the tissues and the area of involvement.

A **first-degree burn** damages the epidermis. Symptoms are redness and mild pain. An example of a first-degree burn is mild sunburn, which typically heals in 2 to 3 days.

A **second-degree burn** damages the epidermis and the upper layers of the dermis. Some symptoms associated with second-degree burns are swelling, blistering, and pain. Hair follicles and sweat glands usually remain functional. Healing time can be from 7 days to 4 weeks. Once the burn heals, a mild scar may remain.

A **third-degree burn** destroys the epidermis, dermis, hair follicles, and associated glands. Because of the damage to the glands and follicles, the functions of the skin are reduced or nonexistent. Because of injury of the lymphatics and nerve endings, very little swelling and pain occur. A client with third-degree burns may experience limited mobility because of the restrictive effect of scar tissue. Almost all third-degree burns require skin grafting. *Obtain physician clearance for recent fully healed burns. Once granted, use lighter pressure (including healed skin graft) and techniques that help break up adhesions and increase tissue mobility. All forms of thermotherapy (e.g., hot pack) are contraindicated. All forms of cryotherapy (e.g., cold pack) are contraindicated for third-degree burns*.

Cancer (Skin)

The three most common skin cancers are basal cell carcinoma, squamous cell carcinoma, and malignant melanoma. *Basal cell carcinomas* account for approximately 75% of all cancers of the skin. This cancer is slow growing and characterized by lesions that begin as small raised nodules that ulcerate. Its primary cause is excessive sun exposure. Basal cell carcinoma is the least dangerous and rarely metastasizes.

Squamous cell carcinoma accounts for approximately 20% of all cases of skin cancer, and it begins as a scaly pigmented area that may develop into an ulcerated crater. This type of cancer is common on sun-exposed areas or in the mouth (tobacco chewers) or on the lips (cigarette and cigar smokers).

One of the most malignant and lethal skin cancer types, *melanoma,* is a group of melanocytes that has mutated into cancer. Accounting for approximately 5% of all skin cancers, it typically begins as a raised dark lesion with irregular borders and appears uneven in color. It typically occurs in light-skinned people who are exposed to UV radiation over many years. Melanoma is more likely to metastasize than any other form of cancer and can kill within months of diagnosis. *Obtain physician consent. Once granted, adjust massage according to cancer treatment that the client is undergoing (e.g., surgery, radiation therapy, chemotherapy, bone marrow transplant). If the client has a low platelet count, then use lighter pressure. If the client is nauseated, then avoid aromatherapy or pressure and speed that rock the client (e.g., joint mobilizations, stretches, jostling). Adjust massage to client's stamina and vitality (i.e., slower, gentler, shorter duration, assist client on and off table). Avoid massage over intravenous insertion sites, catheters, surgical wounds over radiation burns, or known tumors sites*.

Cellulitis

Cellulitis is an acute infection of the subcutaneous tissues caused by staphylococci or streptococci bacteria. It is characterized by localized swelling, redness, abscess formation, and warm and tender skin. Bacteria often enter the skin by a wound and spread to surrounding tissues. *Local contraindication of infected area if contained to a small area. Otherwise, massage is contraindicated*.

Contact Dermatitis

Contact dermatitis is a skin irritation often due to an allergic reaction when the skin comes into *contact* with various substances, creating an inflammatory response. *Local contraindication of infected area if contained to a small area. Otherwise, massage is contraindicated*.

Corns or Calluses

A corn or callus is thickened cone-shaped skin involving the uppermost layer of epidermis. It forms because of repeated friction or pressure and occurs primarily over toe joints and between the toes. *Avoid affected area if pressure causes pain*.

Decubitus Ulcers

Decubitus ulcers are caused by local ischemia of tissues that have been subjected to prolonged pressure. Restriction of blood supply to the skin results in cell necrosis (death). The weight of the body puts pressure on the skin (especially over bony projections). As cells die, ulcers form. Decubitus ulcers occur in bedridden patients who are not turned regularly and in people who use wheelchairs or braces or have casts. *Local contraindication of involved area*.

Eczema

Eczema is an acute or chronic inflammatory disorder of the skin characterized by redness, watery discharge, crusting, scaling, itching, and burning. This disorder has no known cause, and it may be hereditary. Eczema is not contagious. *Avoid affected area if open or accompanied by watery discharge or if pressure causes pain.*

Folliculitis

When hair follicles become inflamed, the condition is referred to as *folliculitis*. It is often caused by the bacteria *Staphylococcus aureus*. A form of folliculitis, folliculitis barbae, can develop on the bearded areas of male clients. *Local contraindication of infected area.*

Herpes Simplex

Herpes simplex is a highly contagious viral infection that has the ability to remain dormant within the dorsal nerve root ganglion corresponding to the site of infection for extended periods without expressing any signs or symptoms of disease. Flare-ups are characterized by cold sores on the skin and mucous membranes. The appearance of cold sores can be triggered by stimuli such as UV radiation from the sun, hormonal changes that occur during menstruation and pregnancy, or emotional upset. *Massage is contraindicated.*

Hives

Hives are an inflammatory disorder consisting of localized edema, with development of wheals. The presence of hives is often due to an allergic reaction to food, insect bites or stings, or medications. Hives may be either acute and transient or chronic; the former evolves over a few hours and lasts less than 24 hours, and the latter is continuous or persists episodically for 6 weeks or more. *During acute phase, massage is contraindicated. Otherwise, local contraindicated where wheals are still visible but not inflamed.*

Impetigo

Impetigo is an inflammatory skin infection caused by staphylococci or streptococci bacteria. It is characterized by raised, fluid-filled sores that itch or burn. This condition is most common in children, and it occurs mainly around the mouth, nose, and hands. Impetigo is highly contagious and can be spread by hand contact and handling contaminated objects such as linens, doorknobs, and toothbrushes. *Massage is contraindicated.*

Lice

The body louse is a parasitic insect that is highly contagious. Lice present on pubic hair are commonly called *crabs*. Lice are typically found in hair and are diagnosed with the presence of egg sacs, called *nits*, on the hair shaft. *Massage is contraindicated.*

Pigmentations (Skin)

Skin pigmentations include age spots, albinism, birthmarks (Café au lait and port wine spots, strawberry and cherry hemangiomas), chloasma, freckles, and vitiligo. Some pigmentations are congenital; some are a response to hormones (i.e., the mask of pregnancy); others appear as a result of age or UV light such as sun exposure. *Massage is fine.*

Psoriasis

Psoriasis is characterized by red, flaky skin elevations covered by thick, dry, silvery scales. A chronic form of dermatitis, it is characterized by periods of remission and exacerbation. In severe forms, psoriasis is a disabling and disfiguring disorder and can involve the scalp, elbows, knees, back, and buttocks. The condition is often genetic. Psoriasis has no known cause and is not contagious. Stress can exacerbate the condition. *Avoid affected areas if pressure causes pain. Scales may dislodge during treatment.*

Ringworm

Ringworm is not a worm at all but rather a group of contagious fungal diseases characterized by itching, scaling, and sometimes painful lesions exhibited as a raised red-ringed patch. *Massage is contraindicated.*

Rosacea

A chronic inflammatory disorder affecting the blood vessels and hair follicles of the face, rosacea is characterized by persistent redness and swelling. Usually, only the middle third of the face is involved. *Avoid hot immersion baths, and use light pressure on affected areas.*

Scabies

Scabies are a highly contagious infestation caused by parasitic mites that burrow and crawl under the skin's surface. The mites cannot be seen by the naked eye. The female mite excretes a material that causes intense itching (typically at night). *Massage is contraindicated.*

Scars

Scar tissue is the result of the healing process. A cicatrix is a scar with substantial constriction because of the natural healing process, as in a burn, or by the way it was sutured. A keloid is a large smooth scar and may be pink in color as a result of the presence of blood vessels. Scar tissue often creates pain and discomfort, stiffness, weakness, and loss of function. *Obtain physician clearance for recent fully healed scars. Once granted, use cross-fiber and chucking friction and myofascial release directly on the scar to increase tissue flexibility.*

Scleroderma

Scleroderma is an autoimmune disorder affecting blood vessels and connective tissue. Excessive collagen production of the connective tissue of the skin, lungs, and internal organs occurs. The skin tightens and becomes fixed to underlying tissues. Scleroderma is most common in middle-age women. Death may occur because of cardiac, renal, pulmonary, or intestinal involvement. Localized forms occur with just small patches of the skin involved. Scleroderma is not contagious. *Obtain physician clearance. Once granted, massage is fine if symptoms are not severe. Use techniques to help reduce adhesions and increase local circulation. Passive and active stretches and joint mobilization help retain mobility.*

Sebaceous Cysts

A sebaceous cyst is a common benign swelling beneath the skin lined by keratinizing epithelium and filled with material composed of sebum and epithelial debris. These cysts are mobile but attached to the skin by the remains of a sebaceous gland duct. Sebaceous cysts frequently become infected. Treatment is surgical excision. *Local contraindication of affected area.*

Seborrheic Dermatitis

Seborrhea, also known as *dandruff* and *cradle cap*, is dry, scaly material from the scalp or any excessive scaly material from the skin that may not be associated with disease. Seborrheic dermatitis has no known cause. *Massage is fine, unless due to a contraindicated disease. If that is the case, local and possibly general massage is contraindicated.*

Shingles

Shingles is an acute infection of the peripheral nervous system caused by the reactivation of a latent herpes zoster (chickenpox) virus. Affecting mainly adults, shingles produces painful, blister like eruptions in a strip pattern along the affected nerves of a dermatome. These blisters eventually dry up and form scabs that resemble shingles. Scarring may result. The distribution of the blisters is usually unilateral, typically affecting the thoracic area and sometimes the face, although both sides of the body may be involved. The skin in the area of the blisters is hypersensitive. *Local contraindication of infected area. General massage is fine, if client feels up to it.*

Skin Tags

Skin tags are tiny flaps of skin. These tags are most common in middle-aged men and women and are typically located around the neck, upper chest, armpit, and groin. Some skin tags are genetic; others are a result of friction, such as clothes rubbing on skin. *Avoid the area if it is sensitive. Take care not to pull skin tags during treatment.*

Stretch Marks

Stretch marks are tearing, thinning, or overstretching of skin that actually reduces its thickness. They begin as red to pink streaks that eventually fade to silvery white. These streaks often result from extreme stretching of the skin. This stretching can be a result of pregnancy, body building, sudden weight gain, or severe swelling caused by an accident or surgical complications. *Avoid affected areas if pressure causes pain. Deep pressure is contraindicated over affected areas.*

Warts

A wart is a thickening of the epidermis resulting in a mass of cutaneous elevations caused by a contagious virus, papillomavirus. *Local contraindication of affected area.*

> ### TABLE TALK
>
> Transdermal patches are used for conditions such as hormone replacement therapy and by clients who are trying to stop using tobacco products. Because the massage lubricant will weaken the adhesive, avoid its use up to 2 inches around the patch area.
>
> If an area of complaint is under the transdermal patch, consult with the client's physician and obtain permission to remove the patch. Proceed with the massage as usual. After the massage, clean the area with alcohol and reapply the patch.

SUMMARY

The skin is so much more than an external covering. It is a highly sensitive boundary between our body and the environment. It offers protection, heat exchange, vitamin synthesis, and waste removal, and it serves as a membrane of interfacing. We can survive without sight, taste, smell, or hearing, but to lose our sense of touch would leave us walled off from our environment and from contact with others.

Regions of the skin include the epidermis and the dermis. A layer called the *subcutaneous layer* lies beneath the dermis. Skin appendages include hair, nails, and glands.

evolve

Go to *Chapter Extras* on Evolve for additional illustrations and resources for this chapter. *Extras* for this chapter include:

1. Crossword puzzle (downloadable form)

MATCHING

Place the letter of the answer next to the term or phrase that best describes it.

A. Arrector pili   E. Hair follicles   I. Nails
B. Cuticle   F. Keratin   J. Sebaceous glands
C. Dermis   G. Melanin   K. Sudoriferous glands
D. Epidermis   H. Melanocytes   L. Superficial fascia (subcutaneous layer)

_____ 1. The tough ridge of skin that grows out over the nail's base

_____ 2. True skin, containing adipose tissue, blood vessels, and nerve endings

_____ 3. A tough, fibrous protein that provides protection by waterproofing the skin

_____ 4. Tiny muscles that pull the hair upright

_____ 5. Skin layer that contains melanocytes, nails, and pore openings

_____ 6. Granules that gives color to the skin, hair, and the iris of the eye

_____ 7. Glands whose primary functions are to regulate temperature and eliminate wastes

_____ 8. Connective tissue layer that connects the dermis to underlying structures

_____ 9. Specialized cells in the epidermis where skin pigment is synthesized

_____ 10. Thin hard plates found on the distal ends of the fingers and toes

_____ 11. Can become irritated during a massage because of allergies, hair pulling, and inadequate amount of lubricant

_____ 12. Glands that secrete a fatty substance, lubricating both hair and epidermis

INTERNET ACTIVITIES

Visit http://www.melanomafoundation.org/prevention/sun.htm and write five tips on sun protection.

Visit http://www.hsph.harvard.edu/headlice.html and write a short report on head lice.

View the amination at http://www.mydr.com.au/default.asp?Article=4139 to understand how pigment protects your skin and how UV radiation damages your skin.

Bibliography

Abrahams P, Marks S, Hutchings R: *McMinn's color atlas of human anatomy,* St Louis, 2003, Mosby.

Applegate EJ: *The anatomy and physiology learning system,* ed 3, Philadelphia, 2006, Saunders.

Beers MH, Berkow R: *The Merck manual of diagnosis and therapy,* Whitehouse Station, NJ, 2006, Merck Research Laboratories.

Clarke AM, Clarke AD: *Early experience: myth and evidence,* London, 1979, Open Books.

Como D, editor: *Mosby's medical, nursing, and allied health dictionary,* ed 6, St Louis, 2002, Mosby.

Crawley J, Van De Graaff KM: *A photographic atlas for anatomy and physiology,* Englewood, Colo, 2002, Morton.

Damjanov I: *Pathophysiology for the health-related professions,* ed 3, Philadelphia, 2006, Saunders.

Ferri FF: *2003 Ferri's clinical advisor, instant diagnosis and treatment,* St Louis, 2003, Mosby.

Frazier MS, Drzymkowski JW: *Essentials of human diseases and conditions,* ed 3, Philadelphia, 2004, Saunders.

Gerson J: *STD textbook for professional estheticians,* ed 9, Albany, 2003, Delmar Learning.

Goldberg S: *Clinical anatomy made ridiculously simple,* Miami, 2004, Medmaster.

Gould BE: *Pathophysiology for the health professions,* ed 3, Philadelphia, 2006, Saunders.

Grafelman T: *Graf's anatomy and physiology guide for the massage therapist,* Aurora, Colo, 1998, DG Publishing.

Guyton A: *Human physiology and mechanisms of disease,* ed 6, Philadelphia, 1996, Saunders.

Haubrich WS: *Medical meanings: a glossary of word origins,* New York, 1984, Harcourt Brace Jovanovich.

Huether SE, McCance KL: *Understanding pathophysiology,* ed 3, St Louis, 2004, Mosby.

Jacob S, Francone C: *Elements of anatomy and physiology,* Philadelphia, 1989, Saunders.

Juhan D: *Job's body: a handbook for bodyworkers,* ed 3, Barrington, NY, 2003, Station Hill Press.

Kalat JW: *Biological psychology,* ed 8, Belmont, Calif, 2003, Wadsworth.

Kapit W, Macey R, Meisami E: *The physiology coloring book,* ed 2, New York, 1999, HarperCollins.

Kapit W, Elson LM: *The anatomy coloring book,* ed 3, New York, 2002, Benjamin Cummings.

Kendall F, McCreary E: *Muscles: testing and function,* Baltimore, 1983, Williams and Wilkins.

Kordish M, Dickson S: *Introduction to basic human anatomy,* Lake Charles, La, 1985, McNeese State University.

Krieger D: Therapeutic touch: the imprimatur of nursing, *Am J Nurs* 75(5):784-787, 1975.

Kumar V, Abbas A, Fausto N: *Robbins and Cotran physiologic basis of disease,* ed 7, St Louis, 2005, Mosby.

Marieb EN: *Essentials of human anatomy and physiology,* ed 8, New York, 2005, Benjamin Cummings.

Martini FH, Bartholomew EF: *Essentials of anatomy and physiology,* ed 3, New York, 2003, Benjamin/Cummings

McAleer N: *The body almanac,* Garden City, NY, 1985, Doubleday.

McCance K, Huether S: *Pathophysiology: the biological basis for disease in adults and children,* St Louis, 2006, Mosby.

Merck manual, ed 17, Whitehouse Station, NJ, 1998, Merck and Company.

Montagu A: *Touching: the human significance of the skin,* ed 2, New York, 1978, Harper and Row.

Moore KL: *Clinically oriented anatomy,* ed 5, Baltimore, 2005, Lippincott Williams & Wilkins.

Netter FH: *Atlas of human anatomy,* ed 3, Teterboro, NJ, 2003, Icon Learning Systems.

Newton D: *Pathology for massage therapists,* ed 2, Portland, Ore, 1995, Simran.

Olsen A, McHose C: *Bodystories: a guide to experiential anatomy,* Barrytown, NY, 1991, Station Hill Press.

Premkumar K: *Pathology A to Z: a handbook for massage therapists,* Baltimore, 1999, Lippincott Williams & Wilkins.

Salvo SG, Anderson SK: *Mosby's pathology for massage therapists,* St Louis, 2004, Elsevier Mosby.

Skin Cancer Foundation: *The ABCD's of moles and melanomas,* New York, 2005, The Foundation.

Solomon EP, Phillips GA: *Understanding human anatomy and physiology,* Philadelphia, 1987, Saunders.

Thibodeau G, Patton K: *Anatomy and physiology,* ed 6, St Louis, 2006, Mosby.

Thibodeau G, Patton K: *Structure and function of the body,* ed 12, St Louis, 2004, Mosby.

Tortora GJ: *Introduction to the human body: the essentials of anatomy and physiology,* ed 3, New York, 1994, HarperCollins.

Tortora GJ, Derreckson B: *Principles and human anatomy and physiology,* ed 11, New York, 2006, John Wiley & Sons.

Venes D, Thomas CL, Taber CW: *Taber's cyclopedic medical dictionary,* ed 20, Philadelphia, 2005, FA Davis.

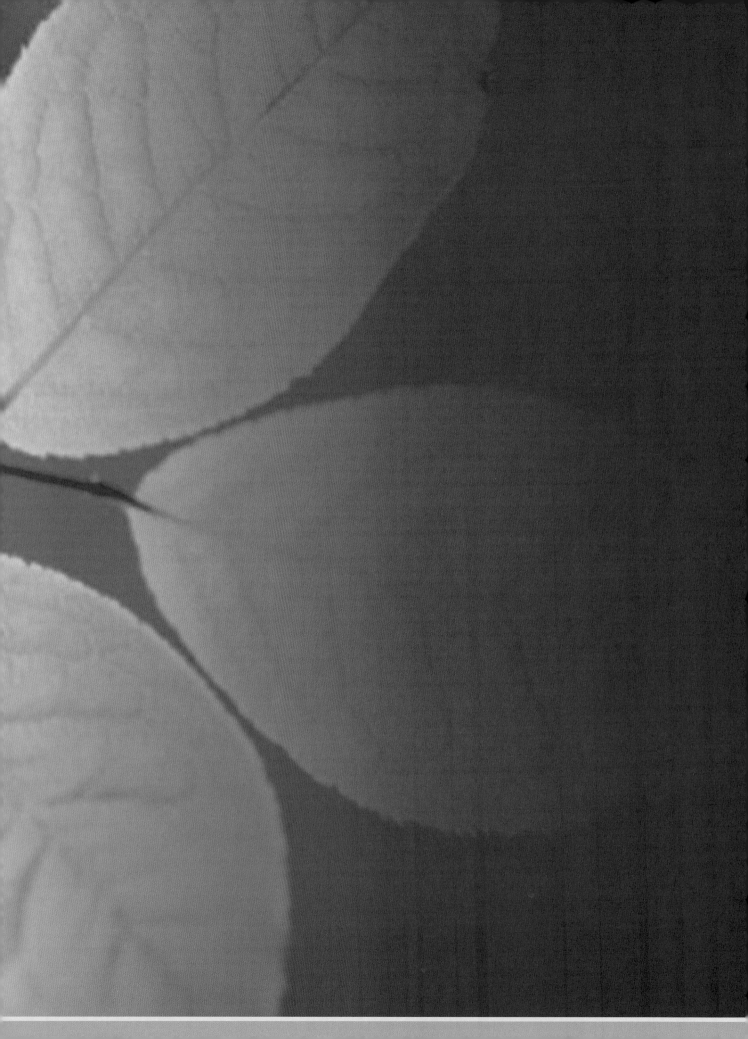

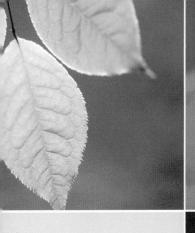

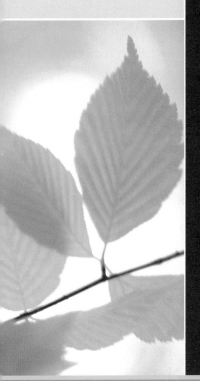

CHAPTER 13

Skeletal System and Joint Movements

"Curiosity is a willing, a proud, and eager confession of ignorance."
—Leonard Rubenstein

STUDENT OBJECTIVES

After completing this chapter, the student should be able to:

- List the anatomical structures, and describe the physiological properties of the skeletal system
- Group the bones into classifications according to their shape
- Classify bones according to their shape
- Name the structures associated with long bones
- State the two types of bone identified by its texture and density
- Compare and contrast osteoblasts and osteoclasts
- Discuss the effects of aging and exercise on bone strength
- Determine if a particular bone is a member of the axial skeleton or the appendicular skeleton
- Name and describe surface markings located on bones
- Compare synarthrotic, amphiarthrotic, and diarthrotic joints
- List the structures associated with synovial joints
- Describe the synovial joint types, giving examples of each
- Demonstrate all the possible movements of synovial joints
- State the three classes of levers, giving examples of each
- Name types of pathological skeletal conditions, giving characteristics and massage considerations of each

INTRODUCTION

The intricate structures of bone, cartilage, ligament, and joints compose the skeletal system. Not only do they provide protection and support movement, they also produce blood cells and store minerals such as calcium and phosphorus.

Bone is living tissue. The skeletons in anatomy classes, laboratories, and museums are the mineral salts that remain after death. Bones are among the hardest materials in the body, yet they are relatively light, somewhat flexible, and able to resist tension and other forces of stress.

The human body has 206 bones. Bones are the steel girders of the body, forming its internal framework. Mammals ranging from humans to bats to elephants have remarkably similar skeleton systems. For example, seven vertebrae are in the human cervical spine and are also in the long-necked giraffe and the no-necked whale.

The skeletal system is of the utmost importance to the massage therapist because it constitutes the road map for locating muscles. Muscles attach to bones at various bony markings known as *origins* and *insertions*. Because bones are hard, most markings are easy to palpate. Learn your bony markings well because they will guide you into locating the muscles that are causing your clients the most difficulty. Muscles are located between their attachment points.

The study of the skeletal system is multifaceted. Besides the basic structure and function of bone, we will also study movement and leverage, types of joints and articulations, pathological skeletal conditions, and the general bony markings.

ANATOMY

Areas of discussion in this chapter include:
- Bones
- Cartilage
- Joints
- Ligaments

PHYSIOLOGY

The skeletal system serves a wide variety of functions that include the following:
- Supports the rest of the body systems through a bony framework
- Protects the body's vital organs
- Provides movement by giving leverage through muscle attachments
- Produces blood cells in the red marrow of long bones, a process called **hemopoiesis** (blood cell formation), producing both red and white blood cells
- Stores fats in yellow bone marrow and releases them when needed
- Stores vital minerals such as calcium phosphate, calcium carbonate, phosphorus, magnesium, and sodium, which are stored and released when the body needs them and is accomplished through vascular interfacing with the bones

Terms and Their Meanings Related to the Skeletal System

Term	Meaning
Amphi	*Gr.* on both sides
Arthr-, arthro-	*Gr.* joint
Blast	*Gr. germ cell or bud*
Bursa	*Gr.* a leather sac
Clast	*Gr.* to break
Condyle	*Gr.* knuckle
Crepitus	*L.* crackling or a rattle
Diarthrotic	*Gr.* two; joint
Epiphysis	*Gr.* upon, over; to grow
Facet	*Fr.* small face
Foramen	*L.* a hole
Fossa	*L.* ditch or depression
Haversian	British physician and anatomist (1650-1702)
Circumduction	*L.* around; to lead
Ligament	*L.* to bind or a band
Ossicle	*L.* little bone
Meatus	*L.* a passage
Ossification	*L.* bone; to make
Osteo, osseo	*L.* bone
Periosteum	*Gr.* around, about; *L.* bone
Process	*L.* going before
Ramus	*L.* a branch
Sesamoid	*Gr.* sesame seed–like; shaped
Skeleton	*Gr.* dried up
Symphysis	*Gr.* together with, joined; to grow
Synarthrotic	*Gr.* together; joint
Trochanter	*Gr.* a wheel or runner
Tubercle	*L.* swelling
Tuberosity	*L.* swelling
Volkmann	German physician (1800-1877)

Fr., French; *Gr.*, Greek; *L.*, Latin.

CLASSIFICATION OF BONES

Bones are classified according to their shape. These categories are long bones, short bones, flat bones, irregular bones, and sesamoid bones (Figure 13-1). A brief description follows.
- **Long.** These bones are longer than they are wide. Examples are the humerus, radius, ulna, femur, tibia, fibula, metacarpals, metatarsals, and phalanges.
- **Short.** Short bones are generally small and cuboidal and contain multiple articulating surfaces, such as the carpals and tarsals.
- **Flat**. These bones possess a broad flat surface for muscle attachment or protection of underlying organs. The sternum, ribs, scapula, and certain skull bones are flat bones.
- **Irregular.** Consider this a catch-all category for bones that do not fit in other categories. Irregular bones are certain cranial bones, facial bones, the vertebrae, and the hyoid bone.
- **Sesamoid.** Sesamoid bones are small, round bones that are embedded in certain tendons. They are often found in the hands and feet. The largest sesamoid bone is the patella (kneecap), which is embedded in the quadriceps tendon.

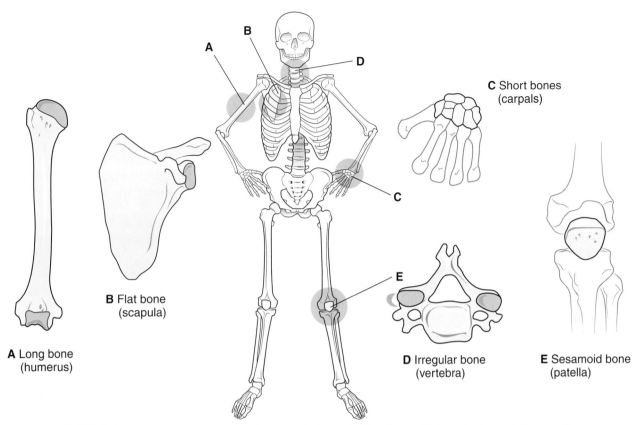

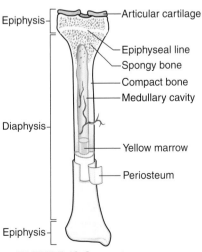

C Short bones
(carpals)

B Flat bone
(scapula)

A Long bone
(humerus)

D Irregular bone
(vertebra)

E Sesamoid bone
(patella)

FIGURE 13-1 Examples of bones. **A**, long bone. **B**, Flat bone. **C**, Short bones. **D**, Irregular bone. **E**, Sesamoid bone.

ANATOMY OF A LONG BONE

A typical long bone has two main regions: (1) the *diaphysis* and (2) the *epiphysis*. These and their associated structures are listed here (Figure 13-2).

Diaphysis: This region is the long cylindrical shaft of the bone.

- **Medullary cavity**: The medullary cavity is the hollow space within the center of the diaphysis. It contains *yellow marrow,* which is filled with fat. Blood cells formed in the cavity can exit the bone and enter the general circulation through the two types of canal systems.
  - **Haversian canals**: minute vascular canals that run longitudinally through the bone
  - **Volkmann's canals**: canals that connect the Haversian canals, running horizontally through the bone
- **Periosteum**: The fibrous, dense, vascular tissue sheath that surrounds the diaphysis and is noticeably absent on the epiphyses. It is the bone's life-support system, containing blood and lymphatic vessels, nerves, and bone-forming cells (osteoblasts) for growth and fracture healing.
- **Interosseous ligament**: A tough membrane that interconnects select bones (i.e., the ulna and radius, tibia and fibula) by attaching to their periosteum. It also provides muscle attachment. This structure is also referred to as the *interosseus membrane.*

Epiphyses: The two ends of a long bone, which are usually wider than the diaphysis, are the epiphyses (singular: epiphysis). The epiphyses are also where the bone grows in length.

- **Articular cartilage**: Articular surfaces, such as the epiphysis, are covered with articular cartilage. The cartilage type is hyaline.

FIGURE 13-2 Long bone anatomy.

- **Metaphysis**: The metaphysis contains the growth portion of the bone and are located where the diaphysis and epiphysis converge. Depending on the bone's age, it can contain the epiphyseal plate or the epiphyseal line.
  - **Epiphyseal plate**: In an immature bone, the epiphyseal plane is a thin layer of cartilage between the epiphysis and the diaphysis where new bone is formed. This is also known as the *growth plate* or *epiphyseal disk*.
  - **Epiphyseal line**: Replaces the epiphyseal plate when bone growth is complete.

HISTOLOGY

The microscopic cells within the skeletal system are the:
- **Osteoblasts:** bone-forming cells found in the periosteum
- **Osteoclasts:** cells in bone that break down bone tissue to maintain homeostasis of calcium and phosphates and to repair bone
- **Osteocytes:** mature osteoblasts or bone cells that soon become embedded in the bone's matrix

The skeletal system is composed of five different types of connective tissue: (1) osseous tissue, (2) cartilage, (3) ligaments, (4) periosteum, and (5) bone marrow. These tissue types have been introduced in Chapter 11. Osseous tissue can be classified according to its texture, differing only in bone density (Figure 13-3). These categories include spongy and compact bone.

Spongy bone: The lighter of the two, spongy bone is a latticelike network found in the center of long bones that are typically filled with red and yellow bone marrow. Bone marrow is where blood cells are made. Spongy bone makes up most of the inside of short, flat bones and is inside the ends of long bones.

Compact bone: The denser of the two types for added strength, compact bone tissue consists of bones cells almost completely surrounded by dense material made of calcium and phosphate. Few spaces are in compact bone

tissue. It forms the periphery of all bones and a portion of the shaft bulk of long bones such as the humerus. It provides protection and support and resists the stresses of weight and movement.

BONE DEVELOPMENT

The processes of bone development, or **ossification,** begin between the sixth and seventh week of embryonic life and continues throughout adulthood. Both of these mechanisms of ossification replace preexisting connective tissue with osseous connective tissue. The two types of ossification are:
- *Intramembranous ossification:* This process involves bone formation from membranes and is found on the roof and sides of the skull.
- *Intracartilaginous ossification:* This type of bone formation begins from cartilage and is found in the bones of the extremities.

BONE HEALTH, EXERCISE, AND AGING

During exercise, the skeletal system becomes stressed as a result of pulling forces (e.g., gravity, tendons, ligaments). The body responds to the demands of physical activity by secreting a hormone (calcitonin), which moves blood calcium into the bones. Osteoblasts are stimulated to create more bone tissue, thus stronger bones. The fact that bones must be physically stressed to remain strong and healthy cannot be overemphasized. When we remain physically active, when muscles and gravity exert force on skeletal bones, they respond by becoming stronger.

To maintain mineral homeostasis, the osteoclasts break down the bone's minerals and move them into the blood while osteoblasts replace the bone lost to metabolism. Both processes occur at approximately the same rate; thus bone density is relatively constant.

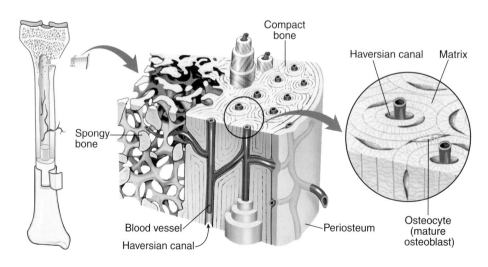

FIGURE 13-3 Spongy and compact bone.

As women and men age, they produce much smaller amounts of estrogen (estrogen helps keep calcium in bones). The decreased hormone level causes osteoblasts to become less active. As a result, osteoclasts break down bone faster than osteoblasts can rebuild it; therefore a decrease in bone mass occurs. Bone mass becomes so depleted, the skeleton can no longer withstand mechanical stress. This lack of bone replacement makes the bones porous (osteoporosis).

SKELETAL DISTRIBUTION

To make the study of the skeletal system easier, it can be divided into the following two distinct regions (Figure 13-4): (1) *axial skeleton,* consisting of the bones associated with the central axis of the body (skull, vertebrae, sternum, ribs); and (2) *appendicular skeleton* composed of the extremities (arms, legs, and girdles).

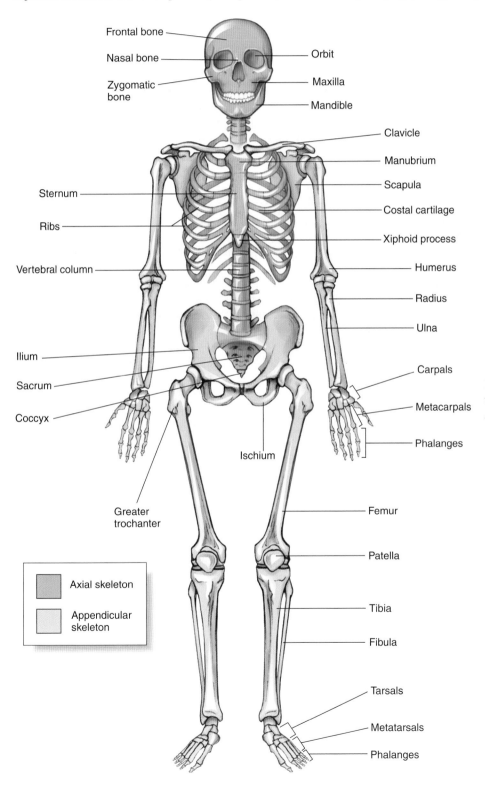

Frontal bone
Nasal bone
Zygomatic bone
Orbit
Maxilla
Mandible
Clavicle
Manubrium
Scapula
Sternum
Ribs
Costal cartilage
Xiphoid process
Vertebral column
Humerus
Radius
Ulna
Ilium
Sacrum
Carpals
Coccyx
Metacarpals
Phalanges
Ischium
Greater trochanter
Femur
Patella

Axial skeleton
Appendicular skeleton

Tibia
Fibula
Tarsals
Metatarsals
Phalanges

A   ANTERIOR VIEW

FIGURE 13-4 Axial and appendicular divisions of the skeletal system **A**, Anterior view. **B**, Posterior view.
Continued

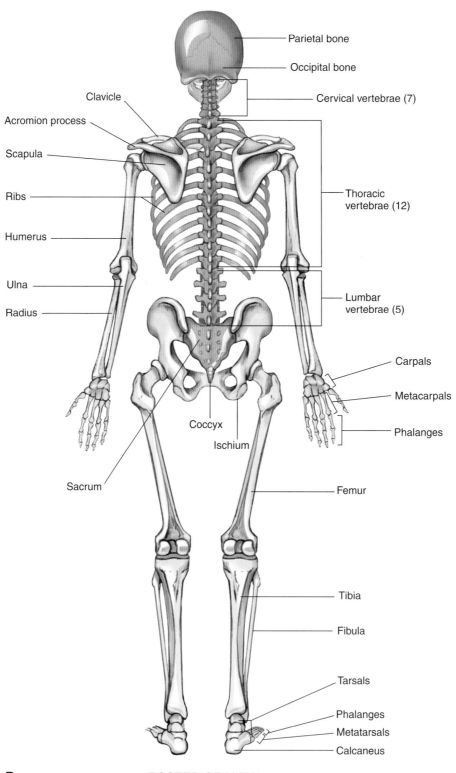

Parietal bone

Occipital bone

Cervical vertebrae (7)

Clavicle

Acromion process

Scapula

Ribs

Humerus

Ulna

Radius

Thoracic vertebrae (12)

Lumbar vertebrae (5)

Carpals

Metacarpals

Phalanges

Coccyx

Ischium

Sacrum

Femur

Tibia

Fibula

Tarsals

Phalanges

Metatarsals

Calcaneus

B

POSTERIOR VIEW

FIGURE 13-4, cont'd

Axial Skeleton

The axial skeleton contains 80 bones, including the following:
- **Skull:** total of 29 bones
  - 8 bones in the cranium
  - 14 bones in the face
  - 6 ear ossicles
  - 1 hyoid bone
- **Vertebral column:** total of 26 in an adult and 31 or 33 unfused bones in the embryo, depending on how many bones are present in the coccyx
- **Sternum:** one fused bone in the adult and three unfused bones in the embryo
- **Ribs:** total of 24 bones or 12 pairs of bones, located in the thorax

Extremities or Appendicular Skeleton

The appendicular skeleton contains 126 bones, including the following:
- **Shoulder girdle:** Often referred to as the *pectoral girdle,* the shoulder girdle contains the right and left clavicle and scapula, totaling four bones.
- **Pelvic girdle:** Consisting of a left and right ilium, ischium, and pubis, the adult pelvic girdle contains two bones, which are the aforementioned three bones fused together; total of two bones.
- **Upper limbs:** Each upper limb contains 30 bones, totaling 60 bones. Each upper limb contains a:
  - Humerus
  - Ulna
  - Radius
  - 8 carpals
  - 5 metacarpals
  - 14 phalanges
- **Lower limbs:** Each lower limb contains 30 bones, totaling 60 bones. Each lower limb contains a:
  - Femur
  - Patella
  - Tibia
  - Fibula
  - 7 tarsals
  - 5 metatarsals
  - 14 phalanges

BONY MARKINGS

Bones are not smooth but are marked with bumps, holes, and depressions. These markings are located where muscles, tendons, and ligaments attach and where nerve and blood vessels pass. These marks are called **bony markings,** *bony landmarks,* or *surface markings.* Because bones are among the hardest substances in the body, bony marking are fairly easy to locate beneath the skin. These landmarks assist the therapist in locating structures such as muscles, endangerment sites, and trigger points.

Even though specific bony markings are not yet identified, examples for each are listed so the therapist can make a connection between the description of the bony marking and its example (Table 13-1). Use this information to remember specific markings on bones when presented in Chapter 14.

TABLE 13-1   **List of Bony Marking Types**

BONY MARKING	DESCRIPTION	EXAMPLE
Angle	Projecting corner of a bone	Mandibular angle
Border	Linear bony ridge, often the edge of a bone	Medial border of the scapula
Condyle	Rounded projection that forms a joint; knuckle shaped	Lateral condyle of the femur
Crest	Very prominent linear elevation	Iliac crest
Epicondyle	Projection over a condyle	Medial epicondyle of the humerus
Facet	Small, smooth, shallow depression articulating with another bone	Vertebral articular facet
Foramen	Hole or opening for blood vessels and nerves to pass	Foramen magnum of the occipital bone
Fossa	Shallow depression in a bone	Glenoid fossa of the scapula
Groove	Depression that accommodates a structure	Intertubercular groove
Head	Rounded end of a bone	Fibular head
Line	A narrow bony ridge that is less prominent than a crest	Superior nuchal line
Meatus	Tubelike opening in a bone that forms a tunnel or canal	External auditory meatus of the temporal bone
Notch	Deep indention or a narrow gap in a bone	Trochlear notch
Process	General term for any prominence or prolongation from a bone	Styloid process of the radius
Protuberance	Knoblike protrusion of a bone	External occipital protuberance
Ramus	Long branchlike bony prolongation of a bone	Superior pubic ramus
Ridge	Elongated projection from a bone	Supracondylar ridge
Spine	Sharp, slender projection of a bone	Spine of the scapula
Trochanter	Large rough process found only on the femur	Greater trochanter
Tubercle	Rounded projection usually blunt and irregular	Lesser tubercle of the humerus
Tuberosity	Large, rounded rough projection	Deltoid tuberosity

IDA PAULINE ROLF, PhD

Born: May 18, 1896; died: March 19, 1979.

"God didn't come down and tell me; I had to find it out through many years of experience. The work came first; the inspiration came later."

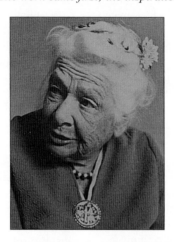

It was the middle of World War II, and most of America's men were far from home. Women began to fill roles they had never dreamed they would. One such young woman, Ida Pauline Rolf, accepted a position with the Rockefeller Institute, even though her father was dead set against it. War or peace, a proper lady stayed home where she belonged. After all, her family had money; she did not need to earn her way.

Rolf had a mind of her own. She earned a doctorate in biochemistry. She was just as passionate about philosophy and general semantics as she was about studying the science of the body; thus she explored homeopathy, was heavily influenced by osteopathy, and practiced yoga under the direction of a tantric yogi. Perhaps even more integral to her success than any other factor was that she was not afraid to pursue new directions.

Rolf's studies led her to Amy Cochran, an osteopath who claimed to have received her special abilities through a psychic encounter with Dr. Benjamin Rush, the physician who signed the Declaration of Independence. When Rolf returned to New York, she began work on a 45-year-old woman who had physical disabilities since the age of 8 years. Within a few years, the woman was up and walking.

Rolf believed that bodies are created balanced and comfortably supported by gravity, but injuries, overwork of one muscle group, or other postural dysfunctions result in fascia that are too tight or loose. Thus our bodies expend energy inefficiently and fight gravity rather than allow it to support us. She also believed that anything that made individuals feel fear or guilt could exhibit itself in bad physiological characteristics. For her, both mental and physical health make up two sides of the same coin.

Rolfing methodically restructures connective tissue through work on one body section at a time, gradually working deeper and deeper. The massage that we know today as *rolfing* was first called structural integration. When the container is aligned properly, the *stuff* inside functions as it should. Structural integration helps achieve homeostasis. Rolf's vision went beyond physi-

cal change because she believed that this tissue reorganization of the body was necessary to achieve spiritual growth.

Rosemary Feitis, Rolf's longtime assistant, writes, "[Ida] was not interested in curing symptoms; she was after a bigger game. She wanted nothing less than to create new, better human beings. The ills would cure themselves; the symptoms would melt as the organisms became balanced."*

To achieve this nirvana, Rolf used her fingers, elbows, and forearms to loosen myofascial restrictions, moving tissue until it was *in the right place*. Then she would proceed to the next problem area, asking for feedback as she went along. Eventually, she developed a sequence of 10 progressive sessions now referred to as the *Basic Ten*.

One of the most lasting impressions of rolfing seems to be that sessions must be painful to be effective. This was never Rolf's goal, and because of the body's reactive mechanism to pain, too much force may have a negative effect on results. In fact, Feitis quotes her as saying, "Don't just go in there as though you were a locomotive charging in at a 100 miles an hour. In general, if there is trouble going on inside the body, fascia on the outside will be so tight it will tend to protect the area that's in trouble. So don't barge through fascia. If you are doing the right thing, and there isn't some deep pathology, the fascia will let go—let you in."

Rolf tried to teach others what she had discovered and, at the same time, attempted to preserve the integrity of her work, but her commitment was singular. Not everyone shared her enthusiasm, work ethic, or understanding of the body. According to Feitis, Rolf did not want *mechanicalness*. She taught whomever she could and cautioned them to wait until they were experienced before considering themselves *rolfers*.

Eventually, an invitation to present her work at Esalen, a California resort proving ground for new movements, landed Rolf in the midst of a new type of student. She began to teach her work to those with no preconceived notions and a variety of backgrounds. The world began to take notice of her work. Research established its effectiveness. Articles

IDA PAULINE ROLF, PhD (*continued*)

were published. The Rolf Institute, formerly the Guild for Structural Integration, was created in the early 1970s.

Today, rolfing has undergone some change. Not all practitioners accept Rolf's notion of the perfect or ideal body. Others plan sessions according to clients' needs in-stead of the *Basic Ten*. It is hard to say what Rolf would think about this evolution.

---

*From Feitis R: *Ida Rolf talks about rolfing and physical reality*, New York, 1978, Harper and Row.

ARTICULATIONS

Articulations, or joints, are the meeting places for bones. Where bones come together, a joint or articulation is formed. Another term for a joint is an **arthrosis** (*pl.* arthroses).

Every bone in the human skeleton articulates with at least one other bone, except the hyoid bone. Where a joint exists so does joint movement. This movement may be limited, such as sutures in the cranium, or it may be highly mobile, such as the ball-and-socket joint of the shoulder.

Joints serve the following two purposes:
• They hold the bones together through the ligaments.
• They allow a rigid skeletal system to become somewhat flexible by changing their relative positions to one another when acted on by muscles or outside forces.

Joints can be classified according to the structure of the joint (specifically, what fills the joint cavity) and the amount of movement allowed.

Three Types of Articulations

The following list classifies joints based on the range or degree of movement that is allowed physiologically with its corresponding classification based on structure in italics (Figure 13-5).

Synarthroses

Movement in synarthrotic joints, also known as *fibrous joints,* is absent or extremely limited. Examples of synarthrotic joints are those between skull bones and sutures in the cranium, and between the tooth socket and the teeth.

Amphiarthroses

Also known as *cartilaginous joints,* these joints are slightly movable, such as the tibiofibular just below the knee, the costochondral joints of the ribs, and the pubic symphysis, where the hip bones join anteriorly, and the intervertebral joints, and move apart only a few millimeters. Some amphiarthrotic joints may be classified as gliding diarthrotic joints such as the sternoclavicular joints.

Diarthroses

Also known as *synovial joints,* these joints are freely movable joints. Synovial joints differ from synarthrotic and amphiarthrotic joints in that they have a space between the articulating bones called the *joint cavity.* Diarthrotic joints allow movement in one, two, or three dimensions. Many synovial joints also feature associated structures such as bursa sacs (bursae) filled with synovial fluid. Examples of synovial joints include knees, elbows, hips, shoulders, wrists, and knuckle joints of the fingers and toes.

TABLE TALK

Crepitus is a noisy discharge that may resemble a cracking sound and is produced by the body. Examples of crepitus are popping joints, rubbing of bone fragments, and flatulence. It can be the result of air present in subcutaneous tissue and can often be palpated.

Synovial Joints

Synovial joints are responsible for movements of the body. The following structures are associated with synovial joints (Figure 13-6):
• **Articular cartilage:** Synovial joints have articular cartilage that covers the epiphyses of the articulating bones. It is smooth and slippery, decreases friction, and helps absorb shock when the bones in the joint move. *Menisci* are pads of fibrocartilage found in the knees and other joints to help them fit together better and to absorb shock.
• **Joint capsule:** A joint capsule forms a sleeve around the synovial joint. It is actually a continuation of the periosteum of the bones involved in the joint. The outer layer is fibrous and forms ligaments, which connect the bones in the joint together.
  • **Joint cavity:** The inner region of the capsule is called the *joint cavity.* It is lined with a synovial membrane and filled with lubricating (synovial) fluid.
  • **Synovial membrane:** Synovial membranes line the joint cavity, synovial sheaths, and bursae. They secrete synovial fluid.

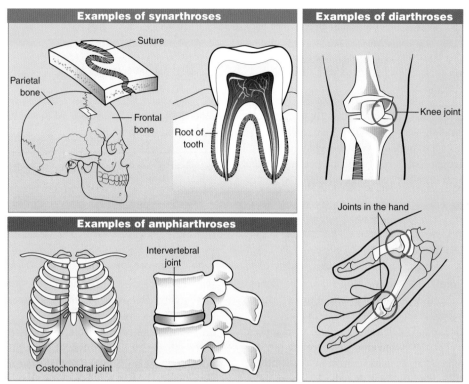

FIGURE 13-5 Classification of joints.

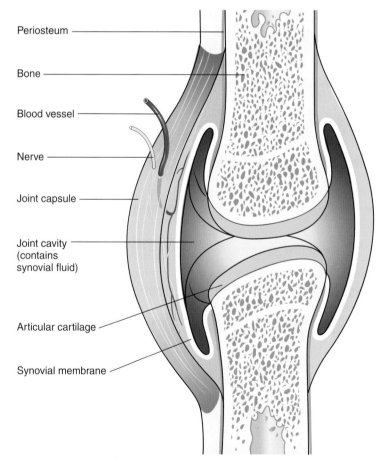

FIGURE 13-6 Synovial joint structure.

- **Synovial fluid:** Also known as *synovia*, this viscous fluid is found in synovial joints, sheaths, and bursae. Synovial fluid provides nutrition and lubrication so the joint can move freely without undue friction. The amount produced depends on the physical activity of the joints.
- **Accessory ligaments:** Many synovial joints have accessory ligaments that further stabilize the joint. Bursae can be found between ligaments and joint capsules. Functionally, ligaments are an extension of the bone to allow lightness, flexibility, and added strength.

The following structures are associated features of synovial joints and are not present in all synovial joints:

- **Bursae:** A bursa is a collapsed saclike structure with an interior lining of synovial membrane containing synovial fluid. It provides a cushion that protects a muscle's tendon from rubbing against the bone during muscular contraction. Many bursae also have villi (additional folds within the bursae to increase the surface area). Not all synovial joints have bursae (for example, the joints located in the ankles, fingers, and toes).
- **Synovial sheaths:** Synovial sheaths are similar to bursae in that they are lined with synovial membranes. However, instead of being flat, they are tubular. These structures surround long tendons and increase the gliding capacity of the tendons and are mainly found in the hands and feet.

ACTION TERMINOLOGY

The following movements are provided by the synovial joints of the body. An action refers to movement in anatomical position. Use the activity at the end of this section as an educational dramatization to assist you in learning joint movements.

Flexion bends or decreases the angle of a joint. *Lateral flexion* refers to the direction of flexion.
- Digital (Figure 13-7, *A* and *B*)
- Elbow (Figure 13-7, *C*)
- Hip (Figure 13-7, *D*)

- Knee (Figure 13-7, *E*)
- Neck (Figure 13-7, *F*)
- Shoulder (Figure 13-7, *G*)
- Spinal (Figure 13-7, *H*)
- Wrist (Figure 13-7, *I*)
- Neck: lateral (Figure 13-7, *J*)
- Spinal: lateral (Figure 13-7, *K*)

Extension straightens or increases the angle of a joint. *Lateral extension* refers to the direction of flexion. *Hyperextension* is a continuation of extension beyond the anatomical position, as in bending the head backward, and may or may not be used by some textbook authors.
- Digital (see Figure 13-7, *A* and *B*)
- Elbow (see Figure 13-7, *C*)
- Hip (see Figure 13-7, *D*)
- Knee (see Figure 13-7, *E*)
- Neck (see Figure 13-7, *F*)
- Shoulder (see Figure 13-7, *G*)
- Spinal (see Figure 13-7, *H*)
- Wrist (see Figure 13-7, *I*)
- Neck: lateral (see Figure 13-7, *J*)
- Spinal: lateral (see Figure 13-7, *K*)

Abduction is movement away from the median plane. *Horizontal abduction* refers to the direction of abduction.
- Digital (Figure 13-7, *L* and *M*); the median plane for finger abduction is the middle digit.
- Hip (Figure 13-7, *N*)
- Shoulder (Figure 13-7, *O*)
- Wrist, also referred to as *radial deviation* or *radial flexion* (Figure 13-7, *P*)

Adduction is movement toward the median plane. *Horizontal adduction* refers to the direction of adduction.
- Digital (see Figure 13-7, *L* and *M*); the median plane for finger abduction is the middle digit.
- Hip (see Figure 13-7, *N*)
- Shoulder (see Figure 13-7, *O*)
- Wrist, also referred to as *ulnar deviation* or *ulnar flexion* (see Figure 13-7, *P*)

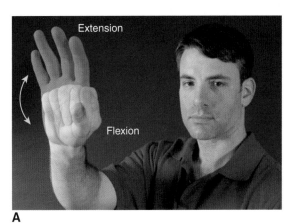
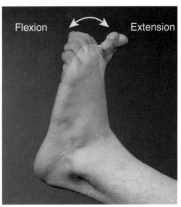

FIGURE 13-7 **A**, Finger flexion and extension. **B**, Toe flexion and extension.

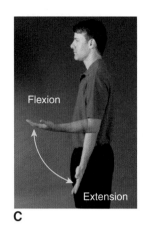
C

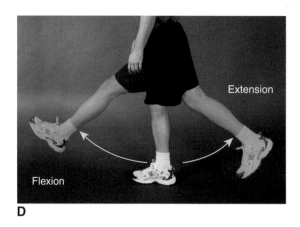
D

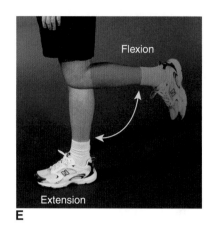
E

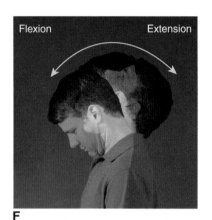
F

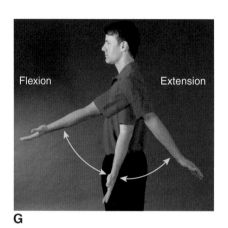
G

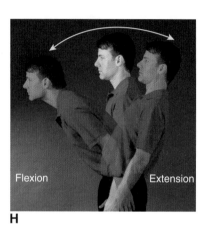
H

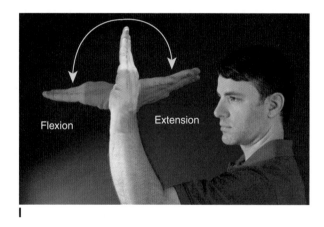
I

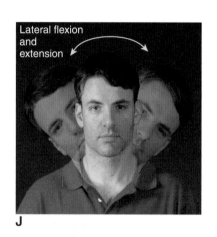
J

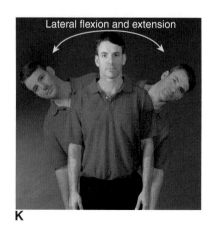
K

FIGURE 13-7, **cont'd C**, Elbow flexion and extension. **D**, Hip flexion and extension. **E**, Knee flexion and extension. **F**, Neck flexion and extension. **G**, Shoulder flexion and extension. **H**, Spinal flexion and extension. **I**, Wrist flexion and extension while elbow is flexed. **J**, Neck lateral flexion and extension. **K**, Spinal lateral flexion and extension.

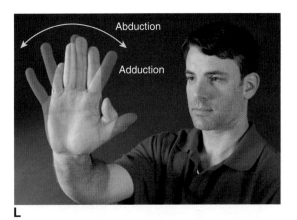

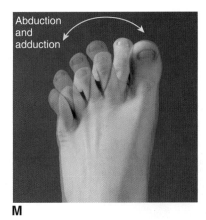

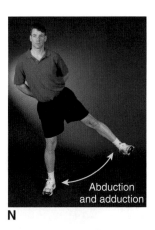

L   M   N

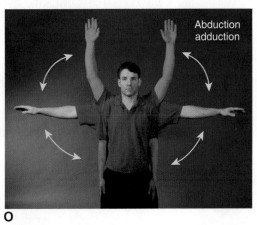

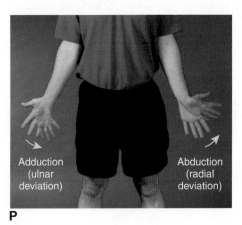

O   P

FIGURE 13-7, **cont'd L**, Finger abduction and adduction. **M**, Toe abduction and adduction. **N**, Hip abduction and adduction. **O**, Shoulder abduction and adduction. **P**, Wrist abduction and adduction.

> **TABLE TALK**
>
> Both ulnar and radial deviations occur around an axis that passes through the capitate.

> **TABLE TALK**
>
> To help remember the difference between radial and ulnar deviation, note that the letter *L* is in both *ulnar* and *little finger*. Hence, during u*l*nar deviation, the *L*ittle finger moves toward the ulna.

Supination is a lateral (outward) rotation of the forearm; the palm is turned up so it can hold a cup of soup (Figure 13-7, *Q*).

Pronation is medial (inward) rotation of the forearm; the palm is turned down and therefore prone to spill (see Figure 13-7, *Q*).

Plantar flexion is extension of the ankle so that the toes are pointing downward, increasing the ankle angle anteriorly (Figure 13-7, *R*).

Dorsiflexion is flexing the ankle dorsally so that the toes are moving toward the shin, as in walking on the heels (see Figure 13-7, *R*).

Inversion is elevation of the medial edge of the foot so that the sole is turned inward (or medially). When both feet are inverted, the soles of the feet face each other (Figure 13-7, *S*).

Eversion is elevation of the lateral edge of the foot so that the sole is turned outward (or laterally). When both feet are everted, the soles of the feet do not face each other (see Figure 13-7, *S*).

Circumduction occurs when the distal end moves in a circle and the proximal end is relatively fixed; it can be described as cone-shaped range of motion but is actually a combination of several movements such as flexion, extension, adduction, and abduction.

- Shoulder (Figure 13-7, *T*)
- Hip (Figure 13-7, *U*)
- Digital (Figure 13-7, *V*)

Rotation is circular movement when a bone moves around its own central axis. *Left* and *right* rotation refers to the direction of rotation and is reserved for joints that lie within the median axis, such as the head, neck, and spine. *Lateral* and *medial rotation* refers to direction of rotation and is used for joints that lie outside of the median axis, such as the shoulder, hip, and knee (the knee can be rotated slightly when flexed). *Upward (lateral)* and *downward (medial)* rotation are terms reserved for the scapula. In scapular rotation, the point of reference is its inferior angle. When the inferior angle slides laterally, it also slides upward. When the inferior angle slides medially, it also slides downward.

- Neck (Figure 13-7, *W*)
- Spinal (Figure 13-7, *X*)
- Shoulder (Figure 13-7, *Y*)
- Hip (Figure 13-7, *Z*)
- Knee (Figure 13-7, *AA*)
- Scapular (Figure 13-7, *BB*)

Elevation is raising or lifting a body part, moving superiorly.

- Mandibular (Figure 13-7, *CC*; mandibular elevation and depression)
- Scapular (Figure 13-7, *DD*; scapular elevation and depression)

Depression is lowering or dropping a body part, moving inferiorly.

- Mandibular (see Figure 13-7, *CC*)
- Scapular (see Figure 13-7, *DD*)

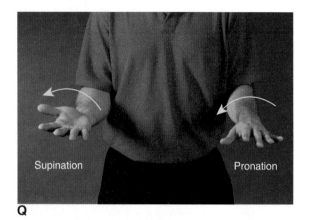

Q

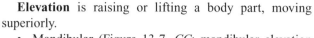
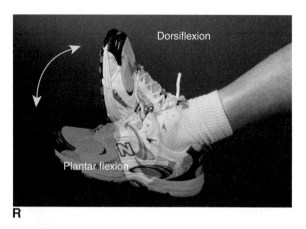

R

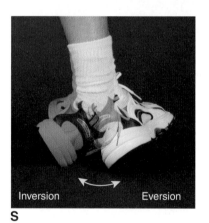

S

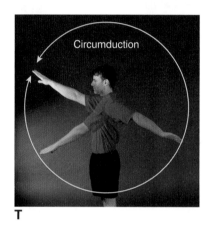

T

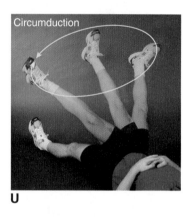

U

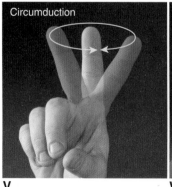

V

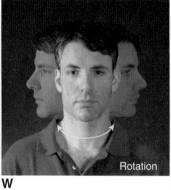

W

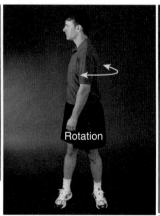

X

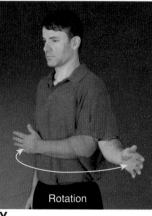

Y

FIGURE 13-7, cont'd Q, Supination and pronation. **R**, Plantar flexion and dorsiflexion. **S**, Inversion and eversion. **T**, Shoulder circumduction. **U**, Hip circumduction. **V**, Finger circumduction. **W**, Neck rotation. **X**, Spinal rotation. **Y**, Shoulder rotation with elbow flexed.

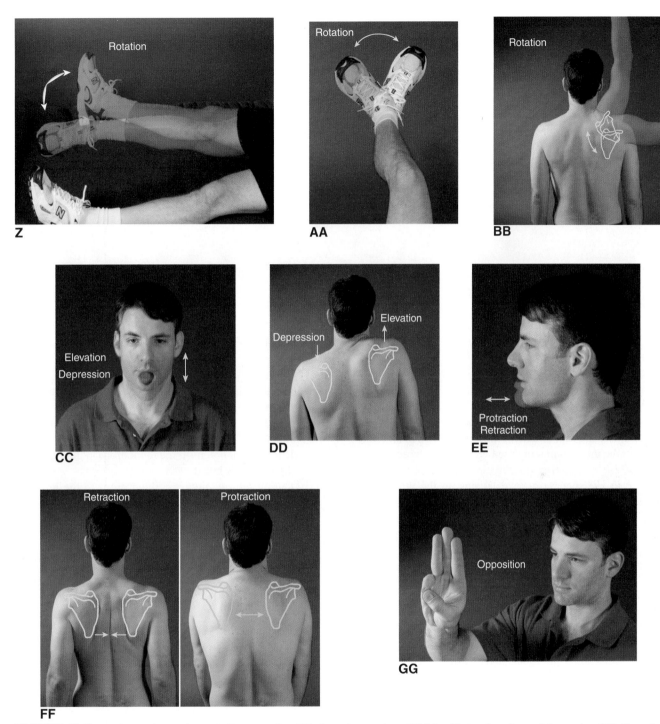

FIGURE 13-7, **cont'd Z**, Hip rotation. **AA**, Knee rotation. **BB**, Scapular rotation. **CC**, Mandibular elevation and depression. **DD**, Scapular elevation and depression. **EE**, Mandibular protraction and retraction. **FF**, Scapular protraction and retraction. **GG**, Thumb opposition.

Protraction is movement forward or anteriorly.
- Mandibular (Figure 13-7, *EE*)
- Scapular (Figure 13-7, *FF*)

Retraction is movement backward or posteriorly.
- Mandibular (see Figure 13-7, *EE*)
- Scapular (see Figure 13-7, *FF*)

Opposition is movement in which the tip of the thumb comes into contact with the tip of any other digit on the same hand (Figure 13-7, *GG*).

Lateral deviation, or side-to-side movement, in the transverse plane is often used when discussing mandibular movements (Figure 13-7, *HH*).

---

evolve *To play a "Match It" game using the action terms above, log on to the Evolve website and go to the course materials for Chapter 13. This fun game can be played to learn, review, or study.* ■

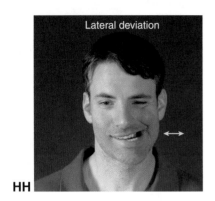

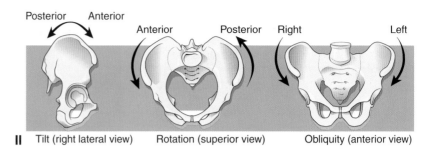

II   Tilt (right lateral view)   Rotation (superior view)   Obliquity (anterior view)

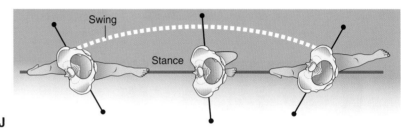

FIGURE 13-7, **cont'd HH**, Lateral deviations of the mandible. **II**, Pelvic tilts, rotations, and obliquities. **JJ**, Pelvic rotations during walking.

Pelvic Angles

Three terms are used to describe pelvic angles: (1) *tilt*, (2) *rotation*, and (3) *obliquity* (Figure 13-7, *II*). Tilt and rotation are the most commonly used terms. In all three categories, the point of reference is the ilium. Some kinesiologists choose to use specific bony markings on the ilium, such as the anterior and posterior iliac spines or the iliac crest. Caution is needed when applying these terms because they do not always delineate whether they are describing pelvic displacement or joint movement.

A pelvic **tilt** refers to an anterior or posterior tilting of the *entire* pelvis in the frontal plane. When describing anterior or posterior pelvic tilts, the reference point is the ilium (Figure 13-7, *JJ*).

- During an *anterior tilt*, the iliums are tilted forward. A common example is a person with lordosis, giving the lumbar spine an exaggerated anterior curve.
- During a *posterior tilt*, the iliums are tilted backward. A common example is a person who is seated, slouched in a chair.

During **rotation**, *one side* of the pelvis is further forward, or more anteriorly, than the other around a central axis. Again, the reference point is the ilium. If an ilium is rotated on one side, then the other ilium will be rotated in the opposite direction. Pelvic rotations occur as part of a normal gait pattern, ceasing when the subject is stationary (Figure 13-7, *JJ*).

- During an *anterior rotation*, the ilium is rotated forward.
- During a *posterior rotation,* the ilium is rotated backward.

With pelvic **obliquity,** *one side* of the pelvis is higher than the other side in the horizontal plane. The terms *right* or *left* are used to indicate the side that has lowered or dropped. Once

more, the ilium is the reference point. Some kinesiologists prefer to use the terms *hike* and *drop* or *lateral tilts*. Some level of pelvic rotation is found in individuals who have pelvic obliquity.

- During *right obliquity,* the ilium drops to the right, and the left hip is hiked.
- During *left obliquity,* the ilium drops to the left, and the right hip is hiked.

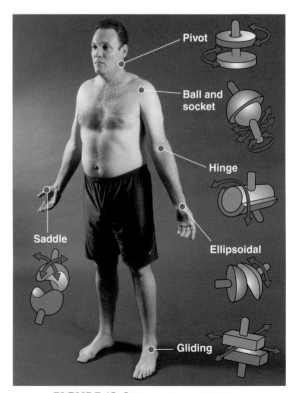

FIGURE 13-8 Types of synovial joints.

MINI-LAB

Perform the different joint movements, such as abduction of the arm and hip, rotation of the cervical region, flexion of the elbow and knee, and so on, until all joint movements have been experienced. Shout each movement as it is performed.

TYPES OF SYNOVIAL JOINTS

Synovial joints are the largest joint classification. The following six joint types allow different ranges of movement in one or all three known dimensions: hinge, pivot, ellipsoidal, saddle, gliding, and ball-and-socket (Figure 13-8). Note

that included in the discussion is whether joints are uni- or monoaxial, biaxial, or triaxial, referring to the number of axes or planes in which movement occurs (Figure 13-9). The following describes each synovial joint.

Hinge (monoaxial) joint movements are limited to flexion and extension, as in the knees, elbows, and interphalangeal joints. These joints possess one concave and one convex articular surface.

Pivot (monoaxial) joints allow movement that is limited to rotation, such as the atlantoaxial or the proximal radioulnar joints. Pivot joints possess one conical surface and one depressed surface.

Saddle (biaxial) joints resemble two saddles and allow movements of flexion, extension, abduction, adduction, opposition, reposition, and circumduction, but rotation is not

Types	Examples		Movements
Monoaxial	Around one axis; in one plane		
Hinge	**Elbow joint** (spool-shaped process fits into concave socket) 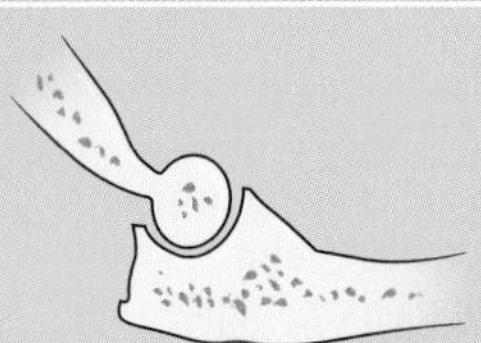	A	Flexion and extension
Pivot	**Joint between first and second cervical vertebrae** (arch-shaped process fits around peg-like process) 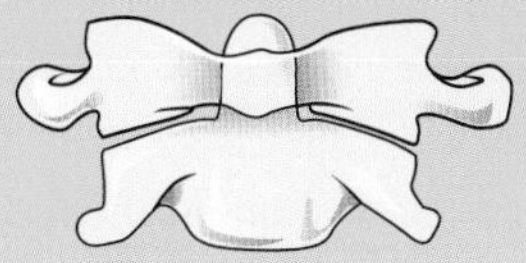	B	Rotation
Biaxial	Around two axes, perpendicular to each other; in two planes		
Saddle	**Thumb joint between metacarpal and carpal** (saddle-shaped bone fits into socket that is concave-convex-concave)	C 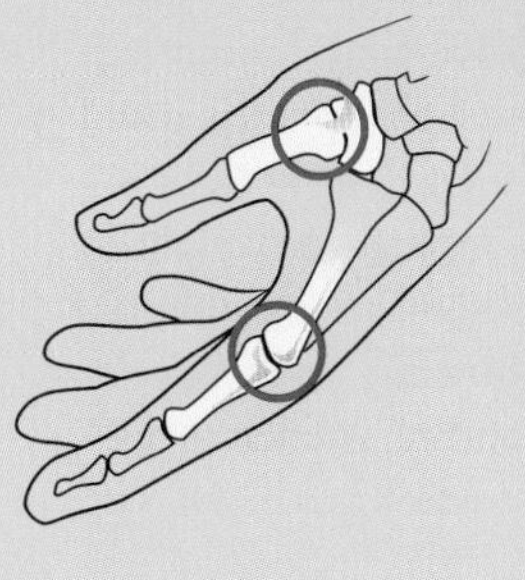	Flexion, and extension in one plane; abduction; adduction in other plane; circumduction, opposing thumb to fingers
Ellipsoidal	**Joint between metacarpal and phalanges** (oval condyle fits into elliptical socket)		Flexion, extension in one plane; abduction; adduction in other plane
Multiaxial	Around many axes		
Ball and socket	**Hip joint** (ball-shaped process fits into concave socket) 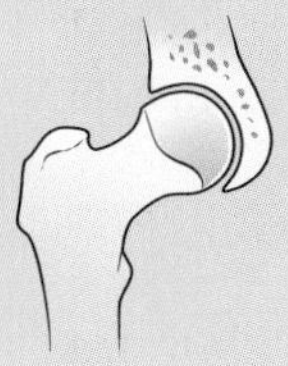	D	Widest range of movements; flexion, extension, abduction, adduction, rotation, circumduction
Gliding	**Joints between articular facets of adjacent vertebrae** (relatively flat articulating surfaces) 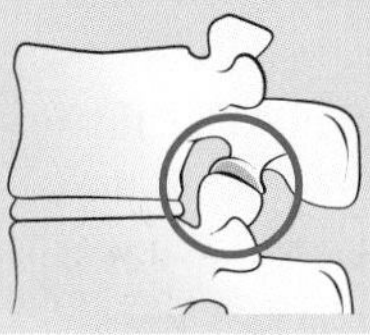	E	Gliding movements without any angular or circular movements

FIGURE 13-9 Classification of levers.

permitted. The articulating surfaces are concave in one direction and convex in the other. The only saddle joints are the carpometacarpal of the thumb. The joint between the malleus and incus in ear canal is structurally a saddle joint, but it is not a synovial joint.

Ellipsoidal (biaxial) joints are essentially reduced ball-and-socket joints. Ellipsoidal joints contain one oval convex surface and one concave surface, allowing flexion, extension, abduction, and adduction, but rotation is not permitted. Examples of ellipsoidal joints are radiocarpal joints located in the wrist and joints between the metacarpals and metatarsals and the phalanges.

Ball-and-socket (triaxial) joints, such as the hips and shoulders, permit all movements and offer the greatest range of motion. In these joints, one articular surface is rounded, fitting into a cuplike cavity.

Gliding (triaxial) joints permit all movements but are limited to gliding; gliding is present in acromioclavicular and intertarsal joints, to name a few. Both articular surfaces are nearly flat.

MINI-LAB

Flex your right elbow 90 degrees and affix your upper arm to your torso so it does not move. Place your left hand on your right ulna. Begin to pronate and supinate your right hand. Notice how your ulna never moves. Also notice how the thumb moves 180 degrees. Pronation and supination result from the radius rotating over the distal end of the ulna. The hand follows the movement of the radius.

CLASSIFICATION OF LEVERS

For the muscular system to produce movement at joints, it uses the skeletal system for leverage. A lever (bone) is a rod that is moved by use of a fulcrum (joint). For a lever to be set in motion, two forces must act on it: (1) resistance (weight of body and/or an object) and (2) effort (muscular contraction).

Levers are categorized into the following three classes according to how the fulcrum, effort, and resistance are arranged (Figure 13-10).

Class-1 Levers

Class-1 levers resemble a seesaw. The fulcrum is positioned between the effort and the resistance. The cranium sitting on top of a vertebra is an example of a class-1 lever. This lever is the least common type of lever in the body.

Class-2 Levers

Class-2 levers function as would a wheelbarrow. The fulcrum is at one end, the resistance is in the middle, and the effort is at the opposite end. One example of a class-2 lever is rising up on the toes.

Class-3 Levers

Class-3 levers are the most common and resemble sweeping with a broom. The fulcrum is at one end, the effort is located in the central portion, and the resistance is at the opposite end. Two examples of a class-3 lever are flexing the elbow.

PATHOLOGICAL CONDITIONS OF THE SKELETAL SYSTEM

Ankylosing Spondylitis

Ankylosing spondylitis is an inflammatory disease leading to calcification and fusion of the joints between vertebrae or in the sacroiliac joint. It is common in men between the ages of 20 and 40 years. Pain and stiffness is present in the hips and lower back and can progress upward along the spine. Inflammation can lead to loss of movement of the joints (ankylosis) and kyphosis. *Position client for comfort. Use techniques to retain joint mobility; do not force ankylosed joints into movement.*

Baker's Cyst

A Baker's cyst is a cyst behind the knee caused by escape of synovial fluid, which becomes enclosed in a membranous sac. It may only appear when the knee is extended. *Local contraindication of involved area.*

Bunion

A bunion is an abnormal medial tilting and enlargement of the joint between the first metatarsal of the great toe and the associated proximal phalanx, but it can also be found on the lateral side of the foot. Bunions are caused by chronic irritation and pressure from poorly fitted shoes or inflammation of the plantar fascia. *Local contraindication if pressure on infected area causes pain.*

Bursitis

Acute or chronic inflammation of the bursae is called *bursitis*. It is most often caused by direct trauma or chronic overuse of the tendon located over the bursae. The most common types of bursitis are subacromial bursitis, subcoracoid bursitis, subscapular bursitis, olecranon bursitis, trochanteric bursitis, ischial bursitis, prepatellar bursitis, and calcaneal bursitis. *Local contraindication of infected area during acute stage. Cold packs can be applied to reduce swelling while in acute phase. If chronic, assess joint mobility and pain with movement, and, if indicated, use joint mobilizations, stretches, and friction to maintain joint mobility. Ice after treatment.*

Dislocation

A dislocation (luxation) occurs when bones are forced out of their normal joint position. Accessory ligaments, tendons, joint capsules, and blood vessels are torn in the process. *Local*

MECHANICAL ASPECT   COMMON EXAMPLE   MUSCULOSKELETAL
                                                       COMPONENT

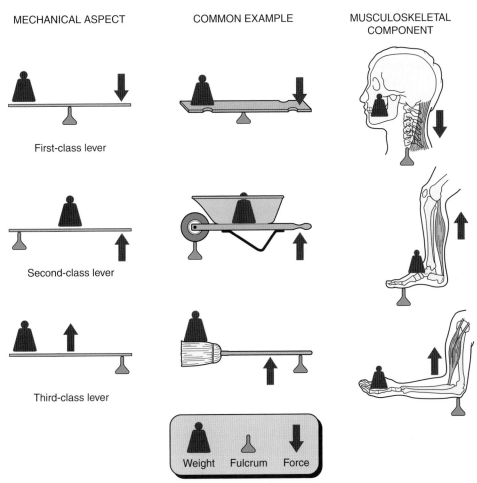

First-class lever

Second-class lever

Third-class lever

| Weight | Fulcrum | Force |

FIGURE 13-10 First-, second-, and third-class levers.

contraindication of involved area, including joint mobilizations. Otherwise, use techniques to increase joint mobility (e.g., stretching, joint mobilizations, cross-fiber friction).

Fractures

A fracture is a break, chip, crack, or rupture in a bone. Bones are highly vascularized, but healing sometimes takes months because calcium and phosphorus are deposited slowly in new bone. The three most common types of fractures are (1) simple (closed) fractures, (2) compound (open) fractures, and (3) stress fractures. *While bone is immobilized, massage near the fracture using techniques to maintain circulation and joint mobility, increase muscle tone, reduce edema, decrease spasms, and reduce pain. Work proximal areas first, then distal areas. Once healed (physician determined), begin slowly for approximately a week, using techniques to help client regain joint mobility and increase tone in muscles that may have atrophied. Then proceed at client's tolerance.*

Gouty Arthritis

Gouty arthritis is characterized by abnormal accumulation of uric acid. Uric acids are produced when nucleic acids are metabolized; uric acids are then converted to monosodium urate crystals. In most cases, uric acids are eliminated in urine. Some individuals, usually men, either produce excessive amounts or are unable to excrete uric acids, resulting in abnormally high levels in the blood. Sodium urate crystals eventually settle in the soft tissue around joints, typically the feet and toes, causing irritation, pain, and swelling. Typically, the first joint affected is the metatarsophalangeal joint of the great toe. Initial bouts may just last a few days; later bouts may last several weeks. *Local contraindication of affected area, which includes joint mobilizations.*

Hammertoe

A hammertoe is a condition in which the proximal phalanx of a toe (most commonly the second toe) is extended and the second and distal phalanges are flexed, causing a clawlike appearance. *Use lighter pressure over the affected area.*

Herniated Disk

Protrusion of the nucleus pulposus from the annulus fibrosus of an intervertebral disk is called a *herniated disk*. The protruding disk may impinge on nerve roots, causing numbness and pain, and may be a result of improper lifting or direct trauma. A herniated disk is also called a *ruptured disk* or a *slipped disk. **Obtain physician clearance. Once granted, use techniques to relieve pain. Focus on iliopsoas, paraspinals, and quadratus lumborum. Use heat first; follow treatment with ice. Avoid traction or mobilization of the involved area.***

Kyphosis

Often called *hunchback* or *hyperkyphosis,* kyphosis is an exaggeration of the normal posterior thoracic curve. Typically, the chest appears caved in, the arms tend to hang in the front of the body, and the head moves forward. Mild to moderate back pain often accompanies this condition. Kyphosis may be caused by rickets (vitamin D deficiency), degeneration of the intervertebral disks in older adults, chronic spasticity of the pectoralis major and minor and serratus anterior muscles, or weak rhomboid major and minor muscles. Rounded shoulders and a dowager's hump are occasionally classified as a mild form of kyphosis. ***Focus on involved muscles (pectoralis major and minor, serratus anterior, rhomboids major/minor), taking care not to over-stretch the spine. If caused by osteoporosis, use light pressure and avoid joint mobilizations.***

Lordosis

Often regarded as *hyperlordosis,* lordosis, or *swayback,* is an exaggeration of the anterior curvature of the lumbar concavity. A tightening of the back muscles followed by a weakening of the abdominal muscles is typical. Increased weight gain or pregnancy may cause or exacerbate this spinal condition. Because of the anterior tilt of the pelvis, hamstring problems are common. ***Focus on muscles of anterior and posterior pelvic tilt (e.g., abdominal muscles, quadratus lumborum, psoas major, paraspinals).***

Lyme Disease

Also called *Lyme arthritis,* Lyme disease is a recurrent form of arthritis caused by the bacterium *Borrelia burgdorferi,* transmitted by a deer tick. This disease usually starts with a bull's-eye rash followed by influenza-like symptoms and joint inflammation. The condition was originally described in the community of Lyme, Connecticut, but has been reported throughout North America and in other countries. ***Adjust massage to client's stamina and vitality (i.e., slower, gentler, shorter duration; assist client on and off table), using techniques to retain joint mobility. Massage is contraindicated if client is experiencing widespread inflammation.***

Osgood-Schlatter Disease

Osgood-Schlatter disease results from overuse of the quadriceps muscle (knee extension). The anterior inferior knee region becomes irritated and inflamed; the tibial tuberosity may even become partially separated. This condition is seen primarily in muscular, athletic adolescents and is marked by swelling and tenderness over the tibial tuberosity that increases with any activity that extends the knee. ***Massage is***

contraindicated during acute phase. Afterward, massage is fine. Focus treatment on reducing adhesion around knee and reducing tension in the quadriceps.

Osteoarthritis

Osteoarthritis (OA) is a chronic, progressive erosion of the articular cartilage resulting from chronic inflammation. OA is often called the *wear-and-tear arthritis.* The most commonly affected areas are weight-bearing joints, which may eventually become immovable. OA, which is more common than rheumatoid arthritis, is most often seen in the elderly population. ***Deep-pressure stretching and joint mobilizations are contraindicated. Use techniques to warm and loosen surrounding tissues.***

Osteoporosis

Osteoporosis is characterized by decreased bone mass and increased susceptibility to fractures. This condition is common in postmenopausal women because of a drop in estrogen (estrogen helps keep calcium in bones). Bone mass becomes so depleted that the skeleton can no longer withstand mechanical stress. Osteoporosis is responsible for hip and other bone fractures, shrinkage of the backbone, height loss, hunched backs, and considerable pain. ***Use light pressure over bones. Limit or avoid joint mobilizations.***

Rheumatoid Arthritis

Rheumatoid arthritis (RA) is a systemic arthritis that destroys synovial membranes, especially in the joints of the hands and feet. These membranes are replaced by fibrous tissues, which add to the joint stiffness already present. This process greatly reduces range of motion of the involved joints. Bilateral involvement is typical with a high incident of crippling deformity. The cause of RA is unknown, but it is believed to be an autoimmune disease. People who have RA experience flare-ups and remissions. ***Massage is contraindicated during flare-ups. Otherwise, use techniques that reduce stress and increase joint mobility.***

Scoliosis

Scoliosis is the lateral deviation or curvature in the normally straight vertical line of the vertebral column, usually in the thoracic region. Causes of scoliosis include congenital malformations of the spine, poliomyelitis, paralysis, chronic spasticity of select muscles, and postural deviations, distorted ribcage, and leg length discrepancy. Unequal position of the hips or shoulders is often an indication of this condition. Early detection and intervention may prevent progression of the curvature. The vast majority of people who have scoliosis are women (80%). ***If not caused by a contraindicated condition, massage is okay. Focus on iliopsoas, quadratus lumborum, and the paraspinal muscles. Position client for comfort. Avoid overstretching the spine.***

Separation

A separation is almost the same as a dislocation, but joint structures are simply pulled and stretched; the bone is not displaced out of the joint capsule. *Position client for comfort. Avoid undue pressure over separated bones. Avoid joint mobilizations until condition is completely healed.*

Spondylolisthesis

Spondylolisthesis is an anteriorly displaced vertebra, usually the fifth lumbar vertebra over the first sacral vertebra. This condition can range from mild to severe. Severe cases deform the spine. *Massage is fine if symptoms are not severe. Use strokes to loosen tight paraspinals and latissimus dorsi. Tight muscles in the area can be stretched but should not be forced.*

Spondylosis

Spondylosis, a general term for degeneration of the spinal column resulting from OA, is often called *arthritis of the spine. Position client for comfort.*

Sprain

Joint trauma that stretches or tears the ligamentous attachments without bone displacement is called a sprain. Sprains cause pain and possible temporary disability. Depending on the severity of the injury, taking 6 months to a year to completely rehabilitate is not uncommon for a ligamentous sprain because ligaments have few blood vessels. Acute ligament sprains can be classified into three grades or degrees of severity: first, second, and third degree. *Obtain physician clearance. Once granted, avoid stretching the injured area.*

Temporomandibular Joint Dysfunction

Temporomandibular joint (TMJ) dysfunction is a common ailment afflicting the jaw joint, its musculature, or both. The chief symptoms of TMJ are pain (e.g., jaw pain, toothache, headache, earache), clicking of the joint, and limited range of motion. Causes of TMJ dysfunction include trauma to the joint; chewing hard objects, especially if only on one side of the mouth; biting fingernails; teeth clenching or grinding (bruxism) whether awake or asleep; poor alignment of the upper and lower teeth; and emotional stress. *Treat involved muscles (i.e., masseter, temporalis, medial and lateral pterygoids, trapezius, rhomboids, levator scapula, scalenes, splenius muscles, suboccipitals).*

Whiplash

Whiplash is a sprain or strain of the cervical spine and spinal cord at the junction of the fourth and fifth cervical vertebrae, usually resulting from sudden acceleration (causing extension) or deceleration (causing flexion). This condition can occur in a rear-end vehicle collision that causes violent back and forth movement of the head and neck. Because of their greater mobility, the four upper vertebrae act as the lash, and the lower three act as the handle of the whip. Symptoms may include headaches, dizziness, pain, and inflammation. *Obtain physician clearance. Once granted, rule out other prevailing disorders (e.g., vertebral luxation). For anterior-posterior whiplash, focus on longus colli, scalenes, splenius muscles, sternocleidomastoid, levator scapula, and upper trapezius. For lateral whiplash, focus on scalenes and sternocleidomastoid. End session with ice.*

BOX 13-1

Effects of Massage on Connective Tissues

Reduces keloid formation. Massage applied to scar tissue helps reduce keloid formation in scar tissue beneath the site of massage application.

Reduces excessive scar formation. Deep massage reduces excessive scar formation, thereby helping create an appropriate scar that is strong yet does not interfere with the muscle's ability to broaden as it contracts.

Decreases adhesion formation. Deep, specifically applied massage helps decrease adhesions, which, in turn, facilitates normal, pain-free motion of the affected muscles and joints.

Releases fascial restrictions. Pressure and the heat it produces convert fascia from a gel state to a sol state (thixotropy), thereby reducing hyperplasia. Softening of the fascia surrounding muscles allows them to be stretched to their fullest resting length, thereby increasing joint range of motion and freeing the body of restricted movements.

Increases mineral retention in bone. Massage increases the retention of nutrients such as nitrogen, sulfur, and phosphorus in bones.

Promotes fracture healing. When a bone is fractured, the body forms a network of new blood vessels at the break site. Massage increases circulation around the fracture, thereby promoting fracture healing. Increased circulation around a fracture leads to increased deposition of callus to the bone. Callus is formed between and around the broken ends of a fractured bone during healing and is ultimately replaced by compact bone.

Improves connective tissue healing. Occurring only with deep pressure massage, proliferation and activation of fibroblasts were noted. Fibroblasts generate connective tissue matrix, which promotes tissue healing by increasing collagen production and increasing the tensile strength of healed tissue.

Reduces surface dimpling of cellulite. Massage flattens out fat deposits located under the skin and makes the skin seem smoother. Cellulite, a type of fat, appears as groups of small dimples or depressions under the skin caused by an uneven separation of fat globules below the skin's surface, which are displaced by manual manipulation. Massage does not reduce the amount of cellulite below the skin; instead, it temporarily alters the shape and appearance of cellulite.

---

evolve On the Evolve website, download and print out the crossword puzzles to reinforce the important terms and concepts from this chapter. ∎

SUMMARY

The intricate structures of bone, cartilage, ligament, and joints are what compose our skeletal system. The skeleton acts as a supportive framework for the rest of our body systems. It protects our delicate internal organs and acts as a storehouse for fats, vital minerals, and blood cell production.

Bones are living tissue that is strong, flexible, and relatively light. The bones of the human body number 206. The study of the skeletal system is not limited to bone alone. It includes the tissue of the bone itself, types of joints, movement, leverage, pathological skeletal conditions, and the specific bony markings.

Finally, bones are the massage therapist's landmarks to muscle location. Although the various soft tissues are at times indistinguishable from one another, bone is easily palpated. Because muscle attachment is fairly consistent from one person to the next, the bones act as reference points for locating muscles.

evolve

Go to *Chapter Extras* on Evolve for additional illustrations and resources for this chapter. *Extras* for this chapter include:

1. Drag and drop (online game)
2. Action terms (worksheet)
3. Microscopic image of Haversian and Volkmann canals within long bones (illustration)
4. Anterior pelvic tilt (photograph)
5. Left hip obliquity (photograph)

MATCHING I

Place the letter of the answer next to the term or phrase that best describes it.

A. Arthrosis
B. Bony markings
C. Cavity
D. Diaphysis

E. Diarthroses
F. Epiphysis
G. Hemopoiesis
H. Medullary

I. Metaphysis
J. Osteoblast
K. Periosteum
L. Sesamoid

_____   1.   Process of blood cell formation occurring in red marrow of long bones

_____   2.   Small, round bone found in tendons

_____   3.   Cylindrical shaft of a long bone

_____   4.   Cavity located within the center of a diaphysis

_____   5.   Dense, fibrous sheath surrounding a diaphysis

_____   6.   End of a long bone

_____   7.   Grown portion of a long bone

_____   8.   Bone-forming cell

_____   9.   Synonymous with the word *joint*

_____   10.   Places on bones where muscles, tendons, and ligaments attach and where nerve and blood vessels pass

_____   11.   Inner region of a joint capsule lined with synovial membranes

_____   12.   Freely movable joints

MATCHING II

Place the letter of the answer next to the term or phrase that best describes it.

A. Abduction   E. Dorsiflexion   I. Protraction
B. Adduction   F. Inversion   J. Retraction
C. Ball-and-socket   G. Pivot   K. Rotation
D. Circumduction   H. Plantar flexion   L. Supination

_____ 1. Lateral rotation of the forearm so that the palm is turned up

_____ 2. Movement toward the median plane

_____ 3. Extension of the ankle so that the toes are pointing downward

_____ 4. Flexing the ankle dorsally so that the toes are moving toward the shin

_____ 5. Movement backward

_____ 6. Elevation of the medial edge of the foot so that the sole is turned inward

_____ 7. Occurs when distal end of a joint moves in a circle and the proximal end is relatively fixed

_____ 8. Movement away from the median plane

_____ 9. Movement occurring when a bone moves around its own central axis

_____ 10. Movement forward

_____ 11. Joint where only rotation is permitted

_____ 12. Joint with the greatest range of movement

INTERNET ACTIVITIES

Visit http://www.spineuniverse.com and click on What Causes Sciatica? Share your findings with classmates.

Visit http://www.spineonline.com/ and watch one of the videos or animations on spinal surgery. Make a note of all the structures you recognize.

Visit http://www.frontiernet.net/~imaging/gait_model.html and visually study human gait patterns.

Bibliography

Abrahams P, Marks S, Hutchings R: *McMinn's color atlas of human anatomy,* St Louis, 2003, Mosby.

Applegate EJ: *The anatomy and physiology learning system,* ed 3, Philadelphia, 2006, Saunders.

Beers MH, Berkow R: *The Merck manual of diagnosis and therapy,* Whitehouse Station, NJ, 2006, Merck Research Laboratories.

Como D, editor: *Mosby's medical, nursing, and allied health dictionary,* ed 6, St Louis, 2002, Mosby.

Crawley J, Van De Graaff KM: *A photographic atlas for anatomy and physiology,* Englewood, Colo, 2000, Morton.

Damjanov I: *Pathophysiology for the health-related professions,* ed 3, Philadelphia, 2006, Saunders.

Dominguez R, Gajda R: *Total body training,* New York, 1984, Warnerbooks.

Ferri FF: *2003 Ferri's clinical advisor, instant diagnosis and treatment,* St Louis, 2003, Mosby.

Frazier MS, Drzymkowski JW: *Essentials of human diseases and conditions,* ed 3, Philadelphia, 2004, Saunders.

Goldberg S: *Clinical anatomy made ridiculously simple,* Miami, 2004, Medmaster.

Gould BE: *Pathophysiology for the health professions,* ed 3, Philadelphia, 2006, Saunders.

Grafelman T: *Graf's anatomy and physiology guide for the massage therapist,* Aurora, Colo, 1998, DG Publishing.

Guyton A: *Human physiology and mechanisms of disease,* ed 6, Philadelphia, 1996, Saunders.

Haubrich WS: *Medical meanings, a glossary of word origins,* New York, 1984, Harcourt Brace Jovanovich.

Huether SE, McCance KL: *Understanding pathophysiology,* ed 3, St Louis, 2004, Mosby.

Jacob S, Francone C: *Elements of anatomy and physiology,* Philadelphia, 1989, Saunders.

Kapandji IA: *The physiology of the joints,* ed 5, New York, 1988, Churchill Livingstone.

Kapit W, Elson LM: *The anatomy coloring book,* ed 3, New York, 2002, Benjamin Cummings.

Kapit W, Macey R, Meisami E: *The physiology coloring book,* ed 2, New York, 1999, HarperCollins.

Kordish M, Dickson S: *Introduction to basic human anatomy,* Lake Charles, La, 1985, McNeese State University.

Kumar V Abbas A, Fausto N: *Robbins and Cotran physiologic basis of disease,* ed 7, St Louis, 2005, Mosby.

Luttgens K, Wells K: *Kinesiology: scientific basis of human motion,* ed 7, Philadelphia, 1990, Saunders College Publishing.

Marieb EN: *Essentials of human anatomy and physiology,* ed 8, New York, 2005, Benjamin Cummings.

Martini FH, Bartholomew EF: *Essentials of anatomy and physiology,* ed 3, New York, 2003, Benjamin Cummings.

McAleer N: *The body almanac,* Garden City, NY, 1985, Doubleday.

McAtee R: *Facilitated stretching,* ed 2, Colorado Springs, Colo, 1999, Human Kinetics.

McCance K, Huether S: *Pathophysiology: the biological basis for disease in adults and children,* St Louis, 2006, Mosby.

Merck manual, ed 17, Whitehouse Station, NJ, 1998, Merck and Company.

Moore KL: *Clinically oriented anatomy,* ed 5, Baltimore, 2005, Lippincott Williams & Wilkins.

Netter FH: *Atlas of human anatomy,* ed 3, Teterboro, NJ, 2003, Icon Learning Systems.

Newton D: *Pathology for massage therapists,* ed 2, Portland, Ore, 1995, Simran Publications.

Platzer W: *Color atlas and textbook of human anatomy: locomotor system,* vol 1, ed 3, New York, 1984, Thieme.

Premkumar K: *Pathology A to Z, a handbook for massage therapists,* Baltimore, 1999, Lippincott Williams & Wilkins.

Salvo SG, Anderson SK: *Mosby's pathology for massage therapists,* St Louis, 2004, Elsevier Mosby.

Solomon EP, Phillips GA: *Understanding human anatomy and physiology,* Philadelphia, 1987, Saunders.

Southmayd W, Hoffman M: *Sports health: the complete book of athletic injuries,* New York and London, 1981, Quick Fox.

Souza TA: *Differential diagnosis and management for the chiropractor,* ed 2, Gaithersburg, Md, 2001, Aspen Publications.

Thibodeau G, Patton K: *Anatomy and physiology,* ed 6, St Louis, 2006, Mosby.

Thibodeau G, Patton K: *Structure and function of the body,* ed 12, St Louis, 2004, Mosby.

Tortora GJ: *Introduction to the human body: the essentials of anatomy and physiology,* ed 5, Hoboken, NJ, 2000, Wiley, John & Sons.

Tortora GJ, Grabowksi SR: *Principles of anatomy and physiology,* ed 11 New York, 2005, John Wiley & Sons.

Venes D, Thomas CL, Taber CW: *Taber's cyclopedic medical dictionary,* ed 20, Philadelphia, 2005, FA Davis.

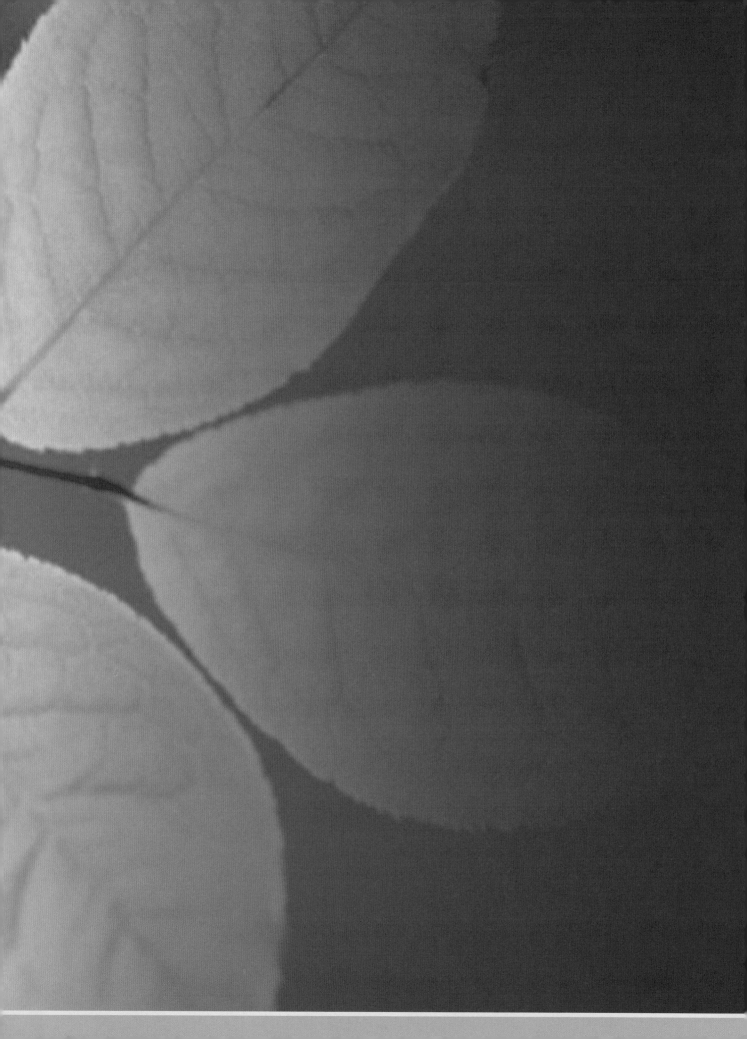

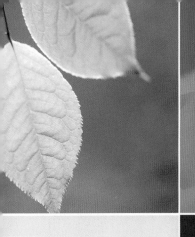

CHAPTER 14

"The map is not the territory."
—Alfred Korzbyski

Skeletal Nomenclature

STUDENT OBJECTIVES

After completing this chapter, the student should be able to:

- Describe the general locations of each bone listed in the chapter
- Distinguish between the right and the left in most bones of the appendicular skeleton
- Locate each bony marking listed in the chapter
- Define each bony marking according to its significance in massage therapy
- Identify bony markings that are endangerment sites in massage therapy
- Distinguish between the proximal and the distal ends of longs bones of the appendicular skeleton
- Under teacher supervision, examine the bony markings on yourself or a classmate
- Name and locate each joint listed in Lesson V of this chapter

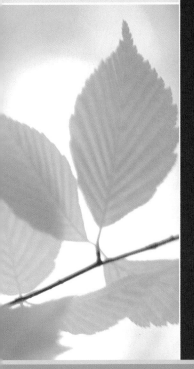

INTRODUCTION

Massage therapists come to know the skeleton well. Bones are landmarks for locating muscles and other soft tissues. Bony structures may also be areas to avoid in massage therapy (endangerment sites). Many of the terms in earlier chapters are repeated here. For example, the thighs are called the *femoral region* because the thigh bones are the femurs. This information is a prerequisite to learning muscular nomenclature, which is one of the main focuses for the study of massage therapy.

This chapter is divided into the anatomical regions of the body, and each region is subdivided into the bones of that region or a discussion on joints (Figure 14-1). Along with the bone names and locations are bony markings. Not all of the bones and their surface markings or joints are listed—only those that are the most important in the practice of massage therapy. Each bone is listed in chart form, with the bony markings on the left and its significance on the right. When a structure such as the head, breastbone, or foot bone is discussed, the bones are listed to the left, with important information to the right. Illustrations are included to locate the markings. Use anatomical models and a classmate to locate these bones and markings in class (Figure 14-2).

Your own body and all the bodies with which you will be working are the best teachers. Instead of thinking, "I am massaging the arm," repeat to yourself the terms *humerus, radius,* and *ulna.* This exercise continually reinforces your new vocabulary. Try using *scapula* instead of *shoulder blade* or *olecranon process* instead of *tip of the elbow.* The sooner you begin to incorporate this new language into your massage work, the sooner you will have the confidence to progress into the world of muscles.

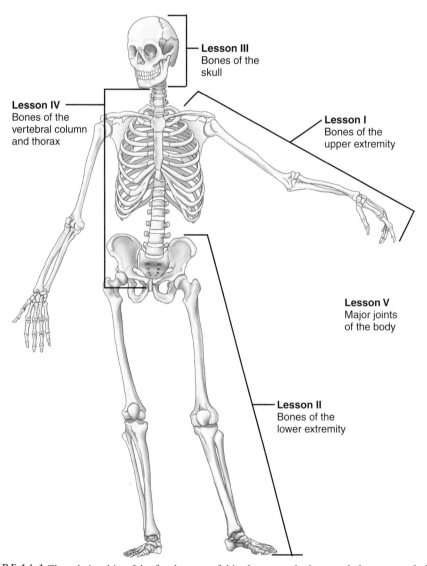

Lesson III
Bones of the skull

Lesson IV
Bones of the vertebral column and thorax

Lesson I
Bones of the upper extremity

Lesson V
Major joints of the body

Lesson II
Bones of the lower extremity

FIGURE 14-1 The relationship of the five lessons of this chapter to the human skeleton as a whole.

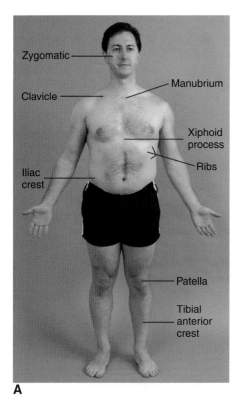

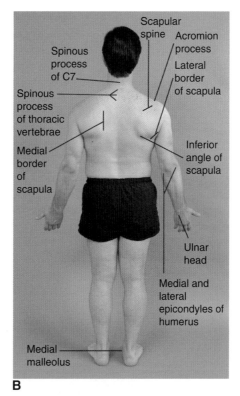

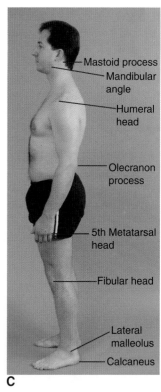

FIGURE 14-2 Miscellaneous bony marking locations. **A,** Anterior view. **B,** Posterior view. **C,** Lateral view.

Terms and Their Meanings Related to the Skeleton

TERM	MEANING	TERM	MEANING	TERM	MEANING
Acetabulum	L. vinegar, saucer, or bowl; small	Humerus	L. shoulder	Pedicle	L. small foot
		Hyoid	Gr. U shaped	Pelvis	L. a basin
Acromion	Gr. extremity; topmost; the shoulder	Ilium	L. flank	Phalanx	Gr. a line of soldiers
		Ischium	L. hip	Pisiform	L. pea shaped
Atlas	Gr. to bear; as the giant of Greek mythology holding up the world	Lambdoidal	Gr. shaped as the Greek letter A	Poples	L. ham
				Prominens	L. prominent or projecting
		Lamina	L. a plate	Pterygoid	Gr. shaped as a wing
Axis	Gr. an axis; an axle	Linea	L. line	Pubic	L. grownup
Bifid	L. cleaved or split in two; twice	Malleolus	L. hammer or mallet; small	Sacrum	L. sacred
		Mandible	L. to chew	Sagittal	L. an arrow
Carpus	Gr. wrist	Manubrium	L. a handle	Scaphoid	Gr. shaped as a boat
Calcaneus	L. heel	Mastoid	Gr. breastlike; shaped	Sinus	L. a hollow or cavity
Clavicle	L. little key	Meniscus	Gr. crescent; small	Sphenoid	Gr. shaped as a wedge
Coracoid	Gr. as a crow's beak	Metacarpal	Gr. after or beyond; wrist	Spine	L. spiny or thorny plant
Coronal	L. shaped as a corona or crown around the head	Metatarsal	Gr. after or beyond; foot	Stapes	L. a stirrup
		Navicular	A ship; small	Suture	L. to sew; a seam
Costal	L. rib	Obturator	L. to obstruct, close, block up, or plug	Styloid	Gr. shaped as a pillar
Crural	L. leg			Talus	L. ankle
Cuneiform	L. wedge shaped	Odont	Gr. toothlike	Tarsal	L. broad, flat surface; foot
Digit	L. resembling a finger or toe	Olecranon	Gr. skull or tip of the elbow	Temporal	L. time
Dens, dent	L. toothlike	Ossicle	L. small bone	Ulna	L. elbow
Ethmoid	Gr. sievelike; shaped	Parietal	L. a wall or partition	Vertebrae	L. turning joint
Femur	L. thigh	Patella	L. a little dish	Xiphoid	Gr. shaped as a sword
Glenoid	Gr. shaped as a socket	Pectoral	L. breast or chest	Zygomatic	Gr. a yoke or bar
Hamate	L. to possess a small hook				

L., Latin; Gr., Greek.

LESSON I—BONES OF THE UPPER EXTREMITY

This lesson examines the clavicle, scapula, humerus, ulna, radius, carpals (pisiform, triquetrum, lunate, scaphoid, hamate, capitate, trapezoid, trapezium), metacarpals, and phalanges.

Shoulder Girdle

The bones of the shoulder (pectoral) girdle are the clavicle and scapula (Figure 14-3). The shoulder girdle lacks a posterior attachment to the axial skeleton, which allows for wider range of motion. The shoulder girdle and the adjoining arm articulate with the axial skeleton at its anterior aspect and the medial end of the clavicle. Its primary function is to allow attachment areas for numerous muscles that move the shoulder and elbow.

Clavicle

The clavicle, shaped like *f* in italics, acts as a brace to hold the arm away from the top of the thorax. A helpful mnemonic to recall these two bones is *C and C* (the *c*ollarbone is the *c*lavicle). The clavicle's medial end articulates with the sternum, and its lateral end articulates with the scapula. The most commonly fractured bone is the clavicle. When the clavicle is broken, the entire shoulder region caves in medially. This consequence demonstrates its function as a brace (Table 14-1).

Scapula

The scapula is a triangular bone located between the second and seventh ribs. When the scapula is set in motion, it floats against the posterior aspect of the rib cage. A helpful mnemonic to recall these two bones is *S and S* (the *s*houlder blade is the *s*capula). It articulates with the clavicle and humerus at the shoulder (Table 14-2).

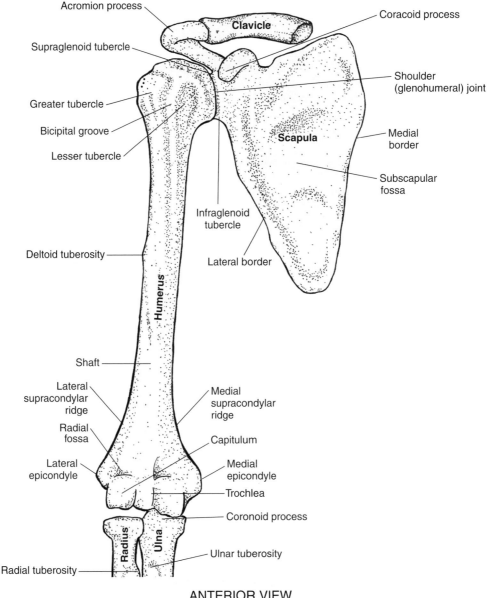

ANTERIOR VIEW

A

FIGURE 14-3 Right scapula, right clavicle, and right humerus. **A**, Anterior view. **B**, Posterior view. **C**, Lateral view.

Arm—Humerus

The humerus is the arm bone, which is also known as the *funny bone* or *crazy bone* because hitting the elbow in a certain way makes it feel funny, or *humorous*. The sensation felt when hitting the funny bone is caused by stimulation of the ulnar nerve as it passes posterior to the medial epicondyle of the humerus. The proximal end of the humerus articulates with the scapula at the shoulder, and the distal end of the

TABLE 14-1 Clavicle

BONY MARKING	SIGNIFICANCE
Sternal (medial) end	Joint formation
Acromial (lateral) end	Joint formation

TABLE 14-2 Scapula

BONY MARKING	SIGNIFICANCE
Medial (vertebral) border	Muscle attachment
Lateral (axillary) border	Muscle attachment
Superior angle	Muscle attachment
Inferior angle	Muscle attachment
Scapular spine	Muscle attachment
Root of spine	Muscle attachment
Acromion process	Muscle attachment and joint formation
Coracoid process	Muscle attachment
Supraglenoid tubercle	Muscle attachment
Infraglenoid tubercle	Muscle attachment
Glenoid fossa	Joint formation
Supraspinous fossa	Muscle attachment
Infraspinous fossa	Muscle attachment
Subscapular fossa	Muscle attachment

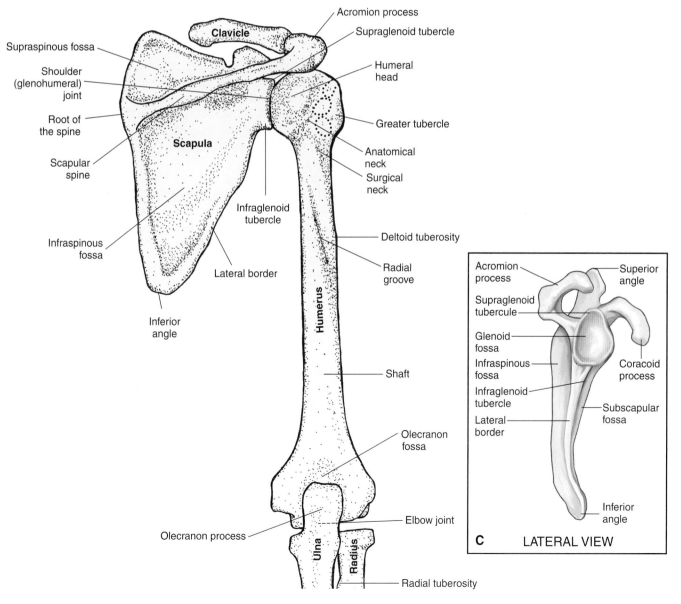

B POSTERIOR VIEW
FIGURE 14-3, cont'd

TABLE 14-3 Humerus

BONY MARKING	SIGNIFICANCE
Humeral head	Joint formation
Surgical neck	Where most fractures occur
Humeral shaft	Muscle attachment
Greater tubercle	Muscle attachment
Lesser tubercle	Muscle attachment
Intertubercular (bicipital) groove	Muscle attachment (medial and lateral lips)
Deltoid tuberosity	Muscle attachment
Radial fossa	Joint formation
Olecranon fossa	Joint formation
Coronoid fossa	Joint formation
Capitulum	Joint formation
Trochlea	Joint formation
Medial epicondyle	Muscle attachment
Lateral epicondyle	Muscle attachment
Supracondylar ridge	Muscle attachment (medial and lateral sections)
Anatomical neck	Nonapplicable
Radial (spiral) groove	Direct trauma to this area on the humerus can damage the radial nerve

humerus articulates with the radius and the ulna at the elbow (Table 14-3).

Forearm

Ulna

In the anatomical position, the ulna is located on the medial, or little finger, side of the forearm (Figure 14-4). The ulna articulates with the humerus at its wider proximal end, a carpal bone (triquetrum via a disk) at its narrower distal end (Table 14-4).

Radius

The radius is the lateral forearm bone, located on the thumb side of the arm. To differentiate the radius from the ulna, locate the radial pulse. You palpate the radial pulse by gently pressing the radial artery onto the distal radius. Another way to remember the name of this bone is to remember that the *r*adius always *r*otates (*r* and *r*) on the ulna (during supination and pronation). The radius articulates with the humerus and the ulna at its proximal end and with the carpal bones (lunate and scaphoid) at its wide distal end (Table 14-5).

An interosseous membrane weaves the ulna and the radius with bands of tough connective tissue. This anatomical arrangement gives the forearm lightness and mobility and provides attachment sites for the many muscles of the forearm and hand. Imagine how heavy the arm would be if the ulna and radius were just one solid bone!

Wrist and Hand

The wrist and hands contain multiple joints and 29 bones, which lead to high mobility: the distal ends of the ulna and radius (two bones), eight carpals, five metacarpals, and 14

phalanges (Figure 14-5). Opposing thumbs make human hands vastly different from those of other mammals; they can be rotated in front of the palms in the opposite direction of the other four for grasping. This flexibility gives us the ability to create and use tools.

Carpals

The eight carpal bones of the wrist are arranged in two rows of four bones (proximal row and distal row) that are linked together by ligaments and bound in a joint capsule. The carpal bones function as eight ball bearings. For centuries, these bones were simply numbered one through eight. In the early 1800s, each bone was named individually. The names of the carpal bones in the proximal row from medial to lateral are the *pisiform, triquetrum, lunate,* and *scaphoid.* The names of the carpal bones in the distal row from medial to lateral are the *hamate, capitate, trapezoid,* and *trapezium.*

A tunnel, called the carpal tunnel, is produced by the carpal bones and bound by the *transverse carpal ligament,* also referred to as the flexor retinaculum (Figure 14-6). This ligament connects the *scaphoid* and *trapezium* on the hand's radial side with the *hamate* on the ulnar side and creates a flexor pulley system important for hand functions. Many muscles of the thumb and little finger originate on the transverse carpal ligament (Table 14-6).

TABLE TALK

To help you learn the names of the carpal bones, learn the following sentence: *Steve left the party to take Cathy home.* The first letter of each word is also the first letter of each of the names of the carpal bones: Scaphoid—Lunate—Triquetrum—Pisiform—Trapezium—Trapezoid—Capitate—Hamate.

TABLE 14-4 **Ulna**

BONY MARKING	SIGNIFICANCE	BONY MARKING	SIGNIFICANCE
Olecranon process	Muscle attachment	Ulnar tuberosity	Muscle attachment
Trochlear (semilunar) notch	Joint formation	Coronoid process	Muscle attachment
Radial notch	Joint formation	Ulnar head	Joint formation
Ulnar shaft	Muscle attachment	Styloid process	Nonapplicable

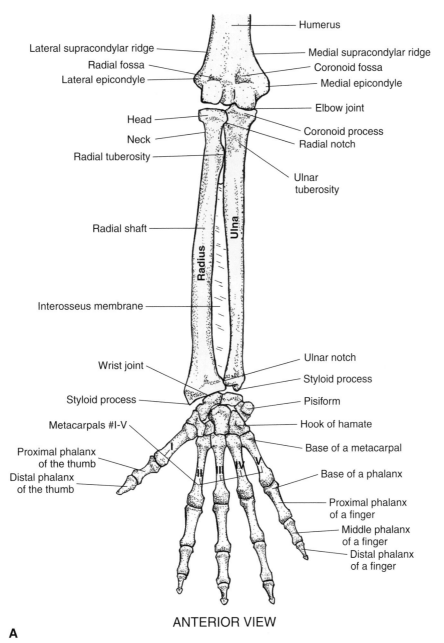

Humerus
Lateral supracondylar ridge
Radial fossa
Lateral epicondyle
Medial supracondylar ridge
Coronoid fossa
Medial epicondyle
Elbow joint
Head
Neck
Coronoid process
Radial notch
Radial tuberosity
Ulnar tuberosity
Radius
Ulna
Radial shaft
Interosseus membrane
Ulnar notch
Wrist joint
Styloid process
Styloid process
Pisiform
Metacarpals #I-V
Hook of hamate
Base of a metacarpal
Proximal phalanx of the thumb
Distal phalanx of the thumb
Base of a phalanx
Proximal phalanx of a finger
Middle phalanx of a finger
Distal phalanx of a finger

ANTERIOR VIEW

A

FIGURE 14-4 Right ulna, radius, and hand. **A**, Anterior view. **B**, Posterior view. *Continued*

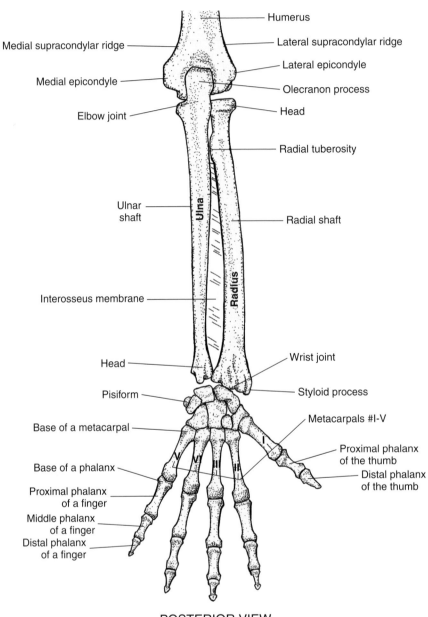

Humerus

Medial supracondylar ridge

Lateral supracondylar ridge

Medial epicondyle

Lateral epicondyle

Olecranon process

Elbow joint

Head

Radial tuberosity

Ulnar shaft

Radial shaft

Interosseus membrane

Head

Wrist joint

Pisiform

Styloid process

Base of a metacarpal

Metacarpals #I-V

Base of a phalanx

Proximal phalanx of the thumb

Proximal phalanx of a finger

Distal phalanx of the thumb

Middle phalanx of a finger

Distal phalanx of a finger

POSTERIOR VIEW

B

FIGURE 14-4, cont'd

TABLE 14-5 **Radius**

BONY MARKING	SIGNIFICANCE	BONY MARKING	SIGNIFICANCE
Radial head	Joint formation	Radial (bicipital) tuberosity	Muscle attachment
Radial neck	Nonapplicable	Ulnar notch	Joint formation
Radial shaft	Muscle attachment	Styloid process	Muscle attachment

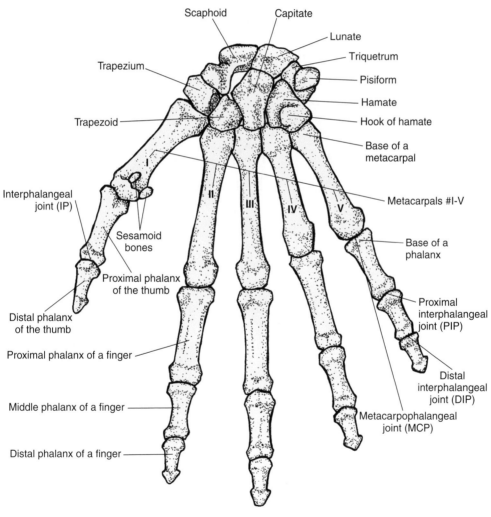

ANTERIOR VIEW

A

FIGURE 14-5 Right hand. **A**, Anterior view. **B**, Posterior view. *Continued*

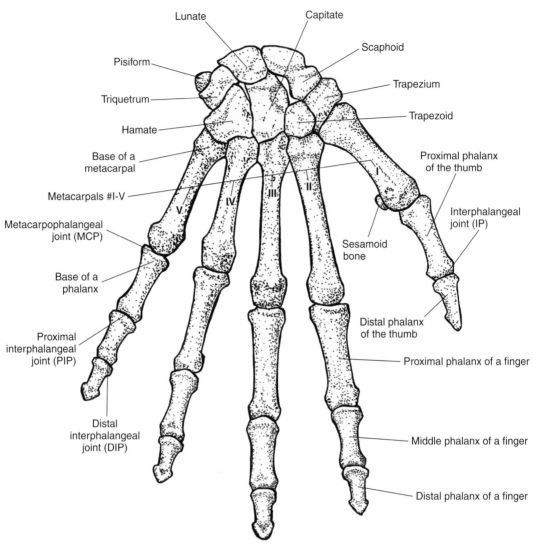

Lunate
Capitate
Pisiform
Scaphoid
Triquetrum
Trapezium
Hamate
Trapezoid
Base of a metacarpal
Proximal phalanx of the thumb
Metacarpals #I-V
Interphalangeal joint (IP)
Metacarpophalangeal joint (MCP)
Sesamoid bone
Base of a phalanx
Distal phalanx of the thumb
Proximal interphalangeal joint (PIP)
Proximal phalanx of a finger
Distal interphalangeal joint (DIP)
Middle phalanx of a finger
Distal phalanx of a finger

B

POSTERIOR VIEW
FIGURE 14-5, cont'd

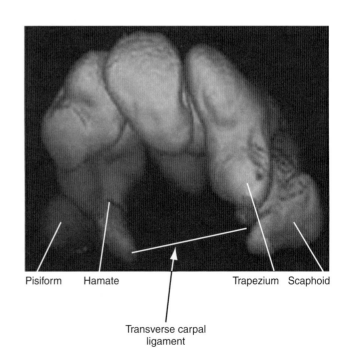

FIGURE 14-6 The carpal tunnel.

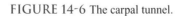

Pisiform   Hamate   Trapezium   Scaphoid

Transverse carpal ligament

TABLE 14-6 **Carpals**

BONY MARKING	SIGNIFICANCE
Scaphoid	Largest bone in the proximal row; most commonly fractured carpal bone
Lunate	Crescent moon–shaped bone; most commonly dislocated carpal and the second most commonly fractured carpal
Triquetrum	Triangular or pyramid-shaped bone
Pisiform	Pea-shaped bone; smallest carpal bone; a sesamoid bone
Trapezium	Triangular bone
Trapezoid	Four-sided bone with two parallel sides
Capitate	Largest carpal bone; has a round head
Hamate	Bone has an anterior hook

Metacarpals

The metacarpals, just distal to the carpals, are also referred to as the *hand bones,* with five in each hand, numbered I through V, starting from the thumb (I) to the little finger (V). When the hand is clenched to make a fist, the distal ends of the metacarpal heads become obvious as the knuckles.

Phalanges

Each hand has 14 phalanges. Each finger has three, and each thumb has two. Depending on their location, the phalanges are referred to as *proximal, middle,* and *distal;* the thumb is also referred to as *pollicis.*

LESSON II—BONES OF THE LOWER EXTREMITY

This lesson examines the ilium, ischium, pubis, femur, patella, tibia, fibula, tarsals (talus, cuneiforms, navicular, cuboid, calcaneus), metatarsals, and phalanges.

Pelvic Girdle

The pelvic girdle is also known as the *os coxa, coxal bones, hip bones,* or *innominate bones.* Each pelvic bone is made up of three embryonic bones: ilium, ischium, and pubis. These bones are totally fused by puberty to form the pelvic bone. In contrast, the pelvis is formed by the two matched pelvic bones articulating anteriorly with the pubic bones at the pubic symphysis, and the sacrum posteriorly with the iliums (Figure 14-7). The sacrum is not part of the pelvic girdle, but is included when discussing the pelvis. The pelvic girdles can move only as one unit, unlike the right and left shoulder girdles, which can move independently of each other.

The *acetabulum,* or hip socket, provides a deep socket for the femoral head. The ilium, ischium, and pubic bones all contribute equally to its makeup. This arrangement allows equal force from all three dimensions to pass into the acetabulum. The *obturator foramen* is located inferior to the acetabulum. The obturator membrane *obstructs* the foramen in a living skeleton. This membrane provides attachment sites for the muscles of the hip and thigh. The superior opening

of the pelvis is called the *pelvic inlet,* and the *pelvic outlet* is the inferior opening of the pelvis. The digestive, urinary, and reproductive systems use the latter opening to empty their products externally.

Ilium

The ilium is the most superior pelvic bone in the pelvic girdle and resembles a broad, expanding blade (Table 14-7).

Ischium

The ischium is the most inferior and most posterior part of the pelvic girdle. Correcting sitting posture involves the ischial tuberosity (Table 14-8).

Pubic Bone

In the most anterior portion of the pelvis, each of the two pubic bones resembles a wishbone, and they are collectively referred to as the *pubis* (Table 14-9).

Thigh

Femur

The femur (thigh bone) is the longest, heaviest, and strongest bone in the body. It has a ball-like head at the proximal end and two ball-like condyles at its distal end. The femur articulates proximally with the acetabulum, forming the hip joint, and distally with the patella and the tibia, forming the knee joint. When looking at the femur, you will notice a distinct slant to the bone. The medial course of the femoral shaft is necessary to bring the hips in line with the knee and lower leg bones. This medial direction of the femur is more noticeable in women because of the wider pelvis. Most of a child's production of red blood cells occurs in the femur (Table 14-10).

Patella

The patella, or kneecap, is the largest sesamoid bone in the body and articulates with the distal end of the femur. It is located within the tendon of the quadriceps femoris muscle and provides additional leverage for knee extension. However, the patella is not always considered part of the knee joint. Its main function is to provide stabilization and protect the knee by shielding it from impact.

Leg

Tibia

The tibia, or shin bone, is the most stout and straight long bone in the body and is located below the femur on the medial side of the leg (Figure 14-8). The proximal aspect of the tibia articulates with the femur, and its distal end articulates with the talus bone. The superior of the tibia is relatively flat, and the shaft is triangular (Table 14-11).

Fibula

The fibula is located on the lateral side of the leg and is about the same length as the tibia. The fibula is much smaller in diameter than the tibia and supports only approximately 10% of the body's weight. The proximal end of the fibula articulates with the tibia inferior to the tibial plateau and is not involved with the knee joint. The distal end of the fibula articulates with the talus bone and the distal end of the tibia. Similar to the ulna and radius of the

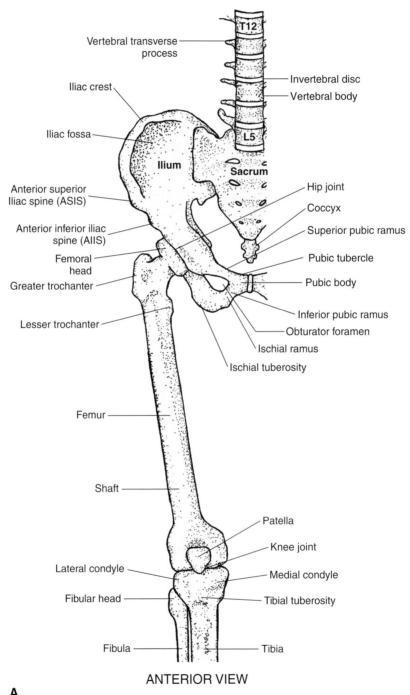

ANTERIOR VIEW

A

FIGURE 14-7 Right pelvis, femur, and patella. **A**, Anterior view. **B**, Posterior view.

upper extremity, an interosseous membrane connects the tibia and the fibula (Table 14-12).

Ankle and Foot

Each ankle and foot contains numerous joints and 28 bones: the distal ends of the tibia and fibula (two bones), seven tarsals, five metatarsals, and 14 phalanges (Figure 14-9). The main functions of the foot are to provide a stable platform, to generate propulsion, and to absorb shock.

Ankle—Tarsals

Each tarsal is an irregularly shaped short bone that slides minutely over the next tarsal bone to collectively provide motion. This characteristic is similar to the way the spine creates movement. In massage therapy, range-of-motion

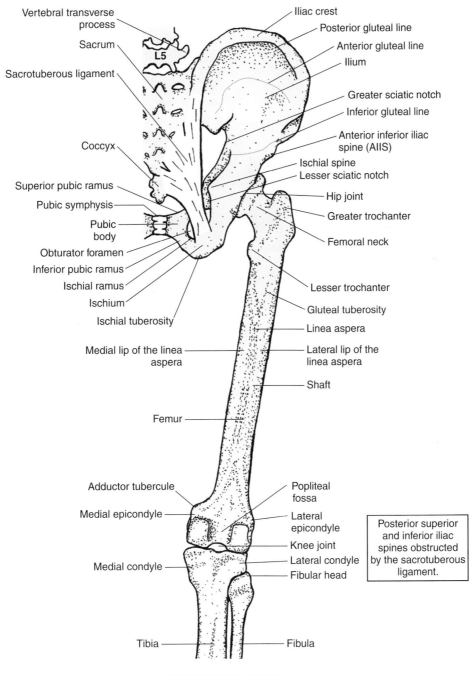

Vertebral transverse process — Sacrum — Sacrotuberous ligament — Coccyx — Superior pubic ramus — Pubic symphysis — Pubic body — Obturator foramen — Inferior pubic ramus — Ischial ramus — Ischium — Ischial tuberosity — Medial lip of the linea aspera — Femur — Adductor tubercule — Medial epicondyle — Medial condyle — Tibia

L5

Iliac crest — Posterior gluteal line — Anterior gluteal line — Ilium — Greater sciatic notch — Inferior gluteal line — Anterior inferior iliac spine (AIIS) — Ischial spine — Lesser sciatic notch — Hip joint — Greater trochanter — Femoral neck — Lesser trochanter — Gluteal tuberosity — Linea aspera — Lateral lip of the linea aspera — Shaft — Popliteal fossa — Lateral epicondyle — Knee joint — Lateral condyle — Fibular head — Fibula

Posterior superior and inferior iliac spines obstructed by the sacrotuberous ligament.

POSTERIOR VIEW

B

FIGURE 14-7, **cont'd**

exercises can help keep the tarsal bones mobile. If the tarsal bones become immobile or stuck, then the foot cannot move properly or absorb shock (Table 14-13).

Foot—Metatarsals

Five metatarsals, numbered I through V, are in each foot starting from the great toe (I) to the little toe (V). The length of the metatarsals determines shoe size. When you flex your toes dorsally and look at your knuckles, you are actually looking at the heads of the metatarsals. The metatarsals articulate proximally with cuboid and cuneiforms and distally with the phalanges.

Phalanges

The phalanges are also known as the *digits,* or *toes.* Each toe has three digits, and the great toe has two. Depending on their location, the phalanges are referred to as *proximal, middle,* and *distal.* The great toe is also referred to as the *hallux.*

"As we acquire more knowledge, things do not become more comprehensible, but more mysterious."
Will Durant

Foot Arches

For walking, running, and jumping to be springy, our feet must absorb shock. To help accomplish this task, the foot uses a system of arches to prevent the plantar surface of the foot from becoming flat (Figure 14-10).

The posterior bones of the foot lie over each other, and the anterior and middle bones of the foot lie side to side. This arrangement produces the three arches of the foot. Together, these three arches resemble a geodesic dome.

The three bony points that are in contact with the ground are (1) the calcaneal tuberosity, (2) the head of the first metatarsal, and (3) the head of the fifth metatarsal. The three points of contact make the shape of a triangle (Figure 14-11).

Because the names of the arches are descriptive, they are easy to learn. Weak arches are referred to as *fallen arches* or *flat feet* (pes planus). To strengthen these arches and the intrinsic muscles of the foot, pick up marbles or rocks with your toes. The three arches are the (1) *medial longitudinal arch,* (2) *lateral longitudinal arch,* and (3) *transverse (metatarsal) arch.*

TABLE 14-7 Ilium

BONY MARKING	SIGNIFICANCE
Iliac crest	Muscle attachment
Iliac fossa	Muscle attachment
Anterior superior iliac spine (ASIS)	Muscle attachment
Anterior inferior iliac spine (AIIS)	Muscle attachment
Posterior superior iliac spine (PSIS)	Muscle attachment
Posterior inferior iliac spine (PIIS)	Muscle attachment
Anterior gluteal line	Nonapplicable
Posterior gluteal line	Nonapplicable
Greater sciatic notch	Passage of sciatic nerve

TABLE 14-8 Ischium

BONY MARKING	SIGNIFICANCE
Ischial tuberosity	Muscle attachment
Ischial spine	Muscle attachment
Ischial ramus	Muscle attachment
Lesser sciatic notch	Passage of obturator internus

TABLE 14-9 Pubis

BONY MARKING	SIGNIFICANCE
Superior pubic ramus	Muscle attachment
Inferior pubic ramus	Muscle attachment
Pubic tubercle	Muscle attachment
Pubic body	Joint formation
Pubic symphysis	Joint formation

TABLE 14-10 Femur

BONY MARKING	SIGNIFICANCE
Femoral head	Joint formation
Femoral neck	Where most fractures occur
Femoral shaft	Muscle attachment
Greater trochanter	Muscle attachment
Lesser trochanter	Muscle attachment
Gluteal tuberosity	Muscle attachment
Linea aspera	Muscle attachment
Adductor tubercle	Muscle attachment
Medial condyle	Joint formation
Lateral condyle	Joint formation
Medial epicondyle	Muscle attachment
Lateral epicondyle	Muscle attachment
Popliteal fossa	Joint formation

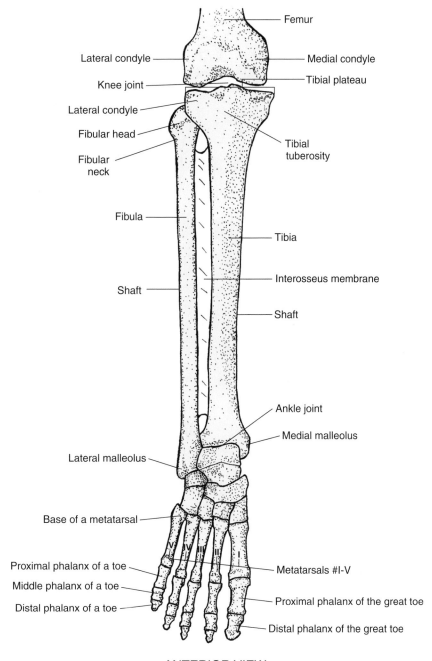

ANTERIOR VIEW

A

FIGURE 14-8 Right tibia, fibula, and foot. **A**, Anterior view. **B**, Posterior view. *Continued*

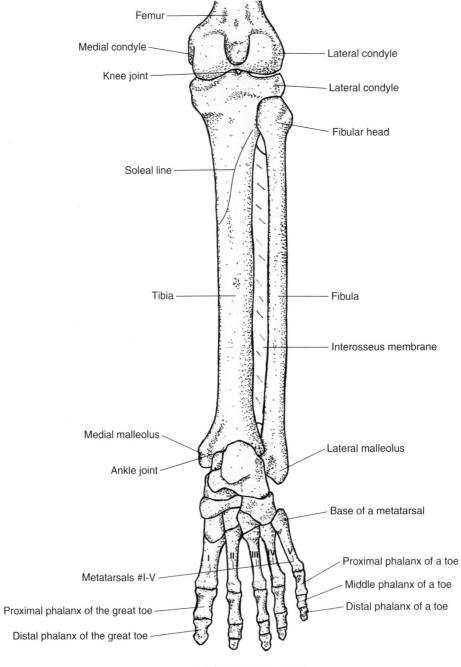

Femur

Medial condyle

Knee joint

Lateral condyle

Lateral condyle

Fibular head

Soleal line

Tibia

Fibula

Interosseus membrane

Medial malleolus

Ankle joint

Lateral malleolus

Base of a metatarsal

Proximal phalanx of a toe

Metatarsals #I-V

Middle phalanx of a toe

Distal phalanx of a toe

Proximal phalanx of the great toe

Distal phalanx of the great toe

POSTERIOR VIEW

B

FIGURE 14-8, cont'd

TABLE 14-11 Tibia

BONY MARKING	SIGNIFICANCE
Tibial plateau	Joint formation
Tibial shaft	Muscle attachment
Anterior crest	Nonapplicable
Tibial (patellar) tuberosity	Muscle attachment

TABLE 14-12 Fibula

BONY MARKING	SIGNIFICANCE
Fibular head	Muscle attachment
Fibular neck	Nonapplicable
Fibular shaft	Muscle attachment
Lateral malleolus	Joint formation

- Medial longitudinal arch: The calcaneus, talus, navicular, cuneiform I and medial metatarsals (I through III) contribute to this arch.
- Lateral longitudinal arch: The calcaneus, cuboid, and lateral metatarsals (IV and V) make up this arch.
- Transverse arch: This arch exists across all metatarsals.

  The imprint of a healthy foot arch is shown in Figure 14-12, *A* and *B*. If the imprint is wide and flattened, then the arches, namely the medial longitudinal arch, have *fallen,* often as a result of overextension of foot ligaments and weakness of the deep (intrinsic) plantar musculature (Figure 14-12, *C*).

If the imprint shows only two unconnected sections, then the foot arches are *high,* (pes cavus), often as a result of the positions of foot bones rather than weak foot muscles and ligaments (Figure 14-12, *D*).

LESSON III—BONES OF THE SKULL

This lesson examines the frontal, parietal, temporal, ethmoid, sphenoid, occipital, hyoid, nasal, vomer, zygomatic, lacrimal, inferior nasal concha, palatine, maxilla, and mandible.

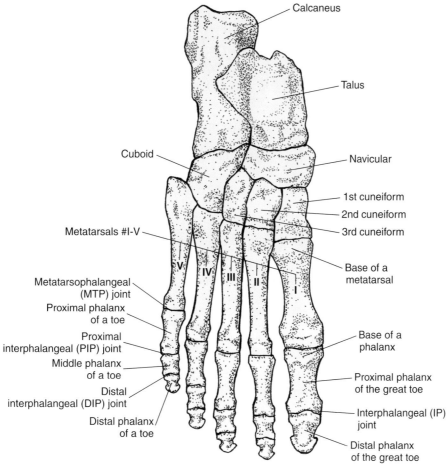

DORSAL VIEW

A

FIGURE 14-9 Right foot. *Continued*

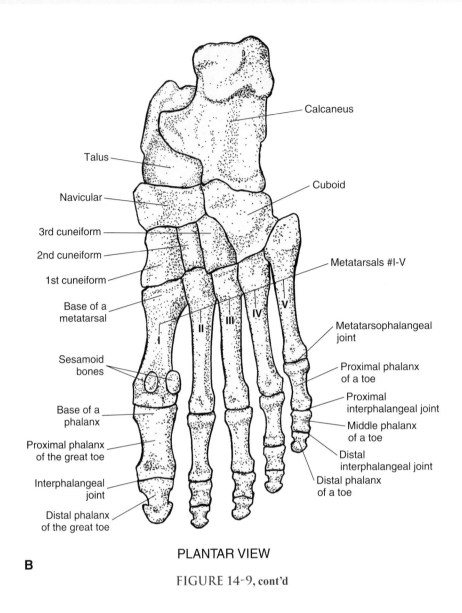

PLANTAR VIEW

B

FIGURE 14-9, cont'd

TABLE 14-13 **Tarsals**

BONES	SIGNIFICANCE
Talus (astragalus)	Joint formation
Cuneiforms: I (medial), II (intermediate), III (lateral)	Muscle attachment and joint formation
Navicular	Muscle attachment and joint formation
Cuboid	Muscle attachment and joint formation
Calcaneus	Muscle attachment and joint formation
Peroneal tubercle	Acts a pulley for tendons of peroneus longus and brevis

Cranial Bones

The cranial vault contains eight bones: frontal bone, two pa-rietal bones, two temporal bones, ethmoid bone, sphenoid bone, and occipital bone (Figure 14-13). This bony region protects the brain and related nerves; it also provides a bony passageway for the organs of sight, taste, hearing, and smell. Except for one synovial joint located at the jaw, all skull bones and facial bones are joined by sutures (Table 14-14). The eye sockets, or *eye orbits*, are where the eyeballs sit.

evolve *Log on to the Evolve website to see an exploded view of the cranial bones.* ∎

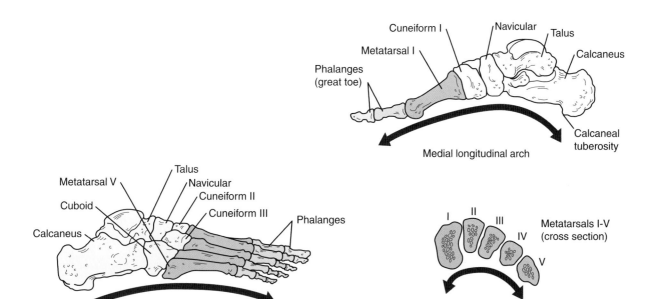

FIGURE 14-10 Arches of right foot.

Sutures are located anywhere cranial bones join and are classified as synarthrotic joints. Very little movement exists in these sutural regions. Sutures may be named by the bones between which they sit (e.g., temporoparietal suture), but some have specialized names.
- The **sagittal suture** joins the two parietal bones.
- The **coronal suture**, shaped as a corona, or crown, around the head, separates the frontal bone from the parietal bones.
- The **lambdoidal suture** separates the parietal bones from the occipital bone.
- The squamosal suture separates the parietal bones and temporal bones.

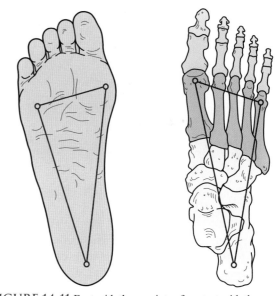

FIGURE 14-11 Foot with three points of contact with the ground.

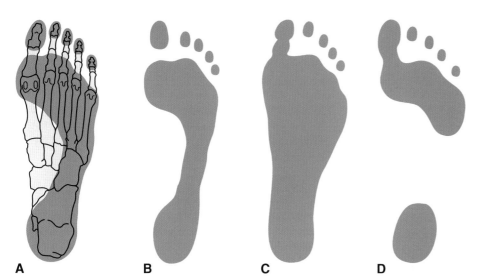

FIGURE 14-12 **A**, Footprint with skeletal overlay. **B**, Imprint of a healthy foot arch. **C**, Imprint of a person with a flat foot. **D**, Imprint of a person with a high arch.

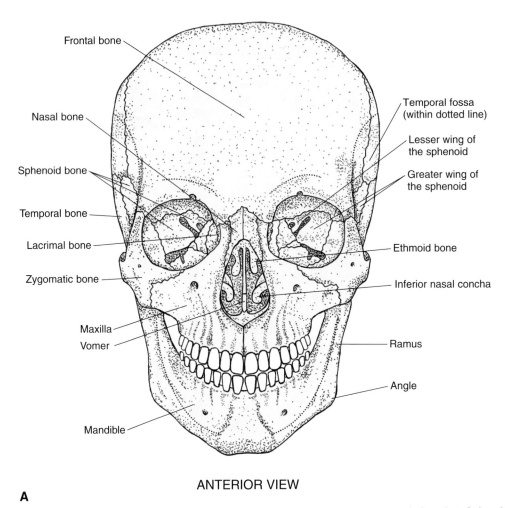

ANTERIOR VIEW

A

FIGURE 14-13 Cranial bones viewed from different angles. **A,** Anterior view. **B,** Lateral view. **C,** Inferior view.

The fontanels are located in the fetal and neonatal cranium in the sutural regions. These membrane-covered spaces allow the head to be compressed during delivery and permit rapid growth of the brain. The anterior and posterior fontanels are also called *soft spots.* Obstetricians and midwives find these areas helpful in determining the position of babies during delivery. Although many fontanels exist in the newborn's head, the following two are the most prevalent:

- The **anterior fontanel** is diamond shaped and is the largest of all the fontanels. It is located where the coronal suture and sagittal sutures meet. The anterior fontanel completely ossifies by 18 to 24 months. You can often see a pulse under the membrane in this region of the head.
- The **posterior fontanel** is located where the sagittal and lambdoidal sutures meet. It typically closes by the time the infant is 2 months of age.

The sinuses are air-containing spaces in the skull and face that lighten the head, provide mucus, and act as resonance chambers for sound. These sinus cavities are named for the cranial bones or facial bones by which they are located. They are the *frontal, sphenoidal, ethmoidal,* and *maxillary*

sinuses. The mastoid process contains air cells that drain into the middle ear (Figure 14-14).

Related Skull Bone—Hyoid

The hyoid bone is shaped as a miniature mandible with two incisor teeth and is usually found at the level of C3. This bone does not articulate directly with any other bone and, as such, is really not a skull bone even though it relates to the skull because it is suspended from the styloid process of the temporal bone by ligaments. These ligaments serve as support for the tongue and provide muscle attachments for the tongue, neck, and pharynx. This bone is important in forensic medicine. When it is found broken, it usually means the victim was strangled or hanged.

TABLE TALK

Dr. William Sutherland, a student of Dr. Andrew Still (father of osteopathy), became convinced through study and practice that the bones of the skull do not completely fuse but rather retain a small, yet significant, degree of motion relative to one another.

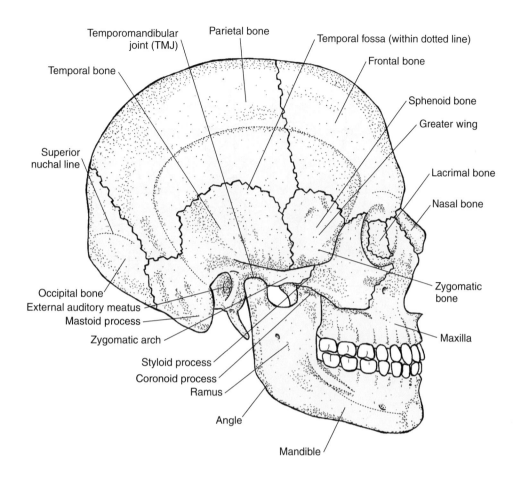

LATERAL VIEW

B

FIGURE 14-13, cont'd   *Continued*

TABLE 14-14 **Cranial Bones**

BONES	BONY MARKING AND/OR SIGNIFICANCE
Frontal bone (1)	Muscle attachment
Parietal bones (2)	Muscle attachment
Temporal bones (2)	Styloid process (ligament attachment and endangerment site)
	External auditory meatus (ear ossicles)
	Mastoid process (muscle attachment)
Ethmoid bone (1)	No relevant bony marking or endangerment site
Sphenoid bone (1) (articulates with all other cranial bones)	Sella turcica (pituitary location)
	Pterygoid plate (muscle attachment)
	Greater wings (muscle attachment)
Occipital bone (1)	Foramen magnum (passage for spinal cord)
	Superior nuchal line (muscle attachment)
	Inferior nuchal line (muscle attachment)
	External occipital protuberance or *inion* (muscle attachment)
	Occipital condyles (joint formation)

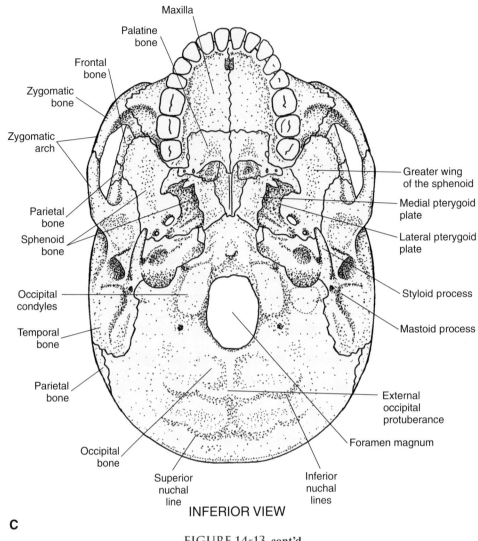

FIGURE 14-13, cont'd

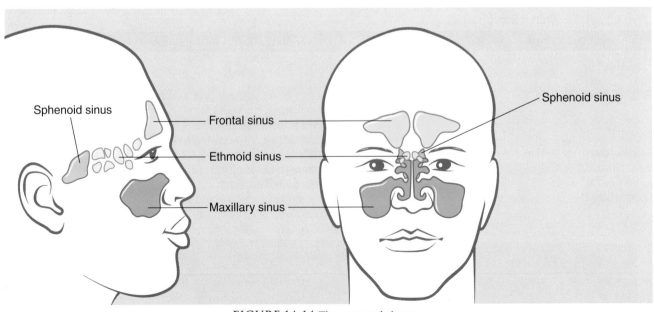

FIGURE 14-14 The paranasal sinuses.

TABLE 14-15 Facial Bones

BONES	BONY MARKINGS AND SIGNIFICANCE
Nasal bones (2)	No relevant bony marking or endangerment site
Vomer bone (1)	No relevant bony marking or endangerment site
Zygomatic bones (2)	Muscle attachment
Lacrimal bones (2)	No relevant bony marking or endangerment site
Inferior nasal concha bones (2)	No relevant bony marking or endangerment site
Palatine bones (2)	No relevant bony marking or endangerment site
Maxillae (2)	Muscle attachment
Mandible (1)	Mandibular ramus (muscle attachment)
	Mandibular angle (muscle attachment)
	Coronoid process (muscle attachment)
	Condylar process (muscle attachment and joint formation)

Facial Bones

The face has 14 bones: the vomer bone, two nasal bones, two zygomatic bones, two lacrimal bones, two inferior nasal concha bones, two palatine bones, two fused maxillae, one mandible. Facial features are largely a result of facial bone and cartilaginous structures. High cheekbones, a prominent nose, or a pointed chin are all representative of facial bones (Table 14-15). Facial bones also articulate with one another by means of sutures named by the bones between which they sit, such as the zygomaticomaxillary suture.

LESSON IV—BONES OF THE THORAX AND VERTEBRAL COLUMN

Thorax

The thorax, or chest cavity, consists of the sternum, 12 thoracic vertebrae, and 24 ribs. These bony structures support the body and protect the organs inside the thorax.

Sternum

The sternum, or breastbone, forms the central portion of the anterior chest wall. In the adult, the sternum is a single bone made up of three fused bones (Figure 14-15). These bones are the manubrium (located superiorly), sternal body, and xiphoid process (located inferiorly). Not only does the sternum protect the chest organs, it also provides a place where the clavicle and most ribs attach (Table 14-16).

Ribs

The ribs are 24 individual (12 pairs) long, slender, curved bones that articulate posteriorly with the thoracic vertebrae. Mobility of the ribcage is a precursor for proper respiration. Anteriorly, the first seven pairs of ribs have their costal cartilages articulate directly with the sternum and are known as the *true ribs*. The next three pairs of ribs attach to the sternum by borrowing the costal cartilage of the seventh rib and are called the *false ribs*. The last two pairs of ribs do not attach to the sternum at all. These ribs are known as the *floating ribs*. The first rib is short and thick, and the great vessels and main nerves run over it (Table 14-17).

Vertebral Column

The vertebral (spinal) column consists of 26 individual bones in the adult and 32 to 34 embryonic vertebrae. The spine offers many functions. It provides stability, it permits movements in all directions, it supports a structure of considerable weight (e.g., head), it provides attachment sites for muscles and ligaments; it acts as a shock absorber; and it protects a vital organ, (i.e., spinal cord).

As previously stated, the vertebral column permits movements. It allows us to bend forward and backward, lean sideways, and twist or rotate through the three planes of movement. All these spinal movements are a result of collective action. The spinal column of an infant is U-shaped, arching posteriorly. It soon becomes S-shaped when learning to walk on two feet. This S-shaped curve is required for a functional upright posture, and provides better balance and better shock absorption qualities.

The bones of the vertebral column are called the *vertebrae*. They differ slightly in their shape and size from region to region (e.g., cervical versus thoracic). Each weight-bearing portion of the vertebra gradually increases in size so that the larger lumbar vertebrae and sacral vertebrae form a stable base. The *supraspinous ligament* connects the spinous process of C7 to L5 and offers strength and stability. The vertebral column encloses the spinal cord and provides support for the spinal cord and the head, articulates with the ribs, and provides attachment sites for muscles of the back. Located in the posterior region of the neck, the *nuchal ligament* attaches from the occipital bone at the external occipital protuberance to all the spinous processes of the cervical vertebrae and offers the neck both stability and muscle attachment sites. In reference, the supraspinous ligament lies superficial to the nuchal ligament and extends to L5.

Parts of a Typical Vertebra

All vertebrae (except C1) have two main regions: the vertebral body and the arch. Collectively, these regions possess eight basic vertebral elements. They are the vertebral body, two pedicles, two transverse processes, two laminae, and the spinous process (Figure 14-16). Each vertebra varies only in location, shape, and size. The circle of bone

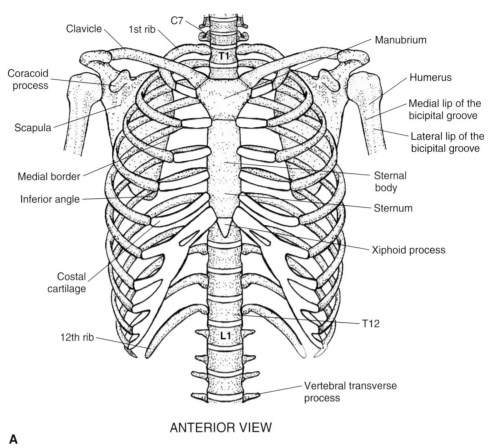

A

ANTERIOR VIEW

FIGURE 14-15 The thorax. **A,** Anterior view. **B,** Posterior view.

that extends out from the body of the vertebra is known as the *vertebral arch,* which is formed by the pedicles and the laminae on either side. The transverse process projects laterally from the arch, and the spinous process projects posteriorly (Table 14-18).

Between each unfused vertebral body is a fibrocartilage disk called the *intervertebral disk.* The functions of these disks are to maintain the joint spaces, assist with spinal movements, and absorb vertical shock. Weight and gravity compresses these disks, and once they are released, they

regain their original shape. The disk has two parts: *annulus fibrosus* (outer ring for shock absorption) and *nucleus pulposus* (soft, gel-like center that adjusts to weight distribution throughout the column). The disk can lose some of its elasticity with age; it can also become compressed and herniate. Just posterior to the intervertebral disk is a large central hole, or canal, for the spinal cord to pass. This opening in the vertebrae is known as the *vertebral canal.* Each vertebra articulates to other vertebrae by *articular facets.* As vertebrae are stacked as a column, an opening is created at the pedicles for spinal roots to pass. This area is called the *intervertebral foramen.* These stacked vertebrae also create a trench in the lamina region of the spine, or the *lamina groove.*

Atypical Vertebrae

C1 – The first cervical vertebra, also known as the *atlas,* or *C1,* is shaped as a bony ring. The atlas possesses no body, pedicles, or laminae. The spinous process has been reduced to a

TABLE 14-16 Sternum

BONY MARKING	SIGNIFICANCE
Manubrium	Muscle attachment and joint formation
Sternal body	Muscle attachment and joint formation
Xiphoid process	Muscle attachment and endangerment site

TABLE 14-17 Ribs

BONY MARKING	SIGNIFICANCE
True ribs (7 pairs)	Attach directly to sternum
False ribs (3 pairs)	Attach to costal cartilage, which attaches to sternum
Floating ribs (2 pairs)	Do not attach to sternum and endangerment site

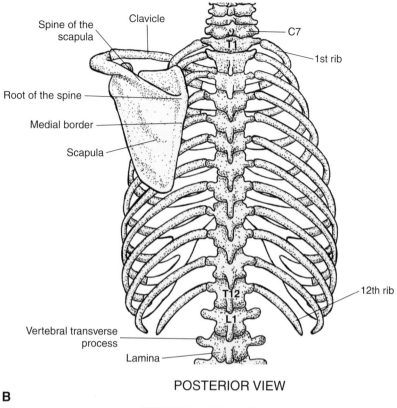

POSTERIOR VIEW

B

FIGURE 14-15, cont'd

posterior tubercle. Facets on the superior surface articulate with the occipital bone and permit head nodding. On the inferior surface, facets articulate with the second cervical vertebrae.

C2 – The second cervical vertebra is often referred to as the *axis,* or *C2.* The axis has a spinous process that is thick and strongly bifurcated (forked). The odontoid process, or dens, is a bony extension that projects superiorly through the ring of the atlas and permits rotation of the head (Figure 14-17). Theories suggest that the dens evolved from the old body of the atlas.

C7 – The *vertebra prominens,* typically *C7,* approximately 70% of the time, has a spinous process that is long and projects posteriorly. The vertebral prominens can be easily palpated at the base of the neck (Figure 14-18). This vertebra is the only cervical vertebra that does not possess a *transverse foramen* (holes in the transverse processes for the passage of blood vessels located in most cervical vertebrae); blood vessels pass directly over the transverse process.

The vertebral prominens is occasionally C6 approximately 20% of the time and T1 approximately 10% of the time.

T1-T12 – Located on the body and transverse processes of the thoracic vertebrae is an extra pair of facets called *demifacets* for articulating ribs.

L1-L5 – The large lumbar vertebrae contain a spinous process and transverse processes that are short and thick.

Divisions of the Vertebral Column

The five regions of the vertebral column are illustrated in Figure 14-19. Each region has unique characteristics. The vertebral column bends anteriorly to posteriorly and back to anteriorly a total of four times (in normal spines). Many liga-

ments join the vertebrae to other structures. The *sacrotuberous ligament,* running from the sacrum to the ischial tuberosity, provides stability to the vertebrae and the pelvis, and the *iliolumbar ligament,* running from the ilium to the transverse process of L5, also provides stability. The different vertebral regions are listed in Table 14-19.

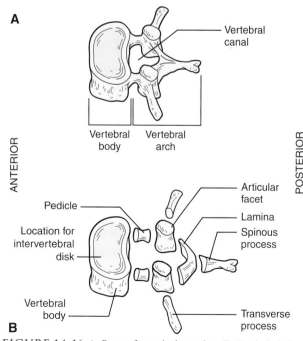

FIGURE 14-16 **A**, Parts of a typical vertebra. **B**, Exploded view.

TABLE 14-18 **Vertebral Components**

BONY MARKING	SIGNIFICANCE
Vertebral body	Joint formation
Pedicle	Attaches arch to body
Transverse processes	Muscle attachment
Lamina	Lamina groove
Spinous process	Muscle attachment
Intervertebral disks	Cartilage between vertebral bodies; contains annulus fibrosus and nucleus pulposus
Vertebral canal	Passage for spinal cord
Articular facet (superior and inferior)	Joint formation
Intervertebral foramen	Passage of spinal roots

TABLE TALK

One way to remember the number of vertebrae in each region is breakfast at seven (7 cervical vertebrae), lunch at twelve (12 thoracic vertebrae), and dinner at five (5 lumbar vertebrae).

MINI-LAB

Obtain an articulated skeleton and a disarticulated skeleton. Most high schools, colleges, or universities use them in biology classes. Working in groups of two or three, locate all the bones, bony markings, and joints discussed in this chapter. Your instructor may add or delete particular structures to suit the needs of the class.

LESSON V—MAJOR JOINTS OF THE BODY

This lesson examines the glenohumeral, iliofemoral, temporomandibular, humeroulnar, humeroradial, tibiofemoral, talocrural, interphalangeal, atlantoaxial, radioulnar, carpo-

metacarpal, radiocarpal, metacarpophalangeal, metatarsophalangeal, atlantooccipital, intervertebral, acromioclavicular, sternoclavicular, intercarpal, pubic symphysis, sacroiliac, lumbosacral, patellofemoral, tarsometatarsal, tibiofibular, costovertebral, and intertarsal.

Articulations

Articulations, also known as *joints,* are the connections between the bones (Figure 14-20). Joints provide a space where one bone articulates with another for the transfer of weight and energy. Joints not only help us move but also help us keep our skeletal system together.

The shape of a joint affects how it functions. As massage therapists, we often have problems in the joints of our hands because we expect them to function in ways for which they were not designed. For example, the wrist is not a weight-bearing structure. When a massage therapist spends too much time with the weight of his or her body on a flexed wrist, it gets injured. This concept is explained in greater detail in Chapter 6. Feet, by contrast, are designed to bear the body's weight. The feet contain many joints for movement and shock absorption, and they provide a stable base.

All the body's articulations have an inverse relationship regarding stability and mobility in which one function is sacrificed for the other. The more secure the joint is, the more stable it will be; however, it is less mobile. For example, the shoulder is the most flexible joint in the body. The joint structure has a shallow socket and hence sustains a greater incident of shoulder dislocations. The hip, by contrast, has a deep socket. The hip joint does not have the flexibility that the shoulder possesses, but it is rarely dislocated. The femur often fractures before the hip joint is affected.

Each joint contains nerve receptors that constantly give us proprioceptive information. These proprioceptive nerves detect stimuli originating from within the body regarding spatial position, muscular activity (motion and resistance), or activation of sensory receptors (see Chapter 17).

ANTERIOR

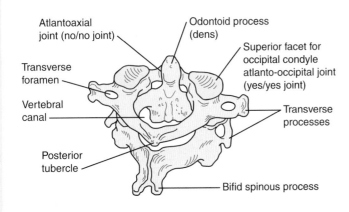

Atlantoaxial joint (no/no joint)

Odontoid process (dens)

Superior facet for occipital condyle atlanto-occipital joint (yes/yes joint)

Transverse foramen

Vertebral canal

Transverse processes

Posterior tubercle

Bifid spinous process

POSTERIOR

FIGURE 14-17 The atlas and axis—atlantoaxial joint.

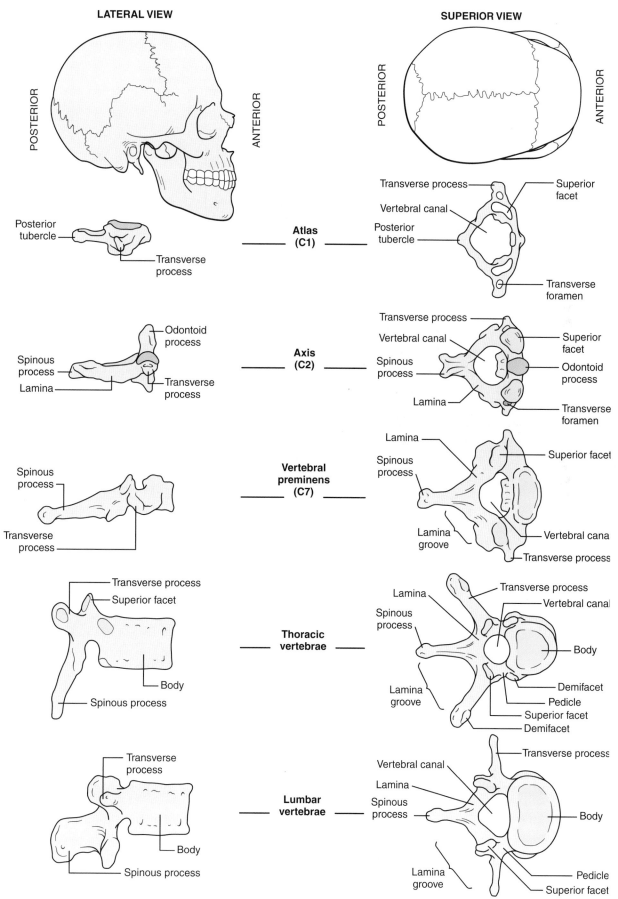

LATERAL VIEW

POSTERIOR

ANTERIOR

Posterior tubercle

Transverse process

SUPERIOR VIEW

POSTERIOR

ANTERIOR

**Atlas
(C1)**

Transverse process

Vertebral canal

Posterior tubercle

Superior facet

Transverse foramen

Odontoid process

Spinous process

Lamina

Transverse process

**Axis
(C2)**

Transverse process

Vertebral canal

Spinous process

Lamina

Superior facet

Odontoid process

Transverse foramen

Spinous process

Transverse process

**Vertebral preminens
(C7)**

Lamina

Spinous process

Lamina groove

Superior facet

Vertebral cana

Transverse process

Transverse process

Superior facet

Body

Spinous process

Thoracic vertebrae

Lamina

Spinous process

Lamina groove

Transverse process

Vertebral canal

Body

Demifacet

Pedicle

Superior facet

Demifacet

Transverse process

Body

Spinous process

Lumbar vertebrae

Vertebral canal

Lamina

Spinous process

Transverse process

Body

Lamina groove

Pedicle

Superior facet

FIGURE 14-18 Vertebrae within the column.

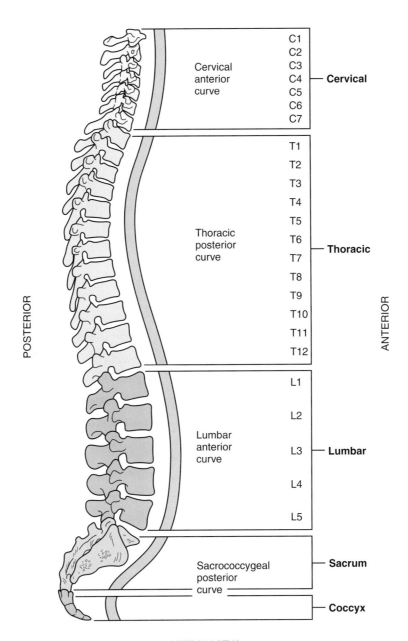

LATERAL VIEW

FIGURE 14-19 The vertebral column with its curves and divisions.

TABLE 14-19 **Vertebral Column**

REGIONS	TRAITS
Cervical (C1-C7)	Curves anteriorly; most possess bifid spinous processes and transverse foramina
Thoracic (T1-T12)	Curves posteriorly; possess demifacets for articulating ribs
Lumbar (L1-L5)	Curves anteriorly; large vertebral bodies
Sacrum (S1-S5—fused)	Curves posteriorly; triangular
Coccyx (Co1-Co3 to Co5—fused)	Curves posteriorly; tail shaped

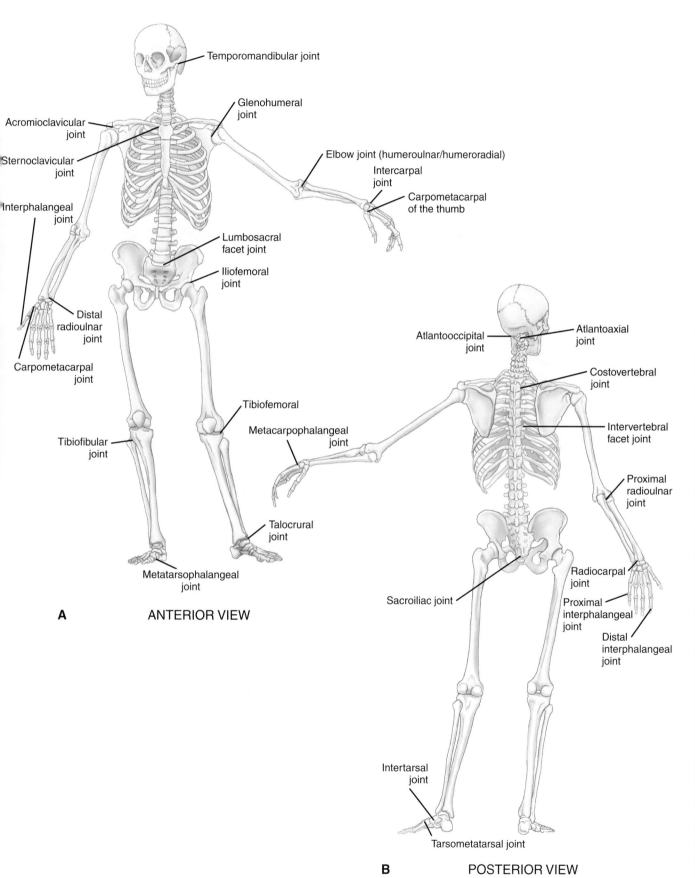

Temporomandibular joint

Glenohumeral joint

Acromioclavicular joint

Sternoclavicular joint

Elbow joint (humeroulnar/humeroradial)

Intercarpal joint

Carpometacarpal of the thumb

Interphalangeal joint

Lumbosacral facet joint

Iliofemoral joint

Distal radioulnar joint

Carpometacarpal joint

Tibiofemoral

Metacarpophalangeal joint

Tibiofibular joint

Talocrural joint

Metatarsophalangeal joint

A   ANTERIOR VIEW

Atlantooccipital joint

Atlantoaxial joint

Costovertebral joint

Intervertebral facet joint

Proximal radioulnar joint

Radiocarpal joint

Proximal interphalangeal joint

Distal interphalangeal joint

Sacroiliac joint

Intertarsal joint

Tarsometatarsal joint

B   POSTERIOR VIEW

FIGURE 14-20 Synovial joints of the body. **A**, Anterior view. **B**, Posterior view.

MINI-LAB

Proprioceptive awareness can be brought to our attention by focusing on the position of our joints and their relative positions in space. Close your right hand into a fist, and place it behind your head. Now open any one finger of this closed fist. Which finger did you open? Can you see the finger? Then how do you know which one you opened? The answer is proprioception. Proprioception allows awareness of the position of each joint of the body.

This section features most of the body's major joints (Table 14-20). The synovial type (ball and socket, hinge, pivot, saddle, ellipsoidal, gliding) classifies each joint. Common names are given along with the joints' scientific names, when applicable. As you learn about each joint, touch and set into motion each joint while imagining the internal joint structures. This learning method will help you understand the mechanisms involved. If additional information is desired on joints, check the references at the end of the chapter.

TABLE 14-20 Articulations

SCIENTIFIC NAME	COMMON NAME	LOCATION
Ball and Socket		
Glenohumeral (scapohumeral) joint	Shoulder joint	Shoulder
Iliofemoral (coxal) joint	Hip joint	Hip
Hinge		
Temporomandibular joint	TMJ	Face/jaw
Humeroulnar/humeroradial joint	Elbow joint	Elbow
Tibiofemoral joint	Knee joint	Knee
Talocrural joint	Ankle joint	Ankle
Interphalangeal joint	IP joint	Fingers and toes
Interphalangeal joint (proximal)	PIP joint	Fingers and toes
Interphalangeal joint (distal)	DIP joint	Fingers and toes
Pivot		
Atlantoaxial joint	*No-no* joint	Upper neck
Radioulnar joint (proximal)	Nonapplicable	Elbow
Radioulnar joint (distal)	Nonapplicable	Wrist
Saddle		
Carpometacarpal joint of the thumb	Nonapplicable	Thumb
Ellipsoidal		
Temporomandibular joint	TMJ	Face/jaw
Radiocarpal joint	Wrist joint	Wrist
Metacarpophalangeal joint	MCP joint	Hand
Metatarsophalangeal joint	MTP joint	Foot
Gliding		
Intervertebral facet joint	Facet joints	Spinal column
Temporomandibular joint	TMJ	Face/jaw
Atlantooccipital joint	Nonapplicable	Upper neck
Acromioclavicular joint	AC joint	Shoulder
Sternoclavicular joint	SC joint	Upper chest
Intercarpal joint	Wrist joint	Wrist
Carpometacarpal joint	CM joint	Hand
Sacroiliac joint	SI joint	Low back
The SI joint is both synovial (gliding) and amphiarthrotic.		
Lumbosacral facet joint	Nonapplicable	Low back
Patellofemoral joint	Nonapplicable	Knee
Tarsometatarsal joint	TM joint	Foot
Intertarsal joint	Nonapplicable	Foot
Tibiofibular joint (proximal)	Nonapplicable	Leg
Costovertebral joints	Nonapplicable	Posterior thorax

Some joints listed previously also contain a disk or meniscus: tibiofemoral (knee); sternoclavicular (SC); the temporomandibular (TMJ) joint; and the joint between the ulna and the triquetrum, which actually has a very cumbersome name, the unlomeniscotriquetral joint.

MINI-LAB

Nod your head slowly as if to say *yes,* and then shake your head slowly as if to say *no.* Now repeat these movements while concentrating on the cervical-occipital area at the back of the neck. Which movement feels higher? Which one feels lower? Is the atlantooccipital joint, also known as the *yes-yes* joint, more superior, or is the atlantoaxial joint, also known as the *no-no* joint, more superior?

evolve *Use your student account via the Evolve website to read an interesting essay on the arthrometric model of the human body.* ∎

Knee Joint

The knee has an internal and external ligament system (Figure 14-21). The internal ligament system is composed of the anterior and posterior cruciate ligaments; they are named for their relative attachment points on tibia. The external ligament system is the medial (tibial) collateral ligament and the lateral (fibular) collateral ligament. The internal and external ligament systems are for static stabilization. Muscles and related tendons are dynamic stabilizers, supporting the knee joint in motion. Although many ligaments are in the joint capsule of the knee, the focus here is on the most important ones (Table 14-21).

evolve *The Evolve website for Chapter 14 is loaded with fun and helpful activites such as "drag and drop" exercises. Check it out!* ∎

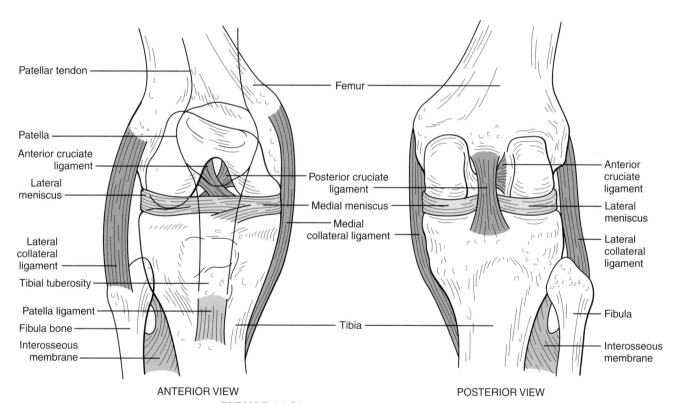

ANTERIOR VIEW   POSTERIOR VIEW

FIGURE 14-21 The knee joint with its ligaments.

TABLE 14-21 Connective Tissue Structures of the Knee

STRUCTURE	COMMENTARY
Patellar (quadriceps) tendon	Attaches the quadriceps femoris muscle to the patella; the entire patella is embedded in this tendon, which continues to the tibia as the patellar ligament.
Patellar ligament	Ligament between the patella and the tibia.
Meniscus (medial and lateral)	Each concave meniscus is composed of half-ring fibrocartilage attaching to the tibia; the two femoral condyles are convex and articulate with the medial and lateral menisci during knee movements.
Collateral ligaments (medial [MCL] and lateral [LCL])	Provide external support and help prevent side-to-side movements; MCL connects the femur to the tibia and may tear during lateral blows to the knee; MCL and the medial meniscus are commonly torn together. LCL connects the femur to the fibula.
Cruciate ligaments (anterior, or ACL, and posterior, or PCL)	Provide internal support and help prevent front to back movements; anchor the tibia to the femur; cross in the middle of the knee joint. ACL often torn in knee injuries.

BOX 14-1

Effects of Massage on Connective Tissues

- **Reduces keloid formation.** Massage applied to scar tissue helps reduce keloid formation in scar tissue.
- **Reduces excessive scar formation.** Deep massage reduces excessive scar formation, thereby helping create an appropriate scar that is strong yet does not interfere with the muscle's ability to broaden as it contracts.
- **Decreases adhesion formation.** The displacement of scar tissue during massage helps reduce formation of adhesions, which, in turn, facilitates normal, pain-free motion of the affected muscles and joints.
- **Releases fascial restrictions.** Pressure, and the heat it produces, converts fascia from a gel state to a sol state (thixotropy), thereby reducing hyperplasia. Fascia loosens and melts, becoming more flexible and elastic. Softening of the fascia surrounding muscles allows them to be stretched to their fullest resting length, thereby increasing joint range of motion and freeing the body of restricted movements.
- **Improves connective tissue healing.** Occurring only with deep pressure massage, proliferation and activation of fibroblasts were noted, which lead to improved tensile strength of healed tissue.

SUMMARY

Skeletal nomenclature is the prerequisite to the muscular system and therefore fundamental to the study of massage. The bony skeleton provides a road map to the muscles, with its signs being the bony markings that are the sites of tendon attachment. The 206 bones of the skeleton have been divided regionally: bones of the upper extremity, bones of the lower extremity, bones of the skull, bones of the vertebral column and thorax, and major joints of the body. In each region, the specifics of each bone are detailed with regard to name, location, joint involvement, and important bony markings.

evolve

Go to *Chapter Extras* on Evolve for additional illustrations and resources for this chapter. *Extras* for this chapter include:

1. Crossword puzzles (downloadable forms)
2. Palpatory anatomy (worksheet)
3. Arthrometric model (illustration)

MATCHING I

Place the letter of the answer next to the term or phrase that best describes it. Some answers may be used more than once.

A. Carpals   D. Metacarpals   G. Scapula
B. Clavicle   E. Phalanges   H. Ulna
C. Humerus   F. Radius

_____ 1.   Greater tubercle

_____ 2.   Lateral forearm bone

_____ 3.   Capitulum

_____ 4.   Trochlea

_____ 5.   Bicipital tuberosity

_____ 6.   Collarbone

_____ 7.   Acromion process

_____ 8.   Ulnar tuberosity

_____ 9.   Deltoid tuberosity

_____ 10. Rotates on the ulna

_____ 11. Glenoid fossa

_____ 12. Supraglenoid tubercle

_____ 13. Medial forearm bone

_____ 14. Collective term for wrist bones

_____ 15. Olecranon process

_____ 16. Hand bones numbered I through V

_____ 17. Shoulder blade

_____ 18. Located in the fingers and thumb

_____ 19. Coracoid process

_____ 20. Infraspinous fossa

MATCHING II

Place the letter of the answer next to the term or phrase that best describes it. Some answers may be used more than once.

A. Femur
B. Fibula
C. Ilium
D. Ischium

E. Metatarsals
F. Patella
G. Phalanges

H. Pubis
I. Tarsals
J. Tibia

_____ 1. Greater trochanter

_____ 2. Bones located in the toes

_____ 3. Talus, cuneiforms, calcaneus

_____ 4. Lateral malleolus

_____ 5. Most superior pelvic bone

_____ 6. Longest bone in the body; thigh bone

_____ 7. Most inferior pelvic bone

_____ 8. Soleal line

_____ 9. Anterior gluteal line

_____ 10. Sesamoid bone

_____ 11. Lateral leg bone

_____ 12. Tibial tuberosity

_____ 13. Iliac fossa

_____ 14. Anterior superior iliac spine

_____ 15. Linea aspera

_____ 16. Foot bones numbered I though V

_____ 17. Ischial tuberosity

_____ 18. Medial malleolus

_____ 19. Gluteal tuberosity

_____ 20. Most anterior pelvic bones

MATCHING III

Place the letter of the answer next to the term or phrase that best describes it. Some answers may be used more than once.

A. Frontal   D. Maxilla   G. Sphenoid
B. Hyoid   E. Occipital   H. Temporal
C. Mandible   F. Parietal   I. Zygomatic

_____ 1. Foramen magnum

_____ 2. Condylar process

_____ 3. External auditory meatus

_____ 4. Styloid process

_____ 5. Bones that are joined with the sagittal suture

_____ 6. Superior nuchal lines

_____ 7. Bone located in the forehead area of the face

_____ 8. Sella turcica

_____ 9. Mandibular angle

_____ 10. Usually located at the level of C3

_____ 11. Mastoid process

_____ 12. Bones located in the cheek area of the face

_____ 13. Coronoid process

_____ 14. Does not join directly with a bone

_____ 15. Bone located in the upper jaw of the face

_____ 16. Mandibular ramus

_____ 17. External occipital protuberance

_____ 18. Bone where the sphenoidal sinuses are located

_____ 19. Pterygoid plate

_____ 20. Occipital condyles

SELF TEST

MATCHING IV

Place the letter of the answer next to the term or phrase that best describes it. Some answers may be used more than once.

A. Atlas
B. Axis
C. Cervical
D. Coccyx
E. False ribs
F. Floating ribs

G. Laminae
H. Lumbar
I. Pedicles
J. Ribs
K. Sacrum
L. Spinous processes

M. Sternum
N. Thoracic
O. Transverse processes
P. True ribs
Q. Vertebrae
R. Vertebral body

_____ 1. Xiphoid process

_____ 2. Spinal region that contains demifacets

_____ 3. Posterior projections of vertebrae

_____ 4. C2

_____ 5. Superior region of spinal column

_____ 6. Joins the vertebral body to the lamina

_____ 7. Ribs that attach by costal cartilage

_____ 8. Long, slender, curved bones

_____ 9. Part of pelvis

_____ 10. Lamina groove

_____ 11. Bones of the spinal column

_____ 12. Ribs that do not attach to sternum at all

_____ 13. Attaches to the intervertebral disk

_____ 14. Possesses the odontoid process

_____ 15. Inferior bone of spinal column

_____ 16. Ribs that attach directly to sternum

_____ 17. Breastbone

_____ 18. Low back region of spinal column

_____ 19. C1

_____ 20. Lateral projections of vertebrae

MATCHING V

Place the letter of the answer next to the term or phrase that best describes it. Some answers may be used more than once.

A. Ball and socket   C. Gliding   E. Pivot
B. Ellipsoidal   D. Hinge   F. Saddle

_____   1.   Atlantooccipital joint

_____   2.   Humeroulnar joint

_____   3.   Talocrural joint

_____   4.   Iliofemoral joint

_____   5.   Metatarsophalangeal joint

_____   6.   Radiocarpal joint

_____   7.   Costovertebral joints

_____   8.   Intercarpal joint

_____   9.   Sternoclavicular joint

_____ 10.   Atlantoaxial joint

_____ 11.   Carpometacarpal of the thumb

_____ 12.   Tibiofemoral joint

_____ 13.   Interphalangeal joint

_____ 14.   Intervertebral facet joint

_____ 15.   Radioulnar joint

_____ 16.   Lumbosacral facet joint

_____ 17.   Metacarpophalangeal joint

_____ 18.   Glenohumeral joint

_____ 19.   Humeroradial joint

_____ 20.   Acromioclavicular joint

INTERNET ACTIVITIES

Visit http://www.arthritis.org/conditions/51_ways/lose_weight.asp to find 51 Ways to be Good to Your Joints. Write down three of the suggestions.

Visit http://www.skeletaldrawing.com and choose a dinosaur from the skeletal drawing gallery and color in the bones. Once colored, contrast and compare your creation with that of a human skeleton. Write down your findings.

Visit http://www.healthpages.org and click on Atlanta Health Pages. Choose Library, and then choose Health Topics. Read about hip and knee replacements. How does your new knowledge of skeletal anatomy help you understand this discussion?

Bibliography

Abrahams P, Marks S, Hutchings R: *McMinn's color atlas of human anatomy,* St Louis, 2003, Mosby.

Ardoin W: From a lecture on temporomandibular joint dysfunction given at the Louisiana Institute of Massage Therapy, Lafayette, La, 1994, personal contact.

Biel A: *Trail guide to the body: how to locate muscles, bones, and more,* ed 3, Boulder, Colo, 2005, Books of Discovery.

Bowden B, Bowden J: *An illustrated atlas of the skeletal muscles,* Englewood, Colo, 2002, Morton.

Brossman AB: *Some of the finer points about temporomandibular joint anatomy and physiology,* Wheeling, W.Va, 1997. Available at: *http://www.ovnet.com/userpages/rebross/tmjoints.html*

Como D, editor: *Mosby's Medical, Nursing, and Allied Health Dictionary,* ed 6, St Louis, 2002, Mosby.

Crawley J, Van De Graaff KM: *A photographic atlas for anatomy and physiology,* Englewood, Colo, 2002, Morton.

Goldberg S: *Clinical anatomy made ridiculously simple,* Miami, 2004, Medmaster.

Grafelman T: *Graf's anatomy and physiology guide for the massage therapist,* Aurora, Colo, 1998, DG Publishing.

Gray H, Pick TP, Howden R: *Gray's anatomy,* ed 29, Philadelphia, 1974, Running Press.

Guyton A: *Human physiology and mechanisms of disease,* ed 6, Philadelphia, 1996, Saunders.

Haubrich WS: *Medical meanings: a glossary of word origins,* New York, 1984, Harcourt Brace Jovanovich.

Hoppenfeld S: *Physical examination of the spine and extremities,* Norwalk, Conn, 1976, Appleton-Century-Crofts.

Jacob S, Francone C: *Elements of anatomy and physiology,* Philadelphia, 1989, Saunders.

Juhan D: *Job's body: a handbook for bodyworkers,* ed 3, Barrington, NY, 2003, Station Hill Press.

Kapandji IA: *The physiology of the joints,* ed 5, New York, 1988, Churchill Livingstone.

Kapit W, Elson LM: *The anatomy coloring book,* ed 3, New York, 2002, Benjamin Cummings.

Kordish M, Dickson S: *Introduction to basic human anatomy,* Lake Charles, La, 1985, McNeese State University.

Marieb EN: *Essentials of human anatomy and physiology,* ed 8, New York, 2005, Benjamin Cummings.

Martini FH, Bartholomew EF: *Essentials of anatomy and physiology,* ed 3, New York, 2003, Benjamin Cummings.

McAleer N: *The body almanac,* Garden City, NY, 1985, Doubleday.

Merck manual, ed 17, Whitehouse Station, NJ, 1998, Merck and Company.

Moore KL: *Clinically oriented anatomy,* ed 5, Baltimore, 2005, Lippincott Williams & Wilkins.

Muscolino JE: *The muscular system manual: the skeletal muscles of the human body,* ed 2, St Louis, 2005, Elsevier Mosby.

Muscolino JE, *Kinesiology: the skeletal system and muscle function,* St Louis, 2006, Mosby.

Netter FH: *Atlas of human anatomy,* ed 3, Teterboro, NJ, 2003, Icon Learning Systems.

Olsen A, McHose C: *Body stories: a guide to experiential anatomy,* Barrytown, NY, 2004, Station Hill Press.

Platzer W: *Color atlas and textbook of human anatomy: locomotor system,* vol I, ed 5, New York, 2003, Thieme.

Souza TA: *Differential diagnosis and management for the chiropractor,* ed 2, Gaithersburg, Md, 2001, Aspen Publications.

Thibodeau G, Patton K: *Anatomy and physiology,* ed 6, St Louis, 2006, Mosby.

Thibodeau G, Patton K: *Structure and function of the body,* ed 12, St Louis, 2004, Mosby.

Tortora GJ: *Introduction to the human body: the essentials of anatomy and physiology,* ed 5, Hoboken, NJ, 2000, Wiley, John & Sons.

Tortora GJ, Grabowksi SR: *Principles of anatomy and physiology,* ed 11, New York, 2005, John Wiley & Sons.

Travell JG, Simons D: *Myofascial pain and dysfunction, the trigger point manual,* Baltimore, 1992, Lippincott Williams & Wilkins.

Venes D, Thomas CL, Taber CW: *Taber's cyclopedic medical dictionary,* ed 20, Philadelphia, 2005, FA Davis.

Wilson JM: *Doctoral dissertation: a natural philosophy of movement styles for theatre performers,* Madison, Wis, 1973, University of Wisconsin-Madison.

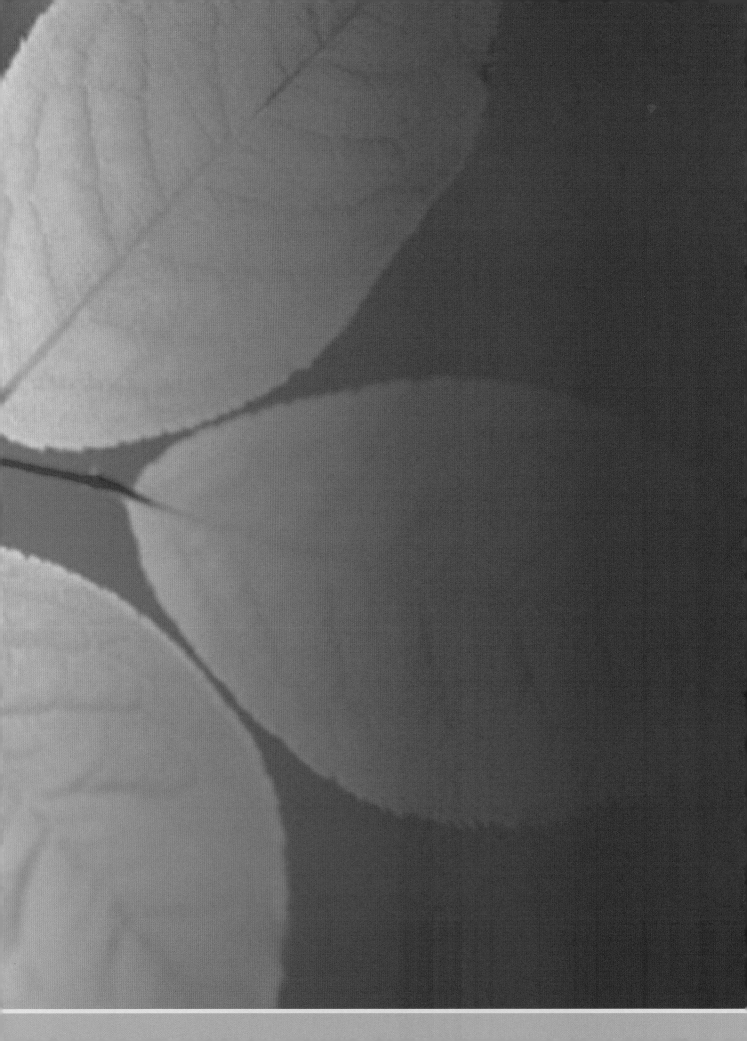

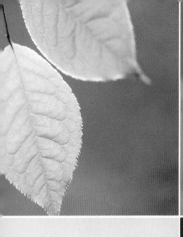

CHAPTER 15

"Perhaps all pleasure is only relief."
—William S. Burroughs

Muscular System

STUDENT OBJECTIVES

After completing this chapter, the student should be able to:

- List the anatomy and describe the physiology of the muscular system
- Describe how muscle cells contribute to the development of muscle organs
- Categorize the connective tissue components of the muscular system
- Identify all characteristics and properties of muscle cells
- Explain the mechanisms involved in muscle contraction
- Describe how a muscle goes from contraction to relaxation
- List and discuss a muscle's energy source
- Identify the parts and possible fiber arrangements of skeletal muscles
- State how skeletal muscles act together to coordinate movement
- Contrast and compare slow-twitch, fast-twitch, and intermediate fibers
- Discuss the receptors involved in stretching
- Demonstrate and explain types of skeletal muscle contraction
- Distinguish between eccentric and concentric contractions
- Discuss the importance of good posture and muscle tone
- Name types of pathological muscular conditions, giving characteristics and massage considerations of each

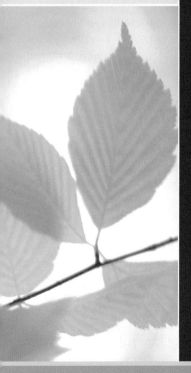

INTRODUCTION

Everything you have learned until now from this text was in preparation for learning and understanding the muscular system. The integument is the primary means of taking messages of touch to the brain, and we certainly treat connective tissue as well because it is found everywhere in the body. However, most clients come to us complaining about muscle tension or soreness somewhere in their bodies. The muscular system is essential to massage therapists because the muscles and the related connective tissues (fascia) are the primary focus of massage. The last two chapters examined the body's framework and the joints that allow movement. However, bones cannot move themselves; they must be moved by something, by skeletal muscles. This chapter examines the muscular system, explores the muscle cells, and the mechanism of skeletal muscle contraction. The individual origin, insertion (muscle attachments), and action of the muscles are discussed in Chapter 16.

The thought of being alive brings to the forefront the idea of movement—the heartbeat, facial expression, and the rise and fall of the chest with each breath. These visible signs of life are all created by muscle contractions.

Years ago, physiologists believed that skeletal muscles contracted by folding, similar to an accordion, or by changes in the diameter of each cell. Some researchers hypothesized that muscles just grew or perhaps moved the way springs move. In 1969 Hugh Huxley discovered that contraction does not occur by folding or springing. Shortening or lengthening of a muscle results from a change in the relative positions of one muscle fiber to another. To understand this shortening, or contractile mechanism of the muscle, we will examine the muscle fibers themselves.

In massage schools, the depth of knowledge regarding the muscular system exceeds that of many other health care fields. Beyond a basic understanding of the anatomy and physiology of the muscles, considering a broad spectrum of information is necessary. This information includes the histological mechanisms of muscle tissue, connective tissue components, structures of skeletal muscles, energy sources for muscular contraction, muscular relaxation, types of skeletal muscle, muscle stretching, types of skeletal muscle contractions, muscle fiber arrangement, parts of a skeletal muscle, how the body coordinates movement, and pathological muscular conditions. This comprehensive study of muscles provides the massage therapist with a complex array of information that can be used to address muscular dysfunction resulting from stress, illness, or injury.

ANATOMY

Areas of discussion in this chapter include:
- Skeletal muscles
- Related fascia
- Tendons

PHYSIOLOGY

- **External mobility.** Skeletal muscles create visible movement. This movement includes both motion and locomotion. *Motion* is defined as the body moving its parts, as compared with *locomotion,* which is defined as the body moving as a whole.
- **Internal mobility.** Internal mobility refers to the movement resulting from the contraction of smooth muscles. An example is peristalsis of the intestines. The special name given to the movement resulting from smooth muscle contractions is *motility.*
- **Heat production.** All muscle contractions produce and release heat. Skeletal muscles are the most metabolical structures in the body and produce a significant amount of heat. This physiological mechanism of thermogenesis is also important to maintain internal body temperature. Additionally, when the body becomes chilled, skeletal muscles contract rapidly (shivering) to produce additional heat.
- **Posture maintenance.** To maintain static positions such as sitting and standing, the skeletal muscles periodically contract to hold us in these postures. Muscles also contribute to joint stability.

MUSCLE CELLS INTO MUSCLE ORGANS

Muscle cells are referred to as **muscle fibers** because of their threadlike, slender shape, and they usually run the length of the muscle. Muscle fibers are generally arranged in parallel rows. Some individual muscle fibers may be more than 12 inches long. Each muscle fiber contains **myofibrils,** very fine longitudinal fibers, consisting of thick and thin myofilaments.

Muscles are considered to be tough, but muscle fibers are quite fragile. Therefore they are arranged and protected by a series of connective tissue wrappings. A connective tissue layer called *endomysium* covers the muscle fibers (Figure 15-1). This important fascial covering allows for muscular vascularization and innervation. Groups of muscle fibers are called **fasciculi** and are bound by a tougher connective tissue envelope called *perimysium*. Groups of fasciculi (*sing.* fascicle) compose a muscle or muscle organ, which is bound by a coarse sheet of connective tissue called *epimysium*. Fibrous bands of connective tissue that surround muscle groups are called *fascia,* more specifically, *deep fascia*. **Myofascial** refers to the skeletal muscles and related fascia in the muscular

---

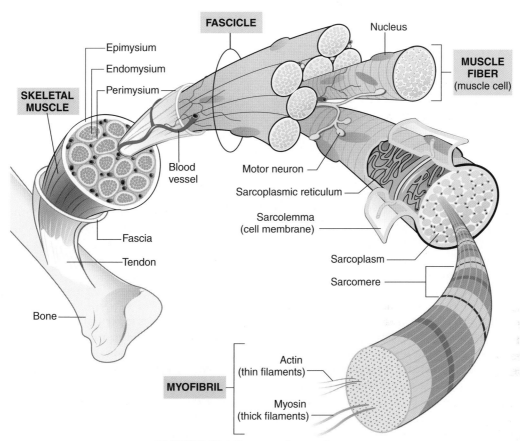

FIGURE 15-1 Structure of a muscle organ.

system. The progression from microscopic to macroscopic is as follows:

Myofilaments → myofibril → muscle fiber (cell) → fascicle → muscle

Let us also review the connective tissue coverings of muscle cells and actual muscles:

Endomysium (wraps around muscle fibers) → perimysium (wraps around fasciculi) → epimysium (wraps around entire muscle) → deep fascia (wraps around muscle groups)

When organization of deep fascia forms a cord, anchoring the ends of muscle to bone, it is called a **tendon.** A broad, flat tendon is called an **aponeurosis** and attaches skeletal muscle to bone, another muscle, or skin. Tendons and aponeuroses are both tough, collagenous structures and differ only in shape; tendons are cords, whereas aponeuroses are sheetlike. When tendons cross multiple joints, as in the hands and feet, they are wrapped in *tendon sheaths*. These tubular structures resemble little sleeves lined with a synovial membrane. Synovial fluid secreted by this membrane reduces friction as the tendons glide back and forth within the sheath. To keep tendons and tendon sheaths in place, **retinacula,** bandagelike retaining bands of connective tissue, are found primarily around the elbows, knees, ankles, and wrists. The retinaculum may also act as a pulley for tendons.

TABLE TALK

If the connective tissue component were removed from skeletal muscles, then it would resemble a mound of jelly without form or functional ability.

MUSCLE CELLS

The three parts of a cell discussed in Chapter 11 (membrane, cytoplasm, organelles) are all present in muscle cells, but they have specialized names and functions. The cell membrane is called the **sarcolemma** (Figure 15-2), and it encases the cytoplasm and organelles. The cytoplasm is called the **sarcoplasm** and surrounds the organelles. The **sarcoplasmic reticulum** is similar to, but not identical with, the endoplasmic reticulum. The sarcoplasmic reticulum is a fluid-filled system of cavities that contain sarcomeres. The sarcoplasmic reticulum plays a crucial role in muscular contraction by storing and releasing calcium ions. Skeletal muscle cells also contain many mitochondria and many nuclei.

evolve *To see a muscle cell from microscopic progressing up to a macroscopic image, log on to the Evolve website and access the course materials for Chapter 15 using your student account.* ■

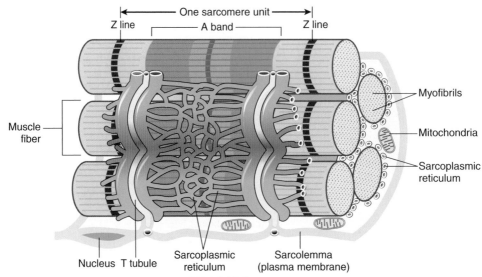

FIGURE 15-2 Muscle cells.

Another structure that is unique to a muscle cell is a system of transverse tubules, or T-tubules, so named because they run transversely across the sarcoplasmic reticulum at the level of the Z-lines (mentioned in the section Sarcomere) and form inward channels of the sarcolemma. The T-tubules spread the nerve impulse by transporting stored ions into and out of the cell.

Myofilaments

Each muscle fiber contains myofibrils. Inside each myofibril are thousands of thick and thin myofilaments. Four different kinds of protein molecules make up myofilaments: (1) actin, (2) myosin, (3) tropomyosin, and (4) troponin. Thin filaments are made of a combination of three proteins, actin, tropomyosin, and troponin. *Actin* molecules are strung together, resembling a twisted double strand of beads to form two fibrous strands that twist around each other (Figure 15-3). Actin (thin myofilaments) and myosin (thick filaments) have a chemical attraction to one another. While the muscle is at rest, binding sites located on actin myofilaments are covered by long *tropomyosin* molecules, blocking entry. Tropomyosin seems to be held in place by *troponin* spaced at intervals along actin filaments. Here they wait for calcium ions to move them off, which exposes the binding sites.

The thick filaments are made almost entirely of myosin protein. Myosin molecules are shaped as golf clubs with the golf shafts bundled together, making up the bulk of the thick filament. Sticking out of the golf club is a structure called a *myosin head*. These heads angle toward the covered binding sites located on actin myofilaments.

Sarcomeres

Sarcomeres, composed of myosin and actin filaments, are present in segments along myofibrils. Defining the ends of the sarcomere are *Z-lines*, thin membranous rows seen as longitudinal sections in skeletal muscle. Z-lines are so called because of their jagged appearance. Actin filaments attach to both Z-lines of a sarcomere, and they extend partway toward the center of the sarcomere. The central region of a resting sarcomere is devoid of actin filaments, gives it a lighter color, and is known as the *H-band* (Figure 15-4). Each myofibril consists of many sarcomeres, each one functioning as a contractile unit.

Sarcomeres are bundled together and lie in parallel rows in a honeycomb arrangement (see Figure 15-3). They are stacked end to end in a continuous chain of repeating compartments. Myosin filaments do not run the entire length of

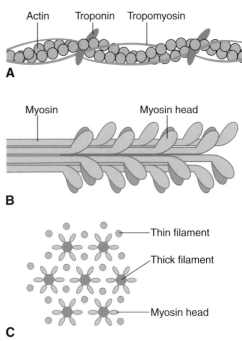

FIGURE 15-3 Myofilaments **A**, Thin myofilament. **B**, Thick myofilament. **C**, Cross-section of several myofilaments to show relative positions and myosin head extensions.

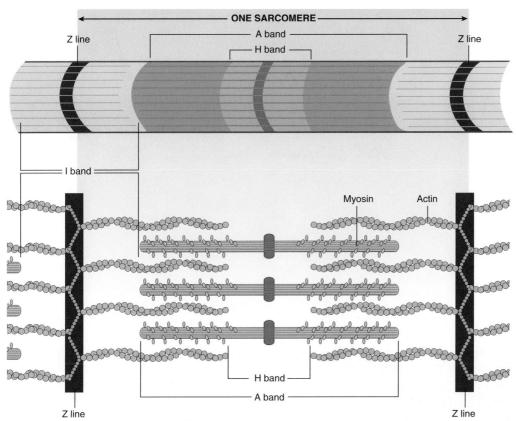

FIGURE 15-4 Sliding filament theory.

the sarcomere. Because the filament arrangement is slightly staggered, the myofilaments overlap in some areas (dark stripe) and not in others (light stripe), which gives it a striated appearance. The dark red area on either side of the H-band contains both actin and myosin and is known as the *A-band.* The absence of the myosin filament at either end of the sarcomere is known as the *I-band,* which has a light appearance. As the muscle contracts and the filaments slide, the H- and I-bands become narrow.

To review:

Z-line: ends of the sarcomere
H-band: center of sarcomere, myosin only
A-band: actin and myosin overlapping
I-band: actin only

> ### TABLE TALK
>
> An easy way to remember that actin is the thinner myofilament and myosin is the thicker myofilament is that actin is a shorter, thinner word. Myosin is a longer, thicker word and is the thicker myofilament.

Muscle Cell Properties

Muscles possess the following characteristics that give them the ability to move:

- **Excitability**: ability to respond to a stimulus
- **Contractility**: ability of muscle fibers to shorten
- **Extensibility**: ability of muscle fibers to lengthen
- **Elasticity**: ability of muscle fibers to return to their original shape after movement

MECHANISM OF CONTRACTION

Excitation of the Sarcolemma

The contraction of skeletal muscle begins with a nerve impulse stimulating the muscle fibers into action. Either a reflex or a conscious desire to change the body's position may initiate this nerve impulse. A special type of neuron, a **motor neuron,** is responsible for sending the impulse to the muscle cell (see Chapter 17). Motor neurons are responsible for carrying messages of contraction (or in some cases, inhibition of contraction) to a muscle. One motor neuron may branch off and connect to 10 or 1000 individual muscle fibers. A single motor neuron plus all the muscle fibers to which it attaches constitute a functional unit called a **motor unit** (Figure 15-5). A single muscle is composed of many motor units.

Motor neurons connect to folded sections of the sarcolemma called a *motor end plate*. The junction between the motor neuron and the motor end plate is called the **neuromuscular junction** (Figure 15-6). This space occupying the junction is called a *synapse,* characterized by a narrow gap or cleft, across which neurotransmitters or chemical messengers such as acetylcholine, diffuse.

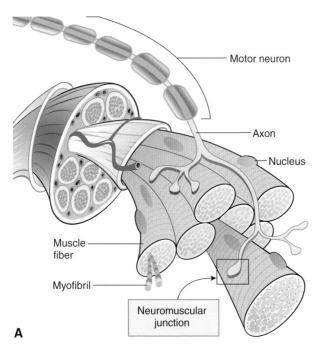

A

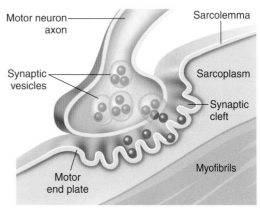

FIGURE 15-6 Neuromuscular junction.

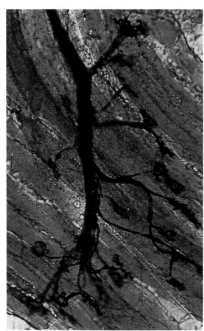

B

FIGURE 15-5 Motor unit. **A,** Motor unit with neuromuscular junction. **B,** Photograph using electron microscope of a motor unit.

The processes involved with the release of neurotransmitters initiated by a nerve impulse entering the sarcolemma are called *excitation*.

Synaptic Transmission

When the nerve impulse travels through a motor neuron axon and enters the neuromuscular junction, neurotransmitters stored in vesicles are released. The principle neurotransmitter involved in muscle contraction is **acetylcholine** (ACh). When ACh crosses the synaptic cleft to the sarcolemma, it

binds with receptor sites on the motor end plate, similar to a key in a lock. When this connection is made with the sarcolemma, the next phase of muscular contraction begins.

Propagation of the Nerve Impulse

The impulse travels across the surface of the sarcolemma and is carried into the cell through the T-tubules. The propagation of the nerve impulse into the cell via the T-tubules triggers the release of a flood of calcium ions from the adjacent sacs in the sarcoplasmic reticulum. Calcium ions are the chemical driving force behind contraction because they assist actin and myosin to connect so contraction can occur.

Contraction

To review, positioned on the actin filaments are two protein molecules, troponin and tropomyosin. Recall that troponin normally holds tropomyosin strands in place and covers myosin binding sites. Without these regulatory proteins, muscles would be in a constant state of contraction. When calcium binds to tropomyosin, it alters them in a way that troponin slides off and exposes the site for a myosin head to attach. The connection between the myosin heads and the actin filaments creates a *cross-bridge* effect. The *power stroke* is the stage of muscle contraction when the cross-bridge myosin heads, which are hinged at their base, toggles similar to a light switch. This action causes the actin filaments to slide past the myosin filaments. Remember that actin filaments attach to the Z-lines (ends of a sarcomere). During the power stroke, the sarcomere shortens, causing the muscle fiber to contract. If adenosine triphosphate is present, each head then detaches itself, binds to the next exposed site, and pulls again (Figure 15-7). Actin filaments sliding toward the sarcomeres center (the H-band) quickly shorten the myofibril and thus the entire muscle fiber. This model of muscle contraction was appropriately named the **sliding filament theory**. Muscle contraction has occurred, taking just a few thousandths of second.

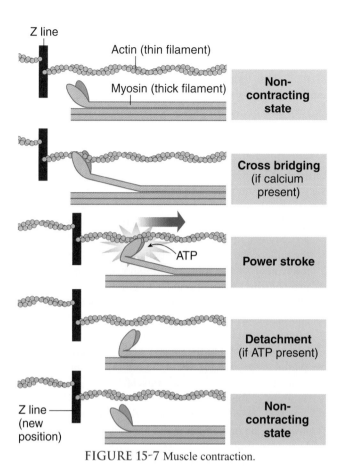

Z line

Actin (thin filament)

Myosin (thick filament)

Non-contracting state

Cross bridging (if calcium present)

ATP

Power stroke

Detachment (if ATP present)

Z line (new position)

Non-contracting state

FIGURE 15-7 Muscle contraction.

THRESHOLDS AND STRENGTH OF CONTRACTION

When a motor neuron delivers a stimulus, all the muscle fibers of the motor unit receive the signal to contract at the same time. If the stimulus lacks sufficient intensity (subthreshold stimulus), motor neurons will not activate, and contraction does not occur. In the absence of sufficient stimuli, each muscle fiber relaxes to its full resting length. Conversely, each individual muscle fiber, when sufficiently stimulated, contracts to its fullest extent. Within the muscle fibers of motor units, no partial contraction takes place. This is known as the **all-or-none response.**

This all-or-none response is true only for motor units, not the entire muscle. Thousands of motor units are in a single muscle. The nervous system regulates the amount of muscular contraction by activating only the motor units needed to perform a given action. If more strength is required, additional motor units are then stimulated, and the muscle contraction is stronger. More motor units are required to pick up a hammer than to pick up a nail. This process of motor unit activation based on need is known as **recruitment.**

RELAXATION

Almost immediately after the sarcoplasmic reticulum releases calcium ions into the sarcoplasm, it begins to actively pump them back into its sacs. Within a few milliseconds,

much of calcium is recovered. Freed from its chemical bond with the calcium ions, the troponin slides back the binding sites on the actin filaments. This action releases the myosin heads and returns them to their precontraction state. The muscle is now at rest.

TABLE TALK

A goal in massage is to release muscular spasm. One of the components of a spasm is a leak of calcium from the sarcoplasmic reticulum without nerve stimulation, which can occur as a result of a tear from an injury or exercise. The calcium triggers contraction, and this action sets up a condition of spasm, unless something flushes the calcium out of the cells. Massage creates a flushing affect and may remove not only calcium but also metabolic wastes. As an added bonus, massage also brings oxygen and other essential nutrients to the tissues.

MINI-LAB

Hold your hands 18 inches from your face, palms facing you. Extend your thumbs up and interlace your fingers. Let your thumbs represent the Z-lines, and your fingers represent thick and thin myofilaments. Slide your fingers toward the middle. Notice how the space between your thumbs, or Z-lines, move closer together. As the spaces between the thumbs shorten, do your fingers shorten? This exercise illustrates how the sarcomere within a muscle creates movement by shortening.

ENERGY SOURCES FOR CONTRACTION

Adenosine Triphosphate

The energy needed for contraction comes from a compound called **adenosine triphosphate** (ATP), which is produced by the body's cells. When ATP's energy bonds are broken, the energy required for myosin heads to toggle back toward their original positions is obtained.

Between contractions, myosin is in a cocked position, ready for action. When calcium ions move troponin from the actin binding sites, the sites become exposed. Myosin then binds to actin, releases ATP's stored energy, and causes the myosin head to spring back to its original or cocked position. Once the myosin head is released, it moves into its resting position again—all set for the next pull. Another ATP molecule binds to the myosin head, ATP's energy is released, and the myosin head toggles and pulls actin toward the center of the sarcomere, which shortens the sarcomere and ultimately the muscle itself. This cycle repeats as long as ATP is available and actin's binding sites are exposed.

Oxygen and Glucose

Skeletal muscle contraction also requires two essential ingredients, glucose and oxygen.

During rest, oxygen is stored in muscle cells. The storage is due to oxygen's binding to a large protein molecule called *myoglobin*. Myoglobin is a red respiratory pigment similar to hemoglobin in red blood cells. Like hemoglobin, myoglobin contains iron that attracts oxygen and holds it temporarily.

When oxygen within muscles cells decreases rapidly, as it does in exercise, it is quickly replenished as a result of myoglobin. Muscle fibers that contain large amounts of myoglobin take on a deep red appearance and are often called *red muscle*. Muscle fibers with little myoglobin are lighter in color and are often called *white muscle*. Most muscles contain a mixture of red and white fibers. Additional information can be found in the section Types of Skeletal Muscle Fibers.

Normal ATP concentration in muscle cells is very small; ATP can sustain approximately 10 to 15 additional seconds of muscle activity. Significant energy-producing mechanisms in the body require the breakdown of the sugars, namely glucose. Glucose is stored as glycogen predominantly in liver and muscle cells. Muscle cells can also receive glucose from the blood supply.

The complete breakdown of glucose occurs in two stages. The first stage of glucose utilization is called *anaerobic* because oxygen is not used. The second stage, when physical activity becomes even more vigorous, is called *aerobic respiration* because oxygen is used to produce even more energy. Let us discuss each step individually.

Almost as soon as muscle contraction starts, the anaerobic process also begins. Anaerobic glycolysis does not contribute a large amount of energy (energy equivalent to two ATP molecules), and its contribution is likely to last from 30 to 60 seconds. Lactic acid is formed as the end product of anaerobic glycolysis. Lactic acid may accumulate in muscle tissue during exercise, causing local fatigue and a burning sensation. Some of the lactic acid eventually diffuses into the blood and is delivered to the liver, where an oxygen-consuming process later converts it back into glucose. This process is one of the reasons that, after heavy exercise, a person may still continue to breathe heavily. The body is repaying the so-called *oxygen debt* by using the extra oxygen gained by heavy breathing to process the lactic acid that was produced during exercise.

The second stage is aerobic glycolysis, creating the equivalent to 36 ATP molecules. Oxygen is brought in and carbon dioxide is expelled from the muscle cell through cellular respiration (see Chapter 20). This process of energy production can continue as long as enough oxygen is available through cellular respiration.

PARTS OF A SKELETAL MUSCLE

The gross structures of a skeletal muscle come in a wide range of shapes and sizes, but all possess a central portion of the muscle and at least two points of attachment.

Most skeletal muscles cross at least one joint and attach to articulating bones. At the simplest level, when contraction

occurs and a muscle shortens, one bone moves while the other stays fixed.

Terms used to indicate attachment sites are *origin* and *insertion*. These terms provide useful points of reference. Generally, insertion moves toward origin; however, the roles can be reversed. Some muscles possess a property of *functional reversibility*. For example, you can lean over, bringing your torso toward your lower extremity, or you can lift your thigh, bringing your lower extremity toward your torso. Thus the terms *origin* and *insertion* do not always provide the necessary information needed to ascertain a muscle's action. Following are the parts of a muscle:

Belly. The belly of the muscle is also referred to as the *gaster* (Figure 15-8). This wide central portion makes up the bulk of the muscle. The belly of the muscle produces movement of the joint by the shortening of its fleshy mass during contraction. This action pulls the tendons attaching the muscle to the bone closer together. The tissue of the muscle belly contains sarcomeres, the functional contractile unit of the muscle discussed earlier. The arrangement of the muscle belly is dependent on the available space, typically in the central portion of a limb. Long tendons attached to muscle bellies are advantageous if a shortage of space exists, such as the hands and feet. Hence the muscle bellies that have the most influence on movement in the hands and feet are located in the forelimbs.

Origin. The tendinous attachment of the muscle on the less movable bone or attachment during contraction is its origin. It is usually located on the medial or proximal end of the skeleton.

Insertion. The insertion, usually located lateral or distal, is the muscle attachment on the more movable bone or at-

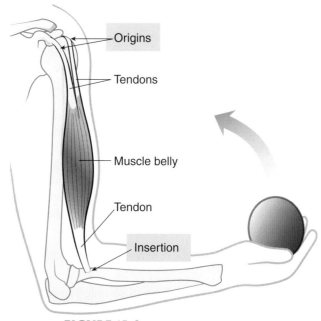

FIGURE 15-8 Parts of a skeletal muscle.

tachment during contraction. When a muscular contraction occurs, the insertion commonly moves toward the origin. As you learn individual skeletal muscles, the origins and insertions will help you to think about muscles causing a desired action. When a muscle crosses a joint, it acts on that joint. Muscles may cross one or more joints and are referred to as *uniarticular*, *biarticular*, and *multiarticular*.

Uniarticular: Muscles that cross one joint.

Biarticular: Muscles that cross two joints, acting on both joints.

Multiarticular: Muscles that cross more than two joints.

MUSCLE FIBER ARRANGEMENT

Muscle fibers are arranged in several ways, typically because of the relationship between the muscle fibers and its tendons.

Some muscles have their fibers running parallel to a bone's long axis. Some muscles converge to a narrow attachment. Their fibers can be obliquely arranged or curved, as in sphincters on the face. Other muscle fibers are arranged as feathers, coming off one or both sides of its plume.

The differences between muscle fiber arrangements affect their shape and the resulting strength (Figure 15-9). Parallel muscle fiber arrangements have greater range of motion but are less powerful. The multipennate shape allows more force in contraction but offers less range of motion. Muscle fiber arrangements are as follows:

- **Parallel:** The fibers in this arrangement run in a parallel arrangement down a long axis. These arrangements can be quadrilateral (four sided) or triangular (fan shaped).
- **Convergent:** These muscles converge at one or both ends. When they converge at one end, they become spindle shaped, fibers tapering at both ends. This muscle shape is also called *fusiform*.
- **Circular:** Muscles that form a circular arrangement describe this arrangement.
- **Pennate:** These muscles are short and are arranged with a central tendon and muscle fibers extending from

the tendon diagonally, giving the muscle a feather-like appearance. Types of penniform muscles are *unipennate* (fibers come off one side of the tendon), *bipennate* (fibers are arranged on both sides of a central tendon), and *multipennate* (having several tendons within the belly with fibers run diagonally between them).

HOW DOES THE BODY COORDINATE MOVEMENT?

Almost all skeletal muscles work in groups instead of separately. Most skeletal muscles are arranged in pairs; some muscles are contracting to perform a specific action, whereas others are relaxing. Muscles do not simply contract simultaneously to achieve motion. Even the simplest movements would be impossible with all the muscles fully contracted. Instead, muscles assume different responsibilities to carry out a variety of movements. In this way, muscles can be functionally classified. Each term suggests an important concept that is vital for understanding how muscles participate in actions such as flexion, extension, abduction, and adduction discussed in Chapter 13 and to be further discussed in Chapter 16. A muscle may function as agonist, antagonist, synergist, or fixator, depending on its role in performing a particular task.

The muscle that is responsible for causing a specific or desired action is the **agonist,** also called a *prime mover*. The opposing muscle, or **antagonist,** must relax and lengthen or eccentrically contract to allow the actions of the agonists to occur. The antagonist usually lies on the opposite side of the joint and causes the opposite joint action. Imagine what movement would resemble without the antagonist opposing the pull of the prime mover. The upper fibers of the trapezius muscle would contract, creating extension of the head. When the movement task is fulfilled, your head would fall, uncontrolled, in response to the pull of gravity.

Therefore the term antagonist is misleading because it does not properly describe its role. These muscles serve a function of cooperation and provide precision and control during contraction. Examples of an agonist-antagonist

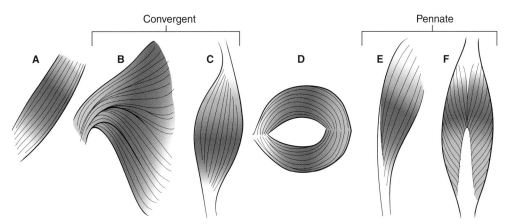

FIGURE 15-9 Muscle fiber arrangement. **A**, Parallel. **B**, Convergent. **C**, Fusiform. **D**, Circular. **E**, Unipennate. **F**, Bipennate.

relationship are the biceps brachii–triceps brachii (see Chapter 16).

To help things run smoothly, other muscles, called **synergists,** aid by contracting at the same time as prime movers, helping to produce more effective movement. For example, the peroneus longus and peroneus brevis are synergistic, as are the gastrocnemius and soleus.

Fixators are specialized synergists and are also referred to as *stabilizers.* They stabilize the joint over which the prime mover exerts its action, which allows the prime mover to perform a motion efficiently. For example, the postural muscles stabilize the vertebral column so the iliopsoas and the rectus femoris can flex the thigh.

To review:

- **Agonist (prime mover):** muscle causing a specific action
- **Antagonist:** muscle opposing the agonist
- **Synergist:** muscle aiding by causing same movement as the agonist

- **Fixators:** muscle acting as joint stabilizer so agonist can exert its action

When the nervous system sends a message for the agonist (muscle causing movement) to contract, the tension in the antagonist (muscle opposing movement) is inhibited by impulses from motor nerves and thus must simultaneously relax. This neural phenomenon is called *reciprocal inhibition* (Sherrington's law).

This information can be used to ease the pain of an acute muscle spasm or cramp. Contract the muscle opposite (antagonist) of the muscle spasm. This conscious contraction may have to be repeated several times, and the contraction must be isometrically resisted. The brain is turning off the message of contraction, and relaxation is the result. A further discussion can be found in Chapter 17.

Strain between body segments alters patterns of movement. Tight muscles can affect movement partly because antagonists cannot fully elongate. Any given movement evokes a response not only from the prime movers, but also from

JON ZAHOUREK

Born: January 5, 1940.

"The mind cannot forget what the hands have learned."

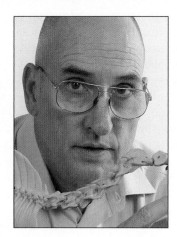

Artists dream of creating a work designed to last. Jon Zahourek is no exception. What makes him unique, however, is that his masterpiece might influence the way future generations learn how the body works—especially how muscles work.

The process was painful for Zahourek, but it was not your typical artistic angst. For years, Zahourek, a sculptor, artist, and Parson's School of Design instructor, was plagued with debilitating back pain. As a drawing teacher, he taught a detailed anatomy class. "The names of some of the muscles scared me to death," he laughs. Therefore, as was the case with a lot of teachers, he would gloss over these and go on. However, a new way to teach anatomy led to a revelation for Zahourek, who began building clay muscles—layer by layer—on a model skeleton.

"It was like 'whoosh,' a wind rushed through me, and suddenly everything that I had been trying to teach about how the muscles work became integrated within me. I spent all weekend trying to understand what happened," he says. "What most of us grasp about how our bodies work is either very childlike or dead wrong."

However, Zahourek was unable to see this—or feel it in his own body—until he actually modeled each muscle in space. By building each muscle, one by one, and learning how it connected to bone and how it worked with or against other muscles, Zahourek moved from the ability to point to a muscle, name it, and tell his students which action it performed to a deeper level of knowing. Suddenly, his body *understood* and *felt* how each muscle worked. "It set me free physically! My back problems of 20 years were gone. It wasn't the pain that was disabling me. It was the fear and lack of knowledge. I didn't understand what was causing the pain until I began to see the conflicts between the muscles."

If this effect could be so liberating on him, it could also help others. Thus what started as the perfect way to instruct art students became a creative work in itself. At first, Zahourek intended to build clay muscles on a life-size wooden skeletal model. Then, realizing that the weight would be not only unwieldy but also downright deadly if it toppled over on someone, he began to create scaled-down models. When these models were

the antagonists, synergists, and fixators. Imagine watching a baseball player throw a baseball. The player's foot goes forward, one hip swings back, then forward, as the entire upper torso and arm are propelling the baseball. Full, powerful motion is a synchronized wave of smaller motions rather than a single movement.

TABLE TALK

One rehabilitative approach for musculoskeletal problems is to strengthen the antagonist. This method corrects positional and postural distortions by creating balanced motion on both sides of the joint. For example, if poor posture is due to hypercontracted back muscles, then strengthening the abdominals can create a change in the resting length of these tight muscles. Do not be surprised if a client with a low back condition comes home from a physician's appointment with a recommended daily routine of proper abdominal exercises.

TYPES OF SKELETAL MUSCLE FIBERS

Smooth and cardiac muscle tissue is the same throughout the body; no variations are evident. However, skeletal muscle can be classified into three types according to its structural and functional characteristics: slow (red), fast (white), and intermediate (pink). Each type is best suited to a particular type of contraction. Although each muscle organ contains a mix of all three, the ratio of slow twitch to fast twitch is unique to each individual, but some commonalities exist, as is described in the following:

Slow twitch: Also known as *red muscle,* slow-twitch fibers are fatigue resistant. They react at a slow rate, and because they contract so slowly, slow-twitch fibers are usually able to produce ATP quickly enough to keep up with the muscle's energy needs and thus avoid fatigue. This effect is enhanced by a good blood supply, a large number of mitochondria, and the rich oxygen supply through myoglobin. Most postural muscles are slow-twitch muscles. A high

JON ZAHOUREK (*continued*)

perfected, Zahourek Systems, Inc., was born. A complete system package contains detailed videos, workbooks, clay, sculpting tools, and mannequins (skeletons of varying degrees of complexity and price ranges).

Zahourek began marketing his entire *learning process* package to anyone who might benefit from understanding how the body works, including physical therapists, college anatomy students, even elementary-age children, massage therapy students, and of course, massage therapists.

For massage therapists, Zahourek's model and ideas have several implications. For massage schools that use the system, it is a guaranteed method to learn—really learn—the musculoskeletal system, not just about where a muscle is and its name and shape. The system is a hands-on system, which benefits all massage students, especially those who are tactile learners, as many massage therapists are. Otherwise, a therapist may complete a degree program and merely work on a very surface level—literally, as well as figuratively—and that is often not enough for a client with a specific problem.

Additionally, the chance exists that, as Zahourek, the massage therapist will somehow have his or her own chance for the great *a-ha* to rush through his or her body and experience the opportunity to travel from a conceptual understanding of how the muscles work to a deeper, cognitive level—to know the body from the inside out.

Massage therapists who are lucky enough to have had this experience can often tell, from the moment the client walks into the office, what is happening with his or her body. The therapist does not just see it; he or she senses it or even feels it.

Massage therapists absolutely and unequivocally must understand their own bodies. Massage therapy can be such physically demanding work that many therapists do not last for more than 5 years. Failing to understand their own bodies—and their hands in particular—is occupational suicide. As Zahourek says, "It's like working hard for a diploma and someone telling you, 'Congratulations, in 4 years you'd better find something else to do.'" Massage therapists need to understand how it all works. Zahourek offers the analogy: If you were a runner and you woke up one morning and your legs were sore, you would not stop running, would you?

One way to stay strong? "Socrates was right," says Zahourek. "Know thyself." As massage therapists, we must return again and again to the learning laboratory—our own minds and bodies, peeling layer from layer, then rebuilding layer on layer until we get it right. Jon Zahourek, in his attempt to teach art students how to draw more lifelike figures, stumbled on a new lease on life for himself and a model that allows massage therapists to learn how the body works in a way that will never be forgotten.

ratio of slow-twitch muscles is present in the legs of world-class long-distance runners.

Fast twitch: Also known as *white muscle,* fast-twitch fibers possess the largest diameters, contain very little myoglobin, few mitochondria, and few capillaries; thus they appear white. White muscles contract more rapidly than slowly because they possess a type of myosin that moves faster and because their system of T-tubules and sarcoplasmic reticulum is more efficient at quickly delivering stored calcium. The price of a more rapid contraction is a quick depletion of ATP and fibers that fatigue quickly. Muscles of the arm contain many fast-twitch fibers.

Intermediate: Intermediate fibers are classified in between the two extremes of slow and fast fibers and are referred to as *pink muscle.* They contain large amounts of myoglobin, many mitochondria, and numerous capillaries. These fibers also generate copious amounts of ATP aerobically. However, they break down ATP quickly. They are more fatigue resistant than fast twitch and can generate more force more quickly than slow twitch. This muscle type predominates in muscles that both provide postural support and are occasionally required to generate rapid powerful contractions. Many world-class sprinters have a high ratio of intermediate fibers in their leg muscles, and world-class boxers have a high ratio in their arms.

TABLE TALK

The presence of myoglobin in skeletal muscles makes them appear darker. Notice that the dark meat of chickens is the legs and the thighs. Ducks, by contrast, have dark breast meat. This difference is because, in general, chickens run around a chicken yard, and ducks fly powered by their breast muscles.

STRETCHING

The opposite of muscular contraction is stretching. Although stretching is covered in Chapter 7, it is important enough to warrant another brief mention here. Stretching a muscle extends it to its full length and elongates both muscle and connective tissue. How far you can stretch a muscle depends on several factors. Most factors are out of our control (e.g., genetics, movement capability of a joint). What can be changed is the amount of tension in a muscle during a voluntary stretch.

Extensibility, the ability of muscles and other soft tissues to lengthen, can be improved by regular stretching. Stretching can also improve the range of movement of a joint because it influences the physiological characteristics of the muscle, tendons, ligaments, and other structures surrounding the joint. Hyperflexibility (hypermobility) is flexibility beyond a joint's normal range of motion and contributes to joint instability.

Proprioceptors are sensory receptors located in muscles, tendons, and joints (see Chapter 17). They send information into the nervous system about muscle length, muscle tension, and joint movements. One of the two proprioceptors that can be stimulated during a stretch is the **muscle spindle** located within the muscle belly (see Figure 17-23 for image of

muscle spindles). If the muscle is stretched too rapidly (ballistic stretch), then the muscle spindles detect the sudden motion, and the nervous system responds by reflexively contracting the muscle. This reflex is a protective mechanism that is intended to safeguard the muscle from overstretching. This reflex is also important for maintaining posture, which is mediated by muscle spindles.

Other proprioceptors stimulated during a stretch are **Golgi tendon organs,** located in the musculotendinous junction (see Figure 17-24 for an image of a Golgi tendon organ). These receptors detect tension applied to the tendon during a slow, static stretch. The nervous system responds by inhibiting muscle contraction, which allows the muscle to relax and stretch. It works the exact opposite of the stretch reflex mentioned previously and represses contraction to prevent tearing of a muscle or avulsion of the tendon from its attachment.

Massage therapists can use this information when applying or instructing clients in stretching. To enhance flexibility, apply only slow, static stretches. Movements that are perceived by the nervous system as dangerous will be met with resistance.

MINI-LAB

Hold a shoestring by the two coated ends with both of your hands. Slowly begin to pull the ends apart. Watch what happens to the individual strands in the string. Do the fibers spread apart or draw closer together? Imagine that this string is a muscle and the two ends are tendinous attachments. Within this muscle is a spasm. Pull the ends again. As the muscle is being stretched, is the spasm released? Note that separation in the muscle fibers does not occur when the muscle is stretched, which explains why stretching does not release local muscle spasms.

TYPES OF SKELETAL MUSCLE CONTRACTIONS

Isotonic Contractions

During isotonic, or *dynamic,* contractions, the tone or tension within a muscle remains the same as the length of the muscle changes. The energy of contraction is used to pull on the thin myofilaments, causing change in the length of a fiber's sarcomere. Isotonic contractions are the most common type of muscle contraction. When a muscle is involved in isotonic contractions, it can shorten or lengthen. In fact, lengthening contractions are as much a part of coordinated motion as shortening contractions. Without the ability of a muscle to shorten and lengthen during contractions, we would be unable to lower objects after we lifted them. Shortening contractions are called *concentric,* and lengthening contractions are called *eccentric* (Figure 15-10).

Concentric Contraction

This type of isotonic contraction occurs when contraction results in shortening of the muscle. An example of a concentric contraction is the lifting phase of a biceps curl (flexing the elbow) to raise a load. Muscles involved in concentric contractions

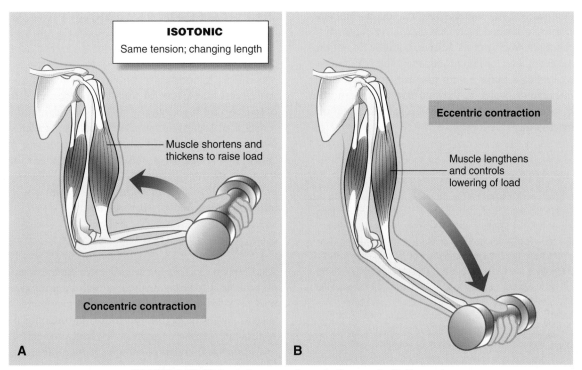

FIGURE 15-10 Isotonic contractions. **A**, Concentric. **B**, Eccentric.

are also known as *accelerators* or *spurt muscles*. They may provide a forward acceleration in locomotion.

Eccentric Contraction

Eccentric contractions, or lengthening contractions, occur when muscle experiences resistance as it is lengthening. For example, during the lowering phase of a biceps curl, the biceps brachii muscle will be eccentrically contracted as you extend the elbow to lower the load. The biceps brachii is contracting, but it is getting longer. Repeated eccentric contraction causes more muscle damage and muscle soreness than concentric

contraction, such as running downhill. These muscles are also known as decelerators or shunt muscles because they slow down the powerful concentric contractors. Unless the body compensates with some corrective braking action, injuries are likely to occur.

Isometric Contractions

Muscles do not always shorten or lengthen when they contract (Figure 15-11). If you attempt to pick up a weight that is too heavy, do the muscles still shorten? No. In isometric

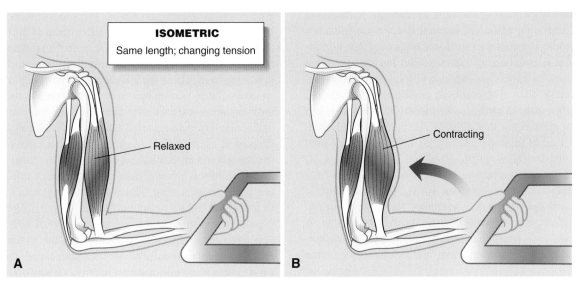

FIGURE 15-11 Isometric contraction. **A**, Relaxed. **B**, Contracting.

muscle contractions, the muscle length remains the same while the muscle tension increases. Isometric contractions do work by *tightening* to resist a force, but they do not produce movements. The tension produced by the *power stroke* of the myosin heads pulling actin filaments toward a sarcomeres center cannot overcome the load placed on the muscle. Isometric contractions are important because they stabilize some joints as others are moved.

TABLE TALK

Isometrics are the therapy of choice when a client fears pain during movement or refuses to move an injured part. However, they only strengthen muscles in the position of the actual contraction. Isometric contractions are the key component of muscle energy techniques. Isometrics are great for building muscle bulk or increasing strength in certain positions, but these exercises do not increase the efficiency or endurance of skeletal muscles.

Isometric contraction can also be used clinically to reset tone on muscles that are weak from nonuse. It is often the first method of rehabilitation after surgery or injury because isometric contractions are relatively painless and increase local blood circulation without stretching tissues.

"Pain is inevitable. Suffering is optional."
Kathleen Casey Theisen

POSTURE AND MUSCLE TONE

Posture is basically maintaining an optimal body position. Good posture implies many concepts. Good posture reduces strain on muscles, ligaments, and bones. Good posture helps keep the body's center of gravity over its base. Poor posture places stress on most body structures and leads to a feeling of soreness and fatigue. As a massage therapist, you should demonstrate good body mechanics that reflect good posture.

Muscles work most of the time to maintain posture and to help keep joints stabilized because muscles must exert a pull on bones to counteract the force of gravity. The continued partial contraction of many skeletal muscles is called *muscle tone*, or *tonus*. Muscle tone enables us to stand, sit, and maintain relatively stable body positions while walking, running, hopping, skipping, and so forth. Muscles with less tone than normal are described as *flaccid* and are often in the first stage of muscular atrophy. Muscles with more than normal tone are called *spastic*.

Tonus is a characteristic of the muscles that normal individuals have when they are awake. However, muscle tone is lost during sleep; we cannot sleep standing up. Hence good posture while asleep is also important. A neutral sleeping posture is best maintained by using pillows to support the neck and extremities to keep the spine straight.

PATHOLOGICAL CONDITIONS OF THE MUSCULAR SYSTEM

Atrophy

A decrease in the size of muscle fibers or a wasting away of muscles from poor nutrition, lack of use, motor unit dysfunction, or lack of motor nerve impulses is called *muscular atrophy*. The opposite of atrophy is *hypertrophy*, or the increase of the size of a muscle, usually caused by weight training. ***Massage using strokes that are slow, superficial, and soothing, with intermittent use of manual vibration and cross-fiber hacking percussion.***

Contracture

Also known as *ischemic contracture*, contracture is an abnormal, usually permanent condition of a joint in which the muscle is fixed in a flexed position. It may be the result of spasm, paralysis, or fibrotic tissue surrounding a joint. A contracture can be brought on by heat or medication. ***Use techniques to increase blood flow, reduce adhesions, stretch and release fascia, and elongate muscles.***

De Quervain's Tendonitis

de Quervain's tendonitis is a type of tendonitis caused by narrowing of the tendon sheath surrounding abductor pollicis longus and extensor pollicis brevis. This condition usually occurs after repetitive use of the wrist. The major symptoms are usually pain at the wrist and thumb and tenderness just distal to the radial styloid process. ***The inflamed area is a local contraindication.***

Fibromyalgia

Also known as *fibrositis*, or *muscular rheumatism*, fibromyalgia is a chronic inflammatory disease that affects muscle and related connective tissues. Pain, joint stiffness, and the presence of *tender points* and *trigger points* are involved in this condition. During the diagnosis, the physician evaluates 18 tender points on the body; if 11 of these 18 points are painful, the diagnosis of fibromyalgia is then often made. However, keep in mind that the symptoms of fibromyalgia are very similar to those of more serious conditions such as rheumatoid arthritis, lupus, and other arthritic conditions. These more serious conditions must be ruled out before fibromyalgia can be diagnosed. Fibromyalgia frequently develops after emotional trauma (client may not have dealt with an emotional situation and it exhibits as physical pain), local or general infections, or even changes in climate. The symptoms vary from individual to individual and may range from pain, insomnia, headaches, depression, gastrointestinal and urinary disturbances, to lethargy. Fibromyalgia may go into remission, only to flare up at a later date. ***Adjust massage to client's stamina and vitality (i.e., slow, gentle, short duration; assist client on and off table).***

Ganglion Cyst

A ganglion cyst is a benign tumor occurring on a tendon such as in the wrist or dorsum of the foot; it consists of a thin fibrous capsule enclosing a clear fluid. *Local contraindication of affected area.*

Headaches

Headaches are a pain in the head from any cause. Types of headaches are muscular contraction or tension headaches, cervicogenic headaches, sinus headaches, posttraumatic headaches, pathological headaches, cluster headaches, and migraine headaches. Migraine headaches and cluster headaches are addressed in the circulatory chapter. *If not caused by a contraindicated disease, then massage is okay. If caused by muscular contraction or tension, then focus on muscles of the neck, shoulder, and back (e.g., trapezius, levator scapulae, splenius capitis and cervicis, suboccipitals, scalenes, sternocleidomastoid). Use moist heat.*

Muscle Spasm

An increase in muscle tension with or without shortening caused by excessive motor nerve activity may result in a rigid zone (knot) in the muscle called a *spasm*. Muscle spasms cannot be alleviated by voluntary relaxation. *Determine cause before treatment. If indicated, use techniques to increase local circulation and to mechanically lengthen and to spread muscle fibers apart.*

Muscular Dystrophy

A collection of genetic diseases, muscular dystrophy is characterized by the progressive atrophy of skeletal muscles without any indication of neural degeneration or damage. All forms of muscular dystrophy involve a loss of muscular strength, disability, and deformity. The most common type of muscular dystrophy is called *Duchenne's muscular dystrophy*. This type, which predominantly affects men, is a condition in which the muscles rapidly deteriorate and the muscle tissue is replaced with fatty deposits and connective tissue. The disease usually begins in the pelvis, hips, and legs and produces a waddling gait. The muscular wasting will eventually progress to the heart muscle and respiratory muscles and lead to death, usually within 10 to 15 years of the onset of symptoms. No cure has been developed for this disease. *Use techniques to increase blood flow, to activate muscle spindles in weak muscles (if they are functional), and to increase colon activity.*

Plantar Fascitis

Plantar fascitis is inflammation of the plantar fascia at the calcaneus, medial aspect of the foot, and insertions of tibialis posterior. Symptoms are pain in the heel, pain on dorsiflexion, or both. Clients will often state that they cannot walk comfortably on their heels for several hours after waking. The pain then goes away, only to return the next morning. *Use techniques to reduce adhesions. Thoroughly massage leg muscles.*

Repetitive Strain Injury

Repetitive strain injuries are self-inflicted and are related to inefficient biomechanics, which includes general posture, sporting movements, and work habits. A repetitive or constant motion, combined with compressive forces or joint hyperextension, causes damage to soft tissues. This injury type encompasses a broad spectrum of injuries. The most common types of repetitive motion injuries are carpal tunnel syndrome, thoracic outlet syndrome, tennis elbow, and rotator cuff problems. The symptoms and damage are progressive, unless the inefficient biomechanics or repetitive strain is altered. The general symptoms are related to the inflammation response: pain, redness, heat, swelling, and limited range of motion. The progression of injury typically starts from muscle soreness and leads to increased tonus to the formation of multiple trigger points and in some cases to nerve entrapment. Chronic repetitive strain injuries may result in neuropathy, subluxation, deterioration, or trauma to the joints, including bursitis, arthritis, and even stress fractures of involved bones. *Tailor massage to type of repetitive strain injury. Avoid area if inflamed.*

Shin Splints

Shin splints are strain of either anterior or posterior tibial muscles marked by pain along the shinbone. The condition is often the result of running or jumping on hard surfaces. During these activities, the tibia and fibula are jarred on top of the talus bone, which causes the tibia and fibula to migrate laterally. This movement tears the interosseous membrane between the two lower leg bones, as well as the muscles attached to all three structures (tibia, fibula, and interosseous membrane). Pain is referred to the anterior tibial shaft (shin). *Avoid massage if condition is acute. If chronic, then massage tibialis anterior and posterior; the latter is accessed through the calf. Use the procedure known as RICE (rest, ice, compression, elevation) on acute cases and ICE (ice, compression, elevation) on chronic cases.*

Spasticity

Spasticity is characterized by increased muscle tone and stiffness and is associated with an increase in tendon reflexes. A spastic muscle will resist stretching and typically involves the arm flexors and leg extensors; effects can range from mild to severe. In severe cases, movement patterns become uncoordinated or impossible and usually involve a neurological dysfunction. *Obtain physician clearance if symptoms are severe. Adjust massage if sensations are impaired. Avoid joint mobilizations. Use techniques to prevent adhesions and contractures.*

Strain

A strain is an injury of a muscle or tendon caused by a violent contraction, forced stretching, or synergistic failure. Most muscle strains occur to the antagonist. When the antagonist is tight or in spasm, it cannot stretch easily and may become injured. Acute muscle strains can be classified into three grades or degrees of severity: *first, second* and *third degree*. First-degree strains involve up to 10% of stretching or a partial tear of fibers with no palpable defects. Mild pain is typically felt at the time of injury, and mild swelling and localized tenderness may occur. The joint structures can maintain efficient motion and hold against resistance.

When the muscle or tendon is torn between 10% and 99%, it is classified as a second-degree strain. A palpable defect is noted, and the joint structures cannot hold against moderate resistance. Edema is typically found, and the muscles surrounding the strain splint to restrict painful movement.

In third-degree tears, 100% of the fibers are torn, and a snap is often heard at the time of injury. Third-degree tears may represent a complete rupture of the involved structures. An avulsion fracture is when a tendon is pulled away from a bone, taking a bone fragment with it. A depression in the area of the torn muscle can be palpated and is usually painful to touch. Function is greatly altered in third-degree tears. *Obtain physician clearance. Once granted, use the RICE procedure for the first 72 hours. Avoid stretching of injured area, and massage distal to the injury site. Use techniques to maintain range of motion and to prevent adhesion formation. Then treatment times should be of shorter duration, becoming longer as the injury heals.*

Tendinitis

Inflammation of the tendon accompanied by pain and swelling is called *tendinitis*. This condition may be a result of chronic overuse, direct trauma, or even a sudden pull of the muscle. When inflammation also involves the tendon sheath, it is referred to as *tenosynovitis*. *Local contraindication for 72 hours if due to injury. Otherwise, use appropriate techniques on involved tendons. End session with ice.*

Torticollis

Torticollis, or wryneck, involves spasms of the sternocleidomastoid muscles (SCMs). The scalenes, trapezius, and splenius muscles may also be involved. This condition may cause vertigo because of the many sensory and positional receptors located in the SCM. Because this muscular condition is often unilateral, a tilt or rotation of the head is often noted. *Focus on the SCM, trapezius, scalenes, and the splenius muscles.*

---

evolve *Use your student account to access the activities for Chapter 15, such as a crossword puzzle.* ∎

BOX 15-1

Effects of Massage on Muscles

Relieves muscular tension. Massage relieves muscular restrictions, tightness, stiffness, and spasms.

Relaxes muscles. Massage reduces excitability in the sympathetic nervous system, thereby relaxing muscles.

Reduces muscle soreness and fatigue. Massage enhances blood circulation, thereby increasing the amount of oxygen and nutrients available to the muscles. Increased oxygen and nutrients reduce muscle fatigue and postexercise soreness. Massage promotes rapid disposal of waste products, further reducing muscle fatigue and soreness. A fatigued muscle recuperates 20% after 5 minutes of rest and 100% after 5 minutes of massage. A reduction in postexercise recovery time was indicated by a decline in pulse rate and an increase in muscle *work* capacity.

Reduces trigger point formation. Trigger point formation in both muscle and fascia is greatly reduced by massage.

Manually separates muscle fibers. Compressive strokes and cross-fiber friction strokes separate muscle fibers, thereby reducing muscle spasms.

Increases range of motion. When muscular tension is reduced, range of motion is improved. The freedom of the joints is dictated by the freedom of the muscles.

Improves performance (balance and posture). Many postural distortions are removed when trigger points and muscle tension are reduced. Range of motion increases, gait becomes more efficient, the posture is more aligned and balanced, and improved performance is the net result.

Lengthens muscles. Massage mechanically stretches and broadens tissue, especially when combined with Swedish gymnastics (joint mobilization and stretches). These changes are detected by Golgi tendon organs, which inhibit contraction signals, further lengthening muscles. Massage retrains the tissue from a contracted state to an elongated state, thereby increasing resting length.

Increases flexibility. By lengthening muscles and promoting relaxation, massage has also been shown to increase flexibility.

Tones weak muscles. Muscle spindle activity is increased during massage strokes (e.g., tapotement, vibration). An increase in muscle spindle activity stimulates minute muscle contractions, thereby helping tone weak muscles. This effect is particularly beneficial in most cases of prolonged bed rest, flaccidity, and atrophy.

Reduces creatine kinase activity in the blood. Creatine kinase is an enzyme that helps ensure enough ATP is available for muscle contraction. By reducing the activity of creatine kinase in the blood, massage indirectly helps decrease muscle spasm, which increases muscle relaxation.

Decreases electromyography (EMG) readings. Lower EMG readings signify a decrease in neuromuscular activity and reduction of neuromuscular complaints.

Terms and Their Meanings Related to the Muscular System

TERM	MEANING	TERM	MEANING
Antagonist	*Gr.* to struggle against	Hypertrophy	*Gr.* over, above, excessive; to grow
Alba	*L.* white	Isometric	*Gr.* same or equal measure
Aponeurosis	*Gr.* away from; nerve; condition	Isotonic	*Gr.* same or equal tension
Atrophy	*Gr.* lacking, without, not; to grow	Myo	*Gr.* muscle
Concentric	*L.* toward the middle	Pennate	*L.* feather
Eccentric	*Gr.* away from the middle	Retinaculum	*L.* a halter
Fatigue	*L.* to tire	Sarco	*Gr.* flesh
Fascia	*L.* strong central structural unit or band	Spasm	*Gr.* a convulsion
Fasciculi	*L.* little bundle	Synergist	*Gr.* together, work
Flaccid	*L.* flabby	Tendon	*L.* to stretch
Golgi tendon organs	Golgi, Italian histologist (1844-1926)		

Gr., Greek; *L.*, Latin.

SUMMARY

The understanding of structures and functions of muscle tissue and its related fascia is vital to the practice of massage therapy. Physiologically, muscles serve four basic functions: They provide external mobility and internal motility, produce heat, and maintain posture. Three different types of muscle tissue are required to perform these various functions: smooth, cardiac, and skeletal.

Each skeletal muscle is composed of bundles of muscle fibers known as fasciculi. These bundles are bound together individually and collectively with layers of fascia, which is a tough, white, protective membrane. The main part of the muscle is the belly, which is attached to the bone by two or more tendons, which are known as its *origin* and *insertion*. The shortening of the muscle belly draws the tendons closer together to produce movement. This shortening is produced by a change in the relative size of the basic contractile unit known as the *sarcomere*. An explanation of the cellular processes of muscular contraction is known as the *sliding filament theory*.

In the coordination of movement, muscles work in pairs or groups. Muscles involved in these groups are classified by function as agonists (prime movers), antagonists, synergists, and fixators (stabilizers). The muscle tissue can also be classified by its chemistry as slow twitch, fast twitch, or intermediate.

Biomechanically, muscles do one of two things: stretch or contract. Muscular contractions can be isometric or isotonic. Isotonic contractions may be further classified as either concentric or eccentric. The opposite of contracting is stretching, which extends the muscle.

With an understanding of the theory and actual mechanics of the muscular system, as well as the structure and location of the individual muscles, the application and effectiveness of the massage strokes can be greatly enhanced.

evolve

Go to *Chapter Extras* on Evolve for additional illustrations and resources for this chapter. *Extras* for this chapter include:

1. Drag and drop (online game)

MATCHING I

Place the letter of the answer next to the term or phrase that best describes it.

A. Actin
B. Aponeurosis
C. Cardiac
D. Contractility
E. Epimysium

F. Extensibility
G. Fasciculi
H. Muscle fibers
I. Myofascial
J. Myosin

K. Retinacula
L. Sarcomere
M. Skeletal muscle
N. Smooth muscle
O. Tendon

_____   1. Muscle found in blood vessels and some organs

_____   2. Thin myofilament

_____   3. Fascial covering of the entire muscle

_____   4. Flat, broad tendon

_____   5. Cordlike structure attaching muscle to bone

_____   6. Groups of muscle fibers

_____   7. Ability of a muscle to shorten

_____   8. Voluntary, striated muscle

_____   9. Muscle of the heart

_____   10. Retaining bands of connective tissue around the elbows, knees, ankles, and wrists

_____   11. Thick myofilament

_____   12. Muscle's contractile unit

_____   13. Synonym for muscle cells owing to their threadlike slender shape

_____   14. Term referring to skeletal muscles and related fascia

_____   15. Ability of a muscle to lengthen

MATCHING II

Place the letter of the answer next to the term or phrase that best describes it.

A. Acetylcholine
B. Agonist
C. All-or-none response
D. Eccentric
E. H-band

F. Insertion
G. Motor unit
H. Muscle spindles
I. Neuromuscular junction
J. Origin

K. Recruitment
L. Sarcolemma
M. Slow-twitch fibers
N. Troponin and tropomyosin
O. Z-lines

_____ 1. Central region of resting sarcomere

_____ 2. Principle neurotransmitter involved in muscle contraction

_____ 3. Fatigue-resistant fibers

_____ 4. Cell membrane of a muscle fiber

_____ 5. Muscle attachment undergoing the greatest movement during contraction

_____ 6. Muscle causing desired action

_____ 7. Defining ends of a sarcomere

_____ 8. Attachment of the muscle that is relatively fixed and immovable during contraction

_____ 9. Lengthening contractions

_____ 10. A single motor neuron plus all muscle fibers to which it attaches

_____ 11. Detects sudden motion, causing reflexive muscle contraction

_____ 12. Junction between a motor neuron and a motor end plate

_____ 13. Muscles contract to their fullest extent or not at all

_____ 14. Process of motor unit activation based on need

_____ 15. Proteins that prevent muscles from being in a constant state of contraction

INTERNET ACTIVITIES

Visit http://www.mayoclinic.com/health/weight-training/HQ01627 and read about how weight training affects muscles. View the slide show and create a personalized fitness program for yourself with weight training.

Visit http://www.mayoclinic.com/health/performance-enhancing-drugs/HQ01105 and read the report on the dangers of steroid use in athletes. Prepare a one-page report.

Visit http://distance.stcc.edu/AandP/AP/AP2pages/Units14to17/unit15/muscle.htm. Contrast and compare Golgi tendon organs with muscle spindles.

Bibliography

Abrahams P, Marks S, Hutchings R: *McMinn's color atlas of human anatomy,* St Louis, 2003, Mosby.

Applegate EJ: *The anatomy and physiology learning system,* ed 3, Philadelphia, 2006, Saunders.

Ardion C: Certified manual lymphatic drainage practitioner, 1996, personal contact.

Beers MH, Berkow R: *The Merck manual of diagnosis and therapy,* Whitehouse Station, NJ, 2006, Merck Research Laboratories.

Como D, editor: *Mosby's medical, nursing, and allied health dictionary,* ed 6, St Louis, 2002, Mosby.

Crawley J, Van De Graaff KM: *A photographic atlas for anatomy and physiology,* Englewood, Colo, 2002, Morton.

Damjanov I: *Pathophysiology for the health-related professions,* ed 3, Philadelphia, 2006, Saunders.

Ferri FF: *2003 Ferri's clinical advisor, instant diagnosis and treatment,* St Louis, 2003, Mosby.

Frazier MS, Drzymkowski JW: *Essentials of human diseases and conditions,* ed 3, Philadelphia, 2004, Saunders.

Goldberg S: *Clinical anatomy made ridiculously simple,* Miami, 2004, Medmaster.

Gould BE: *Pathophysiology for the health-related professionals,* ed 3, Philadelphia, 2006, Saunders.

Grafelman T: *Graf's anatomy and physiology guide for the massage therapist,* Aurora, Colo, 1988, DG Publishing.

Guyton A: *Human physiology and mechanisms of disease,* ed 6, Philadelphia, 1996, Saunders.

Haubrich WS: *Medical meanings: a glossary of word origins,* New York, 1984, Harcourt Brace Jovanovich.

Huether SE, McCance KL: *Understanding pathophysiology,* ed 3, St Louis, 2004, Mosby.

Jacob S, Francone C: *Elements of anatomy and physiology,* Philadelphia, 1989, Saunders.

Juhan D: *Job's body: a handbook for bodyworkers,* ed 3,Barrington, NY, 2003, Station Hill Press.

Kapit W, Elson LM: *The anatomy coloring book,* ed 3, New York, 2002, Benjamin Cummings.

Kapit W, Macey R, Meisami E: *The physiology coloring book,* ed 2, New York, 1999, HarperCollins.

Kordish M, Dickson S: *Introduction to basic human anatomy,* Lake Charles, La, 1985, McNeese State University.

Kumar V, Abbas A, Fausto N: *Robbins and Cotran physiologic basis of disease,* ed 7, St Louis, 2005, Mosby.

Marieb EN: *Essentials of human anatomy and physiology,* ed 8, New York, 2005, Benjamin Cummings.

Martini FH, Bartholomew EF: *Essentials of anatomy and physiology,* ed 3, New York, 2003, Benjamin Cummings.

Mattes A: *Active isolated stretching,* Sarasota, Fla, 1995, self-published.

McAleer N: *The body almanac,* Garden City, NY, 1985, Doubleday.

McCance K, Huether S: *Pathophysiology: the biological basis for disease in adults and children,* St Louis, 2006, Mosby.

Merck manual, ed 17, Whitehouse Station, NJ, 1998, Merck and Company.

Moore KL: *Clinically oriented anatomy,* ed 5, Baltimore, 2005, Lippincott Williams & Wilkins.

Mosby's medical, nursing, and allied health dictionary, ed 6, St Louis, 2002, Mosby.

Muscolino JE: *The muscular system manual: the skeletal muscles of the human body,* ed 2, St Louis, 2005, Elsevier Mosby.

Muscolino JE: *Kinesiology: the skeletal system and muscle function,* St Louis, 2006, Mosby.

Netter FH: *Atlas of human anatomy,* ed 3, Teterboro, NJ, 2003, Icon Learning Systems.

Newton D: *Pathology for massage therapists,* ed 2, Portland, Ore, 1995, Simran.

Platzer W: *Color atlas and textbook of human anatomy: locomotor system,* vol I, ed 5, New York, 2003, Thieme.

Premkumar K: *Pathology A to Z, a handbook for massage therapists,* Baltimore, 1999, Lippincott Williams & Wilkins.

Salvo SG, Anderson SK: *Mosby's pathology for massage therapists,* St Louis, 2004, Elsevier Mosby.

Solomon EP, Phillips GA: *Understanding human anatomy and physiology,* Philadelphia, 1987, Saunders.

Southmayd W, Hoffman M: *Sports health: the complete book of athletic injuries,* New York and London, 1981, Quickfox.

Souza TA: *Differential diagnosis and management for the chiropractor,* ed 2, Gaithersburg, Md, 2001, Aspen Publications.

Thibodeau G, Patton K: *Anatomy and physiology,* ed 6, St Louis, 2006, Mosby.

Thibodeau G, Patton K: *Structure and function of the body,* ed 12, St Louis, 2004, Mosby.

Tortora GJ: *Introduction to the human body: the essentials of anatomy and physiology,* ed 5, Hoboken, NJ, 2000, Wiley, John & Sons.

Tortora GJ, Grabowksi SR: *Principles of anatomy and physiology,* ed 11 New York, 2005, John Wiley & Sons.

Travell JG, Simons D: *Myofascial pain and dysfunction, the trigger point manual,* Baltimore, 1992, Lippincott Williams & Wilkins.

Venes D, Thomas CL, Taber CW: *Taber's cyclopedic medical dictionary,* ed 20, Philadelphia, 2005, FA Davis.

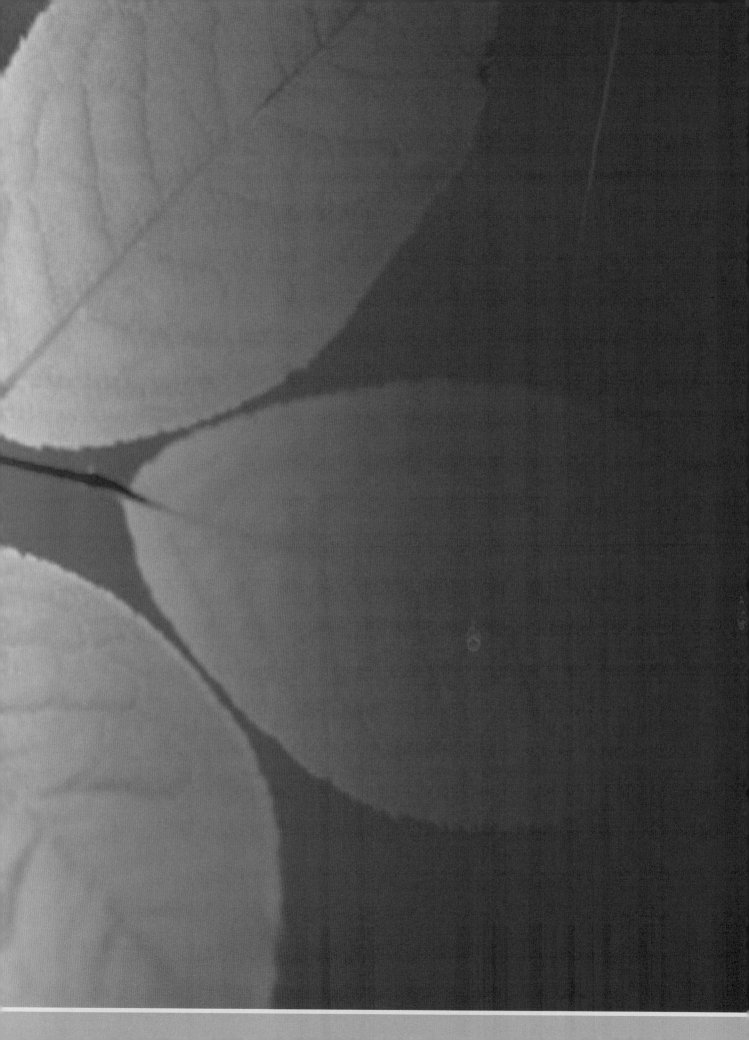

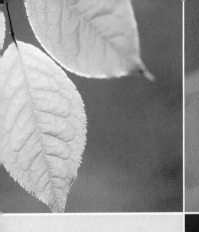

CHAPTER **16**

"I dwell in possibility."
—Emily Dickinson

Muscular Nomenclature and Kinesiology

STUDENT OBJECTIVES
After completing this chapter, the student should be able to:

- Describe the general locations of each muscle listed in the chapter
- Explain the location of each muscle listed in the chapter according to its muscle attachment sites
- Demonstrate the actions of each muscle listed in the chapter
- Apply the knowledge gained in your practice as a massage therapist

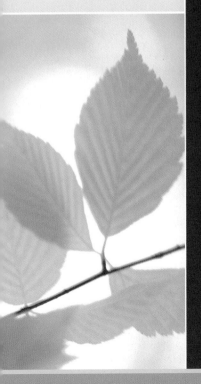

INTRODUCTION

This chapter examines 122 of the major muscles of the body (Figure 16-1). To get the most from this chapter, you must look at how the material is organized. This chapter is divided into two separate sections and nine individual lessons. The first section, Muscles of the Appendicular Skeleton, consists of six lessons: (1) Muscles of Scapular Movement; (2) Muscles of Shoulder Movement; (3) Muscles of Elbow Movement; (4) Muscles of the Forearm, Wrist, and Hand; (5) Muscles of Hip and Knee Movement; and (6) Muscles of Foot Movement.

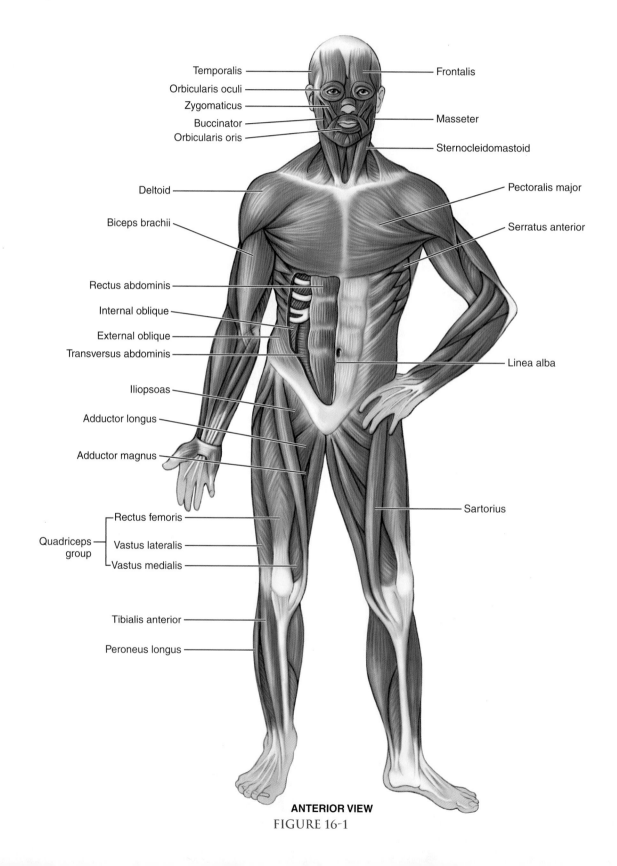

ANTERIOR VIEW
FIGURE 16-1

The second section, Muscles of the Axial Skeleton, consists of three lessons: (1) Muscles of the Head and Neck, (2) Muscles of the Trunk and Vertebral Column, and (3) Muscles of Pulmonary Respiration.

The muscles should be learned in the sequence presented because they are generally the order in which muscles are

addressed during a massage. This system supports students of massage to gain a strong foundation of musculoskeletal anatomy, muscle nomenclature, and kinesiology. **Kinesiology** is the study of human motion.

Muscles commonly attach to the bony markings covered in Chapter 14. However, muscles can also attach to ligaments

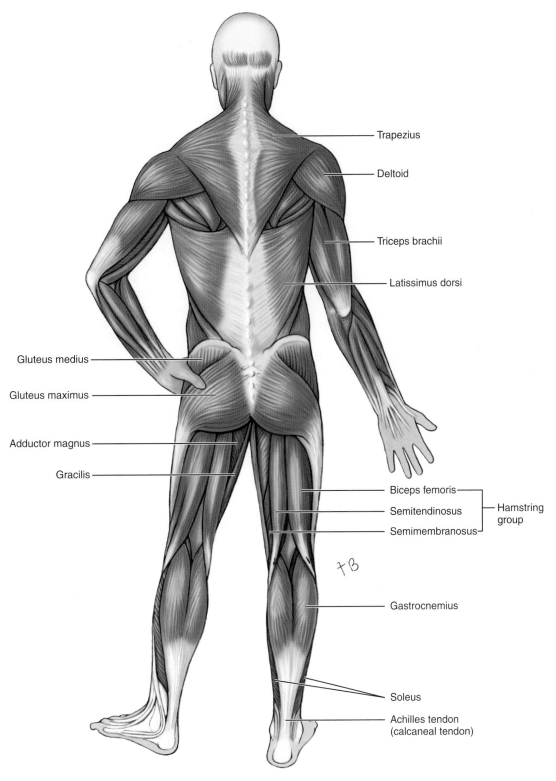

POSTERIOR VIEW
FIGURE 16-1, cont'd

(i.e., nuchal, inguinal, transverse carpal), fascia (i.e., palmar, superficial, abdominal, thoracolumbar, iliotibial band), membranes (i.e., obturator, interosseous), and tendinous structures (i.e., galea aponeurotica, linea alba).

Muscles can be arranged and classified into many groups. They can be grouped regionally (e.g., arm, leg, abdomen), according to their attachment sites (i.e., clavicle, ribs, femur), or by how they move the joints (actions). Muscles in these units are grouped in regions, and the muscles of each lesson are grouped according to actions. Muscles can be examined individually or in the bigger context of motion. At the end of each lesson, a chart is provided to further your study of kinesiology.

One of the best approaches to learning the muscles is to reduce the task into bite-size pieces. Five learning phases are presented to assist you in this endeavor. Understanding is a process similar to learning a new dance. First, you must hear the music, then you observe others, and then you follow them with your body until you are moving through space. This muscle learning system uses the building-block approach to learning on which a foundation is laid before something is built. However, feel free to design your own learning system, and use this system as a starting point for further exploration.

Phase I: Decode muscle names in each lesson and learn pronunciations.

Phase II: Learn general locations of muscles.

Phase III: Learn specific muscle locations using attachment sites.

Phase IV: Study muscle actions using a multisensory approach.

Phase V: Learn the muscle actions.

Phase VI: Apply knowledge and repetition.

In phase I, spend time looking over all the muscles in each lesson of the chapter and learn exactly how they were named. Do not be surprised if it feels similar to a history lesson. Try to imagine a small group of people dissecting a cadaver and having to name all the structures they find. All muscles are named using descriptive words. Read over the information located in Box 16-1 (Muscle Naming) to familiarize yourself with ways muscles are named. Listen to how your instructor pronounces each muscle, and repeat it back to yourself, silently or aloud.

Once you feel comfortable with the language of musculoskeletal anatomy, look at each muscle in each lesson, place your hand on the muscle, and say its name. As your teacher lectures, place your hand on the muscle and repeat its name silently or aloud. Phase II familiarizes you with their general locations on the body.

> **evolve** *While studying individual muscles, use the printable coloring sheets from the Evolve website to understand their positional relationships to neighboring muscles.* ∎

Phase III adds an important dimension to understanding muscle location for a massage therapist by focusing

---

BOX 16-1

Muscle Naming

Muscle names may seem strange, mysterious, and foreign. This unfamiliarity is because they are essentially Latin words (some are Greek). Muscle names seem more logical and therefore easier to learn when the reasons for the names are understood. Following are how most muscles are named.

Attachment sites or origin and insertion: An example of this type is the sternocleidomastoid muscle, which is attached to the sternum, clavicle, and mastoid process.

Action or function: When muscles are named by function, the function is usually named first, and the body part on which the action takes place is usually named second. Examples are flexor pollicis longus (flexes the thumb), levator scapula (elevates the scapula), and erector spinae (keeps the spine erect).

Number of origins: When naming muscles by number of origins, the number of origins, or heads, is given first, and the body part with which it is associated is given second (e.g., biceps femoris [two-headed muscle], triceps brachii [three-headed muscle], and quadriceps femoris [group of four muscles]).

Relative shape and size: Some muscles are named for their geometrical shape or gross size. Examples are gluteus maximus (largest), gluteus minimus (smallest), adductor longus (long), and deltoid (triangular).

Location and direction of fibers: Muscles can be named for where they are located or the direction of the majority of their fibers. Examples are temporalis (temporal bone), frontalis (frontal bone), rectus femoris (straight), internal obliques (slanted), latissimus dorsi (dorsum or posterior), and transverse abdominis (across).

Relative position: Muscles are also named for their relative position. Examples are vastus medialis (toward midline), lateral pterygoid (away from midline), internal intercostal (inward), and obturator externus (outward).

Combinations: Many muscles are named using a combination of the aforementioned (e.g., extensor digitorum longus [long muscle that extends the digits or fingers] and flexor digitorum profundus [deep muscle that flexes the fingers]).

---

on attachment sites. Using an articulated skeleton, find each bony attachment site. Using a piece of colorful yarn or cording, touch the origin and insertion at once. This exercise gives you a graphic idea of the muscles. Make up flash cards; on the front of each card, write the name of the each muscle; the back then states the origin and insertion. Drawing muscles on a real body is helpful; this body may belong to one of your classmates, or you can recruit someone. Use nontoxic, water-soluble markers. Use a plastic model of a skeleton and clay to build the muscles on the model, focusing on attachment sites. A large picture of a skeleton may be used if a skeletal model is not available; use a color marker and draw in the muscle, going from origin to insertion. You can also practice this activity in pairs or groups. As a learning tip, *origins are generally located medial or proximal to their insertions.*

Phase IV is designed to teach the action of muscles. To understand muscle actions, you need to know some things about the muscle. For example, to which bones do the muscles attach? Which joint does it cross? Begin to deduce a muscle's action by applying the principle insertion, or *I*, then moving toward the origin, or *O*. Also remember that the action refers to movement in anatomical position. You can learn actions by rote memory or by a multisensory approach. If you have chosen the latter, go back to the phase III learning strategy; place yarn on the *O* and *I* of an articulated skeleton, and shorten the string. This exercise will produce the action of the muscle because muscles produce movement by contracting their fibers. Another useful technique is to say aloud the name of the muscle while you are doing the action with your own body. You can even touch the muscle, say the muscle name aloud, and perform the action. The muscle producing the action will feel hard and become short and thick. Make up flash cards. On the front, write the name of the muscle; on the back, write the name of the action. To assist you in learning the muscle actions, please review the following information; ask your instructor for additional suggestions:

- Muscles located on the anterior side of the body generally flex (except the thigh).
- Muscles located on the posterior side of the body generally extend (except the thigh).
- Muscles located on the medial side of the body generally adduct.
- Muscles located on the lateral side of the body generally abduct.
- Muscles with fibers running superior to inferior generally flex and extend.
- Muscles with oblique running fibers generally rotate.
- If a muscle crosses two joints, then it has an action on both joints.
- Most muscles have two actions: (1) a primary action and (2) a secondary action.
- The antagonist and agonist are generally situated opposite each other, typically with the same insertion.
- The synergist generally has parallel fiber directions.

Phase V is to APPLY, APPLY, APPLY! With your instructor's help, learn how to palpate these muscles using the information in Box 16-2 (How to Palpate Muscles) wherever possible. Use all of this anatomical information in massage class, and use the names of these muscles with your clients. Use the anatomical terminology as much as you can so it becomes part of *you.* As the names, locations, and actions of the muscles become more fixed in your brain, your confidence will grow. Remember, repetition is the key to learning; repetition is the key to learning; repetition is the key to learning.

BOX 16-2

How to Palpate Muscles

- Locate the bony markings (origin and insertion) of the muscle you are palpating. Repositioning your subject may be necessary to allow neighboring muscles to relax.
- Do not push too hard. In palpation, make contact with the skin and allow your hand to sink into the tissues. Now you can go for depth slowly and with purpose.
- Once you are in the neighborhood of the structure you wish to palpate, allow your fingers to move back and forth. This strumming motion allows for better identification as the structure moves under your fingertips.
- Ask your subject to perform the action of the muscle. The muscle contraction will probably be the muscle you are trying to locate. Apply resistance to the movement. Palpate the muscle in its contracted state. Ask your subject to relax, and repeat the contraction.

Many muscles are part of a larger group. In some instances, the term used to denote the muscle group is more common than the individual muscle name. Examples are the hamstrings, the quadriceps, and the adductors. Because of this regularity, common muscle groups have been featured before their individual muscles. The origins and insertions of the featured muscles are identified in blue. Arrows over the illustrated muscles denote its action. Furthermore, the right side of the body is featured, unless otherwise indicated.

Some muscle names are in a shaded box. These names are commonly used when discussing a group of muscles. An example of muscle groups is the hamstrings and the adductors. The right muscle is featured unless otherwise noted.

All muscles do is contract and relax and contract and relax; therefore relax your brain and enjoy this part of the book by learning through application. The retention of this knowledge comes with reinforcement.

Unit ONE—Muscles of the Appendicular Skeleton

Lesson ONE—**Muscles of Scapular Movement** (Trapezius, Levator Scapulae, Rhomboids Major and Minor, Serratus Anterior, Pectoralis Minor)

Trapezius

Greek:
trapezoeides—tablelike

Origins
external occipital protuberance
superior nuchal lines
nuchal ligament
spinous processes of C7-T12
supraspinous ligament of C7-T12

Insertions
lateral third of the clavicle
acromion process
scapular spine

Actions
extends the neck and head (upper fibers)
elevates the scapula (upper fibers)
upwardly rotates the scapula (upper fibers)
retracts the scapula (middle fibers)
depresses the scapula (lower fibers)
laterally flexes the neck (unilateral contraction)
rotates the head (unilateral contraction)

Nerves
spinal accessory nerve (cranial nerve XI)
third and fourth cervical nerve

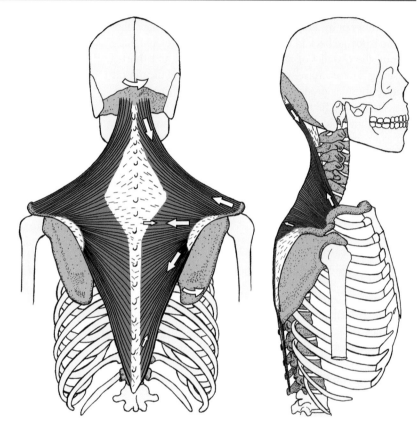

POSTERIOR VIEW   **LATERAL VIEW**

FIGURE 16-2

Notes: Also known as the *coat hanger muscle* because clothes hang from the trapezius, similar to a coat hanger, the trapezius muscle behaves as three muscles in one. Covering more than one half the back, the upper, middle, and lower fibers contract to perform three separate actions. The trapezius, or *traps,* is to the neck and head what the erectors are to the back. Note that this muscle can be an antagonist to itself. This muscle was once called *musculus cucullaris* (Latin for *muscle hood*) because the entire trapezius resembled a monk's hood.

Levator Scapulae

Latin:
levator—a lifter
scapulae—shoulder blade

Origins
transverse processes of C1-C4

Insertion
medial border of the scapula (superior angle to root of spine)

Actions
elevates the scapula
downwardly rotates the scapula
laterally flexes the neck

Nerves
dorsal scapular nerve
cervical nerves

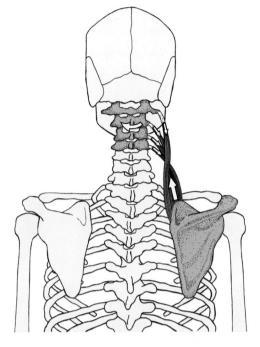

POSTERIOR VIEW
FIGURE 16-3

Notes: This muscle lies between two muscles discussed later, the splenius capitis and the scalenus posterior. The body often shifts its fascial structure from sol state to gel state so as to reinforce this muscle's actions, one of which is stabilizing the scapular, acting as a fixator. In its gel state, it will feel similar to crunches as it is flipped over the insertion. The levator scapulae is the only neck muscle that moves the scapula.

Rhomboids Major and Minor

Latin:
rhombos—all sides even
major—larger
minor—smaller

Origins
spinous processes of C7-T1 (minor)
spinous processes of T2-T5 (major)

Insertions
medial border of the scapula, from root of scapular spine (minor)
   to inferior angle (major)

Actions
retracts the scapula
downwardly rotates the scapula

Nerve
dorsal scapular nerve

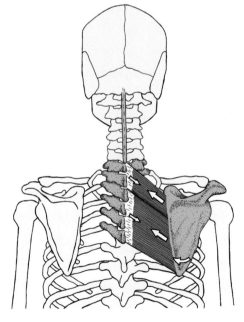

POSTERIOR VIEW
FIGURE 16-4

Notes: *Rhomboids* is the name given for the rhomboid major and rhomboid minor, but they occasionally fuse to form one muscle. Both rhomboids lie deep to the trapezius; the rhomboid minor is superior to the rhomboid major. They are also known as the *Christmas tree muscles* because the fiber direction is obliquely arranged, similar to Christmas tree branches.

Serratus Anterior

Latin:
serratus—notched or jagged, similar to a saw
ante—before

Origins
ribs 1 through 9 (lateral to costal cartilage)

Insertion
anterior medial border of the scapula

Actions
protracts the scapula
upwardly rotates the scapula
depresses the scapula

Nerve
long thoracic nerve

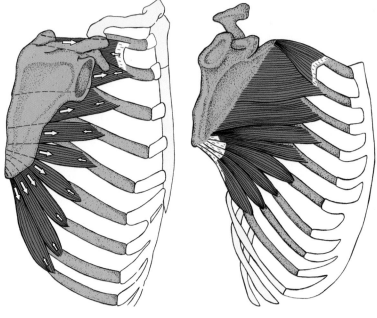

LATERAL VIEW
(the scapula has been lifted
on the right image)

FIGURE 16-5

Notes: This muscle, along with the triceps brachii, is called the *boxer's muscle* because the forward movement of the scapula enables a boxer to deliver a punch. Note that this muscle is antagonist to the rhomboids. The serratus anterior interlaces with the external obliques on the lateral aspect of the trunk. Full or partial paralysis of the serratus anterior produces a *winged scapula,* enabling the person who has this condition to lift the affected arm laterally beyond 90 degrees.

Pectoralis Minor

Latin:
pectoralis—pertaining to the chest
minor—smaller

Origins
ribs 3 through 5 (lateral to costal cartilage)

Insertion
coracoid process of the scapula

Actions
depresses the scapula
protracts the scapula
downwardly rotates the scapula
assists in forced inspiration (elevates ribs)

Nerves
medial pectoral nerves (C8 and T1)

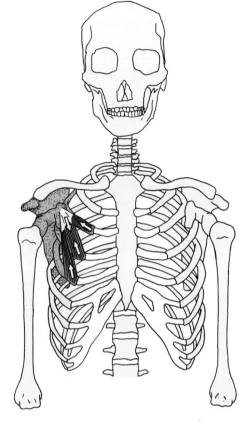

ANTERIOR VIEW
FIGURE 16-6

Notes: Pectoralis minor, along with the scalenes, is known as the *neurovascular entrapper* because the pectoralis minor forms a bridge over the axillary artery and the distal portion of the brachial plexus.

Lesson ONE

Muscles of Scapular Movement

ELEVATION	DEPRESSION	UPWARD ROTATION	DOWNWARD ROTATION	PROTRACTION	RETRACTION
Trapezius (upper fibers)	Trapezius (lower fibers)	Trapezius (upper fibers)	Levator scapulae	Serratus anterior	Trapezius (middle fibers)
Levator scapulae	Serratus anterior	Serratus anterior	Rhomboids	Pectoralis minor	Rhomboids
	Pectoralis minor		Pectoralis minor		

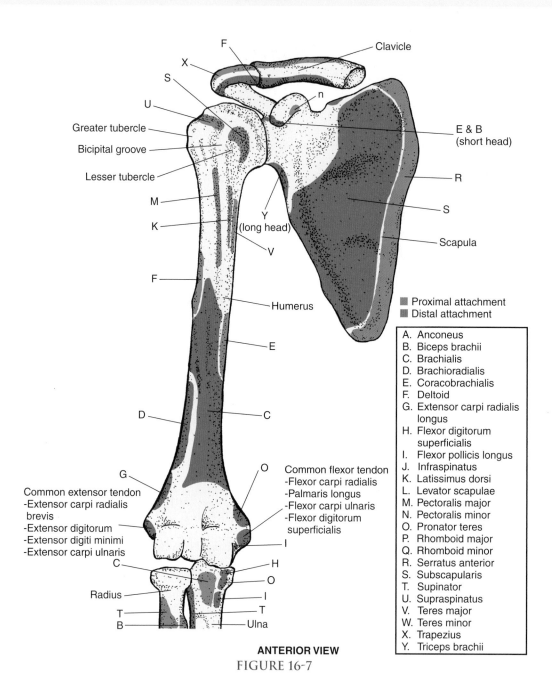

F — Clavicle
X
S
U
Greater tubercle —
Bicipital groove —
Lesser tubercle —
M
K
F
n
E & B (short head)
R
S
Y (long head)
V
Scapula
Humerus
E
■ Proximal attachment
■ Distal attachment

A. Anconeus
B. Biceps brachii
C. Brachialis
D. Brachioradialis
E. Coracobrachialis
F. Deltoid
G. Extensor carpi radialis longus
H. Flexor digitorum superficialis
I. Flexor pollicis longus
J. Infraspinatus
K. Latissimus dorsi
L. Levator scapulae
M. Pectoralis major
N. Pectoralis minor
O. Pronator teres
P. Rhomboid major
Q. Rhomboid minor
R. Serratus anterior
S. Subscapularis
T. Supinator
U. Supraspinatus
V. Teres major
W. Teres minor
X. Trapezius
Y. Triceps brachii

D
C
G
O
Common flexor tendon
-Flexor carpi radialis
-Palmaris longus
-Flexor carpi ulnaris
-Flexor digitorum superficialis

Common extensor tendon
-Extensor carpi radialis brevis
-Extensor digitorum
-Extensor digiti minimi
-Extensor carpi ulnaris
C
H
O
Radius
I
T
B
T
Ulna

ANTERIOR VIEW
FIGURE 16-7

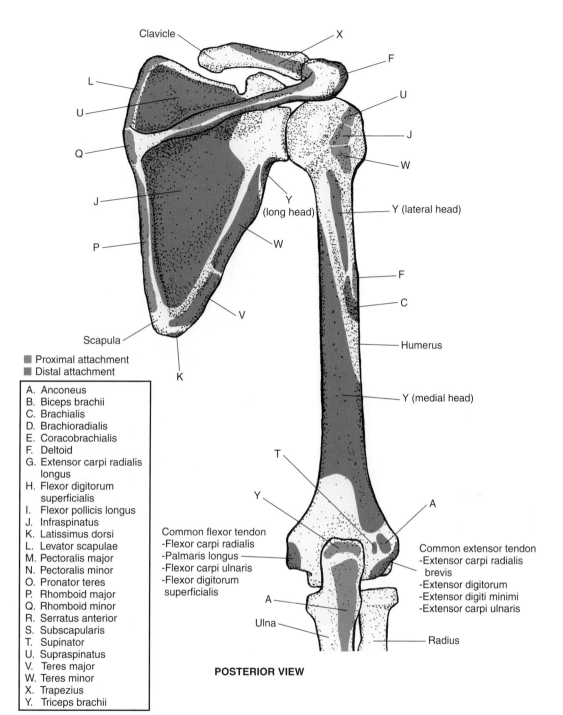

Proximal attachment
Distal attachment

A. Anconeus
B. Biceps brachii
C. Brachialis
D. Brachioradialis
E. Coracobrachialis
F. Deltoid
G. Extensor carpi radialis longus
H. Flexor digitorum superficialis
I. Flexor pollicis longus
J. Infraspinatus
K. Latissimus dorsi
L. Levator scapulae
M. Pectoralis major
N. Pectoralis minor
O. Pronator teres
P. Rhomboid major
Q. Rhomboid minor
R. Serratus anterior
S. Subscapularis
T. Supinator
U. Supraspinatus
V. Teres major
W. Teres minor
X. Trapezius
Y. Triceps brachii

Common flexor tendon
-Flexor carpi radialis
-Palmaris longus
-Flexor carpi ulnaris
-Flexor digitorum superficialis

Common extensor tendon
-Extensor carpi radialis brevis
-Extensor digitorum
-Extensor digiti minimi
-Extensor carpi ulnaris

POSTERIOR VIEW

FIGURE 16-7, cont'd

Unit ONE—Muscles of the Appendicular Skeleton

Lesson TWO—**Muscles of Shoulder Movement** (Latissimus Dorsi, Teres Major, Supraspinatus, Infraspinatus, Teres Minor, Subscapularis, Deltoid, Pectoralis Major, Coracobrachialis, Biceps Brachii [Lesson Three], Triceps Brachii [Lesson Three])

Latissimus Dorsi

Latin:
latus—broad
dorsum—back

Origins
spinous processes of T7-L5
ribs 9 through 12 (posterior surface)
posterior iliac crest
posterior sacrum

Insertion
intertubercular groove of the humerus (middle lip)

Actions
extends the shoulder
medially rotates the shoulder
adducts the shoulder

Nerve
thoracodorsal nerve

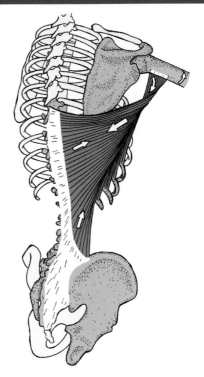

POSTEROLATERAL VIEW
FIGURE 16-8

Notes: The latissimus dorsi is also known as the *swimmer's muscle* because it allows us to extend our arm and propel us in water. The latissimus dorsi is the widest muscle of the body and one of the major muscles involved with back pain. Because of its attachments, improper lifting can cause trauma and tearing in the iliosacral region, resulting in low back pain. Elevation of the hip is assisted with this muscle. The latissimus dorsi interlaces with the external obliques on the lateral aspect of the trunk.

Teres Major

Latin:
teres—round
major—larger

Origin
inferior third of the lateral border of the scapula

Insertion
intertubercular groove of the humerus (medial lip)

Actions
extends the shoulder
medially rotates the shoulder
adducts the shoulder

Nerve
lower subscapular nerve

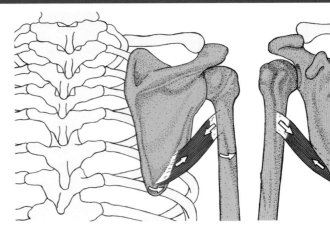

POSTERIOR VIEW   **ANTERIOR VIEW**
FIGURE 16-9

Notes: The teres major muscle is a synergist to the latissimus dorsi muscle and may merge with it. In some cases, it may be completely absent. As a synergist, it is often called *latissimus' little helper*. This muscle also assists in upward rotation of the scapula.

Musculotendinous Cuff

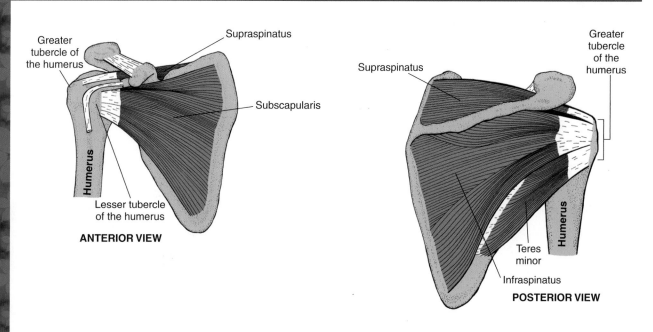

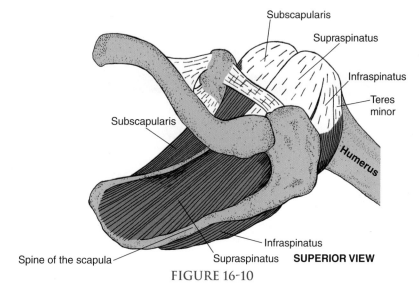

FIGURE 16-10

Notes: Also known as the *rotator cuff,* the musculotendinous cuff is a group of muscles deep to the deltoid. Three of the four muscles arise from scapular fossas (supraspinatus, infraspinatus, subscapularis). Three of the four muscles attach to the greater tubercle (supraspinatus, infraspinatus, teres minor). They do a great deal for the stability of the glenohumeral joint and may function as ligaments. They are also called the *SITS muscles:* **s**upraspinatus, **i**nfraspinatus, **t**eres minor, and **s**ubscapularis.

Supraspinatus

Latin:
supra—above
spinatus—spine

Origin
supraspinous fossa of the scapula

Insertion
greater tubercle of the humerus

Action
abducts the shoulder

Nerve
suprascapular nerve

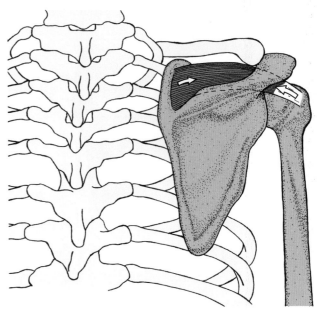

POSTERIOR VIEW

FIGURE 16-11

Notes: The supraspinatus muscle is the only muscle of the musculo-tendinous cuff that does not rotate the humerus. The supraspinatus prevents downward dislocation of the humerus when carrying, for example, a heavy portable massage table.

Infraspinatus

Latin:
infra—beneath
spinatus—spine

Origin
infraspinous fossa of the scapula

Insertion
greater tubercle of the humerus

Action
laterally rotates the shoulder

Nerve
suprascapular nerve

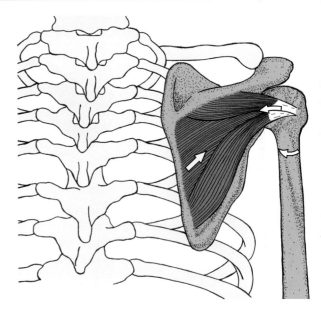

POSTERIOR VIEW

FIGURE 16-12

Teres Minor

Latin:
teres—round
minor—smaller

Origin
superior two thirds of the lateral border of the scapula

Insertion
greater tubercle of the humerus

Actions
adducts the shoulder
laterally rotates the shoulder

Nerve
axillary nerve

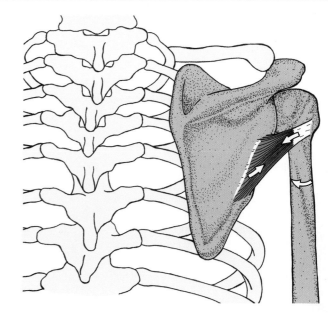

POSTERIOR VIEW

FIGURE 16-13

Notes: The teres minor muscle is the synergist to the infraspinatus muscle and may fuse with it.

Subscapularis

Latin:
sub—below
scapulae—shoulder blade

Origin
subscapular fossa of the scapula

Insertion
lesser tubercle of the humerus

Action
medially rotates the shoulder

Nerve
subscapular nerve

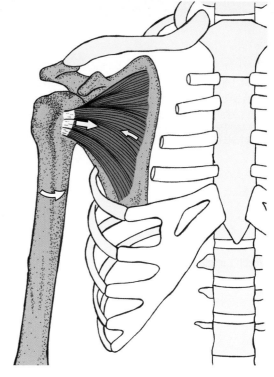

ANTERIOR VIEW

FIGURE 16-14

Notes: Dr. Janet Travell, author of *Myofascial Pain and Dysfunction,* refers to the subscapularis muscle as the *frozen shoulder* muscle.

Deltoid

Greek:
delta—triangular

Origins
lateral third of the clavicle
acromion process
scapular spine

Insertion
deltoid tuberosity

Actions
flexes the shoulder (anterior fibers)
medially rotates the shoulder (anterior fibers)
abducts the shoulder (middle fibers)
extends the shoulder (posterior fibers)
laterally rotates the shoulder (posterior fibers)

Nerve
axillary nerve

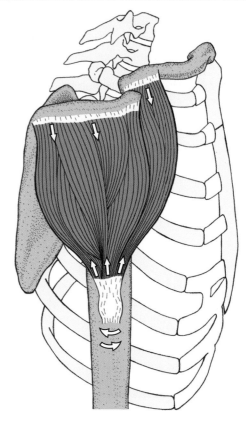

LATERAL VIEW
FIGURE 16-15

Notes: Mary Kordish, a biology professor at McNeese State University, Lake Charles, Louisiana, said that if the deltoid were discovered today, it would be considered three independent muscles. The anterior, middle, and posterior fibers of the deltoid function as three separate muscles. Structurally, they resemble the gluteals. To get a better understanding of this concept, get on your hands and knees and imagine yourself as a four-legged animal. The deltoid is the most important abductor of the shoulder and can be antagonist to itself.

Pectoralis Major

Latin:
pectoralis—pertaining to the chest
major—larger

Origins
medial half of the clavicle
edge of the sternal body
ribs 1 through 7 (costal cartilages)

Insertion
intertubercular groove of the humerus (lateral lip)

Actions
adducts the shoulder
medially rotates the shoulder
flexes the shoulder
extends the shoulder

Nerve
medial pectoral nerve

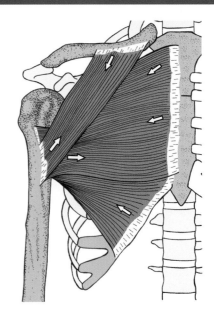

ANTERIOR VIEW
FIGURE 16-16

Pectoralis Major—cont'd

Notes: The pectoralis major muscle, or *pecs,* forms the upper anterior chest wall and anterior axillary fold. This muscle possesses a clavicular, sternal, and costal portions. Tightness in this muscle may cause constriction of chest and angina pectoralis–like pain or postural distortions such as rounded shoulders.

Coracobrachialis

Greek:
korax—crow's beak
Latin:
bracchium—arm

Origin
coracoid process of the scapula

Insertion
medial humeral shaft (middle region)

Actions
flexes the shoulder
adducts the shoulder

Nerve
musculocutaneous nerve

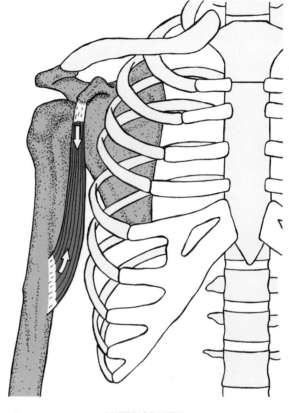

ANTERIOR VIEW
FIGURE 16-17

Lesson TWO

Muscles of Shoulder Movement

FLEXION	EXTENSION	MEDIAL ROTATION	LATERAL ROTATION	ABDUCTION	ADDUCTION
Deltoids (anterior fibers)	Latissimus dorsi	Latissimus dorsi	Infraspinatus	Supraspinatus	Latissimus dorsi
Pectoralis major	Teres major	Teres major	Teres minor	Deltoids (middle fibers)	Teres major
Coracobrachialis	Deltoids (posterior fibers)	Subscapularis	Deltoids (posterior fibers)		Teres minor
Biceps brachii	Pectoralis major	Deltoids (anterior fibers)			Pectoralis major
	Triceps brachii	Pectoralis major			Coracobrachialis
					Triceps brachii

Unit ONE—Muscles of the Appendicular Skeleton

Lesson THREE—**Muscles of Elbow Movement** (Biceps Brachii, Brachialis, Brachioradialis, Triceps Brachii, Anconeus, Pronator Teres [Lesson Four])

Biceps Brachii

Latin:
bis—twice + caput—head
bracchium—arm

Origins
supraglenoid tubercle of the scapula (long head)
coracoid process of scapula (short head)

Insertions
radial tuberosity
bicipital aponeurosis

Actions
flexes the elbow
supinates the forearm
flexes the shoulder

Nerve
musculocutaneous nerve

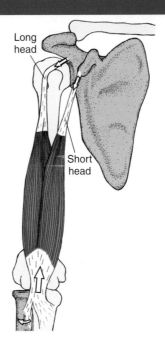

ANTERIOR VIEW
FIGURE 16-18

Notes: The biceps brachii muscle is called the *corkscrew muscle* because two of its actions resemble uncorking a wine bottle. The tendon of the long head passes within the intertubercular groove of the humerus and also passes through the capsule of the shoulder joint itself. This muscle may have an additional head attaching to the midshaft of the humerus (approximately 10% of cadavers).

Brachialis

Latin:
bracchium—arm

Origin
distal anterior humeral shaft

Insertions
ulnar tuberosity
coronoid process of the ulna

Action
flexes the elbow

Nerve
musculocutaneous nerve

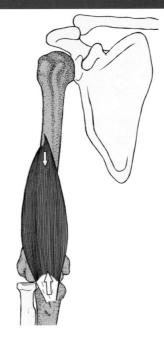

ANTERIOR VIEW
FIGURE 16-19

Notes: The brachialis is the most effective arm flexor because of its mechanical advantage, lying deep to the biceps brachii. Additionally, when you flex your forearm to *show off* your biceps brachii, a great deal of this display is actually the brachialis *pushing up* on the biceps brachii.

Brachioradialis

Latin:
bracchium—arm
radialis—spoke of a wheel

Origin
lateral supracondylar ridge of the humerus

Insertion
styloid process of the radius

Action
flexes the elbow

Nerve
radial nerve

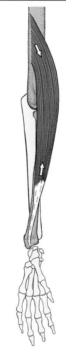

LATERAL VIEW
FIGURE 16-20

Notes: The bulge you can palpate on the radial side of your forearm is the brachioradialis. The radial pulse is located between the tendons of the brachioradialis and the flexor carpi radialis.

Triceps Brachii

Greek:
treis—three
Latin:
bracchium—arm

Origins
infraglenoid tubercle of the scapula (long head)
posterior proximal humeral shaft (lateral head)
posterior distal humeral shaft (medial head)

Insertion
olecranon process

Actions
extends the elbow
extends the shoulder
adducts the shoulder

Nerve
radial nerve

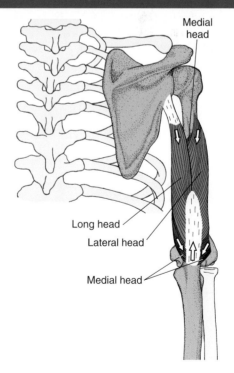

POSTERIOR VIEW
FIGURE 16-21

Notes: This muscle, along with the serratus anterior, is called the *boxer's muscle* because it delivers a straight-arm knockout punch. As the radial nerve passes between the lateral and medial heads on the posterior humerus, it sits virtually on the humerus; because it passes through the radial groove, compression of the radial nerve in this area can cause injury to the radial nerve.

Anconeus

Greek:
angkon—elbow

Origin
lateral epicondyle of the humerus

Insertions
olecranon process
superior eighth of ulnar shaft

Action
extends the elbow

Nerve
radial nerve

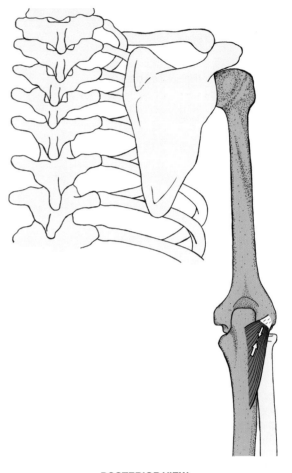

POSTERIOR VIEW
FIGURE 16-22

Lesson THREE

Muscles of Elbow Movement

FLEXION	EXTENSION
Biceps brachii	Triceps brachii
Brachialis	Anconeus
Brachioradialis	
Pronator teres	
Flexor carpi radialis	

Unit ONE—Muscles of the Appendicular Skeleton

Lesson FOUR—**Muscles of the Forearm, Wrist, and Hand** (Pronator Teres, Pronator Quadratus, Supinator, Flexor Carpi Radialis, Flexor Carpi Ulnaris, Palmaris Longus, Flexor Digitorum Superficialis, Flexor Digitorum Profundus, Extensor Carpi Radialis Longus and Brevis, Extensor Carpi Ulnaris, Extensor Digitorum, Extensor Digiti Minimi, Extensor Indicis, Extensor Pollicis Longus and Brevis, Flexor Pollicis Longus and Brevis, Opponens Pollicis, Abductor Pollicis Longus and Brevis, Flexor Digiti Minimi, Abductor Digiti Minimi, Opponens Digiti Minimi, Biceps Brachii [Lesson Three])

Pronator Teres

Latin:
pronus—downward
teres—round

Origins
medial epicondyle of the humerus
coronoid process of the ulna

Insertion
mid lateral radial shaft

Actions
pronates the forearm
flexes the elbow

Nerve
median nerve

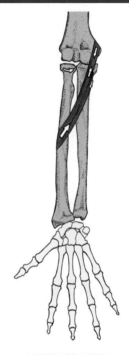

ANTERIOR VIEW
FIGURE 16-23

Pronator Quadratus

Latin:
pronus—downward
quadratus—four sided

Origin
anterior distal quarter of the ulnar shaft

Insertion
anterior distal quarter of the radial shaft

Action
pronates the forearm

Nerve
median nerve

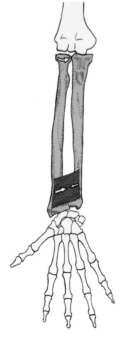

ANTERIOR VIEW
FIGURE 16-24

Supinator

Latin:
supinatus—bent backward

Origins
lateral epicondyle of the humerus
proximal eighth of ulnar shaft
radial collateral ligament
annular ligament

Insertion
proximal lateral radial shaft

Action
supinates the forearm

Nerve
radial nerve

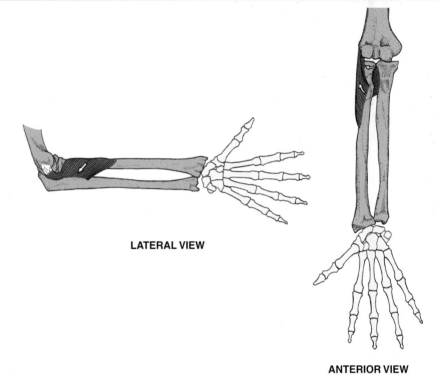

LATERAL VIEW

ANTERIOR VIEW

FIGURE 16-25

Flexor Carpi Radialis

Latin:
flexus—bent
karpos—wrist
radialis—spoke of a wheel

Origin
medial epicondyle of the humerus

Insertions
bases of metacarpals II and III

Actions
flexes the wrist
abducts the wrist
flexes the elbow

Nerve
median nerve

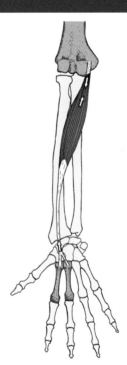

ANTERIOR VIEW
FIGURE 16-26

Notes: Notice how this muscle and the next three (flexor carpi ulnaris, palmaris longus, and flexor digitorum superficialis) all flex the wrist and all originate on the medial epicondyle of the humerus. The flexors lie on the fleshy side of the forearm. In fact, wrist flexion is a more powerful movement than wrist extension, abduction, or adduction. The radial pulse is located between the tendons of the flexor carpi radialis and the brachioradialis.

Flexor Carpi Ulnaris

Latin:
flexus—bent
karpos—wrist
ulna—elbow

Origins
medial epicondyle of the humerus
medial olecranon
posterior proximal two thirds of the ulna

Insertions
metacarpal V
pisiform
hamate

Actions
flexes the wrist
adducts the wrist

Nerve
ulnar nerve

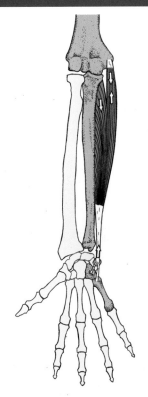

ANTERIOR VIEW
FIGURE 16-27

Palmaris Longus

Latin:
palma—hand
longus—long

Origin
medial epicondyle of the humerus

Insertion
palmar aponeurosis

Actions
flexes the wrist
cups (tenses) the palm

Nerve
median nerve

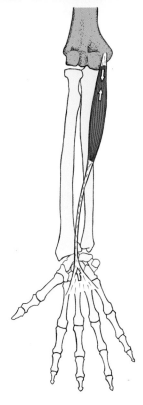

ANTERIOR VIEW
FIGURE 16-28

Notes: This muscle is absent in approximately 10% of cadavers.

Flexor Digitorum Superficialis

Latin:
flexus—bent
digitus—finger
superficialis—toward the surface

Origins
medial epicondyle of the humerus
proximal radial shaft (upper region)
coronoid process of the ulna

Insertions
middle phalanges of digits two through five

Actions
flexes the wrist
flexes the fingers at the proximal interphalangeal (PIP) and
    metacarpophalangeal (MP) joints

Nerve
median nerve

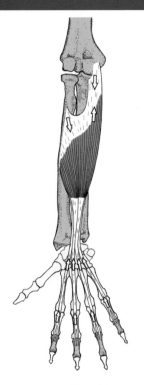

ANTERIOR VIEW
FIGURE 16-29

Notes: Of all the movements allowed at the forearm, wrist, and hand, finger flexion is the most powerful.

Flexor Digitorum Profundus

Latin:
flexus—bent
digitus—finger
profundus—deep

Origins
anterior proximal three fourths of the ulnar shaft
interosseus membrane

Insertions
distal phalanges of digits two through five

Action
flexes the fingers at the distal interphalangeal (DIP), PIP, and
    MP joints

Nerves
ulnar nerve
median nerve

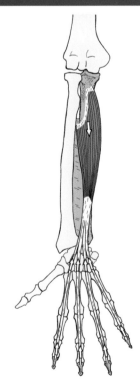

ANTERIOR VIEW
FIGURE 16-30

Notes: Of all the movements allowed at the forearm, wrist, and hand, finger flexion is the most powerful. Flexor digitorum may also flex the wrist.

Extensor Carpi Radialis Longus

Latin:
extensio—to extend
karpos—wrist
radialis—spoke of a wheel
longus—long

Origin
lateral supracondylar ridge of the humerus

Insertion
metacarpal II

Actions
extends the wrist
abducts the wrist

Nerve
radial nerve

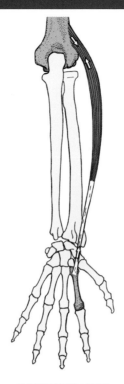

POSTERIOR VIEW
FIGURE 16-31

Extensor Carpi Radialis Brevis

Latin:
extensio—to extend
karpos—wrist
radialis—spoke of a wheel
brevis—brief

Origin
lateral epicondyle of the humerus

Insertion
metacarpal III

Actions
extends the wrist
abducts the wrist

Nerve
radial nerve

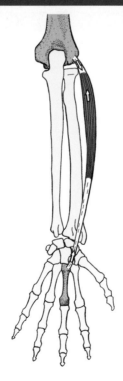

POSTERIOR VIEW
FIGURE 16-32

Notes: Extensor carpi radialis brevis often becomes inflamed at its origin (epicondylitis) in tennis elbow. Notice how these muscles and the next two (extensor carpi ulnaris and extensor digitorum) all extend the wrist and all originate on the lateral epicondyle of the humerus.

The extensors lie on the hairy side of the forearm. These two muscles are also referred to as the *fist clinchers;* for the finger flexors to fully make a fist, the wrist must be slightly extended.

Extensor Carpi Ulnaris

Latin:
extensio—to extend
karpos—wrist
ulna—elbow

Origin
lateral epicondyle of the humerus

Insertion
metacarpal V

Actions
extends the wrist
adducts the wrist

Nerve
radial nerve

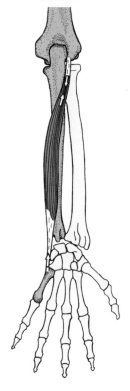

POSTERIOR VIEW
FIGURE 16-33

Extensor Digitorum

Latin:
extensio—to extend
digitus—finger

Origin
lateral epicondyle of the humerus

Insertions
middle and distal digits two through five

Actions
extends the wrist
extends the fingers at the DIP, PIP, and MP joints

Nerve
radial nerve

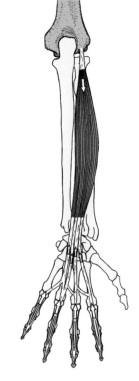

POSTERIOR VIEW
FIGURE 16-34

Notes: Extensor digitorum is sometimes called *extensor digitorum communis.*

Extensor Digiti Minimi

Latin:
extensio—to extend
digitus—finger
minimum—least

Origin
lateral epicondyle of the humerus

Insertions
middle and distal digits of fifth finger

Action
extends the little finger

Nerve
radial nerve

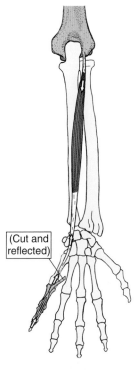

POSTERIOR VIEW
FIGURE 16-35

Notes: The extensor digiti minimi is also known as the *tea drinker's muscle* because it extends the little finger while you raise the teacup to your lips. This muscle may also assist in extending the wrist.

Extensor Indicis

Latin:
extensio—to extend
indices—forefinger

Origins
Distal ulnar shaft
interosseus membrane

Insertions
middle and distal digits of index finger (or second digit)

Action
extends the index finger

Nerve
radial nerve

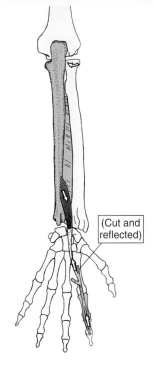

POSTERIOR VIEW
FIGURE 16-36

Notes: This muscle may also assist in extending the wrist.

Extensor Pollicis Longus and Brevis

Latin:
extensio—to extend
pollex—thumb
longus—long
brevis—brief

Origins
posterior ulnar shaft—middle region (longus)
posterior radial shaft—distal region (brevis)
interosseous membrane (brevis and longus)

Insertions
distal phalanx of the thumb (longus)
proximal phalanx of the thumb (brevis)

Action
extends the thumb

Nerve
radial nerve

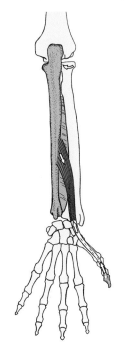
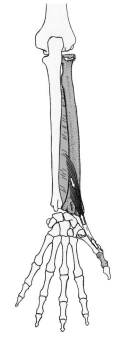

POSTERIOR VIEW
of Extensor Pollicis Longus

POSTERIOR VIEW
of Extensor Pollicis Brevis

FIGURE 16-37

Notes: These muscles may also assist in wrist extension (longus) and abduction (brevis).

Flexor Pollicis Longus and Brevis

Latin:
flexus—bent
pollex—thumb
longus—long
brevis—brief

Origins
anterior radial shaft—middle region (longus)
interosseous membrane (longus)
trapezium (brevis)
transverse carpal ligament (brevis)

Insertions
distal phalanx of the thumb (longus)
proximal phalanx of the thumb (brevis)

Action
flexes the thumb

Nerve
median nerve

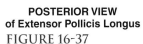
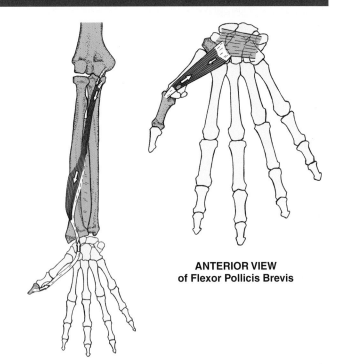

ANTERIOR VIEW
of Flexor Pollicis Brevis

ANTERIOR VIEW
of Flexor Pollicis Longus

FIGURE 16-38

Opponens Pollicis

Latin:
opponens—opposing
pollex—thumb

Origins
trapezium
transverse carpal ligament

Insertion
metacarpal I

Actions
flexes the thumb
adducts the thumb (moves the thumb into opposition)

Nerve
median nerve

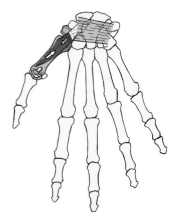

ANTERIOR VIEW
FIGURE 16-39

Abductor Pollicis Longus and Brevis

Latin:
abductus—led away
pollex—thumb
longus—long
brevis—brief

Origins
posterior ulnar shaft—middle region (longus)
posterior radial shaft—middle region (longus)
interosseus membrane (longus)
trapezium (brevis)
scaphoid (brevis)
transverse carpal ligament (brevis)

Insertions
metacarpal I (longus)
proximal phalanx of the thumb (brevis)

Action
abducts the thumb

Nerve
median nerve

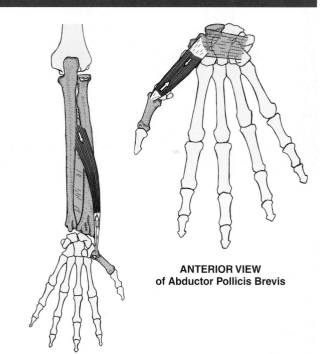

ANTERIOR VIEW
of Abductor Pollicis Brevis

POSTERIOR VIEW
of Abductor Pollicis Longus
FIGURE 16-40

Notes: The abductor pollicis longus also assists in opposition.

Flexor Digiti Minimi

Latin:
flexus—bent
digitus—finger
minimum—least

Origins
hamate
transverse carpal ligament

Insertion
proximal phalanx of the fifth finger

Action
flexion of the fifth (little) finger

Nerve
ulnar nerve

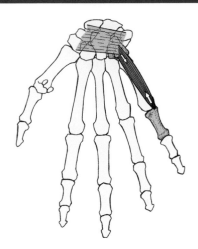

ANTERIOR VIEW
FIGURE 16-41

Notes: Some texts distinguish flexor digiti minimi from the flexor digiti minimi brevis in that the former is in the hand and the latter in the foot. This muscle is often absent.

Abductor Digiti Minimi

Latin:
abductus—led away
digitus—finger
minimum—least

Origins
pisiform
tendon of flexor carpi ulnaris

Insertion
proximal phalanx of the fifth finger

Action
abduction of the fifth (little) finger

Nerve
ulnar nerve

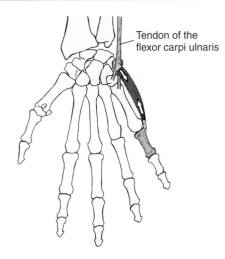

Tendon of the
flexor carpi ulnaris

ANTERIOR VIEW
FIGURE 16-42

Opponens Digiti Minimi

Latin:
opponens—opposing
digitus—finger
minimum—least

Origins
transverse carpal ligament
hamate

Insertion
metacarpal V

Action
adducts the little finger (moves the little finger into opposition)

Nerve
ulnar nerve

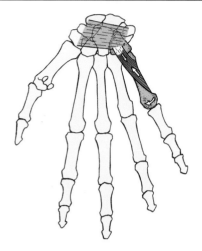

ANTERIOR VIEW
FIGURE 16-43

Thenar Eminence

Greek:
thenar—palm of hand
minere—to hang on

Notes: The thenar eminence is the thumb pad on the anterior surface of the hand. It is made up of three individual muscles called the *opponens pollicis, abductor pollicis brevis*, and the *flexor pollicis brevis*.

Hypothenar Eminence

Greek:
hypo—under
thenar—palm of hand
minere—to hang on

Notes: The hypothenar eminence is the little finger pad on the anterior surface of the hand. It consists of three individual muscles called the *opponens digiti minimi, flexor digiti minimi*, and *abductor digiti minimi.*

Anatomical Snuffbox

Notes: Anatomic snuffbox is a hollow seen on the lateral aspect of the back of the wrist when the thumb is extended fully. It is formed by the tendons of the muscles extensor pollicis brevis and extensor pollicis longus. The reason that it is called the anatomical snuffbox is that snuff (powdered tobacco) could be put there and then inhaled (when this was popular, of course).

The radial artery runs on the floor of the anatomic snuffbox. The carpal bones, scaphoid and trapezium, can be palpated within the snuffbox, as can the styloid process of the radius. Tenderness or pain on contact in the snuffbox is diagnostic of a scaphoid fracture.

Lesson FOUR

Muscles of Forearm, Wrist, and Finger Movements

FLEXION	EXTENSION	ABDUCTION	ADDUCTION	PRONATION	SUPINATION
Flexor carpi radialis	Extensor carpi radialis longus	Flexor carpi radialis	Flexor carpi ulnaris	Pronator teres	Biceps brachii
Flexor carpi ulnaris	Extensor carpi radialis brevis	Extensor carpi radialis longus	Extensor carpi ulnaris	Pronator quadratus	Supinator
Palmaris longus	Extensor carpi ulnaris	Extensor carpi radialis brevis			
Flexor digitorum superficialis	Extensor digitorum				

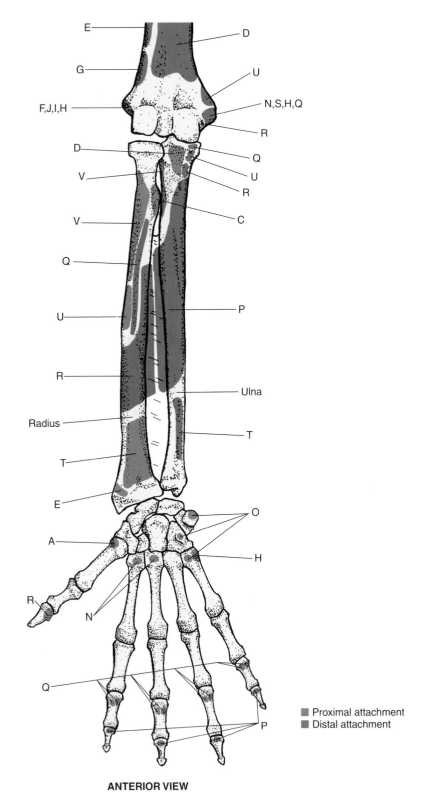

A. Abductor pollicis longus
B. Anconeus
C. Biceps brachii
D. Brachialis
E. Brachioradialis
F. Extensor carpi radialis brevis
G. Extensor carpi radialis longus
H. Extensor carpi ulnaris
I. Extensor digiti minimi
J. Extensor digitorum
K. Extensor indicis
L. Extensor pollicis brevis
M. Extensor pollicis longus
N. Flexor carpi radialis
O. Flexor carpi ulnaris
P. Flexor digitorum profundus
Q. Flexor digitorum superficialis
R. Flexor pollicis longus
S. Palmaris longus
T. Pronator quadratus
U. Pronator teres
V. Supinator
W. Triceps brachii

■ Proximal attachment
■ Distal attachment

ANTERIOR VIEW

FIGURE 16-44

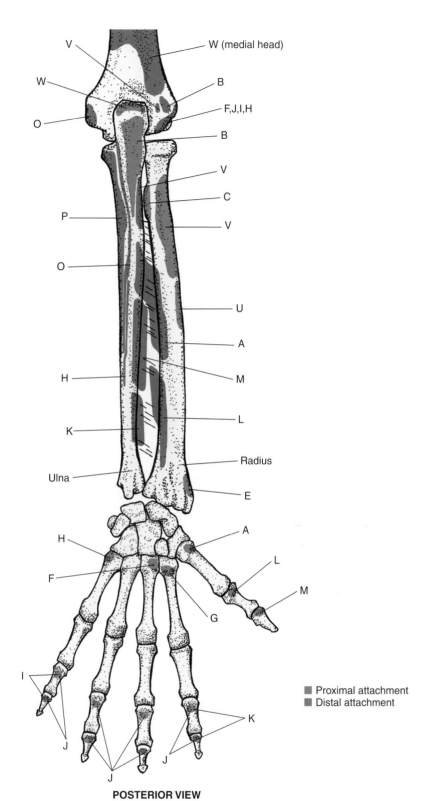

A. Abductor pollicis longus
B. Anconeus
C. Biceps brachii
D. Brachialis
E. Brachioradialis
F. Extensor carpi radialis brevis
G. Extensor carpi radialis longus
H. Extensor carpi ulnaris
I. Extensor digiti minimi
J. Extensor digitorum
K. Extensor indicis
L. Extensor pollicis brevis
M. Extensor pollicis longus
N. Flexor carpi radialis
O. Flexor carpi ulnaris
P. Flexor digitorum profundus
Q. Flexor digitorum superficialis
R. Flexor pollicis longus
S. Palmaris longus
T. Pronator quadratus
U. Pronator teres
V. Supinator
W. Triceps brachii

■ Proximal attachment
■ Distal attachment

POSTERIOR VIEW

FIGURE 16-44, cont'd

Unit ONE—Muscles of the Appendicular Skeleton

Lesson FIVE—**Muscles of Hip and Knee Movement** (Psoas Major, Iliacus, Piriformis, Gemellus Superior, Gemellus Inferior, Obturator Internus, Obturator Externus, Quadratus Femoris, Gluteus Maximus, Gluteus Medius, Gluteus Minimus, Tensor Fascia Lata, Rectus Femoris, Vastus Intermedius, Vastus Medialis, Vastus Lateralis, Sartorius, Semimembranosus, Semitendinosus, Biceps Femoris, Gracilis, Adductor Magnus, Adductor Longus, Adductor Brevis, Pectineus, Gastrocnemius [Lesson Six], Plantaris [Lesson Six], Popliteus [Lesson Six])

Iliopsoas

Latin:
ilium—flank
Greek:
psoa—muscle of the loin

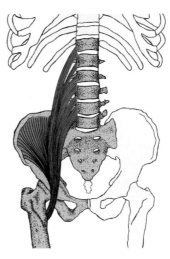

ANTERIOR VIEW
FIGURE 16-45

Notes: The psoas major, psoas minor, and iliacus are usually referred to as the *iliopsoas.* Because the psoas minor is absent in approximately 60% of cadavers, it will not be included for discussion. Tightness in the iliopsoas muscle can play a significant role in functional lordosis and scoliosis. A filet mignon is the iliopsoas muscle of a cow, which is the main flexor of the hip, the muscle that initiates walking (it lifts the leg), and the major cause of muscular low back pain.

Psoas Major

Greek:
psoa—muscle of the loin
major—larger

Origins
transverse processes of T12-L5
vertebral bodies of T12-L5
intervertebral disks of lumbar vertebrae

Insertion
lesser trochanter

Actions
laterally rotates the hip (unilateral contraction)
flexes the hip (uni- or bilateral contraction)
flexes the vertebral column (bilateral contraction)
anteriorly tilts pelvis (bilateral contraction)

Nerves
lumbar plexus

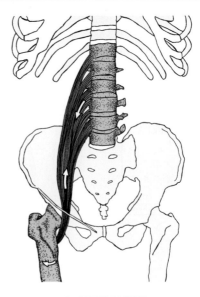

ANTERIOR VIEW
FIGURE 16-46

Notes: The psoas major is the strongest hip flexor.

Iliacus

Latin:
iliacus—ilium

Origins
iliac fossa
anterior inferior iliac spine

Insertion
lesser trochanter

Actions
flexes the hip
laterally rotates the hip
anteriorly tilts pelvis

Nerve
femoral nerve

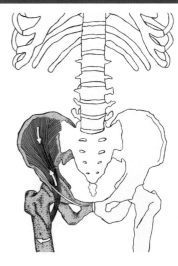

ANTERIOR VIEW
FIGURE 16-47

Deep Hip Outward Rotators

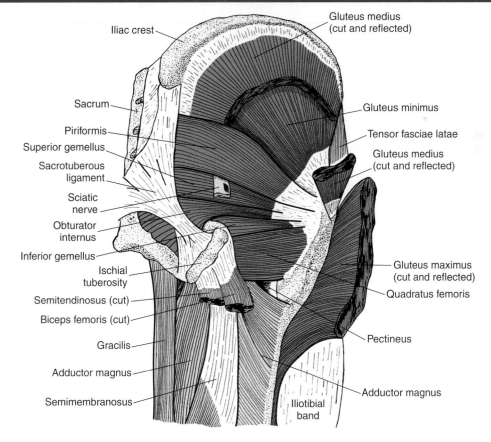

POSTERIOR VIEW
FIGURE 16-48

Notes: The six deep lateral rotators are located beneath the gluteals and correspond to some degree to the rotator cuff muscles of the shoulder joint. Each rotator is synergistic to the other. To help you learn the names of these muscles, from superior to inferior, use the mnemonic phrase, *Pieced goods often go on quilts:* **p**iriformis, **g**emellus superior, **o**bturator internus, **g**emellus inferior, **o**bturator externus, and **q**uadratus femoris. These muscles are the six deep lateral rotators, and all of them have an insertion on the greater trochanter. The hip lateral rotators are stronger than the hip medial rotators. Note how the foot is turned slightly outward when lying down or in normal gait.

Piriformis

Latin:
pirum—pear
forma—shape

Origin
anterior sacrum

Insertion
greater trochanter

Actions
laterally rotates the hip
abducts the hip

Nerve
sciatic nerve

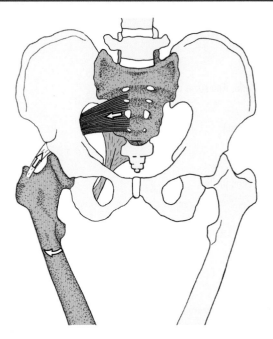

ANTERIOR VIEW

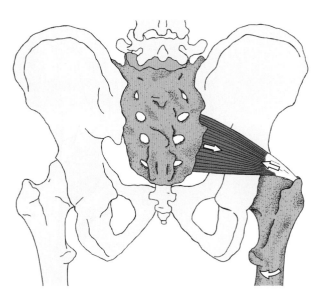

POSTERIOR VIEW

FIGURE 16-49

Notes: The piriformis is the largest of all the lateral rotators and the most likely to become chronically shortened. Of the population, 15% has all or part of the sciatic nerve running *through* this muscle. The piriformis may be in spasm if one or both feet are laterally rotated, in a ducklike position.

Gemellus Superior

Latin:
gemellus—twin
superus—upper

Origin
ischial spine

Insertion
greater trochanter

Action
laterally rotates the hip

Nerve
sciatic nerve

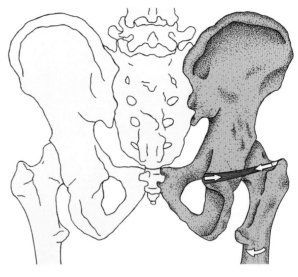

POSTERIOR VIEW

FIGURE 16-50

Notes: This muscle is occasionally absent.

Gemellus Inferior

Latin:
gemellus—twin
inferus—beneath

Origin
superior ischial tuberosity

Insertion
greater trochanter

Action
laterally rotates the hip

Nerve
sciatic nerve

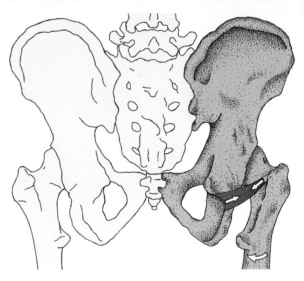

POSTERIOR VIEW

FIGURE 16-51

Notes: This muscle is occasionally absent.

Obturator Internus

Latin:
obturare—obstruct
internus—within

Origins
obturator membrane
obturator margin

Insertion
greater trochanter

Action
laterally rotates the hip

Nerve
sciatic nerve

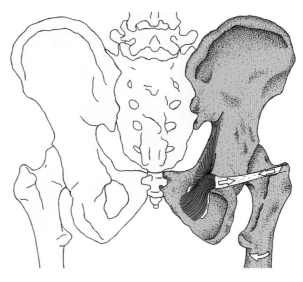

POSTERIOR VIEW

FIGURE 16-52

Notes: The obturator internus passes through and almost fills the lesser sciatic notch.

Obturator Externus

Latin:
obturare—obstruct
externus—outside

Origins
obturator membrane
superior pubic ramus
inferior pubic ramus
ischial ramus

Insertion
greater trochanter

Action
laterally rotates the hip

Nerve
obturator nerve

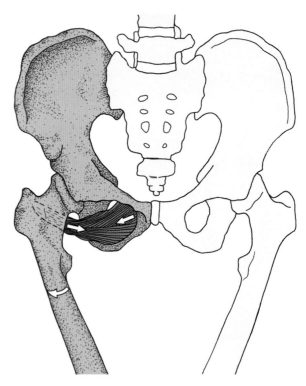

ANTERIOR VIEW

FIGURE 16-53

Notes: This muscle is occasionally absent.

Quadratus Femoris

Latin:
quadratus—four sided
femoralis—pertaining to the femur

Origin
lateral ischial tuberosity

Insertion
greater trochanter

Action
laterally rotates the hip

Nerve
sciatic nerve

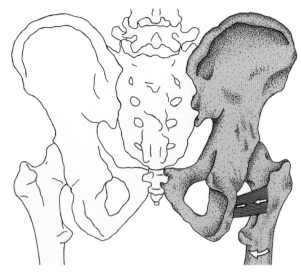

POSTERIOR VIEW

FIGURE 16-54

Notes: This muscle is occasionally absent or fused with the adductor magnus.

Gluteals

Greek:
gloutous—buttock

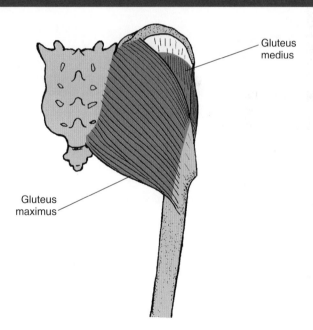

POSTERIOR VIEW

FIGURE 16-55

Notes: The gluteals, or *glutes,* refer to the gluteus maximus, gluteus medius, and gluteus minimus. Note that these muscles can be antagonists to themselves. The iliotibial band is an insertion for both the gluteus maximus and the tensor fascia lata and helps stabilize the knee. Also known as the *iliotibial tract,* the iliotibial band (ITB) is a thickened strap of a fascial tube that surrounds the thigh. The ITB stretches from the iliac crest to the tibia.

Gluteus Maximus

Greek:
gloutos—buttock
Latin:
maximus—greatest

Origins
posterior sacrum
posterior coccyx
posterior iliac crest
external ilium posterior to the posterior gluteal line

Insertions
gluteal tuberosity (25%)
iliotibial band (75%)

Actions
extends the hip
laterally rotates the hip
adducts the hip
posteriorly tilts the pelvis

Nerve
inferior gluteal nerve

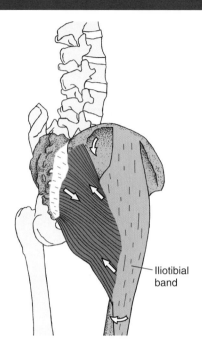

POSTEROLATERAL VIEW
FIGURE 16-56

Notes: The gluteus maximus is the strongest hip extensor and one of the strongest muscles of the body; it is often more than 1 inch thick. This muscle is mainly used for power, as in climbing stairs, rising from a seated position, or running instead of walking. This muscle also helps tense the fascia lata, the fascial tube around the thigh.

Gluteus Medius

Greek:
gloutos—buttock
Latin:
medius—middle

Origin
external ilium between the anterior and posterior gluteal lines

Insertion
greater trochanter

Actions
abducts the hip
medially rotates the hip
laterally rotates the hip
anteriorly rotates the pelvis

Nerve
superior gluteal nerve

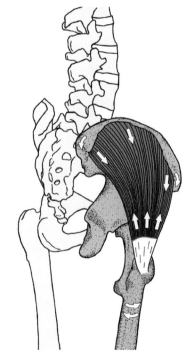

POSTEROLATERAL VIEW
FIGURE 16-57

Notes: This muscle stabilizes the hip to give us the ability to stand on one leg.

Gluteus Minimus

Greek:
gloutos—buttock
Latin:
minimum—least

Origin
external ilium between the anterior and inferior gluteal lines

Insertion
greater trochanter

Actions
abducts the hip
medially rotates the hip
anteriorly rotates the pelvis

Nerve
superior gluteal nerve

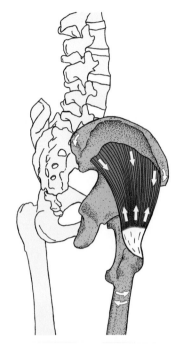

POSTEROLATERAL VIEW
FIGURE 16-58

Notes: The gluteus minimus is the synergist to the gluteus medius and is a weak hip abductor compared with the gluteus medius.

Tensor Fascia Lata

Latin:
tensor—stretching
fascia—band
lata—broad

Origins
anterior iliac crest
anterior superior iliac spine

Insertion
iliotibial band

Actions
abducts the hip
flexes the hip
medially rotates the hip

Nerve
gluteal nerve

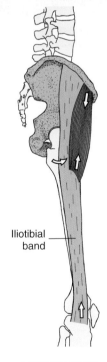

Iliotibial band

LATERAL VIEW
FIGURE 16-59

Notes: As the name implies, this muscle also helps tense the fascia lata, which is the fascial tube around the thigh.

Quadriceps Femoris

Latin:
quattuor—four
caput—head
femoralis—pertaining to the femur

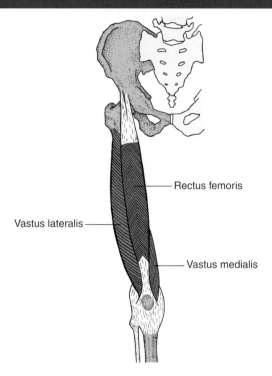

ANTERIOR VIEW

FIGURE 16-60

Notes: The quadriceps femoris is a group of four muscles sharing a common attachment site on the tibia. The four muscle heads, which are often listed as four individual muscles, are the rectus femoris and three vasti—vastus intermedius, vastus medialis, and vastus lateralis.

Lengthening and softening of the quadriceps femoris may provide quick relief from knee problems because the quadriceps tendon crosses the knee joint. Conversely, overuse of quads may create knee problems.

Rectus Femoris

Latin:
rectus—straight
femoralis—pertaining to the femur

Origins
anterior inferior iliac spine
external ilium just superior to the acetabulum

Insertion
tibial tuberosity

Actions
flexes the hip
extends the knee
anteriorly tilts the pelvis

Nerve
femoral nerve

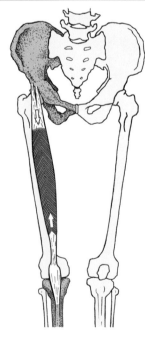

ANTERIOR VIEW
FIGURE 16-61

Notes: The rectus femoris runs in a channel formed by the vastus muscles, and it overlies the vastus intermedius. It is the only muscle in the quadriceps femoris group that crosses two joints (hip and knee) and has several actions.

Vastus Intermedius

Latin:
vastus—immense
inter—internal
medius—middle

Origin
anterior lateral femoral shaft

Insertion
tibial tuberosity

Action
extends the knee

Nerve
femoral nerve

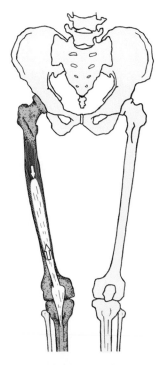

ANTERIOR VIEW
FIGURE 16-62

Vastus Medialis

Latin:
vastus—immense
medius—middle

Origin
linea aspera (medial lip)

Insertion
tibial tuberosity

Action
extends the knee

Nerve
femoral nerve

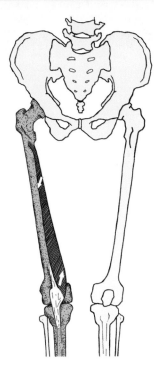

ANTERIOR VIEW
FIGURE 16-63

Notes: The vastus medialis muscle is sometimes called the *teardrop* or *raindrop* muscle because of the way it appears when outlined by the sartorius and rectus femoris.

Vastus Lateralis

Latin:
vastus—immense
lateralis—toward the side

Origins
linea aspera (lateral lip)
gluteal tuberosity

Insertion
tibial tuberosity

Action
extends the knee

Nerve
femoral nerve

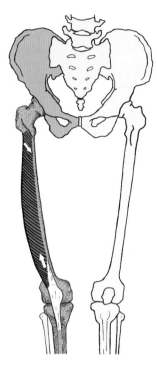

ANTERIOR VIEW
FIGURE 16-64

Sartorius

Latin:
sartor—tailor

Origin
anterior superior iliac spine

Insertion
medial proximal tibial shaft (at pes anserinus)

Actions
flexes the hip
laterally rotates the hip
abducts the hip
flexes the knee
medially rotates the leg (when the knee is flexed)

Nerve
femoral nerve

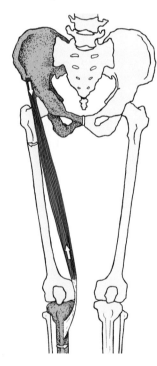

ANTERIOR VIEW
FIGURE 16-65

Notes: Also known as the *tailor's muscle* because, in older times, tailors sat cross-legged while they sewed. The sartorius is the longest muscle in the body, crossing both the hip and knee joints, running superficially and obliquely across the quadriceps femoris muscle.

Hamstrings

Anglo-Saxon:
haun—haunch

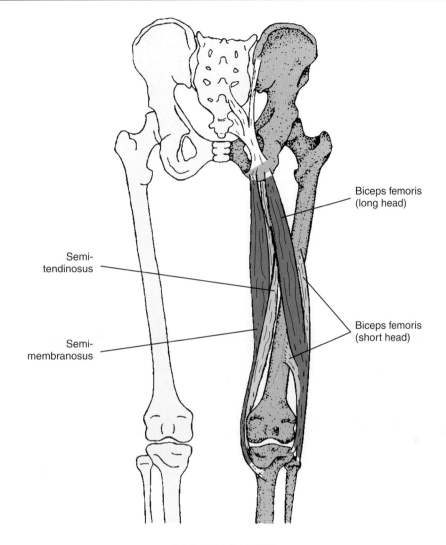

Semi-
tendinosus

Semi-
membranosus

Biceps femoris
(long head)

Biceps femoris
(short head)

POSTERIOR VIEW

FIGURE 16-66

Notes: The term *hamstrings* comes from the fact that butchers in the eighteenth century used the tendons of the thighs and hips of pig carcasses to hang ham. Use the mnemonic BMT to indicate their location on the posterior thigh: *b*iceps femoris, semi*m*embranosus, semi*t*endinosus. Both semimembranosus and semitendinosus occupy the medial posterior thigh, with the biceps femoris occupying the lateral posterior thigh.

Semimembranosus

Latin:
semis—half
membrana—membrane

Origin
ischial tuberosity

Insertion
medial condyle of the tibia (posterior surface)

Actions
flexes the knee
medially rotates the leg (when the knee is flexed)
extends the hip
medially rotates the hip
posteriorly tilts the pelvis

Nerve
tibial nerve

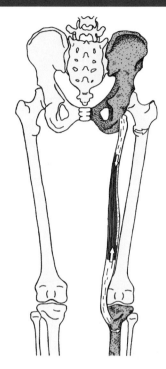

POSTERIOR VIEW
FIGURE 16-67

Notes: Use the mnemonic M&M to remember that the semi*m*embranosus is the most *m*edial hamstring muscle. On rare occasions, this muscle is absent or may fuse with the semitendinosus.

Semitendinosus

Latin:
semis—half
tendinosus—tendinous

Origin
ischial tuberosity

Insertion
medial proximal tibial shaft (at the pes anserinus)

Actions
flexes the knee
medially rotates the leg (when the knee is flexed)
extends the hip
medially rotates the hip
posteriorly tilts the pelvis

Nerve
tibial nerve

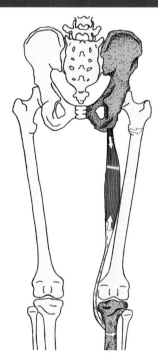

POSTERIOR VIEW
FIGURE 16-68

Notes: The semi*t*endinosus is superficial to, or on *t*op of, the semimembranosus. This muscle may contain obliquely arranged tendinous intersections within its belly.

Biceps Femoris

Latin:
bi—twice
caput—head
femoralis—pertaining to the femur

Origins
ischial tuberosity (long head)
linea aspera; lower lateral lip (short head)

Insertion
fibular head

Actions
flexes the knee
laterally rotates the leg (when knee is flexed)
extends the hip
laterally rotates the hip
posteriorly tilts the pelvis

Nerve
sciatic nerve for long head (tibial division) and sciatic nerve for
   short head (common peroneal division)

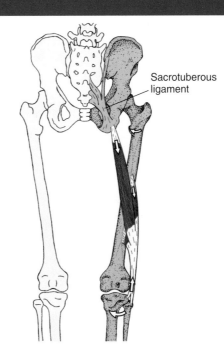

Sacrotuberous
ligament

POSTERIOR VIEW
FIGURE 16-69

Notes: The biceps femoris occupies the lateral side of the posterior thigh. The short head of the biceps femoris does not cross the hip joint and, on rare occasions, is absent.

Adductors

Latin:
adductus—brought forward

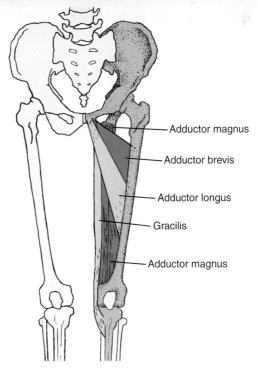

Adductor magnus

Adductor brevis

Adductor longus

Gracilis

Adductor magnus

ANTERIOR VIEW
FIGURE 16-70

Notes: The adductors are a group of muscles forming the inner thigh; all have their origins on the pubis and insertions on the linea aspera except for the gracilis. They are the gracilis, adductor magnus, adductor longus, adductor brevis, and pectineus (shown later).

Gracilis

Latin:
gracilis—slender

Origin
inferior pubic ramus

Insertion
medial proximal tibial shaft (at the pes anserinus)

Actions
adducts the hip
flexes the hip
flexes the knee
medially rotates the leg (when the knee is flexed)

Nerve
obturator nerve

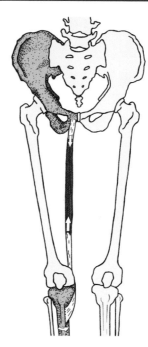

ANTERIOR VIEW
FIGURE 16-71

Notes: The femoral shaft and gracilis form the letter *V*. The gracilis is the most medial adductor and the only adductor that crosses both the hip and knee.

Adductor Magnus

Latin:
adductus—brought toward
magnum—large

Origins
ischial tuberosity
inferior pubic ramus
ischial ramus

Insertions
linea aspera
adductor tubercle of the femur

Actions
adducts the hip
flexes the hip
extends the hip

Nerves
sciatic and obturator nerves

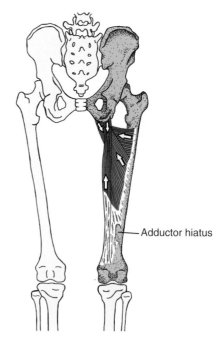

—Adductor hiatus

POSTERIOR VIEW
FIGURE 16-72

Notes: The adductor magnus lies deep to the hamstrings and is divided into two sections: one on the linea aspera and one on the adductor tubercle. Between these two sections is an opening called the *adductor hiatus* for passage of the femoral artery and vein.

Adductor Longus

Latin:
adductus—brought toward
longus—long

Origin
anterior pubic body

Insertion
middle third of the linea aspera (medial lip)

Action
adducts the hip

Nerve
obturator nerve

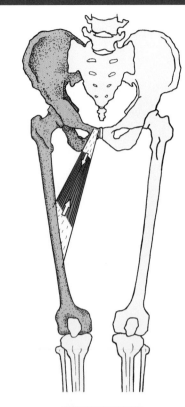

ANTERIOR VIEW
FIGURE 16-73

Adductor Brevis

Latin:
adductus—brought toward
brevis—brief

Origin
inferior pubic ramus

Insertion
proximal third of the linea aspera (medial lip)

Action
adducts the hip

Nerve
obturator nerve

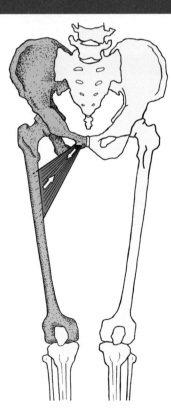

ANTERIOR VIEW
FIGURE 16-74

Pectineus

Latin:
pecten—comb

Origin
superior pubic ramus

Insertion
linea aspera; medial lip (inferior to the lesser trochanter)

Actions
flexes the hip
adducts the hip

Nerve
femoral nerve

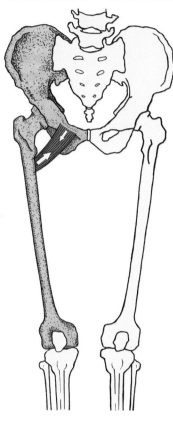

ANTERIOR VIEW
FIGURE 16-75

Notes: In relationship to the pectineus, the femoral artery may lie medial to the muscle; in some cases, it may cross the pectineus superficially. Additionally, this muscle is often regarded as an extension of the iliopsoas muscle because of its insertion and action.

Pes Anserinus

Latin:
pes—foot
French:
anser—a goose

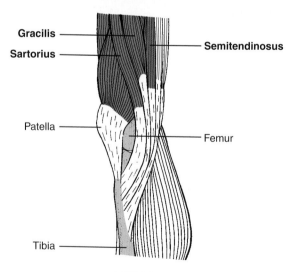

Gracilis

Sartorius

Semitendinosus

Patella

Femur

Tibia

LATERAL VIEW
FIGURE 16-76

Notes: The pes anserinus is the tendinous expansions of the sartorius, gracilis, and semitendinosus inserting at the medial proximal tibial shaft. Use the mnemonic phrase **_S_**ay **_g_**race before **_t_**ea, to assist you in remembering the three muscles that contribute to this structure.

Popliteus

Latin:
Poples—hollow behind the knee

Origin
lateral condyle of femur

Insertion
posterior proximal tibial shaft

Actions
flexes the knee
medially rotates the leg (when the knee is flexed)

Nerve
tibial nerve

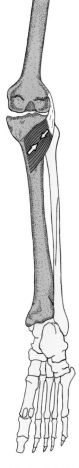

POSTERIOR VIEW
FIGURE 16-77

Notes: The popliteus is a weak knee flexor, but its function of unlocking the extended knee to bring flexion is vital to the other stronger knee flexors. For this reason, it gets the nickname *the key that unlocks the knee.*

Lesson FIVE

Muscles of Hip Movement

FLEXION	EXTENSION	MEDIAL ROTATION	LATERAL ROTATION	ABDUCTION	ADDUCTION
Psoas major	Gluteus maximus	Gluteus medius	Psoas major	Piriformis	Gluteus maximus
Iliacus	Semimembranosus	Gluteus minimus	Iliacus	Gluteus medius	Gracilis
Tensor fascia lata	Semitendinosus	Tensor fascia lata	Piriformis	Gluteus minimus	Adductor magnus
Rectus femoris	Biceps femoris	Semimembranosus	Gemellus superior	Tensor fascia lata	Adductor longus
Sartorius	Adductor magnus	Semitendinosus	Gemellus inferior	Sartorius	Adductor brevis
Gracilis			Obturator internus	Pectineus	
Adductor magnus			Obturator externus		
Pectineus			Quadratus femoris		
			Gluteus maximus		
			Sartorius		
			Biceps femoris		

Lesson FIVE

Muscles of Knee Movement

FLEXION	EXTENSION
Sartorius	Rectus femoris
Semimembranosus	Vastus medialis
Semitendinosus	Vastus lateralis
Biceps femoris	Vastus intermedius
Gracilis	
Gastrocnemius	
Plantaris	
Popliteus	

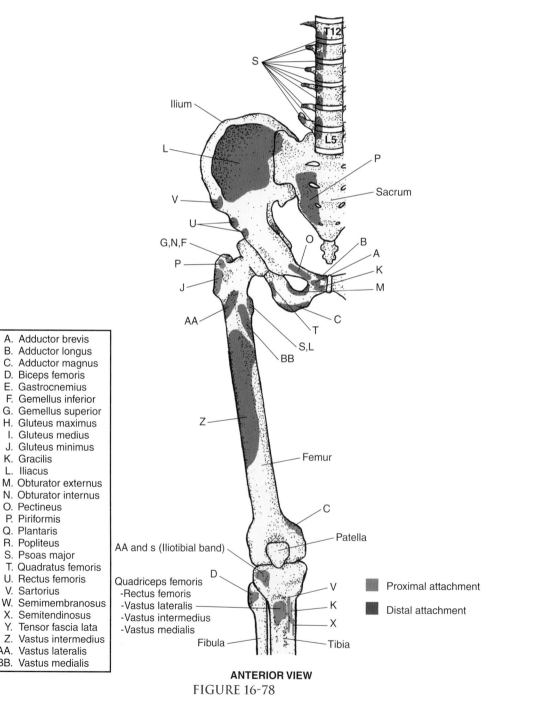

A. Adductor brevis
B. Adductor longus
C. Adductor magnus
D. Biceps femoris
E. Gastrocnemius
F. Gemellus inferior
G. Gemellus superior
H. Gluteus maximus
I. Gluteus medius
J. Gluteus minimus
K. Gracilis
L. Iliacus
M. Obturator externus
N. Obturator internus
O. Pectineus
P. Piriformis
Q. Plantaris
R. Popliteus
S. Psoas major
T. Quadratus femoris
U. Rectus femoris
V. Sartorius
W. Semimembranosus
X. Semitendinosus
Y. Tensor fascia lata
Z. Vastus intermedius
AA. Vastus lateralis
BB. Vastus medialis

Proximal attachment
Distal attachment

ANTERIOR VIEW

FIGURE 16-78

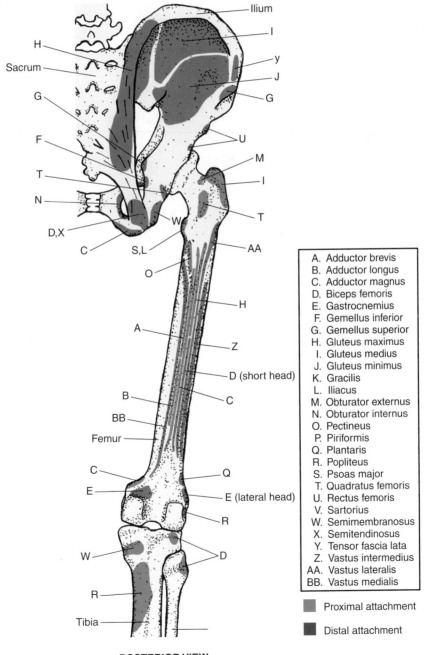

Ilium
H
Sacrum
G
F
T
N
D,X
C
S,L
O
A
B
BB
Femur
C
E
W
R
Tibia

I
y
J
G
U
M
I
T
AA
H
Z
D (short head)
C
Q
E (lateral head)
R
D

A. Adductor brevis
B. Adductor longus
C. Adductor magnus
D. Biceps femoris
E. Gastrocnemius
F. Gemellus inferior
G. Gemellus superior
H. Gluteus maximus
I. Gluteus medius
J. Gluteus minimus
K. Gracilis
L. Iliacus
M. Obturator externus
N. Obturator internus
O. Pectineus
P. Piriformis
Q. Plantaris
R. Popliteus
S. Psoas major
T. Quadratus femoris
U. Rectus femoris
V. Sartorius
W. Semimembranosus
X. Semitendinosus
Y. Tensor fascia lata
Z. Vastus intermedius
AA. Vastus lateralis
BB. Vastus medialis

▨ Proximal attachment

▨ Distal attachment

POSTERIOR VIEW
FIGURE 16-78, cont'd

Unit ONE—Muscles of the Appendicular Skeleton

Lesson SIX—**Muscles of Ankle and Foot Movement** (Tibialis Anterior, Extensor Digitorum Longus and Brevis, Extensor Hallucis Longus, Fibularis Longus, Fibularis Brevis, Gastrocnemius, Plantaris, Soleus, Tibialis Posterior, Flexor Digitorum Longus, Flexor Hallucis Longus)

Tibialis Anterior

Latin:
tibialis—shinbone
ante—before

Origins
proximal half of the lateral tibial shaft
interosseous membrane

Insertions
metatarsal I
cuneiform I (plantar surface)

Actions
dorsiflexes the ankle
inverts the foot

Nerve
deep peroneal nerve

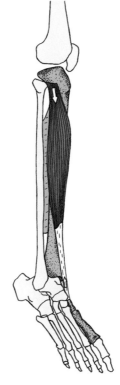

ANTEROLATERAL VIEW
FIGURE 16-79

Notes: The tibialis anterior muscle is strengthened after an inversion sprain is healed to aid in rehabilitation. It is referred to as the *stirrup muscle,* along with fibularis longus.

Extensor Digitorum Longus and Brevis

Latin:
extensio—to extend
digitus—finger or toe
longus—long
brevis—brief

Origins
inferior fibular head (longus)
proximal two thirds of the fibular shaft (longus)
lateral condyle of the tibia (longus)
interosseus membrane (longus)
calcaneus (brevis)

Insertions
middle phalanges of toes 2–5 (longus)
distal phalanges of toes 2–5 (longus)
tendons of extensor digitorum longus to toes 2–4 (brevis)

Actions
extends toes 2–5; dorsiflexes ankle and everts foot (longus)
extends toes 1–4 (brevis)

Nerve
deep peroneal nerve

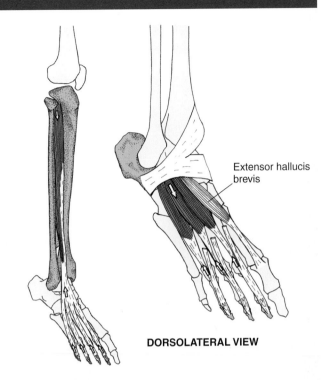

Extensor hallucis
brevis

DORSOLATERAL VIEW

ANTEROLATERAL VIEW
FIGURE 16-80

Notes: Individual tendons may be absent. The tendon for the fifth phalanx is only occasionally present.

Extensor Hallucis Longus

Latin:
extensio—to extend
hallux—large toe
longus—long

Origins
anterior fibular shaft (middle region)
interosseous membrane

Insertion
distal phalanx of the great toe

Actions
extends the great toe
dorsiflexes the ankle

Nerve
deep peroneal nerve

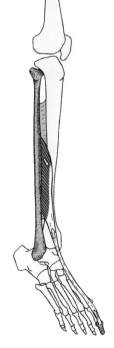

ANTEROLATERAL VIEW
FIGURE 16-81

Fibularis Longus

Greek:
fibula—pin
Latin:
longus—long

Origins
fibular head
lateral proximal half of the fibular shaft

Insertions
metatarsal I
cuneiform I (plantar surface)

Actions
everts the foot
plantar flexes the ankle

Nerve
superficial peroneal nerve

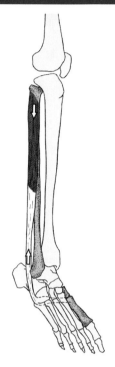

ANTEROLATERAL VIEW
FIGURE 16-82

Notes: The fibularis longus is also known as *peroneus longus* and is referred to as the *stirrup* muscle along with tibialis anterior. This muscle's tendon now lies behind the lateral malleolus but originally lay in front. The latter tendon arrangement is present in predators.

Fibularis Brevis

Greek:
fibula—pin
Latin:
brevis—brief

Origin
lateral distal half of the fibular shaft

Insertion
metatarsal V

Actions
everts the foot
plantar flexes the ankle

Nerve
superficial peroneal nerve

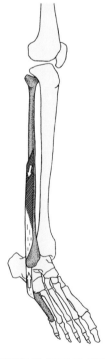

ANTEROLATERAL VIEW
FIGURE 16-83

Notes: The fibularis brevis is also known as *peroneus brevis*. This muscle's tendon now lies behind the lateral malleolus but originally lay in front. The latter tendon arrangement is present in predators.

Triceps Surae

Greek:
treis—three
Latin:
sura—pertaining to the calf of the leg

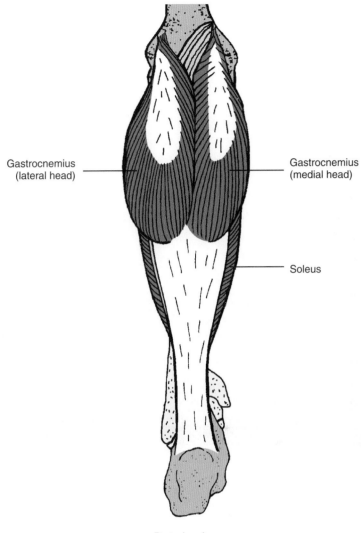

Gastrocnemius
(lateral head)

Gastrocnemius
(medial head)

Soleus

Posterior view

FIGURE 16-84

Notes: The triceps surae is another name for the gastrocnemius and soleus (some references include plantaris). These muscles share a common tendon and are viewed as the triceps brachii of the lower extremity. The triceps surae lift the weight of the body when moving forward, as in walking or running, and make up the superficial layer of the posterior leg.

Gastrocnemius

Greek:
gaster—belly
kneme—leg

Origins
medial epicondyle of the femur
lateral epicondyle of the femur

Insertion
calcaneus via the Achilles tendon

Actions
plantar flexes the ankle
flexes the knee

Nerve
tibial nerve

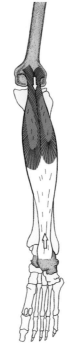

POSTERIOR VIEW
FIGURE 16-85

Notes: The gastrocnemius is also known as the *toe dancer's muscle* because it helps a ballerina stand on the toes. The two actions of this muscle, ankle plantar flexion and knee flexion, are an *either-or* situation—the gastrocnemius cannot perform both actions simultaneously. Occasionally, origins of this muscle are found on the joint capsule of the knee.

Plantaris

Latin:
planta—sole

Origin
lateral epicondyle of the femur

Insertion
calcaneus via the Achilles tendon

Actions
plantar flexes the ankle
flexes the knee

Nerve
tibial nerve

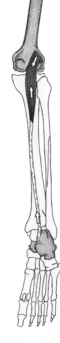

POSTERIOR VIEW
FIGURE 16-86

Notes: The plantaris is regarded as a mini-gastrocnemius because of a common insertion and is occasionally missing in cadavers (approximately 10%). The plantaris tendon may be removed for grafting during reconstructive surgery of tendons of the hand.

Soleus

Latin:
solea—sole of the foot

Origins
superior posterior third of the fibular shaft
soleal line of the tibia

Insertion
calcaneus via the Achilles tendon

Action
plantar flexes the ankle

Nerve
tibial nerve

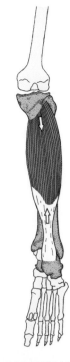

POSTERIOR VIEW
FIGURE 16-87

Notes: According to one source, the soleus was so named because it resembled a sole fish from the Mediterranean Sea.

Tibialis Posterior

Latin:
tibialis—shinbone
posterus—behind

Origins
posterior tibial shaft
posterior fibular shaft
interosseous membrane

Insertions
tuberosity of navicular (plantar surface)
cuneiform I, II, and III
cuboid
calcaneus
navicular
bases of metatarsals II, III, and IV

Actions
inverts the foot
plantar flexes the ankle

Nerve
tibial nerve

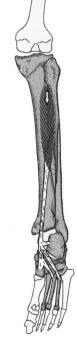

POSTERIOR VIEW
FIGURE 16-88

Notes: This muscle may be completely absent.

Flexor Digitorum Longus

Latin:
flexus—bent
digitus—finger or toe
longus—long

Origin
posterior tibial shaft—middle region

Insertions
distal phalanges 2–5 (plantar surface)

Actions
flexes digits 2–5 at the DIP, PIP, and MP joints
plantar flexes the ankle
inverts the foot

Nerve
tibial nerve

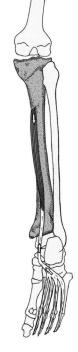

POSTERIOR VIEW
FIGURE 16-89

Flexor Hallucis Longus

Latin:
flexus—bent
hallux—large toe
longus—long

Origins
posterior fibular shaft—middle region
interosseus membrane

Insertion
distal phalanx of the great toe (plantar surface)

Actions
flexes the great toe
plantar flexes the ankle
inverts the foot
supports the longitudinal arch

Nerve
tibial nerve

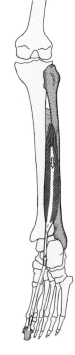

POSTERIOR VIEW
FIGURE 16-90

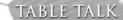

> **TABLE TALK**
>
> Three muscles and one nerve pass behind the medial ankle. Use the expression *Tom, Dick, and Harry* as a mnemonic phrase for learning these muscles *T*om for *t*ibialis posterior, *D*ick for flexor *d*igitorum longus, and *H*arry for flexor *h*allucis longus.

> **TABLE TALK**
>
> The plantar aspect of the foot contains four layers of muscles. Please note the following:
> First (superficial) layer:
>   Abductor hallucis
>   Flexor digitorum brevis
>   Abductor digiti minimi
> Second layer:
>   Quadratus plantae
>   Lumbricals
>   (Flexor hallucis longus tendon)
>   (Flexor digitorum longus tendon)
> Third layer:
>   Flexor hallucis brevis
>   Adductor hallucis
>   Flexor digiti minimi brevis
> Fourth layer:
>   Dorsal interossei
>   Plantar interossei
>   (Fibularis longus tendon)
>   (Tibialis posterior tendon)

Lesson SIX

Muscles of Ankle and Foot Movement

PLANTAR FLEXION	DORSIFLEXION	INVERSION	EVERSION
Fibularis longus	Tibialis anterior	Tibialis anterior	Fibularis longus
Fibularis brevis	Extensor hallucis longus	Tibialis posterior	Fibularis brevis
Gastrocnemius		Flexor digitorum longus	
Plantaris		Flexor hallucis longus	
Soleus			
Tibialis posterior			
Flexor digitorum longus			
Flexor hallucis longus			

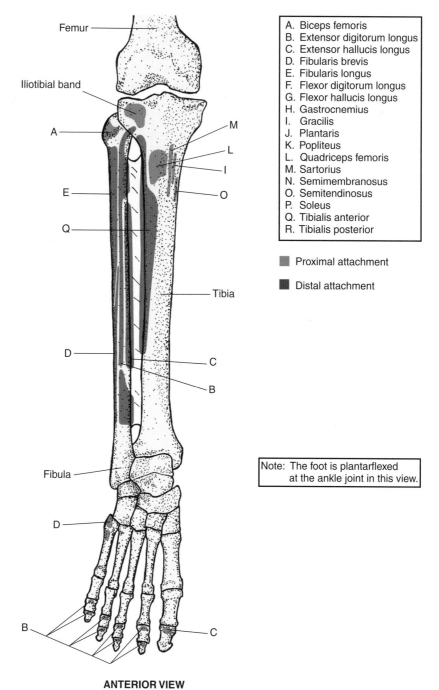

A. Biceps femoris
B. Extensor digitorum longus
C. Extensor hallucis longus
D. Fibularis brevis
E. Fibularis longus
F. Flexor digitorum longus
G. Flexor hallucis longus
H. Gastrocnemius
I. Gracilis
J. Plantaris
K. Popliteus
L. Quadriceps femoris
M. Sartorius
N. Semimembranosus
O. Semitendinosus
P. Soleus
Q. Tibialis anterior
R. Tibialis posterior

Proximal attachment

Distal attachment

Note: The foot is plantarflexed
at the ankle joint in this view.

ANTERIOR VIEW

FIGURE 16-91

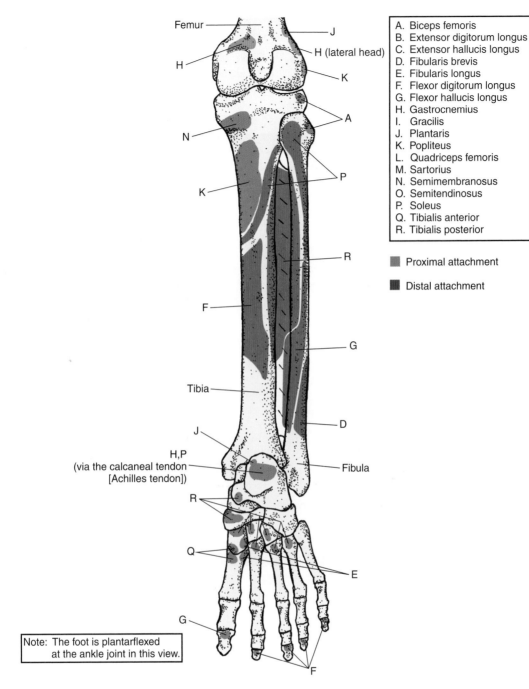

A. Biceps femoris
B. Extensor digitorum longus
C. Extensor hallucis longus
D. Fibularis brevis
E. Fibularis longus
F. Flexor digitorum longus
G. Flexor hallucis longus
H. Gastrocnemius
I. Gracilis
J. Plantaris
K. Popliteus
L. Quadriceps femoris
M. Sartorius
N. Semimembranosus
O. Semitendinosus
P. Soleus
Q. Tibialis anterior
R. Tibialis posterior

▨ Proximal attachment

▨ Distal attachment

Femur

J

H (lateral head)

H

K

A

N

P

K

R

F

G

Tibia

J

D

H,P
(via the calcaneal tendon
[Achilles tendon])

Fibula

R

Q

E

G

F

Note: The foot is plantarflexed
at the ankle joint in this view.

POSTERIOR VIEW
FIGURE 16-91, **cont'd**

Unit TWO—Muscles of the Axial Skeleton

Lesson SEVEN—**Muscles of the Head and Neck** (Frontalis, Occipitalis, Orbicularis Oculi, Orbicularis Oris, Zygomaticus Major and Minor, Buccinator, Platysma, Temporalis, Masseter, Lateral Pterygoid, Medial Pterygoid, Longus Capitis, Longus Colli, Sternocleidomastoid, Scalenus Anterior, Scalenus Medius, Scalenus Posterior, Splenius Capitis, Splenius Cervicis, Rectus Capitis Posterior Major, Rectus Capitis Posterior Minor, Oblique Capitis Superior, Oblique Capitis Inferior, Levator Scapula [Lesson One], Trapezius [Lesson One], Spinalis [Lesson Eight], Longissimus [Lesson Eight])

Occipitofrontalis

Latin:
occipitalis—pertaining to the back of the head
frons—brow or referring to the frontal bone

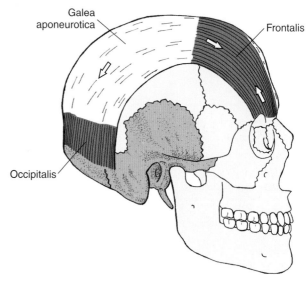

LATERAL VIEW

FIGURE 16-92

Notes: The occipitofrontalis, or epicranius, is a two-bellied muscle containing the occipitalis and the frontalis and is connected by an extensive network of cranial fascia called the *galea aponeurotica*. The galea aponeurotica is firmly connected to the hypodermis and slides over the periosteum of the cranium.

Frontalis

Latin:
frons—brow or referring to the frontal bone

Origin
galea aponeurotica

Insertion
superficial fascia beneath the eyebrows

Actions
elevates the eyebrows
horizontally wrinkles skin on your forehead

Nerve
facial nerve (cranial nerve VII)

Notes: The frontalis muscle contributes to tension headaches. Contraction of many muscles of the head and neck simply displace skin, which is the basis of facial expression. The frontalis muscle produces the expression of worry or concern. See Figure 16-92 (above) for an illustration of this muscle.

Occipitalis

Latin:
occipitalis—pertaining to the back of the head

Origin
lateral two thirds of the superior nuchal line (occipital and
    temporal bones)

Insertion
galea aponeurotica

Action
moves scalp over the cranium

Nerve
facial nerve (cranial nerve VII)

Note: See Figure 16-92 (previous page) for an illustration of this muscle.

Orbicularis Oculi

Latin:
orbiculus—little circle
oculus—eye

Origin
orbital margin

Insertion
superficial fascia beneath the upper eyelids

Actions
closes the eyelids
folds the skin around the orbit (to protect eyeball and assist in
    tear transport)
squints the eyelids

Nerve
facial nerve (cranial nerve VII)

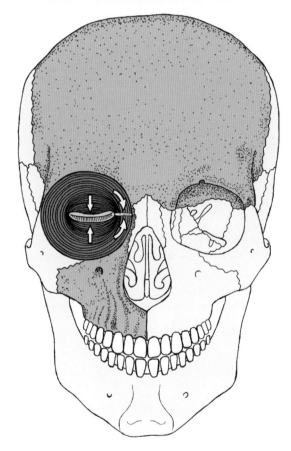

ANTERIOR VIEW

FIGURE 16-93

Notes: Also known as the *winking* or *blinking muscle*, as it closes the eyelid.

Orbicularis Oris

Latin:
orbiculus—little circle
oris—mouth

Origins
maxilla
mandible
buccinator

Insertions
mucous membranes of the lips
muscles inserting into the lips

Actions
closes the lips
protrudes and protracts the lips
assists in dozens of activities such as eating, drinking, talking,
    and sucking

Nerve
facial nerve (cranial nerve VII)

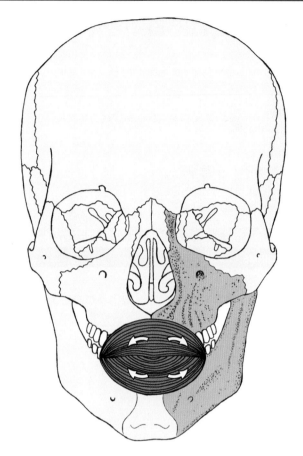

ANTERIOR VIEW

FIGURE 16-94

Notes: Also known as the *kissing muscle,* it protrudes the lips for a kiss.

Zygomaticus Major and Minor

Latin:
zygotos—yoked or to connect
major—larger
minor—smaller

Origins
zygomatic arch (major)
zygomatic arch; just medial to the attachment of zygomaticus
    major (minor)

Insertions
lateral angle of the mouth (major)
lateral angle of the mouth (minor)

Action
elevates corners of the mouth upward and outward

Nerve
facial nerve (cranial nerve VII)

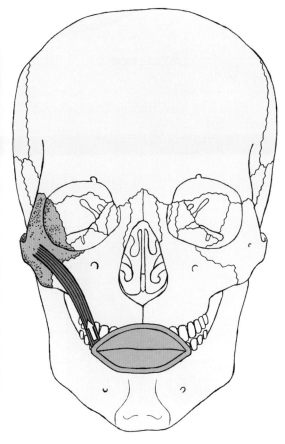

ANTERIOR VIEW
of Zygomaticus Major

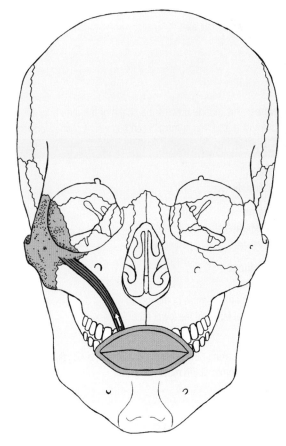

ANTERIOR VIEW
of Zygomaticus Minor

FIGURE 16-95

Notes: Contraction of these muscles produces the facial expression of a smile and are called the *smiling* or *laughing muscles*. The zygomaticus minor inserts just medial to the zygomaticus major.

Buccinator

Latin:
buccinator—trumpeter

Origins
maxilla
mandible

Insertion
orbicularis oris

Action
compresses the cheeks

Nerve
facial nerve (cranial nerve VII)

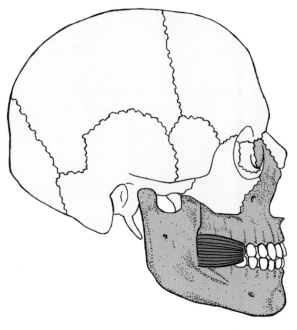

LATERAL VIEW

FIGURE 16-96

Notes: This muscle creates the shape of the mouth for the action of blowing. It also aids in mastication because it pushes food toward the teeth. Because of this action, buccinator is often referred to as an *accessory muscle of mastication*.

Platysma

Greek:
platysma—plate

Origins
superficial fascia of the deltoid
superficial fascia of pectoralis major

Insertions
mandible
muscles around angle of the mouth
superficial fascia of the lower face

Actions
tenses the skin of the anterior neck (creating ridges)
pulls the corner of the mouth down
depresses the mandible

Nerve
facial nerve (cranial nerve VII)

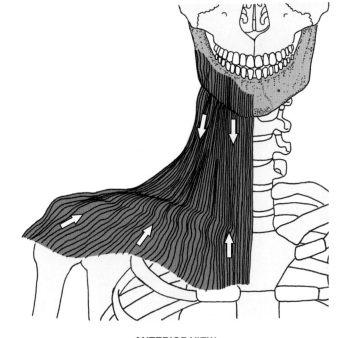

ANTERIOR VIEW

FIGURE 16-97

Notes: This muscle is the most superficial muscle of the anterior neck. The platysma produces the facial expression of pouting and is often called the *pouting muscle*. Additionally, this muscle is often referred to as the *lizard muscle* because when you contract the platysma fully, you give the appearance of a lizard (this is enhanced if you dart your tongue in and out of your mouth quickly).

Muscles of Mastication (Temporalis, Masseter, Medial and Lateral Pterygoids)

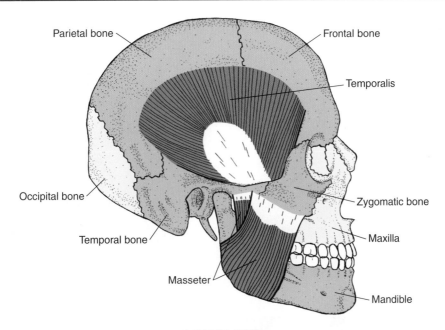

LATERAL VIEW

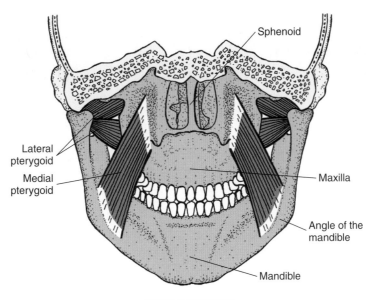

POSTERIOR VIEW

FIGURE 16-98

Temporalis

Latin:
temporalis—pertaining to the temporal bone

Origin
temporal fossa (frontal, parietal, and temporal bones)

Insertion
coronoid process of the mandible

Actions
elevates the mandible
retracts the mandible

Nerve
trigeminal nerve (cranial nerve V)

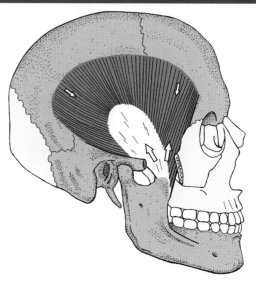

LATERAL VIEW
FIGURE 16-99

Masseter

Greek:
masseter—chewer

Origin
zygomatic arch (zygomatic and temporal bones)

Insertions
mandibular angle (superficial layer)
mandibular ramus (deep layer)

Actions
elevates the mandible
protracts the mandible

Nerve
trigeminal nerve (cranial nerve V)

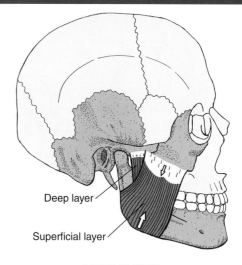

Deep layer
Superficial layer

LATERAL VIEW

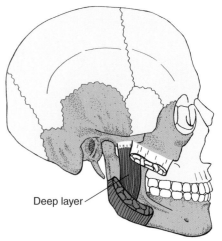

Deep layer

LATERAL VIEW
FIGURE 16-100

Notes: The zygomatic arch (see origin) is formed by two processes extending from the zygomatic and temporal bones.

Lateral Pterygoid

Latin:
lateralis—toward the side
Greek:
pterygodes—a wing

Origins
pterygoid plate of the sphenoid bone (lateral surface)
greater wing of the sphenoid bone

Insertions
condylar process of the mandible
temporomandibular joint capsule

Actions
produces lateral mandibular movements (unilateral contraction)
depresses the mandible (bilateral contraction)
protracts the mandible (bilateral contraction)

Nerve
trigeminal nerve (cranial nerve V)

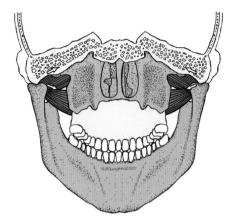

POSTERIOR VIEW
FIGURE 16-101

Medial Pterygoid

Latin:
medialis—toward the midline
Greek:
pterygodes—a wing

Origin
pterygoid plate of the sphenoid bone (lateral surface)

Insertions
mandibular angle (interior surface)
mandibular ramus (interior surface)

Actions
produces lateral mandibular movements (unilateral contraction)
elevates the mandible (bilateral contraction)
protracts the mandible (bilateral contraction)

Nerve
trigeminal nerve (cranial nerve V)

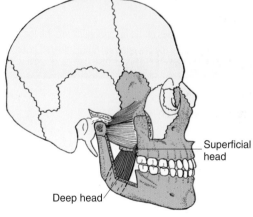

Superficial head
Deep head

LATERAL VIEW

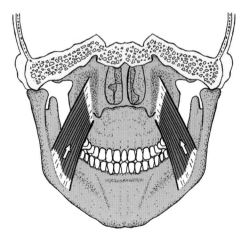

POSTERIOR VIEW
FIGURE 16-102

Notes: The medial pterygoid is the mirror image of the masseter.

Longus Capitis and Longus Colli

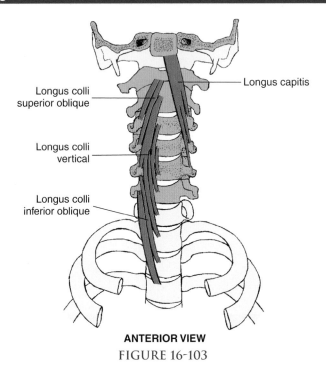

Longus colli
superior oblique

Longus capitis

Longus colli
vertical

Longus colli
inferior oblique

ANTERIOR VIEW
FIGURE 16-103

Notes: Two important muscles of the anterior neck are the longus capitis and longus colli. Part of the prevertebral group, they help maintain an anterior curve of the cervical spine.

Longus Capitis

Latin:
longus—long
caput—head

Origins
transverse processes of C3-C5

Insertion
occipital bone (anterior surface)

Actions
Laterally flexes the neck
flexes the neck

Nerve
anterior rami

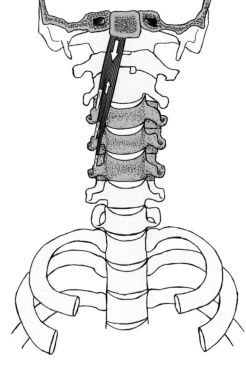

ANTERIOR VIEW
FIGURE 16-104

Longus Colli

Latin:
longus—long
colli—collar

Origins
anterior transverse processes of C3-C5 (superior oblique part)
bodies of T1-T3 (inferior oblique part)
vertebral bodies of C5-T3 (vertical part)

Insertions
anterior tubercle of C1 (superior oblique part)
anterior transverse processes C5-C6 (inferior oblique part)
vertebral bodies C2-C4 (vertical part)

Actions
rotates the head
flexes the neck
laterally flexes the neck

Nerve
anterior rami

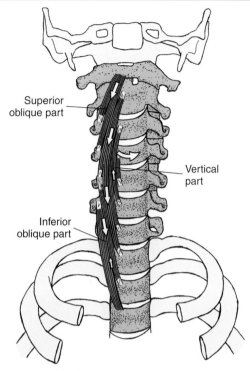

Superior oblique part

Vertical part

Inferior oblique part

FIGURE 16-105

Notes: The longus colli, similar to the iliopsoas of the lower extremity, contains three different muscles: longus colli superior oblique, longus colli inferior oblique, and longus colli vertical.

Sternocleidomastoid

Greek:
sternon—sternum
cleido—clavicle
mastos—breastlike

Origins
manubrium of the sternum
medial third of the clavicle

Insertions
mastoid process
lateral half of the superior nuchal line

Actions
laterally flexes neck (unilateral contraction)
rotates head to opposite side (unilateral contraction)
flexes the neck (bilateral contraction)
assists in forced inspiration (bilateral contraction)

Nerve
spinal accessory nerve (cranial nerve XI)

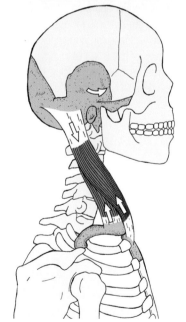

FIGURE 16-106

Notes: The sternocleidomastoid (SCM) feels similar to a cable on both sides of the neck. A condition called *torticollis,* or *wryneck,* involves spasms of the SCM. Spasm in this muscle may also cause vertigo because of the many sensory and positional receptors located here. The SCM is the only muscle that moves the head but does not attach to any vertebrae. The carotid artery lies deep and medial to the SCM and the external jugular vein superficially. SCM is the mirror image of splenius capitis.

Contraction of both muscles on either side of the neck brings the head down in a bow, as in the position assumed while praying. Because of this action, the SCM is also called the *praying muscle.*

Scalenes

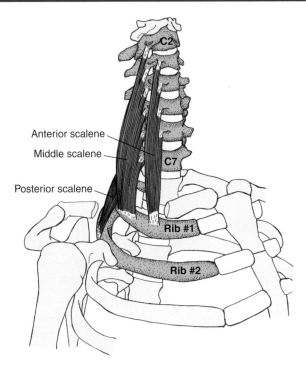

ANTEROLATERAL VIEW

FIGURE 16-107

Notes: The scalenes are a group of muscles consisting of the scalenus anterior, scalenus medius, and scalenus posterior. These muscles, along with the pectoralis minor, are known as the *neurovascular entrappers* because the subclavian artery and brachial plexus pass between the scalenus anterior and the scalenus medius. All scalene muscles are palpable in the posterior triangular of the neck between the SCM and the trapezius. Place your hands in this triangle, and inhale deeply. At the end of the inhalation, gasp very quickly. This action forces the muscles into a very noticeable contraction. Because of the relationship to breathing, the scalenes represent the cranial continuation of the intercostals. Acting unilaterally, they mobilize the neck; acting bilaterally, they actively aid in inhalation.* Additionally, when the body is in motion, the scalenes stabilize the neck by preventing side swaying.

In approximately 30% of all cadavers, another scalene muscle, the scalenus minimus, is found.

*Platzer, 1977

Scalenus Anterior

Greek:
skalenos—uneven
Latin:
ante—before

Origins
transverse processes of C3-C6

Insertion
rib 1 (superior surface)

Actions
laterally flexes the neck (unilateral contraction)
rotates the head (unilateral contraction)
elevates the first rib during inspiration (bilateral contraction)

Nerves
posterior rami of C3-C8

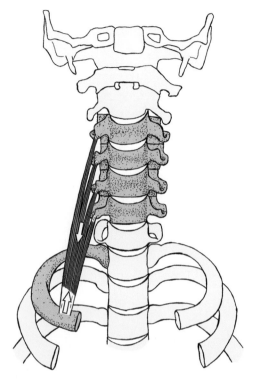

ANTERIOR VIEW
FIGURE 16-108

Scalenus Medius

Greek:
skalenos—uneven
Latin:
medialis—toward the midline

Origins
transverse processes of C2-C7

Insertion
rib 1 (superior surface)

Actions
laterally flexes the neck (unilateral contraction)
rotates the head (unilateral contraction)
elevates first rib during inspiration (bilateral contraction)

Nerves
posterior rami of C3-C8

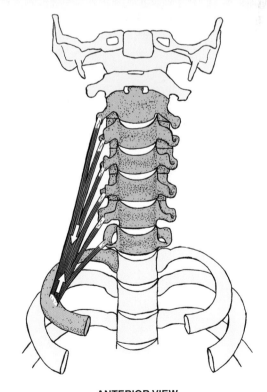

ANTERIOR VIEW
FIGURE 16-109

Scalenus Posterior

Greek:
skalenos—uneven
Latin:
posterus—behind

Origins
transverse processes of C5-C7

Insertion
rib 2 (superior lateral surface)

Actions
laterally flexes the neck (unilateral contraction)
elevates the second rib during inspiration (bilateral contraction)

Nerves
posterior rami of C3-C8

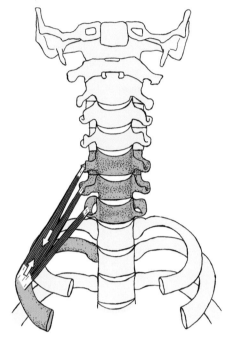

ANTERIOR VIEW
FIGURE 16-110

Splenius Capitis

Greek:
splenion—splint or bandage
caput—head

Origins
inferior nuchal ligament
spinous processes of C7-T4

Insertions
mastoid process
superior nuchal line—lateral region

Actions
rotates the head (unilateral contraction)
laterally flexes the neck (unilateral contraction)
extends the head (bilateral contraction)

Nerves
posterior rami of the middle lower cervical nerves

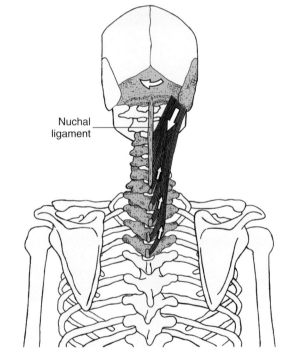

Nuchal
ligament

POSTERIOR VIEW
FIGURE 16-111

Notes: The splenius capitis is the mirror image of the sternocleidomastoid.

Splenius Cervicis

Greek:
splenion—splint or bandage
cervicalis—neck

Origins
spinous processes of T3-T6

Insertions
transverse processes of C1-C3

Actions
rotates the head (unilateral contraction)
laterally flexes the neck (unilateral contraction)
extends the head (bilateral contraction)

Nerves
posterior rami of middle lower cervical nerves

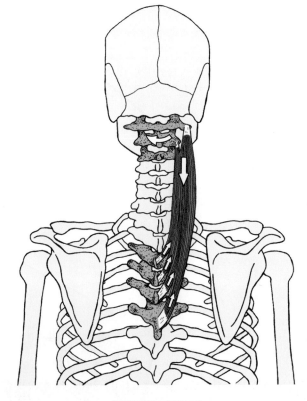

POSTERIOR VIEW

FIGURE 16-112

Suboccipitals

Latin:
sub—below
occipitalis—pertaining to the back of the head

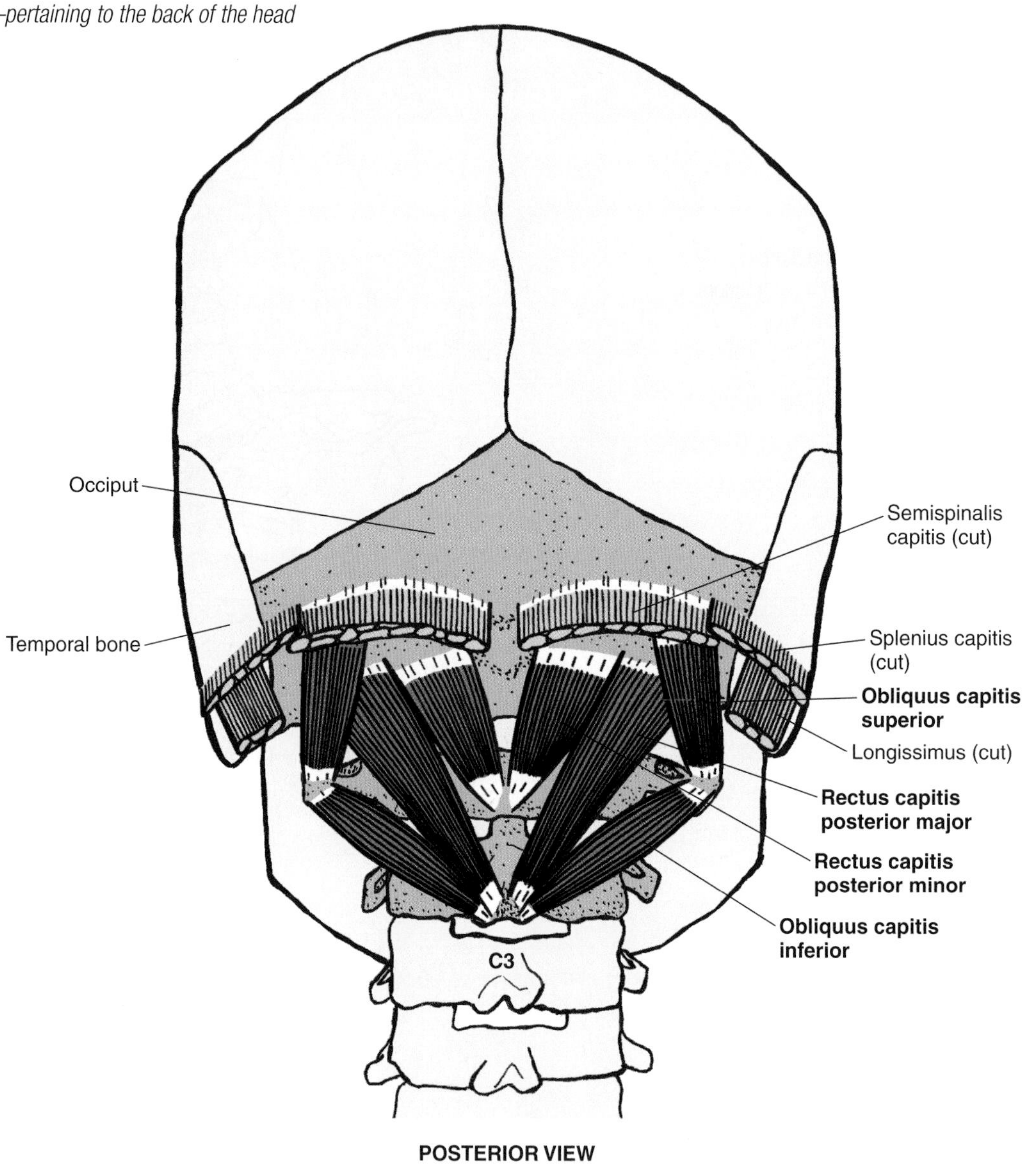

Occiput

Temporal bone

Semispinalis
capitis (cut)

Splenius capitis
(cut)

**Obliquus capitis
superior**

Longissimus (cut)

**Rectus capitis
posterior major**

**Rectus capitis
posterior minor**

**Obliquus capitis
inferior**

C3

POSTERIOR VIEW
FIGURE 16-113

Notes: The suboccipital muscles include the rectus capitis posterior major, rectus capitis posterior minor, obliquus capitis inferior, and obliquus capitis superior. Dr. Janet Travell (see her biography in Chapter 18) refers to the suboccipitals as the *ghost headache muscles* because the pain referred from these muscles seems to penetrate the skull and is difficult to locate. All suboccipitals attach on C1 and C2 and are responsible for initiating most of the head movements.

Rectus Capitis Posterior Major

Latin:
rectus—straight
caput—head
posterus—behind
major—larger

Origin
spinous process of C2

Insertion
inferior nuchal line

Actions
extends the head
rotates the head

Nerve
suboccipital nerve

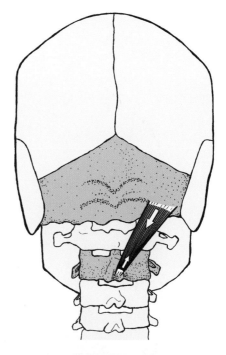

POSTERIOR VIEW
FIGURE 16-114

Rectus Capitis Posterior Minor

Latin:
rectus—straight
caput—head
posterus—behind
minor—smaller

Origin
posterior tubercle of C1

Insertion
inferior nuchal line

Action
extends the head

Nerve
suboccipital nerve

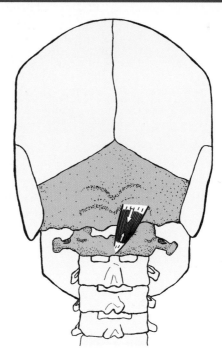

POSTERIOR VIEW
FIGURE 16-115

Notes: This muscle also attaches to the dura mater. Tension in this muscle may cause headaches of a vascular and neurological nature.

Oblique Capitis Superior

Latin:
obliquus—slant
caput—head
superus—upper

Origin
transverse process of C1

Insertion
inferior nuchal line

Actions
extends the head
laterally flexes the head

Nerve
suboccipital nerve

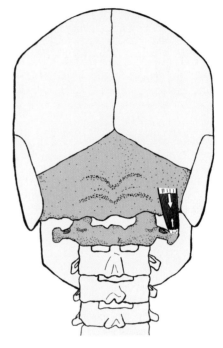

POSTERIOR VIEW
FIGURE 16-116

Oblique Capitis Inferior

Latin:
obliquus—slant
caput—head
infra—beneath

Origin
spinous process of C2

Insertion
transverse process of C1

Action
rotates the head

Nerve
suboccipital nerve

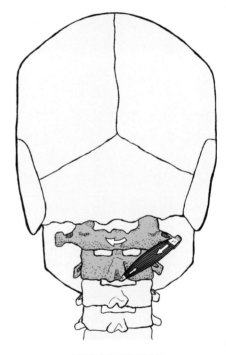

POSTERIOR VIEW
FIGURE 16-117

Notes: Although the muscle includes the word *capitis*, it does not attach to the cranium.

Lesson SEVEN

Muscles of Mandibular Movement

ELEVATION	DEPRESSION	PROTRACTION	RETRACTION	LATERAL MOVEMENTS
Temporalis	Platysma	Masseter	Temporalis	Lateral pterygoid
Masseter	Lateral pterygoid	Lateral pterygoid		Medial pterygoid
Medial pterygoid		Medial pterygoid		

Lesson SEVEN

Muscles of Head and Neck Movement

FLEXION	EXTENSION	LATERAL FLEXION	ROTATION
Longus capitis	Trapezius	Trapezius	Trapezius
Longus colli	Splenius capitis	Levator scapula	Longus capitis
Sternocleidomastoid	Splenius cervicis	Longus colli	Longus colli
	Rectus capitis posterior major	Sternocleidomastoid	Sternocleidomastoid
	Rectus capitis posterior minor	Scalenus anterior	Scalenus anterior
	Oblique capitis superior	Scalenus medius	Scalenus medius
	Spinalis	Scalenus posterior	Scalenus posterior
	Longissimus	Splenius capitis	Splenius capitis
		Splenius cervicis	Splenius cervicis
		Oblique capitis superior	Rectus capitis posterior major
			Oblique capitis inferior

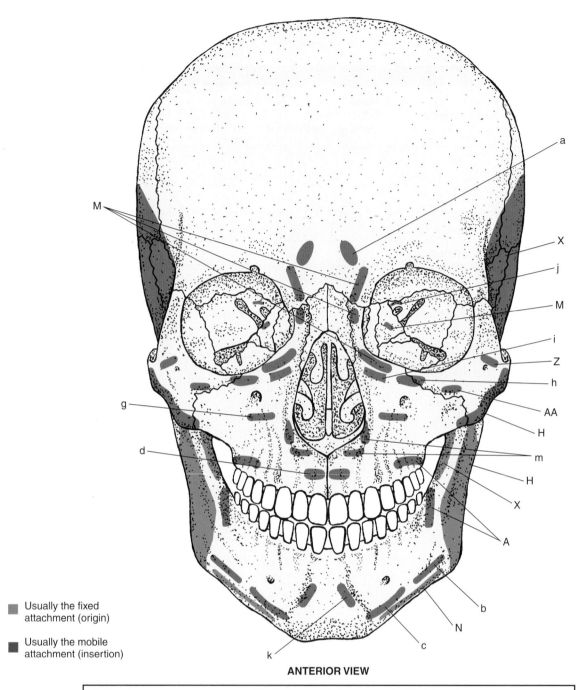

Usually the fixed attachment (origin)

Usually the mobile attachment (insertion)

ANTERIOR VIEW

A. Buccinator	Q. Scalenus anterior	f. Geniohyoid
B. Frontalis	R. Scalenus medius	g. Levator anguli oris
C. Lateral pterygoid	S. Scalenus posterior	h. Levator labii superioris
D. Levator scapula	T. Semispinalis	i. Levator labii superioris alaeque nasi
E. Longissimus	U. Splenius capitis	j. Levator palpebrae superioris
F. Longus capitis	V. Splenius cervicis	k. Mentalis
G. Longus colli	W. Sternocleidomastoid	l. Myohyoid
H. Masseter	X. Temporalis	m. Nasalis
I. Medial pterygoid	Y. Trapezius	n. Omohyoid
J. Oblique capitis inferior	Z. Zygomaticus major	o. Posterior auricular
K. Oblique capitis superior	AA. Zygomaticus minor	p. Rectus capitis anterior
L. Occipitalis	a. Corrugator supercilli	q. Rectus capitis lateralis
M. Orbicularis oculi	b. Depressor anguli oris	r. Sternohyoid
N. Platysma	c. Depressor labii inferioris	s. Sternothyroid
O. Rectus capitis posterior major	d. Depressor septi nasi	t. Stylohyoid
P. Rectus capitis posterior minor	e. Digastric	u. Thyrohyoid

FIGURE 16-118

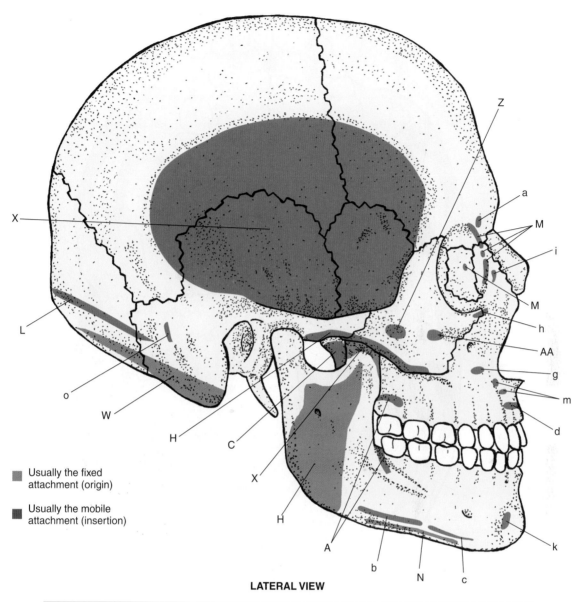

LATERAL VIEW

■ Usually the fixed attachment (origin)

■ Usually the mobile attachment (insertion)

A. Buccinator	Q. Scalenus anterior	f. Geniohyoid
B. Frontalis	R. Scalenus medius	g. Levator anguli oris
C. Lateral pterygoid	S. Scalenus posterior	h. Levator labii superioris
D. Levator scapula	T. Semispinalis	i. Levator labii superioris alaeque nasi
E. Longissimus	U. Splenius capitis	j. Levator palpebrae superioris
F. Longus capitis	V. Splenius cervicis	k. Mentalis
G. Longus colli	W. Sternocleidomastoid	l. Myohyoid
H. Masseter	X. Temporalis	m. Nasalis
I. Medial pterygoid	Y. Trapezius	n. Omohyoid
J. Oblique capitis inferior	Z. Zygomaticus major	o. Posterior auricular
K. Oblique capitis superior	AA. Zygomaticus minor	p. Rectus capitis anterior
L. Occipitalis	a. Corrugator supercilli	q. Rectus capitis lateralis
M. Orbicularis oculi	b. Depressor anguli oris	r. Sternohyoid
N. Platysma	c. Depressor labii inferioris	s. Sternothyroid
O. Rectus capitis posterior major	d. Depressor septi nasi	t. Stylohyoid
P. Rectus capitis posterior minor	e. Digastric	u. Thyrohyoid

FIGURE 16-118, cont'd

Continued

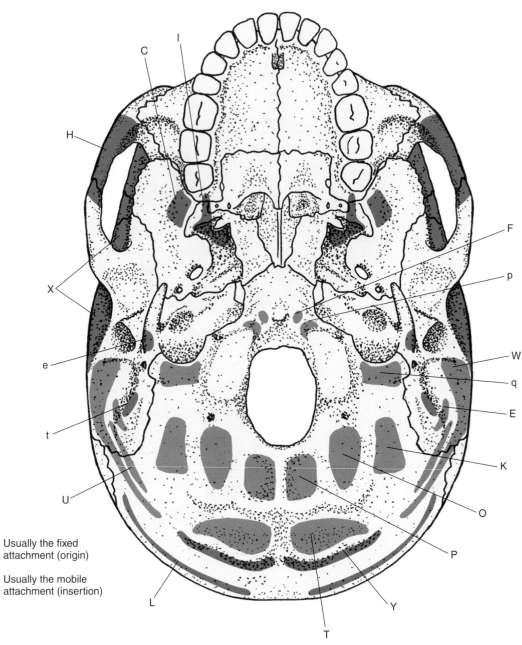

INFERIOR VIEW

Usually the fixed attachment (origin)

Usually the mobile attachment (insertion)

A. Buccinator	Q. Scalenus anterior	f. Geniohyoid
B. Frontalis	R. Scalenus medius	g. Levator anguli oris
C. Lateral pterygoid	S. Scalenus posterior	h. Levator labii superioris
D. Levator scapula	T. Semispinalis	i. Levator labii superioris alaeque nasi
E. Longissimus	U. Splenius capitis	j. Levator palpebrae superioris
F. Longus capitis	V. Splenius cervicis	k. Mentalis
G. Longus colli	W. Sternocleidomastoid	l. Myohyoid
H. Masseter	X. Temporalis	m. Nasalis
I. Medial pterygoid	Y. Trapezius	n. Omohyoid
J. Oblique capitis inferior	Z. Zygomaticus major	o. Posterior auricular
K. Oblique capitis superior	AA. Zygomaticus minor	p. Rectus capitis anterior
L. Occipitalis	a. Corrugator supercilli	q. Rectus capitis lateralis
M. Orbicularis oculi	b. Depressor anguli oris	r. Sternohyoid
N. Platysma	c. Depressor labii inferioris	s. Sternothyroid
O. Rectus capitis posterior major	d. Depressor septi nasi	t. Stylohyoid
P. Rectus capitis posterior minor	e. Digastric	u. Thyrohyoid

FIGURE 16-118, **cont'd**

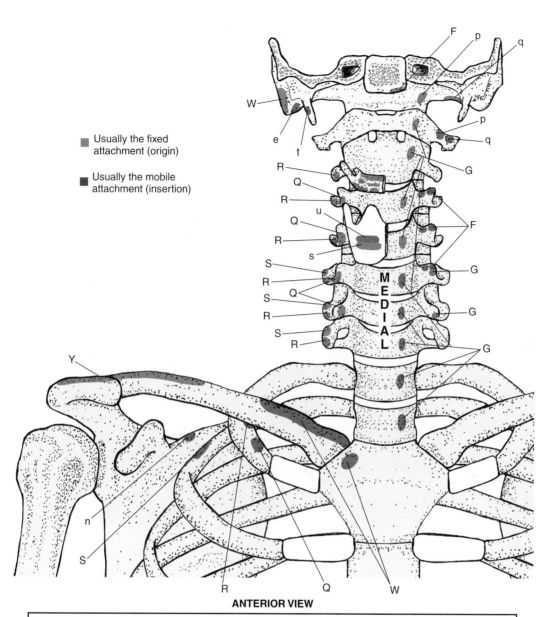

■ Usually the fixed attachment (origin)

■ Usually the mobile attachment (insertion)

ANTERIOR VIEW

A. Buccinator	Q. Scalenus anterior	f. Geniohyoid
B. Frontalis	R. Scalenus medius	g. Levator anguli oris
C. Lateral pterygoid	S. Scalenus posterior	h. Levator labii superioris
D. Levator scapula	T. Semispinalis	i. Levator labii superioris alaeque nasi
E. Longissimus	U. Splenius capitis	j. Levator palpebrae superioris
F. Longus capitis	V. Splenius cervicis	k. Mentalis
G. Longus colli	W. Sternocleidomastoid	l. Myohyoid
H. Masseter	X. Temporalis	m. Nasalis
I. Medial pterygoid	Y. Trapezius	n. Omohyoid
J. Oblique capitis inferior	Z. Zygomaticus major	o. Posterior auricular
K. Oblique capitis superior	AA. Zygomaticus minor	p. Rectus capitis anterior
L. Occipitalis	a. Corrugator supercilli	q. Rectus capitis lateralis
M. Orbicularis oculi	b. Depressor anguli oris	r. Sternohyoid
N. Platysma	c. Depressor labii inferioris	s. Sternothyroid
O. Rectus capitis posterior major	d. Depressor septi nasi	t. Stylohyoid
P. Rectus capitis posterior minor	e. Digastric	u. Thyrohyoid

FIGURE 16-118, **cont'd**   *Continued*

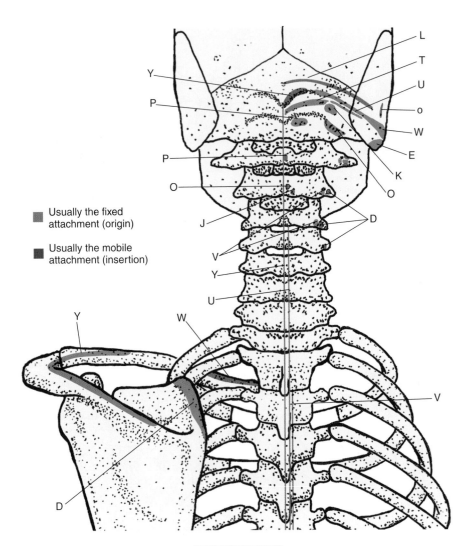

Usually the fixed attachment (origin)

Usually the mobile attachment (insertion)

POSTERIOR VIEW

A. Buccinator	Q. Scalenus anterior	f. Geniohyoid
B. Frontalis	R. Scalenus medius	g. Levator anguli oris
C. Lateral pterygoid	S. Scalenus posterior	h. Levator labii superioris
D. Levator scapula	T. Semispinalis	i. Levator labii superioris alaeque nasi
E. Longissimus	U. Splenius capitis	j. Levator palpebrae superioris
F. Longus capitis	V. Splenius cervicis	k. Mentalis
G. Longus colli	W. Sternocleidomastoid	l. Myohyoid
H. Masseter	X. Temporalis	m. Nasalis
I. Medial pterygoid	Y. Trapezius	n. Omohyoid
J. Oblique capitis inferior	Z. Zygomaticus major	o. Posterior auricular
K. Oblique capitis superior	AA. Zygomaticus minor	p. Rectus capitis anterior
L. Occipitalis	a. Corrugator supercilli	q. Rectus capitis lateralis
M. Orbicularis oculi	b. Depressor anguli oris	r. Sternohyoid
N. Platysma	c. Depressor labii inferioris	s. Sternothyroid
O. Rectus capitis posterior major	d. Depressor septi nasi	t. Stylohyoid
P. Rectus capitis posterior minor	e. Digastric	u. Thyrohyoid

FIGURE 16-118, cont'd

Unit TWO—Muscles of the Axial Skeleton

Lesson EIGHT—**Muscles of the Trunk and Vertebral Column** (Rectus Abdominis, External Obliques, Internal Obliques, Transverse Abdominis, Quadratus Lumborum, Semispinalis, Rotatores, Multifidus, Spinalis, Longissimus, Iliocostalis)

Abdominals

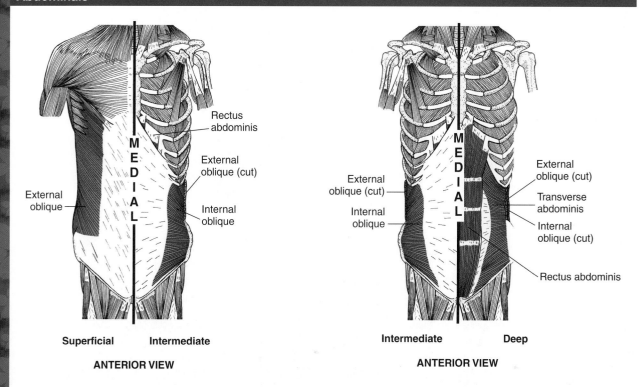

Superficial   Intermediate
ANTERIOR VIEW

Intermediate   Deep
ANTERIOR VIEW

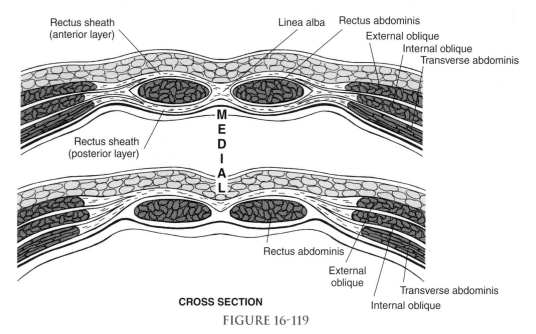

CROSS SECTION

FIGURE 16-119

Notes: The abdominal muscles are the rectus abdominis, external and internal obliques, and transverse abdominis. The fiber arrangement of the abdominal muscles runs in four different directions. Think of this organization as the *plywood* principle of anatomy, used for added strength to hold in internal abdominal organs. You can feel how these muscles compress the abdominal contents by placing your hands on your belly while you laugh, cough, defecate, or vomit. The abdominals are also involved in forced expiration. The rectus sheath is formed by the aponeurosis of the three lateral abdominal muscles.

Rectus Abdominis

Latin:
rectus—straight
abdomen—belly

Origins
pubic symphysis
pubic tubercle

Insertions
ribs 5 through 7 (costal cartilage—anterior surface)
xiphoid process

Actions
flexes the vertebral column
laterally flexes the vertebral column
compresses abdominal contents
posteriorly tilts the pelvis

Nerves
anterior rami of intercostal nerves (T7-T12)

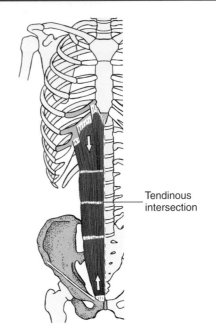

Tendinous intersection

ANTERIOR VIEW
FIGURE 16-120

Notes: The rectus abdominis goes a long distance without any skeletal attachment; thus the physiological properties have provided a way of keeping its length constant by including a horizontal layer of connective tissue every few inches. This band of connective tissue is called a *tendinous intersection*. Separation of this muscle, which may occur during advanced pregnancy, is called *rectus diastasis*.

External Obliques

Latin:
externus—outside
obliquus—slant

Origins
iliac crest
abdominal fascia
linea alba

Insertions
ribs 5 through 12 (anterior lateral surface)

Actions
laterally flexes the vertebral column
rotates the vertebral column
flexes the vertebral column
compresses abdomen contents
posteriorly tilts the pelvis

Nerves
anterior rami of intercostal nerves (T7-T12)

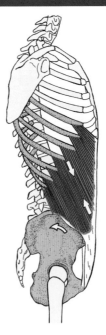

LATERAL VIEW
FIGURE 16-121

Notes: The fiber direction of this muscle is similar to the direction of your fingers when your hands are in the pockets of a jacket. The pockets of most jackets do not reach the midline. Similarly, the external obliques do not reach the midline. They join the rectus sheath instead.

Tendinous intersections such as those in the rectus abdominis may be present.

The external obliques interlace with the serratus anterior and latissimus dorsi on the lateral aspect of the trunk.

Internal Obliques

Latin:
internus—within
obliquus—slant

Origins
iliac crest (anterior portion)
thoracolumbar fascia
inguinal ligament (lateral half)

Insertions
lower ribs 3 and 4 (anterior lateral surface)
linea alba

Actions
laterally flexes the vertebral column
rotates the vertebral column
flexes the vertebral column
compresses abdominal contents
posteriorly tilts the pelvis

Nerves
anterior rami of intercostal nerves

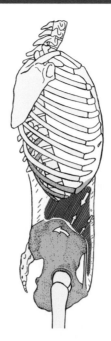

LATERAL VIEW
FIGURE 16-122

Notes: The fiber direction of the internal obliques comes up in a fan-shaped pattern, with the majority of the fibers lying in the direction of your fingers when your thumbs are hooked behind suspenders and your fingers are resting on your chest.

Transverse Abdominis

Latin:
transversus—lying across
abdomen—belly

Origins
ribs 7 through 12 (costal cartilage—inner surface)
iliac crest
thoracolumbar aponeurosis
inguinal ligament

Insertions
abdominal aponeurosis
linea alba

Action
compresses abdominal contents

Nerves
anterior rami of intercostal nerves

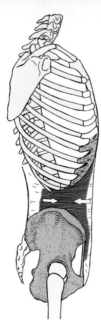

LATERAL VIEW
FIGURE 16-123

Notes: The transverse abdominis is the deepest abdominal muscle and wraps around the internal organs, similar to a cummerbund, and helps stabilize the lumbar spine. The lower fibers of the rectus abdominis are enclosed by the transverse abdominis, probably for added strength. The inferior portion of this muscle may fuse completely with the internal obliques. Because of its frequent variance, the transverse abdominis is often called the *complex muscle*.

Quadratus Lumborum

Latin:
quadratus—four sided
lumbus—loins

Origin
posterior iliac crest

Insertions
rib 12 (inferior surface)
transverse processes of L1-L4

Actions
laterally flexes the vertebral column (unilateral contraction)
elevates the hip (unilateral contraction)
extends the lumbar spine (bilateral contraction)
anteriorly tilts pelvis (bilateral contraction)

Nerves
thoracic nerve
lumbar nerve

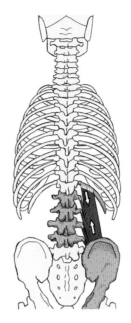

POSTERIOR VIEW
FIGURE 16-124

Notes: Also known as the *hip hiker muscle*, it hikes up the hip.

Paraspinals

Greek:
para—beside
Latin:
spinatus—spine

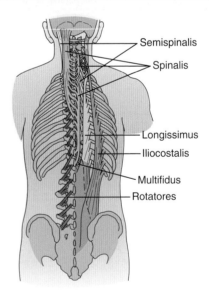

Semispinalis
Spinalis
Longissimus
Iliocostalis
Multifidus
Rotatores

POSTERIOR VIEW
FIGURE 16-125

BOX 16-3

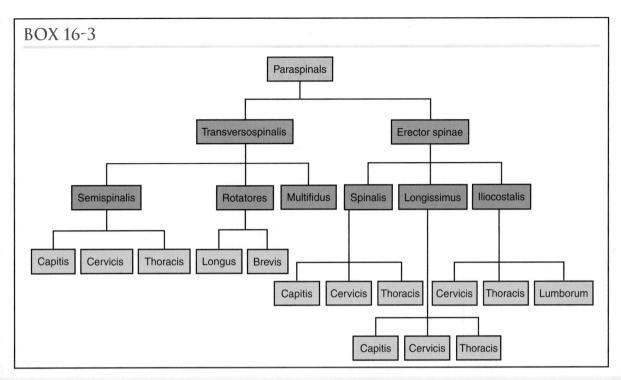

Notes: The *paraspinals* is the collective term given to a group of back muscles composed of two groups: the transversospinalis (deep paraspinals) and erector spinae (superficial paraspinals). Important in maintaining the posture, each muscle group can be subdivided into smaller branches (Box 16-3). Transversospinalis' subgroups are semispinalis, rotatores, and multifidus. Erector spinae's subgroups are spinalis, longissimus, and iliocostalis.

Transversospinalis

Latin:
transversus—lying across
spinatus—spine

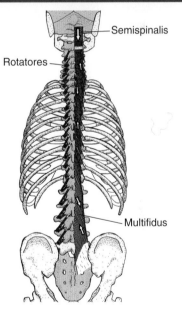

Semispinalis

Rotatores

Multifidus

POSTERIOR VIEW
FIGURE 16-126

Notes: The term *transversospinalis* refers to the vertebral processes to which most of the muscles in this group attach; all originate on the transverse processes and insert on the spinous processes. The muscles of the transversospinalis are the semispinalis, rotatores, and multifidus. Two of the three muscle groups, the semispinalis and rotatores, can be further subdivided. These subgroupings are the semispinalis capitis, semispinalis cervicis, semispinalis thoracis, rotatores longus, and rotatores brevis.

The multifidus has no subgroup. All of these muscles are stacked on top of one another and are composed of many short diagonal fibers.

Two other muscles, called *segmental muscles,* lie deep in the back. These muscles are the interspinales and intertransversarii. They are called *segmental muscles* because they traverse a single vertebral segment. The interspinales attach to the spinous processes, and the intertransversarii attach to the transverse processes.

Semispinalis

Latin:
semis—half
spinatus—spine

Origins
transverse process of one vertebral segment (cervical and
    thoracic regions)

Insertions
spinous processes of the fifth, sixth, and seventh vertebral
    segments above (cervical and thoracic regions except C1)

Actions
rotates the vertebral column (unilateral contraction)
extends the vertebral column (bilateral contraction)

Nerves
posterior rami of spinal nerves

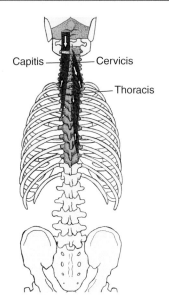

POSTERIOR VIEW
FIGURE 16-127

Notes: This group of muscles runs in only the thoracic and cervical regions of the vertebral column. This muscle is the most superficial of the transversospinalis and is one of the strongest muscles of the neck. It contains the subgroupings of capitus, cervicis, and thoracis. Semispinalis capitis often blends with the medial part of spinalis capitis of the erector spinae group.

Rotatores

Latin:
rotare—to turn

Origins
transverse process of one vertebral segment

Insertions
spinous process of the first or second vertebral segment above

Actions
rotates the vertebral column (unilateral contraction)
extends the vertebral column (bilateral contraction)

Nerves
posterior rami of spinal nerves

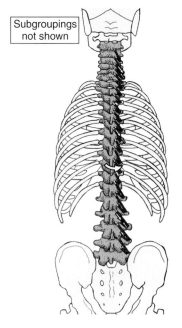

POSTERIOR VIEW
FIGURE 16-128

Notes: The rotatores span one to two vertebrae. This muscle is the deepest of the transversospinalis group. It contains the subgroupings of longus and brevis.

Multifidus

Latin:
multus—many
fidus—to split

Origins
transverse process of one vertebral segment

Insertions
spinous processes of the second, third, and fourth vertebral
   segments above

Actions
rotates the vertebral column (unilateral contraction)
laterally flexes the vertebral column (unilateral contraction)
extends the vertebral column (bilateral contraction)

Nerves
posterior rami of spinal nerves

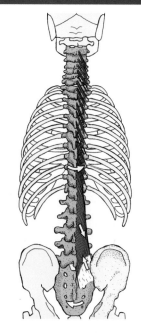

POSTERIOR VIEW
FIGURE 16-129

Notes: The multifidus spans two to four vertebrae and lies over the rotatores.

Erector Spinae

Latin:
erigere—to erect
spinatus—spine

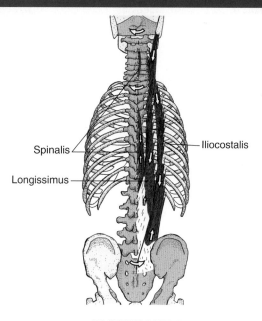

POSTERIOR VIEW
FIGURE 16-130

Notes: The term *erector spinae* refers to the action of this muscle group—erection of the spine. The muscles of the erector spinae are the spinalis, longissimus, and iliocostalis. These muscles fill the osseous canal formed by the vertebral arches (lamina groove). Each subgroup (spinalis, longissimus, iliocostalis) can be further subdivided. These groups are the spinalis capitis, spinalis cervicis, spinalis thoracis, longissimus capitis, longissimus cervicis, longissimus thoracis, iliocostalis cervicis, iliocostalis thoracis, and iliocostalis lumborum.

Also known as the *sacrospinalis muscle,* the erector spinae runs parallel to the spine and erects it, similar to a silo. The word *silo* can be used as a mnemonic to recall the names of the erector spinae muscles: **s**pinalis, **i**liocostalis, and **lo**ngissimus. These muscles lie next to one another, compared with the transversospinalis, which lie on top of one another.

Spinalis

Latin:
spinatus—spine

Origins
spinous processes of C4-T12
nuchal ligament

Insertions
spinous processes of C2-T8
occipital bone (between the superior and inferior nuchal lines)

Actions
laterally flexes the vertebral column (unilateral contraction)
extends the vertebral column (bilateral contraction)
extends the head (bilateral contraction)

Nerves
posterior rami of spinal nerves

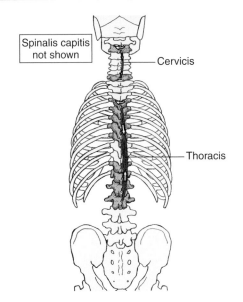

POSTERIOR VIEW
FIGURE 16-131

Notes: The spinalis is the medial tract of the erector spinae. The spinalis *hugs the spine* and lies in the lamina groove. The muscle's sub- groupings are the capitis, cervicis, and thoracis.

Longissimus

Latin:
longus—long

Origins
posterior sacrum
spinous processes of T1-L5
transverse processes of C4-T12

Insertions
mastoid process
transverse processes of C2-T12
ribs 4 through 12 (posterior surface)

Actions
laterally flexes the vertebral column (unilateral contraction)
rotates the vertebral column (unilateral contraction)
extends the vertebral column (bilateral contraction)
extends the head (bilateral contraction)

Nerve
posterior rami of spinal nerves

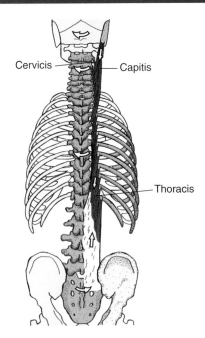

POSTERIOR VIEW
FIGURE 16-132

Notes: The longissimus is the intermediate tract of the erector spinae and covers a *long* territory stretching from sacrum to skull. This muscle's subgroupings are the capitis, cervicis, and thoracis.

Iliocostalis

Latin:
ilium—flank
costae—rib

Origins
posterior iliac crest
posterior sacrum
ribs 1 through 12 (posterior surface)

Insertions
ribs 1 through 12 (posterior surface)
transverse processes of C4-C7

Actions
laterally flexes the vertebral column (unilateral contraction)
extends the vertebral column (bilateral contraction)

Nerves
posterior rami of spinal nerves

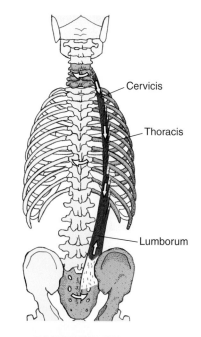

Cervicis

Thoracis

Lumborum

POSTERIOR VIEW
FIGURE 16-133

Notes: The iliocostalis is the lateral tract of the erector spinae. The iliocostal is hugs the costals (ribs). This muscle's subgroupings are the cervicis, thoracis, and lumborum.

Lesson EIGHT

Muscles of Vertebral Column Movement

FLEXION	EXTENSION	LATERAL FLEXION	ROTATION
Psoas major	Quadratus lumborum	External obliques	External obliques
Rectus abdominis	Semispinalis	Internal obliques	Internal obliques
External obliques	Rotatores	Quadratus lumborum	Semispinalis
Internal obliques	Multifidus	Spinalis	Rotatores
	Spinalis	Longissimus	Multifidus
	Longissimus	Iliocostalis	
	Iliocostalis		

Unit TWO—Muscles of the Axial Skeleton

Lesson NINE—**Muscles of Pulmonary Respiration** (Diaphragm, Internal Intercostal, External Intercostal, Serratus Posterior Superior, Serratus Posterior Inferior, Pectoralis Minor [Lesson One], Scalenes [Lesson Seven], Sternocleidomastoid [Lesson Seven])

Diaphragm

Greek:
diaphragma—a partition

Origins
L1-L3
lower six costal cartilages
xiphoid process

Insertion
central tendon (cloverleaf-shaped aponeurosis)

Action
expands the thoracic cavity during inspiration

Nerve
phrenic nerve

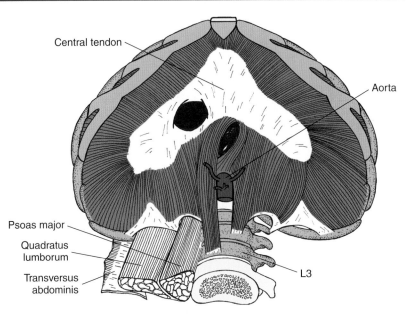

INFERIOR VIEW

FIGURE 16-134

Notes: The diaphragm divides the thoracic from the abdominal cavity and is the prime mover of inspiration. Because of its origins, the diaphragm possesses lumbar, costal, and sternal portions.

Internal Intercostal

Latin:
internus—within
costae—rib

Origins
superior border of rib (below)

Insertions
inferior border of rib (above)

Actions
depresses the ribcage during expiration
maintains intercostal spaces

Nerves
intercostal nerves

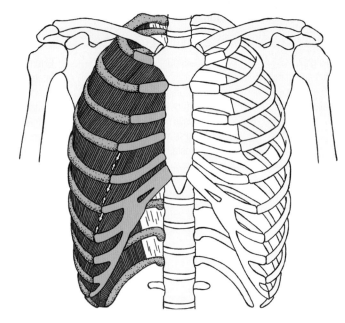

ANTERIOR VIEW

FIGURE 16-135

Notes: The fiber direction of the internal intercostals is the same as the internal obliques.

External Intercostal

Latin:
externus—outside
internus—within
costae—rib

Origins
inferior border of rib (above)

Insertions
superior border of rib (below)

Actions
elevates the ribcage during inspiration
maintains intercostal spaces

Nerves
intercostal nerves

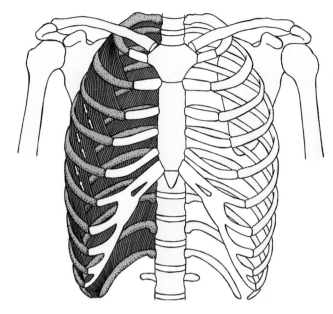

ANTERIOR VIEW

FIGURE 16-136

Notes: As the name implies, the external intercostals are external, or superficial, to the internal intercostals and in between the ribs. The fiber direction of this muscle is the same as the external obliques.

Serratus Posterior Superior

Latin:
serratus—notched or jagged, as a saw
posterus—behind
superus—upper

Origins
nuchal ligament
spinous processes of C7-T3

Insertions
ribs 2 through 5 (posterior surface)

Action
elevates ribs during inspiration

Nerves
intercostal nerves

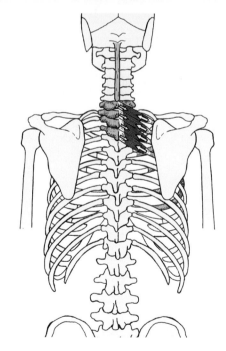

POSTERIOR VIEW

FIGURE 16-137

Notes: Deep to the rhomboids, this and the following muscle aid in the process of labored breathing.

Serratus Posterior Inferior

Latin:
serratus—notched or jagged, as a saw
posterus—behind
infra—beneath

Origins
spinous processes of T11-L2

Insertions
ribs 9 through 12 (posterior surface)

Action
depresses ribs during expiration

Nerves
intercostal nerves (T9-T12)

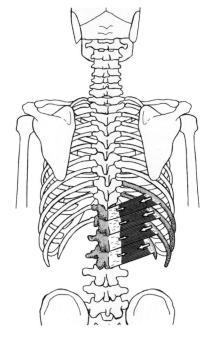

POSTERIOR VIEW

FIGURE 16-138

Lesson NINE

Muscles of Pulmonary Respiration

INSPIRATION	EXPIRATION
Pectoralis minor	Internal intercostal
Scalenes	Serratus posterior inferior
Sternocleidomastoid	Abdominals (forced)
Diaphragm	
External intercostal	
Serratus posterior superior	

evolve *Log on to your student account using the Evolve website for a humorous look at some of the muscles' nicknames, such as the* tailor's *and* swimmer's *muscle.* ■

SUMMARY

Muscular nomenclature deals with the names, locations, attachment points, actions, and nerve supply of individual skeletal muscles. The muscles of the appendicular skeleton are divided into the following groups: muscles of scapula movement; muscles of shoulder movement; muscles of elbow movement; muscles of the forearm, wrist, and hand; muscles of the hip and knee movement; and muscles of foot movement. The muscles of the axial skeleton are broken down into the following groups: muscles of the head and neck, muscles of the trunk and vertebral column, and muscles of pulmonary respiration.

For each muscle in these groups, the origin of its name is broken down; synonyms are listed; and specific actions, origins, and insertions are detailed.

evolve

Go to *Chapter Extras* on Evolve for additional illustrations and resources for this chapter. *Extras* for this chapter include:

1. Drag and drop (interactive game)
2. Crossword puzzle (downloadable form)
3. Muscle trivia (text)
4. Muscles of pelvic tilt (box)

MATCHING—LESSONS ONE, TWO, AND THREE

Place the letter of the answer next to the term or phrase that best describes it. Some answers may be used more than once.

A. Biceps brachii
B. Brachialis
C. Coracobrachialis
D. Deltoid
E. Latissimus dorsi

F. Levator scapula
G. Pectoralis major
H. Pectoralis minor
I. Rhomboids major and minor

J. Serratus anterior
K. Subscapularis
L. Supraspinatus
M. Trapezius

_____ 1. Swimmer's muscle; action of shoulder extension

_____ 2. Corkscrew muscle; flexes the elbow and supinates the forearm

_____ 3. Contractions of this muscle may cause angina-like pain

_____ 4. Frozen shoulder muscle

_____ 5. Neurovascular entrapper

_____ 6. Christmas tree muscle; oblique fiber arrangement

_____ 7. One of the boxer's muscles

_____ 8. Muscle that attaches to the coracoid process of the scapula and ribs 3 through 5

_____ 9. Coat hanger's muscle

_____ 10. Most effective arm flexor because of its mechanical advantage

_____ 11. Muscle that attaches to the deltoid tuberosity

_____ 12. Muscle named for elevating the scapula

_____ 13. Musculotendinous cuff muscle that does not actually rotate

_____ 14. Musculotendinous cuff muscle that attaches on the lesser tubercle of the humerus

_____ 15. Most superficial muscle of the posterior upper back

_____ 16. Muscle that attaches to the coracoid process and the humerus

MATCHING—LESSON FOUR

Place the letter of the answer next to the term or phrase that best describes it. Some answers may be used more than once.

A. Extensor carpi ulnaris   D. Flexor carpi radialis   G. Pronator quadratus
B. Extensor digiti minimi   E. Flexor digiti minimi   H. Supinator
C. Extensor indicis   F. Opponens pollicis

_____ 1.   Only muscle listed in this group that supinates the forearm

_____ 2.   Muscle that extends the index finger

_____ 3.   Muscle that flexes the wrist

_____ 4.   Muscle that pronates the hand

_____ 5.   Tea drinker's muscle; extends the little finger

_____ 6.   Muscle that performs abduction of the wrist

_____ 7.   Muscles that moves the thumb into opposition

_____ 8.   Muscle that extends the wrist

_____ 9.   Muscles that adducts the wrist

_____ 10.   Muscle that flexes the little finger

MATCHING—LESSONS FIVE AND SIX

Place the letter of the answer next to the term or phrase that best describes it.

A. Adductor magnus
B. Biceps femoris
C. Fibularis longus
D. Gastrocnemius
E. Gluteus maximus

F. Gracilis
G. Iliopsoas
H. Piriformis
I. Plantaris
J. Popliteus

K. Rectus femoris
L. Sartorius
M. Semitendinosus
N. Soleus
O. Tibialis anterior

_____ 1. Tailor's muscle

_____ 2. Hamstring that attaches to the fibular head

_____ 3. Quadriceps femoris muscle that crosses two joints

_____ 4. Muscle that initiates walking

_____ 5. Largest outward rotator of the hip

_____ 6. Strongest extender of the hip

_____ 7. Hamstring that is also part of the pes anserinus

_____ 8. Adductor that forms the letter V with the femoral shaft

_____ 9. Mini-gastrocnemius; missing in approximately 10% of cadavers

_____ 10. Muscle that dorsiflexes the ankle and inverts the foot

_____ 11. Muscle that plantar flexes the ankle and everts the foot

_____ 12. Muscle described as *the key that unlocks the knee*

_____ 13. Muscle of plantar flexion that attaches below the knee joint

_____ 14. Toe dancer's muscle

_____ 15. Adductor muscle that attaches to the linea aspera and the adductor tubercle

MATCHING—LESSON SEVEN

Place the letter of the answer next to the term or phrase that best describes it.

A. Buccinator
B. Frontalis
C. Lateral pterygoid
D. Masseter

E. Orbicularis oculi
F. Orbicularis oris
G. Platysma
H. Rectus capitis posterior minor

I. Scalenus medius
J. Sternocleidomastoid
K. Temporalis
L. Zygomaticus major and minor

_____ 1. Muscle for blowing

_____ 2. Winking muscle

_____ 3. Muscle of mastication attaching to the coronoid process of the mandible

_____ 4. Muscle involved in torticollis

_____ 5. Muscle of mastication that attaches to the temporomandibular joint capsule

_____ 6. Muscles that lifts the corners of the mouth into a smile

_____ 7. Muscle of mastication that is the mirror image of the medial pterygoid

_____ 8. Scalene muscle that runs behind the brachial plexus

_____ 9. Muscle that is described as the *pouting muscle*

_____ 10. Muscle that lies across the frontal bone and contributes to tension headaches

_____ 11. Muscle that attaches to the dura mater

_____ 12. Kissing muscle

MATCHING—LESSONS EIGHT AND NINE

Place the letter of the answer next to the term or phrase that best describes it.

A. Diaphragm
B. External obliques
C. Iliocostalis
D. Internal intercostal

E. Longissimus
F. Multifidus
G. Quadratus lumborum

H. Rectus abdominis
I. Rotatores
J. Spinalis

_____ 1. Hip hiker muscle; elevates the hip

_____ 2. Deepest transversospinalis muscle

_____ 3. Most medial erector spinae muscle

_____ 4. Abdominal muscle with oblique fiber arrangement

_____ 5. Main muscle of inspiration

_____ 6. Most lateral erector spinae muscle

_____ 7. Abdominal muscle that attaches to the xiphoid process and the ribs

_____ 8. Part of the transversospinalis named for the muscle's many attachments

_____ 9. Muscle that depresses the rib cage during expiration

_____ 10. Intermediate tract of the erector spinae group that attaches to the occipital bone

INTERNET ACTIVITIES

Visit http://www.sportsinjuryclinic.net and click on Sports Injuries. Scroll down and, on the left, click on the link to Rotator Cuff Injuries/Rotator Cuff Strain. What are symptoms of a rotator cuff strain?

Visit http://www.rice.edu/~jenky/sports/piri.html and read the web page on piriformis syndrome. How is piriformis syndrome diagnosed?

Visit http://www.spine.org/articles/whiplash.cfm and, after reading, answer the following questions: What are some common symptoms of whiplash? How is whiplash diagnosed? How is it treated?

Bibliography

Abrahams P, Marks S, Hutchings R: *McMinn's color atlas of human anatomy,* St Louis, 2003, Mosby.

Applegate EJ: *The anatomy and physiology learning system,* ed 3, Philadelphia, 2006, Saunders

Biel A: *Trail guide to the body: how to locate muscles, bones, and more,* ed 3, Boulder, Colo, 2005, Books of Discovery.

Bowden B, Bowden J: *An illustrated atlas of the skeletal muscles,* Englewood, Colo, 2002, Morton.

Como D, editor: *Mosby's medical, nursing, and allied health dictionary,* ed 6, St Louis, 2002, Mosby.

Crawley J, Van De Graaff KM: *A photographic atlas for anatomy and physiology,* Englewood, Colo, 2002, Morton.

Goldberg S: *Clinical anatomy made ridiculously simple,* Miami, 2004, Medmaster.

Grafelman T: *Graf's anatomy and physiology guide for the massage therapist,* Aurora, Colo, 1998, DG Publishing.

Guyton A: *Human physiology and mechanisms of disease,* ed 6, Philadelphia, 1996, Saunders.

Haubrich WS: *Medical meanings: a glossary of word origins,* New York, 1984, Harcourt Brace Jovanovich.

Hoppenfeld S: *Physical examination of the spine and extremities,* Norwalk, Conn, 1976, Appleton-Century-Crofts.

Jacob S, Francone C: *Elements anatomy and physiology,* Philadelphia, 1989, Saunders.

Juhan D: *Job's body: a handbook for bodyworkers,* ed 3, Barrington, NY, 2003, Station Hill Press.

Kapit W, Elson LM: *The anatomy coloring book,* ed 3, New York, 2002, Benjamin Cummings.

Kapit W, Macey R, Meisami E: *The physiology coloring book,* ed 2, New York, 1999, HarperCollins.

Kendall FP, McCreary EK: *Muscles: testing and function,* ed 3, Baltimore, 1983, Williams and Wilkins.

Kordish M, Dickson S: *Introduction to basic human anatomy,* Lake Charles, La, 1985, McNeese State University.

Lauderstein D: *Putting the soul back in the body: a manual of imaginative anatomy for massage therapists,* Chicago, 1985, self-published.

Lowe WW: *Functional assessment in massage therapy,* Corvallis, Ore, 1995, Pacific Orthopedic Massage.

Marieb EN: *Essentials of human anatomy and physiology,* ed 8, New York, 2005, Benjamin Cummings.

Martini FH, Bartholomew EF: *Essentials of anatomy and physiology,* ed 3, New York, 2003, Benjamin Cummings.

Mattes A: *Active isolated stretching,* Sarasota, Fla, 1995, self-published.

McAleer N: *The body almanac,* Garden City, NY, 1985, Doubleday.

McLaughlin C: *The bodyworker's muscle reference guide,* Bellevue, Colo, 1996, Bodyguide.

Merck manual, ed 17, Whitehouse Station, NJ, 1998, Merck and Company.

Moore KL: *Clinically oriented anatomy,* ed 5, Baltimore, 2005, Lippincott Williams & Wilkins.

Muscolino JE: *The muscular system manual: the skeletal muscles of the human body,* ed 2, St Louis, 2005, Elsevier Mosby.

Muscolino JE: *Kinesiology: the skeletal system and muscle function,* St Louis, 2006, Mosby.

Myers TW: *Anatomy trains: myofascial meridians for manual and movement therapists,* New York, 2001, Churchill Livingstone.

Netter FH: *Atlas of human anatomy,* ed 3, Teterboro, NJ, 2003, Icon Learning Systems.

Olsen A, McHose C: *Body stories: a guide to experiential anatomy,* Barrytown, NY, 1991, Station Hill Press.

Platzer W: *Color atlas and textbook of human anatomy: locomotor system,* vol I, ed 5, New York, 2003, Thieme.

Rolf IP: *Rolfing: the integration of human structures,* New York, 1977, Harper and Row.

Sieg K, Adams S: *Illustrated essentials of musculoskeletal anatomy,* ed 3, Gainesville, Fla, 1996, Megabooks.

Solomon EP, Phillips GA: *Understanding human anatomy and physiology,* Philadelphia, 1987, Saunders.

Souza TA: *Differential diagnosis and management for the chiropractor,* ed 2, Gaithersburg, Md, 2001, Aspen Publications.

St. John P: *St. John neuromuscular therapy seminars: manual I,* Largo, Fla, 1995, self-published.

Thibodeau G, Patton K: *Anatomy and physiology,* ed 6, St Louis, 2006, Mosby.

Thibodeau G, Patton K: *Structure and function of the body,* ed 12, St Louis, 2004, Mosby.

Tortora GJ: *Introduction to the human body: the essentials of anatomy and physiology,* ed 5, Hoboken, NJ, 2000, John Wiley & Sons.

Tortora GJ, Grabowksi SR: *Principles of anatomy and physiology,* ed 11, New York, 2005, John Wiley & Sons.

Travell JG, Simons D: *Myofascial pain and dysfunction, the trigger point manual,* Baltimore, 1992, Lippincott Williams & Wilkins.

Venes D, Thomas CL, Taber CW: *Taber's cyclopedic medical dictionary,* ed 20, Philadelphia, 2005, FA Davis.

Warfel JH: *The extremities: muscles and motor points,* ed 6, Baltimore, 1992, Lippincott Williams & Wilkins.

Warfel JH: *The head, neck, and trunk,* ed 6, Baltimore, 1993, Lippincott Williams & Wilkins.

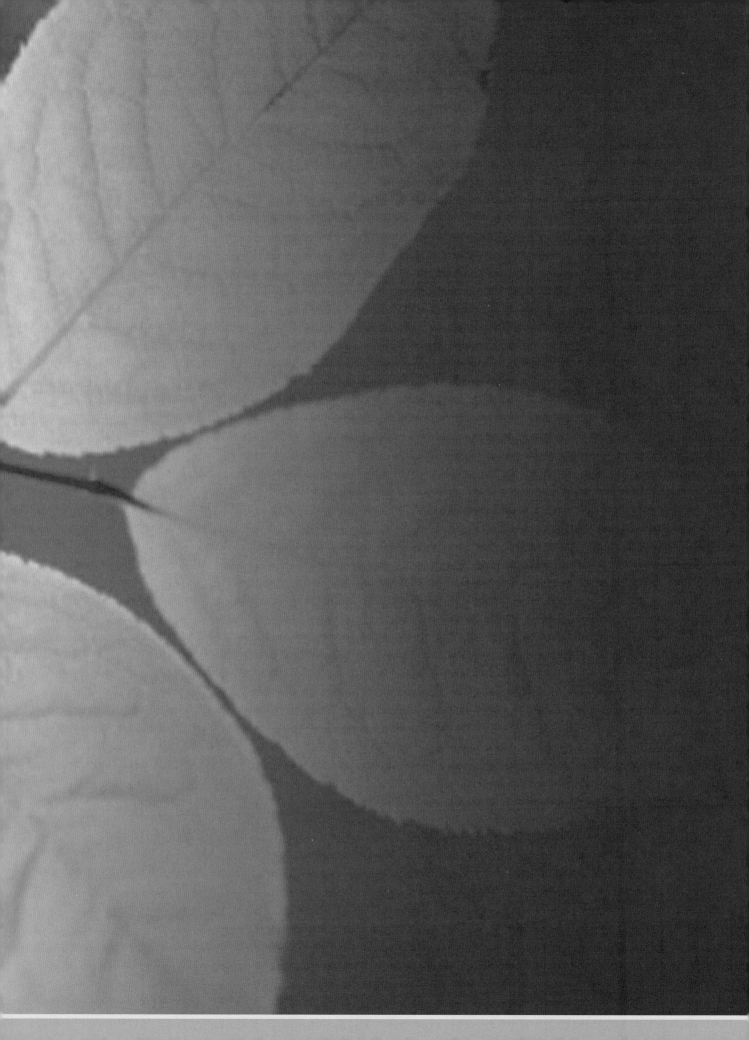

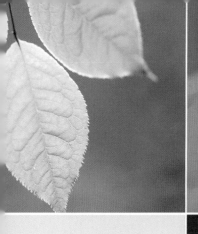

CHAPTER 17

Nervous System

STUDENT OBJECTIVES

After completing this chapter, the student should be able to:

- List anatomical structures and describe the physiological properties of the nervous system
- Discuss basic organization of the nervous system, outlining structures in both the central and the peripheral nervous systems
- Contrast and compare the somatic and autonomic divisions of the peripheral nervous system
- Label parts of a neuron
- Classify neurons according to their function
- Explain the mechanisms involved in a reflex arc
- Discuss nerve impulses, including resting and action potentials
- Label the steps in action potential conduction
- Contrast and compare continuous and saltatory conductions
- Outline the steps in synaptic transmission
- Define thresholds and summation in the nervous system
- List structures of the central nervous system, identifying regions of the brain and spinal cord
- Contrast and compare the left and right cerebral hemispheres according to their specializations
- Identify structures of the peripheral nervous system
- Name the cranial nerves
- Identify cranial and spinal nerves relevant for massage therapists
- Contrast and compare parasympathetic and sympathetic divisions of the autonomic nervous system, listing the physiological effects of each
- Briefly discuss the special senses (taste, smell, hearing, and vision)
- Name and discuss sensory receptors as classified by the stimuli detected
- Name types of pathological conditions of the nervous system, giving characteristics and massage considerations of each

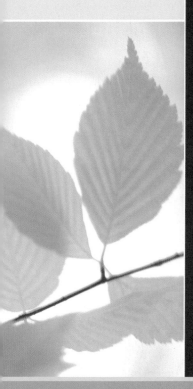

INTRODUCTION

The human body has two specialized centers of control that make important adjustments to maintain homeostasis. The endocrine system, which is discussed in the next chapter, responds slowly and uses hormones as chemical messengers to cause physiological changes in body cells. The nervous system responds to changes in the body rapidly and uses nerve impulses to cause changes in the body. The nervous system is the body's master controlling and communicating system; it even monitors and regulates aspects of the endocrine system. Every thought, action, and sensation reflects its activity. We are what our brain has experienced. If all past sensory input could be completely erased, we would be unable to walk, talk, or communicate; we would remember no pain or pleasure.

The study of the functions and disorders of the nervous system is referred to as *neurology*. This chapter explores neurology and examines the structural and functional classifications of the nervous tissue. It begins with an overview of nerves, the chemistry behind nerve impulses and synaptic transmissions, and then examines the two divisions of the nervous system itself—the central and peripheral nervous systems. Nerves may also be areas to avoid in massage therapy

(endangerment sites) and are also discussed here. Finally, the chapter reviews specialized nerve receptors that provide the five senses and pathological conditions of the nervous system, some of which may affect the application of massage.

ANATOMY

Areas of discussion in this chapter include:

- Brain
- Cerebrospinal fluid
- Cranial nerves
- Meninges
- Special sense organs
- Spinal cord
- Spinal nerves

PHYSIOLOGY

- **Sensory input:** Sensory receptors are either dendrites of neurons or separate, specialized cells. They detect changes, or *stimuli*, inside the body, such as lowered blood sugar levels, or outside the body, such as an increase in temperature. Sensory receptors respond to stimuli by generating nerve

Terms and Their Meanings Related to the Nervous System

TERM	MEANING	TERM	MEANING
Arachnoid	*Gr.* spider; shaped	Neuro	*Gr.* sinew
Autonomic	*Gr.* self; law	Neuroglia	*Gr.* sinew; glue
Axon	*Gr.* axis	Neurotransmitters	*Gr.* sinew; *L.* a sending across
Baroreceptor	*Gr.* weight; *L.* to receive	Nociceptor	*L.* hurt; to receive
Broca's area	Broca, French surgeon (1824-1880)	Nodes of Ranvier	Ranvier, French pathologist (1835-1922)
Cauda equina	*L.* tail-like; horse	Oligodendrocytes	*Gr.* little; tree; cell
Cerebellum	*L.* little brain	Otolith	*Gr.* ear; stone
Cerebrum	*L.* brain	Parasympathetic	*Gr.* by the side of, sympathetic
Chemoreceptors	*Gr.* chemical; *L.* to receive	Photoreceptors	*Gr.* light; *L.* to receive
Cochlea	*L.* snail shell	Pia mater	*L.* tender, soft; mother
Conduction	*L.* to lead together	Plexus	*L.* braid
Corpus callosum	*L.* body; hard or callused	Presbyopia	*Gr.* old man; eye
Cortex	*L.* bark or rind	Proprioceptor	*L.* one's own; a receiver
Cyton	*Gr.* cell	Pons	*L.* bridge
Dendrites	*Gr.* treelike	Reciprocal inhibition	*L.* to move backward; to restrain
Diencephalon	*Gr.* two or second; brain	Reflex	*L.* bent back
Dura mater	*L.* hard or tough; mother	Retina	*L.* a net
Encephalic	*Gr.* brain	Saltatory	*L.* to dance or leap
Extrafusal	*L.* outside of; spindle	Schwann cell	Schwann, German anatomist (1810-1882)
Filum terminale	*L.* threadlike; at the end	Soma	*Gr.* body
Ganglion	*Gr.* knot	Stapes	*L.* stirrup
Gyri	*Gr.* circle	Stimuli	*L.* to incite
Incus	*L.* anvil	Sulci	*L.* groove or furrow
Internuncial	*L.* between; together, amidst; messenger	Summation	*L.* total
Intrafusal	*L.* within; spindle	Sympathetic	*Gr.* to feel with
Macula	*L.* spot	Synapse	*Gr.* to join
Mechanoreceptors	*Gr.* machine; *L.* to receive	Thalamus	*Gr.* chamber
Medulla oblongata	*L.* marrow or middle; long	Thermoreceptors	*Gr.* heat; *L.* to receive
Meninges	*Gr.* membrane	Tympanic	*Gr.* drum
Myelin	*Gr.* marrow	Vagus	*L.* wandering
Neurilemma	*Gr.* sinew; husk	Wernicke's area	Wernicke, German neurologist (1848-1905)

Gr., Greek; *L.,* Latin.

impulses along sensory or afferent neurons that travel into the spinal cord and brain.

- **Interpretive functions:** The spinal cord and brain integrate or process sensory information. They analyze it, store some of it, and decide on an appropriate response. Interneurons are found between sensory and motor neurons (discussed next), and they participate in integrative functions. Most of the neurons of the body are interneurons

- **Motor output:** The motor function of the nervous system is to respond to integrative decisions. Motor or efferent neurons carry nerve impulses from the brain and spinal cord to smooth muscle, cardiac muscle, skeletal muscle, and glands. These impulses are called *effectors*.

- **Higher mental functioning and emotional responsiveness:** The nervous system is also responsible for mental processes (cognition and memory) and emotional responses (joy, excitement, anger, anxiety, and so forth).

BASIC ORGANIZATION OF THE NERVOUS SYSTEM

The nervous system is complex. Divisions exist that possess unique structural and functional characteristics.

The **central nervous system** (CNS) occupies a central or medial position in the body. It is primarily concerned with interpreting incoming sensory information and issuing instructions in the form of motor responses. It is also the major control center for thoughts and emotional experiences. The major components of the CNS include the brain (cerebrum, cerebellum, diencephalon, and brainstem), meninges, cerebrospinal fluid, and spinal cord. These structures are surrounded by the bones of the skull and spinal column.

The **peripheral nervous system** (PNS) is composed of the cranial and spinal nerves emerging from the CNS. **Cranial nerves** originate from the brain, and **spinal nerves** exit the spinal cord. The PNS has 43 pairs of nerves: 12 pairs of cranial nerves and 31 pairs of spinal nerves.

The PNS can be further subdivided into the somatic nervous system and the autonomic nervous system. The **somatic nervous system** (SNS) has sensory neurons that carry information from bones, muscles, joints, and the skin, as well as from sensory receptors for the special senses of vision, hearing, taste and smell, into the CNS. Motor neurons in the SNS carry impulses from the CNS out to skeletal muscles. Because these motor responses can be consciously controlled, they are considered *voluntary*. The **autonomic nervous system** (ANS) is an *involuntary* system, supplying impulses to smooth muscle, cardiac (heart) muscle, and glands. The ANS consists of a sympathetic and parasympathetic division, each of which possesses complementary responses. For example, if the sympathetic nervous system speeds up heart rate, the parasympathetic nervous system then slows it down to a normal heart rate (Figure 17-1).

The nervous system has a highly organized structure. It is made up of billions of neurons (nerve cells) and supporting cells called *neuroglia*.

evolve To view a drawing of the two divisions of the nervous system, log on to the Evolve website. Don't forget to print out the crossword puzzle for this chapter and use it to reinforce important terms related to the nervous system. ■

CELLS OF THE NERVOUS SYSTEM

Neuroglia

Neuroglia, or glia, is connective tissue that supports, nourishes, protects, insulates, and organizes neurons. Because it is not neural tissue, neuroglia is unable to transmit impulses. However, cells are able to replicate themselves through cell division. For this reason, most brain tumors are made up of glial cells. Neuroglia cells are smaller and more numerous

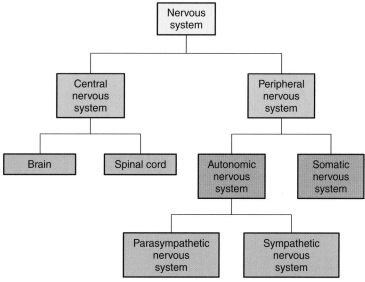
FIGURE 17-1 Nervous system divisions.

than neurons. In fact, more than 50% of the CNS is made up of these cells.

Six types of neuroglia exist; four types are located in the CNS (astrocytes, ependymocytes, microglia, oligodendrocytes), and two are located in the PNS (satellite cells and Schwann cells).

Supporting Cells of the Central Nervous System
- **Astrocytes** are used for structural support of delicate CNS neurons and are part of the blood-brain barrier.
- **Ependymocytes,** or ependymal cells, line the cranial ventricles and central canal of the spinal cord and assist in circulating cerebrospinal fluid.
- **Microglia** protects the CNS by destroying pathogens and removing dead neural tissue.
- **Oligodendrocytes** form a myelin sheath that surrounds some axons in the CNS.

Supporting Cells of the Peripheral Nervous System
The following supporting cells of the PNS are very similar and differ mainly because of their location.
- **Satellite cells** are used for structural support of the PNS, are delicate neurons, and are only found surrounding neuron cell bodies within ganglia. Ganglia are simply a knot-like mass of neuron cell bodies in the PNS.
- **Schwann cells,** or neurolemmocytes, form a myelin sheath that surrounds only axons in the PNS. A layer of this myelin sheath, called the neurilemma, or sheath of Schwann, and plays an important role in the regeneration of PNS neurons.

Neurons

The human body contains an estimated 100 billion neurons. **Neurons** are the basic impulse-conducting cells possessing the following two properties:
- **Excitability:** ability to respond to a stimulus and convert it to a nerve impulse
- **Conductibility:** ability to transmit the impulses to other neurons, muscles, and glands

Parts of a Neuron

Even though neurons vary widely in shape and size to accommodate a large number of neural connections, they all have three basic parts: a cell body, dendrites, and a single axon (Figure 17-2).

Long axons are often referred to as the *nerve fibers.*

Dendrites
Dendrites are typically short, narrow, and highly branched extensions of the nerve cell. These extensions receive and transmit stimuli toward the cell body.

Cell Body
The cell body, or *cyton,* contains the nucleus, ribosomes, and other organelles. In addition to the usual organelles, neurons possess a rough endoplasmic reticulum called *Nissl bodies,* which make protein for the cell. These Nissl bodies are uniquely named because they have a colorful stain under a microscope. Neural cell bodies are the gray matter of the nervous system. In the brain, gray matter is found on the outer layer, or *cortex,* and in the very deep part of the brain; in the spinal cord, it is centrally located and forms regions called *horns.*

Axons
Axons carry the nerve impulse away from the neuron toward another neuron, a muscle cell, or a gland. They may possess infrequent branches, called *collaterals.* Several structures are associated with axons.
- **Synaptic bulbs:** Each axon terminal ends with a small bud, or *synaptic knob* or *end bulbs,* which contain synaptic vesicles.
- **Telodendria:** These clusters of short, fine filaments are located at the distal end of each axon.
- **Synaptic vesicles:** These saclike structures are located within the synaptic bulbs. They produce and store *neurotransmitters,* which are chemicals that facilitate, arouse, or inhibit transmission of nerve impulses.
- **Myelin sheath:** The myelin sheath is actually white in color; therefore myelinated axons are known as *white*

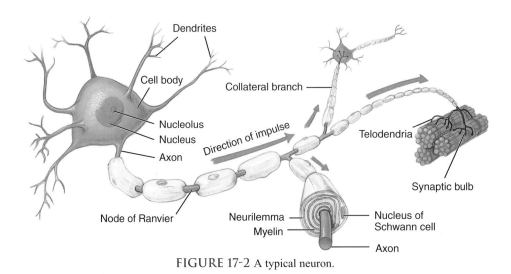

FIGURE 17-2 A typical neuron.

matter. Myelin not only electrically insulates the neuron (preventing signal leakage to adjacent neurons), but also increases nerve impulse speed. Myelin sheaths found in the PNS are formed by *Schwann cells* and is a fatty insulating sheath surrounding most axons. The nucleus, cytoplasm, and cell membrane of these cells form a tight covering around the axon. These coverings are called the *neurilemma.* In the CNS, oligodendrocytes produce myelin but not neurilemma. This characteristic is significant when we explore the regeneration of nerves in the PNS verses nerves in the CNS.

- **Nodes of Ranvier:** These structures are gaps located at intervals (between each Schwann cell) along a myelinated axon. Nerve impulses can jump from one node to another, resulting in an increased rate of conduction.

CLASSIFICATION OF NERVES

Nerves can be classified functionally (based on the direction nerve impulses are traveling in relation to the CNS) as sensory, interneurons, or motor.

- **Sensory (afferent) nerves:** Sensory nerves are said to be afferent because they carry impulses to the brain or spinal cord. Sensory nerves receive stimuli through sensory receptors. Some sensory receptors are close to the surface of the skin, such as Meissner corpuscles. Some sensory receptors lie deep within the body, such as proprioceptors.
- **Interneurons:** Interneurons, or *association nerves,* connect sensory nerves to motor nerves and vice versa. They process sensory information, analyze and store some of it, and then make decisions about appropriate responses. Interneurons make up most of the nerves in the body and are found in both the brain and spinal cord.
- **Motor (efferent) nerves:** Motor nerves are classified as efferent, which means that they carry messages from the brain or spinal cord to activate or inhibit a muscle or gland.

Reflex Arc

Neurons are often arranged in a pattern called a *reflex arc.* Although the neuron is the simplest structural unit of the nervous system, the simplest functional component of the nervous system is the reflex arc. The most common **reflex arc** consists of three neurons: afferent, interneuron, and efferent. It is essentially a conduction route to and from the CNS.

A **reflex** is an instantaneous, automatic response to a stimulus from either inside or outside the body. The reflex provides a short, quick response because the action of the reflex bypasses the brain (Figure 17-3).

When certain stimuli (e.g., contact with direct heat) enter a sensory nerve, it travels into the posterior horn of the spinal cord, excites interneurons (internuncial pool), generates a response out a motor nerve, and causes retraction from the injurious stimuli. This information does not reach the brain until after the motor responses have responded to the stimulus.

Reflexes are essentially a protective reaction to stimuli such as pain, pressure, or even loud noises. **Somatic reflexes** are those that are responsible for contraction of skeletal muscles, such as the patellar tendon tapped with a rubber hammer (knee-jerk or patellar reflex). Examples of somatic reflexes are muscle spindles and Golgi tendon organs; both will be discussed later in this chapter. **Visceral (autonomic) reflexes** maintain homeostasis through coughing, sneezing,

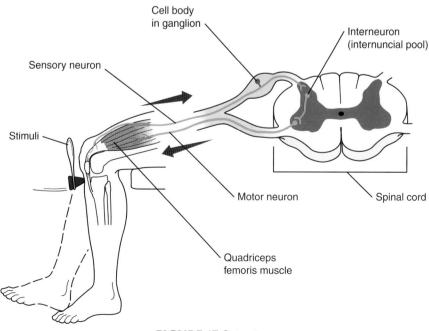

FIGURE 17-3 A reflex.

blinking, and correcting the heart rate, respiratory rate, and blood pressure.

An abnormal arc, or **physiopathological reflex arc,** is caused by increased stimuli or an increase in the amount of afferent impulses entering the cord. The increased stimuli might be the result of pain from an accident, emotional stress, biomechanical dysfunction, or poor posture. For instance, poor posture might cause increased muscle tonus, which, in turn, causes vasoconstriction and begins to starve the muscles of oxygen and nutrition by limiting their blood supply. This ischemic condition generates cellular waste products, many of which are irritants to the tissues, and increases the perception of pain. Trigger points form in the tissues. Pain from the trigger points is referred to adjacent tissues, and the pain-spasm-pain cycle continues. This circumstance is an example of a physiopathological reflex arc.

> ### TABLE TALK
>
> Massage therapy aids in breaking the physiopathological reflex arc and helps reestablish equilibrium and a normal reflex arc. As the tissues are warmed, the fascia, which encases the muscle, is softened, allowing the muscles to more easily lengthen. As the muscles lengthen, the intrajoint pressure is decreased. Massage stimulates increased local circulation by forcing blood through dormant capillary beds. This action brings oxygen and nutrition and removes accumulated waste products and toxins. Massage can also stimulate the release of natural painkillers in the body, such as endorphins. It can also inhibit the sensation of pain by activating the gate theory, in which the experience of one type of stimulation (pressure, cold, heat) can act to exclude the experience of other sensations (pain) that are all vying for the same gate to the brain.

Neurons to Nerves

Nerves are bundles of neurons held together by several layers of connective tissue. A layer of endoneurium wraps each neuron. A bundle of neurons (nerve fibers), each wrapped with its own endoneurium and filled with lymph, form *nerve fascicles.* Nerve fascicles are bound together by a connective tissue layer called *perineurium.* Nerves are bound together by a connective tissue layer known as the *epineurium* (Figure 17-4).

Hence each neuron, nerve fascicle, and nerve has a series of connective tissue wrappings as muscles do. To review:
Neuron (nerve cell) → nerve fascicle (bundles of neurons) → nerve (bundles of nerve fascicles).
Endoneurium (wraps neurons) → perineurium (wraps nerve fascicles) → epineurium (wraps nerves).

NERVE IMPULSES

Neural cell membranes possess potentials, or opportunities. They can be either resting or conducting nerve impulses. A **nerve impulse,** or *action potential,* is an electrical fluctuation that travels along the surface of a neuron's cell membrane. These electrical fluctuations are caused by the movement of charged particles, or ions, moving across the cell membrane.

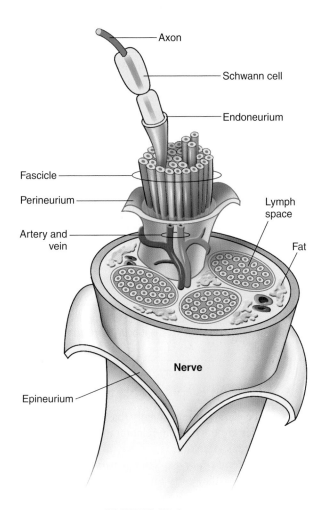

FIGURE 17-4 A nerve.

When a cell membrane is not conducting an impulse, it is at rest. Let us look at membrane potentials in more detail.

Resting Potentials

When a neuron is not conducting electrical signals, it is said to be resting. The method that produces and maintains the resting potential is an active transport system called the **sodium-potassium pump.** This mechanism located in the plasma membrane transports sodium ions (Na^+) and potassium ions (K^+) in opposite directions at an unequal rate. It moves three Na^+ out of the cell for every two K^+ it moves into the cell (3:2). As this pump operates, very little sodium enters the cell. Because very little sodium enters the cell with diffusion, this also helps maintain the imbalance or resting potential.

The concentration of Na^+ outside creates a positive (+) charge, and the concentration of K^+ inside creates a negative (−) charge.

Action Potentials

An action potential is, as the term suggests, an active neuron or one conducting an impulse. The action potential, or nerve impulse, is an electrical fluctuation that travels along the surface of a neuron's plasma membrane.

Action Potential Conduction

The following is a brief description of how a neuron conducts nerve impulses, or action potentials.

- When a stimulus is added to a neuron, Na^+ channels open, permitting N^+ to flow into the cell. This flow creates a differential in charge.
- Other channels across the cell membrane sense the fluctuation in electrical charge and open in response, moving even more Na^+ into the cell. This reverses the charge; the inside of the cell is now positive, and the outside is now negative, creating a nerve impulse. This impulse is conducted along the entire neuron at maximum capacity. The principle that states that an impulse can be conducted only at maximum capacity and never at partial capacity is referred to as the *all-or-none response.*
- The reverse polarization in the initial section of the cell membrane acts as the stimulus for the adjacent sections of the neuron. As Na^+ rushes inward, this next segment is stimulated (Figure 17-5).

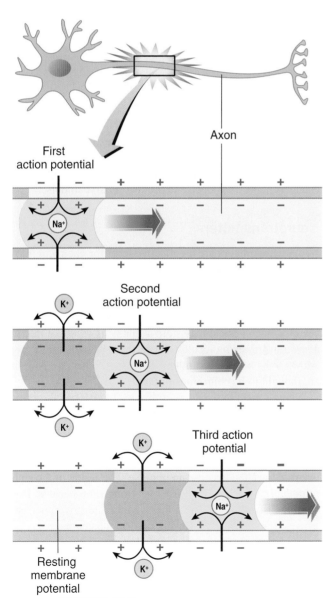

FIGURE 17-5 Action potential conduction.

- Because each action potential is an all-or-none phenomenon, the fluctuations in membrane potential move along the membrane without any decrement, or decrease, in magnitude. The action potential never moves backward, which would restimulate the region from which it just came.
- After the impulse has been conducted, the resting membrane potential is reinstated by the sodium-potassium pump, transporting Na^+ and K^+ in opposite directions at unequal rates. The outside of the cell is once again positively charged, and the inside is negatively charged.

Therefore the nerve impulse is simply a matter of ions changing places and creating different electrical charges along the cell membrane.

Nerve impulses can be conducted along unmyelinated and myelinated axons. Nerve impulse conduction along unmyelinated axons is called *continuous conduction.* Nerve impulses conducted along myelinated axons, which is the faster of the two, are called *saltatory conduction.*

Saltatory conduction – In myelinated fibers, the insulating properties of the myelin sheath resist ionic movement and the resultant flow of current. Impulses can occur only at gaps in the myelin sheath, or the nodes of Ranvier. Most of the electrical current of the nerve impulse flows under the myelin sheath to the next node. This flow stimulates an action potential at that node. Thus the action potential seems to *leap* from node to node along the myelinated fiber.

> **evolve** *To see an image of saltatory conduction or how nerve impulses are transmitted on myelinated axon, look up the course materials for Chapter 17's* Massage Therapy: Principles and Practice, 3e, *on the Evolve website.* ■

The fastest fibers, such as those that innervate the skeletal muscles, can conduct impulses up to approximately 130 meters per second (close to 300 miles per hour). The slowest fibers, such as sensory receptors in the skin, may conduct impulses at only 0.5 meters per second (little more than 1 mile per hour).

SYNAPSE AND SYNAPTIC TRANSMISSION

The junction between two neurons or between a neuron and a muscle or gland, where transmission of nerve impulses takes place, is a **synapse.** Neurons do not actually touch the other neuron, muscle, or gland (Figure 17-6).

Two types of synapses exist: (1) electrical and (2) chemical. *Electrical synapses* occur between cardiac muscle cells and some smooth muscle cells. *Chemical synapses,* the more common, are made up of three structures: (1) a synaptic bulb, (2) a synaptic cleft, and (3) the plasma membrane of a postsynaptic neuron. Each *synaptic bulb* contains many small sacs, or vesicles. Each vesicle contains neurotransmitters. A *synaptic cleft* is the space between the synaptic bulb and the *plasma membrane of the postsynaptic neuron.* The postsynaptic neuron contains receptor sites embedded in it opposite each synaptic bulb. These structures serve as sites where neurotransmitters bind.

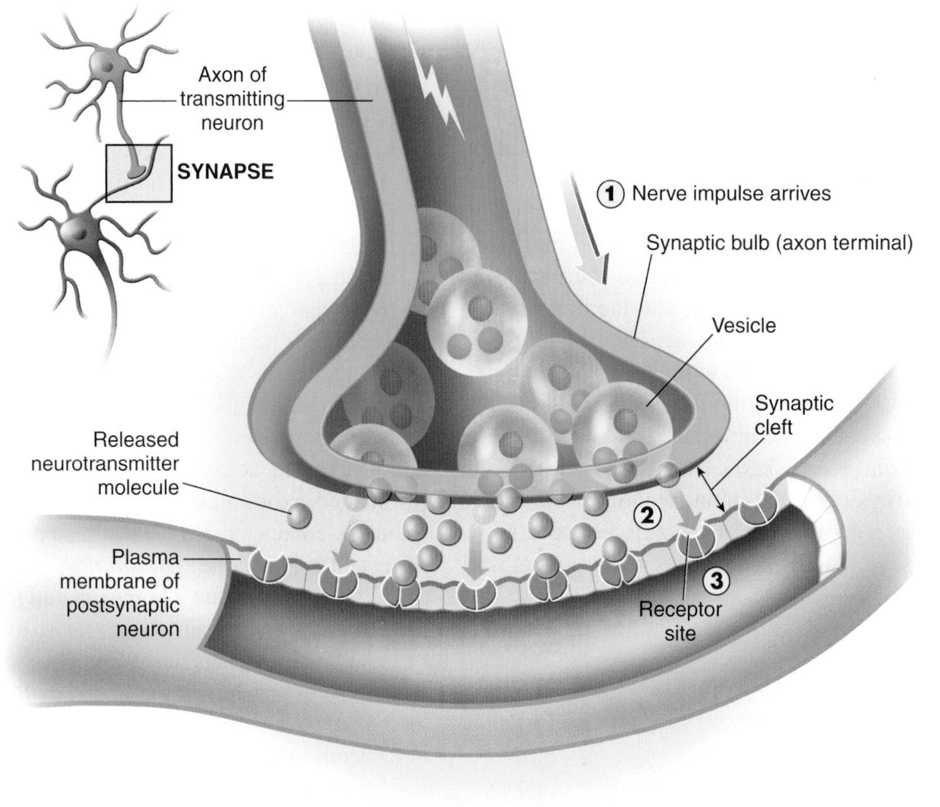

FIGURE 17-6 The synapse.

Synaptic transmission is a one-way process. Let us examine the process in simple steps.

1. Once a nerve impulse has traveled the length of a neuron, it stops at its axon terminal (synaptic bulbs). Nerve impulses cannot cross synaptic clefts; instead, neurotransmitters are released from the synaptic bulb. Thousands of neurotransmitters spurt out of the open vesicles into the synaptic cleft.
2. The released neurotransmitter molecules travel across the synaptic cleft and make contact with the postsynaptic neuron's plasma membrane.
3. The neurotransmitters bind with receptor sites on the postsynaptic neuron, muscle, or gland. This binding brings about a response by the postsynaptic neuron. The response depends on the neurotransmitters being excitatory or inhibitory.

Thresholds

The strength and frequency of stimuli determine whether a nerve impulse is generated. When the stimulus is of sufficient intensity to generate a nerve impulse, threshold stimulus is the result. Any single stimulus below the threshold level does not result in the creation of a nerve impulse.

Summation

In some cases, a subthreshold stimulus (one lower than the threshold) is repeated in succession, and they may add together, or summate. The summation of these small stimuli may act cumulatively to create a nerve impulse. Summation is the amount of stimuli needed (both in frequency and number of fibers stimulated) to reach threshold stimulus; voltage-gated channels in the axon open and produce a nerve impulse.

Neurotransmitters

Neurotransmitters are a collective term for chemical messengers involved in nerve impulse transmission; it is how neurons talk to one another. Presynaptic neurons release neurotransmitters that facilitate, stimulate, or inhibit postsynaptic neurons and effector cells. They are stored in presynaptic vesicles; each vesicle may store as many as 10,000 different neurotransmitter molecules. More than 50 compounds are known to be neurotransmitters. At least 50 other compounds are thought to be neurotransmitters.

Neurotransmitters can be either excitatory or inhibitory. *Excitatory neurotransmitters* decrease the membrane potential (the charge difference across the membrane), thereby increasing the impulse rate. *Inhibitory neurotransmitters* increase the membrane potential, thereby increasing the threshold needed to cause an impulse. The action of the neurotransmitter does not persist for a long time because it is continuously removed from the synaptic cleft by either enzymes or reuptake (the drawing up of a substance).

Types of Neurotransmitters

The following is a list of some of the more important neurotransmitters.

- **Acetylcholine** (ACh), the most common neurotransmitter, is vital for stimulating muscle contraction and is found in junctions between motor nerves and muscles (neuromuscular junction). It is also found between motor nerves and glands, as well as in many parts of the brain. ACh can be excitatory or inhibitory and is also involved with memory.
- **Catecholamines** are a chemical family containing norepinephrine, epinephrine, and dopamine. The major functions of catecholamines include excitation and inhibition of certain muscles, cardiac excitation, metabolic action, and endocrine action. Catecholamines act directly on the sympathetic nervous system.
  - **Epinephrine** is located in several areas of the CNS and in the sympathetic division of the ANS. This neurotransmitter can be either excitatory or inhibitory and acts as a hormone when secreted by cells of the adrenal medulla.
  - **Norepinephrine**, similar to epinephrine, is both a hormone and a neurotransmitter secreted by the adrenal medulla. This neurotransmitter is located in several areas of the CNS and in the sympathetic division on the ANS. Norepinephrine can be excitatory or inhibitory. It mediates several physiological and metabolical responses that follow the stimulation of the sympathetic effectors in the brain; it is also involved in arousal, dreaming, mood regulation, and emotional responses.
  - **Dopamine** is a neurotransmitter found in the brain and ANS. It is mostly inhibitory and is involved in emotions, moods, and in regulating motor control. Dopamine is also implicated in attention and learning. A depletion of dopamine produces the symptoms of rigidity, tremors, and uncoordinated and slower-than-normal movement, such as that seen in Parkinson's disease.
- **Serotonin,** a naturally occurring derivative of tryptophan (an amino acid), is found in several regions of the CNS. It is mostly inhibitory and is important for sensory perception, mood regulation, and normal sleep.
- **Histamine,** found in the brain, is mostly excitatory and is involved in emotions and regulation of body temperature and water balance. Histamine stimulates inflammatory responses when not acting as a neurotransmitter.
- **Enkephalins** and **endorphins** are located in several regions of the CNS, the retina, and the intestinal tract. These neurotransmitters are mostly inhibitory and act similarly to opiates to block pain.

CENTRAL NERVOUS SYSTEM

The spinal cord and brain together comprise the CNS. The brain is housed in the skull, and the spinal cord is housed inside the vertebral column. In addition to this bony protection, the brain and spinal cord are protected by meninges and cerebrospinal fluid.

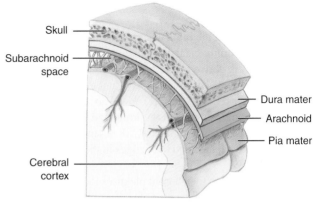

FIGURE 17-7 Cranial meninges.

Meninges

Connective tissue coverings deep in the skull and spine surrounding the brain and spinal cord are called **meninges.** In between each layer is a fluid-filled space (Figure 17-7).
- **Pia mater:** The innermost layer, the pia mater, is delicate, transparent, and vascular and is attached to the surface of the CNS.
  - **Subarachnoid space:** Between the pia mater and the arachnoid is the subarachnoid space, filled with cerebrospinal fluid and an arrangement of collagen and elastic fibers that resembles a spider's web. These extensions extend into the arachnoid.
- **Arachnoid:** The middle layer, the arachnoid or arachnoid mater, forms a loose covering around the CNS.
  - **Subdural space:** The subdural space, filled with circulating serous fluid, lies between the dura mater and the arachnoid.
- **Dura mater:** The outermost layer, the thick and dense dura mater, lies against the bone and contains a double layer of connective tissue, with the outer layer resembling periosteum. The dura mater surrounding the brain dips down between the cerebral hemispheres, creating the *falx cerebri,* dips across between the cerebrum and cerebellum, creates the *tentorium cerebelli,* dips down between the paired cerebellar hemispheres, and creates the *falx cerebelli.*
  - **Epidural space:** The epidural space lies between the dura and the vertebral canal. This space, which is the safest place for injections such as saddle blocks, contains adipose tissue, connective tissue, and blood vessels.

---

evolve *For some nice images of spinal meninges and cranial partitions created by the meninges, log on the Evolve website for this text under Chapter 17's course materials. Be sure and take time to see them.* ■

TABLE TALK

A mnemonic device to recall the three layers of the meninges, from deep to superficial is *PAD: p*ia mater, *a*rachnoid, and *d*ura mater.

Cerebrospinal Fluid

Circulating around the brain and spinal cord within the sub-arachnoid space is a clear fluid called **cerebrospinal fluid** (CSF), which is derived from blood, supplies the tissues of the brain and spinal cord with oxygen and nutrients, and carries away wastes. It also acts as a shock absorber. After CSF circulates through cavities in the brain and spinal cord, it is reabsorbed into the bloodstream. CSF is sensitive to glucose and electrolyte balance and to changes in the carbon dioxide content.

CSF is formed in the choroid plexuses located in the ventricles of the brain. The choroid plexuses are clusters of thin-walled capillaries surrounded by ependymal cells. Water and certain important ions are filtered out of the blood and into the ventricles to form CSF.

Spinal Cord

The **spinal cord** exits the skull through the foramen magnum and extends to approximately the second lumbar (L2) region. In addition to being an integrating center, the spinal cord acts as an information highway. It conveys sensory information from peripheral nerves up to the brain, and it conveys motor information from the brain out to peripheral nerves.

Two enlargements are located in the length of the spinal cord: one in the cervical region and one in the lumbar region. The lower end of the spinal cord is marked by the threadlike fibrous extension of the pia mater called the *filum terminale,* which is anchored to the coccyx. The ends of the cord fan out, resembling a horse's tail, and form a structure appropriately called the *cauda equina.*

The spinal cord consists of 31 segments, each of which gives rise to a pair of spinal nerves. Beginning at the top of the cord are 8 cervical nerves, 12 thoracic nerves, 5 lumbar nerves, 5 sacral nerves, and 1 coccygeal nerve.

A cross-section of the spinal cord reveals white matter on the periphery surrounding gray matter (H-shaped) at the center of the cord. In the center is a structure properly named the *central canal,* which runs the entire length of the spinal cord and contains CSF. The sides of the *H* are called *horns,* which are divided into the anterior, lateral, and posterior horns. White matter is organized into regions called *columns* (anterior, lateral, and posterior). Within the spinal cord is a collection of nerves running up and down in columns called *tracts.* Tracts are divided into two categories: (1) ascending and (2) descending. Sensory or afferent impulses travel up the cord to the brain on *ascending tracts,* and motor or efferent impulses travel down and out of the cord on *descending tracts.*

> *"I happen to feel that the degree of a*
> *person's intelligence is directly reflected*
> *by the number of conflicting attitudes she*
> *can bring to bear on the same topic."*
> Lisa Alter

BRAIN

One of the largest organs in the body, the **brain** contains an estimated 100 billion neurons. The brain is where sensory information is fused into character and behavior. The brain's unimpressive appearance gives no hints of its remarkable abilities. In the embryo, the skull forms before the brain is finished, which results in the forebrain *turning in* on it and mushrooming. *Sulci* are grooves in the outer layer of the brain (cortex), and *gyri* are elevated ridges of tissue. *Fissures* are specialized deep sulci that divide the brain into hemispheres and lobes. Twelve pairs of cranial nerves originate in the brain.

Brain cells can use glucose only as an energy source, and this glucose cannot be stored as glycogen, unlike the glucose stored by liver or muscle cells. Glucose breaks down only by aerobic respiration; thus the brain needs a continuous supply of both glucose and oxygen. The brain uses approximately 20% of the body's oxygen intake. Oxygen deprivation kills brain cells quickly, in as little as 1 to 2 minutes.

The brain consists of four main parts: (1) cerebrum, (2) diencephalon, (3) cerebellum, and (4) brainstem (Figure 17-8).

Cerebrum

Shaped as a boxing glove, the **cerebrum** is the largest part of the brain. This structure is where sensations (e.g., vision, smell, taste, body movements) are consciously perceived, where skeletal muscle motor movements are initiated, and where emotional and intellectual processes occur. This area is also where decisions are made. Sensory areas interpret sensory input, and motor areas control muscular movement. Language centers that interpret written and spoken words, as well as initiating speech, are located in the cerebrum. The limbic system within the cerebrum governs emotional aspects of behavior needed for survival, such as sexual feelings, rage, and docility.

The longitudinal fissure divides the cerebrum into two large (right and left) *cerebral hemispheres.* Connecting the two cerebral hemispheres are large fibrous bundles of transverse fibers, the **corpus callosum,** which provides a communicative pathway for impulses to move from one hemisphere to the other.

The *cerebral cortex* is a thin gray layer covering the outer portion of the cerebrum. White matter, which constitutes most of the cerebrum, lies beneath the cerebral cortex.

Within each hemisphere of the cerebrum are **lobes,** which are named for the bone beneath which each hemisphere lies (Figure 17-9).

White matter makes up the cerebral lobes.

- **Frontal lobe:** The *frontal lobe* regulates motor output, cognition, and speech production (Broca's area; typically the left hemisphere only).
- **Parietal lobe:** The *parietal lobes* govern somatosensory input (namely the skin and muscles) and taste. The postcentral gyrus featured in Chapter 12 in located here (see Figure 12-6).

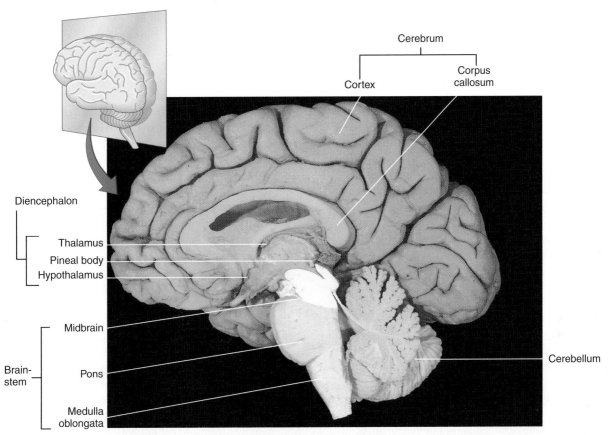

Cerebrum

Cortex

Corpus callosum

Diencephalon

Thalamus
Pineal body
Hypothalamus

Midbrain

Brain-stem

Pons

Medulla oblongata

Cerebellum

FIGURE 17-8 The cerebellum.

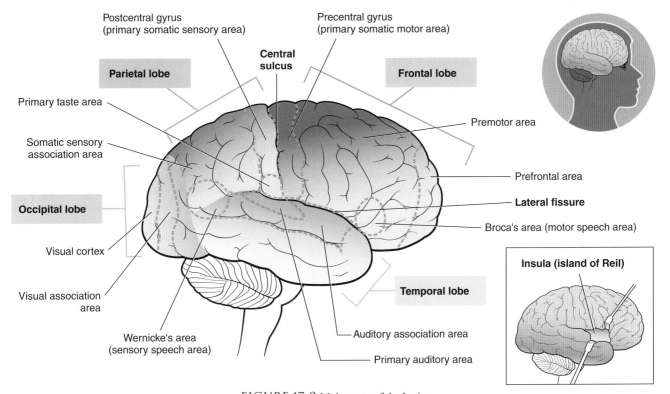

Postcentral gyrus (primary somatic sensory area)

Precentral gyrus (primary somatic motor area)

Central sulcus

Parietal lobe

Frontal lobe

Primary taste area

Premotor area

Somatic sensory association area

Prefrontal area

Occipital lobe

Lateral fissure

Visual cortex

Broca's area (motor speech area)

Visual association area

Temporal lobe

Insula (island of Reil)

Wernicke's area (sensory speech area)

Auditory association area

Primary auditory area

FIGURE 17-9 Main parts of the brain.

- **Temporal lobe:** The *temporal lobes* house an auditory and an olfactory area and Wernicke's area (an area critical to language comprehension that is typically in the left hemisphere only).
- **Occipital lobe:** The *occipital lobe* contains a center for visual input.
- **Insula:** Hidden by parts of the frontal, parietal, and temporal lobes is a structure called the *insula (island of Reil),* which is sometimes considered a fifth lobe of the cerebrum.

The *central sulcus* is located between the frontal and parietal lobes. The *lateral fissure* is located between the temporal lobe and the frontal and parietal lobes.

Specialization of Cerebral Hemispheres

The left and right cerebral hemispheres are similar in appearance. However, research indicates that they possess specialized functions. One of the best-known differences between the two is motor control; the right hemisphere controls the left half of the body, and the left hemisphere controls the right half of the body. These differences were discovered mainly through examination of patients who underwent surgery in an attempt to control seizures by severing the structure that connects the two hemispheres, the corpus callosum.

Several other interesting hemispheric differences were noted in these patients.

- **Left hemisphere:** The left hemisphere specializes in language, both receptive and expressive. It also governs some skilled and general hand movements such as gesturing.
- **Right hemisphere:** The right hemisphere specializes in the perception of nonspeech auditory sounds such as melodies, coughing, crying, and laughing better than the left hemisphere. The right hemisphere may also function better than the left at perceiving and visualizing spatial relationships

Despite the specializations of each cerebral hemisphere, both sides of a normal person's brain communicate with each other via the corpus callosum to accomplish the brain's many complex functions.

Electrical Brain Waves and States of Consciousness

Cerebral activity continues throughout an individual's life. In fact, life ceases when, or just before, cerebral activity ceases.

Brains waves are rhythmic electric impulses produced in the cerebral cortex and are recorded by an electroencephalogram (EEG). Scientists have noted four different types of brain wave patterns based on frequency and amplitude of the waves. Frequency is the number of waves per second and is referred to as *Hertz (Hz). Amplitude* refers to voltage. These waves are associated with various states of consciousness and are identified by Greek letters. Listed in order of frequency from fasted to slowest, these wave patterns are called *beta, alpha, theta,* and *delta.*

- **Beta:** The beta state (13 to 30 Hz) is associated with wakeful consciousness and mental activity. Attention is focused on external surroundings, and rational thinking,

some scattered thought patterns, and occasional distractions typify activity. High-intensity beta waves are associated with extreme stress. Beta waves are *busy* waves. Dreaming while sleeping (rapid eye movement [REM]) appears as beta waves.
- **Alpha:** The alpha state (8 to 12 Hz), in contrast to beta, are *relaxed* waves. The subject is awake but relaxed and nonattentive. Alpha activity is also associated with self-healing, creative processes, and meditation.
- **Theta:** The theta state (4 to 8 Hz) is associated with drowsiness, dreamlike awareness, collective subconscious, and out-of-body experiences. This state of consciousness is used to access deep-rooted memories. Theta waves are *drowsy* waves, but they can be easily aroused.
- **Delta:** The delta state (0.5 to 4 Hz) patterns are *deep sleep* waves from which one is not easily aroused.

Diencephalon

Located in the center of the brain, the **diencephalon** houses two primary structures: (1) thalamus and (2) hypothalamus. Included in the diencephalon are structures such as the pituitary and the pineal glands. The **thalamus,** which is nearly 80% of the diencephalon, relays sensory information (except olfaction) to appropriate parts of the cerebrum.

The **hypothalamus** regulates the ANS and endocrine system by governing the pituitary gland. It also controls behavioral patterns and the person's 24-hour cycle, called the *circadian rhythm.* It controls body hunger, thirst, anger, aggression, hormones, sexual behavior, temperature, and sleep patterns, and, along with the reticular activating system, it maintains consciousness.

The **pituitary gland** is connected to the hypothalamus by a slender stalk (infundibulum). It sits in the sella turcica of the sphenoid bone. The **pineal gland** is located below the corpus callosum. Although its function is not clear, the pineal gland produces and secretes the hormone melatonin. Both of these glands are discussed in the endocrine chapter (Figure 7-10).

Cerebellum

The **cerebellum** is a cauliflower-shaped structure located posterior and inferior to the cerebrum. The cerebellum is the second largest part of the brain and consists of two cerebellar hemispheres (see Figure 17-11).

Similar to the cerebrum, the cerebellum consists of a *cerebellar cortex* (thin outer layer of gray matter). The cerebellum is concerned with muscle tone, coordinates complex movements, and regulates posture and balance.

Brainstem

The **brainstem** is continuous with the spinal cord and has three main divisions: (1) midbrain, (2) pons, and (3) medulla oblongata (Figure 17-12).

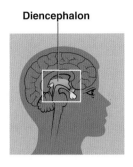
Diencephalon

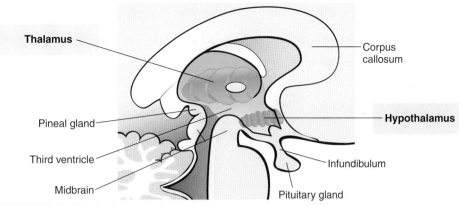

FIGURE 17-10 The diencephalon and surrounding structures.

The **midbrain** conducts nerve impulses from the cerebrum to the pons and sensory impulses from the spinal cord to the thalamus. It also has centers to control movements of the eyes, head, and neck in response to visual and auditory stimuli. The *substantia nigra* in the midbrain helps control movements as well because of its involvement with the release of the neurotransmitter dopamine. An area called the *reticular activating system* is found throughout the entire brainstem. It functions in waking the person up from sleep and maintaining consciousness. Also found in the midbrain is the *cerebral aqueduct,* a narrow canal conveying CSF between the third and fourth ventricles.

The **pons** relays nerve impulses from one side of the cerebellum to another. It also has areas that help control breathing. Four pairs of cranial nerves branch off the pons.

The most inferior portion of the brainstem, the **medulla oblongata,** conducts sensory and motor impulses between other parts of the brain and the spinal cord. The medulla oblongata contains much of the crossing-over fibers that cause the left cerebral hemisphere's association with the body's right side. Conversely, the right hemisphere is associated with the left side of the body.

The medulla, often considered the most vital part of the brain, contains the respiratory, cardiovascular, and vasomotor centers. The medulla also controls gastric secretions and reflexes such as sweating, sneezing, swallowing, and vomiting. Five pairs of cranial nerves branch from the medulla.

Blood-Brain Barrier

The **blood-brain barrier** is a selective semipermeable wall of blood capillaries with a thick basement membrane and neuroglial cells (astrocytes). The function of the blood-brain barrier is to prevent or slow down the passage of some chemical compounds and disease-causing organisms such as viruses from traveling from the blood into the CNS. Blood itself contains chemicals that can damage neurons; if blood comes into contact with neurons, they die.

PERIPHERAL NERVOUS SYSTEM

All nervous tissue outside the CNS is considered part of the PNS. Peripheral nerves arising from the brain are called *cranial nerves*, 12 pairs of them. Peripheral nerves arising from

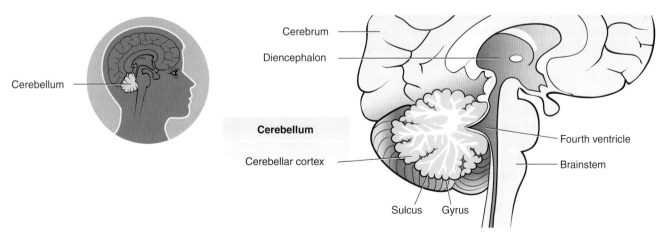

FIGURE 17-11 The cerebellum.

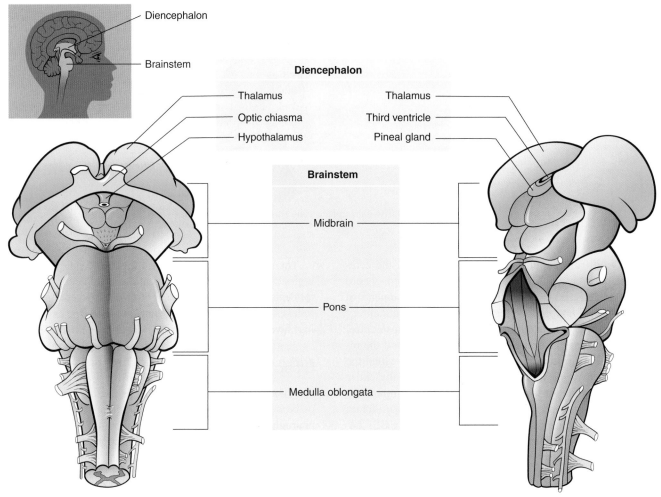

FIGURE 17-12 The brainstem and its relationship to the diencephalon.

the spinal cord are called *spinal nerves*, 31 pairs of them. Most of the peripheral nerves have sensory and motor neurons within them.

Spinal Nerves

Spinal nerves exit the spinal cord at the intervertebral foramen of the spinal column. These areas are openings at the pedicles for spinal roots to pass. Each pair of spinal nerves joins the spinal column at two points, one on the left and another on the right. Each spinal nerve of each pair has anterior and posterior roots. The anterior, or ventral, root contains motor neurons, and the posterior, or dorsal root, contains sensory neurons. A cluster of nerve cell bodies located in the PNS is called a **ganglion.** Most ganglia are located next to the spinal cord. The posterior root of the spinal nerve contains a cluster of sensory nerve cell bodies called the *posterior* or *dorsal root ganglions.*

All spinal nerves have sensory and motor components. When a spinal nerve exits the spinal cord, it divides into two branches: (1) anterior ramus and (2) posterior ramus. The anterior ramus innervates the extremities, lateral and anterior trunk, and superficial muscles of the back; the posterior ramus innervates the skin and deep muscles of the back.

Nerve Plexuses

A network of intersecting nerves in the PNS is called a **plexus.** The body contains many plexuses; the four most important ones are as follows:

- **Cervical plexus** (C1-C5) supplies the head and neck.
- **Brachial plexus** (C5-T1) supplies the arm and hand.
- **Lumbar plexus** (L1-L4) supplies the abdomen, low back, and genitalia.
- **Sacral plexus** (L4-S4) supplies the posterior hip, legs, and feet.

Dermatomes

A **dermatome** is an area of skin that a specific sensory nerve root serves (C2-S5) or one of three branches of the fifth cranial (trigeminal) nerve. Dermatomes are roughly the same from person to person, although sometimes a significant overlap in innervation is found between adjacent dermatomes. A map of the distribution of these nerves is called a *dermatome map* (Figure 17-13).

Myotomes

A **myotome** is a group of skeletal muscles innervated by a single spinal segment. Some overlap exists among myotomes (Figure 17-14).

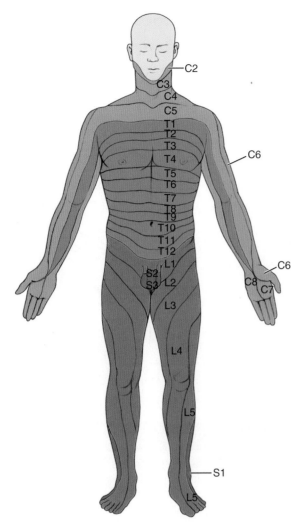

FIGURE 17-13 Dermatome map.

Figure 17-14 illustrates movements produced by skeletal muscles innervated by specific spinal nerves, as indicated by arrows.

Nerves of Importance to Massage Therapists
Some cranial nerves, spinal nerves, and plexuses can be compressed during massage (Figure 17-15).

During manual compression, the client may experience numbness, tingling, burning, or a shooting pain. Whether manual compression will damage the nerve is doubtful, but it may make your client feel uncomfortable. The following list details innervated muscles and organs:
Axillary nerve: deltoids and teres minor
Brachial plexus: C5 to T1 (supplies the arm and hand)
Common peroneal nerve: tibialis anterior, fibularis longus/brevis, extensor digitorum longus/brevis, extensor hallucis longus
Facial nerve: frontalis, occipitalis, orbicularis oris and oculi, buccinator, platysma, zygomaticus major and minor
Femoral nerve: iliacus, pectineus, sartorius fibularis, quadriceps femoris

Median nerve (great flexor): flexor digitorum superficialis/profundus, flexor carpi radialis, pronator teres/quadratus, palmaris longus, flexor pollicis longus/brevis, opponens pollicis, abductor pollicis longus/brevis
Lumbar plexus: L1 to L4 (supplies the abdomen, low back, and genitalia)
Musculocutaneous nerve: biceps brachii, brachialis, coracobrachialis
Obturator nerve: obturator externus, gracilis, adductor magnus, adductor longus, adductor brevis
Radial nerve (great extensor): triceps brachii, anconeus, brachioradialis, extensor carpi ulnaris, extensor carpi radialis longus/brevis, extensor digitorum, extensor indicis, extensor pollicis longus/brevis, extensor digiti minimi, supinator
Sciatic nerve: adductor magnus, bicep femoris (long head), piriformis, quadratus femoris, gemellus superior/inferior, obturator internus
Tibial nerve: gastrocnemius, soleus, plantaris, popliteus, tibialis posterior, flexor digitorum longus, flexor hallucis longus, bicep femoris (short head), semimembranous, semitendinosus
Ulnar nerve (accessory flexor): flexor digitorum superficialis/profundus, flexor carpi ulnaris, flexor digiti minimi brevis, flexor pollicis longus/brevis, opponens digiti minimi, abductor digiti minimi
Vagus nerve: heart, lungs, kidneys, gastrointestinal tract (accessory organs of digestion)

Cranial Nerves
The cranial nerves number 12 pairs. They emerge from the inferior surface of the brain and are named by Roman numerals (I though XII) or the area or areas they supply (Figure 17-16).
The cranial nerves are as follows:
I (olfactory): senses smell
II (optic): employs vision
III (oculomotor): moves the eyeball and eyelid; constricts the pupil
IV (trochlear): moves the eyeball
V (trigeminal) (great sensory nerve of the face and head): contains three branches for chewing, pain, and temperature
VI (abducens): moves the eyeball
VII (facial): makes facial expression; produces saliva and tears
VIII (vestibulocochlear) (auditory or acoustic): conveys messages of equilibrium and hearing (two branches to the inner ear)
IX (glossopharyngeal): produces saliva; employs taste and swallowing
X (vagus): receives sensations from the external ear and external auditory canal and thoracic and abdominal organs; aids digestion; helps regulate heart activity
XI (accessory) (spinal accessory): controls the tongue for speech and swallowing; innervates the trapezius and sternocleidomastoid
XII (hypoglossal): moves the tongue for speech and swallowing

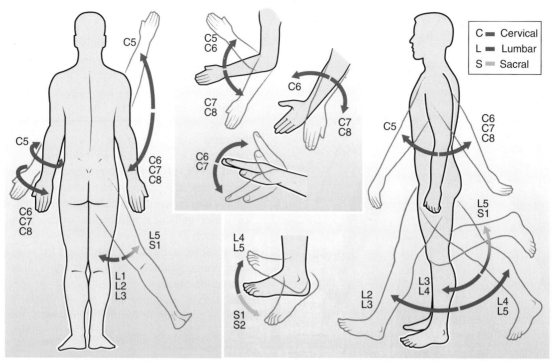

FIGURE 17-14 Myotome map.

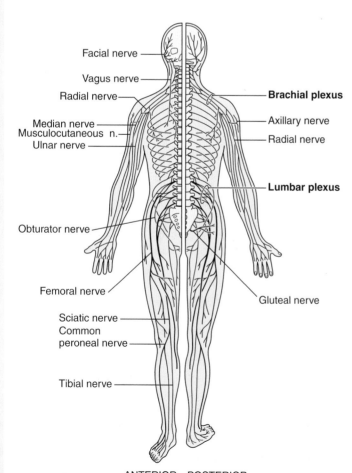

FIGURE 17-15 Nerves of importance to massage therapists.

Facial nerve

Vagus nerve

Radial nerve

Median nerve
Musculocutaneous n.
Ulnar nerve

Brachial plexus

Axillary nerve

Radial nerve

Lumbar plexus

Obturator nerve

Femoral nerve

Gluteal nerve

Sciatic nerve
Common
peroneal nerve

Tibial nerve

ANTERIOR   POSTERIOR

TABLE TALK

The mnemonic device for remembering the names of the 12 cranial nerves is, "Oh, oh, oh! To touch and feel very green vegetables, ah!" (olfactory, optic, oculomotor, trochlear, trigeminal, abducens, facial, vestibulocochlear, glossopharyngeal, vagus, accessory, and hypoglossal), or "On old Olympus's towering tops, a Finn and German viewed some hops" (olfactory, optic, oculomotor, trochlear, trigeminal, abducens, facial, auditory, glossopharyngeal, vagus, spinal accessory, and hypoglossal).

AUTONOMIC NERVOUS SYSTEM: PARASYMPATHETIC AND SYMPATHETIC

As a review, the PNS contains two divisions: (1) the SNS and (2) the ANS. The SNS has sensory neurons that carry information to the CNS. The ANS innervates smooth muscle, cardiac muscle, and glands, and it controls the circulation of blood, activity of the gastrointestinal tract, body temperature, respiration rate, and many other functions (Figure 17-17).

The hypothalamus regulates the activity of the ANS.

Within the ANS are two divisions: (1) the *sympathetic nervous system* and (2) the *parasympathetic nervous system*. The effects of these two systems on the visceral organs are complementary (one system excites, and the other system inhibits) because nerves from both divisions supply many of the same organs. This complementary relationship controls the body's internal organs in a way to maintain homeostasis (Table 17-1).

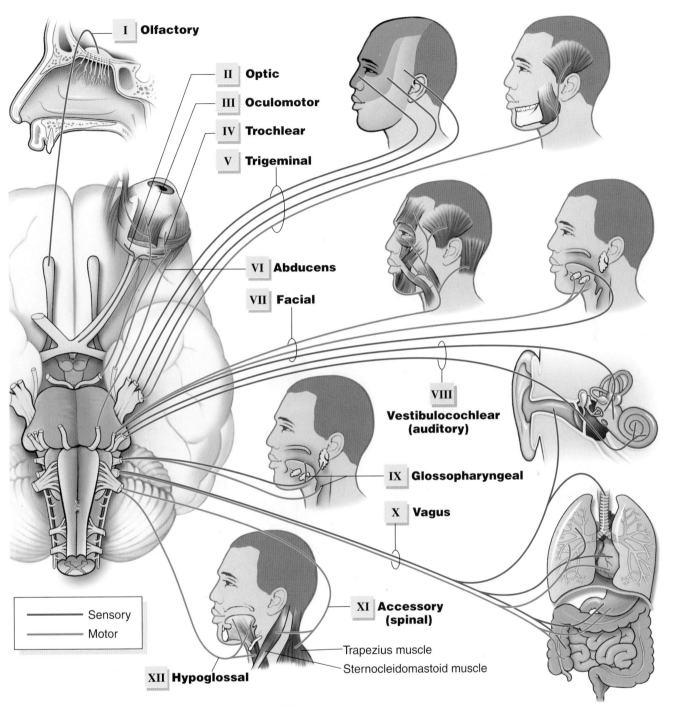

I	**Olfactory**	
II	**Optic**	
III	**Oculomotor**	
IV	**Trochlear**	
V	**Trigeminal**	
VI	**Abducens**	
VII	**Facial**	
VIII	**Vestibulocochlear (auditory)**	
IX	**Glossopharyngeal**	
X	**Vagus**	
XI	**Accessory (spinal)**	
XII	**Hypoglossal**	

Sensory
Motor

Trapezius muscle
Sternocleidomastoid muscle

FIGURE 17-16 Cranial nerves.

Some structures have only sympathetic innervation (adrenal glands and blood vessels); some structures have only parasympathetic innervation (lacrimal apparatus). In extreme fear, both systems may act simultaneously, producing involuntary emptying of the bladder and rectum and a generalized sympathetic response.

Parasympathetic Nervous System

The nickname of the **parasympathetic** division is the *rest-and-digest* division; it dominates at rest and supports body functions that conserve and restore body energy, such as di-

gestion. Because the parasympathetic nervous system is most active under calm conditions and stimulates visceral organs for normal functions as it maintains homeostasis, it is also referred to as the *housekeeping system*. Body processes in parasympathetic mode include salivation, urination, digestive processes, defecation, and storing nutrients to be used later.

The fibers of the parasympathetic nervous system occupy spaces at the spinal cord level S2 to S4 and cranial nerves III, VII, IX, and X. For this reason, the parasympathetic nervous system is often called *craniosacral outflow*.

During stressful situations, the sympathetic nervous system narrows the perceptual field to facilitate the fight-or-flight

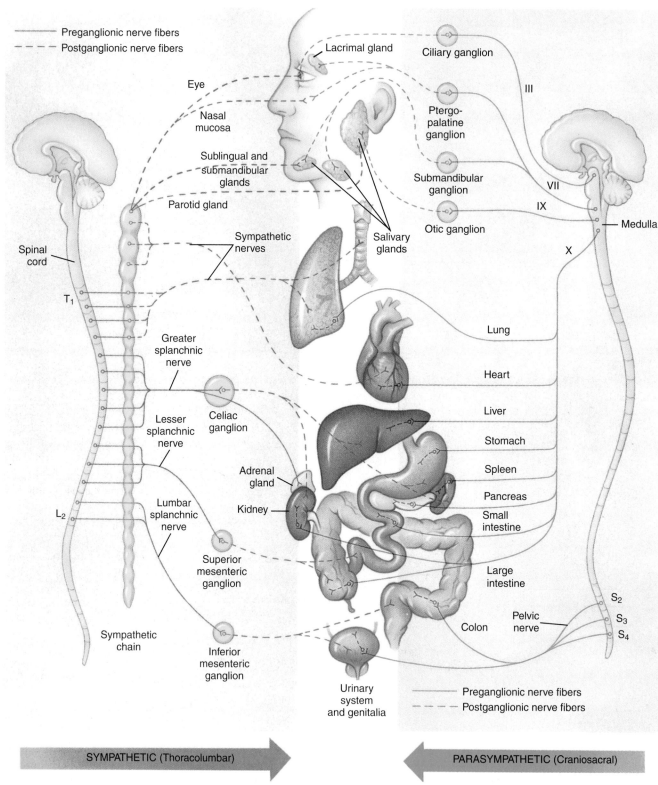

FIGURE 17-17 Divisions of the autonomic nervous system.

fight or flight

Rest + Digest

response. In contrast, during times of rest and relaxation, the parasympathetic nervous system broadens the perceptual field. One gift of parasympathetic response that occurs during a massage is that, in the client's relaxed state, he or she can often contemplate additional options or solutions to life's challenges.

Sympathetic Nervous System

The sympathetic division overrides the parasympathetic division during physical exertion or emotional stress; thus it has the nickname of the *fight-or-flight* division. **Sympathetic** responses require body energy. Effects include pupil

TABLE 17-1 Typical Autonomic Nervous System Reactions

SYMPATHETIC ACTIVITY	PARASYMPATHETIC ACTIVITY
Increases heart rate and strength of contraction	Decreases heart rate and strength of contraction
Increases respiratory rate	Maintains resting respiratory rate
Facilitates bronchiolar dilation	Facilitates bronchial constriction
Releases glucose from liver; raises blood sugar	No effect
Facilitates blood vessel constriction (skin and viscera); raises blood pressure and loss of skin color	No effect
Facilitates blood vessel dilation (skeletal muscles and heart)	Facilitates coronary blood vessel dilation; no effect on skeletal muscle blood vessels
Facilitates blood vessel dilation of external genitalia, causing erection	Facilitates blood vessel contraction of external genitalia
Facilitates pupillary dilation; accommodates far vision	Facilitates pupillary constriction; accommodates near vision
Increases perspiration	No effect
No effect on tearing of eyes	Stimulates tearing of eyes
Inhibits salivation	Stimulates salivation
Inhibits pancreatic secretions	Stimulates pancreatic secretions and that of insulin
Decreases gastrointestinal motility (inhibits digestion)	Increases gastrointestinal motility
Facilitates constriction of gastrointestinal tract sphincters	Facilitates relaxation of gastrointestinal tract sphincters
Inhibits urination	Stimulates urination
Facilitates stimulation of adrenal glands to release epinephrine and norepinephrine	No effect

dilation; an increase in heart rate, force of heart contraction, and in blood pressure; dilation of airways; and constriction of blood vessels in the digestive tract so more blood can be moved to dilated blood vessels in the active skeletal muscles and the heart. All reactions of the sympathetic division occur quickly. Processes that are not needed for meeting the stressful situation, such as movements and secretions of the digestive tract, are suppressed.

The nerves of this divisions cause the adrenal gland to secrete epinephrine, which sustains the actions of the sympathetic nervous system through the endocrine system.

Most of the cell bodies of the sympathetic system lie in a paravertebral chain of ganglia at the level of T1 to L2. For this reason, the sympathetic nervous system is often called *thoracolumbar outflow.*

> *"The word* crisis *is written with two characters in Chinese. One symbol represents danger and the other stands for opportunity."*
> Robert Cantor

SENSE ORGANS

All receptors for sense organs arise from ectoderm (the cellular layer from which the brain and spinal cord arise). Aristotle was the first to enumerate the five senses. Four of the five senses reside in the head and are called *special senses.* Touch, also known as a *general sense,* involves the entire body. In this section, the sense organs are briefly discussed.

General Sense Organs

The sense of touch is an amalgamation of specialized receptors found in the skin. The skin can perceive heat, cold, pressure, pain, and movement. Indeed, touch is not one sense

but many. Specific receptors are discussed in the section on mechanoreceptors.

Touch is the most primitive of all sensations. Among the many studies that have been conducted, touch is the earliest sensory system to become functional in the human embryo. When the embryo is less than 6 weeks of age, measuring less than an inch long from crown to rump, light stroking of the upper lip or wings of the nose will cause bending of the neck and trunk away from the source of stimulation. At this stage of gestation, neither the eyes nor ears have developed.

Taste

Mediated by taste buds *(gustatory organs),* taste is a collection of chemosensitive receptors concentrated on projections on the tongue called *papillae.* Within each papilla are *taste hairs* extending from *taste pores* (Figure 17-18).

These hairs are attached to a *taste cell* that supports chemoreceptors, which become aroused when a molecule of a particular size and shape enters the receptor site, similar to a lock-and-key mechanism. The taste cell rests in the taste bud surrounded by supporting cells.

Most textbooks assert that these four primary tastes (salty, sweet, bitter, and sour) are localized in specific regions on the tongue, but new research indicates that more taste receptors exist than the four primaries. The perception of taste is a combination of impulses from many taste receptors. The input from one receptor means little without the combined information from other receptors, just as the letter *K* is relatively meaningless without surrounding letters to form a word.

Taste is strongly influenced by the sense of smell. Tasting food without scent molecules is difficult (cold food does not have as much taste as hot food). A condition such as

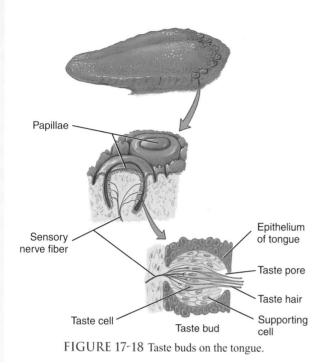

FIGURE 17-18 Taste buds on the tongue.

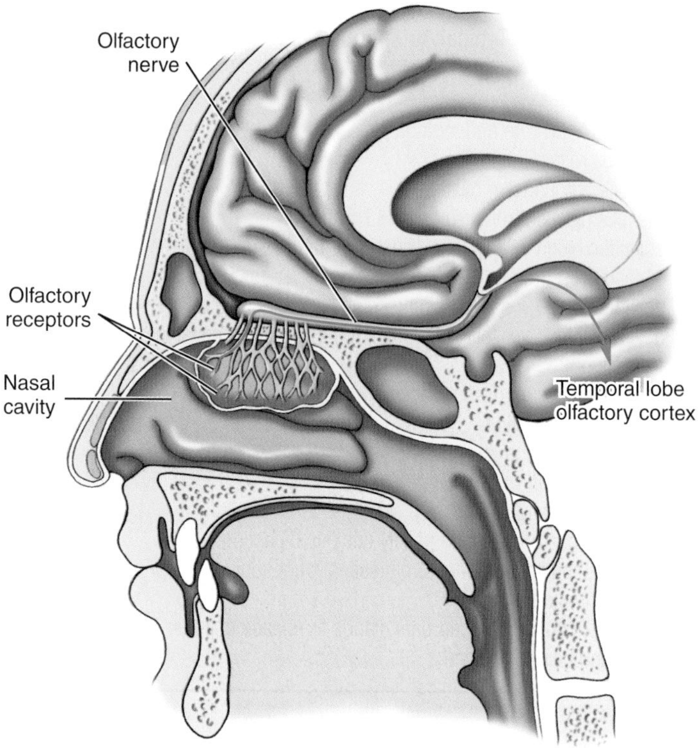

FIGURE 17-19 Olfaction.

a cold often interferes with the sense of smell, and taste is inhibited.

Olfaction

Olfaction (sense of smell) uses chemoreceptors to detect odors. The cell bodies of olfactory receptors are found in the superior nasal cavity, and dendritic extensions are located in the nasal mucosa. Inhalation forces airborne molecules to the mucous layer, where they dissolve and come into contact with the chemosensitive receptors. Once certain gaseous chemical molecules fit into the correct receptor site, nerve impulses are created, and impulses of odor are sent to the olfactory bulb, to the olfactory nerve, and then to the temporal lobe of the cerebrum. Scientists suggest that humans can detect between 7 and 32 primary odors—for example, ether, camphor, musk, floral, mint, pungent, and putrid. Smell plays an important role in sexual behavior for most mammals and is the strongest sense linked to memories (Figure 17-19).

Vision

Vision uses photoreceptors (rods and cones) that are located in the eye. Light enters the eye through the pupil (opening in the center of the iris) and strikes the retina, which is essentially a membranous screen composed of delicate nervous tissue at the rear of the eye (Figure 17-20).

The photoreceptors on the retina convert light energy into nerve impulses, which are transmitted to the brain through the optic nerve for visual interpretation. A point near the thalamus and hypothalamus where portions of each optic nerve cross over is called the *optic chiasm*. A blind spot exists where the optic nerve exits the retina, but this does not affect vision because of the existence of two eyes, and the blind spots do not coincide with each other.

TABLE TALK

Terms of Sight Conditions

Astigmatism: Condition in which the eyeball in not spherical, thus the images and light rays striking the retina are not clearly in focus. Use of vision may cause eye discomfort caused by the blurred vision. Specially ground eye glasses can correct the problem.
Emmetropia: Normal vision
Hyperopia: Farsightedness
Myopia: Nearsightedness
Presbyopia: Farsightedness that often develops with advancing age

Hearing

Hearing is achieved by the detection of sound waves or vibrations via mechanoreceptors. Sound waves hit the *tympanic membrane* (eardrum) at the back of the auditory canal. The membrane, which separates the outer ear from the middle ear, vibrates as a drum at the same frequency as the sound waves striking the membrane. These waves are transmitted through three small bones (ossicles) in the middle ear: (1) malleus (hammer), (2) incus (anvil), and (3) stapes

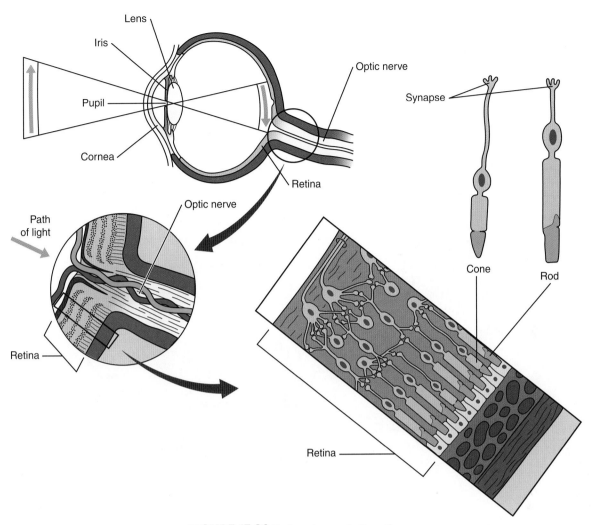

FIGURE 17-20 Rods and cones in the retina.

(stirrup). These bones are the smallest bones in the body. The vibration of these three small bones is relayed to the oval window.

The *oval window* is a membrane that covers the opening to a coiled, fluid-filled cavity (cochlea) of the inner ear. From here, sound waves travel through fluid in the cochlear duct (endolymph). Within the cochlea are three fluid-filled *semicircular canals*. The waves of fluid are interpreted as sound (Figure 17-21).

Two characteristics of sound are pitch and volume. *Pitch* is the quality of a tone or sound, which depends on vibration speed; slow vibrations produce deep sounds, and fast vibrations produce high sounds. The ability to hear high-pitched sounds may decline with age. *Volume* is the loudness of sound and can change without altering pitch.

Ears also play a large part in balance and equilibrium. Within the semicircular canals are gel-filled sacs containing special mechanoreceptors that resemble hair cells. When the sacs of the ear are turned to a new position, the hair cells bend. This action results in an impulse to the vestibulocochlear nerve, notifying the brain of the change of position.

TYPES OF SENSORY RECEPTORS

Special sensory receptors in the body detect certain types of sensory information. They can be classified by location and are exteroceptors, proprioceptors, and interoceptors.

- **Exteroceptors:** These sensory nerve endings are located in the skin, mucous membranes, and sense organs, responding to stimuli originating from outside of the body, such as touch, pressure, or sound.
- **Proprioceptors:** This group is located in the skin, ears, muscles, tendons, joints, and fascia and responds to movement and position.
- **Interoceptors:** Also known as *visceroceptors,* these receptors are located in the viscera and respond to stimuli originating from within the body regarding the function of the internal organs, such as digestion, excretion, and blood pressure.

Sensory receptors can also be classified by the stimuli detected. These receptors are chemoreceptors, mechanoreceptors, thermoreceptors, photoreceptors, and nociceptors (Figure 17-22).

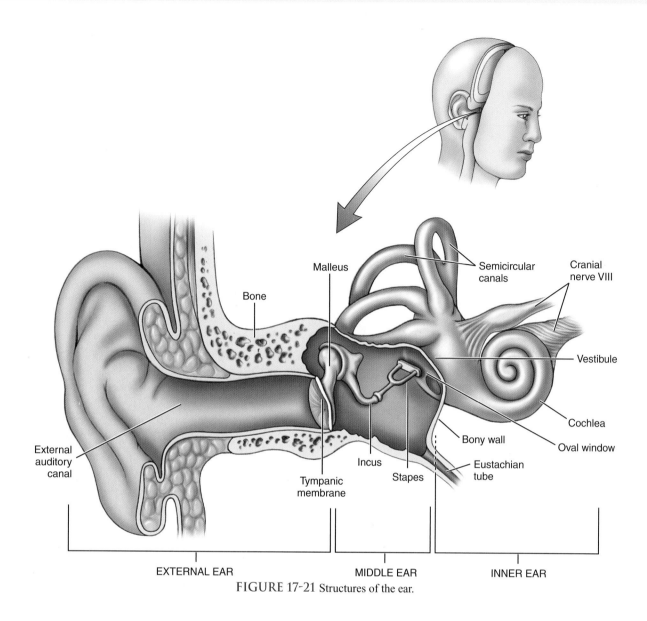

FIGURE 17-21 Structures of the ear.

All initiate nerve impulses but differ in the nature of the stimuli that initiates an impulse (e.g., chemical, pressure, light, heat, pain).

Receptors often exhibit a functional mechanism called adaptation. When a stimulus is constant, over time, **adaptation,** a decrease in sensitivity to a prolonged stimulus, may occur. Adaptation tends to be rapid regarding pressure, touch, and smell. We become accustomed to the weight of our clothes during the day, and an odor that offended us when we first entered the room is no longer detected at the end of the day.

Adaptation occurs slowly with pain and body position. This characteristic is a protective mechanism that prevents us from becoming accustomed to severe pain or from keeping our bodies in awkward, potentially harmful, body positions.

Chemoreceptors

Located in the nose, tongue, within the walls of certain arteries, and in the brain, **chemoreceptors** are activated by chemical stimuli and detect smells, tastes, and changes in blood chemistry.

Chemoreceptors that are sensitive to changes in pH and carbon dioxide concentration are located in the aorta, carotid arteries, and medulla oblongata. If oxygen is low or carbon dioxide is high, the chemoreceptors stimulate the medulla oblongata to increase respiration rate.

Mechanoreceptors

Mechanoreceptors respond to mechanical stimuli and are found in the skin, blood vessels, ears, muscles, tendons, joints, and fascia. They detect sensations such as tactile pressure, blood pressure, vibration, stretching, muscular contraction, proprioception, sound, and equilibrium. Mechanoreceptors include various touch, pressure, and stretch receptors.

- **Touch and pressure receptors:** Examples of these receptors are Meissner, Ruffini's, and Pacinian corpuscles and Krause end bulbs. Also included are Merkel disks and hair root plexus. These structures are discussed in Chapter 12.
- **Stretch receptors:** The most important stretch receptors are muscle spindles and Golgi tendon organs.

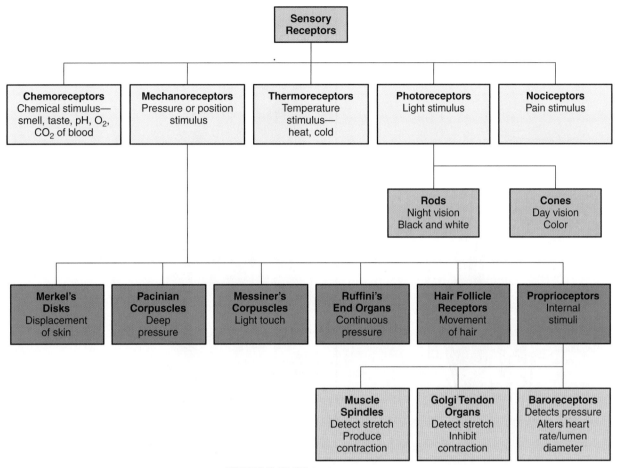

FIGURE 17-22 Sensory receptors.

- **Muscle spindle:** Muscle spindles are stretch-sensitive receptors wrapped around *intrafusal* muscle fibers and monitor changes in muscle length, as well as the rate of this change (Figure 17-23). When muscles are stretched rapidly or are overstretched (ballistic stretches), muscle spindles activate and cause reflexive contraction. Referred to as a *stretch reflex,* this action guards against tissue damage by counteracting sudden muscle lengthening.

A therapist may use the stretch reflex when strengthening a weak antagonist. For example, if a client has rounded shoulders, then the pectoralis major may be tight, whereas the rhomboids are weak. During treatment, use hacking tapotement across the fibers of the rhomboids to create minute muscle contractions. Along with weight training, strengthening of the rhomboids may pull the shoulders back for a more balanced posture.

- **Golgi tendon organ:** Located at musculotendinous junctions are Golgi tendon organs, which are activated by both tension and slow stretch (Figure 17-24).

These organs respond by inhibiting motor neurons if muscle tension is too high. Referred to as a *tendon reflex,* this protective mechanism helps ensure that muscles do not contract too strongly and damage their tendons. The stimulated Golgi tendon organs cause inhibition of contraction throughout the entire muscle.

The tendon reflex may also be used during massage treatment. Plucking the tendons perpendicularly tricks the Golgi tendon organs into thinking a load is present and reduces muscular tension. This technique is also called the *transverse tendon technique (triple T)* and enhances muscular relaxation by inhibiting contraction.

Baroreceptor

Stretch receptors located in the wall of the carotid arteries and aortic arch are called *baroreceptors.* These pressure-sensitive receptor cells affect blood pressure by sending impulses to the cardiac and vasomotor center in the medulla oblongata. Rates of neural firing are determined by pressure exerted on vessel walls. An increase in firing indicates an increase in blood pressure; a decrease in firing indicates decreased blood pressure. The CNS responds by stimulating the ANS; this action either increases or decreases the heart rate and vessel wall diameter.

Photoreceptors

Photoreceptors are sensitive to light. The two types of photoreceptors are rods and cones, which are located in the retina. The **retina** is a delicate nervous tissue membrane of the eye, which is continuous with the optic nerve. Each retina possesses more than 100 million rods and 3 million cones.

- **Rods:** These slender rodlike projections are sensitive to dim light and shades of black, white, and gray. Notice how difficult it is to determine color and detail in dim light.

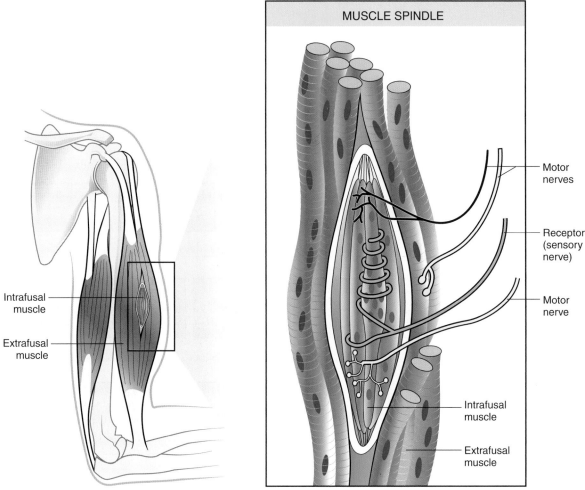

FIGURE 17-23 Muscle spindle.

- **Cones:** These structures are needed for color vision; they are short and thick with blunt projections. Most cones are found in the center of the retina, where very few rod cells are located. This area is designated for acute, detailed vision partly because blood vessels do not exist there and thus color vision is not hindered.

Cones and rods function in a similar way. Three variations of cones exist, and each is sensitive to a different light wavelength (blue, red, and green). Combinations of these three colors give us an entire color spectrum. If all color pigments are activated, then white is perceived; if no color pigments are activated, then black is seen.

Nociceptors

Also referred to as *free nerve endings,* **nociceptors** detect pain and are located in almost every tissue of the body, especially near the surface. The brain lacks nociceptors; however, other tissues of the cranium, such as the meninges and blood vessels, have a large supply of them.

Nociceptors serve a protective function and rarely adapt. If they adapted to pain stimuli, then pain would stop being sensed, and irreparable damage might result. In some cases, nociceptors may continue to fire even after the painful stimulus is removed.

Nociceptors also respond to stimuli that cause tissue damage, to irritants (e.g., ones released by injured cells), and to overstimulation or excessive stimuli (e.g., excessive heat, bright light, loud sound, intense mechanical stimulation such as excessive pressure), which is often the first indication of injury or disease. Pain may cause reflexive withdrawal of the involved body segments. Pain may cause sympathetic arousal, such as changes in heartbeat and blood pressure.

In most instances, pain is felt at the point of stimulation. However, a client may have **referred pain,** which can be experienced as sensations such as tingling, numbness, itching, aching, heat, or cold. Visceral pain may be sensed in the area over the organ or projected to another area of the body. In many instances, the same spinal segment (Hilton's law, Box 17-1) innervates these areas. For example, the pain of angina may cause pain down the left arm resulting from a common spinal nerve connection.

Thermoreceptors

Located immediately under the skin, **thermoreceptors** include two types of free nerve endings: (1) one that detects cold and (2) one that detects heat. Cold receptors are 10 times more numerous than heat receptors and are stimulated by

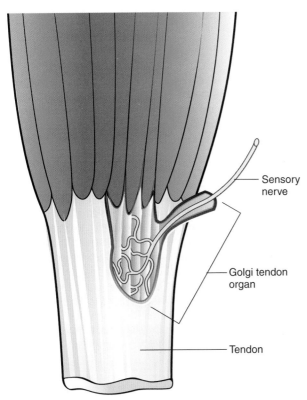

FIGURE 17-24 Golgi tendon organ.

lowering temperatures. Rising temperatures stimulate heat receptors. Once temperature falls below 10° C (50° F) or rises above 45° C (113° F), nociceptors rather than thermoreceptors are activated.

PATHOLOGICAL CONDITIONS OF THE NERVOUS SYSTEM

Pathological conditions involving the special senses are included in this section. Because the nervous system involves cognition, emotional and mental disorders are included in this section as well. Some of these conditions are related to a person's response to life's challenges, some are age related, some are linked to chemical imbalances, and some are associated with genetics.

Alzheimer's Disease

Alzheimer's disease is characterized by confusion, memory failure, disorientation, restlessness, delusions, speech disturbances, and an inability to carry out purposeful movements. Persons with Alzheimer's disease may refuse food, lose bowel or bladder control, and become delirious or violent. The disease usually begins in late middle life, with slight defects in memory and behavior, and then gradually progresses. *Use techniques to prevent joint stiffening and muscle contractures and to maintain mobility. Allow client to determine treatment length, but do not exceed 90 minutes.*

Anxiety Disorders

Acute or generalized anxiety disorders are episodes of severe intense anxiety and panic, with symptoms ranging from tachycardia, chest pains, nausea, and vertigo to faintness, profuse sweating, trembling, chills or hot flashes, and shortness of breath, with feelings of choking or smothering. Attacks typically have a sudden onset, lasting from a few seconds to an hour, and they vary in frequency from several times a day to once a month. Clients with anxiety disorders are often taking prescription medications to treat symptoms. *Massage is indicated. Obtain name and telephone number of contact person and physician in case panic attack occurs during treatment.*

Bell's Palsy

Bell's palsy produces unilateral facial paralysis of sudden onset resulting from inflammation of cranial nerve VII (facial nerve). The cause of the inflammation is usually unknown, but it may be caused by trauma to the nerve, a tumor compressing the nerve, or an unknown infection within the nerve. Paralysis causes distortion of the face and may be so severe that the person may not be able to close an eye or control salivation on the affected side. The symptoms may be transient (lasting only a few months) or permanent. *Use light pressure on face, directed upwards; include strokes used to stimulate muscles contraction.*

Bipolar Disorder

Bipolar disorder is a mood disorder in which both depressive and manic episodes occur. One or the other phase may be predominating. Characteristics of the *depressive phase* are underactivity, fatigue, an increased need for sleep, apathy, feelings of deep loneliness, sadness, guilt, and reduced self-esteem. Characteristics of the *manic phase* are limitless energy, hyperactivity, extreme emotional outbursts, the inability to concentrate, decreased need for sleep, excitement, euphoria, and elation, as well as delusions of grandeur. *Massage is indicated. Obtain name and telephone number of contact person and physician in case panic attack occurs during treatment.*

Carpal Tunnel Syndrome

Carpal tunnel syndrome is a painful repetitive strain injury of the hand and wrist caused by compression of the median nerve by the transverse carpal ligament. Tendinous sheaths may become swollen and irritated through an improper arm-to-wrist angle and overuse. As these tendons become irritated, extra synovial fluid is secreted. The accumulated fluid compresses the median nerve. Chronic inflammation causes the tendon sheath to thicken, compounding the problem. *Local contraindication of inflamed area. If chronic, then use techniques to reduce edema (e.g., elevating the limb, centripetal effleurage, lymphatic drainage). Use moist heat, cross-fiber friction, and passive movement of*

BOX 17-1

Neurological Laws: Presentation and Discussion

Arndt's Law (Rudolf Arndt, German Psychiatrist, 1735-1900)

Weak stimuli excite physiological activity, moderately strong ones favor it, strong ones retard it, and very strong ones arrest it.

Arndt's law applies to the physiological effects of stress and relaxation (massage). Strong stimuli such as pain and trigger points disrupt normal functioning. Muscle tonus may become increased, digestive functions may be inhibited, and blood pressure may rise. Massage, being a weak but pleasurable stimulus, helps return the body to homeostasis.

Davis's Law

If muscle ends are brought closer together, the pull of tonus is increased, thereby shortening the muscle, which may even cause hypertrophy. If muscle ends are separated beyond normal, then tonus is lessened or lost, thereby weakening the muscle.

Davis's law is an example of the body preferring balance to extremes and can be observed in various situations. The increase in muscle tonus gained by weight lifting is the result of repetitive contractions. However, chronic shortening can produce spasms, such as a muscle that has stayed in a shortened position for extended periods (e.g., sleeping on the stomach with ankles in full extension, wearing shoes with high heels). The opposite extreme can occur when muscles have been overstretched in an accident, exceeding their normal limit (e.g., whiplash). The microtrauma of tearing many muscle fibers often causes a loss of strength and increase in muscle flaccidity. Each of these scenarios can effectively be addressed with massage and joint mobilizations.

Hilton's Law (John Hilton, English Surgeon, 1804-1878)

A nerve trunk that supplies a joint also supplies the muscles of the joint and the skin over the insertions of such muscles.

Hilton's law is significant for the massage therapist, especially when combined with Arndt's law. Each nerve trunk supplies both sensory information and motor control for joints, muscles, vessels, skin, and organs in a given area. Pain in this area results in a physiopathological reflex arc, which generates a spontaneous increase in motor impulses, sending signals of the pain to the cord. The increased motor stimuli cause vasoconstriction, a decrease in visceral function, an increase in muscular tonus, and an increase in intrajoint pressure. Arndt's law states that strong stimuli retard or arrest physiological activity.

The advantage of Hilton's law for the massage therapist is that massage not only produces the direct effects of increasing local circulation, relaxing muscle fiber, and calming stimulated nerves, but also has the indirect effect of interrupting the physiopathological reflex arc. As the pain subsides because of disruption of strong stimuli, normal function returns.

Pfluger's Laws (Edward Friederich Wilhelm Pfluger, German Physiologist, 1829-1910)

Although not specifically stated, Pfluger's laws are (1) progressive in nature and (2) dependent on the degree of irritation to the nerve. *Progressive* refers to the fact that the laws are experienced *in order*—that is, a client begins experiencing the *law of unilaterality* and, if left untreated, can proceed through each of the succeeding laws until the *law of generalization* is reached. This concept does not mean that every client experiences the effects of all five laws; progression is dependent on the degree of irritation to the nerve. Clients with minor injuries may experience only the *law of unilaterality*, whereas others may progress to the *law of symmetry*, the *law of intensity*, and so on.

Law of Unilaterality

If a mild irritation is applied to one or more sensory nerves, then the movement takes place usually on one side only—the side that is irritated.

The word *movement* in Pfluger's laws refers primarily to motor reflexes responding to a stimulus. Increased tonus occurs first on the side of the body reporting pain or injury. Motor reflexes tighten muscles on the affected side, limit range of motion as a protective mechanism, and prevent further injury (muscular splinting). Constriction of vessels prevents internal bleeding in muscular tears.

Law of Symmetry

If the stimulation is sufficiently increased, then motor reaction is exhibited not only by the irritated side but also in similar muscles on the opposite side of the body.

When an injury is left untreated on one side of the body, the symptoms begin to migrate to its opposite side. Spasms in the right levator scapulae, if not addressed, increase in intensity. Eventually, the body seeks to reduce some of this sensory input (pain) by directing it to motor nerves on the opposite side of the body. The result is a general

---

the elbow, wrist, and finger joints. Identify and avoid risk factors (e.g., improper arm-to-wrist angle, excessive wrist flexion).

Cataract

Cataracts are a partial or complete lack of transparency in the lens or lens capsule of the eye that can impair vision or cause blindness. A gray-white opaqueness can be seen within the lens and behind the pupil. Most cataracts occur after a person is 50 years of age. The tendency to develop cataracts is inherited. However, trauma, such as a puncture

wound to the eyes or blow to the head, excess exposure to sunlight, and diabetes mellitus, may later result in cataract formation. *If the client is visually impaired, then explain everything that happens during the massage verbally. For more information, see section on visual impairments in Chapter 10.*

Cerebral Palsy

This group of motor disorders produces muscular incoordination and loss of muscle control. It is caused by damage to the brain's motor areas during fetal life, birth, or infancy.

BOX 17-1—cont'd

Neurological Laws: Presentation and Discussion—cont'd

Law of Symmetry—cont'd
increase of tonus in the left levator scapulae and other muscles the nerve innervates.

Law of Intensity
Reflex movements are usually more intense on the side of irritation. At times, the movements of the opposite side equal them in intensity, but they are usually less pronounced.

Pfluger's *law of intensity* states that irritation (pain) increases in intensity on both sides of the body, but the pain is greater on the initial side of irritation and discomfort.

Law of Radiation
If the excitation continues to increase, then it is propagated upward, and reactions take place through centrifugal nerves coming from the cord segments higher up.

Again, if left untreated, the discomfort grows, and the client proceeds from one law to the next. The body seeks to dissipate more sensory input (pain), directing it to motor nerves higher up the cord, such as a tight shoulder radiating to the neck musculature.

Law of Generalization
When the irritation becomes very intense, it is propagated in the medulla oblongata, which becomes a focus from which stimuli radiate to all parts of the cord, causing a general increase of tonus in all muscles of the body.

This law represents a client in chronic pain, having a longstanding history of pain and limited range of motion. The *law of generalization* seldom applies for something similar to a tight levator and is usually reserved for clients with problems such as chronic low back pain. Once the medulla is involved, the internuncial pool of the entire spinal cord is excited, causing pain and increased tonus to all muscles. Clients with chronic pain may experience severe headaches, neck and shoulder stiffness, arm pain, and the expected back and sciatic pain. The goal of the massage therapist is to reduce the sensory stimulation and muscle tonus to a point at which the client begins to back down the scale of Pfluger's laws and symptoms abate. Hydrotherapy, in conjunction with massage therapy, is an excellent modality for clients who have advanced to this stage of pain.

Sherrington's Law (Sir Charles Scott Sherrington, English Physician, 1857-1952)
When a muscle receives a nerve impulse to contract, its antagonist simultaneously receives an impulse to relax.

Sherrington's law is also known as *reciprocal inhibition*. Moving would be difficult if all muscles contracted at the same time. In fact, if opposing muscles were both able to contract simultaneously, the weaker of the two would be torn. Reciprocal inhibition ensures that when an agonist is creating movement, its antagonist cooperates by elongating. In a client with normal neurological function, these two impulses automatically occur simultaneously.

Massage therapists can apply this principle to turn off messages of contraction in acute muscle cramps. For example, when the hamstrings are experiencing a muscle cramp, the cramp might be relieved by forcibly contracting their antagonists, the quadriceps femoris. This task is best accomplished through active resistance (isometric contraction). Maintain the contraction for 10 to 20 seconds, then release. Repeat three times.

Law of Facilitation
When an impulse has passed once through a certain set of neurons to the exclusion of others, it tends to take the same course on future occasions, and each time it traverses this path, the resistance is less.

The repetition of a particular action ingrains a habit between the brain and muscles. Pain from postural distortions and improper movement patterns are often habitual. The best way to break a bad habit is to replace it with a good one. Massage helps reprogram nerves by giving them new information via experience. The client can move differently because he or she has felt something different. The form of massage used really does not matter, as long as it is not perceived as painful to the client because pain triggers a protective response.

A client with a first-degree tear of the right supraspinatus may not be able to raise his or her arm above shoulder level. Even after the tear has healed, the previous experience of pain and limited movement prevents full range of motion. However, if the therapist treats the injury with massage and passively ranges the arm without going through the pain barrier, then the brain is reprogrammed to accept the movement pattern once again. By repeating passive movements several times, neural messages cross certain synapses repeatedly. The message can then easily begin taking that particular route in the future.

Causes include rubella infection, toxemia, or malnutrition during pregnancy or damage during birth in which oxygen to the fetus is reduced. Cerebral palsy is not progressive; however, the damage is irreversible. Intelligence is usually not affected, but speech is impaired. The muscles may be spastic and hyperexcitable. Even small movements, touch, muscle stretch, pain, or emotional stress can increase spasticity. ***Obtain physician clearance if symptoms are severe. Position client for comfort. Do not force muscles into a stretch. If client is unable to speak, then devise a code to communicate. If client uses a wheelchair, then determine if treatment needs to be performed while client is in the chair. For*** *more information, see section on wheelchair-bound clients in Chapter 10.*

Dementia

A cognitive disorder, dementia is characterized by personality disintegration, disorientation, and a general loss of cognitive abilities, including impairment of memory and abstract thinking. The most common cause is Alzheimer's disease. Other causes include cerebrovascular disease, CNS infections, brain trauma and tumors, vitamin deficiencies, certain metabolic and endocrine conditions, immune disorders, multiple sclerosis, Huntington's chorea, and Parkinson's disease. ***Obtain physician clearance. Once granted, see entry under Alzheimer's disease. Adjust massage to client's stamina and vitality (i.e., slow, gentle, short duration; assist client on and off table). If client is unable to speak for himself or herself, then acquire information from client's caregiver.***

Depression

Depression is a mood disorder characterized by feelings of deep sadness, despair, pessimism, low self-esteem, withdrawal from personal contact, decreased energy, and sleep and eating disturbances. It can also include feelings of anxiety and irritability, foreboding, guilt, self-reproach, occasional delusions, hallucinations, and preoccupation with death. Depression, which spans most ages (childhood, adolescence, and adulthood), may develop slowly or suddenly and may last a few days, weeks, or months. Episodes may occur singly or in clusters and be separated by months or even years. By definition, clinical depression is depression that last for periods of 6 months or more. Women are more affected by depression than men. Clients with depressive disorders are often on prescription medications. ***Massage is indicated.***

Encephalitis

Inflammation of the brain, or encephalitis, is an infectious disease typically transmitted by the bite of an infected mosquito. Encephalitis may also be the result of hemorrhage, of lead or other type of poisoning, or as a secondary complication of another condition. This condition is characterized by headaches, fever, vertigo, nausea, and vomiting. In severe cases, encephalitis causes seizures, paralysis, and coma. ***Massage is contraindicated.***

Erb's Palsy

Often caused by birth injury, Erb's palsy is caused by injury to the upper brachial plexus, causing paralysis in the arm. One or more cervical nerve roots may also be involved. ***Position client for comfort, which may include propping up the affected arm. Use light pressure on affected arm, and include techniques to increase muscle function, reduce swelling, and reduce contracture.***

Glaucoma

Glaucoma is a group of eye diseases characterized by an elevated pressure within one or both eyes caused by an obstruction of the outflow of aqueous humor. This increased pressure causes pathological changes in the optic disk and defects in the field of vision. ***Position client for comfort; the face cradle may not be comfortable. If the client is visually impaired, then explain everything that happens during the massage verbally. For more information, see section on visual impairments in Chapter 10.***

Guillain-Barré Syndrome

Guillain-Barré syndrome is a rapidly progressive peripheral nerve paralysis. Although the cause is unknown, many cases followed a viral infection. The accompanying neuritis usually begins in the feet, spreading upwardly to the trunk, down the arms, and then up toward the head. Some people may have minimal symptoms; others have severe symptoms and may require critical care. The disease resolves itself, and recovery may take months or years. ***Obtain physician clearance. Once granted, use techniques to prevent muscle contractures, increase muscle tone of flaccid muscles, reduce adhesions, and improve mobility.***

Lou Gehrig's Disease

A degeneration of motor neurons, Lou Gehrig's disease, or *amyotrophic lateral sclerosis,* is characterized by weakness and muscle atrophy of the hands, forearms, and legs, spreading to involve most of the body. It often begins in life's middle years, progresses rapidly, and causes death within 2 to 5 years. In most cases, the cause is unknown. However, in 5% to 10% of cases, the disease is genetic. ***Obtain physician clearance. Once granted, position client for comfort. If client uses a wheelchair, then determine if treatment needs to be performed while client is in the chair. For more information, see section on wheelchair-bound clients in Chapter 10.***

Macular Degeneration

Associated with the aging process, macular degeneration is a progressive deterioration of the retinal maculae. This condition may also be a secondary complication from other diseases. ***Massage is fine.***

Meningitis

Meningitis is an infection or inflammation of the meninges often characterized by a sudden severe headache, vertigo, stiffness of the neck, and severe irritability. Because the condition progresses, individuals experience nausea, vomiting, and mental disorientation. An elevated body temperature, pulse rate, and respiration rate are often noted. Meningitis can be life threatening. ***Massage is contraindicated.***

Multiple Sclerosis

Multiple sclerosis is an autoimmune disorder in which a progressive destruction of myelin sheaths occurs in the CNS (similar to an electrical wire stripped of its insulation). The myelin sheaths deteriorate to sclerosis (plaques). The symptoms depend on what areas of the CNS are most laden with plaque. It usually begins slowly in young adulthood, worsening throughout life, with periods of flare-ups and remission. Remission occurs because the damaged axons heal, and normal function resumes. Intervals between flare-ups grow shorter as the disease advances. *Adjust massage to client's stamina and vitality (i.e., slow, gentle, short duration; assist client on and off table). Typically, massage is contraindicated during flare-ups. Use techniques to relax client, decrease tone in rigid muscles, and prevent stiffness and contractures. Heat and cold therapies are contraindicated.*

Myasthenia Gravis

Myasthenia gravis is an autoimmune disorder resulting in a loss or impairment of ACh receptors at the junction between the neuron and muscle cell. It is characterized by muscle weakness and fatigue. The onset of myasthenia gravis is gradual, with an initial drooping of the upper eyelids, throat, and facial muscles. The weakness may extend to the respiratory muscles. Muscular exertion may exacerbate this condition and is not advised. Anticholinesterase drugs are the treatment of choice. Anticholinesterase drugs will inhibit the cholinesterase enzyme and will allow acetylcholine to remain in the synaptic cleft for a longer period. This increased period in the synaptic cleft will allow the reduced or impaired ACh receptors more time to bind with ACh to produce a muscle contraction, thus relieving some of the symptoms of weakness. *Obtain physician clearance if symptoms are severe. Use techniques to slow muscle atrophy and to maintain flexibility.*

Nerve Compression

Nerve compression is also known as *nerve impingement* and is caused by pressure against the nerve resulting from contact with hard tissues such as bone or cartilage. Common nerve compressions are found when vertebral discs slip from between the bodies of adjacent vertebrae and migrate into the nerve root branching from the spinal cord. The symptoms of nerve compressions are sharp radiating pain, burning, numbness, tingling, and weakness and may occasionally result in loss of all strength or dexterity. *Obtain physician clearance. Once granted, focus on muscles in area of compression or muscles innervated by the nerve being compressed.*

Nerve Entrapment

Nerve entrapments are a dysfunction of a nerve as a result of pressure against it by adjacent soft tissues such as muscle, tendon, fascia, and ligaments. The entrapment can be caused by muscle tightness and shortening resulting from injury or overuse. These tight soft tissues can affect the nerve two ways. They may press an underlying nerve against hard tissues such as bone, disrupting normal nerve function (e.g., thoracic outlet syndrome caused by either the scalene or pectoralis minor muscles pressing the brachial plexus against the ribcage). The other type of entrapment occurs when a nerve actually passes through the belly of a muscle and is constricted by the tightening muscle, similar to a rubber

band stretched between two fingers (e.g., triceps brachii entrapment of the radial nerve or piriformis entrapment of the sciatic nerve). Both types of entrapment may have symptoms of sharp, radiating pain, especially in the extremities, burning, numbness, pins and needles, or weakness in the affected muscles. *Use techniques to reduce tension in involved muscles. Work deeply but briefly.*

Neuropathy

Neuropathy is a degeneration of the PNS. In many instances, the cause is unknown. Some known causes are chronic inflammation, noninflammatory lesions, complications of diseases such as diabetes, or from harmful substances such as lead. Neuropathic conditions may be specifically named for the nerve (e.g. ulnar neuropathy, femoral neuropathy), for the number of nerves involved (e.g. mononeuropathy, polyneuropathy), or for the specific structures involved (myelopathy). *Obtain physician clearance. Once granted, either avoid massage of affected area, or use light pressure.*

Obsessive-Compulsive Disorder

Obsessive-compulsive disorder is an anxiety disorder characterized by emotionally constricted mannerisms that are overly conventional and rigid. The person has a preoccupation with trivial details, rules and restrictions, order and organization, schedules, and lists. The person also has a tendency to perform repetitive acts, usually as a means of releasing built-up tension or relieving excessive anxiety. *Massage is indicated.*

Paralysis

Paralysis is the loss of muscle function, loss of sensation, or both. This condition can be caused by trauma during a vehicular accident, sporting incidents, gunshot wounds, disease, and poisoning. Paralysis of the lower extremities and trunk is called *paraplegia,* whereas paralysis of the arms and legs is called *quadriplegia.* When the paralysis is restricted to one side of the body, it is called *hemiplegia. Position client for comfort, and use light pressure in areas that lack sensation. Use techniques that increase circulation. Avoid electric vibrators, joint mobilizations, and stretches. If client uses a wheelchair, then determine if treatment needs to be performed while client is in the chair. For more information, see section on wheelchair-bound clients in Chapter 10.*

Parkinson's Disease

Parkinson's disease is a progressive, degenerative neurological disorder marked by the destruction of the dopamine-producing neurons of the brain and depletion of the neurotransmitter dopamine. Symptoms are stooped posture, shuffling gait, and an expressionless face. Muscles may alternately contract and relax, causing tremors, while other muscles contract continuously, causing rigidity in the involved part. ***Obtain physician clearance if symptoms are severe. Use techniques to reduce rigidity. Do not force muscles or joints into movement.***

Pinkeye

Inflammation of the conjunctiva of the eye, or conjunctivitis, is caused by a bacterial or viral infection, allergy, or environmental factors such as debris. Red eyes, a thick discharge, sticky eyelids in the morning, and inflammation are characteristic. ***Massage is contraindicated.***

Poliomyelitis

Poliomyelitis, or *polio,* is an infectious disease transmitted through fecal contamination or nasal secretions. It is caused by one of the three polioviruses and can range in severity from relatively asymptomatic to severe paralysis. Factors that influence the susceptibility to the viruses are gender, stress, and age. In spinal poliomyelitis, the virus replicates in the anterior horn of the spinal cord, causing inflammation and eventual destruction of the spinal neurons. ***If in chronic, noninfective stage, then use light pressure. Use techniques to reduce contractures, retain joint mobility, and loosen adhesions.***

Reflex Sympathetic Dystrophy

Reflex sympathetic dystrophy, also known as *complex regional pain syndrome*, is a disorder or group of disorders affecting the limbs. It may develop as a result of trauma (i.e., accident, repetitive motion, surgery) to bone, soft tissue, or nerves. It is characterized by a chronic pain state, sweating or vasomotor abnormalities, skin atrophy, hair loss, sensory and motor dysfunction, and localized abnormal blood flow. ***Obtain physician clearance if symptoms are severe. Once granted, use light pressure and techniques to increase mobility.***

Sciatica

Inflammation of the sciatic nerve, or sciatica, is a type of neuritis often experienced as a dull pain and tenderness in the buttock region, with sharp radiating pain or numbness down the leg. The pain is felt along the path of the sciatic nerve. As inflammation increases, motor function may be affected, with the knee becoming rubbery or unstable. Sciatica may be a result of nerve compression from bone or cartilage or nerve entrapment from muscle or soft tissues (most likely the piriformis and other hip outward rotators). It may be unilateral or bilateral and can be brought on by injury, overuse, or excessive emotional stress. ***Determine cause of sciatica, and then modify techniques according to cause (e.g., herniated disc, tight piriformis muscle). Modification might include avoiding massage or addressing involved musculature, using techniques to relax muscles, reduce atrophy, prevent spasms, and reduce edema.***

Seizure Disorders

Also referred to as *epilepsy,* seizure disorders are the presence of abnormal and irregular discharges of cerebral electrical activity; billions of neurons in the brain fire at once. During these episodes, the individual may experience sensory disturbances, seizures, abnormal behavior, and loss of consciousness. The causes of most cases are unknown, but it has been linked to cerebral trauma, brain tumors, cerebrovascular disturbances, or chemical imbalances. It is viewed as a *lightning storm in the brain. **Know and limit triggers for seizure. If seizure occurs during treatment, then provide light immobilization to prevent the client from falling off table. Call 911 if seizure lasts more than 5 minutes.***

Spina Bifida

Spina bifida is a congenital defect characterized by a lack of bone development in the lamina (posterior vertebral arch). This condition may be mild (only a small, deformed lamina), or it may be associated with the complete absence of laminae surrounding a large area (usually the lumbar spine). In the more severe cases, the meninges and spinal cord protrude, producing a saclike structure. Severe forms cause weakness or paralysis of the legs. ***Obtain physician clearance. Once granted, position client for comfort. If client uses a wheelchair, then determine if treatment needs to be performed while client is in the chair. For more information, see section on wheelchair-bound clients in Chapter 10. Avoid lumbosacral area and forced stretching of muscles. Use techniques to prevent contractures, prevent pressure ulcers, reduce spasticity, and reduce any edema in the legs. Avoid massage if symptoms are severe.***

Stroke

Also called *cerebrovascular accident*, strokes are caused by an occlusion or blockage of cerebral blood vessels by an embolus, thrombus, or cerebrovascular hemorrhage or vasospasm, resulting in ischemia of brain tissue. Muscular weakness or paralysis, an increase or decrease in sensation, speech abnormalities, or death may result. Subsequent damage depends on the location and extent of neurological damage. ***Obtain physician clearance. Once granted, use techniques to prevent joint stiffness, decrease muscle spasticity, and address postural changes. Adjust massage to client's stamina and vitality (i.e., slow, gentle, short duration; assist client on and off table). Increase treatment time gradually to 1 hour. Deep pressure is contraindicated. Carefully administer joint mobilizations.***

Substance Abuse

Substance abuse is classified as the use of a mood- or behavior-altering substance that results in distress or impairment. These problems can range from failure to fulfill social or occupational obligations or recurrent use in situations in which it is physically dangerous to do so or which end in legal problems. Substances often abused are alcohol and narcotics. *If the therapist suspects that the client is under the influence of a mood-altering substance, then avoid deep pressure because the sensory feedback loop is reduced. Avoid deep pressure during the early stages of withdrawal.*

Thoracic Outlet Syndrome

Thoracic outlet syndrome involves the brachial plexus and is caused by either nerve compression (often between the clavicle and the first rib) or by nerve entrapment (either by the scalenes or pectoralis minor). Pain and weakness down the arm are common symptoms. Some clients also experience pain in the chest and neck. *If caused by nerve compression, then obtain physician clearance. If caused by nerve entrapment, then treat involved muscles (i.e., pectoralis minor, scalenes, muscles of the entire shoulder girdle and arm).*

Trigeminal Neuralgia

Also called *tic douloureux,* trigeminal neuralgia is a neurological condition of the trigeminal nerve characterized by excruciating episodic pain in the areas supplied by the trigeminal nerve, or cranial nerve V. Any one or all three of the nerve branches may be affected. First-branch involvement results in pain around the eyes and over the forehead; second-branch involvement results in pain in the upper lip, nose, and cheek; third-branch involvement results in pain on the side of the tongue and the lower lip. The pain may last only a few seconds to many hours. *Obtain physician clearance if symptoms are severe. Avoid affected area if pressure causes pain. Otherwise, use light strokes over affected area.*

Effects of Massage on the Nervous System

Reduces stress. Activating the relaxation response reduces stress.

Reduces anxiety. Interestingly, a reduction in anxiety is noted in both the person who received the massage and the person who gave the massage.

Promotes relaxation. General relaxation is promoted through activation of the relaxation response. Relaxation has a diminishing effect on pain.

Decreases beta wave activity. Associated with relaxation, a decrease in beta brain wave activity occurred during and after the massage (confirmed by electroencephalogram [EEG]).

Increases delta wave activity. Increases in delta brain wave activity, which occur during massage, are linked to sleep and to relaxation; both are promoted with massage (confirmed by EEG).

Increase in alpha waves. An increase in alpha brain waves during massage indicates relaxation (confirmed by EEG).

Increases dopamine levels. Increased levels of dopamine are linked to decreased stress and reduced depression.

Increases serotonin levels. Increased levels of serotonin suggest a reduction of both stress and depression. One theory suggests that serotonin inhibits pain signals, indicating that increased levels of serotonin also reduce pain.

Reduces cortisol levels. Massage reduces cortisol levels by activating the relaxation response. Elevated levels of cortisol not only represent heightened stress but also inhibit immune functions.

Reduces norepinephrine levels. Massage has been proven to reduce norepinephrine, a stress hormone.

Reduces epinephrine levels. Epinephrine, another stress hormone, is reduced with massage.

Reduces feelings of depression. Both chemical and electrophysiological changes from a negative to a positive mood were noted and may underline the decrease in depression after massage therapy. Depression associated with chronic pain was also reduced.

Decreases pain. Massage relieves local and referred pain, presumably by increasing circulation, which reduces ischemia. Massage also stimulates the release of endorphins (endogenous morphine), enkephalins, and other pain-reducing neurochemicals. General relaxation brought on by massage therapy also has a diminishing effect on pain. The pressure of a massage interferes with pain information entering the spinal cord by stimulating pressure receptors, further reducing pain. Massage interrupts the pain cycle by relieving muscular spasms, increasing circulation, and promoting rapid disposal of waste products. Massage also improves sleep patterns. During deep sleep, a substance called *somatostatin* is normally released. Without this substance, pain is experienced.

Reduces analgesic use. Because pain is reduced with massage, so is the need for excessive use of pain medication.

Activates sensory receptors. Depending on factors such as stroke choice, direction, speed, and pressure, massage can stimulate different sensory receptors, affecting massage outcome. For example, cross-fiber tapotement stimulates muscle spindles, which activates muscular contraction, whereas a slow passive stretch and deep effleurage activate Golgi tendon organs, thereby inhibiting contraction. Activation of pressure receptors reduces pain.

The hippocampal region of the brain develops faster and more elaborately. Part of the limbic system, development of the hippocampal region is related to superior memory performance.

SUMMARY

A study of the nervous system includes the details of the anatomy and physiology of individual nerve fibers and nerve transmission and a look at the system as a whole.

The neurons are an important unit of the nervous system and can be classified according to function (sensory, association, or motor). The interneurons neurons are found in the brain and spinal cord, where they connect the sensory and motor. Sensory nerves run from receptors and enter the posterior horn of the spine. Motor nerves originate at the anterior horn of the same spinal segment and run until they reach their target muscle or gland.

Nerve impulses or action potentials are simply a matter of ions changing places, creating different electrical charges along the cell membrane. Synaptic transmission uses neurotransmitters flowing across gaps between neurons to bind with receptor sites on the postsynaptic neuron, muscle, or gland. The response depends on whether the neurotransmitters are excitatory or inhibitory.

The nervous system as a whole is divided into the CNS and the PNS. The CNS is composed of the brain, spinal cord, CSF, and meninges.

The PNS consists of the intricate network of many millions of branching nerve fibers that leave and return to the brain and spinal cord, some of which are sensory and some of which are motor. Nerves leaving directly from the brain are referred to as *cranial nerves*; spinal nerves are those originating from and terminating at the spine. Types of sensory receptors include chemoreceptors, mechanoreceptors, photoreceptors, nociceptors, and thermoreceptors; these receptors provide the specialized senses of taste, olfaction, vision, hearing, and touch.

A subdivision of the PNS is the ANS, which, in turn, is divided into the sympathetic nervous system and the parasympathetic nervous system.

evolve

Go to *Chapter Extras* on Evolve for additional illustrations and resources for this chapter. *Extras* for this chapter include:

1. Functional classifications of neurons (illustration)
2. Sodium potassium pump (illustration)
3. Biography of John Upledger (box)

MATCHING I

Place the letter of the answer next to the term or phrase that best describes it.

A. Autonomic nervous system
B. Axon
C. Central nervous system
D. Dendrite
E. Myelin

F. Nerve
G. Neuroglia
H. Neurons
I. Neurotransmitters
J. Nodes of Ranvier

K. Parasympathetic
L. Peripheral nervous system
M. Reflex arc
N. Sympathetic division
O. Synapse

_____ 1. Responsible for the body's alarm reaction; also known as *thoracolumbar outflow*

_____ 2. Contains the brain, spinal cord, CSF, and meninges

_____ 3. Nerve cell classified as connective tissue that supports, nourishes, protects, insulates, and organizes neurons

_____ 4. Bundles of neurons held together by several layers of connective tissue

_____ 5. Extensions of a nerve cell that receives and transmits stimuli toward the cell body

_____ 6. Contains cranial and spinal nerves

_____ 7. Impulse-conducting cells that possess properties of excitability and conductibility

_____ 8. Cell extension that transmits impulses away from the cell body

_____ 9. Junction between neurons where transmission of nerve impulses takes place

_____ 10. Chemical messengers involved in nerve impulse transmission

_____ 11. Division of the ANS involved with the relaxation response; also known as *craniosacral outflow*

_____ 12. Subdivision of the PNS that is involuntary and supplies smooth muscles, heart muscle, skin, special senses, some proprioceptors, organs, and glands

_____ 13. Fatty insulating substance around some axons to assist impulse conduction

_____ 14. A conduction route to and from the CNS consisting of at least an afferent, interneuron, and efferent nerve

_____ 15. Gaps located at intervals along a myelinated axon

MATCHING II

Place the letter of the answer next to the term or phrase that best describes it.

A.	Adaptation	F.	Ganglion	K.	Myotomes
B.	Alpha	G.	Golgi tendon organs	L.	Nerve impulse
C.	Cerebellum	H.	Medulla oblongata	M.	Nociceptors
D.	Cerebrospinal	I.	Meninges	N.	Plexus
E.	Dermatome	J.	Muscle spindles	O.	Sodium-potassium pump

_____ 1. Connective tissue membranes surrounding the brain and spinal cord

_____ 2. Part of the brain that governs muscle tone, coordinates complex movements, and regulates posture and balance

_____ 3. An electrical fluctuation traveling along the surface of a neural cell membrane

_____ 4. A cluster of nerve cell bodies located in the PNS, typically next to the spinal cord

_____ 5. Stretch receptors activated by both tension and excessive stretch, responding by inhibiting motor neurons

_____ 6. Part of the brainstem containing respiratory, cardiac, and vasomotor centers

_____ 7. Active transport system that produces and maintains resting potentials of neural membranes

_____ 8. A network of intersecting nerves in the PNS

_____ 9. Area of skin that a specific sensory nerve root serves

_____ 10. Clear fluid circulating around the brain and spinal cord

_____ 11. Receptors for detecting pain

_____ 12. Brain wave pattern present when the subject is awake but relaxed and nonattentive

_____ 13. Stretch receptors that monitor changes in muscle length, as well as the rate of this change, responding by causing reflexive contraction

_____ 14. A decrease in sensitivity to a prolonged stimulus

_____ 15. Group of skeletal muscles innervated by a single spinal segment

INTERNET ACTIVITIES

Visit the Howard Hughes Medical Institute at http://www.hhmi.org and click on Ask a Scientist. Click on *Neuroscience* and locate the answer to this question: What effect does caffeine have on our reaction time?

Visit http://chemistry.about.com/cs/howthingswork/a/aa122703a.htm and read the article on mad cow disease. How can people protect themselves?

Visit http://www.mult-sclerosis.org and click on Explaining Multipile Sclerosis. Scroll down and click on *How does MS do its damage?* What does *demyelination* mean?

Bibliography

Abrahams P, Marks S, Hutchings R: *McMinn's color atlas of human anatomy,* St Louis, 2003, Mosby.

Applegate EJ: *The anatomy and physiology learning system,* ed 3, Philadelphia, 2006, Saunders.

Beers MH, Berkow R: *The Merck manual of diagnosis and therapy,* Whitehouse Station, NJ, 2006, Merck Research Laboratories.

Como D, editor: *Mosby's Medical, Nursing, and Allied Health Dictionary,* ed 6, St Louis, 2002, Mosby.

Crawley J, Van De Graaff KM: *A photographic atlas for anatomy and physiology,* Englewood, Colo, 2002, Morton.

Crooks R, Stein J: *Psychology: science, behavior, and life,* ed 3, Philadelphia, 1993, Harcourt College Publishers.

Damjanov I: *Pathophysiology for the health-related professions,* ed 3, Philadelphia, 2006, Saunders.

Ferri FF: *2003 Ferri's clinical advisor, instant diagnosis and treatment,* St Louis, 2003, Mosby.

Frazier MS, Drzymkowski JW: *Essentials of human diseases and conditions,* ed 3, Philadelphia, 2004, Saunders.

Goldberg S: *Clinical anatomy made ridiculously simple,* Miami, 2004, Medmaster.

Gould BE: *Pathophysiology for the health professions,* ed 3, Philadelphia, 2006, Saunders.

Grafelman T: *Graf's anatomy and physiology guide for the massage therapist,* Aurora, Colo, 1998, DG Publishing.

Gray H: *Gray's anatomy,* ed 29, Philadelphia, 1974, Running Press.

Guyton A: *Human physiology and mechanisms of disease,* ed 6, Philadelphia, 1996, Saunders.

Haubrich WS: *Medical meanings: a glossary of word origins,* New York, 1984, Harcourt Brace Jovanovich.

Huether SE, McCance KL: *Understanding pathophysiology,* ed 3, St Louis, 2004, Mosby.

Jacob S, Francone C: *Elements of anatomy and physiology,* Philadelphia, 1989, Saunders.

Juhan D: *Job's body: a handbook for bodyworkers,* ed 3, Barrington, NY, 2003, Station Hill Press.

Kalat JW: *Biological psychology,* ed 8, Belmont, Calif, 2003, Wadsworth.

Kapit W, Elson LM: *The anatomy coloring book,* ed 3, New York, 2002, Benjamin Cummings.

Kordish M, Dickson S: *Introduction to basic human anatomy,* Lake Charles, La, 1995, McNeese State University.

Kumar V, Abbas A, Fausto N: *Robbins and Cotran physiologic basis of disease,* ed 7, St Louis, 2005, Mosby.

Marieb EN: *Essentials of human anatomy and physiology,* ed 8, New York, 2005, Benjamin Cummings.

Martini FH, Bartholomew EF: *Essentials of anatomy and physiology,* ed 3, New York, 2003, Benjamin Cummings.

McAleer N: *The body almanac,* Garden City, NY, 1985, Doubleday.

McAtee R: *Facilitated stretching,* ed 2, Colorado Springs, Colo, 1999, Human Kinetics.

McCance K, Huether S: *Pathophysiology: the biological basis for disease in adults and children,* St Louis, 2006, Mosby.

Melzack R, Wall PD: *The challenge of pain,* New York, 1996, Basic Books.

Merck manual, ed 17, Whitehouse Station, NJ, 1998, Merck and Company.

Moore KL: *Clinically oriented anatomy,* ed 5, Baltimore, 2005, Lippincott Williams & Wilkins.

Netter FH: *Atlas of human anatomy,* ed 3, Teterboro, NJ, 2003, Icon Learning Systems.

Newton D: *Pathology for massage therapists,* ed 2, Portland, Ore, 1995, Simran.

Premkumar K: *Pathology A to Z, a handbook for massage therapists,* Baltimore, 1999, Lippincott Williams & Wilkins.

Salvo SG, Anderson, SK: *Mosby's pathology for massage therapists,* St Louis, 2004, Elsevier Mosby.

Solomon EP, Phillips GA: *Understanding human anatomy and physiology,* Philadelphia, 1987, Saunders.

St. John P: *St. John neuromuscular therapy seminars,* manual I, Largo, Fla, 1995, self-published.

Taber's cyclopedic medical dictionary, ed 20, Philadelphia, 2005, FA Davis.

Thibodeau G, Patton K: *Anatomy and physiology,* ed 6, St Louis, 2006, Mosby.

Thibodeau G, Patton K: *Structure and function of the body,* ed 12, St Louis, 2004, Mosby.

Tortora GJ: *Introduction to the human body: the essentials of anatomy and physiology,* ed 5, Hoboken, NJ, 2000, John Wiley & Sons.

Tortora GJ, Grabowksi SR: *Principles of anatomy and physiology,* ed 11, New York, 2005, John Wiley & Sons.

Travell JG, Simons D: *Myofascial pain and dysfunction, the trigger point manual,* Baltimore, 1992, Lippincott Williams & Wilkins.

Voss DE, Ionta MK, Myers BJ: *Proprioceptive neuromuscular facilitation,* Philadelphia, 1985, Harper and Row.

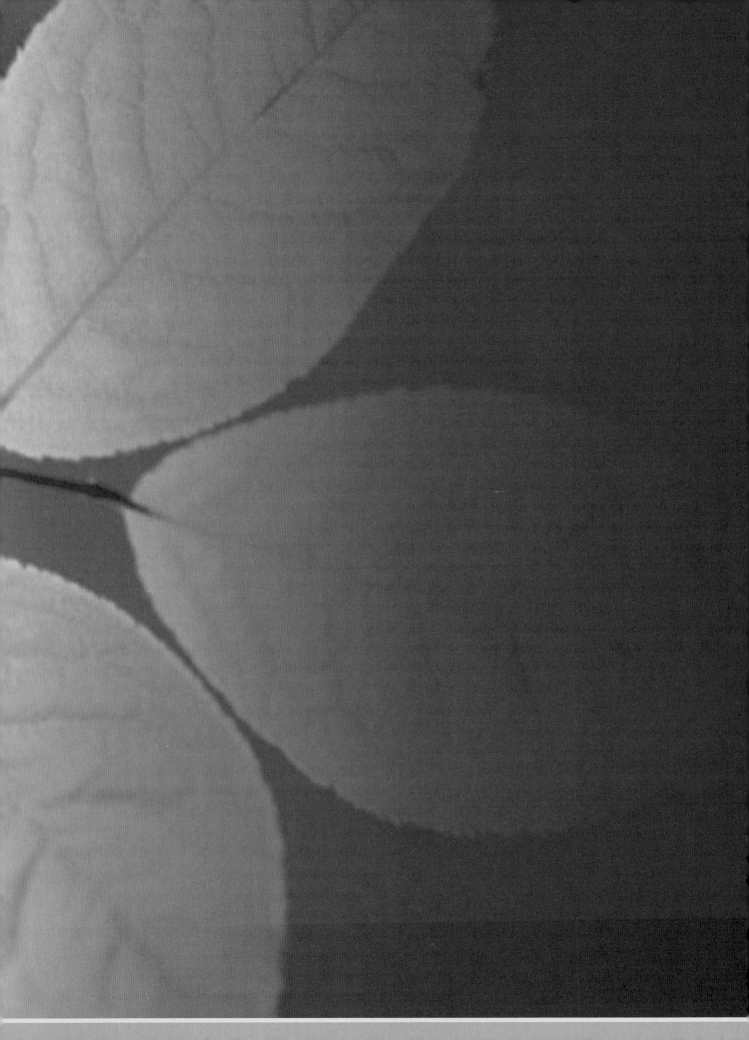

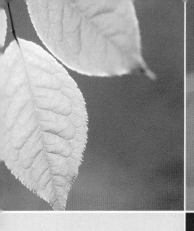

CHAPTER 18

Endocrine Glands and Hormones

STUDENT OBJECTIVES
After completing this chapter, the student should be able to:

- Contrast and compare exocrine and endocrine glands
- List the anatomical structures and describe the physiological properties of the endocrine system
- Define hormones and describe hormone types
- Explain hormonal control systems
- Identify specific endocrine glands
- Name the hormones produced and secreted by each endocrine gland or organs that possess endocrine tissues
- Discuss the function of each individual hormone
- Name types of pathological conditions of the endocrine system, giving characteristics and massage considerations of each

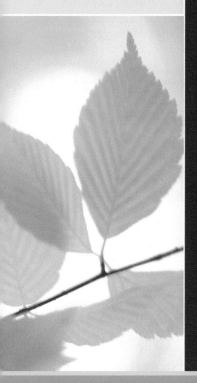

INTRODUCTION

The endocrine system works along with the nervous system to coordinate the functioning of all body systems. Whereas the nervous system uses nerve impulses to communicate, the endocrine system uses chemical messengers called *hormones*. The endocrine system regulates processes that continue for relatively long periods, and its effects are more widespread in comparison with the nervous system (Figure 18-1).

The two types of glands of the body are (1) exocrine and (2) endocrine. **Exocrine glands** secrete their products into ducts that empty into body cavities, the hollow center of an organ, or onto the surface of the body. Examples of exocrine glands are sudoriferous (secretes perspiration), sebaceous (secretes oil), and ceruminous (secretes ear wax). Another example of exocrine glands are digestive glands, which secrete digestive enzymes into the gastrointestinal tract, and mucous glands, which secrete mucus in a variety of areas of the body.

Endocrine glands, or *ductless glands,* have cells that produce glandular secretions called *hormones.* Most hormones are released in one part of the body and travel through the bloodstream, affecting cells in other parts of the body. Some hormones do not enter the bloodstream but work on neighboring cells instead. Endocrine glands include all the structures listed in the next section. Other organs that possess endocrine qualities include the hypothalamus, the thymus, kidneys, the intestinal mucosa, the heart, and the placenta.

Compared with other body systems, which are made up of fairly large organs, the glands of the endocrine system may seem small and unimportant. Although the total weight of all the endocrine glands is less than one half pound, normal functioning of the endocrine system is vital to the body's physiological mechanisms, which becomes apparent when hormone levels are too low or high; drastic changes in the body's metabolism occur when hormonal levels are out of balance.

ANATOMY

Areas of discussion in this chapter include:
- Adrenals
- Gonads
- Hormones
- Pancreatic islets
- Parathyroids
- Pineal
- Pituitary
- Thyroid
- Hormones

PHYSIOLOGY

The endocrine system performs the following actions:
- Produces and secretes hormones
- Regulates body activities such as growth, development, and metabolism
- Regulates the activity of smooth muscle, cardiac muscle, and some glands
- Assists the body to adapt during times of stress, such as infection, trauma, dehydration, emotional stress, and starvation
- Regulates the chemical composition and volume of body fluids and fluids inside cells
- Contributes to the reproductive process

HORMONES

Hormones are internal secretions that are chemical messengers of the endocrine system. They act as catalysts in biochemical reactions and regulate the physiological activity of other cells in the body. The word *hormone* means to set in motion or to arouse. Because hormones circulate freely in the blood, they have the potential of coming into contact with every type of cell in the body. However, hormones *do not affect* every cell they may encounter. Each type of hormone is specifically programmed to seek out a corresponding type of cell, called **target cells** (see Figure 18-1). The target cells contain *receptor sites,* which are chemically compatible with

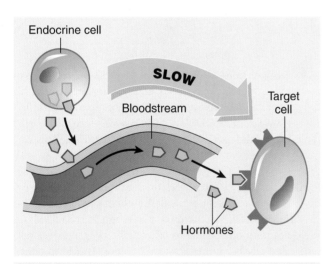

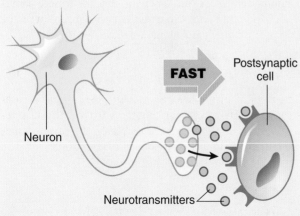

FIGURE 18-1 Comparing endocrine and nervous system functions.

Terms and Their Meanings Related to the Endocrine System

TERM	MEANING
Adenohypophysis	*Gr.* gland; below; to grow
Adrenal	*L.* kidney
Antidiuretic	*Gr.* against; urine; production
Endocrine	*Gr.* within; to separate
Exocrine	*Gr.* away from; to separate
Hormone	*Gr.* to excite, arouse, urge on
Oxytocin	*Gr.* swift; childbirth
Pancreas	*Gr.* all flesh
Pineal	*L.* pine cone
Suprarenal	*L.* above; kidney
Thyroid	*Gr.* shield; shaped

Gr., Greek; *L.,* Latin.

their corresponding hormone. When the hormone comes into contact with the receptor site of the target cell, they lock together as puzzle pieces, and the resulting chemical change produces the desired effect on the cell. This arousal of the target cell usually increases or decreases the rate of its primary metabolic function.

Types of Hormones

Hormones may be grouped according to their chemical makeup. The four most common types of hormones are steroids, peptides, eicosanoids, and biogenic amines.

- **Biogenic amines** function as neurotransmitters. Hormones of the adrenal medulla and thyroid gland are biogenic amines, as well as catecholamines, histamine, serotonin, and dopamine. These substances regulate blood pressure, waste elimination, body temperature, and many other functions.
- **Eicosanoids** alter smooth muscle contractions, blood flow, nerve impulse transmission, and immune responses. Also called *tissue hormones,* eicosanoids are produced by almost every cell in the body.
- **Peptide hormones** introduce a series of chemical reactions to alter the cell's metabolism. Hormones of the pituitary gland, parathyroid glands, and some of the hormones of the thyroid glands are peptide hormones.
- **Steroid hormones** alter cell activity by turning genes on or off. Hormones of the adrenal cortex and gonads are steroid hormones.

Hormonal Control Systems

Generally, negative-feedback systems, other hormones, and the nervous system regulate hormonal secretions.

Negative-Feedback System

Most hormone levels in the body are regulated by a negative-feedback system. Information about blood hormone levels is relayed back to the endocrine gland, and the gland responds by secreting more or less hormone. This process is known as the negative-feedback system because the stimulus triggers the negative, or opposite, response. For example, when a low level of calcium is in the bloodstream, it triggers an increase of parathyroid hormone from the parathyroid gland and releases stored calcium from the bones into the bloodstream. This increase continues until the level of calcium exceeds the target value or becomes high; the parathyroid then responds negatively by decreasing production. Another example of a negative-feedback system involves thyroid hormone from the thyroid gland. Thyroid hormones regulate metabolism. When metabolic needs are low, less thyroid hormone is secreted; when metabolic needs are higher, more thyroid hormones are secreted.

Hormonal Control System

Hormones themselves can stimulate or inhibit the release of other hormones in the endocrine system. An example of hormones controlling the secretion of other hormones is demonstrated by the way the hypothalamus communicates with the pituitary gland. The pituitary gland consists of two parts, an anterior and a posterior portion. The anterior portion secretes hormones in response to hormones that the hypothalamus secretes. Some hypothalamic hormones cause an increase in secretion of anterior pituitary hormones; others cause a decrease in secretion of anterior pituitary hormones.

Neural Control System

Some hormones are secreted as a result of direct nerve stimulation, the most classic example being the release of epinephrine and norepinephrine from the adrenal medulla. Sympathetic arousal, or the *stress response,* releases epinephrine and norepinephrine into the bloodstream. This action helps maintain the fight-or-flight response. The neural control system has a much faster response time than the negative-feedback or the hormonal control systems. How the hypothalamus communicates with the posterior pituitary gland is a demonstration of nerve impulses controlling release of hormones. The posterior pituitary gland does not synthesize any hormones. Instead, it stores two hormones, antidiuretic hormone and oxytocin, that the hypothalamus make. Nerve impulses from the hypothalamus cause the posterior pituitary gland to release these hormones.

INDIVIDUAL ENDOCRINE GLANDS

The endocrine glands are the pituitary, pineal, thyroid, parathyroid, and adrenal glands, as well as pancreatic islets, female ovaries, and male testes (Figure 18-2). Several other organs are featured that possess endocrine qualities.

Pituitary Gland

The bilobed pituitary gland sits in the sella turcica of the sphenoid bone and extends from the hypothalamus by a stalklike structure known as the *infundibulum* (Figure 18-3).

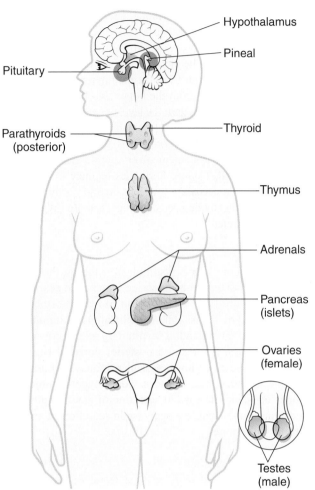

FIGURE 18-2 Location of major endocrine glands.

Approximately the size of a small grape, the pituitary gland is protected on all sides by bone and is considered to be the most protected gland in the body. The pituitary gland was once known as the *master gland* because its hormones control and stimulate other glands to produce and secrete their hormones (Figure 18-4). The pituitary itself also has a master—the hypothalamus, which sends hormones and nerve impulses to control secretions of the pituitary gland; the hypothalamus is the true master gland. The pituitary gland consists of anterior and posterior lobes.

Anterior Lobe

Also known as the *adenohypophysis,* the anterior lobe of the pituitary constitutes approximately 75% of the total weight of the entire gland. Of the nine hormones secreted by the pituitary gland, seven are produced by the anterior lobe. The anterior lobe and the hypothalamus are interconnected by the hypophyseal portal system. Hormones produced by hypothalamic neurosecretory cells travel this vascular network to stimulate or inhibit the release of hormones from the pituitary's anterior lobe (Table 18-1).

---

evolve *Want to see what the hypophyseal portal system looks like? Great! Log on to the Evolve website for Chapter 18's course materials and choose the image.* ■

TABLE TALK

To memorize the hormones of the anterior pituitary, use the mnemonic phrase, *Flat m*iles *p*er *g*allon: *f*ollicle-stimulating hormone, *l*uteinizing hormone, *a*drenocorticotropic hormone, *t*hyroid stimulating hormone, *m*elanocyte-stimulating hormone, *p*rolactin, and *g*rowth hormone.

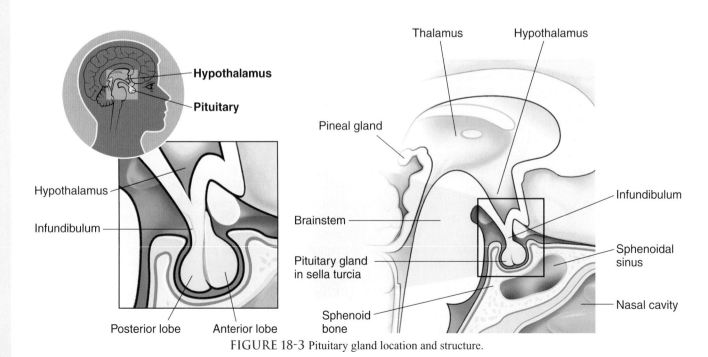

FIGURE 18-3 Pituitary gland location and structure.

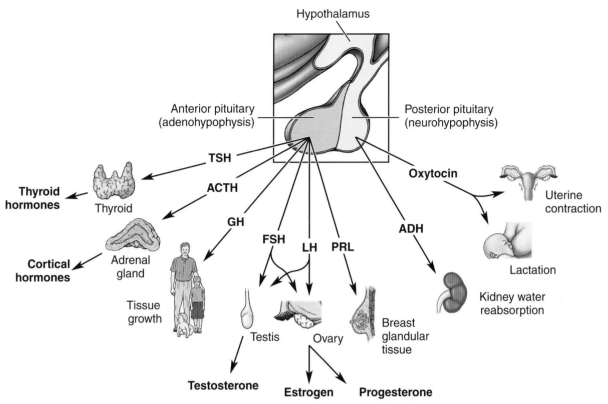

FIGURE 18-4 Some of the major pituitary hormones with their principal target organs.

Posterior Lobe

Also known as *neurohypophysis,* the posterior lobe of the pituitary is not technically an endocrine gland because it does not produce the hormones it releases. It stores and releases hormones produced by the hypothalamus (Table 18-2).

Pineal Gland

The pineal gland, or *pineal body,* is a pinecone-shaped structure in the brain located on the posterior aspect of the brain's diencephalon region. Although its function is not clear, the pineal gland produces and secretes the hormone melatonin (Table 18-3).

Thyroid Gland

Located at the base of the throat, posterior and inferior to the larynx, is the butterfly-shaped thyroid gland (Figure 18-5). The thyroid gland is a bilobed gland connected in the center by a mass of tissue known as the *isthmus* (Table 18-4). The thyroid produces triiodothyronine, thyroxine, and calcitonin.

Parathyroid Glands

Usually four in number, the tiny parathyroid glands are located on the posterolateral surface of the thyroid lobes (see Table 18-4). These glands produce parathyroid hormone.

TABLE 18-1   Hormones of the Anterior Pituitary

HORMONE	ABBREVIATION	ACTION(S)
Adrenocorticotropic hormone	ACTH	Regulates endocrine activity of adrenal cortex, especially cortical hormones
Growth hormone (somatotropin)	GH or STH	Stimulates protein synthesis for muscle and bone growth and maintenance; plays a role in metabolism
Thyroid-stimulating hormone	TSH	Stimulates thyroid gland to produce and secrete its hormones
Follicle-stimulating hormone	FSH	Women: stimulates estrogen production and development of ovarian follicle; men: stimulates sperm production in the testes
Luteinizing hormone	LH	Women: triggers ovulation and development of corpus luteum; men: stimulates production of testosterone
Prolactin	PRL	Stimulates milk production in mammary glands
Melanocyte-stimulating hormone	MSH	Increases skin pigmentation by stimulating distribution of melanin granules

TABLE 18-2 Hormones of the Posterior Pituitary

HORMONE	ABBREVIATION	ACTION(S)	COMMENTARY
Antidiuretic hormone (vasopressin)	ADH	Promotes water retention by kidneys	Alcohol consumption inhibits secretion of ADH, thereby increasing urine production.
Oxytocin	OT	Stimulates uterine contractions and milk expression from mammary glands	A synthetic version of OT, pitocin, is used to stimulate labor in pregnant women.

TABLE 18-3 Hormone of the Pineal Gland

HORMONE	ACTION(S)	COMMENTARY
Melatonin	Involved in the control of circadian rhythms (the body's 24-hours cycle) and in the growth and development of sexual organs	When injected into the body, melatonin produces drowsiness and inhibits the secretion of luteinizing hormone.

Adrenal Glands

The adrenal glands (suprarenals) are located superior to each kidney and are among the most vascular organs in the body. These important glands are divided into two regions and, similar to the pituitary gland, possess two types of tissue, each producing different hormones (Figure 18-6).

Adrenal Cortex

The adrenal cortex is the outer region and makes up most of the gland. It arises from the embryonic tissue endoderm, which is similar to that of the kidneys. The hormones of the adrenal cortex are aldosterone, cortisol, and adrenal androgens and adrenal estrogens (Table 18-5).

Adrenal Medulla

The adrenal medulla is the inner region of the adrenals, which arises from ectoderm. The hormones of the adrenal medulla, also called *neurohormones,* mimic the effects of the sympathetic nervous system and account for the sud-

den emergency energy required for the stress response (see Table 18-5). The hormones of the adrenal medulla are epinephrine and norepinephrine.

> **TABLE TALK**
>
> To memorize the hormones of the adrenal medulla, use the mnemonic phrase, *AMEN*: *a*drenal *m*edulla produces *e*pinephrine and *n*orepinephrine.

Pancreatic Islets

The pancreas, or pancreatic gland, is located inferior to the stomach and is both endocrine and exocrine. Within the pancreas are islands of specialized cells called the **islets of Langerhans**, or **pancreatic islets**. The pancreas contains more than one million islets, each consisting primarily of *alpha* and *beta cells* that function as an organ within an organ. Both hormones of the pancreas help regulate carbohydrate metabolism (Table 18-6). Pancreatic islets also secrete somatostatin

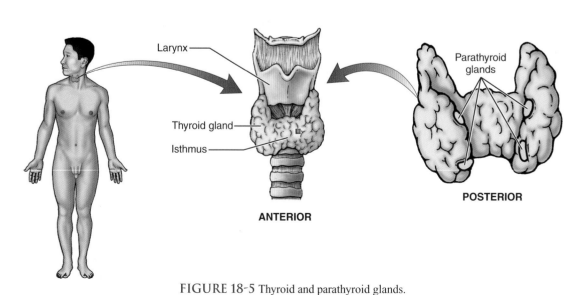

FIGURE 18-5 Thyroid and parathyroid glands.

TABLE 18-4 **Hormones of the Thyroid and Parathyroids**

HORMONE	ABBREVIATION	ACTION(S)	COMMENTARY
Triiodothyronine	T_3	Increases rate of metabolism	T_3 consists of a small peptide molecule bound to iodine; therefore it cannot be made without iodine. Some good sources of iodine are iodized salt and seafood.
Thyroxine (tetraiodothyronine)	T_4	See T_3	See T_3
Calcitonin	CT	Increases calcium storage in bones by stimulating osteoblasts, thereby lowering blood calcium levels	CT production decreases in older adults, which may explain why many older people experience an increase in the decalcification of bones.
Parathyroid hormone (parahormone)	PTH	Decreases calcium storage in bones by stimulating osteoclasts and increases calcium reabsorption from urine and the intestines back into the blood, all to raise blood calcium levels; produces the active form of vitamin D in kidneys.	

and pancreatic polypeptides, but their physiological role is relatively insignificant and not included for discussion.

Gonads

The ovaries and testes, or gonads, are the reproductive glands. Each produces and secretes its own unique set of hormones.

Ovaries

Located in the pelvic cavity of the female body is a set of paired glands called *ovaries*. They produce the hormones progesterone, estrogens, and relaxin. These hormones, along with luteinizing hormone and follicle-stimulating hormone from the anterior pituitary gland, regulate the female reproductive cycle (discussed in Chapter 23). Ovarian follicle cells secrete estrogens, including estradiol and estrone (Table 18-7). Progesterone, the pregnancy-promoting hormone, is se-

creted by the corpus luteum (tissue left behind after rupture of a follicle after ovulation).

Testes

The testes are located in the male scrotum. Composed mainly of coils of sperm-producing seminiferous tubules, a scattering of endocrine interstitial cells is found in areas between the tubules. These *interstitial cells (of Leydig)* produce androgens (male sex hormones); the principal testicular androgen is testosterone (see Table 18-7).

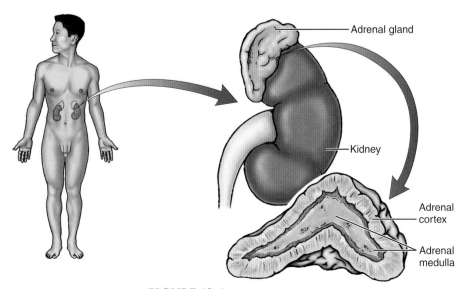

FIGURE 18-6 The adrenal glands.

TABLE 18-5 **Hormones of the Adrenals**

HORMONE	ACTION(S)
Aldosterone	Stimulates kidneys to conserve sodium, which triggers the release of antidiuretic hormone and results in water retention; helps maintain proper mineral balance; monitors blood volume
Cortisol (hydrocortisone)	Affects carbohydrate, protein, and fat metabolism; in large amounts, produces an antiinflammatory response
Adrenal androgen	Though role is uncertain, may support sexual functions
Adrenal estrogens	Believed to be physiologically insignificant
Epinephrine (adrenaline)	Enhances and prolongs effects of the sympathetic division on the autonomic nervous system
Norepinephrine (noradrenaline)	Enhances and prolongs effects of the sympathetic division on the autonomic nervous system

TABLE 18-6 **Hormones of Pancreatic Islets**

HORMONE	ACTION	COMMENTARY
Insulin	Decreases blood glucose levels (hypoglycemic)	Insulin, secreted by beta cells, is the only hormone that decreases blood glucose levels and is necessary for metabolism. Because digestive enzymes deactivate this hormone, it cannot be administered orally. If an individual requires insulin, then it must be given by injection.
Glucagon	Increases blood glucose levels (hyperglycemic)	Glucagon, secreted by the alpha cells, is stimulated by low blood levels of glucose, causing the liver and the skeletal muscles to break down stored glycogen into glucose.

Placenta

The placenta, which serves as a reproductive organ, also contains endocrine tissues. It forms against the uterine lining, and its function is to bring blood and oxygen and remove waste from the developing child. As a temporary endocrine gland, it produces and secretes **human chorionic gonadotropin** (hCG), which is present in the maternal blood and urine. It is known as the pregnancy hormone because, when detected, it means that a woman is pregnant. hCH stimulates the corpus luteum to secrete estrogen and progesterone and to decrease lymphocyte activation. Both factors are important in preparing the uterus to accept the fetus immunologically. The placenta also produces estrogens.

Thymus

The thymus gland is a bilobed gland posterior to the sternum. Although it is considered to be primarily a lymphatic organ, the hormones **thymosin** and **thymopoietin** are produced and secreted, giving the thymus an endocrine gland role. *Thymosin* and *thymopoietin* actually refer to two entire families of peptides that, together, have a critical role in the development of the immune system in that they stimulate the production of specialized lymphocytes involved in the immune response called *T cells*. The role of T cells is discussed in Chapter 19. Large in infancy, the thymus reaches its maximum size at puberty; it then atrophies and is replaced by adipose tissue in adulthood.

Gastric and Intestinal Mucosa

Gastrin, secretin, cholecystokinin-pancreozymin (CCK), and other substances have important regulatory roles in coordinating the digestive process. **Gastrin,** secreted by the gastric mucosa, initiates the production and secretion of gastric juices and stimulates bile and pancreatic enzyme emissions into the small intestines.

Hormones secreted by the intestinal mucosa are cholecystokinin and secretin. **Cholecystokinin** stimulates the gallbladder to release more bile and the pancreas to secrete enzymes. **Secretin** stimulates the pancreas to secrete an alkaline liquid that neutralizes the acid chyme, thereby facilitating the action of the intestinal enzymes. Secretin has a limited stimulating effect on the production of bile. Chapter 21 describes the hormonal control of digestion in the stomach.

Heart

Even though the heart's primary function is to pump blood, it contains some hormone-producing cells in its atrial walls. These cells produce a hormone, **atrial natriuretic hormone** (ANH), which decreases sodium by triggering urine production, or diureses, which additionally decreases blood volume and blood pressure. In this regard, ANH is an antagonist to antidiuretic hormone and aldosterone.

PATHOLOGICAL CONDITIONS OF THE ENDOCRINE SYSTEM

Acromegaly

Acromegaly, or acromegalia, is caused by the overproduction of growth hormone during the adult years. It is characterized by elongation and enlargement of the bones of the extremities, face, and jaw. The condition mainly affects middle-aged and older persons. ***Obtain physician clearance. Once granted, adjust massage if client is in pain.***

TABLE 18-7 **Hormones of the Gonads**

HORMONE	ACTION(S)	COMMENTARY
Estrogen	Responsible for female secondary sex characteristics; during menstrual cycles, triggers the preparation of the female organs for fertilization and implantation of the early embryo; helps keep calcium in bones	Estrogen is also produced in the placenta.
Progesterone	Prepares the endometrium for pregnancy and helps maintain the corpus luteum once conception and implantation occurs; slightly elevates body temperature, creating an incubating effect	One cause of spontaneous abortion (miscarriage) is a drop in progesterone levels.
Relaxin	Facilitates implantation of fertilized ovum; softens connective tissue in pregnant women, especially the pelvic ligaments, for fetal delivery; helps dilate the cervix during labor and delivery	Because relaxin loosens connective tissue during pregnancy, all range-of-motion and stretching activities must be kept to a minimum and performed with caution.
Testosterone	Promotes secondary male sex characteristics, libido (sex drive), and sperm production	

Addison's Disease

Addison's disease, or *hypoadrenalism,* is caused by failure of adrenal functions, often resulting from an autoimmune disease, local or general infection, or adrenal hemorrhage. The disease is characterized by general weakness, reduced endurance, and an increase in pigmentation of the skin and mucous membranes (called *bronzing*). Loss of appetite, anxiety, lethargy, depression, and other emotional disturbances often accompany this disease. *Obtain physician clearance if symptoms are severe. Adjust massage to client's stamina and vitality (i.e., slow, gentle, short duration; assist client on and off table).*

Cretinism

A congenital deficiency in the secretion of thyroid hormones, cretinism is characterized by arrested physical and mental development. This condition is typical in countries where the diet is deficient in iodine and where goiters are common. The addition of iodized salt reduces the occurrence of cretinism. *Obtain physician clearance. Once granted, use light pressure, avoiding neck and throat region.*

Cushing's Disease

Classified as a metabolic disorder, Cushing's disease, or *hyperadrenalism,* is caused by an overproduction of adrenocortical steroids. An overabundance of these hormones causes an accumulation of fluids and fat on the face, neck, and upper back. Other conditions that may develop are muscle weakness, purplish streaks on the skin, acne, osteoporosis, and diabetes mellitus. The person bruises easily, and wound healing is poor. *Obtain physician clearance if symptoms are severe. Use light pressure if client bruises easily or if wound healing is poor.*

Diabetes Insipidus

Diabetes insipidus is caused by a posterior pituitary gland dysfunction that results in deficient production of antidiuretic hormone. Diabetes insipidus has absolutely nothing to do with insulin production or pancreatic dysfunction; however, similar to diabetes mellitus, it results in polyuria, thus reducing fluid volume in the body and increasing thirst. *Adjust massage to client's stamina and vitality (i.e., slow, gentle, short duration; assist client on and off table). Make sure client has necessary medication handy during treatment.*

Diabetes Mellitus

Diabetes mellitus is a group of disorders that leads to elevated blood glucose levels (hyperglycemia). Glucose appears in the urine and is accompanied by polyuria (excessive excretion of urine), excessive eating (polyphagia), polydipsia (excessive thirst), and peripheral neuropathy. Diabetes mellitus is thought to be an autoimmune disease because the beta cells of the pancreas, which produce insulin, are destroyed. Type I diabetes entails a deficiency of insulin, and regular injections of insulin are needed. Type II diabetes represents more than 90% of all cases. Long-term complications such as peripheral vascular disease (decreased circulation in the hands and feet) and neuropathy (decrease or change in sensation in hands and feet) may develop as the disease progresses. Other complications are atherosclerosis, high blood pressure, blindness, and thrombosis. It usually occurs later in life and can be controlled by diet, exercise, and weight loss. *Use light pressure. Avoid vigorous massage (e.g., percussion, vibration). Inform client of any bruises or breaks in the skin, especially in the feet. If client is taking insulin, then avoid injection site for at least 10 days on or around the injection site. Make sure client has necessary medications handy during treatment. Be prepared to make accommodations for client's medication administration or food intake during treatment, such as having drinking water and hard candy available.*

Goiter

An enlarged thyroid gland, or goiter, is associated with hyperthyroidism, hypothyroidism, inflammation, infection, or lack of iodine in the diet. Goiters are more prevalent in countries

JANET TRAVELL, MD

Born: December 17, 1901; died: August 1, 1997.

"It is obvious that our potential for optimal health depends not alone on the pathology of disease, but on the fiber of our personalities."

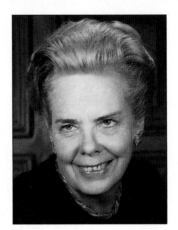

At the 1949 American Medical Association (AMA) convention, a renowned British rheumatologist and author was introduced to Dr. Janet Travell. His response was, "Oooh! Dr. Travell! Soooo, you're the Trigger Queen."

Most massage therapists today are familiar with Travell's groundbreaking work, but mapping previously uncharted patterns of pain is only part of this extraordinary woman's legacy. In addition to her unceasing study of the human body, she was a poet, mother, and the first female physician in the White House.

As a youngster, Travell loved the process of learning but especially enjoyed the sciences. During her school days, one of her roles was to supply the class with earthworms for dissection. Summer months were spent at the farm engrossed in education of a different sort: tree climbing, storm watching, and, of course, earthworm collecting. Her mother taught her basket making, tooling leather, sewing, tatting lace, and knitting.

Her father was responsible for teaching her how to shoot—and how to think. He also showed her how to make the best use of her time. "Over and over, he pointed out the value of time and the importance of concentration," she has been quoted as saying. "If I could do a piece of homework well in fifteen minutes, I should not dawdle over it for thirty. I learned to shut out extraneous matters and to accelerate the pace of my thinking. Another technique of learning that my father taught me to focus on was to focus my attention on things I did not know—new ideas, strange words, and my own mistakes."

Travell wanted to follow in her father's footsteps and become a physician "because he was a magician, and everything he did was wonderful." It did not surprise Travell when she learned through her mother that her father regularly set off giant firecrackers in the fireplace at 3 AM. "I think that he must have been born with a firecracker in one hand and a lighted match in the other," she wrote in her autobiography.

Travell's daughter, Virginia P. Wilson, says this about her grandfather: "I think my mother's energy was inherited from her father, Dr. Willard Travell, an early pioneer in the field of physical medicine. My sister has the same energy. We call it 'the Travell energy' in the family. Those who possess it walk fast so it is difficult to keep up with them, and they get an enormous amount done in a day. They never waste time. They are trim, never overweight, organized people who plan their work, recreation, and activities well."

Travell completed tasks too quickly to suit one of her medical school professors. Again and again, he accused her of hurrying through her dissection. Travell came up with the idea of doing the dissection with her left hand to slow her down enough to match the speed of the rest of the students. Not only did this appease her professor, she also delighted at her newfound ambidexterity.

To better balance career and family, Travell scaled her practice of medicine back to part time. However, it did not really slow her down much; she simply earned less money. Jack Powell, her husband, said that, before they married, he had thought carefully about the consequences of starting a life with someone whose career made her quite different from most of the women of her time. He knew he could not make her into something other than who she was, so he accepted her wholly and completely, including her rigorous daily schedule, offering her support when and where she needed it the most. In a reunion address 45 years after her medical school graduation, Travell commended him and the importance of the man behind every successful woman.

Travell's part-time schedule did give her the freedom to practice at home. Her initial investigation into muscular pain rose out of this additional time to do research, her father's physical medicine experience, and her own shoulder injury at age 38.

When working in a cardiac clinic, Travell had also treated patients with life-threatening pulmonary disease. Common among both the heart and the lung patients were complaints of persistent, acute pain in the shoulder area. Travell came up with enough published findings, mostly from outside the United States, to begin her own study.

Travell researched, ignored skeptics, looked at muscle tissue under a microscope, injected, poked, prodded, and sprayed but did not even stop there. She recognized the role of body mechanics and quizzed patients about how they stood, worked, or turned. She discovered that muscles have memory and can stay contracted for long periods. She found evidence of existing myofascial pain from old

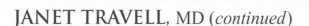

JANET TRAVELL, MD (*continued*)

injuries that responded to trigger point therapy. Although the prevailing protocol in her time was heat for sore muscles, she successfully experimented with the use of cold. She developed a method for painless needle injections and even meandered into chair design for a time. She was a *whole-body practitioner* who listened carefully to her patients, preached preventive medicine, and made pain go away, even for those whose pain had been diagnosed for years as psychosomatic by stumped physicians.

Travell bemoaned the fact that so many of us are willing to accept average health. With this intense dedication and track record for success, not surprisingly, word of her reputation reached the young Senator John F. Kennedy, for whom Travell is credited with getting in good enough shape to launch a presidential race. In return, he appointed her White House physician. After his assassination, Travell remained on staff at President Lyndon Johnson's request. During her tenure in the position, she missed only 1 day because of illness. "Although my health was not a problem, I took the precautions of having thorough medical checkups and of taking a sensi-

ble dose of regular exercise," she stated in her autobiography. On her departure, the Johnsons presented her with a token of their appreciation—a framed "Prescription for Happiness" that stated at the top, "OFFICE HOURS DAY & NIGHT." "That indeed had been my life," she said in the book she later named after the plaque, "and my happiness was founded on hard work."

Travell left the White House in 1965, and although she was 64, she was in no way considering retirement. She published her autobiography in 1968, and in 1992, she and David G. Simons published *The Trigger Point Manuals*.

Wilson describes her mother as "a true humanitarian who wanted to solve the pain problems of as many people as she could and didn't stop answering letters and reading her journals until a few weeks before her death at [age] 95, on August 1, 1997." Richard and Kathryn Weiner of the American Academy of Pain Management wrote a tribute to Travell that included the following line: "She loved those whom she encountered and in return received that special gift of knowing that her life mattered."

where dietary iodine intake is inadequate. *Adjust massage to client's stamina and vitality (i.e., slow, gentle, short duration; assist client on and off table). Avoid neck and throat region.*

Graves' Disease

Hyperthyroidism, related anxiety, fatigue, tremors of the hands, loss of appetite, and increased metabolic rate characterize Graves' disease. An enlarged thyroid and lymph nodes and an unusual protrusion of the eyeballs often accompany this condition. Graves' disease is thought to be an autoimmune disorder. *Adjust massage to client's stamina and vitality (i.e., slow, gentle, short duration; assist client on and off table). Avoid neck and throat region, and any enlarged lymph nodes.*

Hyperparathyroidism

An overproduction of parathyroid hormone results in hyperparathyroidism. It is characterized by an increased reabsorption of calcium from the bones and an increased absorption of calcium by the kidneys and gastrointestinal tract. The client may experience pain and tenderness and even spontaneous fractures. Gastrointestinal symptoms such as loss of appetite, nausea, vomiting, and abdominal pain may also be experienced. *Obtain physician clearance if symptoms are*

severe. Avoid areas of bone fractures or areas where pressure causes pain. Carefully administer or avoid techniques such as stretches or mobilization, and avoid vigorous massage in areas where bones are fragile.

Hyperpituitarism

Hyperpituitarism with overproduction of growth hormone causes acromegaly. Acromegaly occurs during the adult years and is characterized by elongation and enlargement of the bones of the extremities, face, and jaw. Gigantism results from overproduction of growth hormone during childhood and puberty. Hyperpituitarism may also lead to Cushing's disease. *Obtain physician clearance if symptoms are severe. Avoid areas where pressure causes pain. Carefully administer or avoid techniques such as stretches or mobilization, and avoid vigorous massage (if physician approved).*

Hyperthyroidism

Hyperactivity of the thyroid gland, hyperthyroidism is characterized by an enlarged thyroid, nervousness and tremor, heat intolerance, increased appetite with weight loss, rapid forceful pulse, and increased respiration rate. *Obtain physician clearance if symptoms are severe. Adjust massage to client's stamina and vitality (i.e., slow, gentle, short duration; assist client on and off table). Avoid neck and throat region.*

Hypoglycemia

Hypoglycemia is almost the opposite of diabetes, although it too can be related to pancreatic dysfunction. *Hypoglycemia* refers to an excessive loss in blood glucose levels that can result in a variety of symptoms, including weakness, light-headedness, headaches, excessive hunger, visual disturbances, anxiety, and sudden changes in personality. If left untreated, the result may be delirium, coma, and death. Causes of hypoglycemia can be an overdose of prescribed insulin, an excessive level of insulin production by the pancreas, or extreme dietary deficiencies. *Adjust massage to client's stamina and vitality (i.e., slow, gentle, short duration; assist client on and off table).*

Hypoparathyroidism

Hypoparathyroidism is a condition that results from diminished function of the parathyroid gland. It is caused by surgical removal of the glands, an autoimmune disease, or genetic factors. With a fall in calcium levels, the client may experience muscle pain. Other symptoms include tingling in the hands and feet; dry, scaly skin; and a rapid, irregular heartbeat. *Obtain physician clearance if symptoms are severe. Adjust massage to client's stamina and vitality (i.e., slow, gentle, short duration; assist client on and off table). If client has tingling in the hands or feet, then the pressure of massage over these areas needs to be light. Use techniques to maintain flexibility.*

Hypopituitarism

Hypopituitarism is a decrease in the secretion of hormones by the pituitary gland. If it occurs during childhood, then it results in dwarfism; if it occurs during adulthood, then it can result in infertility; lethargy; dry, thick skin; hypoglycemia; loss of appetite; hypotension; abdominal pain; and intolerance

to cold. *Obtain physician clearance if symptoms are severe. Adjust massage to client's stamina and vitality (i.e., slow, gentle, short duration; assist client on and off table, and use of extra drape if client chills easily).*

Hypothyroidism

A deficiency of thyroid activity, hypothyroidism is marked by fatigue and lethargy; weight gain; slowed mental processes; skin dryness; and slow digestive, heart, and respiration rates. More common in women than men, this condition may lead to cretinism. *Obtain physician clearance if symptoms are severe. Adjust massage to client's stamina and vitality (i.e., slow, gentle, short duration; assist client on and off table, and use extra drape if client chills easily). Avoid neck and throat region.*

evolve *There are numerous activites such as labeling sheets and crossword puzzles for your use on the Evolve website that accompanies this text. Be sure to take advantage of them.* ■

Effects of Massage on the Endocrine System

Increases dopamine level. Massage is linked to decreased stress levels and reduced depression.
Increases serotonin level. Research suggests a reduction of both stress and depression. Theories suggest that serotonin inhibits transmission of noxious signals to the brain, indicating that increased levels of serotonin may also reduce pain.
Reduces cortisol level. Research reduces cortisol level by activating the relaxation response. Elevated levels of cortisol represent not only heightened stress, but also inhibited immune functions.
Reduces norepinephrine level. Massage reduces norepinephrine, which is linked to the relaxation response.
Reduces epinephrine level. Massage reduces epinephrine, which is linked to the relaxation response.
Reduces feelings of depression. Both chemical and electrophysiological changes from a negative to a positive mood were noted and may underlie the decrease in depression after massage therapy.

SUMMARY

The endocrine glands and the hormones they secrete make up the endocrine system (Table 18-8). The endocrine glands are ductless, release hormones in one part of the body, travel through the bloodstream, and affect cells in other parts of the body. Some hormones do not enter the bloodstream but work on neighboring cells instead. The functions of the endocrine system are to regulate growth, development, metabolism, and fluid balance and to maintain homeostasis and contribute to the reproductive process.

Hormones are chemical messengers and act as catalytic agents that affect the physiological activity of other cells in the body. Types of hormones are steroids, peptides, biogenic amines, and eicosanoids. Negative-feedback systems, other hormones, and the nervous system govern the amount of hormone secreted.

Hormones are produced by the following glands: adrenals, gonads, pancreatic islets, parathyroids, pineal, pituitary, and thyroid. Abnormal hormone production may result in diseases such as diabetes, hypoglycemia, and obesity.

TABLE 18-8 **Hormonal Functions**

HORMONE	GLAND	PRIMARY ACTION(S)
Adrenocorticotropic hormone	Pituitary (anterior lobe)	Regulates endocrine activity of the adrenal cortex
Aldosterone	Adrenals (cortex)	Stimulates the reabsorption of sodium and water in kidney filtration
Androgen	Adrenals (cortex)	Maintains male sex characteristics
Antidiuretic hormone	Pituitary (posterior lobe)	Decreases urine output and raises blood pressure
Calcitonin	Thyroid	Decreases blood calcium and phosphorus levels
Cortisol	Adrenals (cortex)	Produces an antiinflammatory response and affects carbohydrate, protein, and fat metabolism
Epinephrine	Adrenals (medulla)	Increases blood pressure by stimulating vasoconstriction
Estrogen	Ovaries	Prepares female genital tract for fertilization and implantation embryo and helps keep calcium in bones
Follicle-stimulating hormone	Pituitary (anterior lobe)	Stimulates ovarian egg development and production; stimulates sperm production in testes
Glucagon	Pancreas	Increases blood glucose levels
Human growth hormone	Pituitary (anterior lobe)	Stimulates protein synthesis for muscle and bone growth
Insulin	Pancreas	Decreases blood glucose levels
Luteinizing hormone	Pituitary (anterior lobe)	Stimulates ovulation and production of estrogen and progesterone in ovaries; stimulates testosterone secretion in testes
Melanocyte-stimulating hormone	Pituitary (anterior lobe)	Stimulates distribution of melanin, increasing skin pigmentation
Melatonin	Pineal	Controls circadian rhythms and growth and development of sexual organs
Norepinephrine	Adrenals (medulla)	Helps body maintain the stress response
Oxytocin	Pituitary (posterior lobe)	Involved in milk expression and uterine contractions
Parathyroid hormone	Parathyroid	Increases blood calcium levels
Progesterone	Ovaries	Prepares endometrium for pregnancy
Prolactin	Pituitary (anterior lobe)	Stimulates milk production
Relaxin	Ovaries	Softens connective tissue of a pregnant woman for fetal delivery
Testosterone	Testes	Promotes secondary male sex characteristics, libido, and sperm production
Thymopoietin	Thymus	Play a role in the body's growth and maturation of antibodies
Thymosin	Thymus	Play a role in the body's growth and maturation of antibodies
Thyroid-stimulating hormone	Pituitary (anterior lobe)	Stimulates thyroid to produce and secrete triiodothyronine and thyroxine
Triiodothyronine	Thyroid	Regulates growth and development and influences mental, physical, and metabolic activities
Thyroxine	Thyroid	Regulates growth and development and influences mental, physical, and metabolic activities

evolve

Go to *Chapter Extras* on Evolve for additional illustrations and resources for this chapter. *Extras* for this chapter include:

1. Drag and drop (online game)

MATCHING I

Place the letter of the answer next to the term or phrase that best describes it. Some answers may be used more than once.

A. Adrenal cortex
B. Adrenal medulla
C. Ovaries
D. Pancreatic islets

E. Parathyroids
F. Pineal
G. Pituitary (anterior lobe)
H. Pituitary (posterior lobe)

I. Testes
J. Thymus
K. Thyroid

_____ 1. Prolactin

_____ 2. Contains alpha and beta cells

_____ 3. Insulin

_____ 4. Thyroxin and triiodothyronine

_____ 5. Estrogen and progesterone

_____ 6. Cortisol

_____ 7. Calcitonin

_____ 8. Parathyroid hormone

_____ 9. Adrenocorticotropic hormone

_____ 10. Glucagon

_____ 11. Testosterone

_____ 12. Epinephrine and norepinephrine

_____ 13. Thymosin and thymopoietin

_____ 14. Antidiuretic hormone

_____ 15. Contains neurosecretory cells in pituitary

_____ 16. Melatonin

MATCHING II

Place the letter of the answer next to the term or phrase that best describes it. Some answers may be used more than once.

A. Adrenocorticotropic hormone
B. Antidiuretic hormone
C. Calcitonin
D. Glucagon
E. Growth hormone

F. Insulin
G. Luteinizing hormone
H. Melanocyte-stimulating hormone
I. Oxytocin

J. Parathyroid hormone
K. Prolactin
L. Thyroid-stimulating hormone
M. Thyroxine

_____ 1. Stimulates secretion and production of thyroid hormones

_____ 2. Regulates endocrine functions of the adrenal cortex

_____ 3. Triggers ovulation

_____ 4. Is involved in uterine contractions

_____ 5. Decreases urine output

_____ 6. Decreases blood glucose levels

_____ 7. Stimulates protein synthesis for muscle and bone growth

_____ 8. Stimulates the mammary glands to produce milk

_____ 9. Stimulates milk expression

_____ 10. Increases blood glucose levels

_____ 11. Increases rate of metabolism

_____ 12. Stimulates the distribution of melanin granules in the skin

_____ 13. Increases blood calcium levels

_____ 14. Decreases blood calcium levels

INTERNET ACTIVITIES

Visit the National Institute of Diabetes and Digestive and Kidney Diseases at http://www.niddk.nih.gov. Locate Disease and Nutrition Topics, choose the link to diabetes information, and write a two-page report. Present the report to class.

Visit the http://www.hormone.org and choose Menopause. What are some of the symptoms of menopause? What are *designer estrogens?*

Visit The Obese Society at http://www.naaso.org and choose Information, then Fact Sheets. After reading, find the relationship between obesity and diabetes.

Bibliography

Abrahams P, Marks S, Hutchings R: *McMinn's color atlas of human anatomy,* St Louis, 2003, Mosby.

Applegate EJ: *The anatomy and physiology learning system,* ed 3, Philadelphia, 2006, Saunders.

Beers MH, Berkow R: *The Merck manual of diagnosis and therapy,* Whitehouse Station, NJ, 2006, Merck Research Laboratories.

Crawley J, Van De Graaff KM: *A photographic atlas for anatomy and physiology,* Englewood, Colo, 2002, Morton.

Como D, editor: *Mosby's medical, nursing, and allied health dictionary,* ed 6, St Louis, 2002, Mosby.

Ferri FF: *2003 Ferri's clinical advisor, instant diagnosis and treatment,* St Louis, 2003, Mosby.

Guyton A: *Human physiology and mechanisms of disease,* ed 6, Philadelphia, 1996, Saunders.

Haubrich WS: *Medical meanings: a glossary of word origins,* Philadelphia, 1997, American College of Physicians.

Huether SE, McCance KL: *Understanding pathophysiology,* ed 3, St Louis, 2004, Mosby.

Jacob S, Francone C: *Elements of anatomy and physiology,* Philadelphia, 1989, Saunders.

Kalat JW: *Biological psychology,* ed 8, Belmont, Calif, 2003, Wadsworth.

Kapit W, Elson LM: *The anatomy coloring book,* ed 3, New York, 2002, Benjamin Cummings.

Kordish M, Dickson S: *Introduction to basic human anatomy,* Lake Charles, La, 1985, McNeese State University.

Kumar V, Abbas A, Fausto N: *Robbins and Cotran physiologic basis of disease,* ed 7, St Louis, 2005, Mosby.

Marieb EN: *Essentials of human anatomy and physiology,* ed 8, New York, 2005, Benjamin Cummings.

Martini FH, Bartholomew EF: *Essentials of anatomy and physiology,* ed 3, New York, 2003, Benjamin Cummings.

McAleer N: *The body almanac,* Garden City, NY, 1985, Doubleday.

McCance K, Huether S: *Pathophysiology: the biological basis for disease in adults and children,* St Louis, 2006, Mosby.

Merck manual, ed 17, Whitehouse Station, NJ, 1998, Merck and Company.

Mosby's medical, nursing, and allied health dictionary, ed 6, St Louis, 2002, Mosby.

Netter FH: *Atlas of human anatomy,* ed 3, Teterboro, NJ, 2003, Icon Learning Systems.

Newton D: *Pathology for massage therapists,* ed 2, Portland, Ore, 1995, Simran.

Premkumar K: *Pathology A to Z, a handbook for massage therapists,* Baltimore, 1999, Lippincott Williams & Wilkins.

Salvo SG, Anderson SK: *Mosby's pathology for massage therapists,* St Louis, 2004, Elsevier Mosby.

Solomon EP, Phillips GA: *Understanding human anatomy and physiology,* Philadelphia, 1987, Saunders.

Thibodeau G, Patton K: *Anatomy and physiology,* ed 6, St Louis, 2006, Mosby.

Thibodeau G, Patton K: *Structure and function of the body,* ed 12, St Louis, 2004, Mosby.

Tortora GJ: *Introduction to the human body: the essentials of anatomy and physiology,* ed 5, Hoboken, NJ, 2000, John Wiley & Sons.

Tortora GJ, Grabowksi SR: *Principles of anatomy and physiology,* ed 11, New York, 2005, John Wiley & Sons.

Venes D, Thomas CL, Taber CW: *Taber's cyclopedic medical dictionary,* ed 20, Philadelphia, 2005, FA Davis.

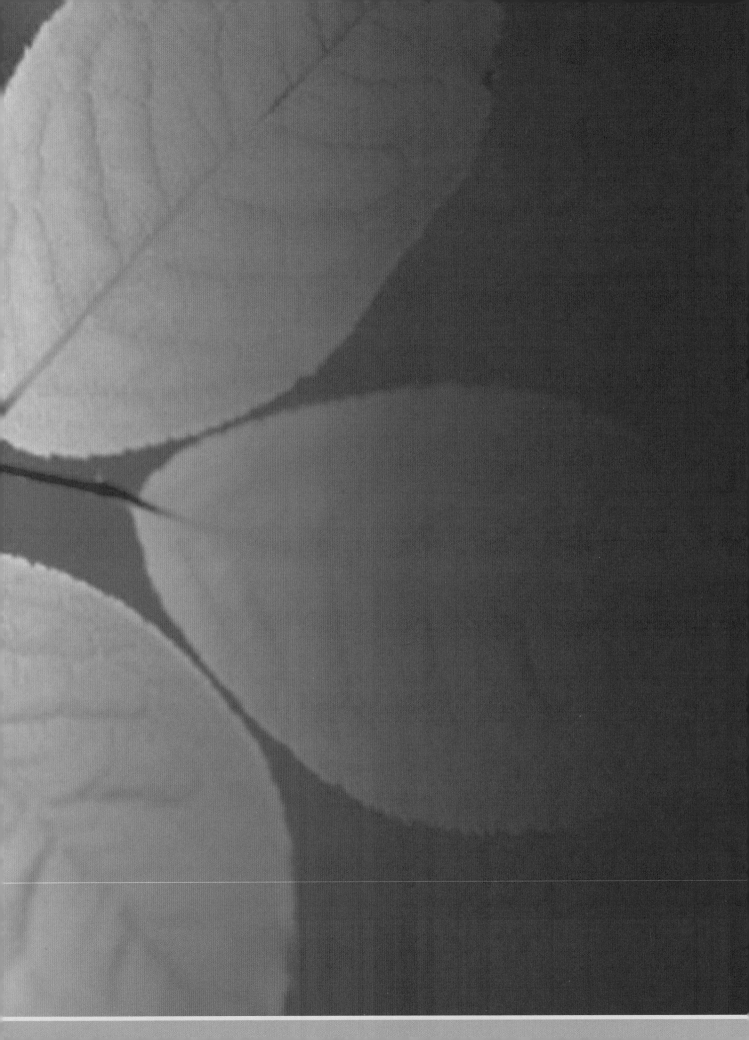

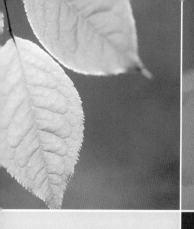

CHAPTER 19

"Be a lamp, a lifeboat, or a ladder."
—Rumi

Circulatory System

STUDENT OBJECTIVES

After completing this chapter, the student should be able to:

- List anatomical structures and describe the physiological mechanisms of the cardiovascular system
- Describe the blood's characteristics and physical composition (plasma and blood cells)
- Identify how oxygen is transported in the blood
- Explain three blood-clotting mechanisms
- Identify and discuss blood types
- Trace blood through the heart, identifying each chamber
- Discuss the heart's conduction system
- List three main types of blood vessels, identifying characteristics of each
- Discuss blood pressure and factors that influence both blood pressure and heart rate
- Name and locate all major arteries, pulse points, and veins of the body
- List anatomical structures and describe the physiological mechanisms of the lymphatic-immune systems
- Identify the lymphatic organs and vessels of the body
- Trace lymph flow from the lymphatic capillaries to the major lymphatic ducts
- Discuss natural and acquired immunity
- Name types of pathological conditions of the cardiovascular and the lymphatic-immune systems, giving characteristics and massage considerations of each

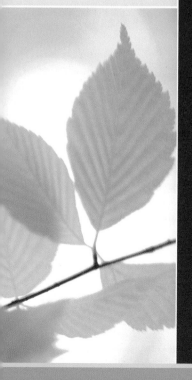

INTRODUCTION

The body is 60% to 80% fluid (by volume). This fluid requires circulation to maintain the body's health. The cardiovascular and lymphatic-immune systems are responsible for fluid movement and maintenance; they are collectively referred to as the *circulatory system*. However, the two divisions will be discussed separately. The cardiovascular system circulates blood, and the lymphatic vascular system circulates lymph. Both subsystems are regarded as *pickup and delivery* systems because their primary function is transportation.

CARDIOVASCULAR SYSTEM

The cardiovascular system consists of the blood, heart, and blood vessels. This section examines the characteristics of blood, such as plasma and blood cells, its clotting function, blood typing, and its main function of transport. Blood is the primary transport medium for a variety of substances that travel through the body. It makes its way through the body in a circular direction because of the pumping action of the heart, traveling through thousands of miles of blood vessels. Some of the blood vessels are areas in which caution needs to be exercised in massage therapy (endangerment sites). Circulation is accomplished by a vast network of vessels, and each vessel plays a different role in the circulatory process.

ANATOMY

Areas of discussion in this part of the chapter include
- Blood
- Blood vessels
- Heart

PHYSIOLOGY

The functions of the cardiovascular system are the following:
1. Transportation and distribution of the respiratory gases, nutrients from the digestive tract, antibodies, waste materials, and hormones from endocrine glands, as well as transportation of heat from active muscles to the skin, where the heat can be dissipated through vasodilation.
2. Protection of the body through disease-fighting white blood cells and the removal of impurities and pathogens
3. Prevention of hemorrhage through clotting mechanisms, including prevention of loss of body fluids from damaged vessels

BLOOD

Blood is a fluid medium containing erythrocytes, leukocytes, and suspended platelets. Blood is classified as a liquid connective tissue and is essential for human life because the body's tissues can get oxygen and nutrients only from its blood supply. Representing approximately 8% of

Terms and Their Meanings Related to the Circulatory System

TERM	MEANING
Aorta	Gr. a strap; to suspend
Atrium	L. corridor
Bicuspid	L. two; pointed
Brady	Gr. slow
Capillary	L. hairlike
Cardio, cardia	Gr. heart
Chordae tendineae	Gr. cordlike; L. tendon
Cisterna chyli	L. a reservoir or cavity; juice
Coagulation	L. to curdle
Coronary	L. shaped as a crown or circle
Cyanosis	Gr. dark blue; condition
Diastole	Gr. to expand
Edema	Gr. swelling
Erythrocyte	Gr. red; cell
Fibrinogen	L. fiber; Gr. to produce
Hemo	Gr. blood
Hemoglobin	Gr. blood; L. globe
Hemorrhage	Gr. blood; to burst forth
Hemostasis	Gr. blood; stopping
Intercalate	L. between; to put in place
Intima	L. innermost
Ischemia	Gr. to hold back blood
Leukocytes	Gr. white; cell
Lumen	L. light
Mediastinum	L. standing in the middle
Mitral	L. headdress
Phagocytosis	Gr. to eat; cell; condition
Pinocytosis	Gr. to drink; cell; condition
Plasma	Gr. a thing formed
Platelet	Fr. flat
Purkinje fibers	Purkyně, Czech anatomist (1787-1869)
Saphenous	Gr. the hidden
Semilunar	L. half; moon
Sphygmomanometer	Gr. pulse; thin; measure
Systole	Gr. contraction
Tachy	Gr. rapid, fast, or swift
Thrombocyte	Gr. clot; cell
Tricuspid	Gr. three; L. pointed
Tunica	L. a tunic
Vascular	L. a vessel or duct
Vasoconstriction	L. vessel; a binder
Vasodilation	L. vessel; to widen
Vena cava	L. vein; cavity
Ventricle	L. little belly

Fr., French; *Gr.,* Greek; *L.,* Latin.

total body weight, blood is composed of a liquid (plasma) in which cells and cell fragments possessing different functions are suspended (Figure 19-1). Blood volume in the average-size man is approximately 5 to 6 liters (L) (6 quarts or 12 pints); blood volume in average-size women is approximately 4 to 5 L. Under normal circumstances, a blood cell makes a round trip through the circulatory system every 60 seconds.

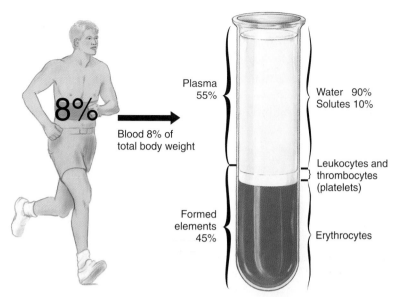

FIGURE 19-1 Composition of blood.

Characteristics of Blood

The following is a list of the characteristics of blood:
- Blood is a viscous fluid that is thicker and more adhesive than water.
- Its pH is slightly alkaline.
- The color varies from bright scarlet red to dull maroon, depending on oxygen content.
- Blood is warmer (100° F) than the rest of the body.

Components of Blood

Plasma

Plasma is a straw-colored liquid that helps transport the blood cells. Approximately 55% of blood is plasma, but plasma itself is 90% water and 10% solutes (substances dissolved in a solution). One of the solutes is *fibrinogen,* which functions in blood clotting. When necessary, fibrinogen is converted to *fibrin* and forms the foundations of a blood clot. Other solutes include plasma proteins, hormones, enzymes, and wastes.

Blood Cells

Blood cells are formed primarily in the red bone marrow of long, flat, and irregular bones. All types of blood cells are produced from a single, undifferentiated cell called a *pluripotent stem cell.* The three blood cells (erythrocytes, leukocytes, and thrombocytes) comprise approximately 45% of blood; each cell performs a different function (Figure 19-2).

   Erythrocytes – The primary function of **erythrocytes**, or red blood cells (RBCs), is to transport oxygen in the blood. They also carry carbon dioxide. RBCs are the most numerous of all cells in the blood, and they are the major factor contributing to blood viscosity. These cells do not have a nucleus, which keeps them from reproducing or carrying out extensive metabolic activities (Figure 19-3). Each functional erythrocyte is biconcave to allow greater surface area

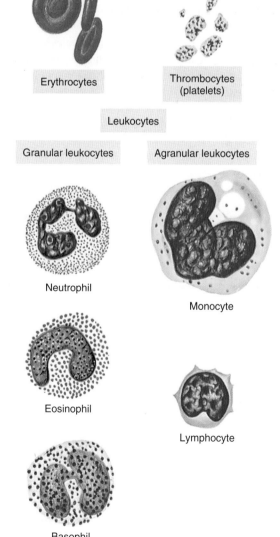

FIGURE 19-2 Types of blood cells.

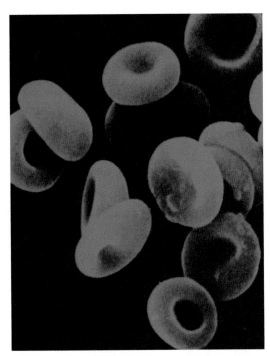

FIGURE 19-3 Erythrocytes.

for more efficient diffusion of oxygen molecules and ease of movement through tiny capillaries (minute blood vessels). Erythrocytes are occupied by a red respiratory pigment called **hemoglobin,** giving blood its characteristically red color. Hemoglobin, an iron-based protein, combines temporarily with oxygen and carbon dioxide so these gases can be transported.

Hemoglobin carries oxygen or carbon dioxide, but not both, at any given time. Special proteins on the surfaces of RBCs determine the different blood types (A, B, AB, or O). The life span of an erythrocyte is between 100 and 120 days, after which it begins to fragment, and the remains are eliminated by the spleen and liver.

TABLE TALK

Cigarette smoking damages approximately 20% of the smoker's hemoglobin because of the presence (and crowding) of carbon monoxide. Carbon monoxide binds to hemoglobin 200 times more strongly than does oxygen, thus leaving no room for oxygen to bind.

Leukocytes – **Leukocytes,** or white blood cells (WBCs), serve as part of the body's immune system by protecting the body from invading bacteria, viruses, and other pathogens. Think of these cells as the blood's defensive *mobile army.* WBCs begin to mobilize and destroy the invader in processes known as *phagocytosis* and *pinocytosis* (see Chapter 11). Some WBCs combat irritants by producing *histamine,* a compound released in allergic, inflammatory reactions that in extreme cases causes dilation of capillaries, decreased blood pressure, and constriction of smooth muscles of the bronchi. Other WBCs produce antimicrobial substances such as antibodies. Antibodies are produced in response to

specific foreign substances such as bacteria, viruses, or an incompatible blood type. **Lymphocytes** are types of WBCs formed in bone marrow, and some mature in the thymus. Whenever WBCs mobilize for action, the body doubles their production within a short time. Their life span varies from a few hours, to a few days, to several years. Specialized leukocytes include basophils, eosinophils, neutrophils, lymphocytes, and monocytes (see Figure 19-2).

Thrombocytes – Also known as **platelets, thrombocytes** are fragmented cells that help repair leaks in the blood vessels through various clotting mechanisms. Their jagged shape helps them adhere to torn surfaces easily, such as from a vessel. The life span of a thrombocyte is approximately 10 days. The three main mechanisms for blood clotting are (1) vascular spasm, (2) a platelet plug, and (3) coagulation.

1. **Vascular spasm:** When the smooth muscle in a vessel is torn, it begins to spasm, reducing the blood flow. This process can continue for up to 30 minutes.
2. **Platelet plug:** When platelets come into contact with the damaged blood vessel, their physical characteristics change by becoming large and sticky, causing them to clump together and form a plug. This plug helps seal damaged vessels.
3. **Coagulation:** Coagulation, or clot formation, is the process of transforming fibrinogen into fibrin threads that trap red blood cells and then tighten the platelet plug into a clot (Figure 19-4). Many plasma proteins are needed to transform fibrinogen into fibrin strands; vitamin K is needed to make many of these proteins. Once a clot is formed, it goes through a process of retraction (tightening) that draws the injured vessel walls closer together for repair and reduces, and later stops, blood loss. At the time a clot is formed, an enzyme is formed, which has the ability to slowly dissolve the clot over time.

evolve Log on to the Evolve website to access a visual representation of blood clotting mechanisms. Be sure to reread the explanation above to review the main processes involved of both the blood and the blood vessel. ■

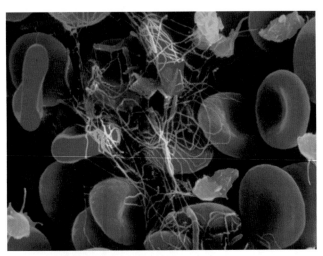

FIGURE 19-4 Fibrin threads creating a clot.

Let us review blood cells:
- Erythrocytes (RBCs) transport oxygen and carbon dioxide.
- Leukocytes (WBCs) fight disease (the body's mobile army).
- Thrombocytes (platelets) clot blood.

TABLE TALK

If your client has clotting difficulties, is on anticoagulant therapy, or is taking prescription or nonprescription blood thinners (e.g., aspirin, ibuprofen, or warfarin [Coumadin]), then deep massage is contraindicated. These clients are prone to bruising, which can result from pressure. Discuss this with your client during the intake before the massage.

BLOOD TYPES

The most common blood typing system is the ABO system, which uses the absence or presence of proteins to classify blood groups. The surfaces of RBCs contain genetically determined proteins called *antigens*. Two blood antigens are A and B. People with antigen A are type A, and those with antigen B are type B. People with both antigens are type AB, and those with neither of the antigens are type O. Additionally, people with type A blood have antibodies against type B in their plasma. People with type B blood have antibodies against type A in their plasma. People with type AB blood do not have antibodies against either type A or type B in their plasma. People with type O blood have antibodies against both type A and type B in their plasma (Table 19-1).

When a foreign antigen is introduced to the body, its corresponding antibody recognizes the foreigner as an intruder and attacks it. This invasion may occur in blood transfusion if the body is given the wrong blood type. If a type A individual is given type B or type AB blood, then the recipient's body recognizes the type B antigens as a foreign protein, attacks it, clumps the foreign cells together, and slices them open. Widespread inflammatory response occurs, and the iron released from the sliced open hemoglobin can cause organ failure and death.

Because type AB has no antibodies for antigen A or B, it can receive all other blood types and is referred to as a **universal recipient.** Type O blood has neither of the antigens and does not react to any other blood types and hence is referred to as a **universal donor.** Blood transfusions must be made with compatible blood types because mismatching can cause severe medical problems or death.

The Rh blood group system depends on the presence or absence of the Rh protein on erythrocytes. Rh factor is so named because the theory was refined in the blood of rhesus

TABLE 19-1 ABO Blood Groups

BLOOD TYPE	ANTIGEN (RBC MEMBRANE)	ANTIBODY (PLASMA)	CAN RECEIVE BLOOD FROM	CAN DONATE BLOOD TO
A (40%)	A antigen	Anti-B antibodies	A, O	A, AB
B (10%)	B antigen	Anti-A antibodies	B, O	B, AB
AB* (4%)	A antigen / B antigen	No antibodies	A, B, AB, O	AB
O† (46%)	No antigen	Both Anti-A and Anti-B antibodies	O	O, A, B, AB

*Type AB: universal recipient.
†Type O: universal donor.

monkeys. Rh positive (approximately 85% of the population) describes the presence of the Rh protein and is not a health problem. Rh negative (approximately 15% of the population) indicates the absence of the Rh protein and can become a problem during pregnancy. If the pregnant mother is Rh negative and the fetus is Rh positive, then blood incompatibility may occur if the blood interacts, such as through a ruptured vessel. The mother's Rh-negative blood develops antibodies against the fetus's Rh-positive blood. These antibodies then attack the fetus's RBCs. Because of medical advances, this situation is now rarely life threatening for the fetus.

JACK MEAGHER, PT, MsT

Born: July 6, 1923; died March 6, 2005.

"Massage is the study of anatomy in Braille."

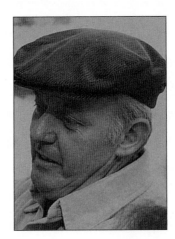

Jack Meagher is the father of sports massage. At age 74, with cancer at the time of this interview, he radiates the energy and demonstrates the quick wit rarely encountered in men half his age.

Before enlisting as a U.S. Army medic for 4 years, Meagher took a course in Swedish massage, hoping eventually to get into physical therapy. When he was in Epernay, France, he experienced a different type of massage than he had learned back home. This massage, performed by a German prisoner of war, made Meagher move markedly better on the baseball field.

After his discharge, Meagher was signed by the Boston Braves as a pitcher, but a wartime shoulder injury threw him a curve that landed him in physical therapy, unable to continue a baseball career. The injury sent him looking for the same kind of massage that he had received in France. He found another German therapist, an instructor at the Viennese Massage School in Connecticut, who relieved his pain to the extent that Meagher was able to play semiprofessional baseball in his hometown of Gloucester, Massachusetts.

The success of his therapy did more than put Meagher's body into motion again; it got him thinking. The result was sports massage, the massage that can enhance athletic performance. Just as Swedish massage uses specific strokes, Meagher classified sports massage strokes as direct pressure, friction, compression, and percussion. He also recommends effleurage and kneading when necessary. "It took me 15 years of putting it together," says Meagher. "I was at a YMCA working on professional athletes and people for whom exercise was a way of life. The sports massage helped them do more before they faded. A loose body uses less energy."

Soon Meagher discovered that what made man go farther and faster might also help horses. That is when sports massage really took off. "In the 1976 Olympics, the horses I'd worked on took two golds and a silver," remembers Meagher. "I was written up and asked to do a book. Then the American Massage Therapy Association became interested, and I was invited to speak at one of their conferences."

The classic sports massage text is *Sports Massage: A Complete Program for Increasing Performance and Endurance in Fifteen Popular Sports* (Doubleday, 1998). It more than introduces a specific massage to the reader; it provides a glimpse into the life of a warm, dedicated, and extremely results-oriented man with a sharp mind, who understands the intricate biomechanics of the body and is able to break it down into simple steps to make his life's work accessible to weekend warriors and professional athletes alike.

Meagher also has a wonderful sense of humor, exemplified in the title of his book, *Never Goose an Appaloosa*. Ticklish himself, he does not even receive Swedish massage, but regarding the horses he massages, Meagher says, "I would not get on a horse, but I do get along with horses. I've never been kicked. Horses understand when you're trying to help them." He is still massaging 40 to 50 horses per week but not the workload he did in his prime. "I used to do 55 people and 30 horses a week," he says.

When asked what characteristics should be present in a successful massage therapist, Meagher says that the desire to help people and the ability to know how to use one's hands are of utmost importance. Additionally, a massage therapist should possess the education for putting it all together.

When asked if he would do it all over again, Meagher says, "I wouldn't do anything differently. It's taken years of hard work. One time a chief of orthopedics told me I had a real gift, and I had to disagree. Gifts come easily. What I do is not a gift. I work hard. I developed my instincts through my failures and my successes."

HEART

The heart is located in the mediastinum region of the thoracic cavity and rests on the diaphragm. Approximately the size of a clenched fist, the **heart** possesses four hollow chambers: two atria (superior chambers) and two ventricles (inferior chambers). A septum separates the ventricles and extends up between the atria (Figure 19-5). These hollow chambers function as a double pump; the right-hand pump forces oxygen-depleted blood to the lungs, whereas the left-hand pump squeezes oxygen-rich blood out to the rest of the body. Pumping blood is the heart's primary function. When the heart contracts, the heart muscle (myocardium) compresses the ventricles, forcing blood out. Valves open and shut to keep the blood on its course. The heart pumps blood intermittently, on the average of 70 beats per minute in a resting person.

TABLE TALK

The heart beats an average of more than 100,000 times a day. The blood is pumped through 60,000 miles of blood vessels, or roughly 2.5 times around the world at the equator.

Heart Coverings and Heart Wall

Surrounding and protecting the heart is a double-layered sac called the *pericardium*. The outer layer of the pericardium is tough, fibrous connective tissue. The inner layer of the pericardium consists of two layers of membrane with serous fluid in between to decrease friction as the heart beats.

The heart wall possesses the following three layers: (1) epicardium, (2) myocardium, and (3) endocardium (Figure 19-6). The *epicardium* is a thin outer layer of serous membrane. This protective layer possesses adipose tissue and the blood vessels that nourish the heart (coronary vessels). The *myocardium* is the thick cardiac muscle layer that makes up the bulk of the heart wall. Contraction of the myocardium forces blood out of the ventricles (see Chapter 11 for a discussion of cardiac muscle). The *endocardium* is the thin, inner lining of the heart and is continuous with the endothelial lining of the heart chambers and blood vessels, as well as the valves of the heart.

"Hippocrates had no means of recognizing the heart as a pump, because there was no such item in his world, and no such word in his vocabulary."
Guido Majno, M.D.

Heart Chambers

The hollow heart is subdivided into four chambers that receive and pump blood. The superior chambers are called the **atria** and take in blood through large veins and then pump it to the inferior chambers. The lower chambers, or **ventricles,** pump blood to the body's organs and tissues (Figure 19-7). The septum separating the right and left atria is called the *interatrial septum,* and the septum separating the right and left

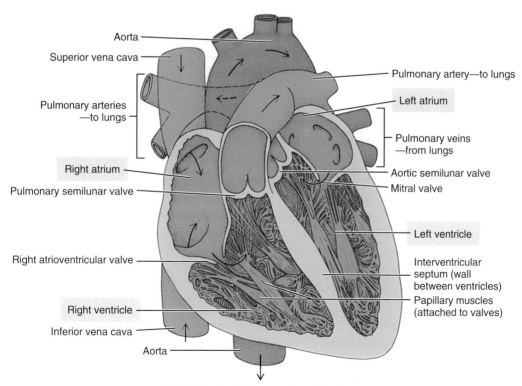

FIGURE 19-5 Cross-section of the heart.

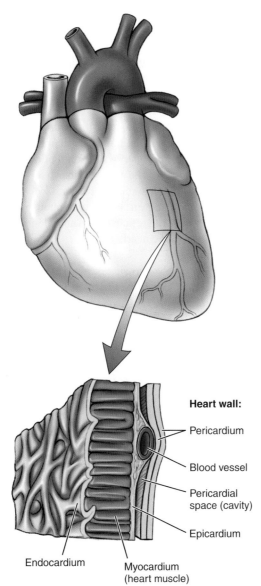

Heart wall:

- Pericardium

- Blood vessel

- Pericardial space (cavity)

- Epicardium

Endocardium Myocardium (heart muscle)

FIGURE 19-6 Cross-section of the heart's wall.

ventricles is called the *interventricular septum*. The heart chambers are described as follows:

- **Right atrium:** Atria, in general, are thin-walled because they need only enough cardiac muscle to deliver the blood into the ventricles. The right atrium receives blood from all parts of the body except the lungs. Blood is received from the superior and inferior vena cava and the coronary sinus. The superior vena cava returns blood from the chest area, arms, and head. The inferior vena cava returns blood from the abdominal area and the legs. The coronary sinus returns blood from the heart itself. Blood from the right atrium is delivered into the right ventricle beneath it.

- **Right ventricle:** The right ventricle receives blood from the right atrium and pumps blood through the pulmonary trunk and into the right and left pulmonary arteries. Blood

is routed to the lungs to release carbon dioxide and pick up oxygen. The oxygenated blood is returned to the heart via the pulmonary veins.

- **Left atrium:** The oxygen-rich blood from the pulmonary veins enters the left atrium. During contraction, blood passes from the left atrium to the left ventricle.

- **Left ventricle:** This ventricular structure has the thickest heart wall because it pumps blood into the aorta and then through miles of blood vessels throughout the body. The amount of blood ejected from the left ventricle during each contraction is called **stroke volume.**

In review, blood travels through the heart as follows:

Blood enters the right atrium,
↓
is delivered to the right ventricle,
↓
moves into the right and left pulmonary arteries,
↓
enters the lungs (releases carbon dioxide [exhale] and obtains oxygen [inhale]),
↓
travels into the right and left pulmonary veins,
↓
moves into the left atrium,
↓
is delivered to the left ventricle,
↓
and flows into the aorta to all parts of the body via the arteries.

Heart Valves

The heart valves are little flaps of endothelium located between the chambers of the heart (atria and ventricles) and between the ventricles and some of the great vessels. These valves keep blood flowing in one direction as the pressure exerted on the blood changes during heart contraction. These valves include the *atrioventricular valves* (AV valves) and the *semilunar valves* (SL valves). The characteristic *lubb-dupp* sound of the heart is from the movement of these valves.

The AV valves separate the atria from the ventricles; these valves are held in place by tendonlike cords called *chordae tendineae,* which attach to the ventricular walls through cardiac muscle projections called *papillary muscles.* The *lubb* sound of the heart is from blood turbulence when the AV valves close. The **tricuspid valve** is the right AV valve and possesses three flaps or cusps. The **mitral valve,** or **bicuspid valve,** is the left AV valve and possesses two flaps or cusps.

The SL valves are located between both ventricles and their adjacent arteries; each valve consists of three half moon–shaped cusps, named for the vessels to which they lead. The *dupp* sound is from blood turbulence when the SL valves close. The **pulmonary SL valve** lies between the

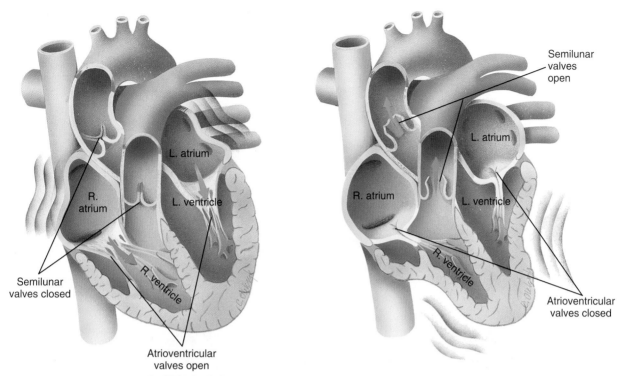

FIGURE 19-7 Heart's chambers and valves during the cardiac cycle.

right ventricle and the pulmonary trunk, and the **aortic SL valve** lies between the left ventricle and the aorta.

Heart Rate and the Heart's Conduction System

The heart's rate of contraction is controlled by a system of modified cardiac cells that conduct impulses through the muscle tissue of the heart. The purpose of this conduction system is to coordinate and synchronize the heart's activity. Cardiac muscle is autorhythmic (capable of self-excitation). Thus the heart has the ability to generate its own independent muscle contraction without outside innervation. The main parts of this system are the *sinoatrial node* (SA node, or pacemaker) and the *atrioventricular node* (AV node), the *bundle of His* (AV bundle), and the *Purkinje fibers,* which are conducting fibers (Figure 19-8).

The SA node lies within the right atrium and initiates the cardiac impulse, stimulating both the right and left atria to contract. It fires an impulse 60 to 100 times a minute (average of 72 times). Because the firing of the SA node sets the rate at which the heart beats, it is called the *pacemaker.*

When the SA node fires, blood in the atria is pushed into the ventricles, and the impulses from the SA node immediately arrive at the AV node. The AV node is designed to work at a slower rate than the SA node to give the atria plenty of time to empty themselves of blood. This brief delay causes the slight pause between two sounds of the heart *(lubb-dupp).* The AV node relays the impulses to the bundle of His. The AV

bundle divides into right and left bundles, which run in the interventricular septum to the right and left ventricles. These bundles branch out to form the Purkinje fibers, the function of which is to spread the impulse throughout the myocardium of the ventricles. This second stimulation through the myocardium causes the ventricles to simultaneously contract, expelling the blood from the ventricles to the arteries.

To review:
- The SA node fires, squeezing the atria to fill the ventricles.
- The signal travels to the AV node, which slows the signal and sends it to the apex of the heart via the bundle of His.
- The Purkinje fibers coordinate the simultaneous contraction of the ventricles.

The cycle of events occurring with each alternating contraction and relaxation of the heart muscle, coordinated by the conducting system, is called the *cardiac cycle.* The firing action of the cardiac cycle remains constant when the SA node acts alone; however, other factors can regulate the cardiac cycle to increase or decrease the output of the heart to meet the demands of the body. A specialized portion of the medulla oblongata known as the *cardiovascular center* controls the majority of heart rate changes. Other influencing factors are as follows:
- Sympathetic division of the autonomic nervous system: Stress increases heart rate.
- Parasympathetic division of the autonomic nervous system: Relaxation decreases heart rate.
- Chemoreceptor input: High carbon dioxide levels increase heart rate, whereas high oxygen levels decrease heart

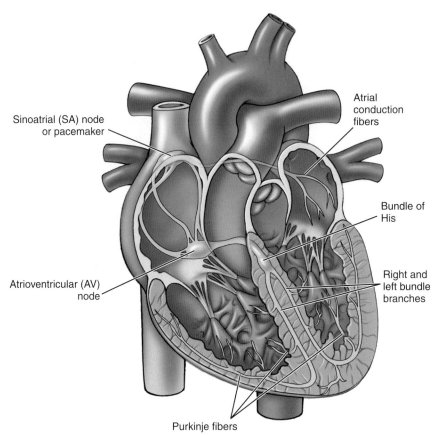

Sinoatrial (SA) node
or pacemaker

Atrial
conduction
fibers

Bundle of
His

Right and
left bundle
branches

Atrioventricular (AV)
node

Purkinje fibers

FIGURE 19-8 Heart's conduction system.

rate; exercise, emotional stress, and altitude changes alter oxygen and carbon dioxide levels.

- Temperature: Elevated temperatures increase heart rates, whereas colder temperatures decrease heart rates.
- Age: Younger people have a higher heart rate than older people.
- General health: Healthier individuals tend to have a lower heart rate than people who are unhealthy.

Any deviation from a normal heart rate pattern is termed **arrhythmia.** The heart rate is the number of ventricular contractions per minute (bpm). Slow heart rate (≤50 bpm) is called **bradycardia.** The condition may be the result of disease; however, it is often normal for people who are physically fit. Rapid heart rate (≥100 bpm) is called **tachycardia.** This condition may be the result of fever, strenuous exercise, or emotions such as anxiety. Tachycardia is the body's response to an increased demand for oxygen by the tissues.

TABLE TALK

Dr. Janet Travell (see the BIO feature in Chapter 18) documents a myofascial trigger point in the right pectoralis major muscle whose pain referral zone refers noxious impulses into the SA node. This trigger point is related to cardiac arrhythmia. Releasing the trigger point with massage techniques can often end symptoms of tachycardia or *runaway* heartbeat. An important point to note is that this procedure is performed only while the client is asymptomatic. A client experiencing tachycardia while in your office should be referred immediately to a physician.

TABLE TALK

An **electrocardiogram** (ECG) is a graphic tracing of the variations in electrical potential caused by the excitation of the heart muscle and detected at the body's surface.

BLOOD VESSELS

Blood vessels are a closed network of tubular structures connected to the heart that transport blood to all the cells of the body. These blood vessels are divided into three main groups based on their structure and function: (1) arteries, (2) veins, and (3) capillaries. The walls of both arteries and veins possess three layers (tunics). The innermost layer is called the *tunica interna,* which is endothelial tissue fused with a small quantity of elastic connective tissue. The middle layer is the *tunica media,* which contains quantities of both connective tissue and smooth muscle. The outer layer, possessing mostly dense connective tissue, is the *tunica externa* (Figure 19-9). Large blood vessels have their own blood supply called the *vasa vasorum,* which are often referred to as the *vessels of the vessels,* and are located in the tunica externa layer.

The walls of arteries and veins, being part muscle, possess two properties: *elasticity* and *contractility.* The levels of these properties differ greatly between the arteries and the

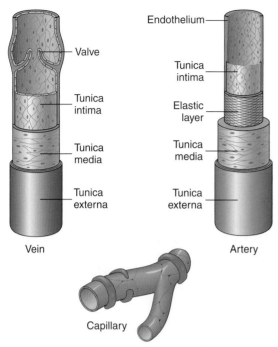

FIGURE 19-9 Blood vessel wall layers.

veins; arterial walls are more elastic than venal walls, and arteries have a thicker muscular layer than veins.

The muscular layer of the arteries and veins can dilate and contract to change the diameter of the vessel. The open space within the blood vessel is known as the *lumen.* When the diameter of the vascular lumen enlarges, the process is called **vasodilation;** when the diameter becomes narrower, the process is called **vasoconstriction.** Vasodilation and vasoconstriction may be initiated by the following two sources: (1) *direct nerve stimulation* from the vasomotor center located in the medulla oblongata and (2) *local reflex response* resulting from a stimulus such as pressure (i.e., massage) or temperature (i.e., heat or cold application).

Arteries

By definition, **arteries** are vessels that move blood away from the heart. In general, blood within the arteries is oxygenated (has already been to the lungs to receive oxygen). The only artery that contains deoxygenated blood is the pulmonary artery, moving blood from the right ventricle of the heart to the lungs; conversely, the pulmonary veins carry oxygenated blood. Because arteries are closer to the pumping action of the heart, their vascular walls are considerably thicker and stronger than veins so as to withstand higher blood pressure and possess a unique elastic layer between tunica interna and media. Arteries continue to branch off into smaller and thinner vessels, becoming **arterioles,** as they lose their two outer layers. When the vessels are one layer thick, they are called *capillaries.*

Because arteries deliver oxygenated blood to the body's tissues, sustained pressure applied on these vessels might interfere with blood delivery and might damage tissues.

Thus the therapist must avoid several important arteries (i.e., endangerment sites; see Chapter 5 for a list of endangerment sites).

Arterial Pulse

The word **pulse** refers to the expansion effect that occurs when the left ventricle contracts, producing a wave of blood that surges through and expands arterial walls. This wave can be felt in the arteries that are located close to the surface of the body or where they lie over bone or other firm tissue. When feeling the pulse, avoid using your thumb or index finger because each contains its own pulse. Each pulse point is named for the region of the body in which it is located. The common pulse points are detailed in the following list (Figure 19-10).

- **Temporal artery:** anterior to the ear; temple region
- **Facial artery:** inferior to the corner of the mouth
- **Common carotid artery:** sides of the throat
- **Axillary artery:** armpit region

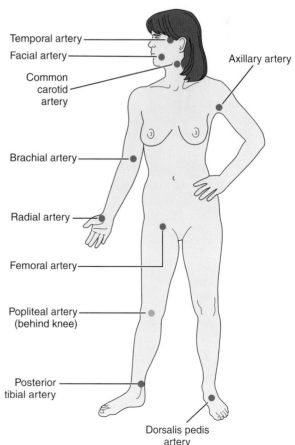

FIGURE 19-10 Pulse points.

- **Brachial artery:** antecubital region
- **Radial artery:** lateral aspect of the wrist
- **Femoral artery:** crease between lower abdomen and upper thigh
- **Popliteal artery:** posterior knee
- **Posterior tibial artery:** behind medial malleolus
- **Dorsalis pedis artery:** anterior medial foot

MINI-LAB

Using the map of pulse points, locate these areas on a partner or on yourself. Note that pressure must be used to feel the pulse, but too much pressure prevents blood from flowing in the vessel.

Capillaries

When the arterioles lose their two outer layers, leaving only endothelium, they become the **capillaries,** which possess a thin, permeable membrane for efficient gas exchange (see Figure 19-9). RBCs carry oxygen in the blood on the hemoglobin molecule; these blood cells must move in a single file to squeeze through each capillary. Capillaries are the functional unit of the cardiovascular system, where gas exchange occurs. The movement of blood in capillaries is the slowest of all the vessels, and its flow is intermittent, providing ample opportunity for exchange to occur. Nutrients and oxygen are provided to the tissues, and waste from cells is removed from interstitial fluid through a process called *capillary exchange*. The exchange of gases is referred to as internal or tissue respiration. Tissues and organs that have extensive capillary networks are the muscles, liver, spleen, adrenals, kidneys, and connective tissue, although cartilage is avascular. Other areas of the body that are devoid of capillaries (and other blood vessels) are the epidermis, hair, nails, and lens and cornea of the eye.

Veins

Veins begin at the capillary level and gradually become larger; small veins are called **venules** (Figure 19-11). **Veins** drain the tissues and organs and return blood, which is now low in oxygen, back to the heart and lungs. Unlike arteries, no pulse is felt in veins, and they are considerably less elastic, possess thinner walls, and are more pliable than arteries. This pliability allows veins to accommodate variations in blood volume. By the time blood leaves the capillaries and moves into the veins, it has lost a great deal of pressure. The blood pressure in veins is usually too low to force the blood back to the heart, and venous return is often flowing against gravity.

To assist venous flow, the lumina in veins are larger than that in arteries, and in small and medium-size veins, folds in the endothelium form numerous valves located at periodic intervals that open in the direction of the heart. This one-way valve system functions to prevent backflow (Figure 19-12). The valve system, combined with the pumping action of muscular contraction in the limbs, is called the **venous pump.** Veins also depend on pressure changes in the thorax and abdomen during breathing (respiratory pump) to push blood back to the heart.

The veins are generally located superficially and near the skeletal muscles so that muscular contraction can assist venous blood flow. This position is why massage movements are performed centripetally (toward the center) to assist the veins in their function.

BLOOD PRESSURE

To understand blood pressure, reviewing some of the basics of physics would be helpful. One law of physics is that pressure of a liquid in a closed system is distributed equally in all directions to the confines of the container. Hence arterial blood pressure is generally consistent throughout the artery in different areas of the body at any given time. Similarly, the same holds true for venous pressure. To distribute itself equally, a liquid always flows from areas of high pressure to areas of low pressure. When a liquid such as blood flows into the heart, it does so because the empty chamber expands and creates a lower pressure or suction effect. Once the blood has filled the chamber, the contraction places force on the blood, and pressure builds. When

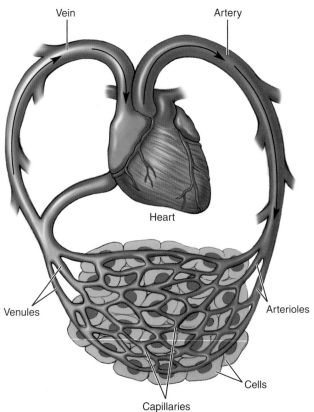

FIGURE 19-11 Blood circulation through vessels.

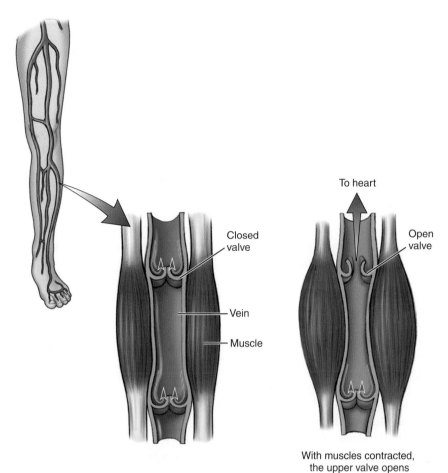

Closed valve

To heart

Open valve

Vein

Muscle

With muscles contracted,
the upper valve opens

FIGURE 19-12 Skeletal muscle pump.

the pressure inside the chamber of the heart overcomes the combination of the pressure outside the heart and the resistance of the valve, blood begins flowing out of the heart. Blood continues to move forward by the one-way action of the valves of the heart.

Blood pressure is the pressure exerted by blood on arterial walls during contraction of the left ventricle. Blood pressure is most often measured in the brachial artery using a *sphygmomanometer,* or blood pressure cuff. The reading gathered during the blood pressure measurement is a fraction or ratio. The top number represents the pressure exerted on the arterial wall during ventricular contraction **(systole).** The bottom number represents the pressure against the arterial wall during the rest or pause between contractions **(diastole).** Blood pressure is measured in millimeters of mercury (mm Hg), which is the pressure required to lift a column of mercury into the gauge to a given height (millimeters). A reading of 120/80 mm Hg is considered to be normal blood pressure for adults. Borderline high blood pressure is above 140/90 mm Hg. Readings over 160/95 mm Hg are considered high, requiring medical attention. The diastolic reading is considered to be the most critical in health considerations. The heart is designed for periodic exertion; it will work hard

to supply the body with blood during times of high demands but cannot keep up a high rate for an extended period without resting. A high diastolic reading may indicate that the heart is working too hard, even during its resting phase. Blood flow, the amount of blood passing through a vessel in a given amount of time, depends on two factors: (1) blood pressure and (2) the resistance of friction between the blood and vessel wall.

When blood pressure rises, the friction resistance rises slightly because of the greater amount of blood being forced through the vessels. The main factor influencing blood flow is the blood pressure. The greater the difference is between systolic and diastolic pressures, the higher the flow rate will be. For example, a blood pressure of 120/80 mm Hg has a pressure difference of 40 mm Hg during the cardiac cycle. If the blood pressure is increased to 140/90 mm Hg because of physical exertion, then the pressure difference has increased to 50 mm Hg. A greater quantity of blood is pushed through the vessel with the higher-pressure drop or greater difference in pressures.

Increased local blood flow is called **hyperemia,** causing the skin to become reddened and warm. This condition often occurs during massage or heat application. Local decrease in blood flow is called **ischemia** and is often marked by pain and tissue dysfunction. Ischemia occurs when blood flow is disturbed, such as a sustained muscular contraction or spasm. Massage therapy, which increases blood flow to an area, reduces ischemia.

Blood flow is influenced by blood pressure. Factors that influence blood pressure itself include resistance, cardiac output, blood volume, homeostatic regulation, and diseases.

- **Resistance.** Resistance is the effect of friction between the blood and vessel walls and is directly influenced by blood viscosity and the diameter of blood vessel.
  - **Viscosity.** The thicker the blood is, the more friction is created, causing blood pressure to rise. Blood thickness may be influenced by medication and by dehydration, which reduces blood plasma, causes blood volume to decrease. An increase in RBC count causes an increase in blood viscosity.
  - **Diameter of the blood vessel.** The smaller the diameter of the blood vessel is, the more resistance it offers the blood, which raises blood pressure.
- **Cardiac output.** Cardiac output represents the blood volume expelled by the ventricles of the heart (stroke volume), multiplied by the heart rate (number of bpm). The ventricles of the heart in a resting adult pump a volume of blood varying from approximately 4 to 8 L of blood per minute. Cardiac output is influenced by the cardiovascular center of the brain, certain blood chemicals, health, and genetics of the person.
- **Blood volume.** As the volume of blood in the body increases, blood pressure increases, which might be the result of a condition such as pregnancy. As blood volume decreases (perhaps because of blood loss by hemorrhage), blood pressure decreases.
- **Homeostatic regulation.** Homeostasis measures and attempts to maintain normal blood pressure through the nervous, endocrine, and urinary systems. These factors include the medulla oblongata (cardiac and vasomotor centers), chemoreceptor input, baroreceptor input, the presence of hormones (epinephrine, norepinephrine, antidiuretic hormone [ADH], aldosterone), and an enzyme (renin).
- **Diseases.** Vascular diseases such as arteriosclerosis may raise systolic blood pressure resulting from the loss of elasticity in arterial walls. Deposits of plaque on the vessel walls may result in an increase of resistance from friction or a diameter restriction and cause an increase in blood pressure. Conditions such as edema may cause extravascular pressure against the vessels, particularly the veins, and may cause the heart to work harder to achieve circulation.

PATHS OF BLOOD CIRCULATION

The primary function of the circulatory system is transportation. Within the cardiovascular system are two paths or circuits based on the areas of the body that are served: (1) pulmonary and (2) systemic (Figure 19-13). In a resting body,

75% of blood volume is located within the systemic system and 25% in the pulmonary system. Looking more closely at blood volume within the systemic system; 20% is arterial, 75% is venous, and the rest is found in the capillaries.

Pulmonary Circuit

The purpose of the pulmonary circuit is to replenish the oxygen supply of the blood and to eliminate gaseous waste products. The **pulmonary circuit** brings deoxygenated blood from the right ventricle to the alveoli of the lungs to release carbon dioxide and regain oxygen. Oxygenated blood returns to the left atrium of the heart and moves into the systemic circuit with the contraction of the left ventricle. When the pulmonary arteries carry blood away from the heart and

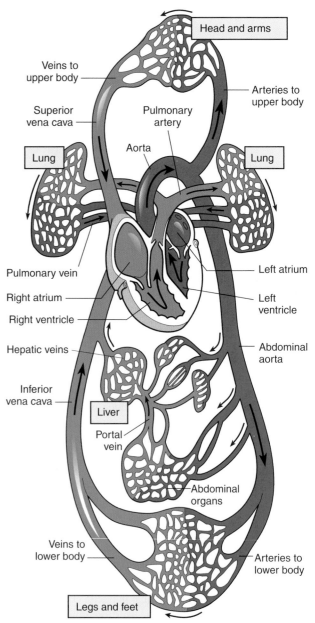

FIGURE 19-13 Pulmonary and systemic circuits.

the pulmonary veins carry blood back to the heart, the oxygen content of the blood is reversed—that is, the pulmonary arteries carry deoxygenated blood away from the heart to the lungs, and the pulmonary veins carry oxygenated blood back from the lungs to the heart.

Systemic Circuit

The **systemic circuit** brings the oxygenated blood from the left ventricle through numerous arteries into the capillaries. From here, blood moves back through the veins and returns the now deoxygenated blood to the right atrium to enter the pulmonary circuit. The function of this circuit is to bring nutrients and oxygen to all systems of the body and to carry waste materials from the tissues for elimination. The systemic circuit is the body's highway system consisting of hollow streets (arteries, capillaries, and veins).

Not all circulation routes begin with arteries and end with veins. Another circulatory network for transporting blood is located within the systemic circuit. *Venous portal systems* start and end with veins. The main venous portal system is the **hepatic portal system,** which collects blood from the digestive organs (stomach, intestines, gallbladder, spleen, and pancreas) and delivers this blood to the liver for processing and storage. The portal vein is a large vein (formed by the union of the superior mesenteric vein and the splenic vein) that carries blood from the organs of digestion to the liver. Because the liver is a key organ involved in maintaining the proper glucose, fat, and protein concentrations in the blood, the hepatic portal system allows the blood from the digestive organs to detour through the liver to process these substances before they enter the systemic circulation (Figure 19-14). The other venous portal system is located between the hypothalamus and the anterior pituitary of the brain.

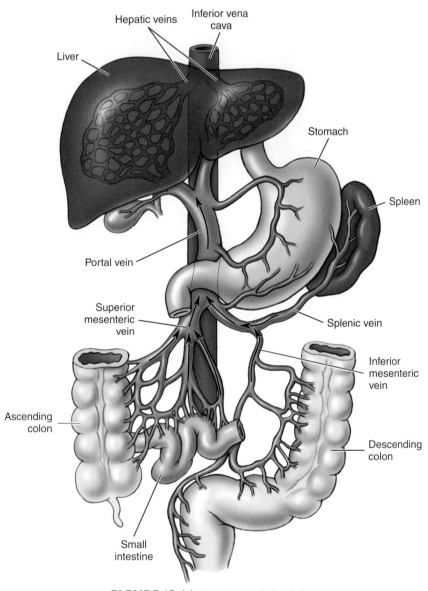

FIGURE 19-14 Hepatic portal circulation.

Major Systemic Arteries

Arteries are named for their locations. Notice how the name of the artery changes as it progresses into a new region of the body, as the name of a road might change as it progresses through a country. It is the same artery, but as it moves down the arm, the name changes from axillary to brachial to radial to ulnar and so on. Arteries generally lie deep and are well shielded within tissues and muscles; however, some are superficial enough that they can be palpated. Figure 19-15 contains names and locations of principal arteries of the body, with the bulleted arteries in the following list in bold type.

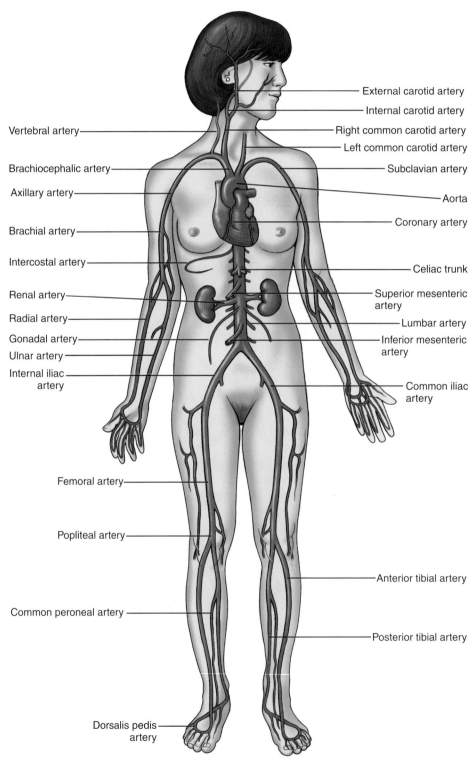

External carotid artery
Internal carotid artery
Right common carotid artery
Left common carotid artery
Subclavian artery
Aorta
Coronary artery
Celiac trunk
Superior mesenteric artery
Lumbar artery
Inferior mesenteric artery
Common iliac artery

Vertebral artery
Brachiocephalic artery
Axillary artery
Brachial artery
Intercostal artery
Renal artery
Radial artery
Gonadal artery
Ulnar artery
Internal iliac artery

Femoral artery
Popliteal artery
Common peroneal artery
Anterior tibial artery
Posterior tibial artery
Dorsalis pedis artery

FIGURE 19-15 Major arteries.

- **Aorta** (aortic arch, ascending, descending [thoracic and abdominal]): the descending and abdominal aorta are endangerment sites
- **Axillary:** this is an endangerment site
- **Brachial:** this is an endangerment site
- **Brachiocephalic**
- **Carotid** (internal, external, and common): external and common are endangerment sites
- **Common peroneal**
- **Coronary**
- **Dorsalis pedis**
- **Femoral:** this is an endangerment site
- **Iliac** (internal, external, and common)
- **Mesenteric** (superior and inferior)
- **Popliteal:** this is an endangerment site
- **Radial:** this is an endangerment site
- **Subclavian:** this is an endangerment site
- **Tibial** (anterior and posterior)
- **Ulnar:** this is an endangerment site

When massaging an area where an arterial endangerment site is located, apply light pressure and feel for a pulse. If a pulse is felt, then avoid prolonged pressure on the specific pulse location.

Major Systemic Veins

Veins, similar to arteries, are also named for their locations. The following list contains the major systemic veins found in the body with endangerment sites noted (notice how the names of the veins, as with the arteries, change as they progress through body). Figure 19-16 contains names and locations of principal arteries of the body, with the bulleted veins in the following list in bold type.

- **Axillary:** this is an endangerment site
- **Brachial:** this is an endangerment site
- **Brachiocephalic**
- **Femoral:** this is an endangerment site
- **Iliac** (internal, external, and common)
- **Jugular** (internal and external): this is an endangerment site
- **Median cubital**
- **Popliteal:** this is an endangerment site
- **Radial:** this is an endangerment site
- **Saphenous** (great and small): this is an endangerment site
- **Subclavian**
- **Tibial** (anterior and posterior)
- **Ulnar:** this is an endangerment site
- **Vena cava** (superior and inferior)

When applying a deep stripping pressure over a superficial vein, always move from distal to proximal, or you may promote varicosities. Varicose veins, or damaged veins, lack a sufficient interior valve system. Pressure in the wrong direction also promotes improper blood flow.

LYMPHATIC SYSTEM

The lymphatic system, or lymphatic-immune system, is a one-way system for drainage of excess fluid from the body's tissues and is a complement to the circulatory system. Similar to the circulatory system, the lymphatic system has disease-fighting functions. The lymphatic system is composed of lymph fluid, lymph vessels, and specialized tissues and organs. **Lymph,** the fluid of the lymphatic system, is transported through progressively larger vessels that drain into two large veins near the neck. This portion of the chapter explores the structures, functions, and pathways of the lymphatic system and the body's immunological responses.

ANATOMY

Areas of discussion in this part of the chapter include:
- Lymph
- Lymph vessels
- Lymph glands
- Lymphocytes
- Lymphatic organs

PHYSIOLOGY

The functions of the lymphatic system are as follows:
1. The lymphatic system drains excess interstitial fluid. Surplus interstitial fluid flows into lymphatic capillaries and becomes lymph. Some of this fluid is returned to the cardiovascular system. This process helps maintain blood volume and pressure and prevent edema (swelling).
2. The lymphatic system transports dietary lipids and lipid-soluble vitamins (A, D, E, and K) from the digestive tract to the blood. Lipids and lipid-soluble vitamins are large molecules that cannot fit into blood capillaries. These specialized lymphatic vessels are called *lacteals.* When the molecules are absorbed from the digestive tract, they move into the larger-diameter lymphatic capillaries instead, entering the blood when lymph drains back into the bloodstream.
3. Through the filtering action of lymph nodes and organs, the lymphatic system provides immunity against disease. Many pathogens and other impurities are removed from the lymph and destroyed by disease-fighting lymphocytes and antibodies.

LYMPH

The body is primarily composed of a base fluid consisting of water with a few proteins and complex sugars. When this fluid is situated between cells, it is referred to as *extracellular fluid.* When it is situated between tissues, it is referred to as

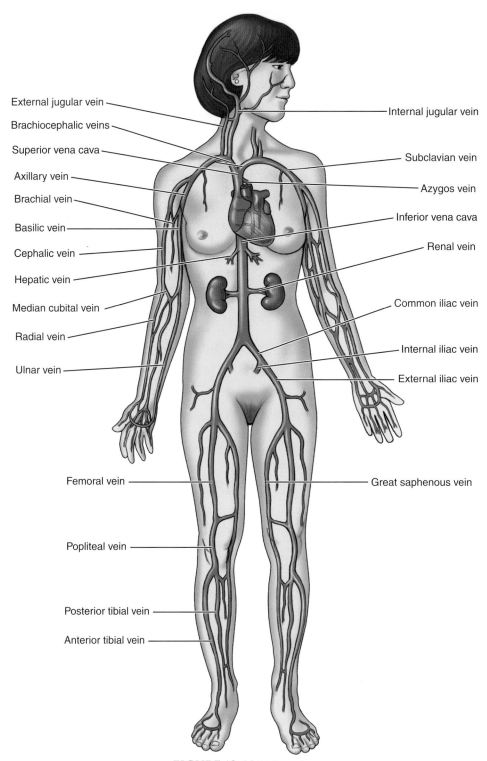

FIGURE 19-16 Major veins.

interstitial fluid. When located in the blood, it is referred to as *blood plasma.* When found in the lymphatic system, it is referred to as *lymph.* Hence the main difference among lymph, blood plasma, extracellular fluid, and interstitial fluid is location.

Unlike the cardiovascular system, which flows in a continuous circle, the lymphatic system moves in only one direc-

tion, toward the subclavian veins (Figure 19-17). Without a pump to assist flow, lymph moves only through pressure gradients from external sources exerted on its vessel walls. This pressure can come from the milking action of skeletal muscle contractions or from the pressure changes in the thorax and abdomen during breathing. Lymph moves slowly when compared with blood circulation. When lymph

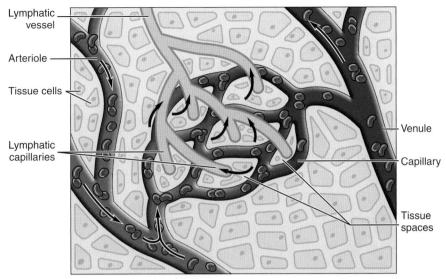

FIGURE 19-17 One-way circulation of lymph.

pools in an area, the condition is referred to as **edema** or *lymphedema*.

LYMPH VESSELS

Lymphatic vessels (lymphatics) include lymph capillaries, lymph vessels, lymphatic trunks, and two main collecting ducts (Figure 19-18). **Lymph capillaries** have the same structures as blood capillaries, but they are larger, more irregular, and more permeable. They start in the tissues and exist in all parts of the body except bone marrow, epidermis, central nervous system (brain and spinal cord), and the eyes. Lymph nodes are located throughout lymphatic tributaries to filter the lymph moving through the system.

Lymph capillaries become larger and are called *lymph vessels*. Compared with veins, lymphatic vessels have thin walls and more valves that open in only one direction. These vessels merge along similar pathways to form region draining **lymphatic trunks,** which join to form one of two lymphatic ducts: right and thoracic. The **right lymphatic duct** drains lymph from the right arm and the right side of the head and the right half of the thorax into the right subclavian vein. The **thoracic duct** drains lymph from all remaining parts of the body into the left subclavian vein. The thoracic duct begins at the *cisterna chyli* (i.e., lymphatic sac located between the abdominal aorta and the second lumbar region) and lies along the thoracic vertebrae.

LYMPH ORGANS

The primary lymphatic structures are the bone marrow and thymus (these are known as the *generative lymphatic organs* because they produce and mature lymphocytes; Figure 19-19). Secondary lymphatic structures include the spleen, lymph nodes, tonsils, Peyer's patches, and the inside of the vermiform appendix. These secondary lymphatic structures

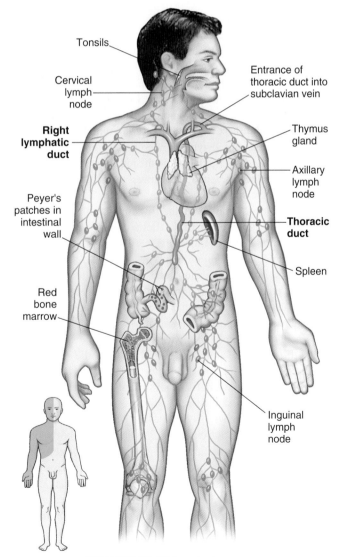

FIGURE 19-18 Lymphatic system.

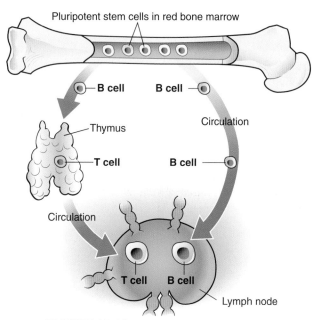

Pluripotent stem cells in red bone marrow

B cell   B cell

Thymus

Circulation

T cell   B cell

Circulation

T cell   B cell

Lymph node

FIGURE 19-19 Development of B and T cells.

are populated by lymphocytes from the bone marrow and the thymus, which are described as follows:

1. **Bone marrow,** located in the hollow cavity of bones, produces precursor blood cells, a *pluripotent stem cell* (see previous section on *Blood Cells*). **Lymphocytes** are a type of WBC that comprises approximately 25% of the total WBC count; these WBCs increase in number in response to infection. Some lymphocytes mature and become B lymphocytes, or B cells, within the red bone marrow. Other lymphocytes differentiate and travel to the thymus, where they mature and become T lymphocytes or T cells.

2. Also an endocrine gland, the **thymus gland** is located in the mediastinal region of the thorax. As stated previously, the thymus receives immature T cells. These lymphocytes complete their maturation and become T lymphocytes or T cells. Both T cells and B cells then travel to secondary lymphatic structures. Large in infants, the thymus reaches its maximum size at puberty and then atrophies and is replaced by adipose tissue in adults.

3. The largest lymphatic organ, the dark purple **spleen** lies within the left lateral rib cage (between the ninth and eleventh ribs) just posterior to the stomach. Functions of the spleen have baffled physiologists for hundreds of years, but recent research indicates that it stores blood cells and destroys old, worn-out RBCs and platelets. Another major activity of the spleen is antibody production. As blood flows into the spleen, antigens are greeted and destroyed by T cells, B cells, phagocytes, and macrophages.

4. **Lymph nodes** are bean-shaped structures located along lymph vessels that collect and filter lymph. Lymph nodes are the only place where lymph is filtered in the lymphatic system. These structures are powerful defense stations that help protect the body from unwanted invaders. These

nodes also house phagocytes and lymphocytes (both B and T cells) that destroy bacteria, viruses, and other foreign substances in the lymph before it is returned to the blood. When the body is experiencing a local infection, the regional lymph nodes enlarge.

> **evolve** *Log on to your student account using the Evolve website and view an image of a lymph node. Practitioners trained in manual lymphatic drainage must have a clear understanding of these structures.* ■

Although lymph nodes are located along all lymphatic vessels, nodes are clustered superficially in three areas on each side of the body and are palpated on routine physical examinations. They are named for their location: cervical nodes, axillary nodes, and inguinal nodes.

5. **Mucosal-associated lymphoid tissue** (MALT) is a collection of lymphoid cells or nodules in the mucosa or submucosa of the digestive tract. These structures are tonsils, Peyer's patches, and the vermiform appendix.

   • **Tonsils** are a group of large specialized lymph tissues embedded in the mucous membranes around the throat. They include the adenoids or pharyngeal tonsils, palatine tonsils, and lingual tonsils. The function of the tonsils is to protect the body from airborne pathogens or other harmful substances that might enter through the nose or mouth. The lymphatic tissues use lymphocytes and macrophages to combat hostile intruders.

   • **Peyer's patches,** or intestinal tonsils, are groups of lymphatic nodules found in the mucous membrane of the small intestine, usually in the ileum and jejunum. These lymphatic cells constitute another member of the body's defense mechanisms by combating ingested pathogens.

   • Located inferior to the cecum, the **vermiform appendix** varies from 3 to 6 inches in length. Similar to other members of the lymphatic system, the appendix helps fight pathogens and other bodily intruders.

PATHS OF LYMPH CIRCULATION

All lymph moves back toward the cardiovascular system. Lymph, which starts out as interstitial fluid, is collected by lymph capillaries and moves into lymph vessels, which become successively larger. Periodically along its one-way path, lymph flows into lymph nodes. Similar to venous blood flow, lymphatic flow is maintained by contraction of skeletal muscles. Ultimately, lymph converges into either the right lymphatic duct or the thoracic duct and then enters the bloodstream through the right and left subclavian veins. The thoracic duct enters only the left venous circulation. In fact, most of the body's lymph empties on the left side. Only the right side of the head and neck, the right upper extremity, and right half of the upper trunk empty into the right lymphatic duct (see Figure 19-18).

The following diagram shows lymph's flow in this pathway:

It starts out as interstitial fluid,

↓

is collected by the lymphatic capillaries,

↓

moves into lymphatic vessels,

↓

moves through lymph nodes,

↓

moves through larger lymph vessels,

↓

collects in lymph trunks (either thoracic duct or right lymphatic duct),

↓

and is dumped in the right or left subclavian veins.

The deeper structures of the thorax, abdomen, pelvis, and perineum drain directly into the larger lymph vessels rather than passing through lymph capillaries.

IMMUNITY

The body has two major categories of defenses. The first is natural immunity and the second is acquired immunity. **Immunity** is an anatomical and physiological defense reaction to invading microorganisms. The key components of this response are lymphocytes and WBCs, although structures (e.g., the skin) and chemicals (e.g., digestive enzymes) are also involved. Immunology is studied in the lymphatic system because lymphoid tissue is the anatomical component of the immune system.

Natural Immunity

Natural immunity refers to the nonspecific responses to invading pathogens. Natural immunity can be affected by diet, mental health, environment, and metabolism. The following are examples of natural immune responses:

Physical barrier: Skin, mucosa, and cilia physically resist invaders.

Chemical barrier: Digestive enzymes, perspiration, vaginal secretions, and acid mantel (on skin) form chemical barriers.

Complement proteins: Proteins found in blood attack foreign agents.

Phagocytes: Cells kill pathogens by approaching their prey and engulfing and digesting them with lysosomal enzymes. Primary phagocytic cells are neutrophils and macrophages. Phagocytes are involved with both natural and acquired immunity.

Fever: Normal body temperature elevates to destroy many disease-producing organisms.

Inflammation: This reaction is a protective mechanism that stabilizes and prepares the damaged tissue for repair and is involved in both natural and acquired immunity. Inflammatory symptoms are local heat, swelling, redness, pain, and decreased function.

Acquired Immunity

If pathogens penetrate the first line of defense, the lymphatic system becomes activated. This process is referred to as acquired immunity. **Acquired immunity** involves diverse but specific responses to invaders employing lymphocytes. The cells involved in acquired immunity are specialized and possess memory (once they encounter and destroy the invader, they remember it and can destroy it more quickly in the future). The two types of acquired immunity based on the type of lymphocyte involved are (1) humoral immunity and (2) cellular immunity. Humoral immunity involves B cells, and cellular immunity involves T cells.

B Cells, T Cells, and Natural Killer Cells

All types of blood cells, including lymphocytes, are formed in the red bone marrow. Two main types of lymphocytes are created: T cells and B cells. To be able to recognize and attack pathogens, the T cells and B cells need to undergo a further maturation. B cells continue to mature in the red bone marrow. T cells go to the thymus gland to complete their maturation.

Once T cells and B cells mature, they travel to areas of lymphatic tissues. These tissues include lymph nodes, the lymphatic tissue inside the spleen, or in the mucous membranes of the respiratory, digestive, urinary, and reproductive tracts (i.e., MALT).

For T cells and B cells to mount an immune response, they need to come in contact and interact with a pathogen. This interaction can occur in three main ways. One way is for the pathogen to travel through the lymph to a lymph node. Another way is for the pathogen to travel through the blood to the lymphatic tissue in the spleen. The third way is for the pathogen to penetrate mucous membranes and come in contract with the embedded lymphatic nodules.

Once the T cells and B cells contact the pathogen, they are activated for that specific pathogen. The T cells and B cells clone themselves by the thousands, which accounts for the swelling of lymph nodes during infection. The T cells leave the lymphatic tissue and kill the pathogen as they come across it. The B cells produce antibodies that leave the lymphatic tissue and circulate in body fluids, such as the blood. The antibodies inactivate pathogens as they come across them.

Helper T cells, cytotoxic T cells, and memory T cells are types of T cells. Helper T cells help both T cells and B cells fight an infection by secreting hormones to stimulate them. Cytotoxic T cells kill body cells infected by pathogens. Memory T cells, similar to memory B cells, stay after the infection is contained to recognize the pathogen if it invades again.

In autoimmune diseases, T cells and B cells are unable to distinguish the body's own tissues from something that is foreign to the body. They then attack the tissues. For instance, in rheumatoid arthritis, the immune system attacks the synovial lining of joints; in multiple sclerosis, the immune system attacks the myelin sheath around neurons in the central nervous system; in type I diabetes mellitus, the immune system attacks the insulin-producing cells of the pancreas.

Natural killer cells are large lymphocytes and are neither B nor T cells. They bind to pathogens and tumor cells to kill them.

PATHOLOGICAL CONDITIONS OF THE CARDIOVASCULAR SYSTEM

Anemia

Anemia is a reduction of the oxygen-carrying capacity of the blood, a decrease in RBCs, or a reduced number of functional hemoglobin in the blood. It is usually a sign of other disorders. Characteristics of anemia include fatigue, vertigo, headaches, insomnia, paleness, and intolerance to cold. *Adjust massage to client's stamina and vitality (i.e., slow, gentle, short duration; assist client on and off table). If anemia is due to a bleeding disorder, then use light pressure.*

Aneurysm

An aneurysm is a weakened section of a blood vessel wall that bulges outward. The most common causes are atherosclerosis, hypertension, and trauma, but it can also be the result of a congenital vascular weakness. The most common areas for aneurysms are the aorta and blood vessels in the brain, but they can occur in the extremities. Aneurysms may burst, causing hemorrhage and possibly death. *Obtain physician consent. If client has been diagnosed with an abdominal aortic aneurysm, then abdominal and psoas massage is contraindicated.*

Angina Pectoris

Often felt as chest pain, angina pectoris is commonly caused by constriction of coronary arteries and myocardial anoxia (lack of oxygen in the heart muscle). The pain originates from the chest and then radiates down the inner side of the left arm. The pain disappears with rest, and no lasting tissue damage occurs. Angina pectoris is often associated with physical overexertion, when the heart needs more oxygen. Emotional stress and exposure to intense cold can also trigger angina pectoris. *Massage is fine. Keep client warm. Avoid using heat or cold packs. If client has an attack during treatment, then assist him or her to a sitting or standing position and call for help. Have necessary medications (e.g., beta-blockers, nitroglycerin) when a client with this condition comes in for treatment in case of medical emergencies. If client takes nitroglycerin while in the office, then make sure he or she sits or lies down for at least an hour.*

Arteriosclerosis

Arteriosclerosis is a group of arterial diseases characterized by a thickening and loss of elasticity, which leads to a hardening of the arterial walls. This condition can result in high blood pressure, and/or in a decrease in blood supply, especially to the brain and lower extremities. The patient is usually given a prescription of adequate rest, moderate exercise, and avoidance of stress. *Physician clearance recommended. Avoid deep-pressure massage.*

Atherosclerosis

A type of arteriosclerosis, atherosclerosis is the narrowing and hardening of arteries caused by the accumulation of lipid plaques in their walls. Atherosclerosis is often associated with obesity, hypertension, and diabetes. The narrowed arteries reduce blood flow, especially to the heart and brain. Because the plaque has a rough surface, platelets can snag on it and rupture, forming clots, which can further impede blood flow. *Physician clearance recommended. Avoid deep-pressure massage.*

Coronary Artery Disease

In coronary artery disease (CAD), the coronary arteries are narrowed, and blood flow to the heart is reduced. CAD is the leading cause of death in the United States, with symptoms ranging from mild angina to a full-scale heart attack. Symptoms usually start when approximately 75% of a coronary artery is blocked. The three main causes are atherosclerosis, coronary artery spasm, and blood clots. *Physician clearance recommended. Use light pressure, and avoid deep-pressure massage if client is prone to thrombosis.*

Embolism

A blood clot, bubble of air, or any piece of debris transported by the bloodstream is an embolus. When an embolus becomes lodged in a vessel and cuts off circulation, it is then called an *embolism*. *Obtain physician clearance. Once granted, avoid deep, vigorous massage. If a client is taking anticoagulants, then use light pressure.*

Heart Murmur

Heart murmurs are abnormal heart sounds caused by problems with the heart valves, which can interfere with blood flow through the heart. They are diagnosed by the sound they create, hence the name *murmur*. The most common heart murmur is a mitral valve prolapse in which the mitral valve is pushed backward into the left atrium during ventricular contraction. It affects 10% of the population, women more often than men. *Obtain physician clearance if murmur is severe. Once granted, use light pressure.*

Hematoma

A localized collection of blood trapped in the tissues of an organ, body space, or the skin is a hematoma. It is often the result of trauma or surgery. If the hematoma is near the skin's surface, then it can be palpated. *Local contraindication of affected area.*

Hypertension

Hypertension is a common, often asymptomatic disorder of elevated blood pressure; 140/90 mm Hg is regarded as the threshold of hypertension, and 160/95 mm Hg is classified as serious hypertension. With sustained hypertension, arterial walls become inelastic and resistant to blood flow, and as a result, the left ventricle may become enlarged to maintain normal circulation. Risk factors for hypertension are cigarette smoking, obesity, lack of exercise, diabetes, and genetic predisposition. *If not controlled by diet, exercise, and/or medication, then client should not receive massage. Otherwise, use stress-reduction techniques to help lower blood pressure. Client may need assistance to get up from table after the treatment.*

Migraine and Cluster Headaches

Also called *vascular headaches,* migraines are caused by dilation of extracranial blood vessels. Migraines may be triggered by foods (carbohydrates, iodine-rich foods, cheese, chocolate), alcohol (red wine), bright lights, loud noises, hormones (pregnancy hormones), or during a period of relaxation after physical or emotional stress. Nausea, vomiting, chills, sweating, irritability, and extreme fatigue may accompany the acute phase. After an attack, the individual often has dull head and neck pains and a great need for sleep. Cluster headaches are somewhat similar to migraine headaches. They occur one after the other for several days in a row. Cluster headaches affect men more often than women. *Do not massage during a migraine or cluster headache. Otherwise, massage is fine between attacks.*

Peripheral Vascular Disease

Peripheral vascular disease affects both blood and lymphatic vessels. Various metabolical disorders such as diabetes, obesity, sedentary lifestyle, and cigarette smoking cause or contribute to this disease. Symptoms include numbness, pain and discomfort, skin discoloration, and elevated blood pressure, *Local contraindication if symptoms are severe (i.e., numbness, severe pain). Use only light pressure in areas that are mildly numb or tingling.*

Phlebitis

Phlebitis, or thrombophlebitis, is an inflammation of the veins, often accompanied by a thrombus (blood clot). Phlebitis usually occurs after acute or chronic infection, surgery, pregnancy and childbirth, or prolonged sitting, standing, or immobilization. The affected area is hypersensitive to pressure and swollen and can be either hot or cold to the touch. It generally affects the arms or the calf area. *Local contraindication of affected area.*

Raynaud's Syndrome

Raynaud's syndrome is periodic attacks of vasospasm of blood vessels in the body's extremities, especially the most distal parts such as the fingers, toes, ears, and nose. It is most commonly caused by exposure to cold, emotional stress, or smoking (nicotine is a powerful vasoconstrictor). This condition can lead to ischemia, tissue necrosis, and nerve damage. *Pressure is determined by client's pain level (light pressure if client is experiencing more pain; moderate pressure if client is experiencing less pain). Use techniques to increase local circulation, reduce stress, and relax muscles. Heat and ice packs are contraindicated.*

Sickle Cell Disease

A genetic disorder, sickle cell disease is characterized by abnormal hemoglobin, which causes red blood cells to take on the shape of a sickle. This shape greatly reduces the amount of oxygen that can be supplied to the tissues, eventually causing extensive tissue damage. Sickle cell anemia is characterized by lethargy, fatigue, pain in the joints, thrombosis, and headaches. *Obtain physician clearance. Once granted, avoid massage during flare-ups. If in remission, then adjust massage to client's stamina and vitality (i.e., slow, gentle, short duration; assist client on and off table).*

Telangiectasia

Telangiectasia is permanent dilation of superficial capillaries or small blood vessels (venules and arterioles). The face is the most common region affected. Common causes are rosacea, elevated estrogen levels, and collagen vascular diseases. *Use light pressure over affected area.*

Thrombophlebitis

Thrombophlebitis is thrombus (blood clot) formation in an unbroken blood vessel, restricting blood flow. The vessel feels hard and thready or cordlike and is extremely sensitive to pressure. The surrounding area may be red and warm to the touch, and the entire limb may be pale, cold, and swollen. Aching or cramping pain, especially in the calf when the patient walks or dorsiflexes the foot (Homan's sign), characterizes deep-vein thrombophlebitis. *Local massage is contraindicated. Avoid deep pressure in the inner thigh areas.*

Transient Ischemic Attack

Transient ischemic attack (TIA) is an event of temporary cerebral dysfunction caused by ischemia or reduced blood flow. TIAs can be characterized by abnormal vision in one or both eyes, vertigo, shortness of breath, general loss of sensation, or unconsciousness. Common causes are occlusion by embolus, thrombus, or atherosclerotic plaque. The attack is typically sudden and brief (lasting only a few minutes) and leaves no long-term neurological damage. TIAs are often recurrent and may be a presage to a stroke. ***Obtain physician clearance. Once granted, use light pressure if client is on anticoagulant therapy. Refer to a physician if client experiences tingling, numbness, or loss of movement during or immediately after the massage session.***

Varicose Veins

Varicose veins are dilated veins resulting from incompetent valves. In veins with weak valves, gravity prevents large amounts of blood from flowing upward. The back pressure overloads the vein and pushes its walls outward. The veins lose elasticity and become stretched and flabby. Thromboses may form in the varicose veins. They are typically caused by a congenital defect or repeated stress from overloading, such as pregnancy or obesity. The condition may worsen if the client is on his or her feet for long periods. ***Local contraindications if blood clots or pain is present. Otherwise, elevate legs during treatment.***

PATHOLOGICAL CONDITIONS OF THE LYMPHATIC-IMMUNE SYSTEM

Acquired Immunodeficiency Syndrome

Acquired immunodeficiency syndrome (AIDS) is a disease caused by the human immunodeficiency virus (HIV). Transmission of the virus occurs through the exchange of bodily fluids such as blood, semen, vaginal secretions, and mother's milk. The average time between exposure to the virus and diagnosis is 8 to 10 years, but the incubation time is much shorter. Generally, lymph nodes may be enlarged, and weight loss, fatigue, night sweats, and fever may be present. An AIDS diagnosis is made when a person has three or more opportunistic infections (e.g., tuberculosis, pneumonia, fungi) and/or a T-cell count below 200/mL^3. A normal T-cell count is 1200/mL^3. ***Adjust massage to client's stamina and vitality (i.e., slow, gentle, short duration; assist client on and off table).***

Allergies

Allergies are a hypersensitivity and overreaction of the immune system to otherwise harmless agents (most are environmental or dietary). The person may experience inflammation or a runny nose from excess mucus secretion or, more seriously, anaphylactic shock, in which air passageways constrict. A local allergic reaction might result in a rash or hives. ***Ascertain and avoid all known and possible allergens (e.g., pet dander, nut oils). Ask client to review lubricant ingredient list.***

Chronic Fatigue Syndrome

Chronic fatigue syndrome (CFS) is characterized by the onset of disabling fatigue, sometimes after a viral infection. CFS is often accompanied by influenza-like symptoms such as low-grade fever, sore throat, and headache. Memory deficits and sleep disturbances are also associated with this condi-

tion. Treatment is geared toward relieving symptoms, which resemble those of fibromyalgia. Counseling is often indicated because depression is common. CFS occasionally resolves spontaneously. ***Treatment should be of short duration if client is currently fatigued.***

Edema

An abnormal accumulation of interstitial fluid tissues is referred to as edema or lymphedema. It is most often the result of lack of muscular activity (e.g., sitting in a car all day) but may be the result of local or general inflammation, obstruction, or removal of lymph vessels. ***Massage is contraindicated if client has a history of heart or kidney disease or if caused by a contraindicated disease. Elevate area and use lymphatic drainage techniques. Work proximal areas first, then distal areas.***

Lupus Erythematosus

Lupus erythematosus is an autoimmune, inflammatory disease of the connective tissues. It is not contagious. The cause of lupus is unknown. Its onset may be abrupt or gradual, but it primarily affects women age 20 to 40 years. A rash develops around the nose and check, resembling a wolf's markings (often called a *butterfly rash*). Symptoms include painful joints, fever, fatigue, weight loss, enlarged lymph nodes and spleen, and sensitivity to light. Periods of remission and exacerbation occur. Triggers for exacerbation include certain drugs, exposure to excessive sunlight, injury, and stress. Serious complications of the disease involve inflammation of the kidneys, liver, spleen, lungs, heart, and central nervous system. The three main types of lupus are as follows:
- **Discoid lupus erythematosus:** a skin disease characterized by the presence of skin rash showing varying degrees of edema, redness, and scaliness
- **Systemic lupus erythematosus:** most serious; body attacks connective tissue in joints, skin, and organs; this is a chronic, remitting, relapsing, inflammatory process and is often a multisystemic disorder
- **Drug-induced:** medications used to treat hypertension and irregular heartbeat can cause the onset of lupus; usually resolves after withdrawal of the medication

Massage is contraindicated during flare-ups. Otherwise, carefully administer stretches and mobilizations. Use lighter pressure if client is taking corticosteroids and antiinflammatory drugs. Avoid exposing clients who are taking immunosuppressants to any form of infection.

Mononucleosis

Infectious mononucleosis is an acute viral infection that results from the Epstein-Barr virus. Symptoms are a slight to high fever, sore throat, red throat and soft palate, stiff neck, enlarged lymph nodes, coughing, and fatigue. It is highly contagious, transmitted by droplets that contain the virus. No cure has been found, and treatment usually involves allowing it to run its course, treating any complications. ***Massage is contraindicated.***

Effects of Massage on the Cardiovascular System

Dilates blood vessels. Superficial blood vessels become dilated as a result of reflex action.

Improves blood circulation. Deep stroking improves blood circulation by mechanically assisting venous blood flow back to the heart. The increase of blood flow is comparable to that of exercise. Research suggests that during a massage, local circulation increases up to three times more than circulation at rest.

Decreases blood pressure. Blood pressure is decreased by blood vessel dilation. Both diastolic and systolic readings decline and last approximately 40 minutes after the massage.

Creates hyperemia. Increased blood flow creates a hyperemic effect, which is visible on some skin types.

Stimulates release of acetylcholine and histamine. These two substances are released as a result of vasomotor activity, thereby helping prolong vasodilation.

Replenishes nutritive materials. Increased circulation aids in the delivery of products such as nutrients and oxygen to cells and tissues.

Promotes removal of waste products. Increased circulation also aids in the removal of metabolic wastes. Therapists often say that massage *dilutes the poisons*.

Reduces ischemia. Massage reduces ischemia. Ischemia is linked to pain and trigger point formation.

Reduces heart and pulse rates. Massage decreases heart rate through activation of the relaxation response.

Increases stroke volume. Stroke volume is the amount of blood ejected from the left ventricle during each contraction. As the heart rate decreases, the time for the heart's ventricles to fill with blood increases. The result is a larger volume of blood being pushed and moving through the heart, thereby increasing stroke volume.

Increases RBC count. The number of RBCs and their oxygen-carrying capacity are increased. This effect is due to (1) promoting the spleen's discharge of RBCs, (2) recruiting blood from engorged internal organs into general circulation, and (3) stimulating stagnant capillary beds and returning this blood into general circulation.

Increases oxygen saturation in blood. When the RBC count rises, oxygen saturation of the blood increases.

Increases WBC count. The presence of WBCs increases after massage. The body may perceive massage as a mild stressor (an event to which the body must adapt) and recruits additional WBCs. The increase in WBC count enables the body to protect itself against disease more effectively.

Enhances the adhesion of migrating WBCs. The surfaces of WBCs become *stickier* following a massage, thereby increasing their adhesive quality and therefore their effectiveness.

Increases platelet count. Massage has been found to increase the number of blood platelets.

Effects of Massage on the Lymphatic-Immune Systems

Promotes lymph circulation. Lymph circulation depends on pressure: from muscle contraction, pressure changes in the thorax and abdomen during breathing, or applied pressure from a massage. Hence massage promotes this circulation.

Reduces edema. Massage reduces edema (swelling) by enhancing lymph circulation.

Decreases the circumference of an area affected with edema. When an area swells, the diameter increases. When the swelling subsides, circumference decreases.

Decreases weight in patients with edema. Fluid retention adds weight to an individual. When edema is addressed with massage, weight is consequently reduced.

Increases lymphocyte count. Lymphocytes are a type of WBC. This effect indicates that massage supports immune functions.

Increases the number and function (or cytotoxicity) of natural killer cells, CD4 cells, and CD4/CD8 ratio. All the aforementioned cells are types of WBCs, further suggesting that massage strengthens immune functions.

SUMMARY

The cardiovascular and lymphatic-immune systems are the main transport mechanisms of the body for various fluids, gases, nutrients, wastes, antibodies, hormones, and heat. These two systems also play an important role in the body's defense system by fighting a variety of invaders. The clotting mechanism of the blood enables the body to make repairs to breaches of its tissues. The circulatory system also plays a part in water and chemical balance of the body. The main components of the cardiovascular system are the blood, heart, and vast network of arteries, capillaries, and veins that make up the circulatory vessels. The two main circuits of the cardiovascular system are pulmonary and systemic.

Although the cardiovascular system provides nourishment to the body's tissues, the lymphatic-immune system collects and recycles fluids back into circulation. Along with fluid conservation, the lymph system also transports fats, vitamins, lost proteins, and cellular debris, in addition to filtering the lymph and combating diseases with its own immune functions. The lymphatic system's major structures include lymph, bone marrow, thymus, spleen, lymph nodes, and MALT (e.g., tonsils, Peyer's patches, the inside of the vermiform appendix). Lymphatic vessels route the collected fluids from all areas of the body and direct it to two main vessels, which return it into the cardiovascular system.

The two types of immunity are natural and acquired. Natural immunity is the nonspecific response to invaders. Acquired immunity involves specific responses to invaders involving lymphocytes, namely B cells and T cells.

evolve

Go to *Chapter Extras* on Evolve for additional illustrations and resources for this chapter. *Extras* for this chapter include:

1. Crossword puzzle (downloadable form)
2. Drag and drop activities (online game)

MATCHING I

Place the letter of the answer next to the term or phrase that best describes it.

A. Antigens
B. Arteries
C. Atrium
D. Blood pressure
E. Carotid
F. Erythrocytes

G. Hemoglobin
H. Hyperemia
I. Ischemia
J. Leukocytes
K. Plasma
L. Platelets

M. Stroke volume
N. Type AB
O. Type O
P. Vasodilation
Q. Veins
R. Ventricle

_____   1.   Local decrease in blood flow

_____   2.   Straw-colored liquid that helps transport blood cells

_____   3.   The amount of blood ejected from the left ventricle during each ventricular contraction

_____   4.   Cells involved in blood clotting

_____   5.   Superior heart chamber

_____   6.   Enlargement of the vascular lumen

_____   7.   Universal blood recipient

_____   8.   Genetically determined proteins on the surfaces of RBCs

_____   9.   Superficial artery in the throat region

_____   10.   Cells that serve as part of the immune system

_____   11.   Most numerous blood cells that possess hemoglobin

_____   12.   An iron-based protein that is the red respiratory pigment in RBCs

_____   13.   Thick-walled inferior heart chamber

_____   14.   Vessels that return deoxygenated blood back to the heart

_____   15.   Increased local blood flow

_____   16.   Vessels that move blood away from the heart

_____   17.   Universal blood donor

_____   18.   Pressure exerted by blood on arterial walls during contraction of the left ventricle

MATCHING II

Place the letter of the answer next to the term or phrase that best describes it.

A. Acquired immunity
B. B cells
C. Bone marrow
D. Cisterna chyli
E. Inflammation
F. Lymph

G. Lymph nodes
H. Mucosal associated lymphoid tissue
I. Natural immunity
J. Right lymphatic duct
K. Spleen

L. T cells
M. Thoracic duct
N. Thymus
O. Tonsils
P. Vermiform appendix

_____ 1. Generative lymphatic structure that produces precursors of all lymphocytes

_____ 2. Lymphatic duct that drains the right arm, right side of head, and right half of thorax, dumping lymph into the right subclavian vein

_____ 3. Groups of specialized lymph tissues embedded in mucous membranes around the throat

_____ 4. Thymus-derived cells that respond quickly to pathogens, which include helper cells, cytotoxic cells, and memory cells

_____ 5. Largest lymphatic organ

_____ 6. A protective mechanism that stabilizes and prepares the damaged tissue for repair, the symptoms of which are local heat, swelling, redness, pain, and decreased function

_____ 7. Type of immunity that is a nonspecific response to invading pathogens

_____ 8. Lymphoid cells in the mucosa or submucosa of the alimentary canal

_____ 9. Filtering stations for lymph

_____ 10. Immunological response that is diverse but specific and involves lymphocytes

_____ 11. Lymphatic structure located inferior to the cecum

_____ 12. Fluid of the lymphatic system

_____ 13. Bone marrow-derived cells secreting antibodies that destroy antigens

_____ 14. Lymphatic duct that drains the majority of the body and dumps lymph into the left subclavian vein

_____ 15. Lymphatic sac located between the abdominal aorta and second lumbar region; inferior portion of the thoracic duct

_____ 16. Generative lymphatic organ receiving immature B cells, maturing them into T cells

INTERNET ACTIVITIES

Visit http://www.americanheart.org and click on Heart Attack/Stroke Warning Signs. List four warning signs of a heart attack.

Visit http://www.eurekalert.org/pub_releases/2004-11/uoc--psa112204.php, and after reading, write a paragraph on how stress affects the immune system.

Visit http://www.givelife2.org and click on About Blood and read the section. Summarize the section in report form.

Bibliography

Abrahams P, Marks S, Hutchings R: *McMinn's color atlas of human anatomy,* St Louis, 2003, Mosby.

Applegate EJ: *The anatomy and physiology learning system,* ed 3, Philadelphia, 2006, Saunders.

Beers MH, Berkow R: *The Merck manual of diagnosis and therapy,* Whitehouse Station, NJ, 2006, Merck Research Laboratories.

Crawley J, Van De Graaff KM: *A photographic atlas for anatomy and physiology,* Englewood, Colo, 2002, Morton.

Como D, editor: *Mosby's medical, nursing, and allied health dictionary,* ed 6, St Louis, 2002, Mosby.

Damjanov I: *Pathophysiology for the health-related professions,* ed 3, Philadelphia, 2006, Saunders.

Ferri FF: *2003 Ferri's clinical advisor, instant diagnosis and treatment,* St Louis, 2003, Mosby.

Frazier MS, Drzymkowski JW: *Essentials of human diseases and conditions,* ed 3, Philadelphia, 2004, Saunders.

Gould BE: *Pathophysiology for the health professions,* ed 3, Philadelphia, 2006, Saunders.

Gray H, Pickering P, Howden R: *Gray's anatomy,* ed 29, Philadelphia, 1974, Running Press.

Guyton A: *Human physiology and mechanisms of disease,* ed 6, Philadelphia, 1996, Saunders.

Haubrich WS: *Medical meanings: a glossary of word origins,* New York, 1984, Harcourt Brace Jovanovich.

Huether SE, McCance KL: *Understanding pathophysiology,* ed 3, St Louis, 2004, Mosby.

Jacob S, Francone C: *Elements of anatomy and physiology,* Philadelphia, 1989, Saunders.

Kalat JW: *Biological psychology,* ed 8, Belmont, Calif, 2003, Wadsworth.

Kapit W, Elson LM: *The anatomy coloring book,* ed 3, New York, 2002, Benjamin Cummings.

Kumar V, Abbas A, Fausto N: *Robbins and Cotran physiologic basis of disease,* ed 7, St Louis, 2005, Mosby.

Marieb EN: *Essentials of human anatomy and physiology,* ed 8, New York, 2005, Benjamin Cummings.

Martini FH, Bartholomew EF: *Essentials of anatomy and physiology,* ed 3, New York, 2003, Benjamin Cummings.

McAleer N: *The body almanac,* Garden City, NY, 1985, Doubleday.

McCance K, Huether S: *Pathophysiology: the biological basis for disease in adults and children,* St Louis, 2006, Mosby.

Merck manual, ed 17, Whitehouse Station, NJ, 1998, Merck and Company.

Moore KL: *Clinically oriented anatomy,* ed 5, Baltimore, 2005, Lippincott Williams & Wilkins.

Netter FH: *Atlas of human anatomy,* ed 3, Teterboro, NJ, 2003, Icon Learning Systems.

Newton D: *Pathology for massage therapists,* ed 2, Portland, Ore, 1995, Simran.

Premkumar K: *Pathology A to Z, a handbook for massage therapists,* Baltimore, 1999, Lippincott Williams & Wilkins.

Salvo SG, Anderson SK: *Mosby's pathology for massage therapists,* St Louis, 2004, Mosby.

Solomon EP, Phillips GA: *Understanding human anatomy and physiology,* Philadelphia, 1987, Saunders.

Thibodeau G, Patton K: *Anatomy and physiology,* ed 6, St Louis, 2006, Mosby.

Thibodeau G, Patton K: *Structure and function of the body,* ed 12, St Louis, 2004, Mosby.

Tortora GJ: *Introduction to the human body: the essentials of anatomy and physiology,* ed 5, Hoboken, NJ, 2000, John Wiley & Sons.

Tortora GJ, Grabowksi SR: *Principles of anatomy and physiology,* ed 11, New York, 2005, John Wiley & Sons.

Travell JG, Simons D: *Myofasical pain and dysfunction, the trigger point manual,* Baltimore, 1992, Lippincott Williams & Wilkins.

Venes D, Thomas CL, Taber CW: *Taber's cyclopedic medical dictionary,* ed 20, Philadelphia, 2005, FA Davis.

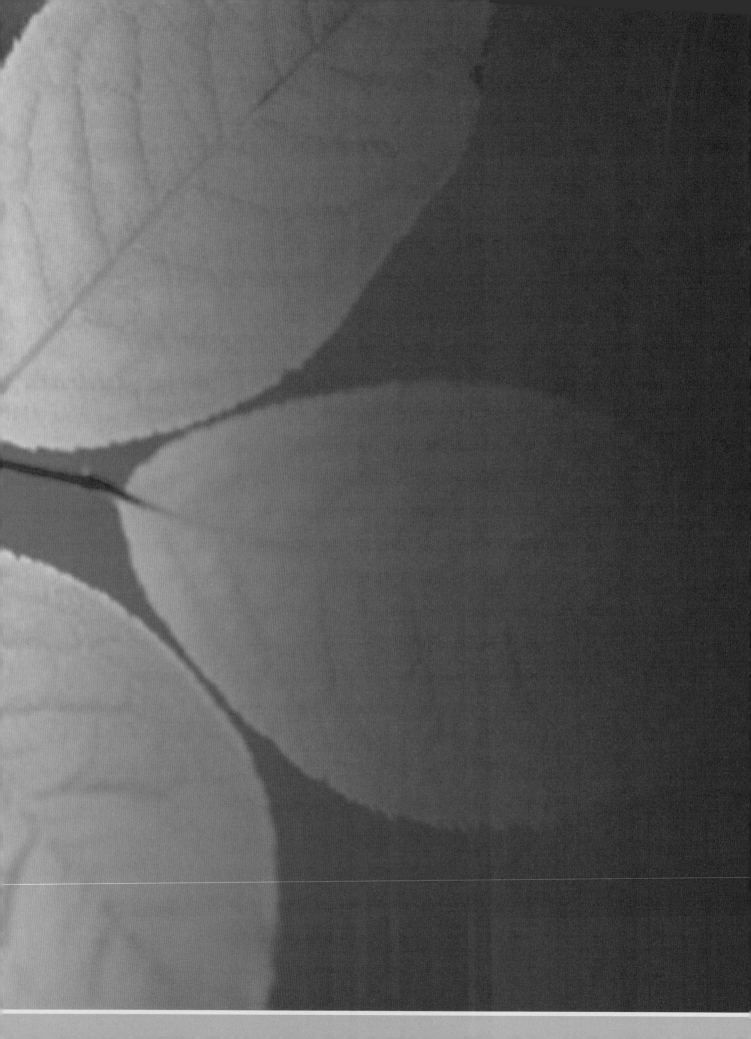

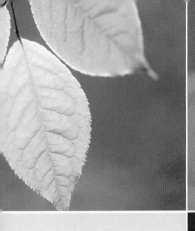

CHAPTER 20

Respiratory System

"Life is known only by those who have found a way to be comfortable with change and the unknown. Given the nature of life, there may be no security, but only adventure."
—Rachel Naomi Remen

STUDENT OBJECTIVES

After completing this chapter, the student should be able to:

- List the anatomical structures of the upper and lower respiratory tracts
- Explain the physiological mechanisms of the respiratory system
- Trace the air-conduction pathway
- Describe mechanisms of breathing, both inspiration and expiration
- Define the terms *dyspnea*, *apnea*, *hypoxia*, *anoxia*, and *vital capacity*
- Contrast and compare internal and external respiration
- Describe modified respiratory air movements
- Name types of pathological conditions of the respiratory system, giving characteristics and massage considerations of each

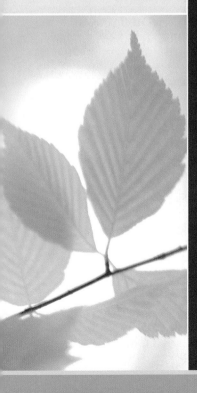

INTRODUCTION

Breathing has long been the inspiration of poets and philosophers. Books have been filled with references such as *his dying breath, her breast rose and fell, his breath quickened,* and *he breathed life into them.* Breath and the breathing process are synonymous with life itself. Breathing is the most easily observable of the body's vital signs. Through respiration, we take in new air, extract oxygen from it, and expel carbon dioxide and other waste gases back into the atmosphere. Every cell of the body needs oxygen, and delivery is accomplished by way of the bloodstream. The respiratory and the circulatory systems both participate in this respiratory process. Failure of either system has the same effect on the body, including disruption of homeostasis and rapid cell death from oxygen deprivation.

The various life-sustaining mechanisms of the respiratory system are discussed in this chapter, along with some of the modified respiratory functions. The following topics are included in discussion: anatomy of the respiratory system, the respiratory system's role in the senses of smell and speech, mechanisms of breathing, internal and external respiration, and how breathing aids massage.

ANATOMY

Areas of discussion in this chapter include
- Alveoli
- Bronchi
- Bronchioles
- Larynx
- Lungs
- Nasal cavity
- Nose
- Pharynx
- Respiratory diaphragm
- Trachea

PHYSIOLOGY

The functions of the respiratory system include the following:
- **Exchange of gases:** Oxygen and carbon dioxide exchange is the primary function of the respiratory system (Figure 20-1). A constant intake of oxygen is essential for maintaining life. Without oxygen intake and the elimination of carbon dioxide, the body's cells would start to perish within 5 minutes. This gas exchange occurs in the lungs and in systemic capillaries.
- **Olfaction:** *Olfaction* refers to the sense of smell. Through the act of inhalation, scent molecules enter the nose and are forced against the nasal cavities' mucosal lining. Chemoreceptors embedded in the nasal mucosa are stimulated and send nerve impulses of scent to the brain.
- **Speech:** The production of speech is a complex coordination of muscles and nerves. Speech and other sounds are produced by air moving over the vocal cords. This action, combined with movements of facial muscles and tongue, forms words.

- **Homeostasis:** The respiratory system helps maintain oxygen levels in the blood. It also helps maintain homeostasis through the elimination of wastes (e.g., carbon dioxide, heat). Excess carbon dioxide in the blood can lead to a dangerous acidic condition. The act of breathing helps regulate blood pH.

> *"All things share the same breath."*
> Chief Sealth, Duwamish tribe, 1885

UPPER RESPIRATORY TRACT

Air is conducted by a pathway of structures in the respiratory system. The following two sections include descriptions of each structure.

Nose

The nose is port of entry for air and the beginning of the air conduction pathway. What we see and feel as the structure of the nose is primarily hyaline and elastic cartilage. The paired nasal bones and process of the maxillae bone form the central region of the nose. The bridge of the nose consists of the nasal bones and the frontal bone. The two external openings are called *nostrils,* or by their technical term, *anterior nares* (*sing.* naris).

Nasal Cavity

Immediately adjacent to the nose is the nasal cavity. The nasal septum, formed by the vomer and the ethmoid bones and hyaline cartilage, divides the nasal cavity into right and left sides. Each nasal cavity is divided into three passageways by projections that form lateral walls. The walls, or *nasal*

Terms and Their Meanings Related to the Respiratory System

TERM	MEANING
Alveoli	*L.* little hollow
Apnea	*Gr.* not; breathing
Auditory	*L.* to hear
Bronchus	*Gr.* windpipe
Cilia	*L.* hairlike
Conchae	*Gr.* shell
Eustachian	Eustachius, Italian anatomist (1524-1574)
Glottis	*Gr.* back of the tongue
Meatus	*L.* passage
Olfaction	*L.* to smell
Phrenic	*Gr.* diaphragm
Pleura	*Gr.* rib; side
Pneumo, pneum	*Gr.* air; lungs
Pulmo	*L.* lung
Trachea	*Gr.* rough
Ventilation	*L.* to air
Volitional	*L.* will

Gr., Greek; *L.,* Latin.

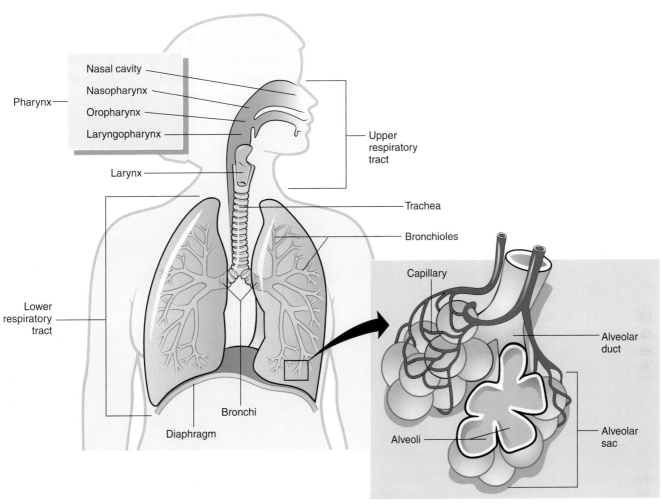

FIGURE 20-1 The respiratory system.

conchae, are individually called the *superior, middle,* and *inferior conchae* and are the ridges that extend out of each lateral wall of the nasal cavity (Figure 20-2). The passage-ways created by the conchae are called *meatuses*. The nasal cavity possesses a superior, middle, and inferior meatus. The inferior meatus terminates just above two funnel-shaped ori-fices called the *posterior nares*.

The mucosal lining of the nasal cavity contains blood capillaries, cells with cilia, and goblet cells. As air flows over the nasal cavity mucosa, it becomes warm and moist. The nasal cavity tries to clean the air before it enters the lungs, thus cilia trap air particles and move them up and out or down the throat. *Cilia* are hairlike projections on the outer surfaces of certain cells. *Goblet cells* produce mucus that moistens the air and traps incoming foreign particles. Because of all of these functions, the nasal cavities are called the *air-conditioning chambers.*

Because the nasal mucosa has such a rich blood supply, nosebleeds, or *epistaxis,* often occur as a result of blows to the nose, weak blood vessels, or high blood pressure. Al-though they are dramatic, nosebleeds are seldom serious.

The paranasal sinuses, also lined with nasal mucosa, have openings into the nasal cavity. Sinuses are air-containing spaces in skull and facial bones that lighten the head and act as resonance chambers for sound. These cavities are named for the bones by which they are located. See Figure 14-14 for a diagram of the sinuses, which are as follows:

- Frontal sinus
- Sphenoidal sinus
- Ethmoidal sinus
- Maxillary sinus

Pharynx

The pharynx, or throat, is a muscular tube approximately 5 inches long that is shared by the respiratory and the diges-tive systems. Located anterior to the cervical vertebrae, the pharynx extends from behind the nasal cavity (nasopharynx) to the back of the oral cavity (oropharynx) and down to the larynx (laryngopharynx). It contains the tonsils (pharyngeal or adenoids, palatine, and lingual), which help our immune system by protecting against inhaled or ingested pathogens (Figure 20-3).

The eustachian tube opens into the nasopharynx. Because of this close proximity, respiratory infections can easily cre-ate middle ear infections and vice versa.

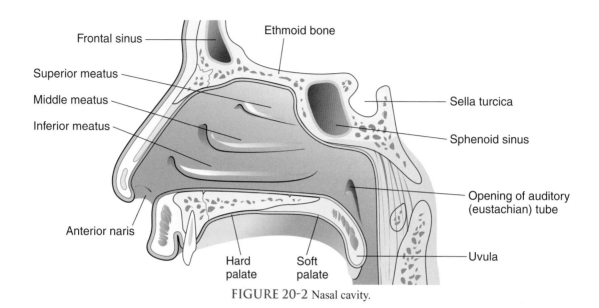

FIGURE 20-2 Nasal cavity.

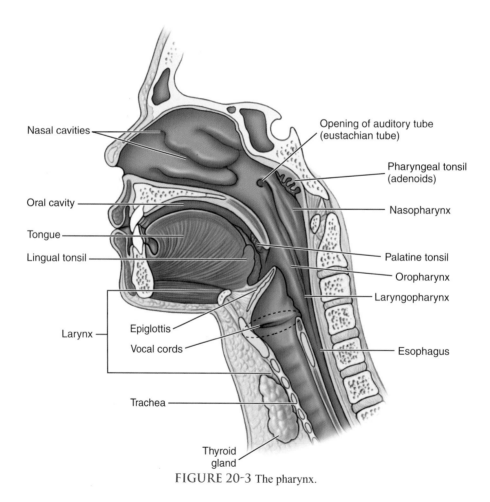

FIGURE 20-3 The pharynx.

Larynx

The larynx, or voice box, a triangle-shaped structure formed by three single and three paired cartilages. The single cartilages are the epiglottis, cricoid, and thyroid (Adam's apple), which is the largest (Figure 20-4). Enlargement of the thyroid cartilage occurs primarily in men because of the presence of testosterone. The three paired smaller accessory cartilages (arytenoid, corniculate, and cuneiform) attach to and support the vocal cords or folds.

The two sets of **vocal cords** are a superior pair called the *false vocal cords* and an inferior pair called the *true vocal cords,* or simply *vocal cords*. The true vocal cords are used for normal voice production; however, a person can train to use the false cords, as is shown in ventriloquism or singers who have two ranges.

The vocal cords are bands of elastic ligaments that are attached to the rigid cartilage of the larynx by skeletal muscle. At the space between the cords, air passes over them, causing vibration and producing sound. The tighter the skeletal muscles pull the vocal cords, the higher is the pitch of the voice.

evolve One of the interesting things about going to massage school is learning about the human body. To view a photograph of a set of vocal cords, log on to the Evolve website for Massage Therapy: Principles and Practice, 3e, and choose course materials for Chapter 20. While there, explore other items of interest for this chapter.

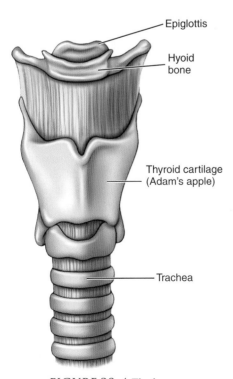

FIGURE 20-4 The larynx.

Epiglottis
Hyoid bone
Thyroid cartilage (Adam's apple)
Trachea

One of the single laryngeal cartilages, the **epiglottis,** closes the trachea during swallowing (deglutition), preventing food from entering the lower respiratory passageways. Because of this function, the epiglottis is referred to as the *guardian of the airways.*

LOWER RESPIRATORY TRACT

Trachea

The trachea, or windpipe, is a tube from the larynx to the upper chest. Located anterior to the esophagus, it measures approximately 9 to 10 inches long and consists of 16 to 21 half-ring hyaline cartilages. These half-ring cartilages serve a dual purpose. The incomplete sections of the ring allow the esophagus to expand into the trachea when a food bolus is swallowed (Figure 20-5). The rings also keep the tracheal wall from collapsing during pressure changes that occur during breathing. The trachea bifurcates at its base into two primary bronchi.

Bronchi

The right and left bronchi are the large air-conduction passageways leading from the trachea to each lung. Each tube-like structure is reinforced with hyaline cartilage, helping keep the airway open. The right primary bronchus is slightly wider and has a slightly steeper downward angle than the left; because of this feature, foreign bodies more often lodge on the right side. Each primary bronchus enters the lungs on its respective side, branching out (similar to tree roots), and becoming smaller or secondary bronchi and then even smaller divisions called *bronchioles*. As the airways branch out, they become smaller, with less cartilage and more smooth muscle. Eventually, bronchioles become microscopic branches that terminate at *alveolar ducts*, leading to alveoli.

Alveoli

Alveoli are tiny sacs attached to alveolar ducts. Groups of alveoli are *alveolar sacs,* which resemble a cluster of grapes. Each alveolus is made of single-layer epithelial tissue; this simple feature makes gas exchange possible. The walls are so thin that imagining their thinness is difficult, but a sheet of notepaper is much thicker. The lungs contain approximately 300 million alveoli, providing an immense surface area of approximately 1000 square feet (ft^2), roughly the area of a handball court. Superficial to the alveoli are numerous capillaries, so many that 900 ml of blood are able to participate in gas exchange at any given time (Figure 20-6).

Each alveolus is coated with fluid-containing surfactants. *Surfactants* are phospholipids that assist in the exchange of gas by reducing surface tension, which contributes to lung elasticity and thereby contributes to its general compliance. Surfactants are also important because they stabilize the alveoli. Lungs are the last organs to develop in utero. Infants born prematurely (before 28 gestational

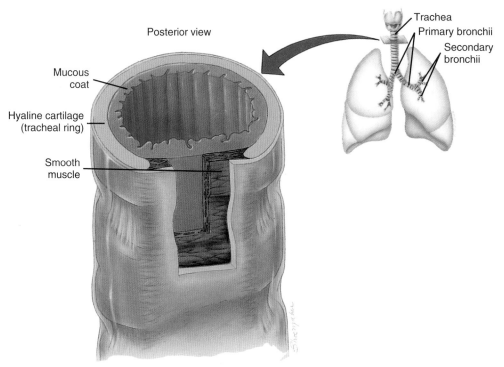

FIGURE 20-5 The trachea.

weeks) may not have produced enough surfactants to assist with gas exchanges. Medical technologies can do much to rectify this problem.

Lungs

Lungs are spongy, highly elastic paired organs of respiration. They extend from the diaphragm to just above the clavicles and lie against the interior portion of the ribcage. Although the lungs fill most of the thoracic cavity, they

weigh less than 1 lb each. The inferior surface of the lungs is broad and concave to match the shape of the superior surface of the respiratory diaphragm. The right lung has three lobes; the left lung has two lobes because the heart is more localized on the left side than the right side. This depression in the left lung to accommodate the heart is called the cardiac notch (Figure 20-7). The external surfaces of the lungs are lined by a serous membrane, and both lungs are encased by a pleural membrane, which secretes a thin serous fluid. This fluid prevents friction, allowing the lungs to move easily in the doubled-walled pleural cavity during respiration.

Respiratory Diaphragm

The respiratory diaphragm is a dome-shaped muscular partition that separates the thoracic cavity from the abdominal cavity. It is the main muscle of respiration. The diaphragm consists of both contractile muscular fibers and resistant, tendinous connective tissues, which serve to increase extensibility and help keep its firm shape. Passing through the transverse plane with an airtight seal and inserting into its central tendon, the diaphragm attaches around the circumference of the lower six ribs, connecting the spine, ribs, and xiphoid process. The opening for the passage of the descending aorta, inferior vena cava, and the esophagus pierces the diaphragm (see Figure 16-134). During contraction, the diaphragm is pulled down, creating a vacuum in the chest cavity, which sucks air down into the lungs. Relaxation of the diaphragm causes it to rise, allows the lungs to deflate, and pushes out air as a result.

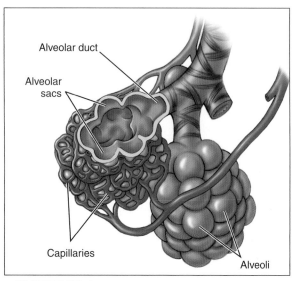

FIGURE 20-6 Alveolar duct, alveolar sac, and alveoli.

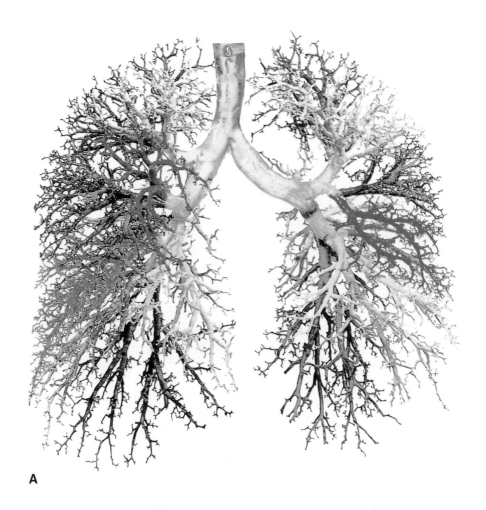

A

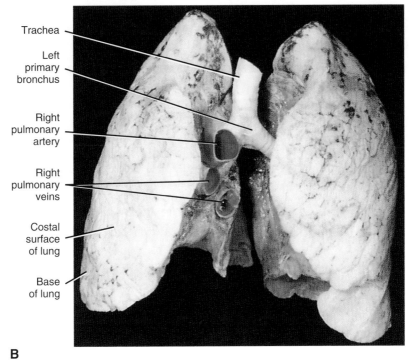

Trachea

Left
primary
bronchus

Right
pulmonary
artery

Right
pulmonary
veins

Costal
surface
of lung

Base
of lung

B

FIGURE 20-7 **A**, Lung air space. **B**, Photograph of the lungs.

ROBERT TISSERAND

Born: November 11, 1948.

"Love what you do. Enjoy listening to people. It can be hard work, but the potential for helping people is tremendous."

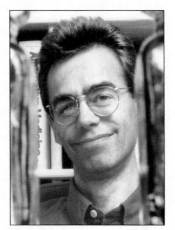

Robert Tisserand, author and aromatherapist, was born in London to a father who made baskets and a mother who "did a little of this and that, but mostly raised three kids." Luckily for his *mum,* the two girls were not quite as inquisitive as Tisserand, who shares his first *taste* of the aromatherapy experience. "Curiously, I did actually drink a bottle of perfume when I was about 2 years old. My father bought it for my mother in a flea market in Paris in 1945, so the perfume would have been about 5 years old at the time. It was called *Creme de Zofali.* I survived, but the bottle has not."

Considering that it is often the smell and not the taste of foods that makes them appealing, it is easy to understand why a little boy would not think twice before turning up a bottle of slightly aged perfume. However, aromas affect more than our appetites. Odors of certain plants have been used to dedicate newborns, banish evil spirits, guide dearly departed souls to the other side, and heal all manner of ills in between. Long before frankincense and myrrh were offered to the Christ child, Egyptian physicians were using it in their practices. Greek mythology includes stories regarding the healing properties of

aromatic plants, and Romans enjoyed massage with wonderfully scented and unbelievably expensive oils.

What has become a popular trend in the last few years was an academic area of study as far back as the Middle Ages. During this time, essential oils were classified according to the four elements or humors, the degree of *hotness* or *coldness,* and by the shape or color of the plant from which it was derived. For example, lungwort resembles lungs; therefore it was used for the respiratory system. Blue is a calming color; thus plants with blue flowers were considered to have sedative properties. This way of cataloging plant essences was called the *doctrine of signatures.* Astronomy also helped play a role in organizing certain scents. Late in the sixteenth century, Nicholas Culpepper, an astrological physician, associated oils with planetary characteristics. For instance, ylang-ylang is identified as having Venus properties because it has a strong, sweet odor and a slightly yellow tint and is considered an aphrodisiac.

The first people to dispense aromatics were the priests. They were the first perfumers, or what we would call an

---

In review, air is conducted by the following pathway of structures:

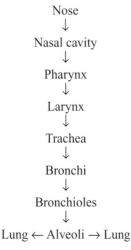

Nose
↓
Nasal cavity
↓
Pharynx
↓
Larynx
↓
Trachea
↓
Bronchi
↓
Bronchioles
↓
Lung ← Alveoli → Lung

TABLE TALK

Because the respiratory diaphragm never stops contracting, the potential for trigger point development is tremendous. Tightening of the diaphragm's fibers can cause torquing of the ribcage around the spine and central tendon, thus limiting the efficiency of inhalation. Some ribcage mobilizations and deep-tissue diaphragmatic releases can actually increase the lung's vital capacity.

MECHANISMS OF BREATHING

Three processes are required to get oxygen from the atmosphere to the body's cells. They are breathing (mechanics of inhaling and exhaling), external respiration (extraction of oxygen and disposal of carbon dioxide), and internal respiration (attaining oxygen to the cells and removing carbon dioxide from the cells).

ROBERT TISSERAND (*continued*)

aromatherapist today. Physicians picked up the practice soon thereafter.

Although aromatherapy (the use of essential oils distilled from plants for certain conditions) has been widely used in England for some time, only recently did its climb in popularity start in the United States. Lately, massage therapists are learning more about how aromatherapy can benefit their practices. At the very least, aromatherapy adds another sensory-pleasing dimension to the pleasure of receiving a massage. However, because of the strong connection between our sense of smell and mood, it can also add other benefits. For instance, lavender is thought to be calming. On the other end of the spectrum, mints and citrus oils have an energizing effect. Mixed with oil or lotion, essential essences are considered by many people to work magic on myriad maladies, from clogged sinuses to diarrhea. Aromatherapy can also be ingested (only by trained aromatherapists) for treatment of some ailments.

When asked which five essential oils are most important for massage therapists to always have on hand, Tisserand hesitates, pointing out that, ideally, no limit should be made. However, if choosing only five is necessary, then he recommends eucalyptus, lavender, rosemary, geranium, and ylang-ylang. He also advises therapists to practice the craft in as professional a manner as possible, experiment, and attend some type of training in aromatherapy. The Tisserand School of Aromatherapy requires 6 months' full-time attendance or 2 years' part-time attendance. Massage therapists should also be aware that some oils do have contraindications. For example, a popular essential oil for muscular aches and pains, bergamot, can cause photosensitivity.

Tisserand's *taste* for aromatherapy piqued around 1967 at age 19, when he attended a lecture on the subject along with his mother. She bought a book and had it signed by the speaker, Dr. Valnet. A couple of years later, Tisserand became interested in bodywork and did some training in that area. He soon made a conscious decision to pursue a career in aromatherapy. "Not for the money," he laughs, "or I would have given up a long time ago. Basically, I starved for 20 years."

Today, Tisserand teaches others the art of aromatherapy. He has also developed and distributes Tisserand essential oil products all over the world. His works include the quintessential *The Art of Aromatherapy* (Beekman, 1977), *Aromatherapy to Heal and Tend the Body* (Lotus Light, 1996), and *Essential Oil Safety* (Churchill Livingstone, 1995).

Tisserand still has his mother's signed copy of Valnet's French aromatherapy book, and after 30 years of hard work, audiences flock to his seminars, buy his books, seek his advice, and ask for his signature. The little boy who could not resist his mother's bottle of flea market perfume is finally able to sit back and enjoy the sweet smell of success.

- **Breathing**, or *pulmonary ventilation,* is a two-phase process: (1) inspiration and (2) expiration. These phases occur as a result of pressure differences, or a pressure gradient, between air in the lungs (more specifically, the alveoli) and air outside the lungs. As the relative size of the thorax changes, pressure differences are created and air moves in and out of the lungs.

  Air moves from an area of higher pressure to an area of lower pressure until the pressures are equalized.

- **Inspiration**, or *inhalation,* is the process that is responsible for drawing air into the lungs. During quiet inspiration, the diaphragm contracts and descends into the abdominal cavity, and the external intercostals contract to raise the ribs and chest. This action increases the size and length of the thoracic cavity and creates a decrease in pressure. Air, moving down the pressure gradient, enters the lungs. Inspiration, an autonomic process, can be intensified such as during exercise or it can be forced. Forced, or volitional, inspiration requires additional muscular contraction by the sternocleidomastoid, scalenes, and pectoralis minor. These muscles are regarded as accessory muscles of respiration (Figure 20-8).

  The ability of the thorax and lungs to stretch during inspiration is called *compliance*. The tendency of the thorax and lungs to return to their pre-inspiration size is called *elastic recoil.*

- **Expiration**, or *exhalation,* is the process that is responsible for expelling air from the lungs. During expiration, the diaphragm relaxes and ascends back up toward the thoracic cavity. This action decreases the size of the thoracic cavity, creating an increase in air pressure (Figure 20-9). Air, moving down the pressure gradient, exits the lungs by moving up and out the airway. Expiration, similar to inspiration, can also be forced. Forced expiration is

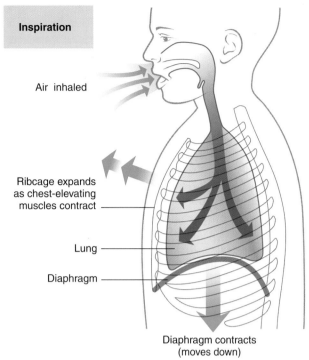

Inspiration

Air inhaled

Ribcage expands
as chest-elevating
muscles contract

Lung

Diaphragm

Diaphragm contracts
(moves down)

FIGURE 20-8 Mechanisms of inspiration.

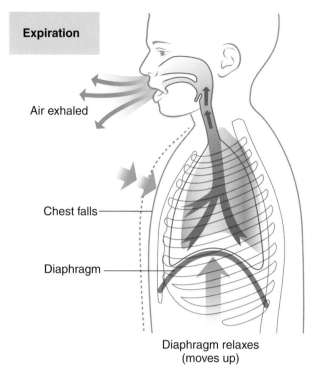

Expiration

Air exhaled

Chest falls

Diaphragm

Diaphragm relaxes
(moves up)

FIGURE 20-9 Mechanisms of expiration.

an active process, using voluntary muscular contractions of the internal intercostals and the abdominal muscles.

At rest, adults respire approximately 15 to 20 times a minute; children breathe twice as fast as adults. *Dyspnea* refers to labored or difficult breathing, and *apnea* refers to the temporary cessation of breathing.

Hypoxia refers to inadequate oxygen at the cellular level. This condition is characterized by cyanosis, tachycardia, hypertension, peripheral vasoconstriction, dizziness, and mental confusion. *Anoxia* is a condition characterized by a lack of oxygen either locally or systemically. This condition may be the result of an inadequate supply of oxygen to the respiratory system, inability of the blood to carry oxygen to the tissues, or inability of the tissues to absorb the oxygen from blood.

The respiratory center in the medulla oblongata controls the basic rhythm of breathing and is influenced by the amount of carbon dioxide in the blood. It operates without conscious control and works by sending nerve impulses down the phrenic nerve to the diaphragm. These impulses are also sent to muscles of respiration.

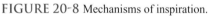

TABLE TALK

If an individual lives to be age 72, then he or she will have taken more than 530 million breaths of air.

Several other factors help regulate the respiratory center; for example, the cerebral cortex can modify our breathing

patterns when laughing or crying and can initiate volitional breathing. Volitional, or voluntary, breathing allows you to hold your breath while swimming under water and to take deep breaths to project your voice during public speaking. However, if you control your breath by rapid breathing (hyperventilation), or if you hold your breath too long, you will become unconscious. How long the breath is held is limited by carbon dioxide buildup in the blood.

An increase in body temperature (e.g., fever, exercise) increases respiration, whereas a decrease in body temperature (e.g., hypothermia, jumping into cool water) decreases respiration. Emotions such as anger or fear can also change respiration rates. A sudden, severe pain can temporarily stop breathing (apnea), and stretching the anal sphincter muscle increases the respiration rate (this technique is sometimes employed to stimulate respiration during medical emergencies).

The total amount of air that can be forcibly inspired and expired from the lungs in one breath is called *vital capacity*. This capacity represents the greatest respiratory volume of an individual. Age, gender, physical fitness, and disease

MINI-LAB

Using a tape measure, note the change in the circumference as you measure the ribcage during inspiration and expiration. Measure parts of the body such as the upper and lower ribs and abdomen.

affect vital capacity. Average values range from 4000 to 5000 ml.

During massage, apply downward pressure for an effleurage during exhalation. When applying sustained pressure over a trigger point, wait for the client to exhale. Follow the wave of the client's breath; release pressure on the inhalation and apply pressure on the exhalation. This process not only gives a sense of rhythm to your massage but also uses the client's natural ability to relax during an exhalation to enhance the effectiveness of your work.

Encourage your client to breathe properly during the massage. Invite the client to focus on breathing by placing your hand just below his or her navel while he or she is lying supine. Ask the client to take a deep breath and to allow his or her belly to elevate your hand. Occasionally, a simple goal such as using the breath to move the therapist's hand helps the client understand the abdominal changes that occur while breathing.

While your client is prone, place your hand on the small of his or her back and ask the client to take a deep breath, elevating your hand during inhalation. After instructing your client how to breathe for relaxation, teach him or her to use this simple technique when feeling stressed or fatigued. These types of client-therapist interactions help teach clients how to relax and how to become aware of their bodies.

> **evolve** *To see an illustration of the breathing wave discussed above, log on to the Evolve website and click on* Breathing Wave *under course materials for Chapter 20. Note both the functional and dysfunctional patterns.* ■

EXTERNAL AND INTERNAL RESPIRATION

Respiration takes place by *diffusion,* or the tendency of molecules to move from an area of high concentration to an area of low concentration. The main functions of the respiratory process are to supply the body with oxygen and dispose of carbon dioxide. Cells need oxygen to sustain life. Respiration occurs through two distinct processes: (1) external respiration and (2) internal respiration.

External (pulmonary) respiration is gas exchange in the lungs, between blood and air in the alveoli that came from the external environment. Oxygen diffuses from the air inside the alveoli across the alveolar walls into the blood capillaries. Oxygen binds to the hemoglobin inside red blood cells and is then transported to cells throughout the body. Carbon dioxide is transported by the blood from the cells of the body to the capillaries covering the alveoli. Carbon dioxide diffuses from the blood across the alveolar walls into the air inside the alveoli, which will then be exhaled (Figure 20-10).

Internal (tissue) respiration is the gas exchange between blood and body's tissues. Oxygen diffuses from the

blood into the cells, and carbon dioxide diffuses from the cells into the bloodstream. Each cell participates in absorption of oxygen and removal of waste materials in connection with this process.

> **evolve** *The difference between internal and external respiration is often a difficult concept for students to grasp. Because most people learn best visually, a diagram is located on the Evolve website under course materials for this chapter. I've drawn this image on the board for years and was delighted to find it in a textbook.* ■

MODIFIED RESPIRATORY AIR MOVEMENTS

Coughing is a sudden expulsion of air to clear the lungs and lower respiratory passageways of irritants or foreign materials. Coughing is a protective reflex but can be voluntarily induced or inhibited. The act of coughing occurs after a brief inspiration. Abdominal muscles contract, which forces air out of the lungs during expiration. Productive coughing helps clear the respiratory tract.

Crying is a response to emotions, such as grief, pain, fear, or joy. A common breath pattern while crying involves a sudden inspiration followed by the release of air in short breaths.

Hiccups, or hiccoughs, are intermittent contractions of the diaphragm followed by a spasmodic closure of the vocal cords. The sound occurs when inspired air hits the closed vocal cords. Hiccups have a variety of causes that appear to be linked to irritation of gastrointestinal sensory nerve endings.

Laughing involves the same modified respiratory patterns as crying and is usually a response to happiness, being tickled, or something that strikes us as funny. During laughter, the mouth is typically open in a grin. Laughing and crying can be so similar in sound that we typically have to look at a person's face to tell which emotion is being expressed.

Sneezing is a forceful involuntary expulsion of air through the nose and mouth to clear the upper respiratory passageways. Most sneezes occur as a result of irritation of the respiratory lining by foreign particles such as dust or pollen.

Snoring is audible breathing during sleep resulting from vibration of the uvula and soft palate. Snoring can be accompanied by harsh sounds and is common among individuals who sleep with their mouths open. When a person who snores sleeps on his or her back, the mouth opens because of gravity, and the tongue may rest in the back of the throat, partly blocking the air passage. In most cases, closing the mouth or simply rolling the snoring individual over stops the snoring.

A **yawn** is a very deep breath, initiated by opening the mouth wide and through movements of the upper torso to expand the chest. Some researchers believe that yawning is triggered by the need to increase the oxygen content and decrease carbon dioxide in the blood or as a result of drowsiness, boredom, or depression, but the precise cause is unknown.

TABLE TALK

Breathing and Relaxation

Breathing not only reflects our physiological and psychological states, it also creates them. Actors have known this for many years. Whenever a particular scene requires them to appear anxious, they take shallow, rapid breaths before the scene. Conversely, when a scene requires that they look calm and relaxed, they use slow, deep breaths to bring them to a state of relaxation. Massage therapists use breathing techniques themselves while they are giving a massage and often teach these techniques to their clients.

The most effective type of breathing to produce relaxation is deep, slow abdominal or diaphragmatic breathing. During deep breathing, the muscles of the abdominal wall expand when the diaphragm moves down during inhalation; the abdominal contents get a massage as they are compressed and released.

When we breathe deeply, it is a total body experience. Deep breathing can ease pain, relax tension, or introduce much-needed energy into the body. Shallow breathing does not encourage relaxation and can create tension in the neck and shoulders.

Breathing creates and reflects our emotional sphere; therefore deep, full breaths positively affect the free expression of our feelings. Restrictive breathing tends to constrict our expressions and wall off our feelings; we feel disconnected from the world around us.

The rhythm of breathing can give us an indication of how we feel about our surroundings. If we observe a slight pause before inhalation, then this may announce a fear of new experiences. People inevitably stop breathing in an attempt to prevent something from happening. Clients hold their breath during a massage when the pressure is uncomfortable. A slight pause before exhalation may indicate a fear of the client's own personal expression.

Imagine that the air around you has a fluid quality. As you inhale, the bottom portion of your lungs fills up first, similar to a glass of water. This filling causes a depression of the diaphragm and an expansion of the abdomen and thorax. As air fills the upper lungs, the ribcage expands and elevates on all sides. The spine also moves to accommodate the thoracoabdominal expansion. To complete your inhalation, puff out your cheeks and tightly close your lips. Allow your breath to burst out of your lips and exhale through your mouth, nose, or both. Although exhalation is typically a passive event, you may force air out of your lungs by contracting your abdominal muscles and *kissing your belly button to your spine*. As you breathe, you should feel your body, especially your spine, ribs, and abdomen, move. Subtle movements may be felt in the extremities.

Children and most animals breathe with their bellies. Observe a sleeping cat or a toddler running around in a diaper. The child's belly moves in a wave as he or she breathes. On mornings when you can wake up naturally (without an alarm), notice how you are breathing; you will probably be doing abdominal breathing. Encourage your body to breathe this way throughout the day.

PATHOLOGICAL CONDITIONS OF THE RESPIRATORY SYSTEM

Apnea

Apnea is a temporary cessation (usually lasting 15 seconds) or absence of spontaneous breathing. Sleep apnea occurs during sleep. *Position client for comfort.*

Asthma

Asthma is a chronic, inflammatory disorder in which the smooth muscles of the smaller bronchi and bronchioles spasm close, completely or partially, causing labored breathing. Asthma usually is preceded by emotional stress, respiratory infections, strenuous exercise, or inhalation of allergens (substances that promote allergic reactions). *Position client for comfort. Ascertain and avoid all known and suspected allergens. If client uses a bronchodilator, then have it handy. Focus treatment on muscles of respiration.*

Bronchitis

Bronchitis is inflammation of the bronchial mucosa that causes the bronchial tubes to swell and extra mucus to be produced. The two types of bronchitis are acute and chronic. Acute bronchitis, caused by an upper respiratory tract infection, results in a productive cough and high fever. Chronic bronchitis involves copious secretions of mucus with a productive cough that typically lasts 3 full months of the year for 2 successive years. Cigarette smoking is the most common cause of chronic bronchitis. *Massage is contraindicated if client has fever or is contagious. Otherwise, position client for comfort, including postural drainage. Percuss and vibrate back and ribcage for 15 to 20 seconds, with pauses of up to 5 seconds, for 5 minutes. Focus on the muscles of respiration.*

Chronic Obstructive Pulmonary Disease

Chronic obstructive pulmonary disease is a group of pulmonary disorders characterized by persistent or recurring obstruction of airflow, such as asthma, emphysema, cystic fibrosis, pneumoconiosis, or chronic bronchitis. The individual is unable to breathe freely. *See entries for Asthma, Emphysema, and Chronic Bronchitis.*

Common Cold

A cold is an acute inflammation of the mucosa of the upper respiratory tract, usually confined to the nose and throat; but the larynx can be involved as well. Symptoms include coughing, sneezing, watery eyes, nasal congestion and discharge, sore throat, and hoarseness. Fever and chills may accompany a cold. *Massage is contraindicated for 2 to 3 days after cold symptoms start. Afterward, massage is fine if symptoms are not severe.*

TABLE TALK

Cigarette smoking eventually destroys alveoli and reduces gas exchange in the lungs (Figure 20-10). Smoking also destroys respiratory cilia that remove particles in the nasal cavity and respiratory tract. As cilia die and the respiratory lining becomes irritated, the body produces excess mucus to trap the foreign particles in the cigarette smoke and to protect these delicate membranes and related tissues. This circumstance is why smokers often cough (trying to expel the extra mucus).

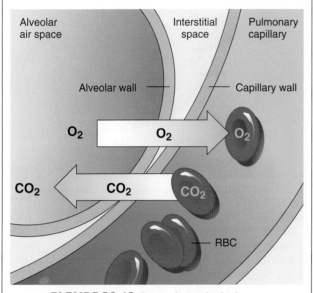

FIGURE 20-10 Gas exchange in the lungs.

Smoking can also inhibit macrophage cells, which increases the likelihood of respiratory infections. The excess mucus is also a breeding ground for bacteria. Hence smokers tend to be sick more often than nonsmokers. A recent medical discovery found that when smoking begins during early teen years, complete maturation of the lungs never occurs, and those additional alveoli are lost forever.

As a result, individuals who smoke one pack of cigarettes a day will statistically take 7 years off their life expectancy. Many respiratory diseases are related to cigarette smoking, including secondhand smoking. These diseases include chronic obstructive pulmonary diseases.

Emphysema

Emphysema involves overinflation and destruction of the alveoli, which produces abnormally large air spaces that remain filled with air during expiration. With the loss of the elasticity of the alveoli, a person may inhale easily but has to labor to exhale. The added exertion increases the size of the ribcage, resulting in a barrel chest. Emphysema is caused by a long-term irritation such as cigarette smoking, air pollution, and exposure to industrial dust. *Position client for comfort. Focus on muscles of respiration. Adjust massage to client's stamina and vitality (i.e., slow, gentle, short duration; assist client on and off table).*

Hay Fever

Hay fever is a general term used to denote any allergic reaction of the nasal mucosa and is characterized by sudden attacks of sneezing, swelling, and profuse water discharge of the nasal mucosa, with itching and watering of the eyes. Often occurring perennially, it is caused by allergens such as house dust, pet dander, and pollen. *Massage is contraindicated during acute allergic attack. Otherwise, massage is fine. Position the client for comfort (lying prone and using face cradle both cause an increase in nasal congestion). Ascertain and avoid all known and suspected allergens.*

Influenza

Influenza is an acute viral infection of the respiratory tract caused by different strains of viruses (influenzaviruses) designated A, B, and C. These viruses have a 3-day incubation period, with the illness lasting between 3 and 10 days. Influenza is characterized by an inflamed nasal mucosa and pharynx with fever and chills. Headaches, muscle aches, and pains may be also noted. *Massage is contraindicated.*

Laryngitis

Laryngitis is inflammation of the larynx that often results in loss of voice. Respiratory infections or irritants such as cigarette smoke cause laryngitis. Most long-term smokers acquire a permanent hoarseness from the damage created by chronic irritation and inflammation. Edema of the vocal cords often accompanies this disorder, with coughing and a scratchy throat. *If not caused by a contraindicated disease, massage is okay*.

Pleurisy

Pleurisy is inflammation of the pleural membranes characterized by stabbing pain during breathing. The painful breathing is caused by friction created as the swollen pleural membranes rub against each other. Chronic pleurisy may result in permanent pleural adhesions. *Obtain physician clearance. If not caused by a contraindicated disease, massage is okay, and treatment should focus on muscles of respiration, if clearance is granted.*

Pneumonia

Pneumonia is an infection or inflammation of the alveoli caused by the bacterium *Streptococcus pneumoniae,* but other infectious agents such as protozoans, viruses, and fungi may be responsible. During pneumonia, the alveoli fill with fluid and exudates such as dead white blood cells and pus. Exudates are substances that have been slowly discharged from cells or blood vessels as waste products. Pneumonia is the most common infectious cause of death in the United States, affecting, in particular, older adults, infants, immunocompromised individuals, and cigarette smokers. *Massage is contraindicated.*

Sinusitis

Sinusitis is an inflammation of the paranasal sinuses. Swelling of nasal mucosa may obstruct the openings from sinuses to the nose, resulting in an accumulation of sinus secretions, causing local tenderness, pain, headache, and fever. *If client has fever, massage is contraindicated. Otherwise, massage is fine. Position client for comfort; lying prone or using the face cradle increases sinus congestion. Moist heat, deep ischemic pressure over the frontal and sphenoidal sinuses, and steam inhalation may help relieve congestion.*

Tuberculosis

Tuberculosis is a chronic lung infection caused by the bacterium *Mycobacterium tuberculosis*. It is typically transmitted by the inhalation and exhalation (or consumption) of infected droplets. Even though the lungs are the primary targets of the disease, the liver, bone marrow, and spleen also may be involved. During tuberculosis, lung tissue is destroyed by bacteria and replaced by fibrous connective tissue, limiting gas exchange. *Massage is contraindicated until client is no longer infective. Check with physician to ascertain this status. Adjust massage to client's stamina and vitality (i.e., slow, gentle, short duration; assist client on and off table).*

See Box 20-1 for massage effects related to the respiratory system.

BOX 20-1

Effects of Massage on the Respiratory System

Reduces respiration rate. Massage slows down breathing because of activation of the relaxation response.

Strengthens respiratory muscles. The muscles of respiration have an increased capacity to contract, thereby helping improve pulmonary functions.

Decreases the sensation of dyspnea. Dyspnea, or short or difficult breathing, is lessened as a result of massage.

Decreases asthma attacks. Through increased relaxation and improved pulmonary functions, a person with asthma experiences fewer attacks.

Reduces laryngeal tension. Laryngeal tension may occur from excessive public speaking or singing. Massage reduces the stress on the larynx and tension on the muscles of the throat.

Increases fluid discharge from the lungs. The mechanical loosening and discharge of phlegm increases with rhythmic alternating pressures. Tapotement (cupping) and vibration on the ribcage are often used to enhance this effect. Phlegm loosening and discharge are further enhanced when combined with postural drainage (promoting fluid drainage of the respiratory tract through certain body positions) and when the client is encouraged to cough.

Improves pulmonary functions. Relaxation plays a big role in how massage improves pulmonary function, but massage also loosens tight respiratory muscles and fascia. Effects include increased vital capacity, increased forced vital capacity, increased forced expiratory volume, increased forced expiratory flow, and improved peak expiratory flow.

A client who is receiving a massage in a recumbent position when he or she is experiencing respiratory congestion compounds the problem. This circumstance is the result of gravity. The following pointers can make the client more comfortable:

1. When the client is in the supine position, elevate the upper body to assist drainage. Dr. Keith De Sonnier, an ear, nose, and throat physician, recommends a 30-degree incline to assist sinus drainage (Figure 20-11).

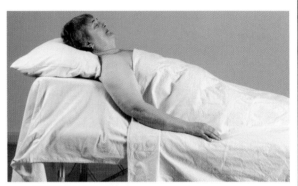

FIGURE 20-11 Client in semireclining position.

2. After massaging in the prone position, lower the upper body by placing pillows or other supportive cushions under the hips and abdomen. Use cupping tapotement, percuss and vibrate the back and ribcage for 15 to 20 seconds, with pauses of up to 5 seconds, for 5 minutes to loosen phlegm. Expect the client to cough as a natural reflex (Figure 20-12). Have tissues handy for client use.

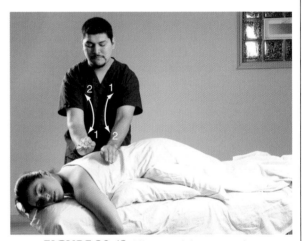

FIGURE 20-12 Client receiving percussion.

3. Adjust the table legs so that you raise the head of the massage table higher than the foot of the table during the massage; then, turning the client 180 degrees while prone, percuss and vibrate the back and ribcage for 15 to 20 seconds, with pauses of up to 5 seconds, for the final few minutes.

4. You may elect not to massage the client in the prone position and instead may choose a side-lying position.

SUMMARY

The respiratory system is physiologically and poetically associated with the very concept of life itself. The main functions of this system include the exchange of gases, homeostasis, olfaction, and production of speech. This method of air movement and chemical exchange is accomplished by the anatomical structures of the respiratory system, including the nasal cavities, pharynx, larynx, trachea, bronchi, alveoli, lungs, and respiratory diaphragm. Breathing, external respiration, and internal respiration are the processes necessary to get oxygen to cells and eliminate gaseous wastes. The main mechanisms of air movement involved in the breathing process are inspiration and expiration. Several modified respiratory air movements are also evident, including yawning, sneezing, coughing, crying, laughing, snoring, and hiccupping. The main purpose of air movement is to take in oxygen, which is vital to sustain life, and to expel carbon dioxide, a waste product.

evolve

Go to *Chapter Extras* on Evolve for additional illustrations and resources for this chapter. *Extras* for this chapter include:

1. Crossword puzzle (downloadable form)

MATCHING I

Place the letter of the answer next to the term or phrase that best describes it.

A. Bronchii
B. Compliance
C. Elastic recoil
D. Expiration

E. External respiration
F. Goblet cells
G. Hypoxia
H. Larynx

I. Nostrils
J. Sinuses
K. Sneeze
L. Vital capacity

_____ 1. Ability of the thorax and lungs to stretch during inspiration

_____ 2. Cells that produce mucus

_____ 3. Tendency of the thorax and lungs to return to their pre-inspiration size

_____ 4. Right and left air-conduction passageways leading to each lung

_____ 5. Voice box housing two sets of vocal cords

_____ 6. Air-containing spaces in skull and facial bones that are named for the bones by which they are located

_____ 7. Total air amount that can be forcibly inspired and expired from the lungs in one breath

_____ 8. Inadequate oxygen supply at the cellular level

_____ 9. A forceful expulsion of air through nose and mouth to clear the upper respiratory tract

_____ 10. Gas exchange in the lungs between blood and the external environment

_____ 11. Two external openings leading to the nasal cavity

_____ 12. Process of expelling air from the lungs

MATCHING II

Place the letter of the answer next to the term or phrase that best describes it.

A. Alveoli	E. Epiglottis	I. Pharynx
B. Cilia	F. Inspiration	J. Respiratory diaphragm
C. Cough	G. Internal respiration	K. Surfactants
D. Dyspnea	H. Lungs	L. Trachea

_____ 1. Fluid-coating phospholipids of the alveoli that assist gas exchange by reducing surface tension and contributing to lung tissue elasticity

_____ 2. Labored or difficult breathing

_____ 3. Tiny sacs attached to alveolar ducts

_____ 4. Referred to as the *guardian of the airways* because it closes the trachea during swallowing

_____ 5. Paired organs of respiration

_____ 6. Muscular tube shared by the respiratory and digestive systems; synonymous with the term *throat*

_____ 7. Process of drawing air into the lungs

_____ 8. Dome-shaped muscle of respiration

_____ 9. Hairlike projections on outer surfaces of certain cells

_____ 10. Tube from larynx to upper chest; synonymous with the term *windpipe*

_____ 11. A sudden expulsion of air to clear lungs and lower respiratory passageways of irritants or foreign materials

_____ 12. Gas exchange between blood and body tissues

INTERNET ACTIVITIES

Visit http://www.lungusa.org and click on Your Lungs. Review the respiratory system by clicking on Human Respiratory System and reading the content.

Visit http://www.medem.com/MedLB/article_detaillb.cfm?article_ID=ZZZ8PPLCGJC&sub_cat=285. Print the diagram of the respiratory system, blocking out all the labels. Using a clean copy, list as many structures as you can from memory. Use the textbook to check your work.

Visit http://www.cdc.gov/tobacco/christy/myths.htm and list the seven deadly myths of smoking. Share this information with your classmates.

Bibliography

Abrahams P, Marks S, Hutchings R: *McMinn's color atlas of human anatomy,* St Louis, 2003, Mosby.

Applegate EJ: *The anatomy and physiology learning system,* ed 3, Philadelphia, 2006, Saunders.

Beers MH, Berkow R: *The Merck manual of diagnosis and therapy,* Whitehouse Station, NJ, 2006, Merck Research Laboratories.

Como D, editor: *Mosby's medical, nursing, and allied health dictionary,* ed 6, St Louis, 2002, Mosby.

Crawley J, Van De Graaff KM: *A photographic atlas for anatomy and physiology,* Englewood, Colo, 2002, Morton.

Damjanov I: *Pathophysiology for the health-related professions,* ed 3, Philadelphia, 2006, Saunders.

Ferri FF: *2003 Ferri's clinical advisor, instant diagnosis and treatment,* St Louis, 2003, Mosby.

Ford CW: *Where healing waters meet: touching mind and emotions through the body,* Barrytown, NY, 1992, Station Hill Press.

Gray H, Pick TP, Howden R: *Gray's anatomy,* ed 29, Philadelphia, 1974, Running Press.

Haubrich WS: *Medical meanings: a glossary of word origins,* New York, 1984, Harcourt Brace Jovanovich.

Huether SE, McCance KL: *Understanding pathophysiology,* ed 3, St Louis, 2004, Mosby.

Jacob S, Francone C: *Elements of anatomy and physiology,* Philadelphia, 1989, Saunders.

Kalat JW: *Biological psychology,* ed 8, Belmont, Calif, 2003, Wadsworth.

Kapit W, Elson LM: *The anatomy coloring book,* ed 3, New York, 2002, Benjamin Cummings.

Kordish M, Dickson S: *Introduction to basic human anatomy,* Lake Charles, La, 1995, McNeese State University.

Kumar V, Abbas A, Fausto N: *Robbins and Cotran physiologic basis of disease,* ed 7, St Louis, 2005, Mosby.

Marieb EN: *Essentials of human anatomy and physiology,* ed 8, New York, 2005, Benjamin Cummings.

Martini FH, Bartholomew EF: *Essentials of anatomy and physiology,* ed 3, New York, 2003, Benjamin Cummings.

McAleer N: *The body almanac,* Garden City, NY, 1985, Doubleday.

McCance K, Huether S: *Pathophysiology: the biological basis for disease in adults and children,* St Louis, 2006, Mosby.

Merck manual, ed 17, Whitehouse Station, NJ, 1998, Merck and Company.

Moore KL: *Clinically oriented anatomy,* ed 5, Baltimore, 2005, Lippincott Williams & Wilkins.

Netter FH: *Atlas of human anatomy,* ed 3, Teterboro, NJ, 2003, Icon Learning Systems.

Newton D: *Pathology for massage therapists,* ed 2, Portland, Ore, 1995, Simran.

Premkumar K: *Pathology A to Z, a handbook for massage therapists,* Baltimore, 1999, Lippincott Williams & Wilkins.

Salvo SG, Anderson SK: *Mosby's pathology for massage therapists,* St Louis, 2004, Mosby.

Solomon EP, Phillips GA: *Understanding human anatomy and physiology,* Philadelphia, 1987, Saunders.

Thibodeau G, Patton K: *Anatomy and physiology,* ed 6, St Louis, 2006, Mosby.

Thibodeau G, Patton K: *Structure and function of the body,* ed 12, St Louis, 2004, Mosby.

Tortora GJ: *Introduction to the human body: the essentials of anatomy and physiology,* ed 5, Hoboken, NJ, 2000, John Wiley & Sons.

Tortora GJ, Grabowksi SR: *Principles of anatomy and physiology,* ed 11, New York, 2005, John Wiley & Sons.

Venes D, Thomas CL, Taber CW: *Taber's cyclopedic medical dictionary,* ed 20, Philadelphia, 2005, FA Davis.

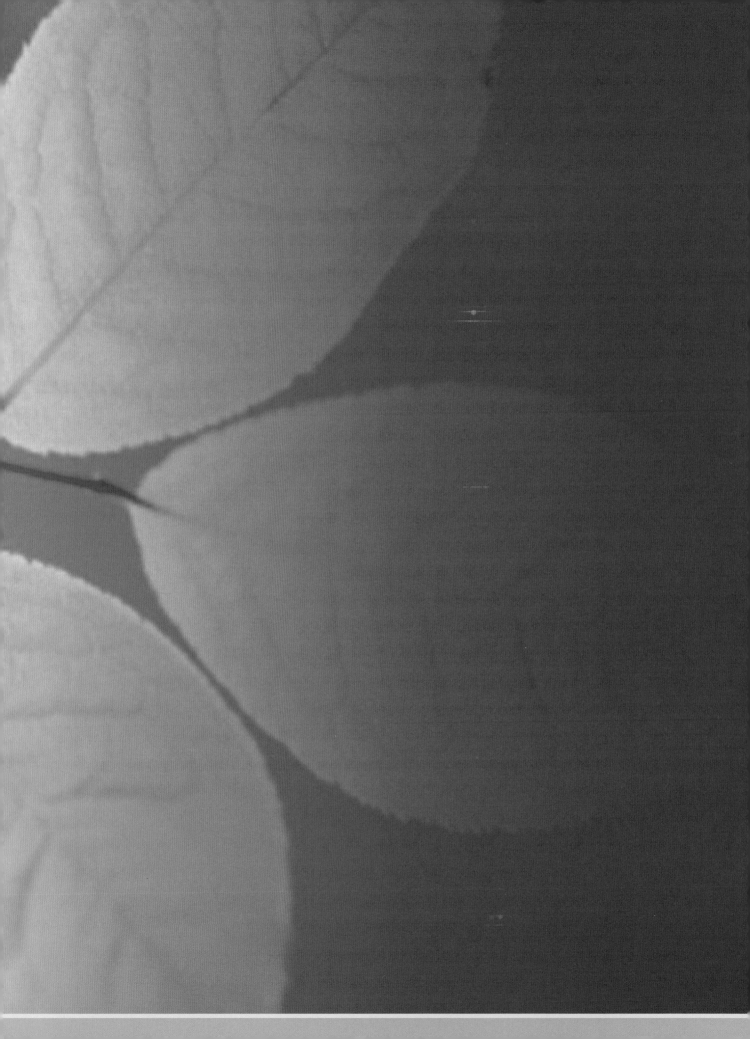

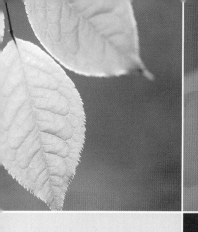

CHAPTER 21

Digestive System

"Be careful about reading health books. You may die of a misprint."

—Mark Twain

STUDENT OBJECTIVES

After completing this chapter, the student should be able to:

- List anatomical structures and describe the physiological mechanisms of the digestive system
- Identify specific divisions of the alimentary canal
- Describe what happens to food when it enters the alimentary canal
- Discuss the specialized cells located in the stomach that contribute to digestion
- Trace the path food takes from the time it enters the mouth to the time wastes are eliminated
- Identify where products of the salivary glands, liver, gallbladder, and pancreas enter the alimentary canal
- Describe the disassembly of foods in the body
- Name types of pathological conditions of the digestive system, giving characteristics and massage considerations of each

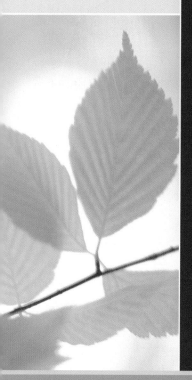

INTRODUCTION

People consume more than 40 tons of food in an average lifetime. The digestive system provides processes by which molecules such as proteins, carbohydrates, and fats are broken down into a state more easily assimilated into the body. Essentially, the digestive process is a *disassembly line*. These digestive processes themselves consume a tremendous amount of bodily resources, but fortunately they produce more energy than they use.

Chapter 17 explained the two divisions of the autonomic nervous system: sympathetic and parasympathetic. Digestive functions are initiated by the parasympathetic nervous system during periods of low stress. Because digestion requires a tremendous expenditure of energy, it occurs during times of low activity. The body can then reallocate energy that would normally be spent on muscular activity and route it to the digestive system. Activation of the parasympathetic nervous system is also known as the relaxation response, or *rest and digest*. Stress and emotions such as anger, fear, and anxiety may slow down digestion because they stimulate the sympathetic nervous system, or stress response. People in high-stress or high-responsibility positions are more likely than normal to have problems with ulcers, heartburn, colitis, irritable bowel syndrome, and constipation because of frequent disruption of the digestive process.

The digestive system may be viewed as a refinery. An industrial refinery takes a product such as raw crude oil from the ground and fractionates or disassembles it into useful components such as gasoline, butane, and diesel. Similarly, the digestive system takes in the raw materials of food and drink and converts them both physically and chemically into highly refined fuel. Just as fuel oil or natural gas is transported to people's homes by pipes, digested materials are delivered to the body's cells through the vessels of the circulatory system. Many unneeded resources can be stored for future metabolism.

Study of the anatomy of the digestive system shows that it is primarily composed of a tube, which is linked to the outside world. This chapter identifies each tube section and organ and describes each by structure and function. Included are the various digestive secretions and the food types on which they act.

ANATOMY

Areas of discussion in this chapter include
- Alimentary canal (tube from mouth to anus)
- Gallbladder
- Liver
- Pancreas
- Salivary glands
- Teeth
- Tongue

PHYSIOLOGY

The four functions of the digestive system are as follows:

Ingestion is the process of orally taking materials into the body. This term applies to taking in food, liquids, and oral medications.

Digestion is the mechanical and chemical process that occurs as food is mixed with digestive enzymes and converted into an absorbable state. Mechanical digestion includes chewing in the oral cavity, churning in the stomach, and the mixing movements of the intestinal tube (peristalsis). After digestion, food is capable of being taken into the bloodstream.

Absorption is the process by which the products of digestion move into the bloodstream or lymph vessels and then into the body's cells.

Defecation is the process of eliminating indigestible or unabsorbed material from the body.

Alimentary Canal

The **alimentary canal**, also referred to as the *gastrointestinal (GI) tract,* is the mostly coiled, muscular passageway leading from the mouth to the anus. The alimentary canal is

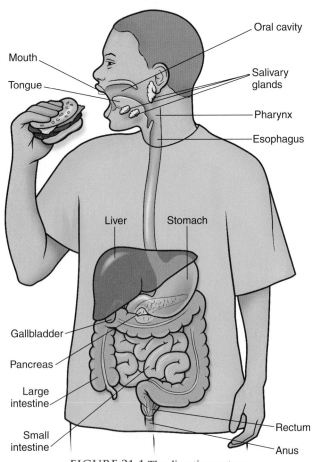

FIGURE 21-1 The digestive system.

approximately 30 feet long and includes the oral cavity, pharynx, esophagus, stomach, small intestine, and large intestine (Figure 21-1). The tube itself has four layers, or *tunics.* From innermost to outermost, the layers are the mucosa, submucosa, muscularis, and serosa, all of which are hosts to blood vessels, lymphatic vessels, and glands that produce and secrete digestive enzymes. An **enzyme** is a catalyst that accelerates chemical reactions. The alimentary canal is primarily smooth muscle, and this muscle tissue is responsible for most of the movement and mixing actions. Skeletal muscle is present only in parts of the pharynx, esophagus, and anus.

Within the muscular layer of the alimentary canal are two types of contractions: (1) *tonic* and (2) *rhythmic.* Tonic contractions are sustained contractions that occur in sphincter muscles. A **sphincter** is a ring of muscle fibers that regulates movement of materials from one compartment of the GI tract to another. Peristaltic contractions are the most common muscular contraction of the digestive system. These wavelike contractions mix and propel materials farther into the GI tract. **Peristalsis** occurs as a contraction just behind a *bolus* (a ball-like, masticated lump of food once swallowed; Figure 21-2). As the bolus approaches, the sphincter relaxes and then opens to allow passage. During mixing movements, peristaltic contractions occur as a rhythmic, sequential contraction of smooth muscle to move the intestinal materials back and forth until they are thoroughly mixed.

Peritoneum

The **peritoneum**, which envelops the entire abdominal wall, is the largest serous membrane in the body. The free surface of the peritoneum is lubricated with a serous fluid, permitting the digestive structures and other visceral organs to glide easily against the abdominal wall without friction. Within

the peritoneum are blood vessels, lymph vessels, and nerves. Sections of the peritoneum include the mesenteries, parietal and visceral peritoneum, and greater and lesser omentum (Figure 21-3). These structures are discussed later in this chapter in the section on the small intestine.

DIVISIONS OF THE ALIMENTARY CANAL

Oral Cavity

Also known as the *mouth,* the **oral cavity** is the port of entry for food and drink. The oral cavity contains the tongue, teeth, gums, and openings from the salivary ducts. Digestion begins in the oral cavity. **Mastication** (chewing) is aided by the tongue; digestive enzymes present in saliva break down food. **Saliva,** containing water, mucus, organic salts, and digestive enzymes, is a clear, viscous fluid secreted by the salivary and mucous glands in the mouth. The functions of saliva are to act as a lubricant and an adhesive by causing food to stick together and to form a bolus for **deglutition** (swallowing). Saliva stimulates the taste buds and protects the mucosa by acting as a buffer. With the exception of several medications, such as nitroglycerin, no absorption takes place in the oral cavity.

Saliva also serves to initiate the digestion of starches and fats through salivary amylase and lingual lipase. Salivary amylase, or ptyalin, begins the digestion of carbohydrates. Lingual lipase, secreted by glands located near the tongue, breaks lipids down into glycerol and fatty acids. Saliva is produced in one of the three pairs of salivary glands: (1) the *submandibular glands,* (2) the *sublingual glands,* and (3) the *large parotid glands.*

The tongue aids in deglutition by directing the bolus toward the back of the throat. Nestled in spherical pockets on the superior and lateral surfaces of the tongue are the **gustatory organs** (taste buds), which are chemoreceptors that detect the primary tastes of sweet, sour, bitter, and salty. However, taste is a response of many neurons and not just a signal from a single gustatory nerve. Even though the tongue is considered the primary organ of taste, the nose and the temperature of food play a significant role in how food tastes. Hot food tastes better than cold food because heat causes the aroma of the food to rise and enter our nose. Food does not taste as good when any type of condition affects the sense of smell.

Within the adult oral cavity are 32 secondary or permanent teeth. Children possess only 20 primary or deciduous teeth that are usually shed between the ages of 6 and 12 years. Enamel, which is the hardest substance in the body, covers each tooth. Teeth are classified according to shape and function: incisors, cuspids (canines), bicuspids (premolars), and multicuspids (molars). The third molars are also called *wisdom teeth* because they evidently erupt when a person is old enough to be wise (usually between the ages of 17 and 25).

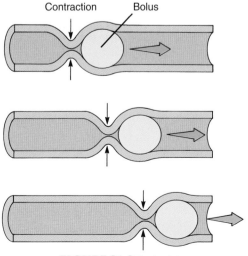

FIGURE 21-2 Peristalsis.

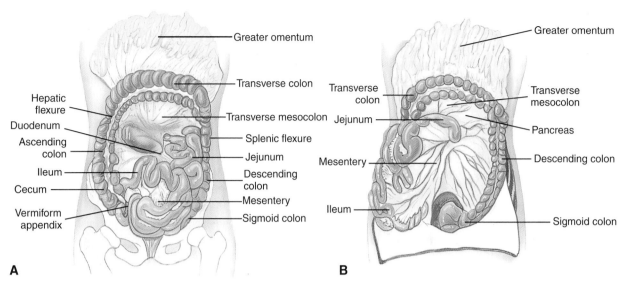

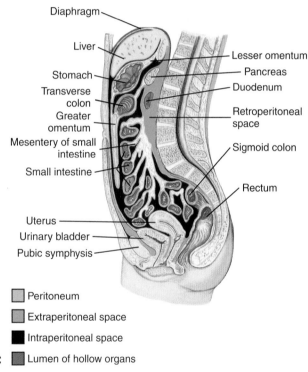

FIGURE 21-3 Peritoneum. **A,** Greater omentum drapes over the intestine, similar to an apron (anterior view). **B,** Greater omentum lifted to show mesenteries, deeper segment. **C,** Peritoneum (lateral view).

- Peritoneum
- Extraperitoneal space
- Intraperitoneal space
- Lumen of hollow organs

MINI-LAB

Most people can recall a biology experiment in elementary school in which different substances were placed on the tongue so as to impart a better understanding of how different parts of the tongue detects tastes.

Gather a small container of sugar, a small container of salt, and a sliced lemon. Apply these foods on different areas of your tongue, and notice the areas that clearly detect the tastes. Can you taste the lemon or the salt on the tip of your tongue? After wetting your finger, apply the sugar on the backside of the tongue. Can you taste the sweetness?

Pharynx

The **pharynx,** or throat, is the tube structure that transports food, liquid, and air to their respective destinations. In the digestive system, the pharynx takes food from the oral cavity to the esophagus during swallowing.

Esophagus

The **esophagus** (gullet) is the muscular tube that connects the pharynx to the stomach by piercing the diaphragm. The esophageal lining secretes mucus to aid in the transport of food. Bypassing the thoracic organs, the esophagus transports food to the stomach.

Stomach

The **stomach** is a J-shaped organ that is essentially an enlargement of the GI tract bound at both ends by sphincters. The superior sphincter, found at the junction between the esophagus and stomach, is the **cardioesophageal sphincter,** or cardiac sphincter. The **pyloric sphincter** is located between the stomach and small intestine. The stomach is situated directly under the diaphragm in the left upper quadrant of the abdomen. The major regions of the stomach include the *fundus,* the *body,* and the *pylorus*. Exteriorly, the shape of the stomach reveals a *greater curvature* and a *lesser curvature* (Figure 21-4).

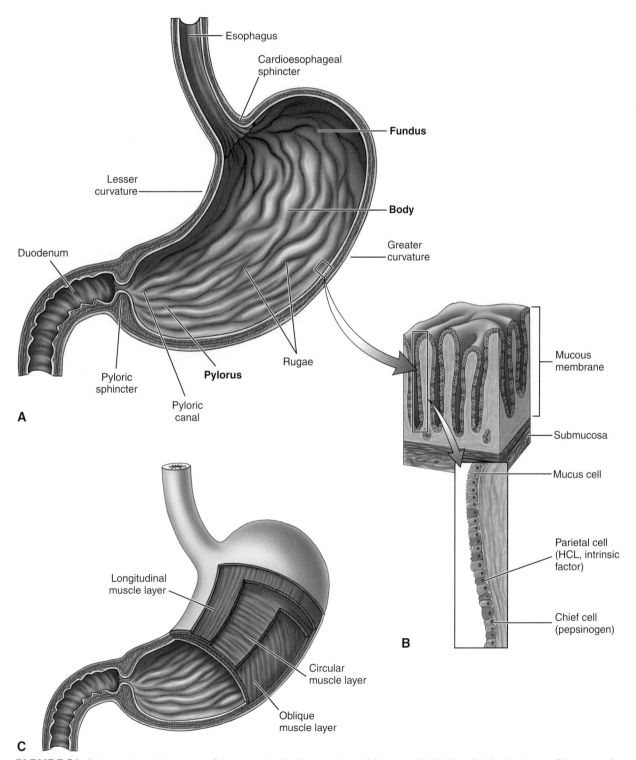

FIGURE 21-4 Stomach. **A**, Structures of the stomach. **B**, Cross section of the stomach's lining. **C**, Muscle layers of the stomach.

The stomach receives partially digested food and drink from the esophagus. When empty, the stomach is approximately the size of a large sausage. Depending on body size, the stomach, when full, can hold up to 1 gallon of food. The longitudinal folds in the lining of the stomach called rugae permit this expansion.

The muscular tunic of the stomach has three layers of muscle: (1) *oblique,* (2) *circular,* and (3) *longitudinal.* The oblique layer adds a new dimension to the churning action of the stomach, giving it an extraordinary ability to mix food. Entering the stomach, food mixes with gastric enzymes to initiate protein digestion. As food is further blended and digested, a bolus of food is reduced to a thin viscous fluid called *chyme.*

The pyloric sphincter opens periodically to allow chyme to enter the small intestine. The process of moving chyme into the small intestine may take up to 4 hours; thus the stomach also serves as both storage tank and digestive chamber. Because of this slow release of chyme into the small intestines, the body is able to maintain energy needs with only two or three meals a day, instead of requiring a steady supply of food, as grazing animals do.

The gastric mucosa possesses both endocrine and exocrine cells. The endocrine cells are called **G cells** and secrete the hormone gastrin, which initiates the production and secretion of gastric juice and stimulates bile and pancreatic enzyme emissions into the small intestines (Table 21-1). The stomach produces approximately 2 to 3 quarts of gastric juice per day. The only substances that are absorbed by the lining of the stomach are water, some minerals, alcohol, and some medications such as aspirin.

Two types of exocrine cells in the stomach are the parietal and chief cells. The **parietal cells** produce intrinsic factor, a substance required for the absorption of vitamin B_{12} from the small intestine to the bloodstream. The parietal cells also produce hydrochloric acid, a compound of hydrogen and chlorine, which breaks down protein and activates many gastric enzymes. Hydrochloric acid, which kills bacteria and other pathogens, is so powerful that it can eat through wood. The gastric lining is protected from this strong acid by a thick layer of alkaline mucus produced by mucous cells within the gastric lining. **Chief cells** produce the gastric enzyme pepsinogen, which is a precursor to pepsin. Pepsin is secreted in an inactive form to prevent the gastric lining from eroding from pepsin's protein digestion. Pepsinogen converts to pepsin when it comes into contact with hydrochloric acid and begins the chemical digestion of proteins.

Chymosin, or rennin, an enzyme found in the gastric juices of infants, is used to aid in milk curdling and is made commercially to produce cheese.

TABLE 21-1 Substances Affecting Digestion

NAME AND SUBSTANCE	LOCATION PRODUCED	ACTION(S)
Bile (emulsifier)	Liver	Physically breaks apart large fat globules into smaller ones
Carboxypeptidase (enzyme)	Pancreas	Breaks down proteins
Cholecystokinin (hormone)	Small intestines	Stimulates the release of bile from the gallbladder and the secretion of pancreatic enzymes
Chymosin/rennin (enzyme)	Stomach (infants only)	Aids in milk curdling
Chymotrypsin (enzyme)	Pancreas	Breaks down proteins
Enterocrinin (hormone)	Small intestines	Stimulates the flow of intestinal juice
Enterokinase (enzyme)	Small intestines	Activates protein enzyme secretion from pancreas
Gastrin (hormone)	Stomach (G cells)	Initiates production and secretion of gastric juice; stimulates release of bile and pancreatic enzymes into the small intestines
Hydrochloric acid (compound)	Stomach (parietal cells)	Breaks down protein and activates gastric enzymes
Intrinsic factor (substance)	Stomach (parietal cells)	Promotes absorption of vitamin B_{12} from the small intestine into the bloodstream
Lactase (enzyme)	Small intestines	Promotes carbohydrate digestion
Lingual lipase (enzyme)	Oral cavity	Breaks lipids down into glycerol and fatty acids
Maltase (enzyme)	Small intestines	Promotes carbohydrate digestion
Pancreatic amylase (enzyme)	Pancreas	Converts polysaccharides into disaccharides
Pancreatic lipase (enzyme)	Pancreas	Converts triglycerides into monoglycerides and fatty acids
Pepsinogen/pepsin (precursor/enzyme)	Stomach (chief cells)	Begins chemical digestion of proteins by converting them into peptides
Peptidase (enzyme)	Small intestines	Promotes the digestion of proteins
Salivary amylase/ptyalin (enzyme)	Salivary glands	Begins carbohydrate digestion
Secretin (hormone)	Small intestines	Stimulates the production and secretion of pancreatic enzymes
Sucrase (enzyme)	Small intestines	Promotes carbohydrate digestion
Trypsinogen/trypsin (precursor/enzyme)	Pancreas	Breaks protein into smaller chains of amino acids

Small Intestine

The **small intestine** is actually the longest section of the alimentary canal and is situated in the central abdomen, framed by the large intestine. This muscular tube is bound at both ends by the pyloric sphincter (at the stomach) and the ileocecal sphincter (at the large intestine). The lumen of the small intestine possesses circular folds called **plicae circulares** (Figure 21-5). The lining of the small intestines contains numerous **villi**, which are fingerlike projections that house blood and lymph capillaries. Mucus-producing *goblet cells* are found in the spaces between some of the villi. The lymph capillaries in the villi are called **lacteals**, which assist in the absorption of fat. Intestinal glands extend downward between adjoining villi. The surfaces of the villi possess microvilli that form a brush border. All three structures (i.e., plicae circulares, villi, microvilla) serve to increase the surface area of the small intestine for more efficient absorption. Layers of smooth muscle, longitudinal and circular, are found in the intestinal wall.

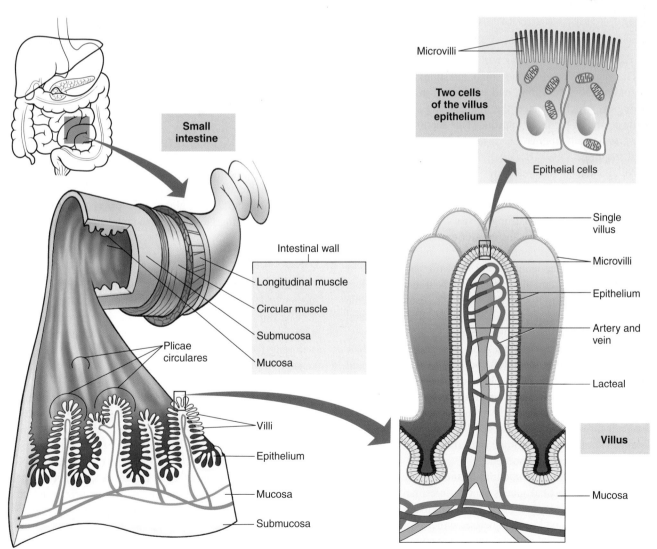

evolve *View a close-up cutaway of the intestines featuring its numerous villi on the Evolve website under course materials for Chapter 21. It is easy to imagine that "it takes a villi" to deal with the absorption issues in the small intestines.* ∎

FIGURE 21-5 Small intestinal wall.

The three divisions of the small intestines, from beginning to end, are (1) the duodenum, (2) the jejunum, and (3) the ileum. The first section of the small intestine, the **duodenum**, is between 10 and 12 inches long and contains the sphincter of Oddi and the major duodenal papilla. The **sphincter of Oddi** regulates the flow of secretions from the pancreas, liver, and gallbladder; the **major duodenal papilla** is the site of entry for these secretions. The major duodenal papilla is a dilation that is formed by the juncture of the pancreatic and common bile ducts as they open into the small intestines.

The intermediate portion of the small intestine, the **jejunum,** runs from the duodenum to the ileum and is approximately 6 feet long. The walls of the jejunum are slightly thicker than those of the ileum, and the jejunum possesses a smaller lumen. The villi are larger in this section, presumably to increase absorption.

TABLE TALK

The word *jejunum* is derived from the Latin adjective *jejunus* (fasting or hungry), meaning being empty or devoid of food. The ancient Greeks, during the practice of necropsy (examination of a dead body), found that the lumen of the middle small intestine was always empty.

The final division of the small intestine, the **ileum,** is approximately 9 feet long and terminates at the **ileocecal sphincter**, which connects the ileum of the small intestine to the cecum of the large intestine. This section of the small intestine contains numerous clusters of lacteals to enhance fat absorption.

All divisions of the small intestines are connected to each other and to the posterior abdominal wall by a section of the peritoneum called the **mesenteries.** The mesentery is a large, fan-shaped structure consisting of two omentums. Also referred to as the *fatty apron,* the **greater omentum** is a double-layered structure that connects to the greater curvature of the stomach and duodenum, drapes down over the coils of the small intestine, and then attaches to the transverse colon. The **lesser omentum** is a fatty, membranous extension of the peritoneum and attaches from the right side of stomach and first section of the duodenum to the liver.

The length of the small intestine is responsible for 90% of all absorption (the other 10% occurs in the stomach and large intestine; Figure 21-6). Digested foodstuffs, absorbed through the intestinal walls, are transported by the blood, which takes care of sugars and proteins, and by lymph, which is responsible for fats. If more food nutrients (e.g., fat, fat-soluble vitamins) are absorbed than the body requires, the extra is then stored until needed.

Brunner's glands (duodenal glands) secrete alkaline mucus. Other intestinal glands secrete intestinal juice containing digestive enzymes such as enterokinase, peptidase, maltase, sucrase, and lactase. These enzymes promote the digestion of proteins and carbohydrates. Hormones secreted by the intestinal mucosa are enterocrinin, cholecystokinin, and secretin. Enterocrinin stimulates the flow of intestinal juice,

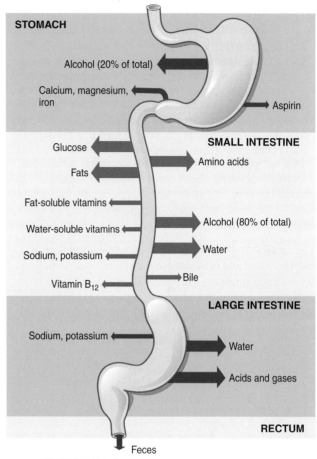

FIGURE 21-6 Absorption sites in digestive tract.

and cholecystokinin stimulates contraction of the gallbladder and pancreatic enzyme secretion. Secretin stimulates the pancreas to secrete an alkaline liquid that neutralizes the acid chyme, facilitating the action of the intestinal enzymes.

Large Intestine

The **large intestine,** or *colon*, is the final stretch that undigested and unabsorbed food takes before the body eliminates it. The lining of the large intestine does not produce digestive enzymes; instead, it produces mucus that allows the developing fecal matter to move down more easily. With the exception of water, vitamins, and minerals, the colon lining absorbs few substances.

The large intestine is characterized by two structures: (1) taenia coli and (2) haustrum. Located in the muscularis tunic of the large intestine are thick, longitudinal bands called the **taenia coli,** which resemble a thread-gathering fabric. The gathers, or tucks, along the length of the colon make a series of pouches, called **haustra.** Once filled, these pouches contract to push the contents to the next haustrum.

The divisions of the large intestine are the cecum, colon proper, rectum, anal canal, and anus. The colon proper is further divided into the ascending, transverse, descending, and sigmoid colons. Flexures exist where the colon turns into an upside-down U shape (Figure 21-7).

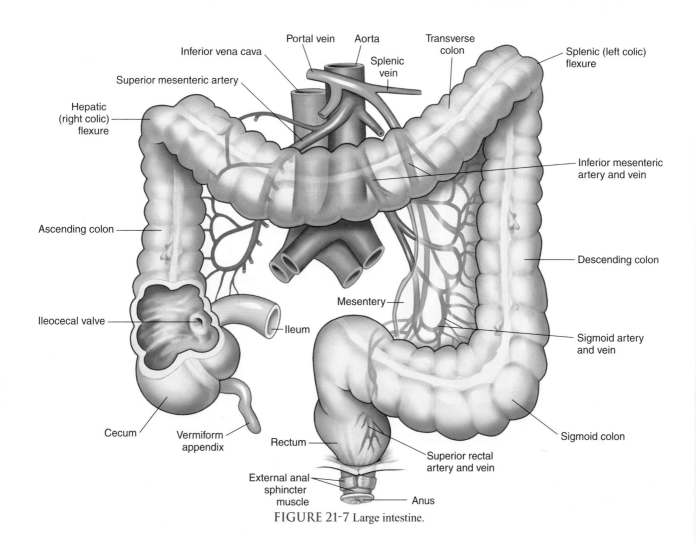

FIGURE 21-7 Large intestine.

The first section of the colon, the **cecum,** is a small saclike structure located in the right lower quadrant of the abdomen. The cecum is attached to the ileocecal sphincter. Suspended from and opening into the inferior portion of the cecum is a lymph gland called the **vermiform appendix.** The wormlike appendix varies from 3 to 6 inches in length and is discussed in Chapter 19.

The next segment of the colon is the ascending colon, continuing from the cecum up the lower right abdomen, turning from the hepatic or right colic flexure. After the hepatic flexure, the colon moves horizontally from right to left, draping to form the transverse colon. The colon proper takes a downward turn at the splenic or left colic flexure and provides the path for the descending colon. At the level of the iliac crest, the descending colon turns back toward the right at the sigmoid flexure to become the sigmoid colon. Then, with a final S-shaped downward curve, the colon reaches the **rectum** and terminates at the **anal canal,** opening to the outside at the **anus.**

The rectum usually contains three circular folds that overlap when empty and grow in size as the rectum fills with waste to be excreted. The main function of the rectum and anal canal is storage.

The anal canal possesses two sphincters: (1) an internal sphincter, containing visceral muscle, and (2) an external sphincter, containing skeletal muscle. As the rectal contents move into the anal canal, the internal anal sphincter muscle distends, stimulating pressure-sensitive receptors and initiating the defecation reflex. If this urge is suppressed, then it may dissipate, and it may be hours before the desire to defecate returns. If the urge to defecate is chronically suppressed, then copious amounts of water are absorbed from the colon, and constipation may result.

evolve *Here's your opportunity to see food's "trail's end." An image of the rectum and anus is located on the Evolve website. Note how the valves go from convoluted to straight before a defecation reflex is experienced.* ■

During defecation, the levator ani muscle raises the anus to eliminate fecal matter. Feces, or stool, are excrement from the GI tract formed in the intestine and released through the anus. Feces consist of indigestible foodstuffs, water, bacteria, and cells sloughed off the walls of the rectum and anal canal.

ACCESSORY DIGESTIVE ORGANS

The accessory digestive organs produce substances that aid digestion in the small intestines. They are the liver, gallbladder, and pancreas (Figure 21-8). The digestive substances produced and secreted by these organs continue the chemical digestion of food.

Liver

The largest internal organ in the body, the **liver,** weighs approximately 3 pounds (lbs). It is located in the upper right quadrant of the abdominal cavity. This reddish-brown organ consists of hepatocytes (liver cells) that are arranged around thousands of specialized venous channels called *sinusoids,* which are larger than ordinary capillaries. Lining the sinusoids of the liver are phagocytic cells called *Kupffer's cells.* These specialized macrophages destroy pathogens and move other foreign material out of the blood before sending it through the hepatic vein. Blood flowing through the sinusoids originates from the stomach and the intestines through the hepatic portal system (see Chapter 19). Because of the vascularity of this organ, the liver holds approximately 1 pint of blood at any given moment.

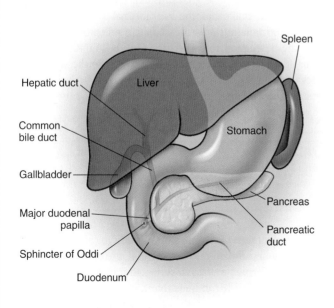

Hepatic duct

Common bile duct

Gallbladder

Major duodenal papilla

Sphincter of Oddi

Duodenum

Spleen

Liver

Stomach

Pancreas

Pancreatic duct

FIGURE 21-8 Accessory digestive organs.

One of the most complex organs of the body, the liver has more than 500 functions. One of its digestive functions is the production of bile—approximately 1 quart of bile per day. **Bile** enters the left and right *hepatic ducts,* which join to form the *common bile duct* that leads to the duodenum of the small intestine. Produced from the hemoglobin in worn-out red blood cells, bile is not an enzyme but an emulsifier. It physically breaks apart large fat globules into smaller ones and provides a larger surface area for the fat-digesting enzymes to work. Bile gives urine and the stool their characteristic colors.

Some other liver functions are the production, storage, and breakdown of glucose and hemoglobin. The liver produces amino acids, blood plasma proteins, fibrinogens (blood-clotting substances), and antibodies. It also processes absorbed nutrients and stores vitamins A, D, E, and K; minerals; iron; copper; and other compounds used by the body.

The liver detoxifies numerous toxic substances such as alcohol, nicotine, and other poisons, into nontoxic materials. Toxic substances that cannot be broken down and excreted are stored. One such substance is dichlorodiphenyltrichloroethane (DDT), which was banned in the United States in 1971.

Gallbladder

The **gallbladder,** which stores bile manufactured by the liver, is a pear-shaped sac located in a depression on the inferior surface of the liver. The sphincter of Oddi controls the release of bile into the duodenum. When the sphincter is closed, bile backs up into the gallbladder, where it is stored until needed. Recall that the intestinal mucosa secretes a hormone, cholecystokinin, which stimulates the release of bile from the gallbladder.

Pancreas

Both an endocrine and exocrine gland, the **pancreas** is a carrot-shaped organ located inferior and posterior to the greater curvature of the stomach. The pancreas is the most important digestive gland because it secretes enzymes that break down all categories of digestible foods, including proteins, carbohydrates, and fats. *Acini cells* secrete pancreatic enzymes. The pancreatic duct runs the length of the organ, draining the smaller ducts and emptying the pancreatic enzymes into the duodenum (Figure 21-9). Pancreatic enzymes are secreted in an alkaline fluid to neutralize the acid chyme from the stomach. Recall that secretin, a hormone produced by the intestinal mucosa, stimulates the production and secretion of pancreatic enzymes.

The pancreas produces approximately 1.0 to 1.5 quarts of digestive enzymes per day, including trypsinogen, chymotrypsin, carboxypeptidase, pancreatic amylase, and pancreatic lipase. Trypsinogen, a protein-splitting enzyme, is converted to trypsin when it enters the duodenum. Trypsin, activated by the intestinal enzyme enterokinase, breaks protein into peptides before the conversion to amino acids. Chymotrypsin and

JOEY ERWIN

February 7, 1976

"If you can't get outside of your own garbage, you will never be able to handle anyone else's."

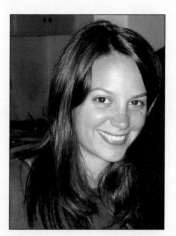

Joey Erwin is a relative newcomer to the field of massage therapy. In a short time, however, Erwin has pioneered a path for herself in the area of oncology massage.

Erwin was born in California in 1976 and, until recently, when she moved to Louisiana, called California her home. Erwin went to massage school with the idea of pursuing oncology massage firmly planted in her mind. The American Cancer Society estimates that more than 10 million patients with cancer are in the United States, but for Erwin, this number is more personal. Instead of a statistic, she sees the face of her stepfather, uncle, and grandmother, all of whom died of cancer.

Erwin studied at the California College of Physical Arts in Huntington Beach, California, before receiving her Holistic Health Practitioner's Certificate in 2003. As a student, she spent a great deal of time outside the classroom, learning as much as she could about the practice of oncology massage. A decade ago, Erwin noted, "There seemed to be a conservative approach to oncology massage," and she had difficulty locating instruction in a field that was at the time predominantly closed to patients with cancer.

Today, this taboo is changing. Erwin had the chance to put her oncology lessons to practice at a weekend retreat for patients with breast cancer. She served as one of a small group of massage therapists on hand to give therapy sessions. Erwin remembers one client in particular who would ultimately shape and define her passion for oncology massage.

"One woman had so many tumors taken out and so many complications, her body looked like a road map of scars. She was so uncomfortable and in so much pain and just wanted massage," Erwin said. As her hands went to work, Erwin said she was able to feel the woman changing under her touch. They both cried. The woman told her that nobody had touched her like that for years.

That moment was a turning point in Erwin's career. She no longer felt fear of sickness or dying but rather had a renewed interest in bringing the healing powers of massage to patients with cancer. Today, Erwin is excited about the future of her profession and hopes that others will follow in her footsteps.

"Lose your fear," she says. "People are scared of scars, sickness, tubes, and bags. It's messy and it's dirty and it's stinky, but when you get the really challenging cases...those are my favorites."

Erwin has returned to school to study nursing. Although oncology massage is her first love, she hopes to combine traditional medicine and medical knowledge with her expertise in massage. As Erwin seeks to bring the practice of massage therapy into the medical world, she says her number-one goal is to work in an oncology ward where massage is part of the protocol.

When the waters rose in New Orleans after hurricane Katrina, Erwin was there. When the floods subsided, she was back, ready to rebuild. As a pioneer in the practice of oncology massage, Erwin hopes to always be on the cutting edge in her field.

carboxypeptidase also assist in the breakdown of proteins. Pancreatic amylase converts polysaccharides into disaccharides (maltose, sucrose, and lactose). Pancreatic lipase helps convert fats into fatty acids.

DISASSEMBLY OF FOODS

The major purpose of eating is to feed the body. This concept sounds simple enough, but the process is not quite so simple. Ultimately, nutrient delivery takes place at the cellular level.

The previous discussion examined the how-to part of getting food broken down, but this next section explores what food becomes and how our cells use these products.

To be beneficial on the cellular level, food must be disassembled into its component parts: proteins, carbohydrates, fats, vitamins, minerals, and water (Table 21-2). Two functions of the digestive system are to disassemble these nutrients and eliminate the unused matter. Nutrients such as vitamins, minerals, and water do not have to be digested before they are used in the body, but proteins, carbohydrates, and

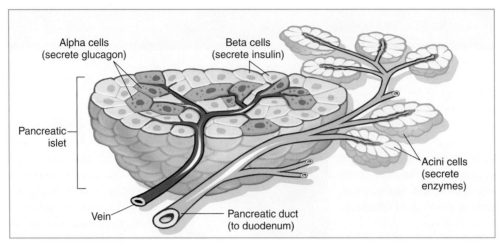

FIGURE 21-9 Exocrine cells of the pancreas and their relationship to endocrine cells.

fats need to be mechanically and chemically broken down (see Appendix D for a discussion on nutrition).

Proteins

Proteins are naturally occurring organic compounds that contain large combinations of amino acids. Twenty-four (24) identified amino acids are vital for proper growth, development, and health maintenance. Ten of the amino acids are classified as nonessential, meaning that the body can synthesize them. The remaining 8 amino acids are essential amino acids, and these must be obtained from dietary sources (Table 21-3). Sources rich in protein are meat, poultry, seafood, eggs, soy products, and dairy products (including yogurt and cheese).

Amino acids are the building blocks of protein and are the major components for building muscles, blood, skin, hair, nails, and visceral organs. Protein is also essential for the formation of hormones, enzymes, and antibodies and is used by the body to repair and rebuild tissues because the body is in a constant state of tearing down and rebuilding.

Carbohydrates

Also known as *starches* and *sugars,* **carbohydrates** are classified according to molecular structure as mono-, di-, and polysaccharides (see Table 21-3). Monosaccharides, simple sugars, are glucose (blood sugar), fructose (fruit sugar), and galactose (milk sugar). Disaccharides, the union of two monosaccharides, are sucrose (table sugar), lactose (milk sugar), and maltose (malt sugar). Polysaccharides (trisaccharides), carbohydrates containing three or more simple sugar molecules, are dextrins, glycogen (stored glucose), cellulose, and gums.

TABLE 21-2 **Nutrients and Their Functions**

NUTRIENT	FUNCTION
Proteins	Building and repairing muscles, blood, skin, hair, nails, and visceral organs
	Formation of hormones, enzymes, and antibodies
Carbohydrates	Preferred source of energy
	Metabolism of proteins and fats
Fats	Maintenance of cell membranes
	Storage and absorption of fat-soluble hormones and vitamins
	Cushioning and insulation of visceral organs
Vitamins	Normal physiological and metabolic function, including the following:
	Antioxidants: vitamins E and C and beta carotene
	Hormones: vitamin D
	Enhances the immune system: vitamin A
Minerals	Building of bone (calcium, magnesium, boron, etc.)
	Muscular activity (calcium and magnesium)
	Support for various organs such as the pancreas (manganese, chromium, and vanadium)
	Transportation of oxygen and carbon dioxide (iron)
Water	Maintenance of proper body pH, nutrient transport, lymphatic transport, and elimination

TABLE 21-3   Selected Nutrient Classifications

NUTRIENT	CLASSIFICATION
Amino acids: building blocks of proteins	Nonessential amino acids (can be synthesized by the body)
	Essential amino acids (must be obtained from dietary sources such as meat, poultry, seafood, eggs, soy products, and dairy products [including yogurt and cheese])
Carbohydrates	Monosaccharides (simple sugars):
	Glucose (blood sugar)
	Fructose (fruit sugar)
	Galactose (milk sugar)
	Disaccharides (union of two monosaccharides):
	Sucrose (table sugar)
	Lactose (milk sugar)
	Maltose (malt sugar)
	Polysaccharides (trisaccharides):
	Dextrins
	Glycogen (stored glucose)
	Cellulose and gums
Fats	Saturated (solid at room temperature):
	Lard (animal fats)
	Processed oils (hydrogenated or partially hydrogenated oils)
	Coconut oil
	Palm kernel oil
	Used restaurant oils
	Unsaturated (liquid at room temperature):
	Olive oil
	Peanut oil
	Flaxseed oil
	Sesame oil
Vitamins	Fat-soluble vitamins can be stored by the body, including vitamins A, D, E, and K
	Water-soluble vitamins must be ingested regularly, including B vitamins and vitamin C

Carbohydrates are the body's preferred source of energy and are required for the metabolism of other nutrients such as proteins and fats. Ingested carbohydrates, mediated by the hormone insulin, are absorbed immediately by the cells of the body or stored as glycogen (stored glucose). Some dietary sources of carbohydrates are grains, cereals, vegetables, fruits, potatoes, and legumes.

Fats

Fats are composed of lipids or fatty acids and can range in consistency from a solid to a liquid. Stored fat (adipose tissue) helps cushion and insulate visceral organs. Fats are classified as saturated or unsaturated, depending on whether they are solid (saturated) or liquid (unsaturated) at room temperature (see Table 21-3). Examples of saturated fats are lard (animal fats), processed oils (hydrogenated or partially hydrogenated), coconut and palm kernel oil, and used restaurant oils. Examples of unsaturated fats are olive, peanut, flaxseed, and sesame oils. The body requires fats to maintain cell membranes. Glycerol and fatty acids make up triglycerides (lipids).

Of all the nutrients, fats are probably the least understood of all. Good and bad fats are known, but discussion about each abounds as if no distinction can be made. Bad fats are saturated and include lard (animal fats), processed oils (hydrogenated or partially hydrogenated oils), and even unsaturated oils that have been used numerous times (many restaurant oils) because repeated heating breaks down their molecular structure. Good fats are unsaturated and include olive oil, peanut oil, flaxseed oil, and sesame oil.

evolve Proteins, carbohydrates, and fats go through a disassembly process while in the digestive tract. Log on to the Evolve website and view three schematic drawings of all three process, taking you on a sort of culinary to chemical journey. Bon appetit! ∎

Vitamins

Vitamins are organic compounds essential for normal physiological and metabolic functioning of the body. Many vitamins act as coenzymes. Most vitamins cannot be synthesized by the body and must be obtained from a healthy diet or vitamin supplements. Vitamins are either fat soluble or water soluble (see Table 21-3). The body can store fat-soluble vitamins, whereas water-soluble vitamins must be ingested regularly. Fat-soluble vitamins are A, D, E, and K; water-soluble vitamins are the B vitamins and vitamin C.

Vitamins have various functions. Vitamin E is an *antioxidant* (a substance that inhibits or retards oxidation), as are vitamin C and beta carotene (a precursor to vitamin A); vitamin D functions as a hormone; and vitamin A enhances the immune system. Vitamins are necessary micronutrients for the body, and the U.S. government has recognized their importance by establishing minimum daily requirements (see Appendix D).

Minerals

Minerals are essential nonorganic compounds found in nature that the body uses. Minerals are needed in trace amounts and are used to build bone (calcium, magnesium, boron, etc.), during muscle activity (calcium and magnesium), to support various organs such as the pancreas (manganese, chromium, and vanadium), and to transport oxygen and carbon dioxide (iron). Minerals also play a vital role in regulating many body functions; many also function as coenzymes.

A mineral is usually referred to by the name of a metal, nonmetal, radical, or phosphate rather than by the name of the compound (e.g., sodium chloride or table salt).

Water

Although water is not often thought of as food, it is an essential nutrient that every part of the body needs. Water-based fluids surround every cell in the body, except the outer layer in the skin, and all nutrients and wastes travel through fluids (blood, lymph, and interstitial fluid). These fluids require a continuous supply of fresh water for proper body pH, nutrient transport, lymphatic transport, and elimination. Each day, a person should drink at least 0.5 ounces (oz) of water per 1 lb of body weight (e.g., 128 lb = 64 oz [½ gallon] of water per day).

MINI-LAB

Calculate your total caloric intake over a 24-hour period by using a simple caloric guide from any drugstore. Look at the distribution of the basic food groups, and write a list of what improvements might (and should) be made in your eating habits.

PATHOLOGICAL CONDITIONS OF THE GASTROINTESTINAL TRACT

Anorexia Nervosa

Classified as both an eating and emotional disorder, anorexia nervosa is the prolonged avoidance of eating. Lack of nutrients results in emaciation, amenorrhea (cessation of menstruation), decreased sleep, and psychological disturbance. Although cases among young men are on the rise, most anorexia nervosa sufferers are young Caucasian women. ***Obtain physician clearance if symptoms are severe.***

Appendicitis

An inflammation of the vermiform appendix, appendicitis is often detected by acute pain in the lower right quadrant of the abdomen, vomiting, fever, and elevated white blood cell count. Intestinal disease, intestinal obstruction or adhesions, or parasites typically cause appendicitis. The most common treatment is an appendectomy. ***Massage is contraindicated.***

Bulimia

Bulimia is characterized by overeating (bingeing) and self-induced vomiting (purging). Similar to anorexia nervosa, bulimia is classified as an eating and emotional disorder. ***Massage is indicated.***

Cholecystitis

Chronic or acute inflammation of the gallbladder is called cholecystitis. Gallstones that cannot pass through the bile duct often cause acute cholecystitis. Pain is felt in the right upper quadrant of the abdomen, accompanied by nausea and vomiting. Chronic cholecystitis is more common than the acute form. Pain is often felt at night following a large, fatty meal and gradually increases in intensity. ***Massage is contraindicated during acute stage. For chronic cholecystitis, massage is fine if symptoms are not severe. Position client for comfort, and avoid abdominal area.***

Cirrhosis of the Liver

Cirrhosis of the liver is a chronic degenerative disease in which the hepatic cells are destroyed and replaced with fibrous connective tissue, giving the liver a yellow-orange color. Liver functions deteriorate as hepatic cells are destroyed. As the disease progresses, GI hemorrhage and kidney failure may also occur. Cirrhosis is usually the result of chronic alcohol abuse or severe hepatitis. The symptoms of cirrhosis are nausea, fatigue, and loss of appetite. ***Massage is contraindicated.***

Colitis

Colitis is an inflammation of the mucosa of the large intestine and rectum and is characterized by weight loss, intestinal ulcerations, diarrhea, and bleeding of the colon wall. The origins of colitis are not known, although it is thought to be an autoimmune disease. ***Position the client for comfort. Abdominal massage is contraindicated if pressure causes pain.***

Constipation

Constipation is infrequent or difficult passing of stools. Common causes of constipation are insufficient intake of fluid or dietary fiber, lack of physical activity, emotional disturbance, diverticulitis, pregnancy, and enema abuse. *If not caused by a contraindicated disease, then massage is okay. Position the client for comfort. Gliding strokes on the abdomen, moving clockwise, may be helpful.*

Crohn's Disease

A disease of unknown origin, Crohn's disease is a progressive inflammatory disease of the colon and/or ileum. Early symptoms are severe abdominal pain, diarrhea, fever, nausea, and loss of appetite. Typically, diseased colon segments are separated by normal colon segments. Crohn's disease is often confused with colitis. *Position the client for comfort. Avoid abdomen if pressure causes pain.*

Diarrhea

The frequent passing of unformed, loose, watery stools is called *diarrhea*. Factors that cause diarrhea are stress, poor diet, infection, medication side effects, or inflammation. The stool may also contain blood, pus, or mucus. Other symptoms are abdominal pain, cramping, and intestinal crepitus. Diarrhea may also lead to dehydration. *If not caused by a contraindicated disease, massage is okay. Avoid abdomen if pressure causes pain.*

Diverticulitis

Diverticula are pouchlike herniations of the colon wall where the muscle has become weak. Diverticulitis is an inflammation of one or more diverticula. This condition can lead to obstruction, perforations, and abscess formation. People with diverticulitis often have pain and/or a mass in the left lower quadrant and a change in bowel habits such as an increase or decrease in constipation or diarrhea or alteration between the two. *Massage is contraindicated if symptoms or pain is severe. Otherwise, position client for comfort, and avoid abdomen if pressure causes pain.*

Diverticulosis

Diverticulosis involves small mucosal herniations through the muscular wall anywhere in the colon but most typically in the sigmoid colon. Other colon changes include bleeding, abscesses, stenosis, and the presence of pericolonic fat. Fistulas may form between the colon and the small intestines. Even though people who have diverticulosis have no symptoms, 15% will develop diverticulitis (inflammation of the diverticula; see prior entry) and associated abdominal pain. *Massage considerations are the same as those as for diverticulitis.*

Gallstones

Gallstones result from the fusion of cholesterol crystals in bile. They gradually grow in size and number and may cause minimal to total obstruction of bile flow into the duodenum. *Massage considerations are the same as those for cholecystitis.*

Gastritis

Inflammation of the stomach's lining is called *gastritis*. It occurs in two forms: acute and chronic. Food poisoning, a virus, bacteria, or a chemical toxin may cause acute gastritis. Chronic gastritis is often the sign of an underlying illness, such as an ulcer. One of the main symptoms of gastritis is pain in the abdominal area. *Massage is contraindicated for acute gastritis. For chronic gastritis, massage is fine. Position the client for comfort. Abdominal massage is contraindicated if pressure causes pain.*

Gastroenteritis

Gastroenteritis is an inflammation of the lining of the stomach and intestines characterized by nausea, vomiting, diarrhea, abdominal pain, lack of appetite, and weakness. *If caused by infectious agent, then massage is contraindicated. If caused by other factors, then massage is fine. Position the client for comfort. Abdominal massage is contraindicated if pressure causes pain.*

Gastroesophageal Reflux Disease

If the lower cardioesophageal sphincter fails to close normally after food has entered the stomach, hydrochloric acid from the stomach can enter the inferior portion of the esophagus. The hydrochloric acid irritates the esophageal wall and causes a burning sensation. This condition is known as *gastroesophageal reflux disease*, also referred to as *heartburn* because the sensation is near the heart, not because of cardiac problems. *Massage is fine if symptoms are not severe. Ask client not to eat a large meal before massage. Position client for comfort, and avoid abdomen if pressure causes pain.*

Hepatitis

Hepatitis is an inflammation of the liver that can be caused by alcohol, drugs, toxins, or infection by the hepatitis virus, of which several viral types are known. Symptoms include muscle and joint pain, fatigue, loss of appetite, nausea, vomiting, diarrhea or constipation, abdominal discomfort, tea-colored urine, white stools, and jaundice. Severity ranges from mild and brief to chronic and life threatening. *Massage is contraindicated during acute phase. If client has chronic hepatitis, then obtain physician clearance. Once granted, avoid abdominal massage. Adjust massage to client's stamina and vitality.*

Hernia

A hernia is a protrusion of an organ or part of an organ through its surrounding connective tissue membranes or cavity wall. The four most common types of hernia are esophageal, hiatal, inguinal, and umbilical. From 75% to 80% of all hernias are inguinal hernias. *If client is in pain from the hernia, then medical attention is needed. If not, position client for comfort, and avoid herniated area. If client has a surgical mesh, then use light pressure over mesh site, especially for first 3 months following surgery. Deep pressure and myofascial release are contraindicated over mesh site.*

Irritable Bowel Syndrome

Also known as *spastic colon,* irritable bowel syndrome is a condition of the large intestine characterized by abnormal muscular contraction (i.e., peristalsis is not working properly) and excessive mucus in stools. It is generally associated with young adults under extreme emotional stress. Early symptoms are diarrhea, nausea, and cramping in the lower abdomen. *Massage is fine if symptoms are not severe. Position the client for comfort, avoiding abdomen if pressure causes pain.*

Obesity

Obesity is characterized by an abnormal increase in subcutaneous fat, primarily in visceral regions of the body. Generally, an individual is regarded as obese if his or her body weight is 30% above desired body weight for his or her age, height, frame size, and sex. Normal (nonathlete) body fat is 18% in men and 25% in women. *Position the client for comfort. Carefully apply pressure in areas containing large amounts of adipose tissue. If client is edematous because of inactivity, then elevate legs during treatment, and use lymphatic massage. If needed, use a sheet or an extra-large towel as a top drape. If needed, be prepared to massage client on the floor.*

Pancreatitis

An inflammation of the pancreas, pancreatitis is usually the result of trauma, alcohol abuse, infection, or certain medications that damage the pancreas. Symptoms may be severe abdominal pain that refers to the back, fever, lack of appetite, nausea, vomiting, and a decreased production of pancreatic enzymes. *Massage is contraindicated if in acute stage. Otherwise, obtain physician clearance. Once granted, massage is fine if symptoms are not severe. Position the client for comfort, avoiding abdomen if pressure causes pain.*

Peritonitis

Bacteria or irritating substances that gain access into the abdominal cavity produce peritonitis, an acute inflammation of the peritoneum. These substances are introduced into the cavity by a ruptured organ, a penetrating wound, perforation of the GI or urogenital tract (e.g., ectopic pregnancy), or a ruptured appendix. *Obtain physician clearance. Once granted, avoid the abdomen. Adjust massage to client's stamina and vitality (i.e., slow, gentle, short duration; assist client on and off table), or do not massage if client is debilitated.*

Pharyngitis

Inflammation or infection of the pharynx is called *pharyngitis* or sore throat. Causes range from viral and bacterial to irritation from nasal secretion. Strep throat, a type of pharyngitis, is caused by *Streptococcus* infection and is accompanied by fever, chills, and enlarged cervical lymph nodes. *If not caused by a contraindicated disease, massage is okay.*

Polyps

Polyps can be single or multiple growths on a mucous membrane, but they most commonly occur in the colon. Most polyps are benign, but their presence is a risk factor for the future development of colon cancer. No symptoms may be present, or rectal bleeding and abdominal pain may occur. *Abdominal massage is contraindicated if pressure causes pain. In the case of cancerous polyps, obtain physician clearance. Once granted, position client for comfort.*

Thrush

Caused by the fungi *Candida albicans,* thrush affects the oral mucosa. It is characterized by white plates of soft curd-like material that may be wiped off, leaving a raw bleeding surface. Thrush usually affects sick or weak infants, individuals in poor health or who are immunocompromised, and occasionally individuals who have been treated with antibiotics. *Massage may be contraindicated, depending on the cause. If not caused by disease, then massage is okay.*

Tonsillitis

Tonsillitis is inflammation of the tonsils, especially the palatine tonsils. Acute tonsillitis, frequently caused by *Streptococcus* infection, is characterized by severe sore throat, high fever, dull headache, difficulty in swallowing, earache, and enlarged lymph nodes in the neck. *Massage is contraindicated.*

Ulcerative Colitis

A type of chronic inflammatory bowel disease, ulcerative colitis is an inflammation of the mucosa of the large intestine and rectum. It is characterized by weight loss, intestinal ulcerations, diarrhea, and bleeding of the colon wall. The origins of ulcerative colitis are not known, although it is thought to be an autoimmune disease. *See entry under colitis.*

Ulcers

An ulcer is a lesion in a membrane. A peptic ulcer can develop in parts of the digestive tract exposed to acidic gastric juice. Ulcers that occur in the first part of the duodenum are called *duodenal ulcers*. Some occur in the stomach and are called *gastric ulcers*. Symptoms of ulcers are a nonradiating pain in the upper abdominal region, dark fecal stools, and bleeding that might lead to anemia. ***Position the client for comfort. Abdominal massage is contraindicated if pressure cause pain.***

TABLE TALK

The generally accepted belief asserts that ulcers are attributed to stress, but the cause of ulcers is an overproduction of gastric enzymes, which is actually a parasympathetic response. Stress does the opposite; it stimulates a sympathetic nervous system response and reduces gastric secretions, making the condition of ulcers seem counterintuitive.

Using monkeys as subjects, several experiments were conducted to study ulcers in 1971 and again in 1979. Situations were set up in which shocks were administered to monkeys at a predictive rate. One monkey, the executive monkey, was able to control whether or not the shock was administered by using a lever. Another monkey, the passive monkey, did not have the same control over the shock. If the executive monkey received a shock, both monkeys were shocked. Similarly, both monkeys were spared the shock if the executive monkey pressed the lever at the appropriate time.

Therefore which monkey got the ulcers? The executive monkey was full of ulcers, but the passive monkey had none. Although this experiment was not perfect, apparently ulcers may develop after periods of emotional strain, excessive responsibility, and worrying. Because gastric enzymes do not freely flow during periods of stress, ulcers seem to form during periods of rest or parasympathetic activity. The body is attempting to *catch up* after frequent and prolonged stress.

"In dwelling, live close to the ground. In thinking, keep it simple. In conflict, be fair and generous. In governing, don't control. In work, do what you enjoy. In family life, be completely present."
Tao Te Ching

Effects of Massage on the Digestive System

Promotes evacuation of the colon. By increasing peristaltic activity in the colon through massage, bowel contents move toward the anus for elimination.

Relieves constipation. Because evacuation of the colon is promoted, constipation is relieved.

Relieves colic and intestinal gas. Increased peristaltic activity also helps relieve colic and intestinal gas.

Stimulates digestion. Massage also promotes activation of the parasympathetic nervous system, which stimulates digestion.

Terms and Their Meanings Related to the Digestive System

TERM	MEANING
Amylase	*Gr.* starch; enzyme
Bolus	*Gr.* a lump
Brunner's glands	Brunner, Swiss anatomist (1653-1727)
Bucca	*L.* cheek
Cecum	*L.* blindness
Chyme	*Gr.* juice
Deglutition	*L.* to swallow
Duodenum	*L.* 12 fingers (refers to its length)
Enzyme	*Gr.* leaven
Fundus	*L.* base
Gingiva	*L.* gums
Gustatory	*L.* to taste
Haustra	*L.* to draw, drink
Hepato	*Gr.* liver
Ileum	*L.* twisted
Jejunum	*L.* empty
Kupffer's cells	Kupffer, German anatomist (1829-1902)
Lacteal	*L.* of milk
Mastication	*L.* to chew
Mesentery	*Gr.* middle; intestine
Omentum	*L.* a covering or apron
Peristaltic	*Gr.* around; contraction
Plicae circulares	*L.* a fold; a little ring
Pylorus	*Gr.* gatekeeper
Rectum	*L.* straight
Rugae	*L.* a crease or fold
Sacchar	*Gr.* sugar
Sigmoid	The Greek letter *sigma,* meaning S-shaped
Sphincter	*Gr.* a binder
Sphincter of Oddi	Oddi, Italian physician (1864-1913)
Taenia coli	Tape; colon
Tonsils	*L.* almond
Vermiform appendix	*L.* wormlike; hanger-on
Villi	*L.* tuft of hair

Gr., Greek; *L.*, Latin.

SUMMARY

The digestive system consists of a series of structures designed to break down food and liquids into usable body fuel by the processes of ingestion, digestion, absorption, and defecation. To carry out these processes, the digestive system uses a series of specialized, interrelated structures collectively known as the *alimentary canal.* These structures include the oral cavity, pharynx, esophagus, stomach, small intestines, and large intestines. The alimentary canal uses a set of accessory organs that aid in the digestive processes. These accessory organs include the liver, gallbladder, and pancreas. The six types of nutrients are proteins, carbohydrates, fats, vitamins, minerals, and water.

evolve

Go to *Chapter Extras* on Evolve for additional illustrations and resources for this chapter. *Extras* for this chapter include:

1. Crossword puzzle (downloadable form)
2. Drag and drop (online game)
3. Digestive system functions (illustration)
4. Peristaltic contractions (illustration)

MATCHING

Place the letter of the answer next to the term or phrase that best describes it.

A. Absorption	G. Esophagus	M. Peristalsis
B. Alimentary canal	H. Gallbladder	N. Plicae circulares
C. Bolus	I. Large intestine	O. Rugae
D. Deglutition	J. Liver	P. Sphincter
E. Digestion	K. Mastication	Q. Stomach
F. Duodenum	L. Pancreas	R. Vitamins

_____ 1. Synonymous with the word *chewing*

_____ 2. The muscular tube connecting the pharynx to the stomach

_____ 3. A muscular ring regulating movement of materials from one compartment of the GI tract to another

_____ 4. The process of moving digested products into the bloodstream and then into the body's cells

_____ 5. The last major section of intestine through which undigested and unabsorbed food travels before it is eliminated by the body

_____ 6. Synonymous with the word *swallowing*

_____ 7. Ball-like, masticated lump of food once swallowed

_____ 8. Organic compounds essential for normal physiological and metabolical functions

_____ 9. The process that occurs as food is mixed with digestive enzymes and converted into an absorbable state

_____ 10. J-shaped organ bound by the cardioesophageal and pyloric sphincters

_____ 11. Fingerlike projections that increase the small intestines' surface area; houses blood and lymph capillaries

_____ 12. The muscular passageway leading from mouth to anus

_____ 13. Rhythmic contractions that mix and propel materials in the GI tract

_____ 14. Stores bile manufactured by the liver

_____ 15. First section of the small intestines

_____ 16. Digestive gland secreting enzymes that break down all categories of digestible foods, including proteins, carbohydrates, and fats

_____ 17. Largest internal organ in the body; carries out more than 500 functions

_____ 18. Longitudinal folds in the stomach's lining that allow expansion

INTERNET ACTIVITIES

Visit http://www.aca-usa.org/faq.htm. Contrast and compare the positive and negative reasons people drink alcoholic beverages.

Visit http://www.gastro.org and click on Patient Center and then on Your Digestive System—At the Core of Good Health. After reading, take the AGA's Core Score Quiz and see how you fare.

Visit the United States Department of Agriculture's website at http://www.mypyramid.gov and click on Tour My Pyramid (animated feature). How has the pyramid changed since it was first introduced in the 1960s?

Bibliography

Abrahams P, Marks S, Hutchings R: *McMinn's color atlas of human anatomy,* St Louis, 2003, Mosby.

Applegate EJ: *The anatomy and physiology learning system,* ed 3, Philadelphia, 2006, Saunders.

Beers MH, Berkow R: *The Merck manual of diagnosis and therapy,* Whitehouse Station, NJ, 2006, Merck Research Laboratories.

Como D, editor: *Mosby's medical, nursing, and allied health dictionary,* ed 6, St Louis, 2002, Mosby.

Crawley J, Van De Graaff KM: *A photographic atlas for anatomy and physiology,* Englewood, Colo, 2002, Morton.

Crooks R, Stein J: *Psychology: science, behavior, and life,* New York, 1990, Harcourt College Publishers.

Damjanov I: *Pathophysiology for the health-related professions,* ed 3, Philadelphia, 2006, Saunders.

Ferri FF: *2003 Ferri's clinical advisor, instant diagnosis and treatment,* St Louis, 2003, Mosby.

Frazier MS, Drzymkowski JW: *Essentials of human diseases and conditions,* ed 3, Philadelphia, 2004, Saunders.

Goldberg S: *Clinical anatomy made ridiculously simple,* Miami, 1984, Medmaster.

Gould BE: *Pathophysiology for the health professions,* ed 3, Philadelphia, 2006, Saunders.

Haubrich WS: *Medical meanings: a glossary of word origins,* New York, 1984, Harcourt Brace Jovanovich.

Huether SE, McCance KL: *Understanding pathophysiology,* ed 3, St Louis, 2004, Mosby.

Jacob S, Francone C: *Elements of anatomy and physiology,* Philadelphia, 1989, Saunders.

Kalat JW: *Biological psychology,* ed 8, Belmont, Calif, 2003, Wadsworth.

Kapit W, Elson LM: *The anatomy coloring book,* ed 3, New York, 2002, Benjamin Cummings.

Kordish M, Dickson S: *Introduction to basic human anatomy,* Lake Charles, La, 1995, McNeese State University.

Kumar V, Abbas A, Fausto N: *Robbins and Cotran physiologic basis of disease,* ed 7, St Louis, 2005, Mosby.

Marieb EN: *Essentials of human anatomy and physiology,* ed 8, New York, 2005, Benjamin Cummings.

Martini FH, Bartholomew EF: *Essentials of anatomy and physiology,* ed 3, New York, 2003, Benjamin Cummings.

McAleer N: *The body almanac,* Garden City, NY, 1985, Doubleday.

McCance K, Huether S: *Pathophysiology: the biological basis for disease in adults and children,* St Louis, 2006, Mosby.

Merck manual, ed 17, Whitehouse Station, NJ, 1998, Merck and Company.

Moore KL: *Clinically oriented anatomy,* ed 5, Baltimore, 2005, Lippincott Williams & Wilkins.

Newton D: *Pathology for massage therapists,* ed 2, Portland, Ore, 1995, Simran.

Premkumar K: *Pathology A to Z, a handbook for massage therapists,* Baltimore, 1999, Lippincott Williams & Wilkins.

Salvo SG, Anderson SK: *Mosby's pathology for massage therapists,* St Louis, 2004, Elsevier Mosby.

Solomon EP, Phillips GA: *Understanding human anatomy and physiology,* Philadelphia, 1987, Saunders.

Thibodeau G, Patton K: *Anatomy and physiology,* ed 6, St Louis, 2006, Mosby.

Thibodeau G, Patton K: *Structure and function of the body,* ed 12, St Louis, 2004, Mosby.

Tortora GJ: *Introduction to the human body: the essentials of anatomy and physiology,* ed 5, Hoboken, NJ, 2000, John Wiley & Sons.

Tortora GJ, Grabowksi SR: *Principles of anatomy and physiology,* ed 11, New York, 2005, John Wiley & Sons.

Venes D, Thomas CL, Taber CW: *Taber's cyclopedic medical dictionary,* ed 20, Philadelphia, 2005, FA Davis.

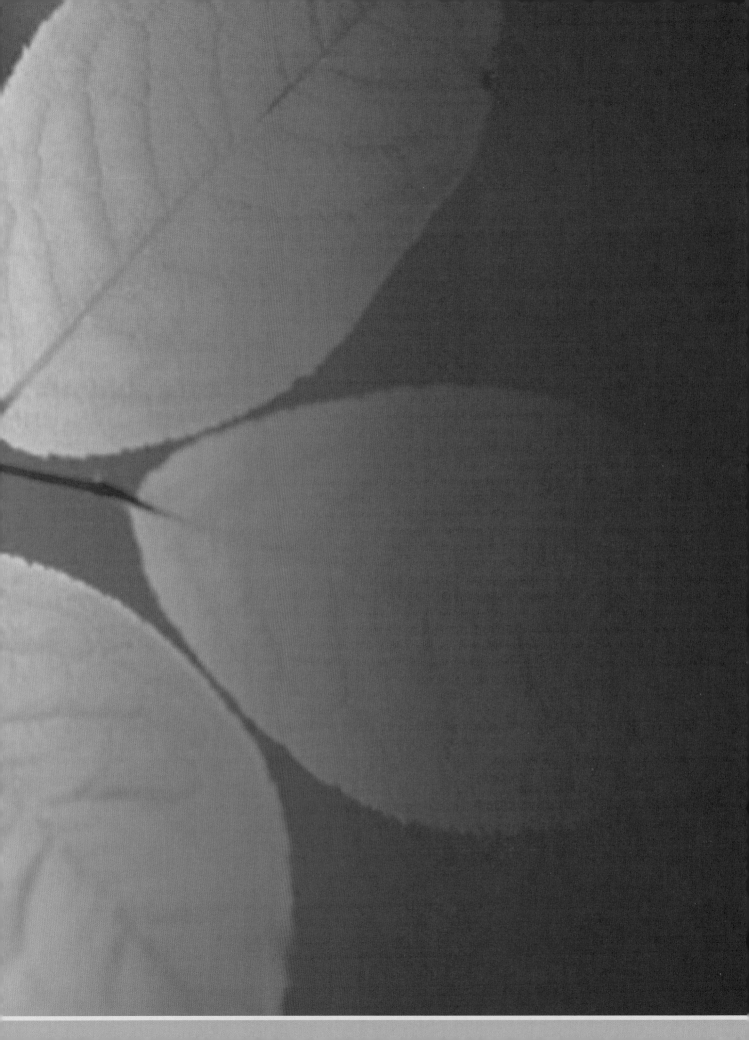

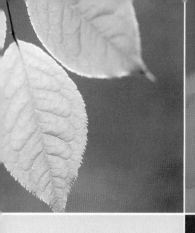

CHAPTER 22

Urinary System

STUDENT OBJECTIVES

After completing this chapter, the student should be able to:

- List anatomical structures of the urinary system
- Describe the physiological mechanisms of the urinary system
- Name parts of the kidney
- Define the kidney's nephron
- Trace the path of fluids that flow in the nephron
- Name and describe parts of a nephron
- Discuss the importance of the juxtaglomerular apparatus
- Identify blood vessels and blood flow through the kidneys
- Explain the processes of filtration, reabsorption, and tubular secretion
- Describe urine formation
- List the urinary system's accessory organs, describing their function
- Explain what urine is and how the body disposes of it
- Identify and discuss how hormones aid in regulating the body's water balance
- Name types of pathological conditions of the urinary system, giving characteristics and massage considerations of each

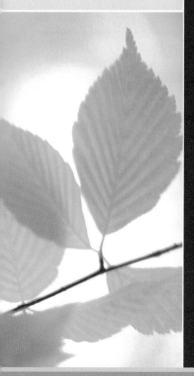

INTRODUCTION

The human body is a complex machine, and as such, it does not perform properly if residues from fuel combustion and other processes are not removed. The cells of the body machine metabolize nutrients, which produce wastes. The breakdown of proteins produces the nitrogen wastes such as ammonia and urea, which are toxic to the system. Sodium chloride, sodium sulfate, phosphate, hydrogen molecules, ions, and other substances also accumulate as a result of metabolical activities. All of these waste materials must be excreted from the body for homeostasis to be maintained and for metabolism to function optimally.

Excretion of waste products is such a large task that no single body system can handle it alone. Several systems contribute to waste elimination.
- **Respiratory.** Waste elimination is done through expiration.
- **Integumentary.** Sweating is a method of eliminating wastes.
- **Digestive.** Solid wastes are eliminated through excretion.
- **Urinary.** Wastes are excreted through urination.

The urinary system consists of two kidneys, two ureters, one urinary bladder, and one urethra. The kidneys are the primary organs of the urinary system. The other parts are mostly passageways and storage areas. The kidneys perform an important function: filtering wastes out of the blood. They also play a significant role in maintaining blood pressure.

ANATOMY

Areas of discussion in this chapter include
- Kidneys
- Ureters
- Urethra
- Urinary bladder
- Urine

PHYSIOLOGY

The six functions of the urinary system are as follows:
1. **Eliminates wastes and foreign substances as urine.** Metabolic wastes include ammonia and urea from protein in metabolism, creatinine from muscle metabolism, and uric acid from metabolism. Foreign substances include drugs and environmental toxins.
2. **Regulates blood's chemical composition.** The kidneys possess specialized cells that monitor the acid-base balance of the blood. Metabolic wastes are laundered from the blood, and substances such as glucose, sodium, vitamins, and minerals are reabsorbed into the blood to adjust its chemical composition. Hydrogen ions are secreted from the blood into the urine as needed to maintain the blood's pH balance.
3. **Regulates blood pH.** Mechanisms in the kidney assist with the regulation of blood pH by eliminating acids and conserving buffers.
4. **Regulates blood volume and fluid balance.** The kidneys adjust blood volume by conserving or eliminating water in the urine. In this way, both the blood volume and the body's water balance are altered. If fluid levels are not regulated, then excess fluids collect in the tissues, producing edema of the hands, feet, face, heart, and other body areas.
5. **Regulates blood pressure.** The kidneys continuously monitor blood pressure and help maintain a normal range by secreting an enzyme that stimulates vasoconstriction. Blood pressure is also kept in balance by the regulation of blood volume. Blood pressure is maintained by interaction of the circulatory, endocrine, and nervous systems.
6. **Maintains homeostasis.** With the removal of metabolic wastes, the body maintains homeostasis by regulating the chemical composition of the blood, by regulating blood volume, and by maintaining fluid balance and blood pressure. Because of these many functions, *the kidneys are the major homeostatic organs of the body*. The cells and tissues of the body are constantly making wastes as byproducts of cellular metabolism. These wastes need to be removed quickly because, if they were to build up, then cell, tissue, and even organ death can occur. In fact, malfunction of the kidneys causes dangerous changes in blood composition, which often lead to death.

KIDNEYS

The **kidneys** are the principal organs of the urinary system, which both processes blood and forms urine to be excreted. These structures are reddish paired organs located bilaterally in the upper lumbar region of the spine (Figure 22-1). They are lima bean–shaped organs (convex laterally and concave medially) and are approximately the size of a bar of bath soap. The kidneys are located behind the abdominal peritoneum

Terms and Their Meanings Related to the Urinary System

TERM	MEANING
Antidiuretic	*Gr.* against or opposed; urine flow
Bowman's capsule	Bowman, English physician (1816-1892)
Calyx	*Gr.* cup
Diuretic	*Gr.* urine flow
Glomerulus	*L.* little ball
Hilum	*L.* a trifle
Juxtapose	*L.* close by, adjacent, side by side
Loop of Henle	Henle, German anatomist (1809-1885)
Macula densa	*L.* spot; thick
Nephro, nephra	*Gr.* kidney
Peritubular	*Gr.* around, about; as a tube
Renal	*L.* kidney
Retroperitoneal	*L.* backward; the peritoneum
Trigone	*Gr.* three-cornered figure

Gr., Greek; *L.*, Latin.

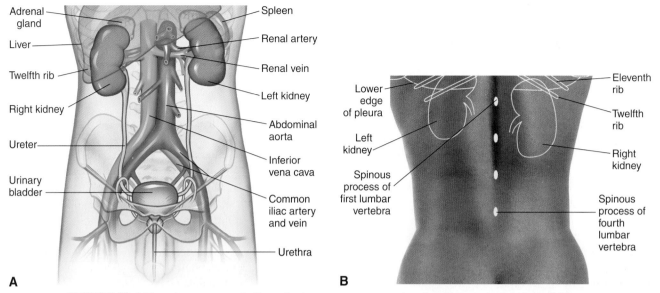

FIGURE 22-1 The urinary system. **A**, General urinary structures; anterior view. **B**, Posterior location of kidneys.

(retroperitoneal) and are surrounded by a fibrous *renal capsule* and are imbedded in adipose tissue called *perirenal fat;* this fat serves as a barrier against trauma and the spread of infection. Because of the presence of the liver, the kidney on the right side of the body is slightly lower than the one on the left. Each kidney is a separate, functioning organ. If one kidney is removed, the other will then increase its filtering capacity so that it will filter at 80% of two normal kidneys.

TABLE TALK

Because the kidneys do not have the extra protection of the abdominal peritoneal lining or the ribcage, massage tapotement (percussion) is contraindicated over the kidney area in the dorsum of the body. Drawing the kidneys on a fellow student with a washable, nontoxic marker may be helpful to identify the location of these structures.

The **hilum** is the indentation located in the medially concave region of the kidney; here is where the renal arteries, renal veins, and the ureters enter and exit.

Each kidney is divided into two major regions: (1) the *cortex* (outer region) and (2) the *medulla* (inner region) (Figure 22-2).

Nephron

The kidneys are composed of filtering units called **nephrons.** Approximately 1.25 million nephrons are found in each kidney. Approximately 85% of all nephrons are located almost entirely in the renal cortex. The remainder lies in the renal medulla. The nephron has three main parts: (1) the glomerulus; (2) the Bowman's capsule; and (3) the renal tubule, which is further divided into the proximal and distal tubule and the loop of Henle (Figure 22-3).

Glomerulus

The glomerulus is formed by the afferent arterioles, which then branch into a tuftlike network of fine capillaries within Bowman's capsules. Between the wall of the glomerulus and the Bowman's capsule is a filtration membrane. This membrane contains pores that allow only certain substances to be filtered out of the blood, such as water, wastes, ions, amino acids, and glucose. Blood cells and large proteins are too large to fit through the filtration membrane. Blood pressure is the force responsible for filtration.

Bowman's Capsule

The hollow cup-shaped mouth of a nephron is called the Bowman's capsule. The filtrate is collected in the *Bowman's capsule* for transport through the nephron. The Bowman's capsule and the glomerulus are often referred to as the *renal corpuscle.*

Renal Tubule

The renal tubule is divided into the proximal and distal tubule and the loop of Henle.

Proximal convoluted tubule: The proximal convoluted tubule is the first part of the renal tubule and is proximal, or nearest to, the Bowman's capsule.

Loop of Henle: Just past the proximal convoluted tubule is the loop of Henle, which consists of a descending limb, a hairpin turn, and an ascending limb. The loop of Henle extends deep into the medulla.

Distal convoluted tubule: The distal convoluted tubule is the portion just beyond, or distal to, the loop of Henle. An important structure, the juxtaglomerular apparatus, is found at the point where the afferent arteriole touches part of the distal convoluted tubule (discussed next section).

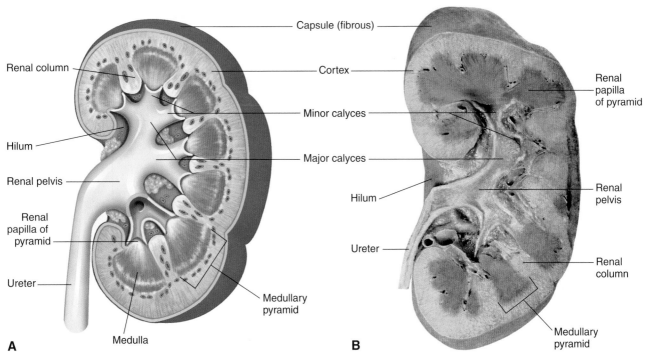

FIGURE 22-2 Cross-section of a kidney. **A**, Illustrated view. **B**, Photographic view.

Numerous collecting tubules that organize themselves into a dozen or so distant triangular wedges make up much of the medullary tissue, called **medullary pyramids.** The narrow base of the pyramid, or *renal papilla,* faces toward the hilum. Cortical tissue dips into the medulla between the pyramids and form areas known as *renal columns*.

Bowman's capsules and both convoluted tubules lie in the cortex. Loops of Henle and collecting ducts extend into the medulla.

Juxtaglomerular Apparatus

Given that blood pressure is the force behind filtration, the kidneys are equipped with cells that measure blood pressure; the **juxtaglomerular apparatus** (Figure 22-4). Recall that this structure is located where the afferent arteriole touches the distal convoluted tubule. Within the juxtaglomerular apparatus are two important structures: (1) the juxtaglomerular cells and (2) the macula densa.

Juxtaglomerular Cells
The juxtaglomerular cells are located in the afferent arteriole. These cells contain renin granules that act as mechanoreceptors. This structure assists in maintaining blood pressure by secreting **renin** when blood pressure drops. Renin converts angiotensinogen from the liver into angiotensin I. Angiotensin I, when transported through the lungs, becomes angiotensin II. Angiotensin II causes the secretion of aldosterone, which increases sodium and water reabsorption. This action increases blood volume and blood pressure. This pathway is called the *renin-angiotensin-aldosterone system*.

evolve The renin-angiotensin-aldosterone system is essential to understand because many medications used to treat high blood pressure act on this system as inhibitors. Log on to the Evolve website to see a schematic drawing of this mechanism. ∎

Macula Densa
The macula densa is located in the ascending limb of Henle's loop and contains dense, tightly packed cells that are chemoreceptors, sensing the concentration of the filtrate as it passing through the tubule. The cells of the macula densa respond to a decrease in sodium by releasing prostaglandins (hormonelike substances), which stimulate the secretion of renin. You already know how renin affects blood pressure.

In review, the juxtaglomerular cells monitor changes in blood pressure in the afferent arteriole, and the macula densa monitors the concentration of the filtrate in the renal tubule. Both respond by secreting renin.

Collecting Duct

The collecting duct is made up of the distal tubules of several nephrons. Collecting ducts join larger ducts and become the renal papilla, the apex of each medullary pyramid. Each renal papilla protrudes into a small, cuplike structure called a **calyx.** The calyces are considered the beginning of the plumbing system because here is where urine leaves the renal papilla and is collected for transport out of the body. Several minor calyces join to form a major calyx. These structures combine together to form a large collection reservoir called the **renal pelvis,** which is the upper region of the ureter.

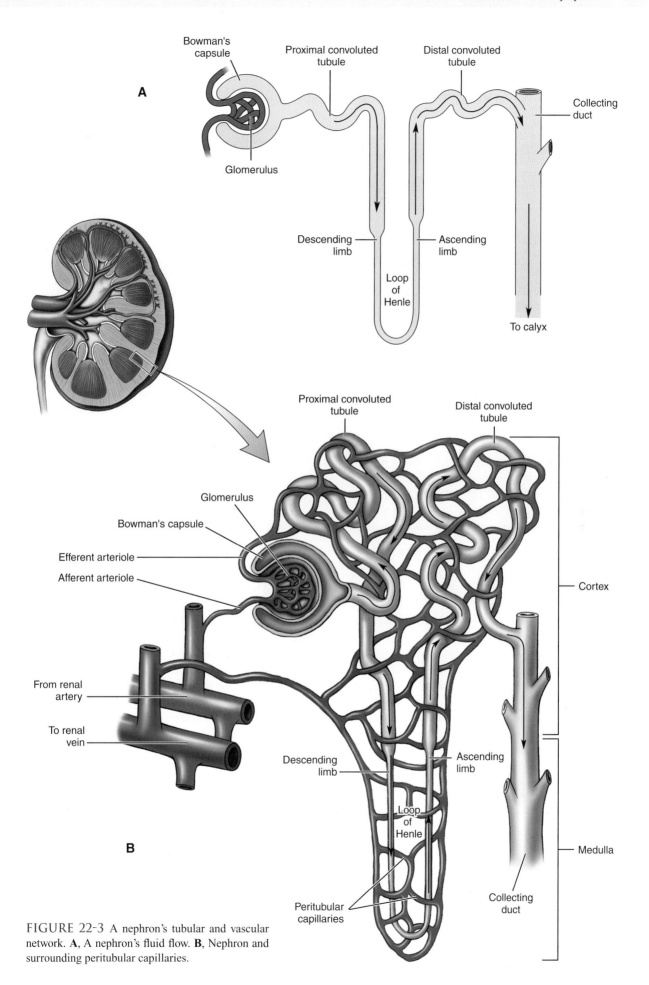

FIGURE 22-3 A nephron's tubular and vascular network. **A**, A nephron's fluid flow. **B**, Nephron and surrounding peritubular capillaries.

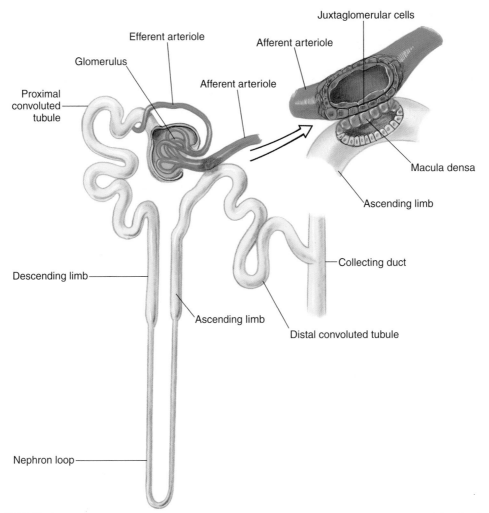

FIGURE 22-4 Juxtaglomerular apparatus: the positional relationship of the afferent arteriole and the distal tubule.

The following diagram represents how fluids flow in nephron.

Bowman's capsule
↓
Proximal convoluted tubule
↓
Loop of Henle
↓
Distal convoluted tubule
↓
Collecting duct
↓
Renal papilla
↓
Minor calyx
↓
Major calyx
↓
Renal pelvis
↓
Ureter

Blood Vessels and Blood Flow in the Kidneys

Oxygen-rich blood enters the kidneys by the renal artery, where it branches off the abdominal aorta. As the renal artery enters the hilum, the artery becomes smaller, turning into the afferent arteriole. The afferent arteriole is a high-pressure vessel that feeds the glomerular capillaries. As stated earlier, the afferent arteriole branches into a tuftlike network of fine capillaries within the Bowman's capsule called the *glomerulus*.

> ### TABLE TALK
>
> The entire blood supply of the body passes through the kidneys every 3 minutes. At rest, a fifth to a fourth of the body's blood can be found in the kidneys. In fact, the body's entire blood volume is filtered 65 times in a 24-hour period.

At this juncture, blood leaves the glomerular capillaries and flows into efferent arterioles (not venules). Blood from the efferent arterioles moves into the peritubular capillaries.

This placement of an arteriole between two capillary beds (glomerular capillaries and peritubular capillaries) is unique and found only in the kidney. The peritubular capillaries surround the renal tubule; this location is where most water reabsorption occurs. The blood peritubular capillaries join the venous system first through the renal venules. The venous structures grow larger, becoming the renal vein, and then flows directly to the inferior vena cava (see Figure 22-3, *B*). To review, the sequence of blood in the kidneys is as follows:

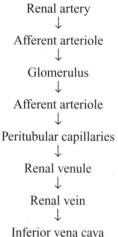

Renal artery
↓
Afferent arteriole
↓
Glomerulus
↓
Afferent arteriole
↓
Peritubular capillaries
↓
Renal venule
↓
Renal vein
↓
Inferior vena cava

Filtration Process

The kidney does not selectively filter out only harmful or excess material. In a sense, it filters out many wanted and unwanted materials in blood plasma. Some important molecules that are filtered are then reabsorbed by the nephron before the filtrate reaches the end of the tubule and becomes urine. This process includes three important and distinct steps for filtration and formation of urine.

Filtration
In the first step of the filtration process, blood enters the renal corpuscle via the glomeruli. Water and other substances from the blood plasma in the glomerulus cross over into the Bowman's capsule. The bloodstream retains proteins and formed elements of the blood that are too large to cross the membrane. Toxins, excess free ions, and nonessential substances such as urea, uric acid, ammonia, drug residue, excess minerals, and water-soluble vitamins (especially B vitamins) are collected and eventually leave the body in the urine. This process explains why your urine turns bright yellow when you take these supplements. The filtration process is so efficient that approximately 45 gallons (180 liters) of filtrate are produced in a 24-hour day. Not all of this water is excreted as urine. Most of it is reabsorbed back into the blood.

Reabsorption
Approximately 99% of the fluids removed from blood plasma are reabsorbed. This process occurs when water and useful substances are reabsorbed from all parts of the renal tubule into peritubular blood. The majority of the body's water, along with much-needed substances such as glucose and amino acids, is retained and returned to the blood through the process of reabsorption.

Tubular Secretion
Tubular secretion means the movement of substances out of the blood and into tubular fluid (called *filtrate*). As you may recall, in the reabsorption phase, water and necessary nutrients are recovered by crossing back from the renal tubules to the bloodstream. In the final phase of the filtration process, wastes are moved in the opposite direction; they are transported from the peritubular capillaries into the renal tubules for excretion.

Tubular secretions rid the body of toxic elements and control blood pH. These toxins may include organic compounds and ions. Toxic organic compounds may occur naturally within the body, or they may be residue from drugs introduced into the body, such as penicillin. Ion levels must be regulated to maintain various bodily functions. The secretion of hydrogen ions is a major factor in the regulation of blood pH. Potassium ion secretion prevents a buildup of ions that would affect heart rhythm.

Let us review the filtration process.
- **Filtration:** Blood plasma enters and is filtered into the renal corpuscle.
- **Reabsorption:** Water, nutrients, ions, and useful substances are reabsorbed into peritubular capillary system from renal tubules.
- **Tubular secretions:** Unwanted elements are discharged back into the tubules to produce urine.

> **evolve** *As simplistic as this system may seem, the filtration process is one of the hardest concepts to teach because it is just short of a miracle. Posted on the Evolve website under course materials for Chapter 22 are illustrated steps of the filtration process. Log on to your student account to view it and other important materials.* ∎

Urine Formation in the Kidneys

Urine production begins in the cortex when blood enters and is filtered in the renal corpuscle (glomerulus and Bowman's capsule). Next, the filtered fluids, known as **filtrate,** enter the first section of the renal tubule, called the *proximal convoluted tubule.*

The proximal convoluted tubule feeds into the loop of Henle, with its sharp turn and descending and ascending limbs. From here, the filtrate flows into the distal convoluted tubule and then into collecting tubules located in the medulla. You might say that the *cortex is the urine-manufacturing facility,* and the *medulla is the urine-collecting facility.*

These collecting tubules route the filtrate into large papillary ducts. When the concentrated filtrate of the kidney reaches the calyces, it is then called *urine.*

Encourage your clients to drink a lot of water (0.5 oz of water per 1 lb of body weight). Without an adequate water intake, kidneys cannot adequately do their job. Increasing water intake often helps kidneys balance electrolytes, which may reduce muscle cramping. Increasing water intake is also good advice for therapists.

After urine is formed in the nephrons, it travels toward the hollow center of each kidney. Urine is drained by peristaltic activity from the major and minor calyces and from the renal pelvis in the kidney down the ureter to the urinary bladder.

URETERS

The **ureters** are two slender hollow tubes approximately 10 inches long that transport urine formed by the kidneys. Similar to the kidneys, the ureters are located bilaterally; each kidney has one ureter. Leaving the kidney at the renal pelvis, the ureters course medially into the pelvis until they reach the lateral angle of the urinary bladder.

Each ureter contains a specialized valve at its distal end, which prevents urine backflow as the bladder contracts and empties. When the bladder is empty, the ureters are spaced ap-

proximately 2 cm apart. However, when the bladder expands, the ureters move approximately 5 cm apart.

URINARY BLADDER

Located in the pelvis behind the pubic symphysis, the muscular **urinary bladder** provides a temporary storage reservoir for urine. In women, it sits on the anterior vagina and in front of the uterus, whereas in men, it rests on the prostate. The floor of the bladder has three openings—two from the ureters and one into the urethra (discussed next). The ureter openings line at the posterior corners of the triangular floor, or *trigone* (Figure 22-5).

The urinary bladder is often filled with and emptied of urine. To allow for expansion, it is lined with mucous transitional epithelium that forms folds called *rugae*. Tissue expansion puts pressure on pressure-sensitive receptors located in the muscular wall, which causes the internal urethral orifice to relax and results in the conscious desire to

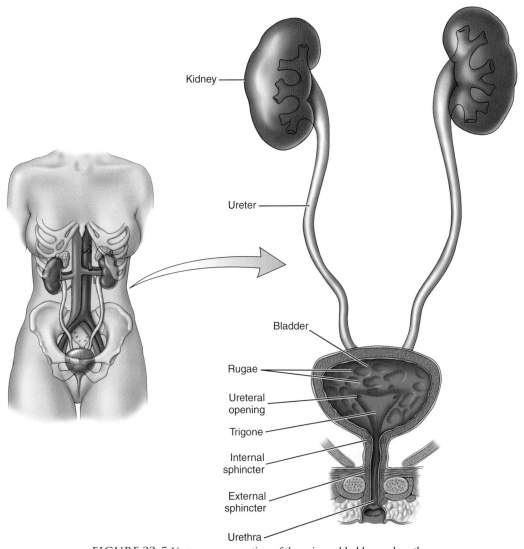

FIGURE 22-5 Ureters, cross section of the urinary bladder, and urethra.

void (urinate). On demand, the cerebral cortex of the brain sends impulses to the external urethral orifice muscle to relax, and urination takes place. The bladder can hold 700 to 800 ml. At 300 ml, the bladder is distended enough that the conscious sensation of needing to urinate arises.

URETHRA

The **urethra** is a small tubular structure that transports urine from the urinary bladder out of the body during *micturition* (urination). The internal sphincter muscle closes the proximal end of the urethra, whereas the external sphincter muscles are located in the wall of the urogenital diaphragm. The internal urethral sphincter contains visceral muscle, and the external urethral sphincter contains skeletal muscle and is typically under voluntary control after the age of 15 months.

The length of the urethra differs in men and women. In women, the path of the urethra is located anterior to the vagina and exits between the vaginal opening and clitoris. The female urethra is relatively short (approximately 1.5 inches). This feature and the fact that the female urinary orifice is close to the anal opening may account for the much higher incidence of bladder infections in women.

The male urethra extends from the center of the prostate and joins the ejaculatory duct and passes through the length of the penis (approximately 8 inches, depending on penile length). Because the male urethra unites with the ejaculatory ducts, it also serves as a pathway for semen as it is ejaculated out of the body through the penis.

TABLE TALK

If water loss exceeds 5% to 10% of total body weight, serious dehydration results. A 20% loss of water is often fatal. Common causes of water loss are infection, fever, severe burns, and diarrhea.

URINE

Urine is concentrated filtrate from the kidneys that is 96% water and 4% dissolved wastes (e.g., urea, creatinine, uric acid, sodium chloride, potassium, sulfates, phosphates, and drug residue). Urine tends to be slightly acidic and has a normal amber color. The more concentrated the urine is, the darker its color will be. Abnormal constituents in urine may include albumin, glucose, red blood cells (uremia), white blood cells, bilirubin, kidney stones, and bacteria.

Micturition, the mechanism for voiding urine, begins with a voluntary relaxation of the external sphincter muscle of the bladder. Parasympathetic fibers transmit the impulses that cause contractions of the bladder and relaxation of the internal sphincter.

The average adult produces 1 to 2 quarts (1000 to 2000 mL) of urine per day. Chemical, nervous, and even physical factors can affect the amount of urine produced and excreted by the body. An example of a chemical factor is the consumption of coffee, tea, and many carbonated beverages. Stimulating the production of urine, these drinks have a diuretic effect on the urinary system. A **diuretic,** or substance promoting the formation and excretion of urine, can increase urine production by increasing the amount of blood fluid crossing the glomerulus, or it can decrease the amount of water reabsorbed from the renal tubule; both processes increase urine production. Anxiety often suppresses the body's urge to void. During periods of physical activity, the heart beats rapidly, moving the blood through the kidney at a fast rate and increasing urine production.

CONTROLLING THE WATER BALANCE OF THE BODY

The bloodstream is responsible for water transfer to and from all the cells of the body and for oxygen and nutrient exchange. The key to the water balance of the entire body is regulating the fluid balance of the blood. The secretion of *antidiuretic hormone* (ADH) regulates the control of water balance of the body. If the bloodstream becomes concentrated as a result of the loss of water through sweat or urination, then the posterior pituitary gland releases ADH, which stimulates the kidneys to reabsorb more water. If the blood is too dilute, the pituitary reduces the production of ADH, and the kidneys begin to produce more urine. Along with the water, important substances such as glucose are reabsorbed into the bloodstream. *Aldosterone,* produced in the adrenal cortex, works in concert with ADH to maintain homeostasis of bodily fluids.

Additionally, specialized cells located in the atrial walls of the heart produce a hormone, *atrial natriuretic hormone* (ANH). This hormone decreases sodium by triggering urine production, or **diureses,** which additionally decreases blood volume and blood pressure. In this regard, ANH is an antagonist to the ADH and aldosterone.

PATHOLOGICAL CONDITIONS OF THE URINARY SYSTEM

Cystitis

Also known as a *bladder infection,* cystitis is an inflammation of the urinary bladder or ureters or both. It occurs more often in women than in men. This condition is often caused by a bacterial infection from neighboring organs such as the kidney or urethra. Cystitis is often characterized by pain, blood in the urine, and by urgency and frequency of urination. ***Position client for comfort, and avoid abdomen if pressure causes pain***.

Glomerulonephritis

Also known as *Bright's disease,* glomerulonephritis is an inflammation of the glomeruli. This disease often follows other infections and is characterized by blood in the urine, edema, and hypertension. ***Obtain physician clearance. Once***

JAN SCHWARTZ

Born: May 12, 1947

"Be the change you want to see in the world"

Jan Schwartz fell into a career in massage therapy, but that has not kept her from making her mark in the industry. Today, Schwartz is widely recognized for her efforts to advance educational standards for massage therapists.

Schwartz was born in Pennsylvania in 1947. She attended Rutgers University and graduated with a bachelor's degree in economics. After a long career with Dale Carnegie, Schwartz was ready for what she called "the proverbial get out of corporate life."

Schwartz moved to Tucson, Arizona, in 1992 with her partner. "As we drove up Sixth Avenue, I saw Desert Institute of the Healing Arts and we stopped. I went in and found out they were a school of massage therapy and I thought, oh, I could do that for a year," recalls Schwartz.

What started out as 1 year turned to 14 with the Desert Institute. After completing her training, Schwartz stayed on as the admissions director for 2 years and spent 12 years as the school's educational director.

While with the Desert Institute, Schwartz also spent time in the classroom, teaching injury management and rehabilitation classes. An avid runner and cyclist, Schwartz dealt with the common aches and pains that come with dedicated athleticism for her entire life. Schwartz has completed the 100-mile Tour de Tucson quite a few times and competed in the Kona half marathon. A bad hamstring injury from cycling that plagued her for 6 years gave Schwartz intimate knowledge from which to teach.

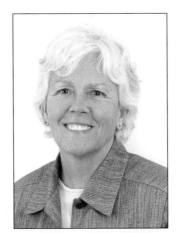

"I love teaching, I like being able to transfer knowledge to other people. I like the excitement when people start to get it," Schwartz said.

Today, Schwartz works with the Cortiva Institute, an education company that currently boasts nine massage therapy schools in 11 different locations around the country. Schwartz took the job with Cortiva to help shape the future of massage therapy and is currently doing just that. She has already co-developed, from the ground up, an 884-hour curriculum and is constantly looking for ways to improve the educational standards and teaching practices for massage therapists.

Schwartz says, "one of the shortcomings of vocational education in this country is that there's the mistaken idea that if you can do something well you can teach something well and the profession of teacher requires a certain skill set that isn't conveyed when you learn massage therapy," said Schwartz.

However, Schwartz's work has not gone unnoticed. The American Massage Therapy Association recognized her for outstanding leadership and distinguished service in 2002 and 2005.

Schwartz hopes to continue her work with Cortiva to improve educational standards and teaching practices for massage therapists. She says, "I love my job, I love the traveling and going to different schools and helping schools to problem solve in the areas of education and faculty development."

granted, use light pressure and massage of only short duration. Do not use lymphatic massage to reduce edema.

Gout

Gout is a condition characterized by high levels of uric acid in the blood as a result of high production or an inability of the kidneys to excrete this substance. The uric acid is converted to sodium urate crystals, which are often deposited in joints, kidneys, and other tissues. Gout is more common in men than in women. The great toe is a common site for the accumulation of sodium urate crystals, causing painful swelling. When gout settles in the joints, it is

called *gouty arthritis*. *Local contraindication of affected area during acute phase; this precaution includes joint mobilizations.*

Kidney Stones

Kidney stones are crystals in the urine, such as uric acid or calcium salts. Causes of kidney stones include an excessive calcium intake, a low water intake, or abnormally alkaline or acidic urine. *Obtain physician clearance if client is taking medication for treatment of kidney stones. Once granted, massage only if symptoms are not severe. Position client for comfort.*

Urinary Incontinence

The inability to control urination is referred to as *urinary incontinence*. This condition may be the result of an infection or damage to the central or peripheral nervous system or injury to the urinary sphincter or perineal structures, which can occur during childbirth. Urinary incontinence is often precipitated by laughing, coughing and sneezing, late stages of pregnancy, or straining while lifting heavy objects. ***Abdominal massage is contraindicated if client is uncomfortable.***

Urinary Tract Infection

Urinary tract infection (UTI) is an infection of one or more structures of the urinary system. Most UTIs are caused by bacteria and are more common in women than in men because women have a short urethra that is located near the anus. Bacteria from feces can be transported to the urethra as a result of improper toilet habits (i.e., wiping from back to front rather than from front to back). The most common symptoms of UTIs are increased urination, burning and pain during urination, and, if the infection is severe, blood and pus in the urine. ***Abdominal massage is contraindicated if pressure causes pain or if symptoms are severe.***

Effects of Massage on the Urinary System

Increases urine output. Massage activates dormant capillary beds and recovers lymphatic fluids for filtration by the kidney, which, in turn, increases the frequency of urination and amount of urine produced. Massage is also relaxing, which promotes general homeostasis, thereby increasing urine output.

Promotes the excretion of nitrogen, inorganic phosphorus, and sodium chloride in urine. Levels of these metabolic wastes are elevated in urine after massage.

SUMMARY

The urinary system maintains homeostasis in the body by accomplishing several functions. This system eliminates metabolic waste; regulates the pH and chemical composition of the blood; and regulates blood volume, fluid volume, and blood pressure. This small system accomplishes these varied functions with only two primary organs and their accessory organs: a pair of kidneys, a pair of ureters, a urinary bladder, and a urethra.

The kidney is a highly complex lima bean–shaped organ located bilaterally in the upper lumbar area. Kidneys have two main divisions—the cortex and the medulla—that are covered with a tough renal capsule. The hilum is the point where the artery and vein connect to permit blood circulation through the kidney and is the origin of the ureters. The cortex carries out the process of urine manufacture, and the medulla houses the urine-collecting apparatus. The chief structural and functional unit of the kidney is the nephron, which is responsible for the filtration process. This task is accomplished by two interlaced networks of vessels—one carrying blood and the other carrying urine. The blood is carried through some specialized vessels known as *glomeruli* and *peritubular capillaries.* In the renal corpuscle, the liquid portion of the plasma filters across into the renal tubules, which are urine-transport structures. Excess water and certain needed elements are reabsorbed from the renal tubules back into the bloodstream in the peritubular capillaries. The product remaining in the renal tubule is known as *filtrate.* Other toxins are secreted into this filtrate, which is collected and becomes urine.

The urine flows out of the kidneys through a pair of ureters and into the urinary bladder, where the liquid is stored until it can be excreted from the body. When full, the bladder is emptied through a tube to the outside known as the *urethra.*

---

evolve

Go to *Chapter Extras* on Evolve for additional illustrations and resources for this chapter. *Extras* for this chapter include:

1. Crossword puzzle (downloadable form)

MATCHING

Place the letter of the answer next to the term or phrase that best describes it.

A. Aldosterone
B. Antidiuretic hormone
C. Glomeruli
D. Hilum
E. Juxtaglomerular apparatus
F. Kidneys

G. Medullary pyramids
H. Micturition
I. Nephron
J. Renal cortex
K. Renal medulla

L. Retroperitoneal
M. Ureters
N. Urethra
O. Urinary bladder
P. Urine

_____ 1.   Basic filtering unit of the kidney

_____ 2.   A small tubular structure that transports urine from the urinary bladder out of the body during urination

_____ 3.   Hormone that promotes the retention of sodium, which stimulates the reabsorption of more water back into the blood plasma

_____ 4.   Two slender hollow tubes that transport urine from the kidneys to the urinary bladder

_____ 5.   Concentrated filtrate from the kidneys that is 96% water and 4% dissolved wastes

_____ 6.   Region of the kidney called the *urine-collecting facility*

_____ 7.   Bean-shaped pair of organs; the major homeostatic organs of the body

_____ 8.   Mechanism monitoring blood pressure consisting of the macula densa and the juxtaglomerular cells

_____ 9.   Indentation in the medial concave region of the kidney where arteries, veins, and the ureters enter and exit

_____ 10. Word meaning urination

_____ 11. Hormone that stimulates the kidneys to reabsorb more water

_____ 12. Bundles of renal tubules in the medulla

_____ 13. Muscular organ providing a temporary storage reservoir for urine

_____ 14. Region of the kidney called the *urine-manufacturing facility*

_____ 15. Loops of minute blood vessels in the glomerular capsule

_____ 16. Word meaning behind the abdominal peritoneum

INTERNET ACTIVITIES

Visit http://www.nephron.org. Under Patient Education, click on How the Kidney Works. Use this section to review the urinary system.

Visit http://www.kidney.org and click on Patients, then on Dialysis. After reading, prepare a report and present it to your class.

Visit http://www.nafc.org and click on Bladder and Bowel Health, then Frequently Asked Questions. Choose three questions, writing down both the question and the answer.

Bibliography

Abrahams P, Marks S, Hutchings R: *McMinn's Color Atlas of Human Anatomy,* St Louis, 2003, Mosby.

Applegate EJ: *The anatomy and physiology learning system,* ed 3, Philadelphia, 2006, Saunders.

Beers MH, Berkow R: *The Merck manual of diagnosis and therapy,* Whitehouse Station, NJ, 2006, Merck Research Laboratories.

Como D, editor: *Mosby's medical, nursing, and allied health dictionary,* ed 6, St Louis, 2002, Mosby.

Crawley J, Van De Graaff KM: *A photographic atlas for anatomy and physiology,* Englewood, Colo, 2002, Morton.

Damjanov I: *Pathophysiology for the health-related professions,* ed 3, Philadelphia, 2006, Saunders.

Ferri FF: *2003 Ferri's clinical advisor, instant diagnosis and treatment,* St Louis, 2003, Mosby.

Goldberg S: *Clinical anatomy made ridiculously simple,* Miami, 2004, Medmaster.

Gould BE: *Pathophysiology for the health professions,* ed 3, Philadelphia, 2006, Saunders.

Gray H, Pick TP, Howden R: *Gray's anatomy,* ed 29, Philadelphia, 1974, Running Press.

Guyton A: *Human physiology and mechanisms of disease,* ed 6, Philadelphia, 1996, Saunders.

Haubrich WS: *Medical meanings: a glossary of word origins,* New York, 1984, Harcourt Brace Jovanovich.

Huether SE, McCance KL: *Understanding pathophysiology,* ed 3, St Louis, 2004, Mosby.

Jacob S, Francone C: *Elements of anatomy and physiology,* Philadelphia, 1989, Saunders.

Kapit W, Elson LM: *The anatomy coloring book,* ed 3, New York, 2002, Benjamin Cummings.

Kordish M, Dickson S: *Introduction to basic human anatomy,* Lake Charles, La, 1995, McNeese State University.

Kumar V, Abbas A, Fausto N: *Robbins and Cotran physiologic basis of disease,* ed 7, St Louis, 2005, Mosby.

Marieb EN: *Essentials of human anatomy and physiology,* ed 8, New York, 2005, Benjamin Cummings.

Martini FH, Bartholomew EF: *Essentials of anatomy and physiology,* ed 3, New York, 2003, Benjamin Cummings.

McAleer N: *The body almanac,* Garden City, NY, 1985, Doubleday.

McCance K, Huether S: *Pathophysiology: the biological basis for disease in adults and children,* St Louis, 2006, Mosby.

Merck manual, ed 17, Whitehouse Station, NJ, 1998, Merck and Company.

Moore KL: *Clinically oriented anatomy,* ed 5, Baltimore, 2005, Lippincott Williams & Wilkins.

Netter FH: *Atlas of human anatomy,* ed 3, Teterboro, NJ, 2003, Icon Learning Systems.

Newton D: *Pathology for massage therapists,* ed 2, Portland, Ore, 1995, Simran.

Premkumar K: *Pathology A to Z, a handbook for massage therapists,* Baltimore, 1999, Lippincott Williams & Wilkins.

Salvo SG, Anderson SK: *Mosby's pathology for massage therapists,* St Louis, 2004, Elsevier Mosby.

Solomon EP, Phillips GA: *Understanding human anatomy and physiology,* Philadelphia, 1987, Saunders.

Thibodeau G, Patton K: *Anatomy and physiology,* ed 6, St Louis, 2006, Mosby.

Thibodeau G, Patton K: *Structure and function of the body,* ed 12, St Louis, 2004, Mosby.

Tortora GJ: *Introduction to the human body: the essentials of anatomy and physiology,* ed 5, Hoboken, NJ, 2000, John Wiley & Sons.

Tortora GJ, Grabowksi SR: *Principles of anatomy and physiology,* ed 11, New York, 2005, John Wiley & Sons.

Venes D, Thomas CL, Taber CW: *Taber's cyclopedic medical dictionary,* ed 20, Philadelphia, 2005, FA Davis.

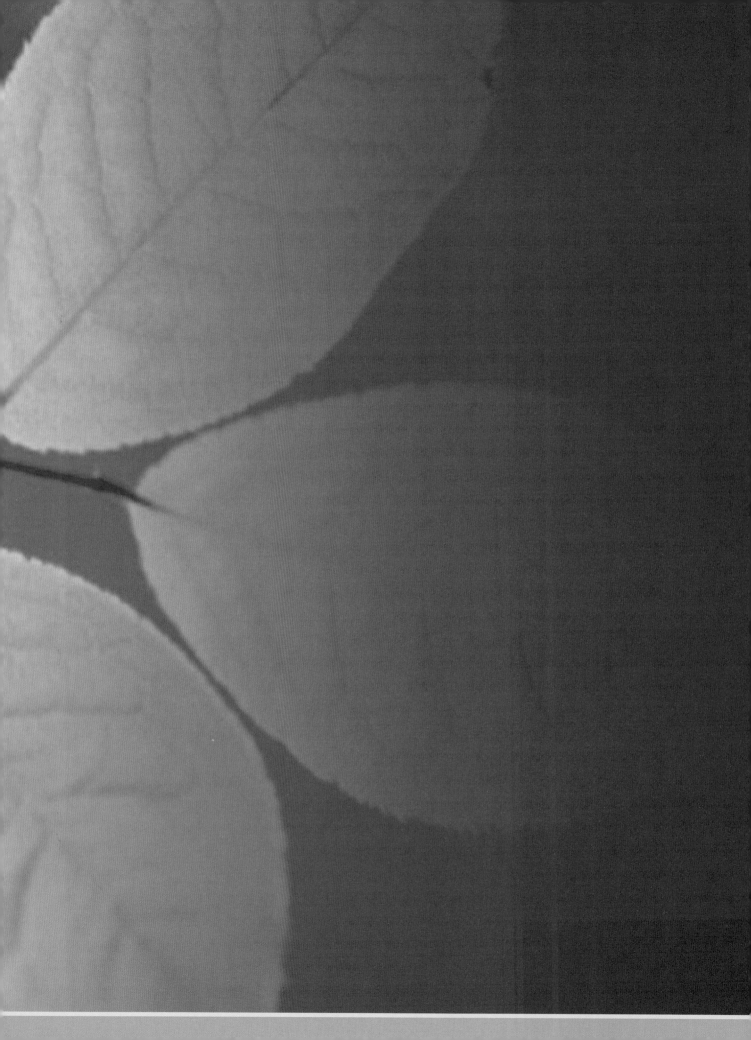

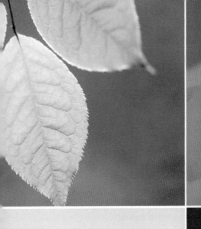

"Sometimes a scream is better than a thesis."
—Ralph Waldo Emerson

CHAPTER 23

Reproductive System

STUDENT OBJECTIVES

After completing this chapter, the student should be able to:

- List anatomical structures and describe the physiological mechanisms of the reproductive system
- Discuss the reproductive cycle, pointing out specific hormonal levels
- Identify stages of human development
- Name the primary germ layers, and give examples of each
- Discuss chromosomal relationships in human genetics
- Contrast and compare normal and abnormal chromosomal pairing
- Identify pathological conditions related to the reproductive system, and ascertain their related massage treatment modifications

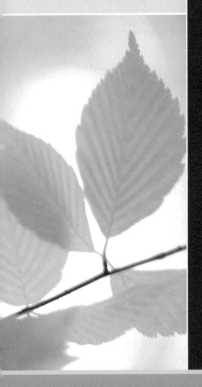

INTRODUCTION

As with most higher forms of life, human beings reproduce sexually. **Sexual reproduction** is the process by which male and female sex cells unite to produce offspring.

ANATOMY

Areas of discussion in this chapter include
- Ducts (fallopian tubes in women and spermatic duct in men)
- Gametes (oocyte in women and spermatozoon in men)
- Gonads (ovaries in women and testes in men)
- Penis, accessory sex glands (prostate, bulbourethral, seminal vesicles) and urethra in men
- Uterus, vagina, and breasts in women

PHYSIOLOGY

The process is one by which new individuals of a species are produced and the genetic material is passed from one generation to another, sustaining continuation of the species.

SEX CELLS

Male and female sex cells are called **gametes.** Female sex cells, called **oocytes** (i.e., eggs; Figure 23-1), carry genetic information from the woman who produced them. An **ovum** is an egg that has ovulated. Male sex cells, called **spermatozooa** (i.e., sperm; Figure 23-2), carry genetic information from the man who produced them.

The number of chromosomes in each egg and each sperm produced is one half that of all other body cells. When the sperm fertilizes the egg, the resulting offspring must contain the same number and kind of chromosomes as the parent cells ($\frac{1}{2} + \frac{1}{2} = 1$). The process of uniting the sperm with an egg is called **fertilization** (Figure 23-3). A *zygote* is a fertilized ovum containing genetic information from each parent.

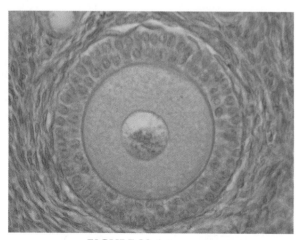

FIGURE 23-1 An oocyte.

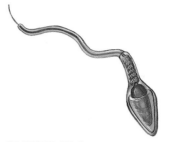

FIGURE 23-2 Spermatozoon.

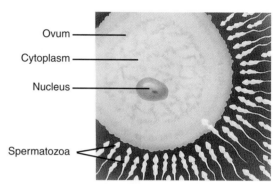

FIGURE 23-3 Fertilization.

evolve *To view a zygote, an embryo in the earliest stages of human development, log on to your student account from the Evolve website and access the course materials for Chapter 23. Keep in mind that, in actuality, a zygote is smaller than the period at the end of this sentence.* ■

REPRODUCTIVE ORGANS

Reproductive organs are divided into two groups, (1) *primary* and (2) *secondary*. The primary reproductive organs are called **gonads.** They produce hormones and the cells necessary for reproduction. In men, they are the testes; in women, they are the ovaries. The secondary set of organs is a combination of ducts used to transport the reproductive cells for possible fertilization and then transport the fertilized ovum (or zygote) to a place of incubation.

Male Reproductive Organs

The primary reproductive organs, or gonads, in men are the testes. The secondary set of organs in the male includes the spermatic duct (epididymis, vas deferens, ejaculatory ducts, and urethra) and the accessory male sex glands (seminal vesicles, prostate gland, and bulbourethral glands). Other supportive structures are the scrotum and the penis (Figure 23-4). Secretions from these glands produce the fluid that becomes semen.

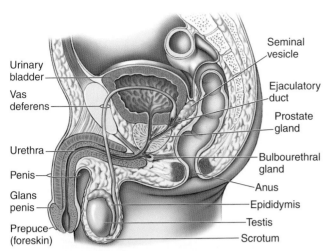

FIGURE 23-4 Male reproductive organs.

and nourished by the surrounding Sertoli cells. By the time sperm cells reach maturity, they are located near the end of the tubule. Then, the cells begin to be moved through a series of ducts for storage and final maturation in the epididymis.

Spermatic Duct

The duct system in the male reproductive system is called the *spermatic duct*. It includes the epididymis, vas deferens, ejaculatory duct, and the urethra. Each duct listed is a pair, except the urethra, of which only one is present.

The convoluted **epididymis** is a comma-shaped, tightly coiled duct located on the posterior border of the testes and is approximately 20 feet long and connects with the vas deferens. The epididymis is the site for final sperm maturation. Sperm can be stored here for up to 4 weeks before they are either expelled to the vas deferens or reabsorbed by the body.

The **vas (ductus) deferens,** or seminal duct, runs from the epididymis into the pelvic cavity where it loops over the side and down the posterior surface of the urinary bladder. The vas deferens carries sperm from the epididymis to the ejaculatory duct. The walls of the vas deferens contain three layers of muscle that undergo peristaltic contractions during ejaculation to propel sperm toward the urethra. A portion of this tube is surgically removed during a sterilization procedure called a vasectomy.

The **ejaculatory duct** is a tube that transports sperm from the vas deferens to the urethra during ejaculation.

The **urethra,** in men, transports urine from the urinary bladder and semen from the male reproductive system to outside the body. The urethra passes through the prostate gland and the penis.

Accessory Male Sex Glands

The accessory male sex glands secrete the liquid portion of the semen. These glands include the prostate gland, bulbourethral glands, and the seminal vesicles. All of these structures

Scrotum

The scrotum is a divided pouch that supports two testes and parts of the duct system. Its primary function is temperature regulation to facilitate sperm production and survival (approximately 4° F cooler than normal body temperature). The scrotum also regulates the testes' temperature by drawing them closer to or away from the body, depending on ambient temperature. The cremaster muscle provides this action. The sac is made of thin, loose, usually wrinkled skin that hangs down behind the penis. The scrotal skin contains kinky hairs and numerous sebaceous glands, which give the scrotum a characteristic odor.

Testicles

Testicles are paired oval glands that descend into the scrotum in the seventh month of fetal life and are the site of spermatogenesis (sperm production). Located within the lobes of the testes are the seminiferous tubules that contain *Sertoli cells,* which are supportive cells that assist in the development of sperm cells. Interstitial cells of Leydig are also found in these lobes in the surrounding connective tissue. Spermatogenesis begins during puberty and continues throughout life. Each day, a man makes millions of sperm. The **interstitial cells of Leydig** (Figure 23-5) produce testosterone. The testes also produce the hormones dihydrotestosterone (DHT) and inhibin. Luteinizing hormone (LH) from the anterior pituitary gland stimulates the production of testosterone. Follicle-stimulating hormone (FSH) from the anterior pituitary gland, testosterone, and inhibin controls spermatogenesis. Testosterone and DHT are responsible for the development of the male sex organs and masculine secondary sexual characteristics that occur at puberty. These characteristics include the muscular and skeletal system growth that results in wide shoulders and narrow hips; facial, axillary, pubic, and chest hair; and deepening of the voice.

Within the testes are tightly coiled tubes called **seminiferous tubules** that produce sperm. Developing sperm go through a progressive series of maturation while still in the walls of the tubules. The developing sperm are supported, protected,

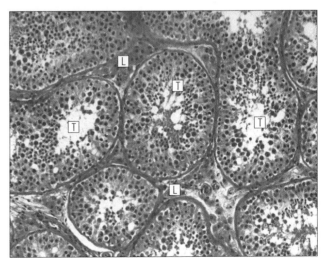

FIGURE 23-5 Interstitial cells of Leydig and their relationship to the seminiferous tubules. *L,* Interstitial cells of Leydig; *T,* seminiferous tubules.

possess ducts that conduct the fluids they secrete into the urethra. The seminal vesicles have ducts that join with the vas deferens into the ejaculatory duct, which then merges into the urethra.

The **prostate** is a firm donut-shaped gland approximately the size of a chestnut located inferior to the urinary bladder and surrounds the superior region of the urethra. It produces an alkaline secretion that makes up approximately 25% of semen volume, which liquefies coagulated semen and contracts to excrete its contents during ejaculation.

The **bulbourethral (Cowper's) glands** are a pea-sized pair of glands located on either side of the prostate. They secrete an alkaline substance, making up approximately 5% of semen, that neutralizes the acidic environment of the urethra and the mucus that lubricates the glans penis during intercourse.

The **seminal vesicles** are paired saclike pouches located posterior to the base of the urinary bladder and anterior to the rectum. They secrete a thick alkaline fluid that makes up 60% of semen volume. This fluid contains a combination of sugar, prostaglandins, and fibrinogen. The alkalinity protects the sperm from the acid environment of the female reproductive tract. The sperm uses sugar as an energy source. Prostaglandins contribute to sperm mobility and stimulate muscle contraction in the female reproductive tract. Fibrinogen helps semen coagulate and then liquefy after ejaculation. Abnormal or delayed liquefaction can completely or partially immobilize sperm and inhibit their movement through the cervix of the uterus.

Semen

Semen is a thick, milky alkaline fluid that is a mixture of sperm (10%) and seminal fluid (90%). Seminal fluid is a transport medium and source of nutrients for sperm. Between 50 and 100 billion sperm cells are found in each cubic centimeter of semen; any level lower than 50 million is regarded as clinically sterile.

Penis

The penis introduces sperm into the vagina. It is composed of three masses of spongy erectile tissue containing blood sinuses (two corpus cavernosum and a corpus spongiosum). Under sexual stimulation, the penile arteries dilate, and large quantities of blood enter these sinuses, resulting in erection. A sphincter at the base of the urinary bladder closes during ejaculation to prevent the mixing of acidic urine with semen in the urethra, which would immobilize sperm; it also prevents semen from entering the bladder. The distal end is called the *glans penis* and is covered by the loosely fitting foreskin (prepuce). This skin is removed in a surgical procedure known as *circumcision*.

Female Reproductive Organs

The primary reproductive organs, or gonads, in women are the ovaries. In women, the secondary organs include the fallopian tubes, uterus, cervix, vagina, and the vulva (mons pubis, labia majora and minora, and clitoris; Figure 23-6). The breasts are also considered accessory organs of reproduction because they produce and secrete the milk that will feed the young.

Ovaries

The ovaries are a pair of glands held in place by ligaments and located in the superior part of the pelvic cavity, lateral to the uterus. Each ovary is normally bumpy (filled with developing follicles and corpus albicans) and resembles an almond in size and shape. The ovaries produce the hormones progesterone, estrogens, relaxin, and inhibin. Progesterone and estrogens are responsible for regulating the reproductive cycle and feminine secondary sexual characteristics that occur at puberty. These characteristics include distribution of adipose tissue in the breasts, hips, and abdomen; a wide pelvis; and

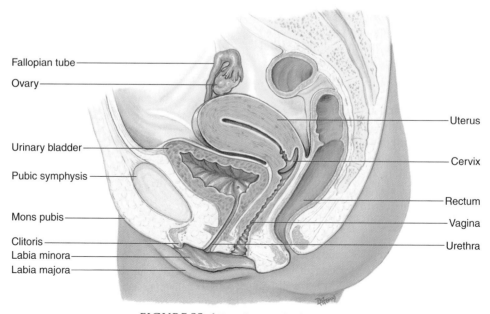

FIGURE 23-6 Female reproductive organs.

pubic and axillary hair. The ovaries contain all the oocytes a woman will ever need at birth—they are arrested in primary follicles until puberty occurs, when hormonal changes stimulate the cycle to begin.

Ovarian follicles contain an immature oocyte surrounded by epithelial cells that proliferate as the follicle develops. The follicle ruptures to release an ovum during ovulation. Ova formation begins during early fetal development as primordial oocytes. At puberty, one follicle is stimulated per month by FSH and LH to cause one oocyte to mature. This cycle of producing mature oocytes continues from the onset of first menstruation until menopause (around the age of 45 to 60).

Fallopian Tubes (Oviducts)

The fallopian tubes extend laterally from the uterus. Each tube serves as a passage through which an ovum move toward the uterus and through which spermatozoa moves toward the ovary. The *infundibulum* is the funnel-shaped end of each tube that lies close to the ovary and is surrounded by fingerlike projections called *fimbriae,* which help draw the ovum into the tube following ovulation. The ovum is moved along the tube by cilia and peristaltic contractions of the muscle layer. The fallopian tubes are also the site of fertilization.

Uterus (Womb)

The uterus is a hollow, pear-shaped internal organ in which the fertilized ovum implants and the fetus develops during pregnancy and from which menses flows if no pregnancy takes place (Figure 23-7).

The uterus contains three layers of the uterus: (1) the endometrium, (2) the myometrium, and (3) the perimetrium. The *endometrium* is a mucous membrane lining of the uterus. The endometrium varies in thickness from approximately 0.05 mm just after menstrual flow to approximately 5 mm near the end of the menstrual cycle. Most of the endometrial lining is shed with each menstrual flow.

The *myometrium* is the muscular layer of the wall of the uterus, with fibers running horizontally, vertically, and diagonally around the uterus. It contracts forcibly to expel a fetus, moving it down and out of the uterus. The perimetrium is the outer uterine layer.

The uterus has three parts: (1) a body, (2) a fundus, and (3) a cervix. The *body* contains a cavity; the walls of the cavity touch, unless the woman is pregnant. The *fundus* is the

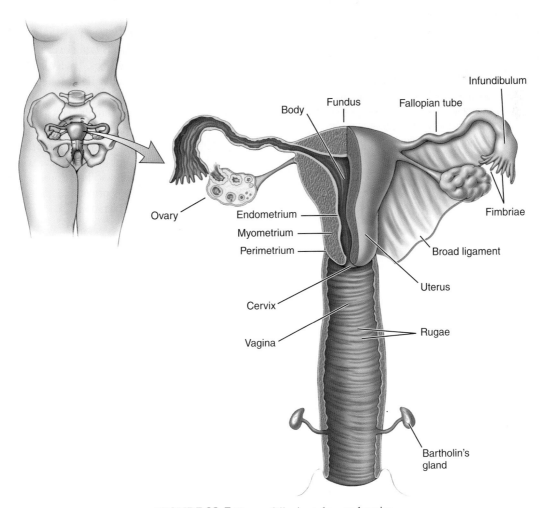

FIGURE 23-7 Uterus, fallopian tubes, and vagina.

uppermost position of the uterus. The *cervix* is located at the base of the uterus and protrudes into the vagina.

Vagina (Birth Canal)

The vagina is a 4-inch-long muscular canal that extends from the uterine cervix to outside the body. It is the passageway for menstrual flow and childbirth and the receptacle for the penis during sexual intercourse. The vagina is located between the bladder and the rectum. The vagina is actually a potential space; its walls possess transverse folds called *rugae,* which permit expansion for intercourse and childbirth. At the vaginal opening, a thin fold of vascularized mucous membrane may be found, called the *hymen,* which may partially cover the opening. Vaginal secretions create an acidic environment, which retards microbial growth (and injures sperm).

On either side of the vaginal opening are located *Bartholin glands.* They produce mucus for lubrication during intercourse and are the equivalent to the bulbourethral glands in men.

Vulva

The **vulva** is the external genitalia in women. It is made up of the mons pubis, the labia majora and minora, and the clitoris.

The **mons pubis** is a mound of adipose tissue covered by skin and pubic hair, cushioning the pubic symphysis. The **labia majora** are two folds of skin extending inferiorly and posteriorly from the mons pubis; they are the equivalent to the scrotum in men. The labia majora contain adipose tissue and oil and sweat glands and are covered with pubic hair. The **labia minora** are two folds of skin inside the labia majora, containing numerous oil glands.

The **clitoris** is a small cylindrical mass of erectile tissue and nerves located at the anterior junction of the labia minora. A small layer of foreskin is formed at the point where the labia minora unites and covers the body of the clitoris. The clitoris and the glans penis in men are equivalent structures.

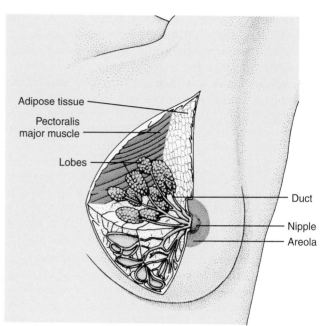

FIGURE 23-8 Female breast.

The clitoris is capable of enlargement following tactile stimulation and assumes a role in sexual excitement.

Breasts (Mammary Glands)

Breasts are specialized glands lying over the pectoralis major and serratus anterior muscles. Each gland consists of 15 to 20 lobes arranged radially. Each lobe has a system of ducts for the passage of milk to the nipple. The pigmented area around the nipple is the areola. The outer portion of the breast is mostly adipose tissue (Figure 23-8). Milk production is called *lactation.* Mammary glands are developmentally controlled by estrogens and progesterone, where estrogens stimulate duct development and progesterone stimulates secretory cells. The hormones prolactin and oxytocin are important for the function of lactation.

FEMALE REPRODUCTIVE CYCLE

At puberty, the woman begins a reoccurring cycle marked by changes in the endometrium of the uterus. This reproductive, or fertility, cycle occurs approximately every 28 days. The cycle is divided into four phases and is dependent on changes in hormones (Figure 23-9). In brief, the endometrium sheds, then re-grows, proliferates, and is maintained for several days; it then sheds again at menstruation. The monthly cycle usually continues until menopause, unless interrupted by pregnancy, disease, or stress.

First Phase (Menstruation)

Day 1-5: Day one of menstruation is day one of the reproductive cycle.

Uterus: Menstruation is the periodic discharge of built-up uterine lining from the previous cycle. The discharge, called *menses,* contains between 50 and 150 ml blood, tissue fluid, mucus, and epithelial cells. It is caused by sudden reduction in estrogens and progesterone, which, in turn, causes constriction of uterine arteries and death of the internal lining. As a result, patch areas of bleeding develop, and small portions of the lining detach. Menstruation lasts approximately 5 days.

Ovary: Follicular development begins during menstruation.

Second Phase (Before Ovulation)

Day 5-14: The production of estrogens by the follicular cells is stimulated by FSH and LH from the pituitary.

Uterus: Estrogens from the ovary stimulate the inner uterine lining to proliferate and thicken with tissue and blood vessels in anticipation of a fertilized ovum (zygote).

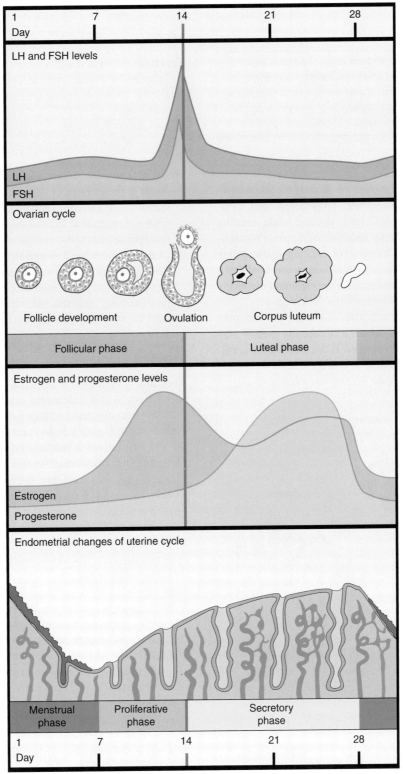

FIGURE 23-9 Female reproductive cycle.

Ovary: In the follicle, the oocyte begins to mature while secretion of estrogens increases after stimulation of pituitary hormones, causing further proliferation of the follicle.

Third Phase (Ovulation)

Day 14: High surge of LH causes rupture of ovarian follicle and release of the egg into pelvic cavity. The follicle then collapses, and the cells develop into the corpus luteum, which also secretes estrogens and progesterone (Figure 23-10).

> **evolve** *Ovulation is controlled totally by hormones. To view a photograph taken at the exact moment of ovulation, log on to the Evolve website. While there, check out the images of a morula and blastocyst, which will be discussed shortly.* ■

Fourth Stage (After Ovulation)

Day 15-28: LH and FSH stimulate the formation of the corpus luteum. The corpus luteum secretes progesterone and estrogens. FSH stimulates new follicles to develop while assisting the corpus luteum to continue secreting estrogens. Progesterone slightly elevates body temperature, creating an incubating effect. The corpus luteum secretes increasing amounts of estrogens and progesterone to maintain the uterine lining in a richly vascular state necessary for implantation and pregnancy.

After ovulation, the ovum is moved down the fallopian tube toward the uterus. If fertilization occurs, then it normally happens in the fallopian tube. If the ovum is not fertilized, then the level of estrogens and progesterone decreases over 2 weeks. This decrease causes the uterine lining to

shrink and die, leading to menstruation, which flushes out the unfertilized ovum. The corpus luteum atrophies, undergoes fibrotic degeneration, and becomes a pale spot on the surface of the ovary called the *corpus albicans.*

SEXUAL INTERCOURSE

The following includes a brief discussion of sexual intercourse.

Men

Erection: Erection is enlargement and stiffening of the penis initiated by stimuli such as anticipation, memory, visual stimuli, or touch. Penile arteries dilate and fill the sinuses with blood.
Lubrication: Bulbourethral glands secrete mucus through the urethra (women produce the majority needed for comfort during intercourse).
Orgasm: Tactile stimulation of the penis brings about peristaltic contraction of (1) the ducts of the testes that propel sperm into the urethra (emission) and (2) the seminal vesicles and prostate to expel their fluids. Rhythmic impulses from the spinal cord stimulate skeletal muscles at the base of the penis to expel semen from the urethra to the exterior (ejaculation). Sensory and motor responses include rapid heart rate, increased blood pressure, increased respiration rate, and the pleasurable sensation associated with orgasm or climax that accompanies ejaculation.

Women

Erection: Stimulation of the female genitalia results in clitoral erection and widespread sexual arousal (dependent on both psychological and tactile responses).
Lubrication: Cervical lining and Bartholin glands are stimulated by nerves to produce mucoid fluid.
Orgasm: Orgasm is the reflex that occurs when genital stimulation reaches maximal intensity. It increases respiration, pulse and blood pressure, and muscular contractions of reproductive organs, which aid in fertilization of the ovum. Female orgasm differs from male orgasm by the possibility of multiple orgasms of varying intensity, with accompanying pleasurable sensations, and no physiological ejaculation occurs.
Approximately 15 minutes after semen is deposited within the vagina, it liquefies to allow sperm to swim into the cervix. These sperm cells are aided by perineal muscle contraction. Prostaglandins in semen and oxytocin released from the pituitary of the woman during orgasm may stimulate uterine contractions to further aid the movement of sperm toward the fallopian tubes.

HUMAN DEVELOPMENT

The joining of egg and sperm takes place at any time up to approximately 24 hours after ovulation. The fertilized ovum, or *zygote,* continues to be swept through the fallopian tube

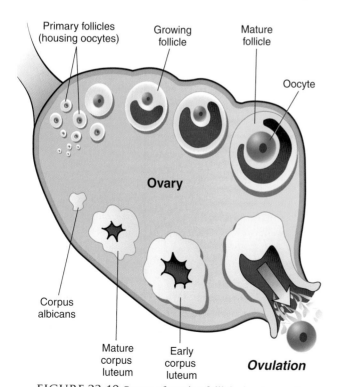

FIGURE 23-10 Stages of ovarian follicle development.

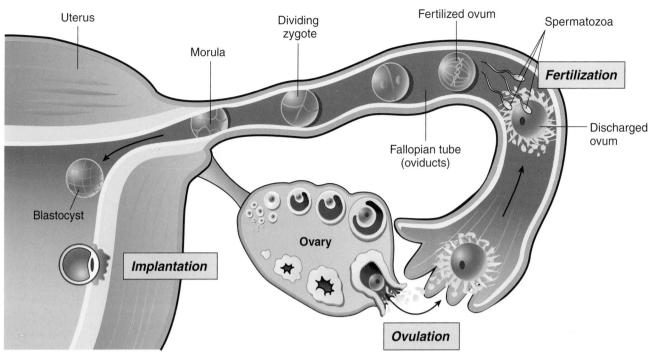

FIGURE 23-11 Ovulation, fertilization, and implantation.

and enters the uterus approximately 7 days after fertilization, where it implants (Figure 23-11). The result is pregnancy, the sequence of events that includes implantation and embryonic and fetal growth and ends in birth approximately 266 day later. Included in these stages is postpartum lactation.

TABLE TALK

Pregnancy may be of a singleton or higher-order multiples; the most likely are twins. *Fraternal twins* are produced from independent release of two ova that are each fertilized by different sperm. They are the same age and develop in the uterus at the same time but are genetically different from other siblings. *Identical twins* develop from a single fertilized ovum that splits at an early stage of development. They contain exactly the same genetic material and are always the same gender.

Approximately 36 hours after fertilization, the zygote undergoes division to form two cells; then the cells divide again to form four cells, then eight cells, then 16, and so forth. Although the number of cells increases, the size of the zygote does not. Finally, a solid mass of tiny cells, the *morula,* is formed 3 to 4 days after fertilization. The solid mass eventually becomes a hollow fluid-filled ball of cells called the *blastocyst.*

Implantation

Approximately 6 to 7 days after fertilization, the blastocyst enters the uterus and burrows into its endometrial lining. The placenta will develop to provide nutrients for the growth of the embryo. Human chorionic gonadotropin (hCG) hor-

mone begins to be secreted by the placenta and increases to a maximum by the ninth week, then decreases. It maintains the corpus luteum, which still produces the progesterone and estrogens necessary to maintain the pregnancy. The high level of this hormone in the bloodstream is one cause of morning sickness. Once the placenta begins to secrete these hormones, the level of hCG declines, allowing the corpus luteum to degenerate.

Embryonic Development

The first 2 months of development is referred to as the *time of the embryo.* By day 14, a connecting stalk forms; this structure will later develop into the umbilical cord. By day 16, the inner cell mass of the blastocyte begins to differentiate into three primary germ layers (Figure 23-12). From superficial to deep, these layers are ectoderm, mesoderm, and endoderm. These layers will develop into all tissues and organs of the body. Fluid-filled spaces form and produce the amnion and yolk sacs. The yolk sac is temporary and provides nutrients to the developing embryonic disc.

The outermost layer, the **ectoderm,** gives rise to the structures of the nervous system, including the special senses (e.g., inner ear, lens), the mucosa of the mouth and anus, the epidermis of the skin, and epidermal tissues such as fingernails, hair, skin glands, and the pituitary.

The middle layer, the **mesoderm,** develops into the muscles and connective tissues of the body such as fascia, tendons, retinaculum, ligaments, cartilage, bone, mesenteries, dermis, and hypodermis that arise from this embryonic cell layer. Blood, lymph and related vessels, as well as the pleurae of the lungs, the pericardium, the peritoneum, and the urogenital tract are all derived from the mesoderm.

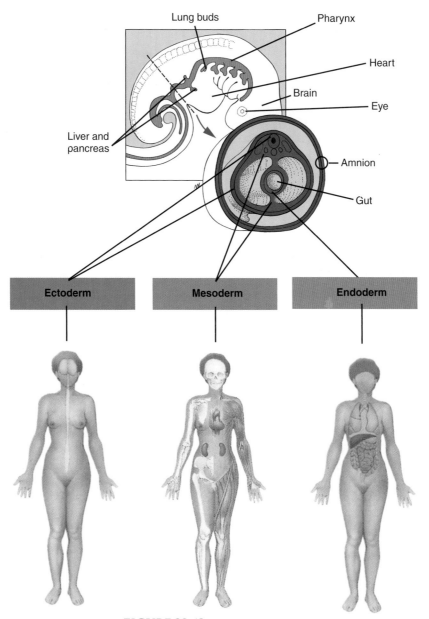

FIGURE 23-12 Primary germ layers.

The innermost cell layer is the **endoderm.** From this embryonic cell layer arise the lining of the gastrointestinal tract, the lining of the respiratory passages, and most tissues of organs and glands. Thus the endoderm comprises the lining of the body's passages and the covering for most of the internal organs.

By day 24, the embryonic disc has developed into a curved embryo with a definitive head and tail end surrounded by amniotic fluid. The gastrointestinal tract, brain, and heart begin to develop. Fingerlike projections on the outside of the developing structure, *chorionic villi*, grow into the uterine lining and absorb nourishment for the embryo from the mother.

By 8 weeks, a section of the villi will develop into the placenta, which allows the developing embryo and the mother to exchange nutrients and wastes; it also secretes hormones required to maintain the pregnancy. The *placenta* serves as a spongelike filter system that allows only small molecules (i.e., glucose, oxygen, nitrogen) to enter. Blood cells are too large to pass through the filter. Unfortunately, many drugs, alcohol, viruses (e.g., Rubella, human immunodeficiency virus), and other toxic substances can pass through this filter from the mother's blood, producing devastating effects on the unborn child.

The developing embryo secretes hCG, stimulating the continual production of estrogens and progesterone, which enables the uterus to maintain pregnancy. The corpus luteum secretes increasing amounts of progesterone. Pregnancy tests detect the presence of hCG in the mother's urine. During pregnancy, the ovaries and placenta produce large amounts of relaxin. This hormone increases flexibility of the pubic symphysis and helps the cervix dilate, assisting in fetal delivery.

Fetal Development

After 8 weeks, the baby is termed a *fetus*. For the remaining 32 weeks of pregnancy, organs established by the primary germ layers grow rapidly, and the fetus takes on a human appearance. The fetus is contained within the fluid-filled amniotic cavity and is joined to the placenta via the umbilical cord.

Birth (Parturition)

After a gestation period of approximately 40 weeks (10 lunar months), the uterus begins a complex process called *labor*. The pituitary hormone oxytocin initiates and strengthens uterine contractions that continue until the baby is expelled through the vaginal opening. The three stages of labor are as follows:

1. **Dilation:** the time from the onset of labor to complete cervical dilation (10 cm or 4 inches). Rupture of the amniotic sac occurs during this stage.
2. **Expulsion:** the time from complete cervical dilation to delivery.
3. **Placental stage:** the time after delivery until the placenta, or *afterbirth,* is expelled by powerful uterine contractions. These contractions also constrict torn blood vessels that occur during delivery to prevent hemorrhage.

Lactation

The secretion and ejection of milk by the mammary glands is called *lactation*. This process is facilitated by the pituitary hormones prolactin (milk production) and oxytocin (milk expression). During late pregnancy and the first few days after birth, the mammary glands secrete fluid called *colostrum* (first milk). True milk appears at approximately the fourth day postpartum. It contains more lactose and fat than colostrum, but both contain antibodies that protect the infant from disease during the first few months of life.

INHERITANCE

Both traits and conditions are passed from one generation to another through sexual reproduction. The expression of this genetic material is called **inheritance.** The study of inheritance is **genetics.**

Each cell in the body (except eggs and sperm) contains 23 pairs, or 46 chromosomes. Each chromosome contains a chemical called **deoxyribonucleic acid** (DNA), which appears as a small-coiled string. Different sections of the DNA strand code for the production of specific substances in the cell called *enzymes* (and other functional proteins or polypeptides). A section of DNA on a chromosome that codes for a specific enzyme is called a **gene.** When reproduction occurs, the offspring receives 23 chromosomes from the father and a corresponding 23 from the mother. They join together in the fertilized egg to reestablish 23 pairs of chromosomes. Combinations of these chromosomes control our traits (e.g., hair and eye color, blood type). Sometimes mistakes, or **mutations,** occur in our gene-coding system so that the message is read wrong by our cells. This circumstance can result in

defects in our body's structure or function. Mutations can occur spontaneously, or they can be passed though generations. These mutations can result in genetic diseases. Mutations happen all the time, many without our knowing. Some of them are harmful or lethal, but most are not.

Kinds of genetic diseases are chromosomal and gene diseases. *Chromosomal diseases* are caused by having too many or not enough chromosomes or by having a broken or missing piece of a chromosome. Examples include Down syndrome (three #21 chromosomes) and Turner's syndrome (only one X chromosome). *Gene diseases* are caused by a mistake in the DNA code of a particular gene on a particular chromosome. Examples include Huntington's disease, cystic fibrosis, sickle-cell disease, muscular dystrophy, and spina bifida. Patterns of inheriting these diseases vary, depending on whether the mutation occurred on a dominant gene, a recessive gene, or on a sex chromosome.

Human Genetics

Chromosomes are made up of DNA. DNA's major function is to store genetic information (heredity). Mutations occur when the genetic code is not perfect. Each parent has 23 pairs of chromosomes (22 autosomes and one sex chromosome). Sperm determines the offspring's gender; all eggs are X, and sperm can be either X or Y. The fertilized egg will be either an XY (male) or an XX (female). Other possibilities include XO, XXX, XXY, and XYY, all of which are abnormalities. Many drugs and x-rays affect chromosomes, which may negatively affect offspring. Three chromosomal diseases are featured in the next section.

XO Female: Turner's Syndrome

Individuals with Turner's syndrome possess 45 instead of 46 chromosomes. They have immature sex organs and cannot reproduce. Persons with this syndrome are characterized by angled elbows and a webbed neck, and they are usually short in stature. They do not possess low IQ scores but typically have personality disorders. One in 5000 births are XO births.

XXY Male: Klinefelter's Syndrome

Men with Klinefelter's syndrome have female characteristics such as hairless chest and very little, if any, facial hair. They do not develop a proper penis and testes and are usually sterile. They usually have low IQ scores and are mentally disturbed. Some have criminal instincts. A surprising number of male infants born are XXY, one in every 500 births.

Down Syndrome (Trisomy 21)

Down syndrome is more common than normal in the offspring of older women (40+). These children have three #21 chromosomes instead of the usual two. They have facial features of the Mongolian race (moon-shaped face, flat profile, slanted eyes) along with a creased tongue; misshaped ears; a single crease in the palm; fat, stubby fingers and toes; and a distinct curve of the pinkie.

PATHOLOGICAL CONDITIONS OF THE REPRODUCTIVE SYSTEM AND SEXUALLY TRANSMITTED DISEASES

Abortion and Miscarriage

The spontaneous or induced termination of pregnancy before the fetus has developed to the stage of viability (24 weeks) is abortion. The symptoms of spontaneous abortion are uterine contractions, uterine hemorrhage, dilation of the cervix, and expulsion of all or part of the fetus. *Avoid deep abdominal massage until client has completely healed*.

Amenorrhea

The absence of menses, or amenorrhea, may be caused by dysfunction of the hypothalamus, pituitary, ovaries, or uterus or by certain medications. This condition is normal before puberty, during pregnancy, after menopause, or after surgical removal of both ovaries or of the uterus (hysterectomy). *Massage is fine unless caused by a contraindicated condition, such as a tumor*.

Benign Prostatic Hypertrophy

Benign prostatic hypertrophy is an enlargement of the prostate gland, which is common among men after age 50. This condition is not malignant or inflammatory, but it is usually progressive and can obstruct the urethra and interfere with the flow of urine. Possible accompanying symptoms include frequency of urination, urge to urinate at night, pain, and urinary tract infections. Treatments include heat pack, medication, balloon dilation, and sometimes surgery. *Position client for comfort. Avoid abdomen if pressure causes pain*.

Chlamydia

Caused by the bacterium *Chlamydia,* this condition is one of the most common sexually transmitted diseases (STDs) in North America and is a frequent cause of sterility. In women, early symptoms are thick vaginal discharge with localized burning and itching. Men with *Chlamydia* infection will experience a penile discharge with painful urination (caused by urethritis), as well as localized burning and itching. The scrotum may be enlarged. Both infected men and women may have swollen lymph nodes. Infants born to an infected mother may acquire this disease during the birth process. *Chlamydia* infection is often called the silent STD because symptoms may be absent and sexual transmission can occur unknowingly. *Chlamydia* infection is the leading cause of pelvic inflammatory disease in women. *Massage is contraindicated*.

Genital or Venereal Warts

Genital or venereal warts are sexually transmitted warts of the genital and perianal area in men and women. They are caused by the *human papillomavirus* (HPV). This virus is the cause of common warts of the hands and feet, as well as lesions of the mucous membranes of the oral, anal, and genital cavities. Transmission has occurred without the presence of warts, which indicates that transmission may occur through body fluids such as semen or cervical secretions. *Position client for comfort. Avoid abdomen if pressure causes pain*.

Dysmenorrhea

Painful menstruation, or dysmenorrhea, is extremely common and occurs at least occasionally in almost all menstruating women. Pain occurs in the abdominopelvic or back region of the body. The sensations are felt as cramps, occurring in successive waves or as a constant cramp. The discomfort usually begins just before or at the start of menstrual flow and may last from 1 day to the entire period. In approximately 10% of women, dysmenorrhea is severe enough to cause episodes of partial or total disability. *Massage is fine if symptoms are not severe. Position client for comfort. Avoid abdomen if pressure causes pain*.

Endometriosis

Endometriosis is a gynecological condition characterized by painful cramping before and during menstruation. It is caused by the growth of the lining of the uterus (endometrial tissue) outside the uterus. Endometriosis is an important cause of infertility. *Massage is fine. Position client for comfort. If client is dealing with infertility issues, then refer to a mental health counselor*.

Fibrocystic Breast Disease

Fibrocystic breast disease consists of the presence of single or multiple cysts that are palpable in the breasts. Cysts can increase or decrease in size with the woman's menstrual cycle. These benign cysts are fairly common yet must be observed carefully for any change in growth, which might be related to a malignancy. Women with fibrocystic breast disease are at increased risk of developing breast cancer later in life. *Massage is fine. Position client for comfort*.

Genital Herpes

Genital herpes is an acute and chronic inflammatory disease of the genitals caused by type 2 herpes simplex virus (HSV2). It is primarily transmitted by sexual contact (via genital secretions). Infection causes painful vesicular eruptions on the skin and mucous membranes of the genitalia of men and women; symptoms are more severe in women than in men. An infected pregnant woman can pass the virus onto the infant either through the placenta or by direct contact with infected tissues during birth. *Position client for comfort. Avoid abdomen if pressure causes pain*.

Gonorrhea

A common STD, gonorrhea is an acute inflammation of the urogenital tract mucosa and occasionally the pharynx, the eyes, and the rectum. In men, infection is characterized by urethritis (inflammation of the urethra), penile discharge, and pain during urination. Women are commonly asymptomatic; however, infection may spread to the peritoneum. It can be passed from the infected pregnant woman to her newborn at birth. ***Massage is contraindicated.***

Mastitis

Mastitis, or inflammation of the mammary gland (breast), is usually caused by a *streptococcal* or *staphylococcal* infection. Acute mastitis is most common in the first 2 months of lactation. It is marked by local redness, pain, swelling, and fever. ***Position client for comfort. Avoid upper chest.***

Menopause

Regarded as a life stage and not a disease, menopause is the cessation of ovarian hormone function and menstruation in the human female. Symptoms include dry skin, vaginal irritation, and hot flashes. ***Massage is fine. Adjust room temperature for client comfort.***

Menstruation

Regarded as a normal physiological process and life stage (not a disease), menstruation is the cyclic discharge of the mucosal lining of the nonpregnant uterus through the vagina. This cycle is under hormonal control and normally occurs approximately every 28 days during the reproductive period (puberty through menopause) of the female human. ***Avoid deep pressure on abdomen; instead, a moist hot pack may be used. Focus on low back (e.g., quadratus lumborum, paraspinals, latissimus dorsi) and gluteals.***

Ovarian Cysts

Ovarian cysts are saclike structures filled with fluid or semisolid material. Most cysts are benign, but they can be painful. ***Position client for comfort and avoid the abdomen if pressure causes pain.***

Pelvic Inflammatory Disease

Caused primarily by a bacterial infection, pelvic inflammatory disease is an inflammatory condition of the female pelvic organs. Fever, foul-smelling vaginal discharge, irregular vaginal bleeding, pain in the lower abdomen, and painful intercourse characterize pelvic inflammatory disease. A mass may be palpated in the lower abdomen if abscesses are present. ***Massage is contraindicated.***

Premenstrual Syndrome

Premenstrual syndrome is a condition that causes nervous tension, irritability, weight gain, edema, headache, and lack of coordination that occurs a few days before the onset of menstruation. The causes range from stress and emotional disturbance to hormonal imbalance and nutritional deficiency. ***Position client for comfort. Abdominal massage is contraindicated if pressure causes pain.***

Prostatitis

Inflammation of the prostate, or prostatitis, is usually the result of an infection and may be chronic or acute. The client with prostatitis usually complains of frequency and urgency of urination and burning during urination. ***Position client for comfort and avoid abdomen if pressure causes pain.***

Syphilis

Syphilis is a subacute to chronic infectious disease transmitted mainly by sexual intercourse. It can travel through the human placenta, producing congenital syphilis in infants. The disease is characterized by distinct stages of effects over a period of years. Any organ system may become involved, including the nervous system. ***Massage is contraindicated.***

Trichomoniasis

Trichomoniasis is an STD that produces a urogenital infection of a parasitic flagellated protozoon. A frothy, pale yellow-to-green, odorous vaginal discharge with local itching and redness characterizes trichomoniasis in women. If the infection is chronic, then symptoms may disappear even though the parasite is still present. Men infected with trichomoniasis are usually asymptomatic, but they may experience persistent or recurrent urethritis. The parasite can be transmitted to a newborn during birth. If sexual partners are not treated simultaneously, then reinfection is common. ***Massage is contraindicated.***

Vaginal Candidiasis

Vaginal candidiasis, or yeast infection, is a vaginal infection caused by the fungus *Candida albicans*. A thick creamy vaginal discharge, local itching, and redness characterize the condition. ***Massage is contraindicated during acute systemic candidiasis.***

Terms and Their Related Meanings

TERM	MEANING	TERM	MEANING
Bulbourethral glands	*L.* swollen root	Labia	*L.* lips
Cervix	*L.* neck	Lactation	*L.* milk; process
Chorion	*Gr.* skin	Mammary	*L.* breast
Chromosome	*Gr.* color; body	Mons pubis	*L.* mountain; grown-up or hair
Corpus albicans	*L.* body; white	Morula	*L.* mulberry or blackberry
Corpus luteum	*L.* body; yellow	Mutation	*L.* to change
Cowper's gland	William Cowper, English surgeon, 1666-1709	Oocytes	*Gr.* egg; cell
		Ovum	*L.* egg
Cremaster	*Gr.* hanging	Parturition	*L.* to desire to bring forth
Ejaculation	*L.* to hurl or throw out	Placenta	*L.* cake
Embryo	*Gr.* in, to grow	Prostate	*Gr.* standing before
Epididymis	*Gr.* upon; pair	Rugae	*L.* ridge
Fallopian tubes	Gabriele Fallopio, Italian anatomist, 1523-1562	Scrotum	*L.* a bag
		Semen	*L.* seed
Fertilization	*L.* fruitful	Seminiferous	*L.* seed; to bear
Fetus	*L.* fruitful	Seminal vesicles	*L.* seed; bladder
Gametes	*Gr.* to marry	Spermatozoa	*Gr.* seed; life
Gene	*Gr.* to produce	Testis	*L.* to bear witness
Glans	*Gr.* acorn	Turner's syndrome	Henry H. Turner, American physician, 1892-1970
Gonads	*Gr.* seed		
Hymen	*Gr.* membrane	Uterus	*L.* womb
Infundibulum	*L.* funnel	Vagina	*L.* sheath
Inheritance	*L.* within; to inherit	Vas deferens	*L.* to lead; to carry away
Interstitial cells of Leydig	Franz von Leydig, German anatomist, 1821-1908	Vulva	*L.* a covering
		Zygote	*Gr.* yoke
Klinefelter's syndrome	Harry F. Klinefelter, American physician, 1912-		

Gr., Greek; *L.*, Latin.

SUMMARY

This chapter discusses the reproductive system, distinguishing male and female anatomy. Among women in their childbearing years, a cycle of reproduction occurs that is hormonally regulated and is associated with ovulation and menses. If ovulation results in ovum fertilization, then a series of miraculous events take place that most often lead to labor and fetal delivery. The resultant offspring possess characteristics of both parents. Although rare, mutations can occur. Also discussed are pathological conditions associated with the reproductive system outlining related massage treatment modifications.

evolve

Go to *Chapter Extras* on Evolve for additional illustrations and resources for this chapter. *Extras* for this chapter include:

1. Crossword puzzle (downloadable form)
2. Male penis (illustration)
3. Tubules of the testis and the epididymis (illustration)
4. Human embryo and fetus (photographic series)
5. Stages of labor and delivery (illustrated series)
6. Delivery of child (photographic series)
7. Gender determination (illustration)

MATCHING I

Place the letter of the answer next to the term or phrase that best describes it.

A. Epididymis
B. Gametes
C. Gonads
D. Interstitial cells of Leydig

E. Penis
F. Prostate
G. Scrotum
H. Semen

I. Sexual reproduction
J. Spermatozoa
K. Testes
L. Urethra

_____   1.   The process uniting male and female sex cells to produce offspring

_____   2.   Male and female sex cells

_____   3.   Male sex cells that carry genetic information from the man who produces them

_____   4.   Primary reproductive organs

_____   5.   Male primary reproductive organs and site of spermatogenesis

_____   6.   Cells that secrete testosterone

_____   7.   The convoluted and tightly coiled duct that houses sperm during final maturation

_____   8.   Pouch that contains the testes

_____   9.   Thick, milky fluid that is a mixture of sperm and seminal fluid

_____   10.   Passageway for semen and urine in men

_____   11.   Contains the urethra in men

_____   12.   Firm, chestnut-sized gland that produces a secretion to liquefy coagulated semen

MATCHING II

Place the letter of the answer next to the term or phrase that best describes it.

A. Cervix
B. Corpus luteum
C. Reproductive cycle
D. Menopause

E. Menstruation
F. Oocyte
G. Ovaries
H. Ovulation

I. Postovulatory phase
J. Preovulatory phase
K. Uterus
L. Vagina

_____   1.   A hollow internal organ in which the fertilized ovum implants, in which the fetus develops, and from which menses flows

_____   2.   Cycle marked by changes in the endometrial lining of the uterus

_____   3.   Houses the oocytes

_____   4.   Cessation of ovarian hormone function and menstruation in the female human

_____   5.   Reproductive cycle phase in which the uterine lining becomes thick and vascular in anticipation of a fertilized ovum

_____   6.   Part of the uterus that protrudes into the vagina

_____   7.   The release of the mature oocyte

_____   8.   Canal that extends from the cervix to the outside of the body

_____   9.   Day 15 to menstruation in the reproductive cycle

_____   10.   The structure left behind by the released ovum

_____   11.   First phase or day one of the reproductive cycle

_____   12.   Female sex cells that carry genetic information from the woman who produces them

INTERNET ACTIVITIES

Visit the President's Council on Bioethics at http://www.bioethics.gov and click on Cloning. Click on Frequently Asked Questions about Human Cloning and the Council's Report. Write down three questions and their answers.

Visit http://www.breastcancer.org and click on Symptoms and Diagnosis. Then click on Screening and Testing and familiarize yourself with the Breast Self Exam for yourself or a loved one.

Visit http://www.cdc.gov/mmwr/preview/mmwrhtml/rr5106a1.htm and read the report on Sexually Transmitted Diseases. Write a short report and present it to your class.

Bibliography

Abrahams P, Marks S, Hutchings R: *McMinn's color atlas of human anatomy,* St Louis, 2003, Mosby.

Applegate EJ: *The anatomy and physiology learning system,* ed 3, Philadelphia, 2006, Saunders.

Beers MH, Berkow R: *The Merck manual of diagnosis and therapy,* Whitehouse Station, NJ, 2006, Merck Research Laboratories.

Como D, editor: *Mosby's Medical, Nursing, and Allied Health Dictionary,* ed 6, St Louis, 2002, Mosby.

Crawley J, Van De Graaff KM: *A photographic atlas for anatomy and physiology,* Englewood, Colo, 2002, Morton.

Damjanov I: *Pathophysiology for the health-related professions,* ed 3, Philadelphia, 2006, Saunders.

Ferri FF: *2003 Ferri's clinical advisor, instant diagnosis and treatment,* St Louis, 2003, Mosby.

Frazier MS, Drzymkowski JW: *Essentials of human diseases and conditions,* ed 3, Philadelphia, 2004, Saunders.

Gould BE: *Pathophysiology for the health professions,* ed 3, Philadelphia, 2006, Saunders.

Gray H, Pick TP, Howden R: *Gray's anatomy,* ed 29, Philadelphia, 1974, Running Press.

Haubrich WS: *Medical meanings: a glossary of word origins,* New York, 1984, Harcourt Brace Jovanovich.

Huether SE, McCance KL: *Understanding pathophysiology,* ed 3, St Louis, 2004, Mosby.

Jacob S, Francone C: *Elements of anatomy and physiology,* Philadelphia, 1989, Saunders.

Kapit W, Elson LM: *The anatomy coloring book,* ed 3, New York, 2002, Benjamin Cummings.

Kordish M, Dickson S: *Introduction to basic human anatomy,* Lake Charles, La, 1995, McNeese State University.

Kumar V, Abbas A, Fausto N: *Robbins and Cotran physiologic basis of disease,* ed 7, St Louis, 2005, Mosby.

Marieb EN: *Essentials of human anatomy and physiology,* ed 8, New York, 2005, Benjamin Cummings

Marieb EN: *Human anatomy and physiology,* ed 7, New York, 2000, Benjamin Cummings.

Martini FH, Bartholomew EF: *Essentials of anatomy and physiology,* ed 3, New York, 2003, Benjamin Cummings

McAleer N: *The body almanac,* Garden City, NY, 1985, Doubleday.

McCance K, Huether S: *Pathophysiology: the biological basis for disease in adults and children,* St Louis, 2006, Mosby.

Merck manual, ed 17, Whitehouse Station, NJ, 1998, Merck and Company.

Moore KL: *Clinically oriented anatomy,* ed 5, Baltimore, 2005, Lippincott Williams & Wilkins.

Netter FH: *Atlas of human anatomy,* ed 3, Teterboro, NJ, 2003, Icon Learning Systems.

Newton D: *Pathology for massage therapists,* ed 2, Portland, Ore, 1995, Simran.

Premkumar K: *Pathology A to Z, a handbook for massage therapists,* Baltimore, 1999, Lippincott Williams & Wilkins.

Salvo SG, Anderson SK: *Mosby's pathology for massage therapists,* St Louis, 2004, Mosby.

Solomon EP, Phillips GA: *Understanding human anatomy and physiology,* Philadelphia, 1987, Saunders.

Thibodeau G, Patton K: *Anatomy and physiology,* ed 6, St Louis, 2006, Mosby.

Thibodeau G, Patton K: *Structure and function of the body,* ed 12, St Louis, 2004, Mosby.

Tortora GJ, Grabowksi SR: *Principles of anatomy and physiology,* ed 11, New York, 2005, John Wiley & Sons.

Tortora GJ: *Introduction to the human body: the essentials of anatomy and physiology,* ed 5, Hoboken, NJ, 2000, John Wiley & Sons.

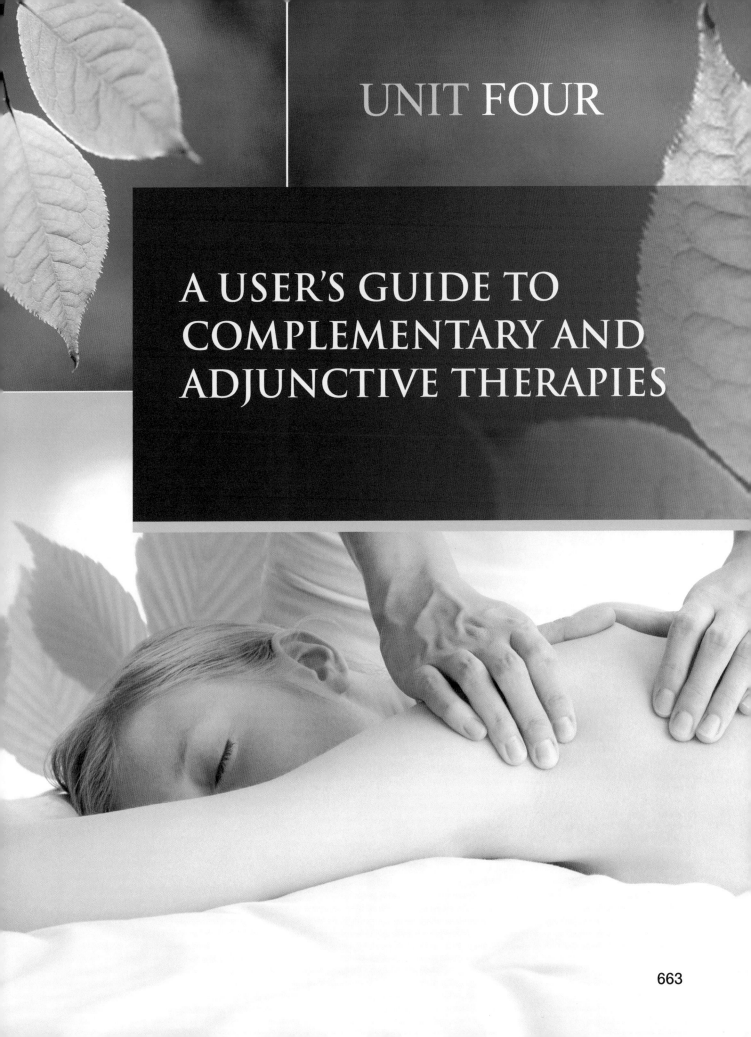

UNIT FOUR

A USER'S GUIDE TO COMPLEMENTARY AND ADJUNCTIVE THERAPIES

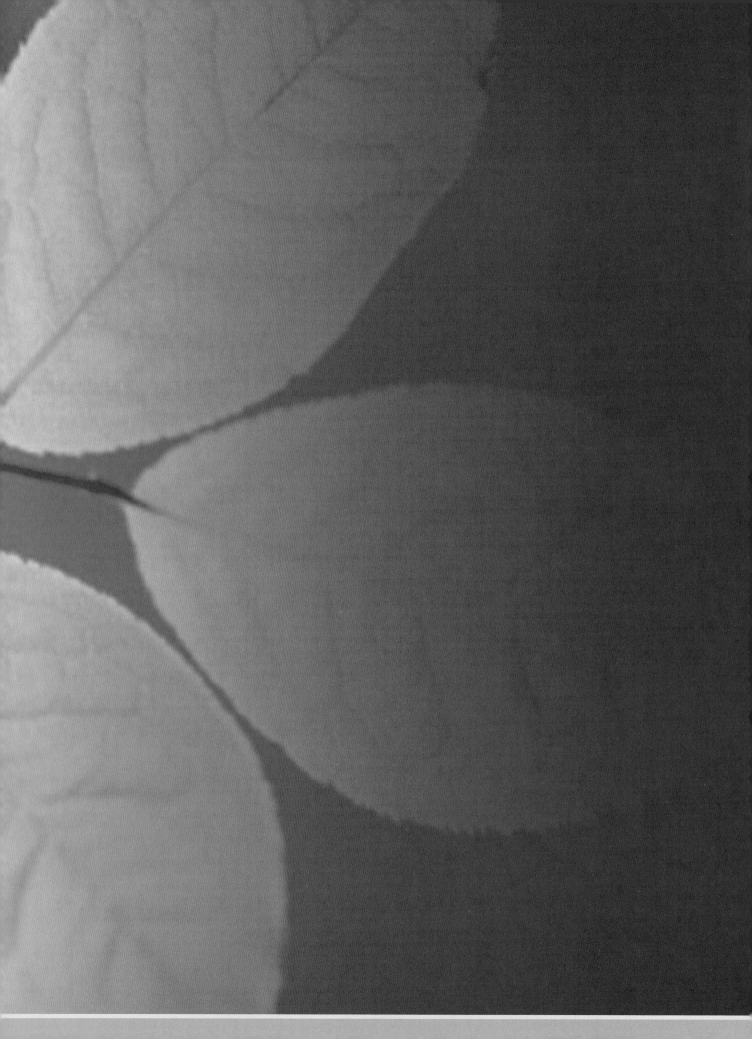

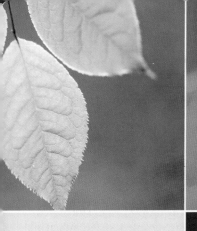

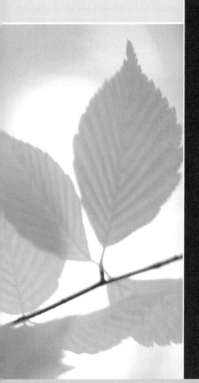

CHAPTER **24**

Hydrotherapy
and Spa Applications

STUDENT OBJECTIVES

After completing this chapter, the student should be able to:

- Define hydrotherapy, thermotherapy, cryotherapy, and spa
- Contrast and compare types of spas
- Describe the factors that contribute to the effects of water on the body
- Define density and hydrostatic pressure and how these affect hydrotherapy treatments
- Contrast and compare the mechanisms of heat transfer
- Name the effects and contraindications of thermotherapy
- Name the effects and contraindications of cryotherapy
- Discuss the hunting response
- List the sensations that the client feels during local ice application
- Discuss guidelines used before, during, and after treatment
- State the significance of the contrast method
- Demonstrate or explain compresses, packs, cryokinetics, body masks, and body wraps
- Demonstrate or explain immersion baths, hot air baths, and various showers
- Demonstrate or explain body shampoos, scrubs, ice massage, and cold-towel friction
- Discuss how aromatherapy works
- Define essential oils
- Exhibit proper storage and handling of essential oils
- Identify characteristics and rationales for the use of essential oil carriers
- Discuss essential oil safety
- Name ways aromatherapy and essential oils are used in massage and spa services

INTRODUCTION

Water, transformational by its very nature, has always been used to maintain health, manage pain, and treat physical and emotional ailments. The Babylonians, Egyptians, Indians, Cretans, Chinese, Japanese, and Mesopotamians advocated and used water's healing effects in the form of various baths and with treatment such as packs and frictions. Water was also an essential component in religious rituals and healing rites of these various cultures (e.g., rites of passage such as baptisms). Hippocrates, the most famous of early physicians, advised both hot and cold bathing. He was the first to record the role of opposites, or contrast, baths.

Although both ancient Greece and Rome had adopted the beliefs that water had healing properties, the Romans were the first to integrate hydrotherapy into their social and political life, building temples and baths near natural springs. Ancient Greek societies built public baths in conjunction with gymnasiums to facilitate sound bodies and sound minds (Figure 24-1). Bath temperatures were adjusted to the needs of each individual bather and to achieve the intended therapeutic outcome. In Sparta, laws were passed that made frequent bathing mandatory.

Hydrotherapy is any therapeutic use of water. By definition, **hydrotherapy** is the internal and external therapeutic use of water and complementary agents. Agents added to the water to enhance its therapeutic value were soaps, essences, aromatics, minerals, seaweed, salt, carbon dioxide, and oxygen. The word *hydrotherapy* finds its roots in the Greek word *hydro,* meaning *water.* Hydro as a prefix is defined as *fluid* or *liquid.* Water is often heated or cooled for use in specific applications. Water, in its various forms, continues to be employed to enhance the health and well-being of individuals and can be used to add therapeutic value to massage therapy. To help students comprehend the scope of hydrotherapy, this chapter introduces the student to the factors that contribute to how water affects the body, the effects of

heat (thermotherapy) and cold (cryotherapy), and numerous application methods. Cold and heat are often combined in the same treatment to induce a more pronounced therapeutic effect. Included in the discussion of thermo- and cryotherapy are contraindications to assist therapists in safely using these powerful modulates in their practices. Hydrotherapy is not only used during treatment, but also suggested as home care for the client.

Father Sebastian Kneipp (1821-1897), from Worshofen, Bavaria, in western Germany, is regarded as the father of hydrotherapy. Father Kneipp possessed exceptional knowledge and skill in using water to heal the ailments that afflicted his community. These treatments, known as Kneipp therapy, are still used today and are found on menus of services at world-class spas. Key components of this therapy are herbal and mineral baths, as well as cold or alternating hot and cold treatments administered by water, stones, or pebbles. Kneipp published his only book on hydrotherapy, *My Water Cure,* in 1886.

SPA

The origin of the word *spa* is uncertain. Some scholars believe the term is derived from the Walloon phrase *espa,* meaning fountain. Most scholars, however, believe that the word comes from the letters *S-P-A* that were scribbled on the marble walls of ancient public baths of Rome. This coded message is translated from the Latin term *sanus per aqua,* meaning *healing through water* or *cure of water.* In those times, the spa was more than just a place to feel good; it was considered a sacred space—a place to experience nurturing, transformation, and healing on both spiritual and physical levels. In the sixteenth century, people traveled to the town of Spa, Belgium, to *take the waters* as a way to rest, retreat, find lost health, preserve vitality, and rejuvenate.

The term **spa** has evolved to describe a place where water therapies are administered. The common denominator for

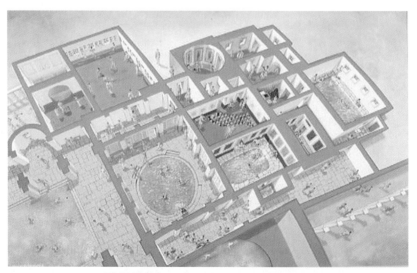

FIGURE 24-1 Ancient Roman public bath.

both massage and water therapies, according to international spa expert Robin Zill, is that the "skin is the portal of entry" for both. **Spa therapies** include a variety of body treatments administered in spas that may or may not incorporate massage, but water is the heart of the spa experience. Massage therapists have begun to add spa services to their repertoire, which can range from hot towels to scrubs to steam baths to body wraps. Clients enjoy these additional ways to relax and revive themselves. This chapter offers exposure and training in several hydrotherapy and spa applications. Additional training in the form workshops is available. See the weblinks on the Evolve website for more information.

Spa esthetics and ambience play an important role because beauty and art go hand in hand with the spa experience. Spas have evolved to include four basic types of facilities: (1) day spas, (2) resort or hotel spas, (3) destination spas, and (4) medical spas. Most spas offer their own signature treatments.

- **Day spa.** Day spas provide beauty, health, and therapeutic treatments, with services varying by provider. As the name suggests, day spas offer their services on a day-use basis. Overnight accommodations are not available.
- **Resort or hotel spa.** These spas are owned by and located within a resort or hotel. These facilities provide professionally administered spa services, fitness and wellness components, and spa cuisine menu choices.
- **Destination spa.** These facilities offer on-site accommodations, professionally administered spa services, physical fitness and wellness elements, educational programming, and spa cuisine to provide their guests with lifestyle improvement and health enhancement.
- **Medical spa.** The primary purpose of a medical spa is to provide medical and wellness care in an environment that integrates spa services. Both conventional and complementary therapies are provided.

WATER AS A HEALING AGENT

Water turns into a solid called *ice* at 32° F and into a vapor called *steam* at 212° F. Heat can be added or removed from water to change its physical state. Adding heat to ice excites the molecules and causes them to move farther apart, changing a block of ice into a puddle of water and a puddle of water into a cloud of water vapor. Removing heat from water turns vapor into liquid and liquid into solid.

The body's ability to maintain homeostasis in a changing environment is the key that unlocks the benefits of hydrotherapy. This process is thermal-dynamic. Many different treatments and effects can be achieved by varying the temperature, the mechanical distribution, the chemical composition of water, or any combination. As the nervous system perceives changes, the body responds as follows with alterations in the flow of blood and lymph:

- *Heat applications* cause an initial action of increasing blood flow to the skin. The skin becomes hyperemic as a result of blood vessel dilation; perspiration is produced in an attempt to cool the body. Prolonged heat application depresses blood flow and increases swelling and inflammation.
- *Cold applications* cause the skin to blanch initially as a result of blood vessel constriction. Prolonged cold application produces a reaction that stimulates dilation of blood vessels and increases blood flow to bring warmth to the area. This application also reduces swelling and decreases inflammation. The skin becomes hyperemic, and sensations may be felt as heat is carried to the application site by the bloodstream.

By increasing and decreasing blood and lymph flow, hydrotherapy can assist the body in detoxifying. Water is the universal solvent, and the electrolytes of the body follow the flow of water. By using water externally, the internal flow of water (blood and lymph) is altered to move oxygen and nutrients to a desired location and remove toxins. Both cold and hot applications reduce pain and discomfort through the gate theory (see Chapter 5). Other physiological effects are listed later in the chapter.

TABLE TALK
In 1785, Antoine Lavoisier proved that water is composed of two parts hydrogen and one part oxygen. (Author C. S. Lewis added "one part magic.")

The four major factors that contribute to the effects of water on the body are its *temperature,* its *moisture* and *mineral content,* and its *mechanical effect.*

Temperature

Temperature variation is the most common tool used in hydrotherapy treatments. The contact point of water is the skin. Maintaining body temperature at a comfortable and consistent level is one of the skin's primary functions (Box 24-1). This function is critical in maintaining homeostasis. Water is an excellent conductor, which allows it to transfer heat effectively and quickly.

BOX 24-1

Temperature Conversion

Fahrenheit to Celsius
Subtract 32, then multiply by $\frac{5}{9}$
$(°F - 32) \times \frac{5}{9} = °C$
EXAMPLE: $(212°F - 32) \times \frac{5}{9} = 100°C$

Celsius to Fahrenheit
Multiply by $\frac{9}{5}$, then add 32
$(°C \times \frac{9}{5}) + 32 = °F$
EXAMPLE: $(0°C \times \frac{9}{5}) + 32 = 32°F$

Water temperature is a stimulus that generates a neurological response, the first being a vasomotor response, or dilation and constriction of vessels. The skin uses circulation of the blood and lymph system to help maintain homeostasis. By increasing or decreasing circulation, water temperature can assist in natural detoxification, cleansing, or elimination processes. The greater the difference is between the body temperature and water temperature, the greater the physiological effect will be. For a more detailed look at the physiological effect of temperature, see Box 24-2 (Water Temperature Ranges and Effects on the Body).

Watsu massage and the LeBoyer method of child birthing use water at nearly skin temperature to relax the body. For more information about Watsu, see page 673 for the biography on its founder, Harold Dull.

Moisture

Moisture content in this context is the amount of humidity or dampness in the air. Steam baths at 100% humidity help moisten the mucous membranes of the nasal passages and throat and help keep the skin supple. However, high-humidity air feels heavier than dry air, often making breathing difficult. In saunas, where humidity ranges from 6% to 20%, breathing is often easier, but low-humidity air can be drying and irritating to skin and mucous membranes.

Mineral Content

The mineral or chemical content of water is another factor that influences the therapeutic effect on the body. Water, being a wonderful solvent, can readily dissolve other substances to form therapeutic solutions. Famous destination spas are often sought out for the health-giving properties of their mineral waters. Three kinds of mineral waters found at these spas are

- **Saline:** These waters containing dissolved salts are used for their purgative effects.
- **Iron oxide:** This rust-colored water is used for its restorative effects.
- **Sulfur:** This water is used for its cleansing effects.

TABLE TALK

Thalassotherapy is a hydrotherapy treatment using seawater and marine byproducts. The term *thalassotherapy* comes from the Greek word for sea. Seawater and blood plasma are remarkably similar in chemistry. Proponents of thalassotherapy often cite this fact. Spa treatments that use thalassotherapy are seawater baths that provide underwater massage using water jets in the tub, seawater massages delivered with a manual hose, and body wrap treatments using seaweed paste.

Adding minerals to water may duplicate the effects of natural springs. The most commonly used substances are sea salt (sodium chloride), Epsom salt (magnesium sulfate), and baking soda (sodium bicarbonate). These minerals draw out toxins as the body attempts to balance the percentages of saline content between the water and skin.

TABLE TALK

A common practice in massage is to recommend that a client soak in a tub with salt and baking soda after the massage to enhance the detoxification process and reduce postmassage soreness. The recipe for the bath is one part salt and one part baking soda (e.g., 1 cup of each) in a tub of warm water and a soaking for 20 minutes. Rinse off after the tub soak.

Mechanical Effect

Water, weighing 8.33 lbs per gallon, is often used for its mechanical effect. Water may be pressurized as in a whirlpool or in a shower. The mechanical effect of water intensifies with increased pressure. The two important mechanical effects of water are density and buoyancy.

Density

The most important mechanical effect in water immersion is the *Principle of Relative Density,* discovered by Archimedes (c. 287-212 BC). This famous discovery, made during a bath, prompted him to run down the street naked shouting, "Eureka," meaning *I found it*. He realized that when a body is immersed in water, it experiences an upward force equal to the weight of water. Relative density of water is set at one. Objects with a density less than one will float, and objects that have a density greater than one will sink. The adult human body has a relative density of 0.97. This ratio varies with age and deposition of fat.

BOX 24-2

Water Temperature Ranges and Effects on the Body

Fahrenheit	Celsius	Description	Effect on the Body
212	100	Boiling point of water	Burn
110+	43+	Painfully hot	Possibly injurious
102-110	40-43	Very hot	Tolerable for short periods
98-102	38-40	Hot	Tolerable, may redden the skin
92-98	33-38	Warm-neutral	Comfortable
80-92	27-33	Tepid	Slightly below skin temperature
65-80	18-27	Cool	Produces goose flesh
55-65	13-18	Cold	Tolerable, but uncomfortable
32-55	0-13	Very cold	Painfully cold
32	0	Freezing point of water	Burn

Because the density of water is near that of the human body, it produces a buoyant effect on immersion equal to the weight of the water displaced. The water pressure exerted against the body when in water offsets some or all of the effect of gravity and allows it to bob or float. This property is particularly useful for paralyzed muscles that are unable to move a heavy limb on dry land; the limb weighs less in the water and takes less muscular effort to induce movement. Similarly, water therapies are highly recommended for patients with chronic pain, such as failed low back surgeries. Although these patients may be unable to walk around without pain on dry land, putting them in waist to chest deep water buoys up some of their weight and takes pressure off the spine and faulty discs.

The density of water depends on whether or not minerals are dissolved in it. The more mineral in the water, the denser it becomes and the greater the upward force. Water in floatation tanks often has up to 100 lbs of salt to create the floating effect.

Hydrostatic Pressure

Hydrostatic pressure is another essential factor in hydrotherapy and bathing. The *Law of Pascal* (1623-1662) states that when a body is immersed in fluid, the pressure exerted on it is equal at a constant depth and is exerted equally in a horizontal direction at any level. In other words, the sideways pressure is equal on all surfaces at certain depths. Hydrostatic pressure increases with depth and increases with fluid density.

For example, when decreasing edema, the limb should be placed deep into the water. This placement will move the fluid upward, eventually to the kidneys. This action, in turn,

increases fluid output (diuresis). Research indicates that when a body is immersed for 1 hour, urination increases by 50%.

Generally, then, the basic tools of the water therapist are water temperature, moisture, and mineral or chemical content, and its mechanical effect.

"Everything flows."
Heraclitus

THERMOTHERAPY

Thermotherapy is the external application of heat for therapeutic purposes. The body can tell whether something is hot or cold only in relation to the skin temperature. Heat is transferred into the body only when the temperature of the water is greater than the body temperature. Heat moves into the tissues using one of the four methods of delivery (Figure 24-2).

- **Conduction** involves the exchange of thermal energy while the body's surface is in direct contact with the thermal agent or conductor (e.g., hot packs, hot stones). Water has 27 times greater capacity for conducting heat than air.
- **Convection** involves transferring heat energy through movement of air or liquid (e.g., sauna, steam bath).
- **Radiation** is the transfer of heat energy in rays (e.g., infrared lamps). Heat transfer occurs without direct contact.
- **Conversion** involves one energy source changing (or converting) into a heat energy source as it passes into the body (e.g., diathermy, ultrasound). This method is generally not used by massage therapists but is within the scope

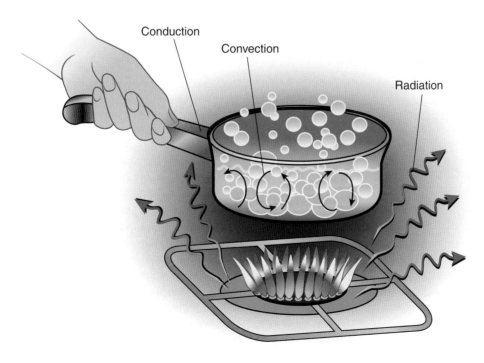

FIGURE 24-2 Examples of conduction, convection, and radiation.

of practice for chiropractic, physical, and occupational therapy.

> **TABLE TALK**
>
> *Heat* is energy resulting from the motion of molecules, atoms, and other subatomic matter. *Temperature* is a measure of this atomic activity.

Effects of Heat Application

In general, short-term applications of heat have a stimulating effect on the body, whereas prolonged applications of heat have a depressing effect on the body. Some physiological effects of heat are as follows:

- Increases sweating so evaporation can create a cooling effect
- Stimulates vasodilation so excess heat is dissipated through the skin
- Increases local blood flow
- Increases oxygen absorption
- Increases blood volume by stimulating circulation in dormant capillary beds
- Increases metabolism
- Reduces pain
- Relieves stiffness and soreness
- Induces relaxation
- Increases joint range of motion
- Increases white blood cell count by producing an artificial fever (heat application must be between 102° and 104° F and maintained for 20 minutes)
- Stimulates the immune system and inhibits growth of many bacteria and viruses (heat application must be between 102° and 104° F and maintained for 20 minutes)
- Reduces muscle spasms by inhibiting motor nerve activity and muscle spindle activity
- Increases extensibility of collagen in connective tissue (e.g., scar tissue, tendons)
- Distends and softens superficial fascia.

> **TABLE TALK**
>
> Heat alters the viscoelastic state of fascia, just as the heat created by handling modeling clay makes it pliable. Massage manipulations are much more effective after the tissues have been prepared by heat.

Contraindications of Heat

Most of the following conditions are contraindicated for thermotherapy because of the effect heat has on the circulation of blood and swelling. Heat may irritate some conditions. Avoid heat application with clients who have the following conditions or who fall into the following circumstances:

- Acute injury
- Autoimmune diseases
- Clients with an aversion to heat
- Area over a fresh bruise or hemorrhaging under the skin

- Recent burns, including sunburn
- Cardiac impairment
- Cerebrovascular accident (CVA, stroke) survivor
- Edematous conditions
- Directly over the eyes
- Fever or systemic inflammation
- Hypertension or hypotension
- Directly over injection sites less than 10 days old
- Area of recent injury (possibility of internal bleeding)
- Directly over areas of local inflammation
- Area over joint prosthetics
- Malignant or chronic illness
- Significant obesity
- Over open wounds, blisters, or abrasion burns
- Over area with phlebitis or thrombophlebitis
- Over implanted devices such as a pacemaker and an implantable cardioverter defibrillator (ICD)
- Pectoralis angina
- Pregnancy, with the exception of paraffin baths on hands, elbows, knees, and feet
- Areas with rosacea
- Sensory impaired individuals who cannot report subjective reactions (e.g., infants, older adults) and clients who are unable to react appropriately to excessive temperature changes (e.g., infants, older adults, people with diabetes, mentally handicapped clients, clients who have multiple sclerosis or Raynaud's syndrome)
- Over areas of skin infections or rashes
- Area directly over a tumor or cyst
- Clients who are weak or debilitated

> **TABLE TALK**
>
> The unit used for measuring heat energy is the calorie. Specific heat of water is 1. It takes 1 calorie of heat to raise 1 gram of water 1° C.

CRYOTHERAPY

Cryotherapy is the external, therapeutic application of cold. As stated earlier, heat moves into the body only when the temperature of the water is greater than the body temperature. Otherwise, heat moves toward cold (or the absence of heat) and will continue until the two are equal or until cold is removed; the body then returns to homeostasis.

Cold application is the safest, simplest, and most effective method for reducing pain and swelling in injuries and has replaced the use of heat in many sports and rehabilitation clinics. The application of cold has several distinct physiological effects. During the first 9 to 16 minutes of cold application, the area undergoes a reduction of blood flow through reflexive *vasoconstriction*. Vasoconstriction causes the skin to appear blanched or pale; local edema is reduced, and hematoma formation is controlled.

If cold application continues beyond this stage, then a sudden deep-tissue *vasodilation* occurs lasting for 4 to 6 minutes. This reaction is a thermoregulatory response to restore homeostasis and raise local temperature. After a few minutes, vasoconstriction resumes, and the cycle continues. One complete rotation of vasoconstriction and vasodilation takes approximately 15 to 30 minutes. This up-and-down cycle is the **hunting response.** Even though the goal is homeostasis, these cycles of vasoconstriction and vasodilation bring blood into and out of the area, flushing out tissue debris and bringing in oxygen. This vascular pumping or gymnastics is one of the most important effects of cryotherapy.

During the cold treatment, a client most likely experiences the following sensations:
- Coldness or cooling
- Burning
- Stinging or aching
- Numbness or reduced sensation

Allow cold application to remain on the body until the fourth and final phase (this may take from 5 to 20 minutes), and then promptly remove it to prevent tissue damage from excessive cold exposure.

Caution must be used when applying cold. If using cryotherapy in conjunction with massage, use it after. Ice before a massage creates an alteration in sensation. When the sensory feedback loop is reduced or lost, the client may be injured because of the inability to feel pressure and discomfort.

If local application is prolonged more than 20 minutes, then tissue damage may result in the form of frostbite. The consequence of prolonged general application is hypothermia.

Additionally, if the client is feeling chilled before cold application, then do not proceed. Instead, attempt to warm the client with warm towels, a warm footbath, immersion bath, or even a vapor bath (steam or sauna). Cold application can then be performed at the therapist's discretion.

Effects of Cold Application

As with heat application, short applications of cold have a stimulating effect on the body, and prolonged applications of cold have a depressing effect on the body. The following are some other effects that occur:
- Reduces acute inflammation
- Reduces swelling
- Reduces muscle spasm
- Reduces pain through reduced nerve conduction velocity
- Reduces muscular spasticity by reducing muscle spindle activity
- Stimulates circulation
- Stimulates vasodilation
- Decreases metabolism
- Temporarily decreases local oxygen supply
- Decreases tissue damage
- Reduces blood clot formation
- Increases urine production

Contraindications of Cold

Contraindications for cold application are as follows:
- Arthritis
- Aversion to cold

- CVA survivor
- Cold or plastic allergies
- Over injection sites that are less than 3 days old
- Open wounds
- Hypertension (cold application may cause a transient increase in blood pressure)
- Over implanted devices such as a pacemaker and an ICD
- Pectoralis angina
- Rheumatoid conditions
- Client with sensory impairments, individuals who cannot report subjective reactions (e.g., infants, older adults), or clients who are unable to react appropriately to excessive temperature changes (e.g., infants, older adults, people with diabetes, those who are mentally handicapped, clients who have multiple sclerosis or Raynaud's syndrome)
- Skin infections or rashes

MINI-LAB

Arrange a meeting with a local physical or occupational therapist. Ask him or her how and why he or she uses ice, heat, and water in rehabilitation. Prepare a summary and present it to the class.

TREATMENT GUIDELINES

Before

- Follow all safety recommendations outlined in Chapter 4.
- Explain to the client any critical safety points such as emergency buttons.
- Maintain hot tubs, spas, steam cabinets, and whirlpools in compliance with public and multiple-use standards.
- Require that spa guests wear waterproof shoes or sandals to prevent infection because chlorine does not kill fungus.
- Require that spa guest take a shower before entering pool to reduce the frequency and severity of waterborne infections.
- Make sure individuals with long hair have it either tied up or secured beneath a cap for hygiene reasons. Long hair might also become trapped in water outlets.
- If hydrotherapy equipment is kept in the massage room, then make sure it is not in a high-traffic region of the room. For example, electrical cords can create a tripping hazard, and a Hydrocollator and units for heating stones can burn.
- Plan ahead and assemble all necessary articles.
- Make sure treatment room is warm.
- Ask the client not to eat at least 1 hour before scheduled appointment.
- As with massage, perform client intake, obtain an informed consent, and conduct a premassage interview (Box 24-3).
- Wash your hands.
- Place a towel on equipment that will be in direct contact with the client, such as stools and benches.
- Use nonslip floor mats.
- Avoid using liniments before treatment.
- Offer water or juice before, during, and after treatment.

BOX 24-3

Questions Relevant to Spa and Hydrotherapy Clients

Along with a thorough but brief intake, the following questions may be added to the premassage interview to provide the client with comfort and safety.

Do you have any allergies? Have an ingredient list that the client can review. Have an alternate product or treatment to substitute if the client is allergic to any ingredients in the products.

Do you suffer from claustrophobia? If the answer is *yes,* then treatments such as body wraps, steam cabinets or canopies, or other spa therapies may be inappropriate or may require creative modifications.

Are you experiencing acute diarrhea? Avoid all water therapies within 48 hours of the symptoms subsiding.

Are you prone to nausea? Avoid all water therapies within 48 hours of the symptoms subsiding.

During

- Check and monitor water temperature. For an accurate reading, use a thermometer, which can be purchased at a pool supply or spa supply store. Although testing the water temperature using your fingertips is helpful, use caution when placing a hand or foot into water of unknown temperature.
- Use a timer to monitor treatment duration. Do not overtreat.
- Ask for client feedback regarding comfort level of water temperature. Adjust temperature as needed.
- Remain with the client or within easy calling distance during treatment.
- If water collects on the wet room or bathroom floor, then wipe it up immediately to prevent accidents (floor drains are helpful).
- In the event of body fluid seepage, glove up and use paper towels to absorb the spill, and then clean the area with mild soap and water. Next, disinfect equipment with a solution of water and chlorine bleach in a 10:1 solution. Discard the contaminated gloves and paper towels in a safe manner (determined by the local department of health). Finally, wash and dry your hands.
- Implements used during the massage such as stones that become contaminated should be immersed in a 10% bleach solution or a 70% alchohol solution for 10 minutes.

After

- Make certain the client's skin is dry.
- Assist the client on and off the table because hydrotherapy treatments may cause client to feel woozy.
- After treatment, allow the client to rest for at least 10 minutes so that body temperature can return to normal.
- Rewash your hands.
- Document the type of treatment, products used, duration of treatment, and the client's reactions.

- Clean all surfaces that come in direct contact with clients and all reservoirs that collect perspiration or exfoliated skin cells.

TABLE TALK

Extreme hot and cold can harm your client; therefore the therapist must always be aware of the temperature of the water. Water temperatures below 32° F or above 124° F can cause tissue damage. Bear in mind when using hot water from a faucet that many water heaters are set at approximately 140° F.

APPLICATION METHODS

When looking at a spa's menu of services, a person can easily become overwhelmed by all the possibilities. To assist the learning process, application methods have been organized into categories. Most hydrotherapy applications can be classified into one of three categories: (1) *packs,* (2) *baths,* and (3) *rubs* (Box 24-4).

A **pack** is a device for the application of heat, cold, or nutrients. It can refer to the actual item (i.e., hot stones, terrycloth), a pouch (i.e., canvas or vinyl bag filled with substances such as silica or gel), or the products themselves (i.e., clay, seaweed).

Baths are a broad category of hydrotherapy application encompassing partial or full immersion in water or vapor. The enveloping substance can also be wax, light, or air that is heated. A range of shower techniques, which is a type of bath, is included in this section.

Hydrotherapeutic **frictions** include all modalities in which the client's skin is stimulated by rubbing. This category encompasses body shampoos, skin brushing, polishes, scrubs, and glows. In most cases, friction includes an applied product. These products range from soap to a grainy agent such as salt or sugar to ice water. Therapists can friction the skin with his or her hands or with a cloth, a brush or sponge, or grainy agent that is rubbed on the skin's surface. A rinse with water and quick, vigorous drying are essential elements.

Note that some category overlap exists, such as in ice massage (using frictional movements to apply an ice pack). Another category overlap is terminology. For example, some spas call a mudpack a *mud bath.* These treatments can be used exclusively or as part of the massage therapy session. When describing the applications that follow, the student will note both definitions and instructions.

Several popular ayurvedic treatments have been included, such as Udvartana (body mask), Swedhana (hot air or steam), Garshana (dry brushing), and Shirodhara (oil over forehead). Also, please note the spa icon to denote a spa treatment.

PACKS

Compress

A compress is a wet cloth, generally a washcloth or towel, that has had water wrung from it and is applied to the skin's surface. The most common types are hot and cold compresses.

HAROLD DULL, MA

Born: December 18, 1935.

"The body is movement. Breath is life. And the base of our being is the support of others."

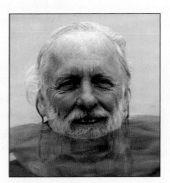

No direct path to a career in facilitating health is evident; thus it is no surprise that a physics major who decided to become a beatnik poet is the man behind one of the latest forms of hands-on therapy. Watsu is the combination of water and shiatsu. The name was coined by wordsmith and bodyworker Harold Dull. Developed 15 years ago, it is a hybrid of Zen shiatsu, flotation, joint mobilization, and stretching.

The oldest of four boys, Harold Dull was born in Seattle to parents in real estate. He attended the University of Washington with the intention of studying physics, prelaw, or philosophy. He wound up studying poetry instead, became a writer, and was part of the poetry renaissance. "At age 40 I had never had a massage," Dull says, "but I decided to begin studying Zen shiatsu in San Francisco with Wataru Ohashi and Reuho Yamada." Dull finally traveled to Japan to complete studies with world-renowned master Shizuto Masunaga. When he returned home, Dull began teaching others the ancient Japanese art and later emphasized how to combine shiatsu with the hot spring therapy he had enjoyed at Harbin Hot Springs Resort in California. In its earlier incarnation, Watsu was dubbed Wassage. Dull used a board set up in a hot tub. In time, however, he began doing his unique form of bodywork in Harbin's hot springs.

In Watsu, the water is the medium as is the message. Its buoyancy helps practitioners and clients by supporting body weight so that small practitioners are able to handle large clients. The water also helps the therapist see, feel, and listen to what is going on with the client's body. As the body rises and falls with each breath, the water helps the practitioner identify areas that need work. The water, maintained at body temperature, also soothes the client, releasing tense muscles, taking the load off joint articulations, and helping increase flexibility and range of motion.

Step into a conventional massage room and you may not feel the result of your massage until after the therapist begins, but immerse yourself in water and you immediately feel different—lighter. As you relax into your breathing pattern, supported by your therapist, you gradually let go as the tickle of the water filling your ears silences a chaotic world and lulls you into a heightened state of relaxation.

One writer describes her experience with Watsu as follows:

"The surprise, for me, was just how profound this was. It has become a cliché to say that a therapy works 'on many different levels,' but that is actually an excellent description of Watsu. Deeply rooted physical tensions and ailments are worked on more easily, while the experience of being safely held and moved through the water also touches profound emotional and spiritual levels."
From Diana Brueton: "Watsu, Flowing Free in Water," Kindred Spirit Quarterly.

Dull notes that it is "the unconditional acceptance that is so powerful. So many injured people are treated as less than what they once were." In addition to its emotional impact, Watsu has reportedly helped headache pain. Muscle spasms disappear, and chronic lower back pain and spine misalignment have been corrected.

Dull's vision is to make the therapeutic value of his work, especially the added benefit of the sense of unconditional acceptance it brings, available to everyone. "From an equipment standpoint, you need a 10-foot diameter pool with about 4 feet of water, which should be maintained at body temperature," he explains, adding that new ways will be discovered to heat water at a lower cost.

Poultices and dressings are other types of compresses but are used as home treatments and not as spa or massage ancillaries.

Hot Compress

Hot compresses are most often laid across the forehead or across the back. Hot compresses are used primarily to soothe, relax, or warm clients during or after massage or during local cold application. Heat moves quickly to the client's skin, causing the hot compress to become cool; therefore refresh it often. An infrared light can be used to keep compresses hot longer. Many therapists use electric hot towel cabinets, to keep hot towels or washcloths readily available.

Cold Compress

Cold compresses are frequently used to help keep clients comfortable during thermotherapy such as hot baths, steam bath, sauna baths, or during body wraps. They can also be styles. The liability for both hot and cold packs is that they block access to and observation of the treatment area, but massage to adjacent areas may be preformed.

Hot Pack

Therapists use hot packs, also known as *fomentation packs,* to prepare an area before massage because heat softens and distends fascia and brings fresh blood into the area. Some hot packs are electrical, some are heated in a microwave oven, and others must be filled with hot water.

A common hot pack uses a *hydrocollator,* a stainless steel kettle that keeps water temperature at approximately 165° F (Figure 24-3). Submerged in the hot water are canvas pouches containing channels filled with silicon granules. To prevent touching the water or the packs, the therapist removes the packs from the unit using a pair of tongs or cloth tabs that extend above water's surface. Because the pack is hot, it must be wrapped in terrycloth before being placed on

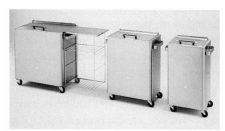

FIGURE 24-3 Hydrocollator unit. (Courtesy of TouchAmerica, Hillsborogh, NC.)

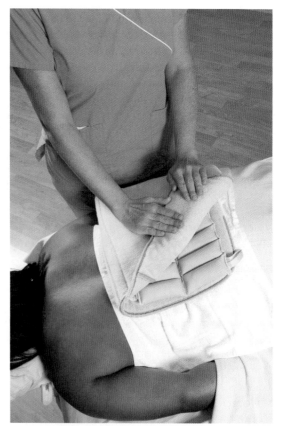

FIGURE 24-4 Hot pack with terrycloth pouch.

used to soothe an area after deep-pressure or aggressively applied massage. As with hot compresses, cold compresses quickly become warm and should be refreshed.

The procedure is as follows:

1. For a hot compress, dip a washcloth in hot water. For a cold compress, dip a washcloth in icy water.
2. Squeeze out excess water.
3. For a small area, layer the cloth by folding.
4. Apply to the desired area.
5. Allow it to remain on the skin until it reaches near body temperature.
6. Remove or replace with a fresh compress (therapist's discretion).

Pack

In this subcategory, hot and cold packs use a pouch to deliver heat or cold. These packs used in professional settings are commercially manufactured and available in a variety of the client's back (Figure 24-4). This pack is placed on top of the client's body and never underneath. These packs can retain heat for up to 30 minutes.

Cold Pack

Most professional cold packs are strong vinyl bags filled with a special gel that does not freeze to a solid block mass and retains cold for approximately 20 minutes (Figure 24-5). Other cold packs must be filled with ice or icy water before use (Figure 24-6). Cold packs are often used to decrease inflammation or to reduce the chance of soreness after deep massage. Some therapists prepare their own cold packs by mixing a solution of two thirds water and one third alcohol. These packs can be kept in the freezer until needed. The alcohol will prevent the water from freezing solid.

The procedure is as follows:

1. Prepare the hot or cold pack.
2. Place the wrapped pack on the client's skin.
   a. If using a Hydrocollator, wrap the hot pack in up to three layers of terry cloth.
   b. If using a cold pack, wrap the pack in a single paper towel or thin cloth such as a pillowcase (if the cloth is too thick, then treatment effectiveness is reduced).
3. Every 5 minutes, lift the pack and observe the skin underneath. If the skin appears puffy or raised, then remove the pack immediately; if not, then continue treatment.
4. If the client begins to perspire or shiver, then place a cold or hot compress, respectively, on the back of the neck.
5. Allow the pack to remain on the treatment area for 20 to 30 minutes.

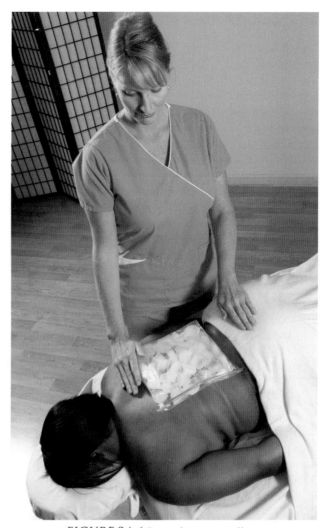

FIGURE 24-6 Ice pack on prone client.

Cryokinetics

The application of a cold pack, ice immersion, or ice massage (the latter two are discussed shortly in the chapter) with or followed by full joint range of motion is **cryokinetics.** The goal of this procedure is full functional use of the affected area. The pain-reducing effect of ice allows the client to move previously uncomfortable movement comfortably. Active range of motion is an important component to rehabilitation because joint movements encourage decongestion of the injured area and stretching of involved muscles.

The procedure is as follows:

1. Use a method of cold application to chill the affected area.
2. Allow it to remain on the treatment area until numb (10 to 15 minutes).
3. Ask the client to actively and slowly move the joint by mirroring back to you demonstrated movements. The therapist may elect to use active-resisted movements or passive movements.
4. Continue movements until feeling is restored (approximately 3 to 5 minutes).
5. Reapply ice until the area is numb.
6. Continue two more cycles of ice and movement, for a total of three cycles.

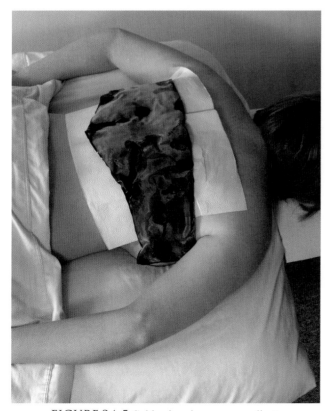

FIGURE 24-5 Cold gel pack on a prone client.

Thermal Mittens and Booties

Thermal mittens and booties are rarely used as an independent treatment. Instead, they add another dimension of luxury and pampering to a massage or spa treatment. Two types of thermal mittens or booties are available for use. The first type is filled with buckwheat or a similar material and warmed in a microwave oven. The second type uses small, electrically warmed sleeves for the hands and feet. If the latter types are used, then make sure the cord is long enough for the client to lie down while in use yet does not create a tripping hazard. In many instances, a moisturizing agent such as Shea or cocoa butter, jojoba oil, or paraffin wax is applied to the skin before the warmed mittens or booties are slipped on. Essential oils are frequently used with the moisturizing agents for their therapeutic effects (see section on Essential Oil).

> **evolve** *I use heated mittens as an add-on service or as a special treat during massage for a client who happens to also be celebrating a birthday or another special event. See a picture of how this is used on the Evolve website that accompanies this text.* ■

The procedure is as follows:
1. Preheat the mitts or boots.
2. Apply product to the hands or feet (if applicable).
3. If product is used, wrap the hands or feet in plastic wrap.
4. Slide the heated mitts or boots on the hands or feet.
5. Slip off after 15 minutes.
6. Remove any excess product (if applicable).

Stones

Stones are used to apply heat or cold or as a massage tool. For this application, the therapist employs smooth stones of various sizes. The size of the stone determines its placement. For example, small stones may be placed on the client's face or between the toes, or both. Hot larger stones are placed in a pattern on the table ready for client to lie supine; additional hot stones can be arranged along the client's midline. For the client lying prone, hot stones are placed along the spine (Figure 24-7). Medium-sized hot stones are often placed in the palms of a client's hands.

Native Americans have been using hot and cold stones for centuries. Teaching application of hot and cold stones began in Arizona by Mary Hannigan, and she called it *la stone therapy*. Since then, other technique strategists have entered the training circuit. Hot stone massage is a popular spa technique, especially in ayurvedic treatments. Basalt is recommended for the *hot* stones, and marble is recommended for the *cold* stones. In most instances, a section of the sheets used to drape either the client or the table is placed between the hot stone and the client's skin.

Exercise caution because hot stones can burn the skin. As with a compress, the temperature of stones changes quickly as heat moves into or out of the body. The procedure is as follows:
1. Heat the basalt stones in water 130° to 140° F, or chill the marble stones in a freezer or icy water for approximately 15 to 20 minutes.
2. Arrange the stones (determined by which treatment is employed).
3. Allow hot stones to remain on the skin until they are cool.
4. Move cool stones across the treatment until the desired effect is achieved.
5. Replace with fresh stones as needed.

Body Mask

A **body mask** is a type of spa treatment in which mud or other products are applied to most of the body. Body masks may be used as an independent treatment or combined with a body wrap (discussed in the next section). Products include moisturizers such as oils, creams, lotions, and natural agents such as moor mud, fango (meaning mud in Italian), paraffin,

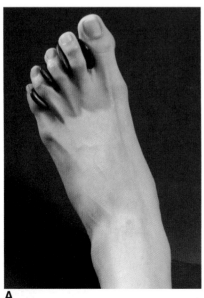
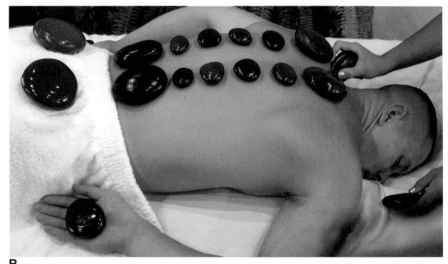

FIGURE 24-7 **A**, Stone placement in between client's toes. **B**, Stones arranged down a client lying prone.

parafango (fango mud and paraffin), clay, volcanic ash, charcoal, seaweed, and algae (see Table Talk Box on moor mud). These agents are known to cleanse, detoxify, nourish, and soothe the skin. Some spas claim that their muds promote the release of toxins and relieve muscular and arthritic pain. Heat is often used to enhance penetration of these products. Some therapists apply the product with a clean paintbrush or with gloved hands for easy clean up. *Udvartnana* is an ayurvedic treatment that uses a thick herbal paste, adding an exfoliating element.

TABLE TALK

Moor mud was formed more than 30,000 years ago and is a complete nourishing matter containing over 800 plants with at least 380 having known medicinal values. Treatments remineralize, hydrate, and exfoliate the skin, leaving it with a vital, healthy glow.

The procedure is as follows:
1. Apply the product to the client's skin according to the manufacturer's recommendations. The client will remain in the supine position. For the back of the legs, flex the hip and knee; for the hip, internally rotate the hip; for the back, help the client up to a seated position (Figure 24-8).
2. Allow it to remain on the skin according to the manufacture's recommendations (usually 20 minutes).
3. If needed, lay hot towels across the client or use a heat lamp to warm the product.
4. Remove the product with warm, wet towels; a Vichy or Swiss shower; or a hand-held hose. If paraffin is used as the applied product, then it must be removed by hand.
5. Apply moisturizer to rehydrate the skin.

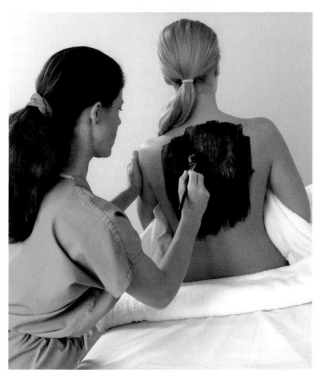

FIGURE 24-8 Therapist applying mud to client's back.

Body Wrap

A body wrap uses large wet or dry sheets or bandages to wrap most of the body. Many types of body wraps are available. Some wraps increase circulation, and some reduce swelling; others soften and nourish the skin, and some help eliminate toxins. These treatments may be followed by a massage, leaving the body totally at ease. Body wraps can be divided into two main categories: (1) compression wraps and (2) cover wraps.

Compression Wraps
This type of body wrap encases selected parts of the client's body in elastic bandages that have been soaked in a special solution. This solution increases circulation, detoxifies, and supposedly helps remove cellulite and fatty deposits. The objective is to contour the body and reduce fluids. The effects are temporary. Avoid misleading the client into thinking that compression wraps are a method of weight reduction.

Cover Wraps
Either wet or dry sheets are used to wrap, or cover, the body (Figure 24-9). Dry sheets are used to wrap the body after applying a body mask product. Wet sheets are soaked in medicinal herbal teas before the body is wrapped.

The principle behind body wraps is simple: to raise the body temperature. With the body covered in sheets, blankets, and other insulating material, the body temperature rises and the body registers a fever. This rise triggers a sweat response, cools the body, and helps eliminate the toxins the body *thinks* is causing the fever. During this process, circulation and metabolism is increased, as well as the opening of the skin's pores. This response encourages absorption of the therapeutic substance (e.g., herbal teas, clay, moor mud, seaweed).

Herbal wrap — For this spa treatment, the body is wrapped in warm sheets that have been soaked in herbal teas—hence the name *herbal wraps*. Select herbs are used to make a tea (decoction or infusion). A **decoction** is a tea made from boiling

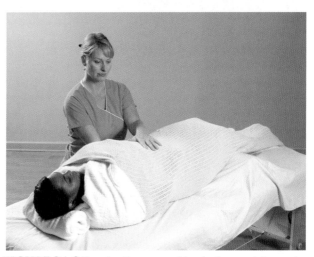

FIGURE 24-9 Female client encased in a body wrap lying supine with a bolster under knees.

parts of the plant (e.g., bark, roots, seeds). An **infusion** is a tea made from steeping the parts of the plant (e.g., stems, leaves).

Paraffin wrap — This body wrap treatment uses hot oil and dry brushing techniques to remove dead skin cells. Then an emollient-heated wax is applied to the skin for an intense hydrating treatment.

Procedures for a wet or dry body wrap are as follows:
1. Layer the following from bottom to top to prepare the table. Make sure the blankets, Mylar foil, and the sheet are lined up at the head of the table (Figure 24-10).
   - Wet sheet or plastic table sheet
   - Washable cotton thermal blanket
   - Washable wool or fleece blanket
   - Mylar foil or thermal plastic wrap
   - Flat full or queen sheet
2. Place a towel at the head of the table. Fold the towel lengthwise, tucking the blankets, foil, and sheet in between. This towel will surround the client's head and neck when the body is wrapped.
3. Ask the client to lie face up on the table, placing his or her head on the towel, and drape using an additional towel.
4. Stimulate the client's skin with dry brush massage (discussed later in the chapter).
5. For a dry wrap, apply a product for a body mask. For an herbal wrap, ask the client to stand briefly, lay the

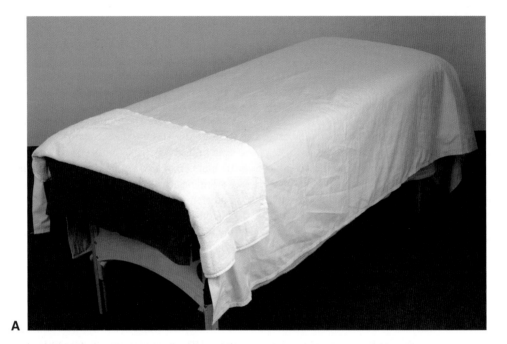

A

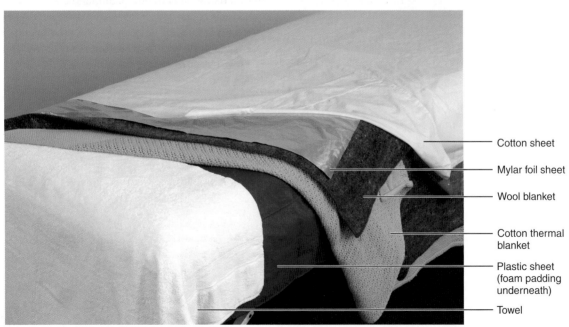

B

Cotton sheet

Mylar foil sheet

Wool blanket

Cotton thermal blanket

Plastic sheet (foam padding underneath)

Towel

FIGURE 24-10 **A**, Table set up for body wrap. **B**, Bottom edge pulled back to reveal layering.

tea-soaked sheet or towels on the table, and ask the client to lie back down.

6. Wrap the client snugly, keeping the face exposed. The client may choose to leave his or her arms unwrapped to avoid feeling claustrophobic. Place bolsters under the neck and knees and a cool compress over the forehead.

7. Allow the client to stay wrapped for up to 15 to 20 minutes. Remain nearby.

8. Unwrap the client.

9. If a body mask product was applied, then remove the product using the suggestions in the prior section on body masks. Showering is optional after an herbal wrap.

TABLE TALK

If a client feels nauseated as a result of a detox treatment such as a body wrap, a cup of cool peppermint tea should help ease the queasiness.

Shirodhara

This ayurvedic treatment uses oil, usually sesame, poured in a steady stream over the client's forehead, particularly the brow and in the region between the eyes (Figure 24-11). The therapist administers the oil from a copper vessel hung above the client's forehead. Shirodhara is suitable as a stand-alone service, or it can be combined with other treatments such as body masks, body wraps, or massage. Essential oils are added to the carrier oil to enhance doshic balance (see Chapter 28 for more information). The client should be advised to plan only light activity for several hours following the treatment. This rest allows the client to integrate the treatment more fully and with more awareness.

1. Cover the client with a drape, and place a bolster under the client's knees.

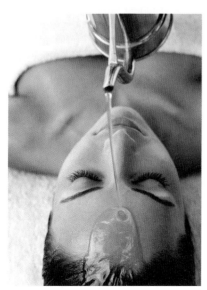

FIGURE 24-11 Shirodhara.

2. Assist the client in tilting his or her head back with the chin toward the ceiling. The top of the head should extend off the table.

3. Position a large bowl on the floor under the client's head to catch the oil as it runs off the forehead.

4. With a copper vessel positioned approximately 6 to 8 inches above the client's forehead, begin the oil steam.

5. Allow the stream to run for approximately 30 minutes. The treatment may last for a shorter time, if needed.

Contrast Pack

One of the most potent techniques in hydrotherapeutics is to combine heat and cold (Box 24-5). This application technique is known as the *contrast packs* or the **contrast method.** Two variations of contrast packs are *alternate* and *simultaneous.*

Alternate Contrast Pack

The *alternate contrast pack* is the most commonly used. This application involves alternating hot and cold packs, which intensify the circulatory effect through cycles of vasodilation and vasoconstriction. The alternate method procedure is as follows:

1. Apply a cold pack on the affected area for 10 to 15 minutes.

2. Remove the cold pack

3. Apply a heat pack for 10 minutes.

4. Remove the heat pack.

5. Repeat this sequence two more times, for a total of three times.

6. End with a cold pack application of 10 minutes.

Simultaneous Contrast Pack

During *simultaneous contrast treatment,* a cold pack is placed on the area of complaint, and a heat pack is placed next to the cold pack at the same time (Figure 24-12). Not only do the heat impulses interfere with the cold impulses, but the sensation of heat also comforts the client and induces relaxation. The simultaneous method procedure is as follows:

1. Place a cold pack on the affected area and a hot pack on the affected areas opposite side or juxtaposed to the cold pack.

2. After 15 to 20 minutes, remove both the cold and hot packs.

BATHS

For centuries, people from all cultures enjoyed the relaxing pleasures and therapeutic benefits of soaking in warm water. Water also has its place in rehabilitation. Baths, or *balneology,* is the art and science of bathing for therapeutic and relaxation purposes. This broad category encompasses submerging all or part of the body in water, wax, light, heated air, or steam. Also included are bath techniques such as showers, sprays, and hoses.

BOX 24-5

Comparative Effects of Cold and Heat

Physiological Response	Initial Effect of Cold	Prolonged Effect of Cold	Initial Effect of Heat	Prolonged Effect of Heat
Heart rate	Increases	Decreases	Decreases	Increases
Vascular response	Vasoconstriction	Vasodilation	Vasodilation	Vasoconstriction
Depth of action	Superficial	Deep	Superficial	Superficial
Effect on pain	Reduces	Reduces	Reduces	Reduces
Fascial response	Unchanged	Softens	Softens	Softens
Tissue damage	Decreases	Decreases	Nonapplicable	Nonapplicable
Analgesic	No	Yes	Yes	Yes
Anesthetic	No	Yes	No	No
Inflammatory response	Decreases	Decreases	Increases	Increases
Renal response	Stimulates	Inhibits	Nonapplicable	Nonapplicable
Digestive response	Stimulates	Inhibits	Inhibits	Inhibits
General response	Stimulates	Depresses	Stimulates	Depresses

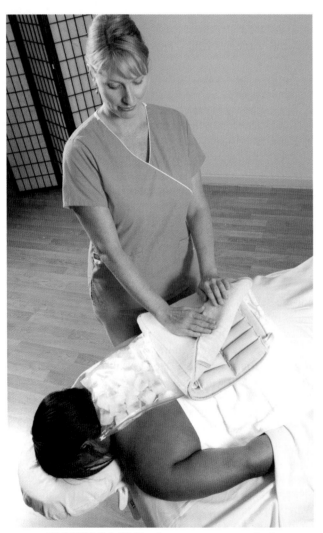

FIGURE 24-12 Simultaneous contrast method.

TABLE TALK

When water immersion is combined with light exercise, a *Hubbard tank* is used. Named after its inventor, Carl Hubbard, this tank is often used in rehabilitation clinics because the buoyancy of the water allows ease of movement and produces a soothing sensation. This type of treatment is indicated for individuals with weak or painful muscles or joints.

Immersion Baths

Immersion baths include spas, hot tubs, whirlpools, herbal baths, footbaths, underwater massage, flotation, and plunges. Immersion baths are best used before a massage session. Hot immersion baths help soften superficial fascia and relax muscles, making them more pliable.

Additives such as minerals, milk, whey, or herbs are added to individualized baths to suit a client's need. Epsom salts (named for the mineral springs in Epsom, England) or commercial bath salts such as Batherapy create a *mineral bath*. Blended herbs in the form of sachets, oils, or extracts create an *herbal bath*. Goat or cow milk added to the water creates a *milk bath*, a luxurious bath choice. The hot water disperses the healing qualities of the minerals and herbs to the skin while opening the pores to facilitate transdermal absorption.

A general rule about bath treatment times is that the greater the difference is between body and water temperatures, the shorter the treatment time will be. Most people believe that 100° to 103° F is a comfortable temperature. If the client becomes too warm during treatment but is not ready to leave the tub, then he or she may lift the arms out of the water, exposing a greater surface area of the skin to allow for evaporative cooling. If the client feels weak or dizzy, then immediately discontinue bathing and assist him or her out of the tub. The procedure for immersion baths is as follows:

1. Ask clients to cleanse themselves in a shower before treatment or perform a body shampoo—the tub is a soaking,

not a cleansing, chamber. Body shampoos are discussed later in this chapter

2. Instruct the client on how to enter and exit the tub safely. Assistance may be required.
3. While the client is in the tub, offer a cup of water in a nonbreakable cup and a cool compress for the face and neck.
4. Soaking time ranges from 1 to 20 minutes, depending on the water temperature and client's comfort level.
5. After treatment, allow the client to take a 2- to 3-minute tepid shower or use a damp cloth applied to the client's skin. Client may also elect to take a plunge.
6. Place the client in a warm, quiet place and allow him or her to rest for 10 to 20 minutes.

Hot Tub

The age-old tradition of barrel making (cooperage) dates back thousands of years and has long been used to hold liquids such as wines and spirits. Cedar and oak are the most popular woods, resulting from their natural resilience to decay and their expansive properties when soaked, which led to the early development of hot tubs. **Hot tubs** are wooden barrels of hot or cool water in which to soak. They can be found at both spas and private residences. The water can be heated using electricity (found in spas), a wood fire, or propane.

Spa Tub

A **spa tub** is a heated pool that uses high-pressure jets to agitate and circulate the water. These jets are positioned on the sides and sometimes the bottom of the tub. Temperatures are maintained between 99° and 104° F. The water is treated to remain clean and sanitary for multiple uses.

Whirlpool

Whirlpools are essentially the same as a spa tub, except the tubs are filled with hot water just before use and drained after each use (Figure 24-13).

Underwater Massage

This treatment involves initial time spent in a warm-water tub. Some tubs are equipped with high-pressure jets and a hand-held hose. The jets deliver a continuous stream of water that massages the neck, shoulders, feet, calves, thighs, and hips intended to induce relaxation. The hose can be operated by the client for self-massage or by a therapist for work on specific problem areas.

Ice Immersion

Ice immersion baths involve soaking the affected area, usually a limb, in icy water. This procedure is ideal for injured or inflamed areas. Because this treatment is often uncomfortable, clients may elect to leave the tips of their fingers or toes out of the icy water. The procedure is as follows:

1. Immerse the affected area in a container of tepid water.
2. Add plenty of ice to the water, enough to chill it quickly.
3. Keep the area immersed in the icy water for 5 minutes.

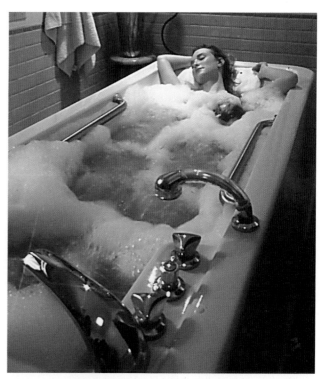
FIGURE 24-13 Client in a whirlpool.

4. Once the immersed area is numb, instruct the client to draw pictures or trace the alphabet in the icy water with his fingers or toes (Figure 24-15). Remove the immersed area from the icy water and dry immediately.

> **evolve** *Mostly used as a rehabilitative tool, ice immersion combines the therapeutic effects of ice with movement. An image of this is located on the Evolve website under Chapter 24's course materials.* ■

Pool Plunge

These applications involve small hot or cold deep-water pools that are used alone or alternately to enhance circulation. The hot water pool is equivalent to a hot tub or spa. The cold plunge follows a sauna, steam, or hot immersion bath. The water is maintained at a chilly 50° to 60° F. Brief submersion causes rapid contraction of the capillaries stimulating circulation after a sauna. Once out of the pool, dry off immediately.

Watsu

During Watsu (water shiatsu), the therapist holds the client in a near-body-temperature pool while, at the same time, massaging and stretching his or her muscles and mobilizing the joints to release and open energy pathways. Warm water and the buoyancy it provides are ideal for reducing mental and physical tension.

Flotation

A sensory deprivation spa technique, flotation uses a tank or capsule close in size to a twin bed. The tank is filled with sterile salt water regulated so that its temperature is precisely the same as body temperature for a sense of buoyancy and weightlessness. Research has shown that sensory deprivation (lack of light, sound, and gravity) combined with the body floating in water at a thermoneutral temperature induces deep relaxation. Total weightlessness is a unique and unforgettable experience. Some clients may feel claustrophobic in the tank or capsule.

Hot Air Baths

Two main types of hot air baths are available: a steam bath and a sauna. Both baths are highly therapeutic and involve sitting in a heated room. Hot air baths are often used before a scrub, a body wrap, massage, or bath technique such as a shower or a hose. Both steam baths and saunas are used to generate perspiration and induce artificial fever. All bathers must be in good health, and if the client feels weak or dizzy, then discontinue treatment immediately. Because these applications are physically demanding, clients need to be monitored through the treatment, and exposure should be limited to once a week. The general procedure follows:

1. Ask the client to shower before treatment.
2. Assist the client into the room, instructing him or her to sit on a towel placed there for comfort and sanitation.
3. Offer a cup of cool water in a nonbreakable cup and a cool compress for the face. Because of the intense heat and minerals lost during the sweating response, clients must be well hydrated before, during, and after treatment.
4. After the initial sweat, which may take from 5 to 15 minutes, have the client take a tepid shower or cool pool plunge.
5. If desired, the client may reenter the steam room or sauna.
6. After the second sweat, allow the client to take another brief tepid shower or cool pool plunge.
7. Place the client in a warm, quiet place and allow him or her to rest and drink water for 10 to 20 minutes.

 Sauna

The **sauna** is a dry heat treatment wherein the client is in a wood-lined room that is able to withstand and insulate intense temperature. Temperature in a sauna ranges from 160° to 210° F (180° to 190° F is ideal) with 10% to 20% humidity. A sauna is indicated for general tension and insomnia, but it also increases metabolism and circulation and aids in the removal of toxins. A Finnish sauna is the type on which most modern saunas are based. In a Finnish sauna, a fire (preferably using birch wood) heats a pile of stones until they are red hot. Water may be thrown on the stones to create steam. The client is then gently beaten with leafy birch twigs to stimulate circulation.

 Steam Bath

A steam bath is conducted in a ceramic-tiled room filled with steam. Temperatures are maintained between 105° and 120° F with 100% humidity. Steam baths, or sweat lodges, are used to decrease stress and assist removal of toxins from the body. Essential oils may be used to create an aromatherapy steam bath. Add lavender for a sedative effect, rosemary to increase circulation, or eucalyptus for a stimulating effect and to increase respiratory drainage.

A *steam canopy* fits over a wet table and is an inexpensive way to offer clients the benefits of a steam bath. It not only can be used in the privacy of a massage room, but it also keeps the head cool and the body supine.

Similar to the canopy, the *steam cabinet,* or *Russian bath,* allows the head to be exposed and remain cool during treatment.

---

evolve *My first experience in a steam cabinet was in a Japanese spa in San Francisco. This, along with a massage, was my way of unwinding after taking the National Certification Exam in the mid 1990s. Shortly thereafter, I purchased one for my practice. To see an illustration of a steam cabinet, access your student account from the Evolve website.* ■

Swedhana, an ayurvedic heat treatment, encourages the client to sweat via a steam bath. The most common and practical option for therapist is a steam canopy or steam cabinet. Using essential oils is recommended. Lavender, lemon, amber, juniper, and eucalyptus are safe choices for most people. It should be preceded by a massage using oil.

> *"Give me the power to create a fever,*
> *and I shall cure any disease."*
> Hippocrates

Paraffin Bath

Paraffin baths are dipped baths in a heated waxy mixture. Paraffin wax treatments are used to apply heat and are particularly useful on angular bony areas such as the hands, wrists, elbows, knees, ankles, and feet. These treatments soften the skin and are used for pain relief. The paraffin wax is kept in a thermostatically controlled container at 125° to 134° F. The molten wax can be painted on the affected part instead of dipped, but the latter is most widely used. Lotion or cream can be applied to the treatment area to assist in hardened wax removal. The procedure is as follows:

1. Clean and dry the treatment area thoroughly before the wax dip.
2. Dip the body part into and out of the wax bath quickly.
3. Repeat the process four to six times or until a thick layer of wax is formed (at least ¼-inch thick). Allow time for the wax to dry between dippings.
4. Wrap the waxed area with a plastic wrap and then with a towel (the towel serves as insulation).
5. Allow the client to rest for up to 15 minutes or until the client reports that he or she can no longer feel heat.
6. Remove the wax covering.
7. Discard the used paraffin wax mixture.

Shower

A bath technique in which water pressure is sprayed in fine streams is a shower. The two most popular varieties of spa showers are Swiss and Vichy showers. The client stands in a Swiss shower and lies down in a Vichy shower.

A type of shower, called a *spray* or a *hose,* is a single fine jet of pressurized warm or cool water. Jet blitz or jet douche treatments use a spray nozzle attached to a rubber hose to deliver a high-pressure stream of water to a standing client. Other treatments use a spray nozzle fastened to a rubber hose. Vichy showers often come with an optional hose attachment to help the therapist more effectively remove body masks and exfoliants. As mentioned earlier, the therapist can use a high-pressure hose to massage a client while he or she is in an immersion bath.

Swiss Shower

The Swiss shower features water sprayed over a standing client from both overhead and side-positioned needlelike jet valves. The water pressure and temperature varies to create a stimulating or invigorating effect (Figure 24-14). It gets its name from its country of origin, Switzerland.

Vichy Shower

Also known as an *affusion shower*, the Vichy shower is taken while a client reclines on a special table as jets of water spray from multiple overhead-mounted showerheads. It gets its name from its city of origin, Vichy, France. In the United States, this shower is used mostly to rinse off treatment products (Figure 24-15). The needlelike streams of water are either warm or alternately hot and cold.

Jet Blitz or Jet Douche

This shower type is received in a standing position performed by a therapist who uses a hose to spray strong jets of water on the client's body. The water temperature alternates from hot to cold at regular intervals. It is a relatively high-pressured hose, used at a distance, and gives an invigorating hydromassage. The therapist begins the treatment at the client's feet and works up toward the neck to stimulate lymphatic flow. This treatment is also known as a *Scotch hose,*

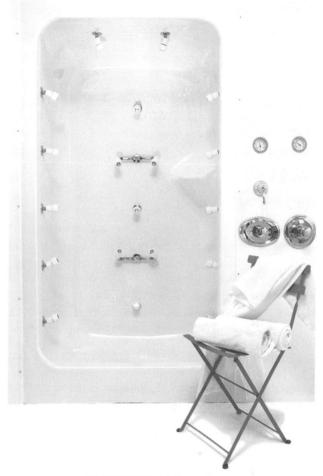

FIGURE 24-14 Swiss shower.

Scottish douche, or a *Blitz Gus. Douche* is a French word meaning *shower*.

Contrast Bath

Combining applications of hot water with cold is called a *contrast bath.* This treatment choice boosts the immune system, tones the body, closes the pores and blood vessels opened with heat treatments, and helps the body get rid of metabolic wastes.

FRICTIONS

Frictions include shampoos, brushings, polishes, scrubs and glows, and is any treatment in which the client's skin is rubbed or frictioned with the therapist hands, a cloth, brush,

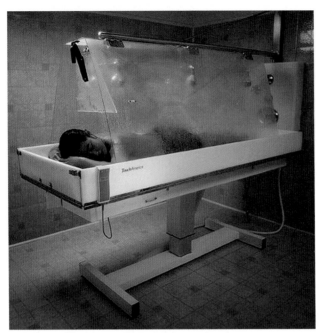

FIGURE 24-15 Vichy shower.

sponge, grainy agent, or ice. **Exfoliation** is the removal of dead skin cells. For exfoliation treatments, once a month is the maximum recommendation time. Avoid using exfoliants (such as salt) that may sting on skin lesions or on areas that have been freshly shaved or waxed. Pressure used during frictions must be monitored because areas may become easily irritated. If brushes, sponges, or loofahs are used during treatment, disinfect them by placing them in a dishwasher's top basket and run through a cleaning and heat dry cycle.

Shampoo

Body shampoos involve gently scrubbing the client's skin using a brush dipped in warm, soapy water. The client may stand, sit on a water-resistant stool, or lie on a wet table. Body shampoos may be administered outdoors.

Swedish Shampoo
Swedish shampoos include a pail of hot water (105° F) over the client's skin.

Turkish Shampoo
A *Turkish shampoo* is the same as a Swedish shampoo except it concludes with a tepid pail pour (90° F) after the hot pail pour.

The procedures are as follows:
1. Dampen the client's skin.
2. Using a mild liquid soap, generate a thick lather using a circular or linear friction.
3. Remove the lather with a shower, hose, or a pail of water poured over the client's skin. Water temperature varies according to Swedish or Turkish shampoos.
4. Dry the client's skin immediately.

Body Scrubs

A **body scrub,** body rub, or glow is any procedure that exfoliates the skin using either a dry natural bristle brush (or loofah) or grainy products. Sugar and salt are commonly used. Body scrubs are most often used before a body mask or body wrap to exfoliate and stimulate the skin. The client may be standing, sitting on a stool or bench, or lying on a table. This treatment is beneficial if the client is undergoing a fast or other self-cleansing regimen. Clients who have fair, ruddy, thin, or fragile skin should use a polish instead of a scrub.

Dry Brush Massage
Highly stimulating to skin glands and circulation, a dry brush massage uses a dry natural bristle brush or loofah to friction massage the skin. The client's skin should turn light pink (relative to client's usual skin color), a sign that the skin has been heated slightly, which promotes the removal of waste products. *Garshana,* an ayurvedic dry brush treatment, is performed with textured cotton gloves, loofah, and wool or raw silk gloves. The procedure is as follows:
1. Use brush strokes that are short and brisk and directed upward to assist lymphatic drainage. Circular brush strokes are used on the soles of the feet, palms, and the hands, and on joints. Linear brush strokes are used on limbs and the back.
2. Start at the soles of the feet and work up the legs, using mild to moderate pressure (client's tolerance level).
3. Avoid the face, but work the neck and scalp.
4. If a burning sensation occurs, then reduce pressure or speed or discontinue treatment altogether.

Body Scrub
Scrub products range from salt, sugar, oatmeal, cornmeal, ground seeds or nuts such as almond or sesame, or sea algae (dulse scrub).

If salt is used, called a *salt glow,* noniodized is recommended because some clients are allergic to iodine.

The procedure is as follows:
1. Dampen the client's skin.
2. Create a thick paste by mixing the exfoliant with either warm mineral water, liquid soap, or cold pressed oil.
3. Use short, brisk back-and-forth friction strokes to apply the compound over the client's body. Use circular friction around joints. If a burning sensation occurs, then reduce the pressure or speed or discontinue treatment altogether.
4. Rinse off the product with a warm shower, nozzle, or pail pour.
5. Dry the client immediately.
6. Apply a body moisturizer.

Body Polish
The use of a fine grainy substance to gently exfoliate, refine, and buff the skin is called a **body polish.** The products used to polish are not as coarse or abrasive as scrubs and glows. Some polishes use a *gommage,* which is a cream-based polishing agent.

The procedure is as follows:

1. Dampen the client's skin.
2. Create a thick paste by mixing the exfoliant with either warm mineral water, liquid soap, or cold pressed oil.
3. Use short, brisk back-and-forth friction strokes to apply the compound over the client's body. Use circular friction around joints. If a burning sensation occurs, then reduce the pressure or speed or discontinue treatment altogether.
4. Rinse off the product with a warm shower, nozzle, or pail pour.
5. Dry the client immediately.
6. Apply a body moisturizer.

Udvartana

Udvartana is a treatment that uses an herbal paste to stimulate lymphatic circulation. The consistency of the paste adds an exfoliating element. Udvartana is usually done before Swedhana (steam therapy) for optimal effects. These Ayurvedic pastes can be customized to suit client needs.

1. Prepare the paste using the following ingredients:
    a. 1½ cups barley flour
    b. 1½ cups chickpea flour
    c. 2 tbs coconut oil
    d. 1¼ cups neem oil
    e. 2 tbs rose petal powder
2. Mix together and heat in a frying pan at medium temperature until a thick oatmeal consistency is achieved.
3. Wait a few minutes to allow the paste to cool slightly.
4. Apply the warm paste to the client, rubbing it in vigorously.
5. Allow it to sit for a few minutes to dry.
6. Rub it off in upward directions towards the heart.

*"The cure for anything is salt water—
sweat, tears, or the sea."*
Isak Dinesen

Ice Massage

Ice massage combines the use of ice with circular friction. Have a 6-oz foam or paper cup filled with water frozen in the freezer ready to go. You may elect to insert a tongue depressor into the cup before freezing to give it a handle. The therapist may elect to combine active range of motion of the affected area after numbness is achieved. See the section on cryokinetics for more information. The basic procedure is as follows:

1. Expose the affected area.
2. Place a towel under the affected area or a rolled-up towel around the affected area to absorb the water from the melting ice.
3. Tear the top edges of the cup to expose the ice, leaving the top or bottom portion of the cup to protect your fingers.
4. Using circular friction, rub the ice on the affected area (Figure 24-16).
5. Continue the ice massage for 5 to 10 minutes or until numb, whichever comes first.
6. Dry the treatment area.

Cold-Towel Friction

Cold-towel friction, also called *cold-mitten friction,* combines ice application through towels dipped in icy water and friction movements. This application is regarded as a tonic treatment because it is thought to aid in the prevention of

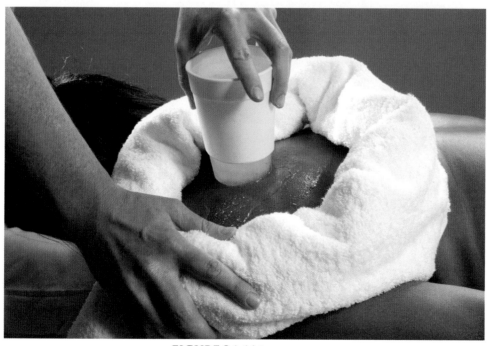

FIGURE 24-16 Ice massage.

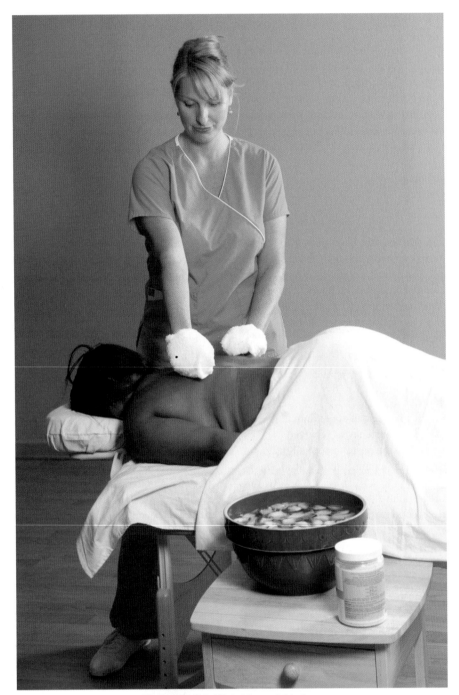

FIGURE 24-17 Cold-towel friction.

colds, low energy and endurance, poor resistance to infections, poor circulation, and anemia (Figure 24-17). Ice application through cold friction causes blood vessels to contract and dilate, promotes heat production, and reduces swelling. The client may stand, sit on a water-resistant stool, or lie on a wet table. Address one area at a time, drying it thoroughly before moving on to the next. The procedure is as follows:

1. Dip two hand towels into icy water. Do not wring the excess water out.
2. Apply to client's skin using vigorous back-and-forth friction movements.
3. Dip the towels again, and repeat the process.

4. Cover the treated area with a towel, and rub vigorously until dry.

AROMATHERAPY

The use of aromatherapy and essential oils dates back over 10,000 years to India. The Indians have used essential oils in their practice of ayurvedic medicine. The Egyptians, dating back to 4500 BC, were experts in the art of aromatherapy, especially with their embalming process.

Aromatherapy, also called essential oil therapy, is the use of plant-derived essential oils for therapeutic purposes.

Aromatherapy can be used in baths, candles, massage lubricants, incense, and specially designed aromatherapy diffusing units. Essential oils are widely used in the spa industry to scent steam baths, in products used for body mask, and in body scrubs. Massage and aromatherapy are often combined to enhance the therapeutic value of each other.

Why then should a therapist use aromatherapy?

- **Enhances treatment effectiveness.** Many spas and massage therapists use aromatherapy as a way of enhancing the effectiveness of their treatments.
- **Creates an inviting atmosphere.** A pleasant aroma will help clients relax and feel welcome the moment they walk into the room.

Aromatherapy and Olfaction

We do not smell with the nose; we smell with our brains. With the sense of smell (olfaction), aromatherapy can be used to relax or stimulate the nervous system. The olfactory bulb, located on the superior surface of the nasal cavity, is the only place in the body where the central nervous system is exposed and in direct contact with the environment. When olfactory receptors are stimulated, impulses travel along olfactory nerves toward the brain.

The olfactory bulb is part of the limbic system, which is regarded as the neurological seat of the emotions. Other parts of the limbic system are the hypothalamus, hippocampus, amygdala, thalamus, and a marginal section of the cerebral hemispheres close to the thalamus. Research indicates that these structures work as a system to regulate emotional behaviors.

In 1937, J. W. Papez identified these structures and stated that the structures of the limbic system responded to smell, taste, sound, sight, and painful stimuli, all of which elicit emotional responses. He found that when these structures are damaged, emotional experience decreases significantly. Conversely, when these structures were stimulated, individuals experience emotions such as anger, aggression, fear, sadness, pleasure, happiness, and sexual arousal. Structures of the limbic system are also associated with memory and hunger.

The easiest way to stimulate the limbic system is through the sense of smell.

Essential Oils

Concentrated essences of aromatic plants are known as **essential oils.** Over 200 pure essential oils are available. These essences are 75 to 100 times stronger than the dried version of the plant. This strength is the primary reason for dilution before its use. In fact, essential oils are so concentrated, only small amounts, or drops, are used. Essential oils enter the body through either absorption through the skin or through inhalation.

Essential oils are extracted from botanicals by several methods, most commonly steam distillation. These precious oils are regarded as the soul of the plant by aromatherapists.

Essential oils can be obtained from many parts of the plants. Examples are as follows:

- Flowers (e.g., lavender, jasmine)
- Fruits (e.g., bergamot, lemon)
- Grasses (e.g., citronella)
- Leaves (e.g., eucalyptus, peppermint)
- Roots (e.g., ginger, vetiver)
- Seeds (e.g., black pepper, fennel)
- Tree blossoms (e.g., ylang-ylang, clary sage)
- Woods and resins (e.g., sandalwood, frankincense)

Storage of Essential Oils

Store essential oils in a dark, airtight container, and place in cool, dry place away from direct sunlight. Make sure the container does not have a rubber cap or rubber squeeze bulbs because these oils will deteriorate the rubber.

If properly cared for, essential oils can have a shelf life up to 7 years. However, when mixed with carrier oils, their shelf life is only as good as the carrier oils.

Although they are oils, their consistency is similar to water. As with water, essential oils are *volatile* (*Fr.* "to fly") and will easily evaporate without a trace when exposed to open air.

Keep out of children's reach.

Carrier Oils

As stated earlier, essential oils must be diluted before use because of their concentration. Not just any substance will do. Essential oils, being *lipophilic* (*Gr.* "fat loving"), require a fatty material not only to dilute it, but also to suspend it. This material is referred to as **carrier oils** because they help to carry the essential oil. Carrier and essential oils also complement one another's effects; the skin easily absorbs them.

Most fatty substances are appropriate as carriers. These include vegetable and nut oils such as olive oil or almond oil. Other fatty products that work well are jojoba oil and Shea butter. Whole milk is also an appropriate carrier because it contains fat. Other carriers are creams, lotions, shampoo, conditioner, and liquid soap.

Generally, the higher the fat content is, the more stable the carrier oil will be. Stability refers to its shelf life and resistance to oxidation and resultant rancidity. Jojoba is very stable. Safflower oil is not very stable and will go rancid quickly. Vitamin E, which helps stabilize carrier oils, can be added to lengthen its shelf life. The two fats that are not appropriate for carriers are lard and mineral oil.

Even though essential oils are not soluble in water, they can be added to water if they are properly dispersed as in shaking a mist bottle, adding to water to be turning into vapor, or water moved through a pump in an immersion bath. If not dispersed, the essential oil will then float, concentrated, on top of the still water.

Essential Oil Safety

- Use only the oils that are familiar to you and that you can use on yourself (you are inhaling and absorbing them too).

- Avoid using on infants.
- Cut the dose for children in half.
- Avoid using essential oils on or near the eyes.
- Always use carrier oil (two exceptions are lavender and tea tree).
- Predetermine possible contraindications such as those for pregnancy or nursing women (see Chapter 9 for more information). Some essential oils are not recommended for certain neurological conditions such as seizure disorders, especially birch, cedar, clary sage, jasmine, juniper, marjoram, peppermint, and rosemary. Research and know your essential oils before use.
- Do not apply angelica, lavender, lemon, orange, tangerine, mandarin, and especially bergamot before direct sun exposure. These essential oils are photosensitive and may cause hypersensitivity in ultraviolet light or sunlight.
- Many essential oils have a high level of toxicity, such as juniper, cinnamon, pennyroyal, fennel, hyssop, and wintergreen. This concern is primarily for the therapist; if he or she is using the aforementioned oils regularly throughout the day, toxicity through frequent exposure may then develop.

Aromatherapy in Massage and Spa

Following are suggested uses in massage and spa settings. Up to four essential oils can be blended in the same treatment.

- **Inhalation:** For inhalation, place 5 to 10 drops of essential oil on the center flap of a face rest cover, on a corner of a pillowcase, or on a tissue placed on the arm shelf while the client is prone.
- **Diffusion:** A diffuser is used to disperse essential oils into the air. Add 10 to 15 drops of essential oils to diffuser. Add more drops as needed.
- **Room mister:** Add 2 to 10 drops per one ounce of water in spray bottle. Shake before use.
- **Baths:** For immersion bath, add 5 to 10 drops of essential oil in a tub for a single user. Make sure the water is moving while the client is in the water. For steam bath, add 5 to 10 drops in the water well.
- **Compress:** Add 2 to 5 drops of essential oil to a small dish of water. Drench washcloth in scented water. Wring out excess water and apply to client.
- **Massage lubricant:** Add 15 to 30 drops of essential oil to a fat-based lubricant for a full-body massage.

- **Body treatment product:** When using essential oils in body masks or body scrubs, mix the essential oil in a carrier, and then add it to the body treatment product.

Essential Oil Starter Kit

The following oils are recommended to begin building a supply of oils. They are chosen for versatility and economic value.

1. **Eucalyptus.** Highly used for respiratory congestion, eucalyptus helps bring comfort when experiencing loss and grief. This oil is also used during periods of physical and mental fatigue and exhaustion.
2. **Lavender.** The most widely used essential oil, it combats insomnia, calms, and balances the mind and emotions, and helps ease irritability.
3. **Lemon.** Lemon is used for added energy to the mind and body and a sense of clarity, which makes it useful during times of indecisiveness. Lemon essential oil may irritate the skin.
4. **Peppermint.** Peppermint adds a sense of excitement and enthusiasm. It is great for a pick-me-up or after a long period of depression. This oil is used for headaches, nausea, and motion sickness. Do not use during pregnancy. If your client is taking homeopathic remedies, then avoid using peppermint because it can act as an antidote.
5. **Rose geranium.** Relaxing and soothing, rose geranium also can enhance sensuality and assist in confidence building.
6. **Rosemary.** Aiding in stimulating mental clarity, concentration, and memory, rosemary promotes cerebral activity (and is used by some students during exams). Rosemary also brings balance by helping detoxify the mind and body. Do not use during pregnancy or on clients with seizure disorders.
7. **Sandalwood.** Sandalwood promotes deep relaxation, abates depression, and quiets the mind and emotions.
8. **Tangerine.** Tangerine is said to clear away negativity and opens up the heart by inspiring sensitivity and empathy. It also helps calm an overactive nervous system.
9. **Tea tree.** Tea tree acts as an antiseptic so it can be used to disinfect contaminated items. It also helps strengthen the immune system.
10. **Ylang-ylang.** This oil can calm the nervous system, ease depression, and reduce frustration. Used topically, ylang-ylang can irritate the skin.

SUMMARY

As long as mankind has known pain, so too have people turned to water for relief from it. Hydrotherapy is the use of water for its healing properties. Each type of application has its own beneficial effects, contraindications, safety issues, and procedures regarding its use. Water can be used for different therapeutic effects by varying its temperature, by its moisture and mineral content, and by use of its mechanical effect. Variations in temperature result in the use of thermotherapy (heat) applications and cryotherapy (cold) applications.

Both thermotherapy and cryotherapy can be applied by means of packs, baths, and frictions. Pack application methods include compresses, packs, thermal mittens and booties, hot or cold stones, body mask, body wraps, and cryokinetics.

Bath application methods include immersion baths, hot air baths, paraffin baths, plunges, showers, sprays, and douches. Friction application methods include shampoos, body scrubs, body polishes, ice massage, and cold-towel friction.

Aromatherapy is used to enhance the therapeutic effect of both spa and massage techniques. Knowledge of these techniques and safe use are important elements.

Today, these varied hydrotherapy applications have become known as spa techniques. Spa techniques can be added to the massage therapist's repertoire of modalities to offer a greater variety of services, increase therapeutic effectiveness and client satisfaction, and make the massage therapist more competitive and marketable.

evolve

Go to *Chapter Extras* on Evolve for additional illustrations and resources for this chapter. *Extras* for this chapter include:

1. Crossword puzzle (downloadable form)
2. Father Sebastian Kneipp (illustration)
3. Udvartana (photograph)

MATCHING I

Place the letter of the answer next to the term or phrase that best describes it.

A. Aromatherapy   E. Essential oil   I. Sauna
B. Body mask   F. Glow   J. Spa
C. Conduction   G. Herbal wrap   K. Spa tub
D. Cryotherapy   H. Hydrotherapy   L. Vichy shower

_____   1. The internal and external therapeutic use of water and complementary agents

_____   2. Place where water therapies are administered

_____   3. Exchange of heat while the body's surface is in direct contact with the thermal agent

_____   4. External, therapeutic application of very cold water or ice

_____   5. Spa treatment in which mud or other products are applied to most of the body

_____   6. Body wrap in which the sheets have been soaked in herbal tea

_____   7. Heated pool with high-pressure jets that agitate and circulate water

_____   8. Dry heat treatment in which the client is in a wood-lined room

_____   9. Shower taken while client reclines on a special table as jets of water spray from multiple overhead-mounted showerheads

_____   10. The use of plant-derived essential oils for therapeutic purposes

_____   11. Concentrated essences of aromatic plants

_____   12. Term that is synonymous with the word *scrub*

MATCHING II

Place the letter of the answer next to the term or phrase that best describes it.

A. Balneology
B. Body shampoo
C. Contrast method
D. Convection

E. Cryokinetics
F. Day spa
G. Exfoliation
H. Father Sebastian Kneipp

I. Hydrostatic
J. Immersion baths
K. Paraffin bath
L. Steam bath

_____ 1. Father of hydrotherapy

_____ 2. Sideways pressure applied to an immersed body

_____ 3. Place that provides beauty, health, and therapeutic treatments on a day-use basis

_____ 4. Transfer of heat energy through movement of air or liquid

_____ 5. Application of cold followed by full joint range of motion

_____ 6. Include spas and hot tubs, whirlpools, herbal baths, footbaths, underwater massage, flotation, and plunges

_____ 7. Term that is synonymous with the word *baths*

_____ 8. Bath conducted in a ceramic-tiled room filled with vapor

_____ 9. Dipped baths in a heated waxy mixture

_____ 10. Gently scrubbing the client's skin using a brush dipped in warm, soapy water

_____ 11. Combining heat and cold in the same treatment

_____ 12. Removal of dead skin cells

INTERNET ACTIVITIES

Using the Internet, locate a copy of the laws governing massage therapist in your area. Is hydrotherapy part of your scope of practice? What specifically does the law say?

Visit http://www.sauna.org and write a report on the history of the sauna. Which cultures used the sauna?

Bibliography

Associated Bodywork & Massage Professionals [ABMP]: *Touch training manual,* Evergreen, Colo, 1998, ABMP.

Arnheim DD: *Modern principles of athletic training,* ed 8, St Louis, 1992, Mosby.

Barnes L: Cryotherapy: Putting injury on ice, *Physician Sportsmed* 7(6):130-136, 1979.

Clark S: *Essential chemistry for safe aromatherapy,* New York, 2002, Churchill Livingstone.

Corio C: *Aromatherapy educational package for the retailer and health practitioner: part one* [self-published manual], 1996, Quality of Life Associates.

Crebbin-Bailey J, Haracup J, Harrington J: *The spa book: the official guide to spa therapy,* London, 2005, Thomson.

De Vierville JP: Taking the waters: a historical look at water therapy and spa culture over the ages, *Massage Bodywork: Nurture Body, Mind, Spirit,* Feb/Mar 2000, pp 12-20.

Drez D: *Therapeutic modalities for sports injuries,* St Louis, 1986, Mosby.

Hannigan MD: *LaStone therapy: the original hot stone massage,* Tucson, Ariz, 1999.

Herriott E: Steam and sauna therapy applications with massage, *Massage Magazine,* May/June 1997, pp 32-35.

Knight K: *Cryotherapy: theory, technique and physiology,* Chattanooga, Tenn, 1985, Chattanooga Corporation.

Lavabre M: *Aromatherapy workbook,* Rochester, Vt, 1990, Healing Arts Press

Lawrence DB: *Waterworks,* New York, 1989, Putnam.

Leibold G: *Practical hydrotherapy,* Wellingborough, England, 1980, Thorson.

Marx L: An odyssey through spa therapies, *Massage Magazine,* May/June 1997, pp 45-48.

Mellion MB: *Sportsmedicine secrets,* Philadelphia, 1994, Hanley and Belfus.

Minton M: Body and spa, *Massage Magazine,* Sept/Oct 2001, pp 89-99.

New Life Systems: *The body book,* Minnetonka, Minn, 2001.

Nikola RJ: *Creatures of water,* Salt Lake City, 1997, Europa Therapeutic.

Northern Lights Cedar Hot Tubs: Cedar Tub History, 2006. Available at: *http://www.cedartubs.com/index.html*

Osborn K: Liquid therapy: pouring water on your routine, *Body Sense: Massage, Bodywork, and Healthy Living Magazine,* Autumn/Winter 2004, pp 34-42.

Price S, Price L: *Aromatherapy for health professionals,* ed 2, New York, 1999, Churchill Livingstone.

Rose J: *The aromatherapy book: applications and inhalations.* Berkley, Calif, 1992, North Atlantic Books.

Salvo SG, Anderson SK: *Mosby's pathology for massage therapists,* St Louis, 2004, Mosby.

Schnaubelt K: *Advanced aromatherapy: the science of essential oil therapy,* Rochester, Vt, 1999, Healing Arts Press.

Tepperman PS, Devilin M: Therapeutic heat and cold: a practitioner's guide, *Postgrad Med* 73(1):69-76, 1983.

Thomas DV: Aromatherapy: mythical, magical, or medicinal? *Hol Nurs Pract* 17(8):8-16, 2002.

Thrash A, Thrash, C: *Home remedies: hydrotherapy, massage, charcoal and other simple treatments,* Seale, Al, 1981, Yuchi Pines Institute.

Tisserard R: *The art of aromatherapy handbook,* Boulder, Colo, 1977, Healing Arts Press.

Tuckerman B: How to add body wraps to your practice, *Massage Magazine,* Nov/Dec 1999, pp 92-96.

Wissell S: *Aromatherapy educational package for the retailer and health practitioner: part two* [self-published manual], 1996, Quality of Life Associates.

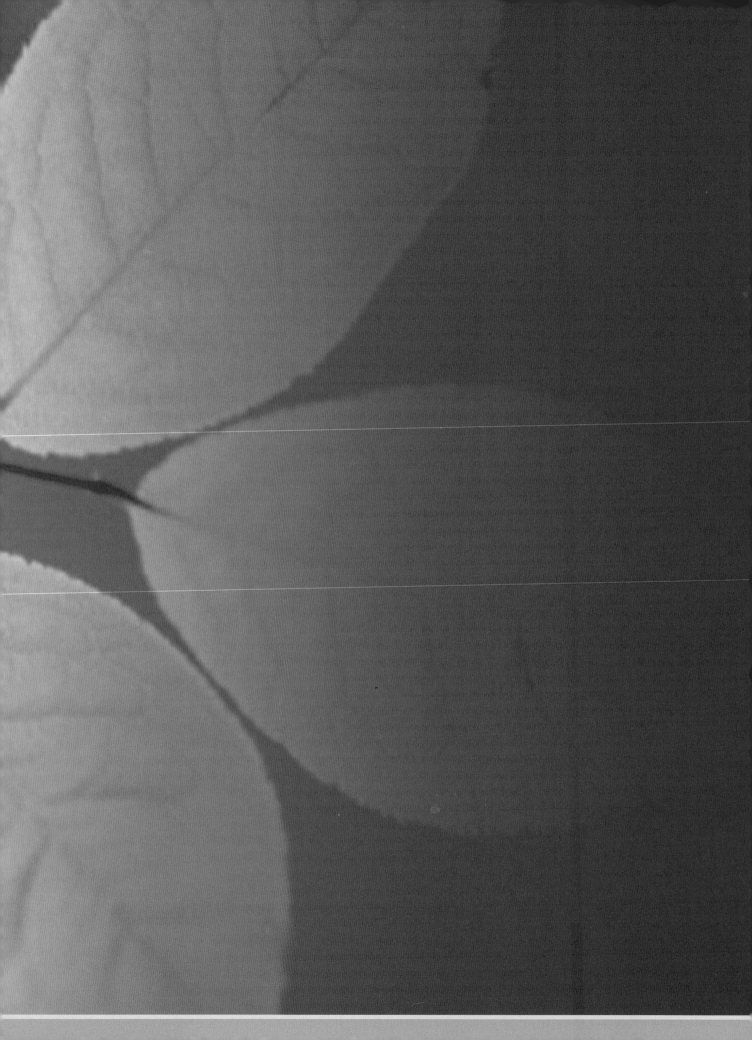

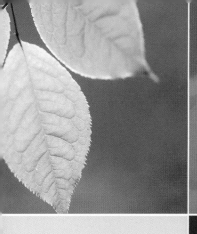

Foot Reflexology

STUDENT OBJECTIVES
After completing this chapter, the student should be able to:

- Discuss the theories of how foot reflexology works
- Identify the 10 zones and the horizontal landmarks on the foot
- Locate all the reflex points on the feet and ankles
- Use the guidelines for reflexology
- Explain the importance of relaxation techniques before the foot reflexology session
- Perform the basic techniques used in foot reflexology

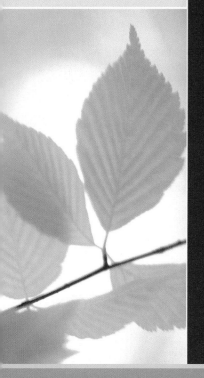

INTRODUCTION

Reflexology originated over 5000 years ago and can be traced back to many countries, including India, Egypt, China, and Japan. Early statues from India of the Hindu god Vishnu depict Sanskrit symbols placed on his feet at the same location where modern reflexologists locate reflex points. One of the earliest pieces of evidence depicting reflexology is an Egyptian tomb that dates back to 2500 BC. It features a physician performing foot reflexology to ease his patient's pain. Underneath the pictograph is carved the words "Do not hurt me." To this statement, the physician replies, "I will act only to help you."

Feet have been revered and considered sacred in many cultures. Jesus washed the feet of his disciples, and Asian students traditionally kissed the feet of their spiritual teacher. Native Americans believed the feet were sacred because they are in contact with the earth's energy; therefore feet should be uncovered to receive life force.

Over centuries, knowledge of this art form spread, and re-flexology was used around the world to ease aches and pains. Modern reflexology developed out of *zone therapy* and the research and writings of Dr. William Fitzgerald in the early 1900s. It was popularized in North America by Eunice Ingham, a physiotherapist, who is affectionately referred to as *the mother of reflexology* (Figure 25-1). She spent most of her life mapping the exact location of reflexes on the feet. Ingham spread her love and knowledge of reflexology through teaching, writing, and demonstrating reflexology on as many people as possible. Her work is still carried on by International Institute of Reflexology through seminars worldwide.

Today in many parts of Europe and China, reflexology is an accepted form of medical treatment that offers health benefits for relief from conditions ranging from a simple headache to diabetes mellitus. In the United States, reflex-ologists can only legally provide clients with stress reduction through relaxation and improved circulation.

One of the reasons why reflexology is so popular is that disrobing is unnecessary, and lubricant is not needed. Fur-thermore, reflexology can be practiced practically anywhere that is comfortable for both the practitioner and the client.

---

evolve *An Egyptian tomb carving that dates back to around 2500 BC can be seen on the Evolve website that accompanies this text. According to the carving, the patient is saying "Do not hurt me." In hearing this, the physician replies, "I will act only to help you."* ■

MINI-LAB

Use a golf ball or tennis ball to stimulate your feet for the times when you are tired and your feet ache. Simply roll the bottom of your foot over a ball placed on the floor, pressing down on areas that feel good. Maintain a comfortable pressure for 15 seconds. Return to these areas for additional work as needed.

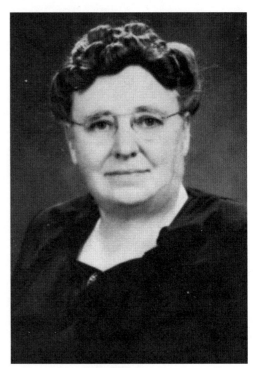

FIGURE 25-1 Eunice Ingham.

MINI-LAB

The following activity is designed to help you achieve self-relaxation and can be used to center yourself before a reflexology session.

Sit comfortably in a chair, feet flat on the floor, sensing the connection between your feet and the earth. Take a few deep breaths through your nostrils, imagining that you are drawing air up from the earth through your feet. As you exhale, allow the breath to exit through your mouth; imagine the exhaled air as it moves out of the top of your head, down your arms, and out through the palms of your hands and your fingertips. In energetic bodywork, the exhaled breath is potential energy.

For the next few minutes, sit and continue to monitor your breathing, anchoring your thoughts in the breath. Sense each inhalation and exhalation as it flows through your nostrils and mouth. When the mind wanders, gently anchor your thoughts with the breath. Your thoughts can be as a playful puppy that cannot be still. Over time, with this simple meditation practice, your mind will become more focused. It is as though you are flexing new muscles. Imagine with each exhalation that the breath traveling down your arms becomes a warm, healing ball of energy in your palms, and the exhalation feeds that ball, sending the flames out through your fingertips.

Having taken the time to center yourself, you can now connect with your client. You may choose to rest the palms of your hands on the client's feet, knowing that you are grounded in the earth's energy and are allowing this energy to flow through your palms and into the client's feet. Imagine the energy continuing out through the top of her head, until both of you are part of a continuous circle of energy, with no beginning and no end.

THEORY OF REFLEXOLOGY

According to ancient Eastern principles, Chi (Ki, Qi) is the life force. All living things are enmeshed in this life force. Chi presents itself as a specific and significant force in the body. In our polarized world, these energy fields flow between North and South poles. Just as iron filings form a specific configuration when a magnet is held over them, this energy travels through the body in a distinct pattern.

In foot reflexology, a mapping technique is used called **zones.** Foot reflexology is basically energy work on the feet (although reflexology principles are applicable to the hands, the focus on this chapter will be on the feet) and is performed with the fingers, thumbs, or knuckles. **Foot reflexology** is based on the theory that our body (e.g., organs, glands, body parts) has reflex points located on the feet and, through applied pressure, energy blocks can be released in corresponding zones to rebalance the entire body. The reflexes in the feet are *reflections* of the body.

Foot reflexologists believe that 10 zones or energy pathways exist in the body, which run vertically from the toes to the head (Figure 25-2). Five zones are found beginning

on each foot, with all ten zones meeting on the head. These zones pass through every part of the body; consequently, all organs, glands, and body parts will fall into one or more of the zones. If you were to draw a line starting at the big toe and continuing straight up to the head, then everything within that line would be considered zone 1. For example, zone 2 is aligned with the second toe; zone 3 the third toe, and so on.

Chi, or life force, travels through these zones. When the body is in a state of health, Chi flows freely. Disease or pain impedes the flow of Chi and represents an imbalance in the life force. Congestion or tension in any part of the zone will affect the entire zone.

During reflexology, sensitivity in a specific zone or reflex point indicates something manifesting in a corresponding organ or body part. Direct pressure will affect the entire zone by directing life force along its natural pathways, untangling *energy knots* caused by physical or emotional stress.

Another theory suggests that by pressing on the feet, toxins and impurities are released by increasing local circulation. The feet are the most distal region of the body. Venous and lymphatic circulation may not be adequate to push these

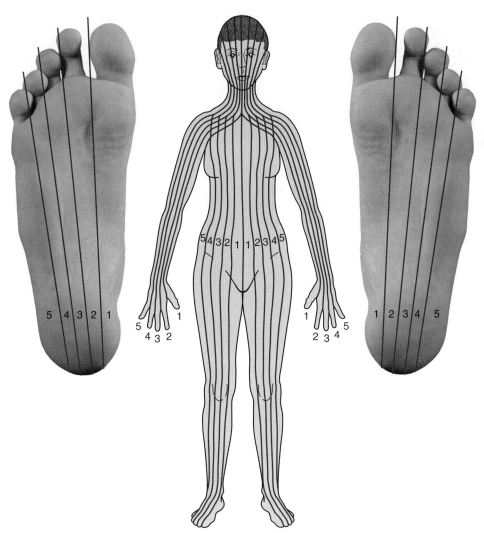

FIGURE 25-2 Zone map of the 10 zones in reflexology.

wastes back to the heart. Reflexology can act to release and return these wastes back into the circulation.

> *"Grow in any dimension and the pain, as well as the joy, will be your reward. The only alternative is not to live fully or not to live at all."*
> M. Scott Peck

Contraindications and Precautions

Reflexology is safe to use with most clients. Contraindications and precautions are the same as with massage clients. For example, do not press on any tumors, cysts, tendons that become prominent when the toes are extended, varicosities, corns, or lesions. The feet are to be avoided when warts, infectious pathological conditions such as athlete's foot, or acute or chronic inflammatory processes such as gouty arthritis are present. If the client is in a weakened state caused by illness, age, or disability, then treatment time is shorter than normal (10 minutes per foot), and the pressure should be considerably lighter than usual. Clients with diabetes and multiple sclerosis often have varying degrees of neuropathy; again, light pressure should be used.

MAP OF THE BODY: ZONES, LANDMARKS, AND REFLEXES

Zones

According to the theory of reflexology, 10 zones exist in the body through which energy travels, five zones on each foot (Figure 25-3). Imagine a line passing from between each toe directly down to the base of the heel and then continuing straight up to your head. Everything in this area in your body, including glands, organs, and body parts, is found in that particular zone located on your foot. If you follow zone 2 from the center of the second toe up through the body, you will pass through the kidneys and eventually the iris of the eyes. Zone 1 passes through the great toe, zone 2 passes

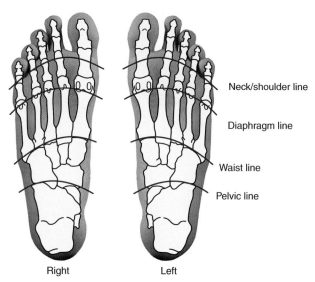

Right   Left

FIGURE 25-3 The four horizontal landmarks in reflexology.

through the second toe, and so on, until you reach the smallest toe, which is classified as zone 5. Each of these zones travels straight up through the body to meet on your head; therefore the head contains all five zones from both feet, totaling ten zones. Any reflexology work done in that zone on the foot affects the entire zone.

Landmarks

The four horizontal landmarks transverses the feet, providing assistance in locating the foot reflexes (see Figure 25-3). They begin at the ball of the foot and work their way down to the heel.

- **Neck and shoulder line**: The first horizontal landmark, which marks the area of the neck and shoulders, is located at the base of the toes, the space where the toes meet the ball of the feet. This area is an important area to work for shoulder or neck pain.
- **Diaphragm line:** The next landmark is located where the ball of the foot meets the arch. In the diaphragm line, you will notice a change in skin texture and color. The edges of the foot rise up until they converge in the center. This line is shaped as the costal arches of the rib cage, which it represents. Just as you can slide your fingers up under the rib cage, you will get the same sensation when working the diaphragm reflex; you can easily slide your fingers up underneath the ball of the foot.
- **Waistline:** To locate the third horizontal landmark, slide your finger down the lateral side of the foot until you feel the tuberosity of the fifth metatarsal. From this spot, trace an imaginary line across to the foot's medial edge.
- **Pelvic line:** The fourth and final landmark is located at the top of the heel.

Reflexes

Once you have an understanding of the zones and horizontal landmarks, you are ready to locate the foot reflexes. Reflex locations and their positional relationships to each other follow a logical anatomical pattern that closely resembles that of the body itself. Glancing at a reflexology chart, imagine that you are laying the feet alongside the body, with the toes next to the head (Figure 25-4).

BASIC TECHNIQUES

Two basic techniques are used in foot reflexology: (1) a general technique called the *walking* and (2) a specific technique called *pointwork*.

Walking Technique

The walking technique is used for working the 10 zones because so many reflexes are along each zone. Typically, the thumb is used when applying the walking technique. To create the *walking* action, bend and straighten the thumb's distal interphalangeal joint. While the thumb of one hand is slowly working the zone, the other is holding the foot

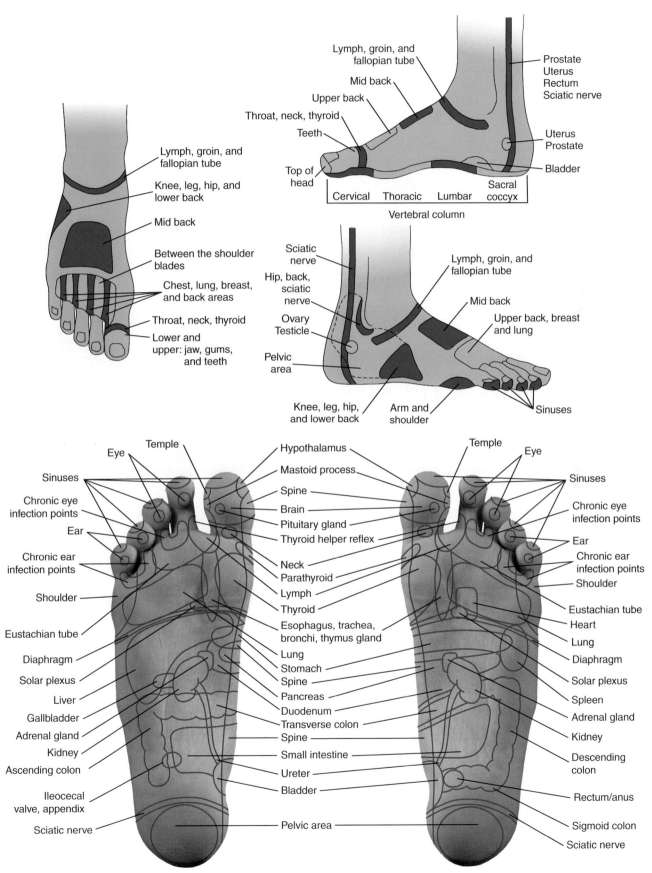

FIGURE 25-4 Reflexology foot map.

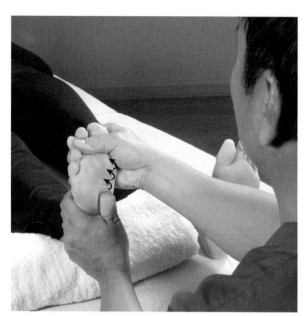

FIGURE 25-5 Thumb walk used to address points in zone.

firmly (Figure 25-5). This strategy ensures that all the reflexes within the zone are stimulated

To find the correct side of the thumb to use, rest your hand on your thigh. The lateral edge of your thumb should be in direct contact with your leg. Begin to walk your thumb from your upper thigh toward your knee, using the technique described in the previous paragraph. As you move your thumb up in small increments, visualize that you are stimulating reflex points (Figure 25-6). Try the walking technique by using your finger. The fingertips are used for hard-to-reach areas such as between the toes, where the thumb is too big.

Pointwork

The second basic technique is pointwork and is used when working specific reflex points. Two methods are used when applying pressure to specific reflexes. The first is *direct pressure*; pressure can be increased by rotating, or flexing, the foot onto the point. The second is called the *hook*; it requires the therapist to apply pressure to the reflex point, then flex and extend the distal joint. This technique can be broken down into three parts. First, locate the desired reflex and apply pressure. Next, bend the distal joint while maintaining contact with the reflex point. Last, straighten the distal joint while maintaining contact. It is as though you are applying the walking technique, only you are not walking to other reflexes (essentially *walking* in place). Pressure is concentrated on one spot, and the movement of the thumb pushes the tissue aside so pressure can be applied more deeply. This technique is used for hard-to-reach areas such as the pituitary reflex, which is deeply embedded in the great toe.

Desserts

Relaxation techniques, also called *desserts,* are used for relaxing the feet before, during, and after a reflexology session. These techniques include shaking the feet and ankles

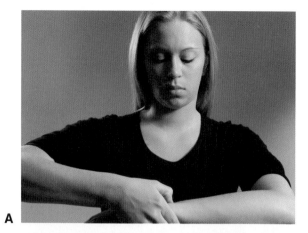

A

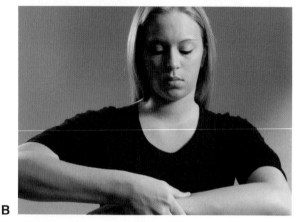

B

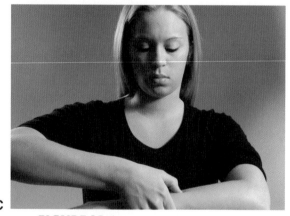

C

FIGURE 25-6 Finger-walking technique.

from side to side (Figure 25-7) and taking the foot through its range of motion (Figures 25-8 and 25-9). If you do whatever feels good to you while you are receiving a reflexology session, it will also feel good to the client. Clients enjoy their feet being kneaded and stroked. Do not be afraid to invent moves. You will discover that your hands and your client's feet work well together.

TREATMENT GUIDELINES

One of the joys of reflexology is that it can be practiced anywhere. Your client may be seated or lying down prone or supine during the session with bare feet.

• Wash your hands before and after each session.

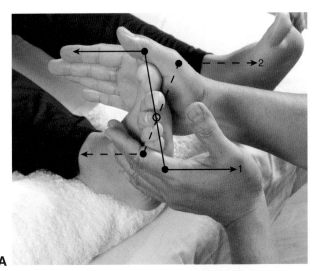

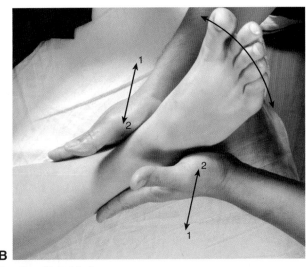

FIGURE 25-7 Desserts. **A,** Foot flop. **B,** Ankle flop.

- To relax the muscles of the feet, begin the session with a footbath; use cool water on a hot day or warm water on a cold day. Use an astringent or a few drops of your favorite essential oil (lavender is good for insomnia or sage for detoxification). An alternative (if you have access to a microwave oven) is to warm two damp hand towels, sprinkle them with the essential oil, then wrap the client's feet. Allow the client to sit back and relax.
- Ideally, the client should remove stockings and his or her feet should be resting on a clean towel.

- The therapist's body should not be unnecessarily bent and contorted or the wrists at extreme angles. The client should not have to hold up his or her body weight but be resting comfortably.
- Do not use oils, gels, creams, or lotions because the foot becomes slippery, and the therapist's fingers and thumbs may slide off reflex points. Additionally, oil often creates the sensation that the therapist's hands are trying to slide over rubber. If any lubricant is used, be sure to wipe off any excess and apply ethyl alcohol before the client

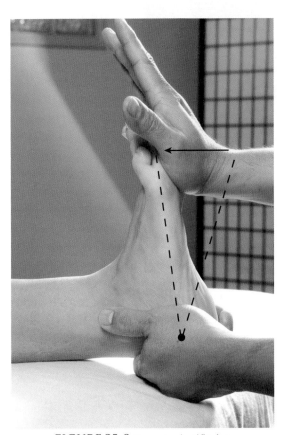

FIGURE 25-8 Desserts: dorsiflexion.

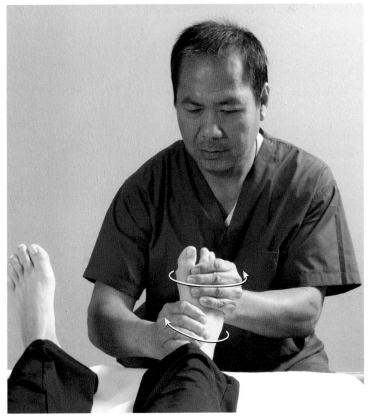

FIGURE 25-9 Desserts: inversion and eversion or *wringing out the foot*.

walks on the floor, which prevents accidents from slips and slides. Keep in mind that ethyl alcohol has a drying effect; avoid using ethyl alcohol or perfumed lubricants if your client has dry or cracked skin on his or her feet.

- Avoid performing reflexology through socks and stockings because the therapist's fingers, thumbs, or knuckles tend to slide off the reflex points, and the client's skin may become irritated from the cloth fibers. Additionally, the reflexes between the toes are difficult to access through socked feet.
- Conduct an interview to rule out any contraindication and to establish client needs.
- Show the client to the area where the reflexology session will take place, and discuss the procedure, answering all questions to the best of your ability.
- Avoid overtreating by working an area too long. Work a reflex point for 15 to 20 seconds.

- You may elect to go back and rework a reflex point.
- Warm up the area well with noninvasive pressure, and increase pressure as the client can tolerate it. Press to the point of dull sensitivity, not pain. Eye contact is a good measuring tool. Watch for signs of tension in the client's face, hand clenching, or body rigidity; ask the client about pressure and adjust it accordingly.
- For pressure on the dorsum (top) of the foot, use the fingertips because less padding is found on the fingertips, and thumb pressure may be too strong. Thumbs are used on the plantar surface of the foot because the thick padding located there requires additional pressure. On the thick skin of the heel, bend your index or middle finger over and use your knuckle.
- If your hands tire, interject dessert strokes.
- After the session, stimulate the feet with a dry brush or dry towel, and dust with a foot powder (Figure 25-10). Help

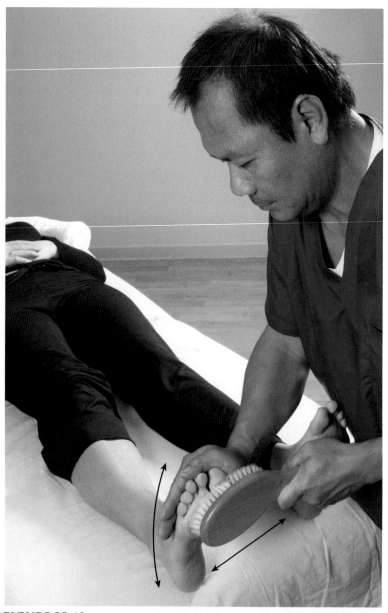

FIGURE 25-10 Therapist stimulating client's feet with dry natural bristle brush.

your client put on shoes and socks or stockings, if appropriate. Asking the client to drink plenty of fluid, namely clean water, for a day or two following the session is helpful.

> **evolve** Watch a therapist performing reflexology by accessing your student account through the Evolve website. Note how the therapist applies direct pressure to the adrenal reflex point while he flexes the client's foot. Included are two figures of how the therapist works on a reflexology client while in supine and prone positions, with the feet placed on a support in the latter position. ■

WHAT TENDERNESS MAY MEAN

Generally speaking, if the client feels only pressure, then his or her reflexes are healthy. When the client feels tenderness, sensitivity, discomfort, or pain during the application of

pressure, it may then mean the reflex or corresponding body area, or both, is under stress or that something is happening in an organ or body part.

Imbalances on the feet can appear in many ways. As the reflex is palpated, the therapist may feel a lumpy or grainy deposit, known as *crunchies*. The general belief asserts that these areas are crystal deposits of uric and lactic acid that accumulate and pool in the feet. These deposits create congestion and blockage around vital nerve functions and interfere with blood circulation to the feet. Also believed is that pressure applied to these areas breaks them down so that the body can more easily reabsorb them into the bloodstream or lymph system, where they can be eliminated.

A client may experience a headache or an increase of elimination through the skin, bowels, or urination. He or she may even experience a flare-up of a current or past illness that had never healed fully. All of these scenarios can be classified as a *healing crisis*; it is the body's way of throwing off

DWIGHT BYERS

Born: February 10, 1929.

"You may be walking on the solution to many of your health problems."

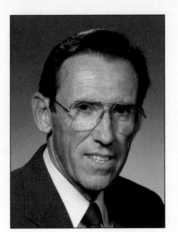

Dwight Byers claims he was one of the guinea pigs for his aunt's early work in reflexology. His aunt, Eunice Ingham, a physical therapist and member of the New York Medical Massage Therapist Association, worked during the early 1930s for a physician who had a passing interest in the art of zone therapy. Zone therapy was a predecessor of reflexology and was introduced in the early 1900s by Dr. William H. Fitzgerald, who successfully used different devices to place pressure on certain points on the hands to relieve pain.

Eunice Ingham took this work a step further and put her own mark on this ancient healing art, which was practiced as far back as 2330 BC. According to Byers, his aunt was strong willed, extremely intuitive, and totally dedicated to easing suffering in her fellow man.

Along with a compassionate heart, Ingham had a keen mind. Her time-honored techniques are the result of experiment, research, and copious notes. She threw out what did not work and perfected what did. Her books, *Stories the Feet Can Tell Through Reflexology* (Ingham Publishing, 1984) and *Stories the Feet Have Told Through Reflexology* (Ingham Publishing, 1984) provide more details on this subject.

Ingham's dedication to helping relieve suffering proved inspirational to her young nephew, who was at first skeptical. His skepticism, along with his hay fever and asthma, vanished after experiencing his aunt's healing touch firsthand.

"At first we kind of laughed at her," remembers Byers, as he shares the stories of traveling with his aunt as she conducted seminars on reflexology across the United States. "I helped her carry her bags and set up. But soon I became fascinated, and eventually my sister and I began helping her teach."

Byers's background as a medic in the U.S. Army and his later experience in mortuary science helped hone some of his anatomy skills as he began practicing reflexology part time. When his aunt died in 1974, Byers formed the International Institute of Reflexology to help preserve the original Ingham method. In 1983, he published his book, *Better Health with Foot Reflexology* (Ingham Publishing, 2001), for the same reason.

This book defines reflexology as "the science that deals with the principle that there are reflex areas in the feet and hands which correspond to all the glands,

(continued)

DWIGHT BYERS (*continued*)

organs, and parts of the body. Reflexology is a unique method of using the thumb and fingers on the reflex areas to help relieve stress and tension, improve blood supply, promote the unblocking of nerve impulses, and help nature achieve homeostasis."

Basically, every aspect of your body can be *found* on the bottom of your feet, and these locations correspond roughly with anatomy, thus the term *zone therapy.* For instance, the gallbladder is located in your upper torso to your right; on the bottom of the right foot, its corresponding point is to the upper portion of the right foot. However, knowing where particular organs are located is not enough. Reflexologists are also trained in physiology to understand how different body systems interface. For instance, while working with someone who might have gallstones, added emphasis is placed on the entire digestive system. Studying the correct pressure and type of motion to employ on the feet or hands is also vital.

"Reflexology sends a message to the organs to normalize, to decrease or increase hormonal levels," explains Byers. His results have been phenomenal, but even he admits that he does not have all the answers to why this method works.

In the foreword of Byers's text, Dr. Ray C. Wunderlich Jr. offers some compelling theories to account for reflexology's success:

"Quite probably, it will eventually be shown that foot reflexology alters energy flow in the body.... There are 7200 nerve endings in each foot. Perhaps this fact, more than any other, explains why we feel so much better when our feet are treated. Nerve endings in the feet have extensive interconnections through the spinal cord and brain with all areas of the body" (From *Better Health with Foot Reflexology,* by Dwight Byers, 1983).

Byers, whose favorite adage is *experience is the father of all knowledge,* claims that the best results are obtained by those who practice, practice, practice. "You've got to work on thousands of feet," he says. "My advice for beginning massage therapists is to master your art. Don't be a jack-of-all-trades and master of none."

Byers believes that the therapist must be the type of person who wants to help people, not someone who thinks of money first. "You've got to give a lot," he says. This statement is not idle lip service from Byers. He has done his share of throwing in an extra free visit for clients and has helped senior citizen clients by providing them with discounted sessions.

Byers is a man who understands people. He is down to earth and pragmatic, and so are his seminars. The final is hands-on, and his feet are up for grabs after a 200-hour program. His criterion for grading: "Would I pay to have this treatment done?"

Massage therapists who become certified in reflexology use it to enhance their business. Beginning the session with reflexology can induce relaxation and increase circulation, which benefits muscles, glands, and internal organs from the inside out.

excess toxins or impurities. More than likely, most of these symptoms will go away in a few days. However, of course, if the client has any questions or concerns, refer the client to his or her physician.

TREATMENT SUGGESTIONS

The foot can be divided into six treatment areas: the head, the chest, the abdominal, the pelvic, the reproductive, and the spinal areas (Figure 25-11). The four horizontal landmarks that transverse the foot previously outlined in the chapter (neck and shoulder, diaphragm waistline, pelvic) are used to delineate five of the six treatment areas; the last area is marked by the foot's medial edge.

Begin by establishing contact with the client. Locate the solar plexus reflexes with your thumbs. Rest your fingers on top of the foot (Figure 25-12). In the body, the solar plexus is often referred to as the *abdominal brain* because it contains a large number of nerves. In reflexology, the solar plexus reflex is referred to as the *key to relaxation.* It is generally located under the ball of the foot between the second and third toes. The client knows exactly when you locate this spot because he or she will often reward you with a generous sigh of relief. Apply pressure with your thumbs in the client's solar plexus reflexes and press while the client inhales; release pressure while the client exhales. Follow the client's breath with our own. As the session proceeds, return to this reflex often because pressing it returns the client to a place of relaxation, especially after deep pointwork. The reflexes will be more accessible if the client is relaxed and if the tissue feels pliable.

> **evolve** *For a sample foot reflexology routine, log on to the Evolve website and choose materials for Chapter 25.* ▪

Next, locate the diaphragm and use a walking technique to help the client breathe with ease, encouraging deeper states of relaxation and a more effective reflexology session.

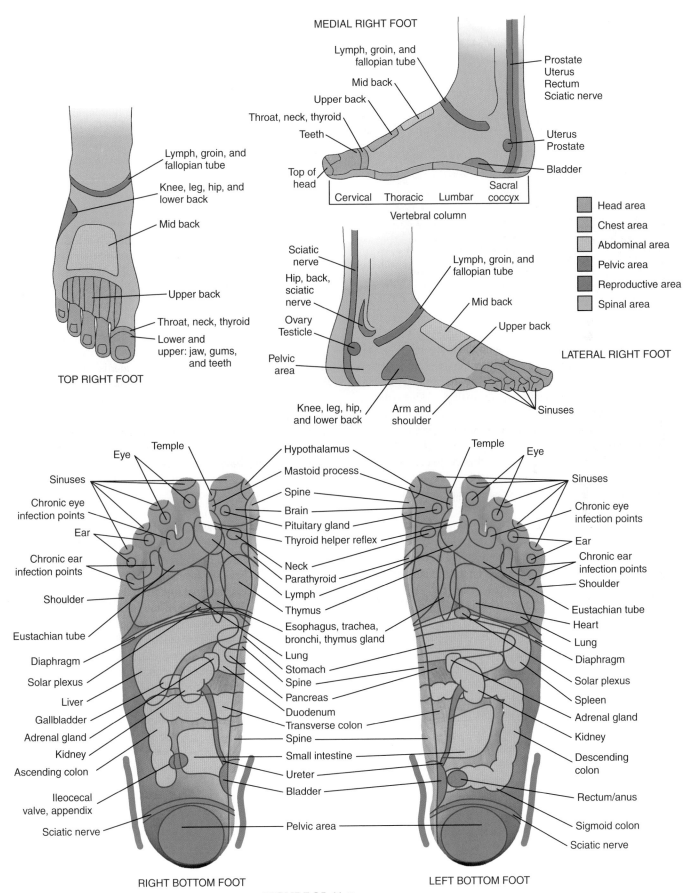

FIGURE 25-11 Six treatment areas.

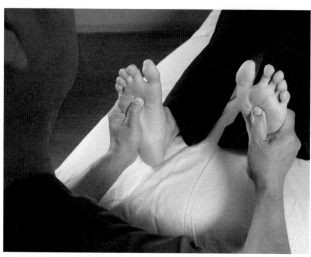

FIGURE 25-12 Therapist holding solar plexus points with the thumbs.

Head Area

The great toe is the head reflex with the brain and pituitary reflexes. Locate the pituitary reflex by looking for the center of the swirl on the big toe and hook into that point with your thumb. It will often feel similar to a small pea. This reflex is an effective reflex to work if a boost of energy is needed or for any glandular problems because of its importance in the endocrine system.

Next, gently squeeze the pads of each toe to stimulate the sinus reflexes. During early spring when the pollen is airborne, this reflex may require additional pointwork.

Chest Area

The ball of the foot is the reflex area for the heart and lungs. In our bodies, the heart is two thirds on the left and one third on the right; this area is represented on the feet. The heart reflex is primarily on the left foot, with a small portion located on the right. The chest area is important to work for asthma and other respiratory conditions. The bronchial reflex is located between the first and second toe. Use a pincer grip and grasp the reflex between your thumb and index finger. Using a thumb-walking technique, work the space between the metatarsals. If the client is congested, then alternately move these metatarsals up and down to enhance the intercostal spaces.

If the client is suffering from shoulder pain, then grasp the lateral side of the ball of the between your thumb and index finger and squeeze firmly. Make sure the client's jaw is unlocked during this technique because this action assists relaxation.

Abdominal Area

The abdomen (in foot reflexology) is located between the diaphragm and the pelvic line. The spleen and stomach reflexes are located on the left foot, and the liver and gallblad-

der reflexes are on the right foot. Work the spleen reflex on individuals who have anemia and who experience blood deficiencies. The liver reflex can be worked for everything from blood sugar to cholesterol to skin problems. Another important reflex to stimulate is the pancreas, located on the right foot just behind the stomach reflex. Both the liver and the pancreas reflexes should be worked thoroughly on anyone with diabetes mellitus. Avoid overworking the reflexes of the abdominal area during the first four sessions because intense reflexology in this area may leave the client feeling overwhelmed and exhausted.

Pelvic Area

Between the pelvic line and the heel is the pelvic area, which houses the organs of the lower abdomen. The right foot contains the reflexes for the ascending colon and part of the transverse colon. The left foot contains reflexes for the rest of the transverse colon and the descending colon. The pelvic area is important to work on individuals experiencing intestinal inflammatory conditions and low back pain.

The reflexes for most of the urinary structures are located here in the pelvic area. The urinary bladder is located where the pelvic line meets the arch of the foot. The kidneys' reflexes are located along the waistline demarcation, between the second and third toes. Because of the kidney's role in filtering toxins from the blood and producing urine, this reflex can be worked for cystitis and blood pressure problems and to encourage the body to rid itself of toxins.

Reproductive Area

One of the last areas worked in reflexology is the reproductive reflex located in the heel. The uterus or prostate reflex is in the medial heel, and the ovaries or testes reflex is in the lateral heel. To locate the reflex for the uterus or prostate, imagine a diagonal line from the high point of the medial malleolus to the base of the heel; in the middle of the line is the reflex point. Use the same measuring procedure to find the ovaries or testes on the lateral heel. Avoid using your thumb to stimulate these reflexes because they are often sensitive. Female clients benefit from work on these areas when they are suffering with emotional imbalances or premenstrual syndrome. Male clients benefit from work on these areas when they are experiencing prostate problems.

The next set of foot reflexes worked is the sciatic nerve. To locate it, imagine a stirrup running from the inside of the calf, medial to the Achilles tendon, to approximately 4 to 6 inches above the anklebone. The client may feel sensitivity if he or she has low back or sciatic pain.

Spinal Area

The last sets of reflexes to be addressed, and one of the most important, are the spinal reflexes, which are located along the medial aspect of the foot. As you look at the arch of the foot, notice how the medial edge possesses four distinct curves, just as does a vertebral column. Because of the importance of these reflexes, they are to be worked in every session. Walk your thumb along the spinal reflexes, pressing on and under the bones of the arch continuously from the base of the heel to the tip of the great toe. If you have only a few minutes to work on the feet, then perform the thumb walk on the entire medial edge of the foot.

"Freedom is what you do with what's been done to you."
Jean-Paul Sartre

.

SUMMARY

The manual manipulation of the feet has been practiced in one form or another for thousands of years. The importance of the feet has been well documented in different customs and cultures throughout the ages. Modern foot reflexology has its roots in the ancient theory and practice of shiatsu, acupuncture, and energy work. The routines we use today were popularized by Eunice Ingham, a physiotherapist of the 1900s. Reflexology postulates that specific points are located on the feet where a reflex mechanism exists for each organ or area on the entire body. Five vertical zone patterns are located on each foot for a total of 10 zones. The reflex for each zone corresponds to the body parts located above, through, or behind it. Problems in an organ are reflected to the reflex point and are exhibited as sensitive *energy knots*. The therapist can act as a catalyst by using reflexology techniques to unblock the river of energy that stagnates at tender reflexes.

One way to locate the foot reflexes is by using a series of horizontal landmarks found on the foot. By using firm but gentle pressure, the reflexologist assists the body to a state of health. Reflexology is a natural addition to the massage therapy practice.

CASE STUDY:

Be Cautious of Labels

Delores has been practicing massage therapy for 10 years. She has a small practice in a local prominent business area. Most of her clients consist of professional men and women who typically have standing appointments. On rare occasions, Delores can work with a new client.

Natalie, the wife of a prominent bank owner, telephoned Delores late one afternoon and requested a massage for 9 AM the next day. Delores had a cancellation and was able to work in a new client on short notice. When Natalie arrived, Delores noted that Natalie was a tall, middle-aged, well-dressed woman adorned with furs and elaborate jewelry. As Delores ushered her to the massage room, Natalie became louder and even more expressive as she discussed the details of her pet poodle, Phoebe. As they sat down to discuss Natalie's health, the stench of whiskey filled the air. Delores realized that her client may be intoxicated and that a dilemma existed.

How should Delores address the situation, if at all?

What risks are involved if Delores decides to massage Natalie in her current state? What modifications should Delores make during the session?

How might Natalie feel if confronted with her alcohol consumption?

What if Delores made an incorrect assumption and Natalie was on prescription medication, was diabetic, or had one small mimosa (i.e., champagne and orange juice) during breakfast?

What if Natalie has received some news that distressed her, such as the death of a loved one, and was doing her best to cope?

What issues might be discussed if the roles are reversed and the therapist showed signs of intoxication?

evolve

Go to *Chapter Extras* **on Evolve for additional illustrations and resources for this chapter.** *Extras* **for this chapter include:**

1. Crossword puzzle (downloadable form)
2. Additional techniques (photograph)

MATCHING

Place the letter of the answer next to the term or phrase that best describes it.

A. Chi
B. Desserts
C. Diabetes mellitus
D. Disrobing or lubricant
E. Egypt
F. Eunice Ingham

G. Fingertips
H. Foot reflexology
I. Landmarks
J. Mother of reflexology
K. Pointwork

L. Ten
M. Walking
N. William Fitzgerald
O. Zone therapy
P. Zones

_____   1. Location of the tomb that features a pictograph dating back to 2500 BC depicting a physician performing foot reflexology to ease his patient's pain

_____   2. Form of therapy out of which modern reflexology developed

_____   3. Person whose research and writings helped develop modern reflexology

_____   4. Physiotherapist who popularized modern reflexology in North America

_____   5. Phrase by which Eunice Ingham is referred

_____   6. Factors that are not required to perform reflexology

_____   7. According to ancient Eastern principles, the term used to describe life force

_____   8. In foot reflexology, the term used to describe the body's energy pathways

_____   9. Term that is based on the theory that our entire body has reflex points located on the feet and, through applied pressure, energy blocks can be release in corresponding zones to rebalance the entire body

_____   10. Total number of zones the body possesses, which run vertically from the toes to the head

_____   11. Condition that requires light pressure

_____   12. Area that runs horizontally and provides assistance in locating the foot reflexes

_____   13. General technique used in reflexology

_____   14. Specific technique used in reflexology

_____   15. A term to denote relaxation techniques that include shaking the feet from side to side and taking the foot through its range of motion

_____   16. What is used to apply pressure on the top of the foot

INTERNET ACTIVITIES

Visit http://www.reflexology-research.com/whatis.htm. Locate the scientific studies regarding reflexology and write a summary of the research.

Visit http://www.reflexology-usa.org and click on Standards and Ethics. Make a poster of the Standards of Practice and display it at your school.

Visit http://www.aboutreflexology.com and click on History. Prepare a one-page report and present it to your class.

Bibliography

Berkson D: *The foot book,* New York, 1977, HarperCollins.
Byers DC: *Better health with foot reflexology: the original Ingham method,* St Petersburg, Fla, 1996, Ingham Publishing.
Dougans I: *The complete illustrated guide to foot reflexology,* Boston, 1996, Element Books.
Norman L: *Feet first,* New York, 1988, Simon & Schuster Publishers.

Additional Resources

American Reflexology Certification Board Study Guide, PO Box 620607, Littleton, CO 81062.
Weil A: *Self-healing newsletter,* 42 Pleasant St., Watertown, MA 02172.

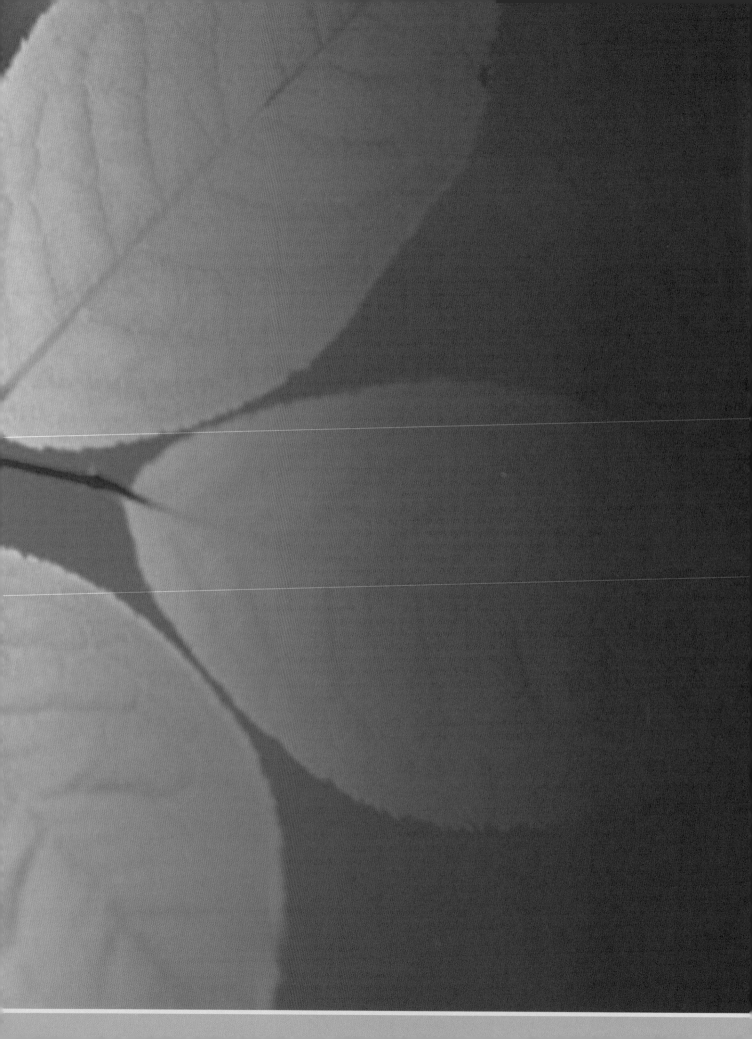

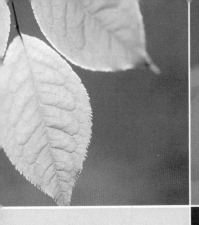

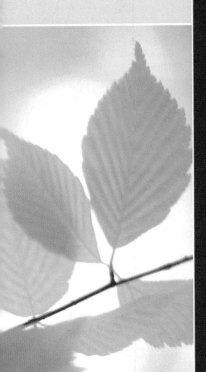

CHAPTER 26

Clinical Massage for Sports and Rehabilitation

Susan G. Salvo, BEd, LMT, NTS, CI, NCTMB
Michael A. Breaux, LMT

"You can't turn back the clock, but you can wind it up again."
—Bonnie Prudden

STUDENT OBJECTIVES
After completing this chapter, the student should be able to:

- Explain the importance of clinical massage
- Contrast and compare a contraction, a spasm, and a trigger point
- Define latent and active trigger points, central and attachment trigger points, and key and satellite trigger points
- Give an example of referred pain
- Define muscle soreness, and list prevailing theories
- Contrast and compare acute and chronic injuries
- Discuss typical causes of sports injury
- List the processes of tissue healing
- Outline factors that affect recovery time
- List stages of rehabilitation and related activities
- Define maximal medical improvement
- Perform a client assessment, and use it to create a plan of care featured in Chapter 8
- Explain and demonstrate techniques used in clinical massage
- Give a brief area-specific clinical massage
- Incorporate an area-specific clinical massage as part of a Swedish massage
- List three client aftercare suggestions
- Explain how to avoid common mistakes of clinical massage
- Explain how to decide which type of sports massage is appropriate for an athlete
- Perform a sports massage routine

INTRODUCTION

Massage therapists are part of a health care team serving clients, most of whom exhibit various injuries and conditions. Research has documented the efficacy of massage. Insurance companies are recognizing massage services as being worthy of payment and reimbursement. The need for rehabilitative massage in clinical and athletic settings has never been greater. For purposes of clarity and consistency, the terms *deep-tissue massage* and *clinical massage* will be used synonymously. Other synonyms are *deep-pressure massage, deep-tissue work, medical massage, neuromuscular therapy,* and *trigger-point work.*

The goal of this chapter is to provide information on trigger points, injuries, tissue healing, rehabilitation, clinical massage techniques, and recommendations for area-specific treatments. These treatment protocols can be used as (1) a stand-alone treatment in a clinical setting (e.g., 15 to 30 minute rotator cuff treatment session), (2) a full-body sports massage session when working with athletes, or (3) a focused segment that constitutes part of a 1-hour massage.

To accomplish these tasks, we will review and develop information that has been covered in other chapters, including assessment, planning, and technique. We also introduce sports massage and how the needs of athletes differ from those of the general public. An **athlete** is someone who possesses natural or acquired abilities such as strength, endurance, or agility required for participating in a sport. The different types of sports massage and their goals are presented.

Several reasons exist for choosing and using targeted techniques. The first reason is *time.* When dealing with prescribed treatments and third-party payers, time is often the limiting factor. In these cases, using techniques designed to rehabilitate the client in a timely manner is important. Recovery time is swifter with deep-tissue techniques compared with other techniques.

The second reason is *effectiveness.* The journal *Medicine and Science in Sports and Exercise* (Gehlsen GM, Ganion LR, Helfst R: Fibroblast responses to variation in soft tissue mobilization pressure, *Med Sci Sports Exerc* 31(4):531-535, 1999) cited a study in which massages were applied with varying degrees of pressure to groups of laboratory rats that had chemically induced Achilles tendonitis. The analysis revealed that the subjects that received *deep-pressure* massage healed faster than those with light or medium pressure. This fact was evidenced by increased fibroblast count in tissue sections taken from the rats' Achilles tendons.

The third reason to learn clinical massage is *need.* Many people who seek massage services have aches and pains and need more than a relaxation massage. Therapists who possess knowledge and skills in both Swedish and clinical massage can address these needs. If you are not prepared to meet their needs, your clients will go to someone who will. Therapists who possess the aforementioned skills are more likely to be hired to work in chiropractic or rehabilitative settings. Therapists deeply interested in clinical massage are encouraged to pursue specialization through continuing education.

Developing precision with your massage skills begins with a solid understanding of anatomy. Repeated opportunities to palpate and compare structures strengthen hands-on anatomy skills immensely. The abnormalities that you encounter most often manifest in the form of muscle spasms, trigger points, and adhesions.

ESSENTIAL INFORMATION

The following information on fascia, muscles, spasms, trigger points, and muscle soreness helps provide a solid foundation for the clinical massage therapist.

Fascia

The most abundant tissue type in the body is connective tissue; one connective tissue type is fascia. According to Juhan, fascias contain a ground substance that possesses two physical states:

- *Sol state:* relatively thin fluid condition that is more pliant and elastic and offers less restriction during movement
- *Gel state:* thicker, more gelatinous fluid condition that is tougher, more inflexible, and can restrict movements

Fascia viscoelastic state can be altered to some degree because it possesses a property called *thixotropism,* the ability to change from one state to the other. Through massage movements that generate heat such as friction, fascia can change from a gel to a sol state. When fascia softens, it becomes flexible and elastic, allowing muscles and trigger points to be manipulated. Thixotropism also occurs during exercise (blood flow increases, and muscle activity generates heat) and with the application of heat such as whirlpool or a hot pack.

> **TABLE TALK**
>
> Effective conversion of fascia, from a gel state to sol state, occur more easily if the body is well hydrated; conversely, the change may not occur as easily if the body is dehydrated. Encourage clients to consume water on a daily basis (i.e., 0.5 oz for every 1 lb of body weight). A 140-lb person should consume 70 oz of pure water each day.

Muscle

As a student moves into the realm of clinical massage, he or she should review basic musculoskeletal anatomy such as origins, insertions, actions, fiber direction, synergist, antagonists, and types of contraction (e.g., concentric, eccentric) from Chapters 13 through 16. Muscles allow our bodies to move, to maintain a position in space (posture), and to produce heat. Muscles receive and respond to signals from the nervous system for movement to occur; skeletal muscle contractions are voluntary.

Spasms

A muscle may experience spasm, often the result of a minor injury such as a strain or contusion. The stress of the injury lowers the threshold (strength of stimuli required to generate a nerve impulse), producing a general or localized contraction; the latter is called a **spasm.** The situation creating the spasm is one of hypersensitivity; the muscle's motor units generate contraction with reduced stimuli.

With increased neurological activity, summation may occur. Recall from Chapter 17 that summation occurs when a subthreshold stimulation is repeated in succession, generating a nerve impulse. The net result may be a rigid zone or knot in part or all of the muscle. Spasms, also known as *tender points*, are basically a neuromuscular event.

Trigger Points

Similar to spasms, **trigger points** are a rigid zone or knot in a muscle, but trigger points can be found in muscle, tendons, fascia, ligaments, and periosteum (Figure 26-1). Unlike spasms, trigger points located in muscles are basically neurochemical events that cause fibers to stick together.

According to Dr. Leon Chaitow, some events leading to trigger point formation in muscle tissue are excessive amounts of acetylcholine (ACh) and calcium, both of which keep calcium-charged gates open on the sarcoplasmic reticulum. This circumstance creates a situation of oxygen-nutrient deficiency, which, in turn, leads to reduced adenosine triphosphate (ATP) production. ATP is needed to release myosin heads and stop contraction. See Chapter 15 for discussion of muscle contraction.

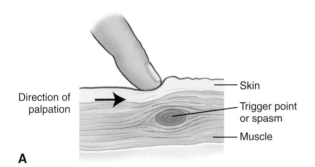

Direction of palpation

Skin

Trigger point or spasm

Muscle

A

What Generates Spasms and Trigger Points?

Some activities that create spasms and trigger points are as follows:

- **Fine-motor movements:** The body is often required to perform movements of constant fine-motor control while maintaining posture, such as computer keyboarding or playing a musical instrument.
- **Gross-motor movements:** These movements occur as large muscle groups generate work to perform activities such as exercise, yard work, or participating in sports.
- **Posture:** Maintaining posture requires constant fine-tuning because the body resists the force of gravity. Muscle contracts to fine-tune the body's position in space as it shifts back and forth. Postural asymmetry such as long leg–short leg and pelvic distortions can stress the musculature and create spasms and trigger points.
- **Stress and fatigue:** This area includes feelings of anxiety and depression, as well as headache. A spasm caused by stress is similar to one caused by injury—the muscle response is the same. Recall that stress produces a response from the body to the demand placed on it. This stress may be emotional *or* physical.
- **Direct trauma:** Tissues can be traumatized directly, as seen in vehicular accidents, slips and falls, or sports injuries. Tissue trauma is always met with inflammation (see section on inflammation later in this chapter).
- **Periods of inactivity:** Oddly, rest does not equate with relaxation, as demonstrated when a person is bedridden for a time. The person who has been lying or sitting for extended periods gets up with pain and stiffness. Hence the adage "the two worst things for your body are overuse and no use."
- **Disease and disorders:** Spasms and trigger points develop in conditions such as fibromyalgia, arthritis, temporomandibular joint disease, and nerve entrapment. Massage is often recommended to reduce the discomfort associated with these and many other conditions, as long as contraindications do not exist.

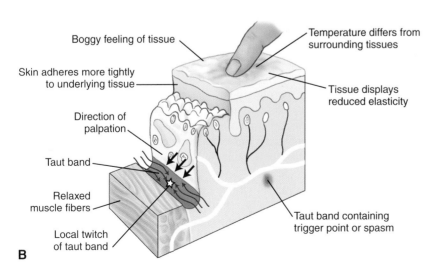

Boggy feeling of tissue

Skin adheres more tightly to underlying tissue

Direction of palpation

Taut band

Relaxed muscle fibers

Local twitch of taut band

Temperature differs from surrounding tissues

Tissue displays reduced elasticity

Taut band containing trigger point or spasm

B

FIGURE 26-1 **A,** Palpation of a trigger point or spasm. **B,** Palpation of a taut band.

- **Miscellaneous factors:** These factors include items such as insufficient strength, lack of flexibility, inadequate hydration, electrolyte imbalance, or lack of proper nutrients.

Repetition of any activity, which involves the law of facilitation, can create a highly synchronized and efficient movement (such as a beautiful golf swing or piano sonata) from hours of practice or dysfunctional, ineffective, and painful conditions (such as stiff neck) from hours in front of computer.

Remember that skeletal muscle contractions are voluntary and stimulated by nerve impulses. Spasm is due to a lowering of the response threshold of the muscle tissue as a result of injury. Trigger points in muscle form as a result of too much calcium and ACh and not enough ATP. We cannot voluntarily shut off the mechanisms of spasm or a trigger point using will power; in most instances, it requires some form of intervention such as massage, stretching, and hydration and, in some cases, the tincture of time. Theories suggest that this spasm reaction to the lower muscular threshold may be involved in the trigger point phenomena in muscle.

Locating Spasms and Trigger Points

Assessment of spasms and trigger points is mainly by palpation. Changes exist in the *feel* of the tissues, and the client will report local tenderness. Additionally, trigger points often induce referred pain phenomena or a local twitch response (see later sections). Both the local pain and referred pain may be either constant or episodic in nature. Not all trigger points refer pain; some are just localized. When locating spasm or trigger points, look for the following:

- Changes in thickness of tissue, resistance to gliding strokes, lumps or strings
- Immobility
- Muscle shortening with weakness
- Edema
- Pain or tenderness
- Hypertonicity
- Temperature changes (area is usually colder)
- Ischemia

When you palpate a possible spasm or trigger point, slide the skin over the underlying tissue while tracing the number *8* or moving in the direction of a compass—north, northeast, east, southeast, south, southwest, west, northwest, north—until the spot of the most tenderness is located (Figure 26-2).

> ### TABLE TALK
>
> According to Travell and Simon's book, *Myofascial Pain and Dysfunction: The Trigger Point Manual,* approximately 75% of pain clinic patients had a trigger point as the sole source of their pain.

Classification of Trigger Points

Trigger points may be classified as active or latent, central or attachment, and key or satellite. Definitions of these terms are listed in the following sections.

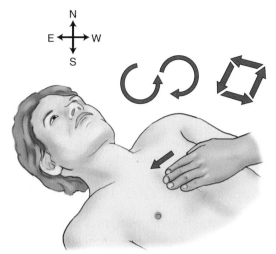

FIGURE 26-2 Compass and figure 8 method for locating trigger points.

Active and Latent Trigger Points

Trigger points can be classified as latent or active, depending on whether they are giving rise to symptoms. All trigger points cause discomfort when compressed, but **active trigger points** cause pain even at rest. An active trigger point may prevent the affected muscle from fully lengthening and may cause it to feel weak. An active trigger point most often refers pain that is remote from the spot compressed. Referred pain is often described as spreading or radiating, and the client recognizes this pattern as part of his or her current symptoms.

Given that an active trigger point refers pain, it may invoke satellite, or secondary, trigger points. As a result, active trigger points can make acute conditions chronic and cause chronic conditions to worsen over time.

A **latent trigger point** has all the same characteristics of an active trigger point, except that it goes unnoticed by the client until pressure is applied. Latent trigger points remain hidden until activated by some stressor such as physical activity, emotional stress, or direct pressure on the muscle. Latent trigger points may be even more important to treat than active trigger points because they are so insidious, lying hidden and dormant and then suddenly producing pain unexpectedly. In many instances, latent trigger points are found during palpation. The client may comment, "I didn't even realize it hurt there."

Central and Attachment Trigger Points

Central trigger points develop almost directly in the center of the muscle, often where the motor end plate innervates it at the neuromuscular junction. **Attachment trigger points** are located at musculotendinous junctions. Attachment trigger points are caused by unrelieved tension characteristic of the taut band that is produced by a central trigger point (see Figure 26-1,*B*).

Therapists who are familiar with muscle fiber direction, as well as the muscle's attachment sites, will easily locate central and attachment trigger points. However, local processes are different and should be addressed differently. Central trigger points should be treated with their contracted central sarcomeres and local ischemia in mind. Hence central trigger points often respond well to heat and compression as a flush of blood irrigates the area and helps remove waste products from injury and inflammation, and attachment trigger points respond well to cross-fiber friction and ice. When possible, treat central trigger points before proceeding to attachment trigger points.

Key and Satellite Trigger Points

Key trigger points are active or latent trigger points that are responsible for activating one or more satellite trigger points. Because a muscle containing trigger points is often weakened by sustained shortening, surrounding muscles are often asked to pick up the slack. This circumstance is one way that satellite points develop.

A **satellite trigger point** is created by key trigger-point activity. A satellite trigger point may arise in pain referral zones of the key trigger point. Satellite points may also arise in an adjacent muscle that works as a synergist or as an antagonist to the muscle harboring the key trigger point.

Clinical experience and research suggest that the deactivation of a key trigger point may relieve activity in satellite trigger points. However, the therapist should treat the satellite trigger points, as well as prevent and arrest the cycle of trigger point referral.

TABLE TALK

Practitioners of medical acupuncture often use trigger points as the basis for their treatment, and studies have shown a considerable similarity between the locations of trigger points and classic acupuncture points.

Referred Pain

When subjected to compression, some trigger points exhibit **referred pain phenomena,** the tendency of trigger points to produce sensations (e.g., pain, tingling, numbness, burning, aching, itching) distal from that of the trigger point. Occasionally, the pain is produced beneath the trigger point itself. According to Dr. Simons, the pain is referred distally from the site of the trigger point 73% of the time, and the pain is produced locally 27% of the time.

Referred pain does not follow segmental, sclerotomal, myotomic, or dermatomal patterns. However, trigger point location and the corresponding zones of referred pain are typically constant from one person to the next. Dr. Janet Travell and Dr. Simons discovered this phenomenon while doing research on myofascial pain syndromes (see Dr. Travell's biography in Chapter 18). Because trigger points and their pain-referral patterns are consistent, we are able to map them.

evolve To gain a better understanding of pain referral patterns of trigger points, access your student account through the Evolve website and click on course materials for Chapter 26. ■

Local Twitch Response and Jump Sign

On application of pressure, the massage therapist may notice two other important symptoms of a trigger point: (1) local twitch response and (2) jump sign. The **local twitch response** is a reflexive impulse that causes the affected muscle or an adjacent muscle to fire or twitch spontaneously.

The **jump sign** is a spontaneous reaction of pain or discomfort that causes a client to wince, jump, or verbalize on application of pressure. Massage therapists should look for jump signs of facial expression, feet leaving the bolster, fist tightening, and so on. When this event occurs, lighten up on pressure, encourage relaxation through deep breathing, and readdress with pressure below the client's pain threshold.

Muscle Soreness

Muscle soreness is a frequent complaint of clients. Two kinds of muscle soreness are (1) immediate and (2) delayed. *Immediate soreness* is experienced during or shortly after exercise or activity, disappearing as soon as the person has rested and blood flow returns to normal (see Mini-Lab).

MINI-LAB

Discontinue this activity immediately if you experience pain. Stand with your arms extended in front of you. With your back straight, slowly lower yourself into a deep knee bend. Stop when your thighs are parallel to the floor. Hold this position, noting where you begin to feel a burning discomfort (it is usually felt in the thigh or the shoulder or both). Maintain this position for a few more moments. Stand up again. Notice how long it takes for this burning sensation to disappear. Normally, when the stress on your muscle ceases and the blood flow returns to normal, the discomfort should subside. This discomfort is an example of immediate muscle soreness.

Delayed-onset muscle soreness (DOMS) is usually not felt until 8 to 14 hours later, reaching a peak 48 hours after activity. Even though DOMS has been under scientific scrutiny since 1902, at present, the actual biological process behind it remains a mystery. Not all theories will be presented, such as lactic acid buildup. Within 1 hour after exercise, most, if not all, of the lactic acid produced is removed. The idea that lactic acid causes DOMS probably evolved from the fact that lactic acid is produced in the muscles during intense exercise and does cause muscle fatigue but not soreness. **Muscle fatigue** is a state of exhaustion or a loss of strength or endurance such as that felt after strenuous physical activity. It occurs from the muscles' use of glucose without adequate oxygen, resulting in a buildup of lactic acid. Muscle fatigue occurs with prolonged contraction; the muscle becomes temporarily weak, unable to generate force. Hence muscle fatigue and soreness are two different processes.

Two prevailing theories of muscle soreness are presented:

1. **Inflammation theory.** Muscles subjected to prolonged periods of work can be damaged, causing microscopic tears within muscles. Pain felt during DOMS is simply part of the inflammatory process as our bodies attempt to repair the damage that has been caused by a workout (e.g., microscopic tears). This circumstance may explain why deep-pressure massage may create soreness in some clients.

2. **Connective tissue damage theory.** A relationship has been established between DOMS and connective tissue damage. A substance called hydroxyproline (OHP) is released into the blood as a result of connective tissue damage (and is excreted by the kidneys). Peak levels of

BONNIE PRUDDEN

Born: January 29, 1914.

"Seeing ahead is fun. But pushing ahead is very hard work."

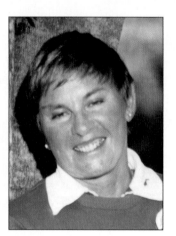

The next time your hands grasp a taut trapezius, remember this: a woman, who, if she had had her way, would have changed our physiological history. At the tender age of 2, your client would have already begun an exercise and strengthening program, supervised by her mother. The body on the table would be flexible, coordinated, and toned—and so would your own.

She is Bonnie Prudden, known in massage circles for her groundbreaking work in myotherapy; but her vision was to change the course of physical education and to develop stronger bodies from the very beginning, rather than provide pain relief for bodies unable to cope with the physical and emotional stress of everyday life.

Why should an individual be so passionate about jumping jacks and push-ups long before fitness became a fad? As a survivor of the Depression, alcoholic and abusive parents, an orphanage, and a stint in Marymount Convent, which she said was similar to trying "to lock a wild horse in a closet," Bonnie Prudden found the outlet she so desperately needed in physical training. She was angry, and that anger fed her boundless, but undisciplined, energy. Prudden says she has physical educators to thank for teaching her the lessons of truth and honor. By contrast, Prudden laughs that her longtime assistant recalls learning nothing more from her physical education classes than the rules for 21 games.

Prudden's fight for better bodies began in the early 1940s. She was part of a team that tested the physical fitness level of children all over the world. The conclusions were frightening. American children were some of the weakest and were getting weaker.

"We are regressing physically," she explains. "Children ride the bus to school, sit down for class, ride the bus home, then sit in front of the TV or play video games until it's time to go to bed. We are a dying nation," Prudden claims, "dying from the inside out."

Ironically, Prudden was unable to recruit physical educators to join her crusade for better health and fitness. However, armed with passion and statistics, she did convince President Eisenhower to start the President's Council on Fitness. (Remember those tests you took in junior high to earn your patch from the president and how you yearned to be the fastest one up and down the rope, the longest distance jumper, or the strongest to throw the softball?)

To some people, implementation of such a program would have been considered a milestone. To Bonnie Prudden, it was a compromise. She knew children could—and should—be stronger. She responded by publishing book after book on the subject and even introduced the first infant exercises in *Sports Illustrated* as early as the 1960s.

However, completely by accident, Prudden came across myotherapy. Through a combination of seeking relief from her own pain after a skiing accident and familiarity with the work of Drs. Hans Kraus, Janet Travell, and Desmond Tivy, myotherapy was born. Travell says it was sheer serendipity.

One morning, Prudden woke up for a mountain climb. She had a neck that was so stiff, it threatened to change her plans. While examining her neck, Dr. Kraus, an associate eager to get on with the climb, grabbed a spot, and Prudden said, "I thought my eyeballs might pop out of my head, it hurt so bad." However, when he let go, her neck was straight.

During work with Dr. Tivy, Prudden's job was to circle the patient's painful area for the physician to inject—a

OHP were measured in urine when peak levels of soreness occurred in individuals. Interestingly, this substance is one of the chemical markers associated the inflammatory response.

DOMS and related inflammation does not result in long-term damage. If it did, we would see declines in the abilities of professional athletes during the course of their careers.

DOMS is not felt at rest. If someone with DOMS were sitting watching television, he or she would not experience DOMS until he or she began to move.

Additionally, DOMS usually follows excessive or difficult exercise or any activity to which the person is not accustomed. For example, if a person worked out in the gym performing exercise at every station for 4 days a

BONNIE PRUDDEN (*continued*)

method pioneered by Janet Travell—then show the client how to exercise the area to prevent further problems. During one of these sessions, Prudden *marked the spot,* and the pressure itself took care of the pain without injection. These events, coupled with her knowledge of anatomy and physiology, led to the study and development of myotherapy.

At the most basic level, myotherapy (*myo,* meaning *muscle; therapy,* meaning *service to*) involves the application of noninvasive pressure to painful muscular areas or specific prescribed points that may cause pain in another location (referred pain or satellite pain). Pressure is applied to these areas—using the finger, elbow, or a special tool—long enough to cut off or limit the oxygen supply to the area or fatigue the muscle, or both, thus effecting change.

These painful areas, or trigger points, are consistently located irritable spots in a muscle that contribute to pain. This recurring pattern allowed Travell and then Prudden to map these points. (Travell laid much of the groundwork for myotherapy. Therapists and students interested in trigger point therapies can benefit from her text, co-authored with Dr. David Simons, *Myofascial and Pain Dysfunction: The Trigger Point Manual,* volumes 1 and 2 [Williams and Wilkins, 1983 and 1992], as well as the medically oriented approach to, and definitions of, myofascial pain disorders.)

Prudden's textbooks on this subject, unlike Travell's, are written in laypeople's terms. Basically, any number of things can cause trigger points. It may have happened the summer you were 8 years of age, and the hay bale came crashing down on your head or just the other day when you lifted the desk to move it a couple of inches away from the wall. It may have even happened during your trip from your mother's womb into your new world. Regardless of the injury or insult to the muscle, trigger points may lie dormant until an emotionally or physically stressful event becomes the proverbial straw that breaks the camel's back. The affected muscle goes into spasm, which splints or guards the area in an attempt to limit usage and prevent further

injury. This spasm-pain-spasm cycle shortens the muscle. Myotherapy returns the muscle to its lengthened, relaxed state.

However, myotherapy does not stop there. Injured and insulted muscles were probably weak or shortened muscles from the start. That is why exercise, which includes stretching, is as integral to the success of myotherapy as the application of pressure to prescribed trigger points.

Massage therapists across the country are beginning to combine different styles of massage, including myotherapy, to address the special needs of clients. For instance, some massage therapists use traditional Swedish massage strokes to warm up the tissue and locate trigger points during the first half of the massage session. Later in the session, they return to these painful areas to apply deeper work, such as myotherapy, concluding with effleurage to flush out toxins that may have been released during the deeper work.

What is Prudden's advice for massage therapists? Exercise and stretch religiously. "You can't help people if you're not in good condition yourself," she warns. She also acknowledges the emotional toll of full-time massage therapy work and recommends a creative outlet such as dance, drawing, or sculpting, which she has incorporated into her school curriculum. She adds that students must get out and teach the community what they have learned about taking care of the body and managing pain.

Today the 93-year-old Prudden takes exercise as seriously as ever, although she has reluctantly heeded her body's message to slow down, which means she does not expect a body with two hip replacements to scale any major mountains. She personally teaches and inspires students at the Bonnie Prudden School for Physical Fitness and Myotherapy in Tucson, Arizona. To learn more about myotherapy, check out Prudden's books on the subject: *http://www.myotherapy.com* and *Pain Erasure* (M Evans, an imprint of The Rowman & Littlefield Publishing Group, Inc., 2002). Prudden has also written the foreword to this edition.

week for the past year, he or she would rarely be sore. However, one fall afternoon, if this person decides to rake leaves for 4 hours, he or she would probably experience DOMS because no exercise in his or her gym mimics raking leaves.

Studies show that the vast majority of pain associated with DOMS is caused by eccentric muscle contraction. Eccentric contractions (or *negatives*, as they are sometimes called in the gym) occur when muscles experience resistance as they lengthen, such as the descending phase of biceps curl.

INJURY

An occurrence that causes tissue damage as a result of violence or accident is an **injury.** The terms *injury* and *trauma* are used interchangeably in this text. You may often see tissue damage referred to as **lesions,** defined as any noticeable or measurable deviation from normal healthy tissue. A lesion can be a mole, wart, or break in the skin; it can also be a tear in the muscle, tumor in the brain, fracture of a bone, or even discoloration of the eye.

Injuries, similar to diseases, are classified according to time of origin, occurrence, and symptom picture. **Acute injuries** begin abruptly; they usually have a recognizable cause (e.g., vehicle accident, slipping or falling) and are characterized by severe symptoms such as pain, swelling, and loss of function. Acute injury management should include protection, rest, ice, compression, and elevation (PRICE). In some cases, rehabilitation of an acute injury was inappropriate or postponed, which may give rise to a chronic injury with accompanying pain, trigger points, muscle spasms, and adhesions.

Chronic injuries develop slowly and persist for long periods, sometimes the reminder of the individual's lifetime. These injuries may be associated with multiple acute episodes, or they may recur because of incomplete recovery from acute injury. Because of the length of time, the original cause may or may not be known. Symptoms of chronic injury are the same as acute injury, just of a lesser degree, with pain being the primary symptom. Chronic injury management includes rehabilitation such as massage, stretching, and physical conditioning and avoiding reinjury (i.e., causative activity).

Working With Athletes: Typical Causes of Sports Injury

The following factors may predispose the athlete to injury; review them with your clients if appropriate.
- *Improper warm-up:* Soft tissues must be warm to achieve optimal elasticity. Failure to properly warm up puts the athlete at risk for muscular tears and fascial restrictions that limit performance. Aerobic activity should be used to raise the heart rate and to get the blood moving through the muscle groups associated with activity. A stretching routine should follow. A min-

imal time frame of 5 to 10 minutes should be spent on warm-up. This time should be increased if the athlete has specific areas of complaint. Warm-up should also be increased as the athlete ages to accommodate the natural loss of flexibility associated with the aging process. Additionally, if competing outdoors, a good rule of thumb is that the cooler the weather is, the longer the warm-up should be.
- *Lack of flexibility:* Muscles that are flexible stretch easily and are injured less. Again, stretching and warm-up is the answer; every athlete should have a stretching schedule in his or her training routine. Remind the athlete that muscles and fascia are similar to clay—they tend to stretch when warm and rupture when cold.
- *Unsuitable equipment:* These items include braces, helmets, or pads that do not fit; worn-out shoes; a bow that is not the right size for the archer; and handlebars and bicycle seats that are not positioned correctly. Unsuitable equipment can damage an athlete's body and his or her performance.
- *Overtraining:* Working too hard or not getting enough rest between sessions can negatively affect health and performance. Look for overtraining symptoms: irritability, fatigue, depression, sleeplessness, weakening of immune system, and DOMS.
- *Miscellaneous factors:* These factors include improper diet and dehydration; competing in abnormal weather conditions such as rain, snow, or extreme temperature and humidity; structural factors such as fallen arches, spinal curvatures, and pelvic distortions; and emotional distractions.

HEALING

Homeostasis is the body's constant migration toward physiological balance. It is a controlled condition, one of relative constancy and equilibrium. When an athlete is injured, homeostasis is disturbed. When tissues are damaged, healing processes are stimulated. Regardless of how much tissue is damaged, our bodies begin immediately to begin repair. Several different methods can be used by which damaged tissue is replaced or repaired. All tissue healing begins with the same initial response—inflammation.

Processes of Tissue Healing

This section introduces the inflammation process followed by the replacement and repair of injured tissues.

Inflammation

Inflammation occurs in response to tissue damage from trauma. Examples of trauma are contusions, burns (chemical and thermal) and radiation, lacerations from injury or surgery, ischemia, allergic reactions, and infection. Inflammation is a protective mechanism; its functions are to stabilize the injured area, contain infection, and prepare the damaged tissue for repair.

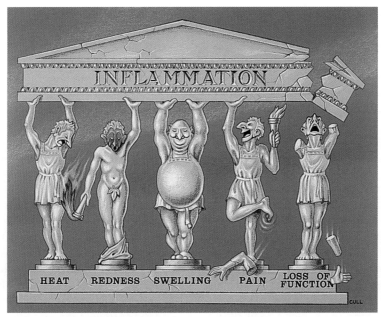

FIGURE 26-3 Cardinal signs of inflammation.

The intensity of the inflammatory response is in direct proportion to the extent of the tissue damage and whether the causative agent remains. The symptoms of inflammation are local heat, redness, swelling, pain, and loss of function (Figure 26-3). The process begins with vasodilation and migration of white blood cells to the site. Vasodilation increases local circulation; thus an increase in heat and redness occurs. Injured tissues respond to injury by releasing histamines and kinins; these chemicals sustain vasodilation and increase permeability in the walls of the local capillaries. These changes allow blood plasma to cross into the interstitial spaces. This excess fluid causes swelling, which results in increased tissue pressure, thereby causing pain. The sensation of pain, combined with swelling and muscle splinting, limits range of motion.

Shortly after the inflammatory response is activated, migrated white blood cells engulf cellular debris, foreign matter, and pathogens. Interstitial fluids cleanse the area and dilute local toxic materials. Clotting proteins located in blood assemble a clot to seal any breaks in vessel walls, to form partitions, and to help isolate the wound. As the inflammatory phase comes to a close (most often between day 4 and 6), other levels of tissue healing begin: resolution, regeneration, fibrosis, and scar maturation.

Resolution

The principal method of tissue replacement is resolution. This process falls in the mild end of the trauma range, such as mild sunburn. As long as cellular membranes are intact and nuclear contents unharmed, the body simply replaces damaged tissue through *resolution*. Most epithelial cells, including the lining of the gastrointestinal tract, undergo daily replacement of aged cells through this process. If tissue damage is between mild and severe, then it must be repaired (and not just replaced) using more involved processes.

Regeneration

Repair of moderately injured tissue occurs by regeneration. *Regeneration* is the process by which damaged tissue is replaced with new tissue of the same type. Naturally, enough healthy undamaged tissue must exist in the area to reproduce itself. In a moderate injury such as a skinned knee, the open wound becomes sealed with a scab, healthy cells underneath the scab divide until the skin has been reproduced completely, and then the scab is sloughed off. No loss of tissue function occurs when an injury is healed through regeneration because the injured tissue has been replaced with the same tissue. When not enough healthy cells are left to replicate, the body then enters a more extreme type of tissue healing—fibrosis.

Fibrosis

If injury is severe enough, the bodily reaction is proportional. In these cases, a repair process is initiated, called *fibrosis* (scar formation). When not enough original tissue is left to repair the wound, fibrosis replaces the original tissue with a *different* kind of tissue, scar tissue. Heat produced from the inflammatory process helps liquefy ground substance in connective tissue's matrix, converting fascia from a gel state to sol state. This process enables specialized cells, called *fibroblasts*, to mobilize and migrate to the area. Fibroblasts secrete collagen fibers, binding wounded tissue to create a scar. In fact, disappearance of fibroblasts at the injury site signifies complete injury repair.

Collagen fibers are formed randomly and are consequently poorly organized. The resulting scar (essentially a patch) is usually stronger than the tissue being replaced. Because scar tissue is not the original tissue type, some loss of function often occurs, such as reduced elasticity. Skeletal and cardiac muscle, as well as central nervous system tissues, are generally repaired by fibrosis.

Fibrosis is often the last stage of tissue healing, but elastic tissues (e.g., muscle, tendon, ligament) undergo a final phase of healing following fibrosis.

Scar maturation — After fibrosis, changes must occur in scars located in elastic tissues to make them pliable. This process is called *scar maturation* or *remodeling*. During this phase, scars are modified by cycles of alternating destruction and creation of collagen fibers. This process occurs naturally with muscle contraction and elongation. Although tissues will heal and scars will mature without any outside intervention, but mobility may be impaired. During fibrosis and scar maturation, an excessive production of collagen often occurs, which infrequently results in irregular, thick, elevated scars called **keloids**. Because much of tissue healing is genetic, the tendency to develop keloids is influenced by heredity.

During fibrosis, adhesions may develop. An **adhesion** is bands of scar tissue binding two or more tissues together that are normally separate. Adhesions may appear as thin sheets of tissue, similar to plastic wrap or as thick fibrous bands. This normal response can occur after surgery, infection, trauma, or radiation. Repair cells within the body cannot tell the difference between one structure and another. If a structure undergoes repair and comes into contact with another part of itself, or another structure, then scar tissue may form to connect the two surfaces.

To review:

Resolution: replacement of aged or mildly damaged tissues

Regeneration: repair of damaged tissue with same tissue type

Fibrosis: repair of damaged tissue with a different tissue type, forming a scar. This process may include a secondary phase called *scar maturation* in which scar tissue is made pliable.

Factors Influencing Recovery Time

The following factors will affect the recovery time and healing rates:

- *Age of patient:* Children typically heal faster than adults. Children have a growth hormone in their systems, which stimulates faster recovery than adults. In cases of bone injury, children have a greater ratio of living bone tissue, periosteum, and blood supply in contrast to adults. Higher amounts of living tissue provide more raw materials for repair. As we progress through the drying-out process that we call aging, tissues such as bone grow brittle and susceptible to fracture.
- *Wound condition:* A clean, sutured wound heals faster than an untreated wound. A sutured wound not only places the edges of the wound in contact with each other for improved healing but it also supports tissue healing by reducing the stress placed on it by the pulling of skin, muscle, or other tissues in different directions. Infection can slow or halt the rate of recovery.
- *Health and habits of the patient:* Healing rates are influenced not only by the health of the patient but also by choices he or she makes. For example, excessive al-

cohol or barbiturate use slows the metabolism. Disease or habits may decrease the supply of oxygen through smoking, sleep apnea, or respiratory illness, or affect the body's metabolism and immune response such as diabetes, autoimmune diseases, or acquired immunodeficiency syndrome.

- *Nutrition:* Good nutrition with an adequate supply of vitamins, minerals, and protein will promote healing. Improper nutrition will retard the healing process.
- *Circulation:* For tissue to heal, oxygen delivery and waste-product removal are necessary to sustain cellular reproduction. Because these prerequisites are all provided by the circulatory system, circulation is probably the most important factor in the rate of tissue healing. Moreover, because blood supply is different for different tissue types, the time factors for healing and recovery will also differ. Lack of adequate circulation and resultant oxygen depletion can cause necrosis. In these cases, surgical débridement is needed before healing can progress.
- *Type of tissue injured:* Different tissue types have varying rates of healing. The cells of epithelial tissue, which make up the skin, are constantly being renewed by cell division. At the opposite end of the spectrum, peripheral nervous tissue regenerates very slowly, if at all. Connective tissue and muscle tissue heal at different rates because of their blood supply. Muscle has excellent blood supply and generally heals faster than an equal section of bone. Bone tissue and adipose connective tissue take a little longer to replace than muscle tissue, and the less vascular forms of connective tissue such as ligaments and tendons are even slower. Cartilage, a relatively avascular tissue, is among the slowest to heal.

"A muscle can never be neutral—if it doesn't work for you, it works against you."
Jack Meagher

REHABILITATION

Rehabilitation is the process of restoration of a person who has had an illness or injury so as to regain maximal self-sufficiency and function in a normal or as near-normal manner as possible. The word *rehabilitation* comes from the Latin word *rehabilitare,* meaning to "make fit again."

Many clients seek out massage services to rehabilitate injuries and address the resulting pain. Some clients are directed to your office by their physicians. Some clients contact their therapist before physician's evaluation. The prudent therapist obtains physician clearance before treatment on clients who present with injury.

Rehabilitation, or recovery, begins after the acute phase, usually day 4. No rehabilitation can take place until redness and swelling are significantly reduced. Getting out of the acute stage as quickly as possible is imperative because being sedentary for longer than 3 days may slow total healing time.

Stages of Rehabilitation

Rehabilitation occurs in three main stages. The first stage's objective must be met before proceeding to the next. Rearranging the order or omitting one of the stages may hinder the rehabilitation process or exacerbate the condition. For example, stretching and strengthening a muscle before eliminating the spasm may interfere with treatment goals.

These stages of rehabilitation are discussed in the following section, highlighting the role of the massage therapist. Reviewing the *principles of neurological law* would be helpful (see Chapter 17). You should also review *mechanisms of the pain cycle* (see Chapter 5).

First Stage: Evaluation

First, the therapist determines which muscles are housing spasms and trigger points and uses appropriate techniques such as effleurage, compression, sustained pressure, and friction. Palpation and client inquiry are the best methods for locating them. Furthermore, taut areas and areas that are sensitive to pressure can lead the therapist to speculate about the client's posture and gait, given that muscle tightness is related to their dysfunction. Massage reduces spasms and trigger-point activity and alleviates ischemia. Massage relieves neurovascular entrapment by relaxing taut muscles and fascia. Muscles in spasm exert a pull on their attachment sites and may rarely cause certain bones to be tractioned out of place; their tightness across a joint may lead to an increased intrajoint pressure. Massage to the muscles crossing the affected joints causes muscles to relax and therefore reduces intrajoint pressure.

Address faulty body mechanics by evaluating shoe wear, dysfunctional postures, and inefficient movement habits (see the section Assessments). These changes may be facilitated by teaching the client new postures for sleeping, sitting, or working, or referring them to other specialists for braces, orthotics, or therapeutic exercise. Many distortions that are longstanding are often taken as normal; the client's discomfort serves as a mystery. Remember that muscle spasms, trigger-points, and faulty body mechanics can block therapy goals and must be addressed first and concurrently. As mentioned earlier, distortions in posture or gait can lead to muscle spasm and trigger points and vice versa. This stage of rehabilitation begins approximately 72 hours after the injury and lasts approximately a week.

This stage also includes suggesting that the client begin or maintain a balanced diet and drink plenty of fluids because these measures will positively influence rehabilitation. This protocol often includes a diet high in protein and reduced alcohol consumption.

Second Stage: Conditioning

Once muscle spasms have been located and reduced with massage, and after dysfunctional biomechanical patterns have been identified and addressed, a period of postinjury conditioning begins. This period includes a regime of stretching, weight training, and aerobic exercise. Notify the client's physician of the plan of care you have devised, and obtain approval and further recommendations before beginning this stage of rehabilitation.

The first activity is stretching. In most cases, the injured area is stretched for five repetitions, two or three times per day. The client increases his or her activity level slowly, adding more repetitions and time each week until a maximal goal is reached (physician or trainer determined). The injury may become irritated as the workload gradually increases, but this irritation is a necessary step toward improvement. The addition of any new therapy (massage, chiropractic, exercise, stretching) may cause a temporary inflammatory response in the tissue. The client usually perceives this inflammation as muscular soreness. The body normally acclimates to the addition of the new treatment by the fourth to sixth session. Remind the client to listen to his or her pain. Soreness is acceptable, but sharp pain is not. If clients are overdoing it and feel increased discomfort, then reduce the repetitions, or take a day off. On the flipside of this situation, also remind the client that being pain free does not equate to being fully healed.

As regular stretching becomes a daily habit, the time comes to begin increasing activity with weight training and aerobic exercise. These and the aforementioned activities are usually done under the supervision of the client's physician or other qualified professional. The second rehabilitation stage begins approximately 1 to 2 weeks after starting the stretching program. To prevent repeated injury, involved muscles and muscles that cross-affect joints must be strengthened. Strength training can be accomplished with rubber tubing, free weights (dumbbells or canned goods), or exercise machines.

Aerobic exercise begins at the same time as weight training. This combination will help build the client's endurance while further building strength. Swimming, walking, running, or biking is great conditioning exercises for building endurance. Classes taught by certified instructors are also excellent choices.

Few people can go from having an injury to a lifestyle that is devoid of some rehabilitation program without having future flare-ups that tend to worsen over time. The massage therapist's role at this stage is to support and encourage the client to follow the prescribed program, along with keeping him or her as pain free as possible with massage. This process will reduce the likelihood of future problems for the client while allowing him or her to lead a lifestyle compatible with his or her wishes and desires.

Third Stage: Maintenance

The third stage is essentially a maintenance stage, with the continuation of the conditioning activities tailored to the client's lifestyle. This stage also includes such modifications as suggesting stress reduction and a massage therapy maintenance plan. The therapist continues to support and encourage the client in his or her quest for health and well-being.

NOTE: Some activities listed in the stages of rehabilitation may be outside a massage therapist's scope of practice. The treatment team may include the client's physician, chiropractor, physical or occupational therapist, a personal or athletic trainer, and a nutritionist.

To review:

- **First stage:** Eliminate spasm and trigger-point activity and address faulty body mechanics.
- **Second stage:** Restore flexibility and strength to muscles and joints and rebuild endurance.
- **Third stage:** Address diet, stress, and emotional well-being.

TABLE TALK

Maximum Medical Improvement

Maximum medical improvement (MMI) refers to a phase or end of recovery. MMI is based either on clinical findings (clinical MMI) or on elapsed time since the injury (statutory MMI). Clinical MMI is based on (1) the client is functional and recovery is complete, or (2) no further recovery from or lasting improvement to an injury can reasonably be expected. The client's physician determines MMI.

The time frame of statutory MMI varies from state to state and is partially based on the nature and the extent of the injury (e.g., ankle vs. spinal injury) and methods used to repair the injury (e.g., physical therapy, surgery).

Working With Athletes: Rehabilitation

Athletes must be handled differently from the average client. Athletes are constantly training their bodies to be strong and function effectively. They tend to fuel them with proper nutrition and stretch to maintain flexibility. For these reasons, the metabolism and hence the healing factors of athletes tend to function more efficiently than those of the average client. Athletes will snap back faster from minor muscular injuries, often in approximately one half the time of sedentary clients. However, damage to ligaments and tendons have a fairly consistent healing time and will heal no faster in athletes.

Another factor to remember is that, although asking the average client to devote some time to rest while recovering from an injury is often necessary, this does not always hold true for athletes. Recommending that they stop exercise is counterproductive to their training and interferes with the trust necessary for the therapeutic relationship to function properly. Athletes generally are more motivated than the average client, and they have to be educated in not overdoing their rehabilitation. Suggest that these clients cut back on their training, either cut back one third on repetitions, or cut back one third on weight, or cut back one third on time spent training.

ASSESSMENTS

Performing assessments is an important component of massage in that it gives direction and purpose to the session while giving the therapist an opportunity to use his or her critical thinking skills. Assessments are performed after using the PPALM method of interviewing (see Chapter 8). The

client's primary concern determines if formal assessments are made and the extent of the assessment. For example, a client who receives a massage to relax does not merit his or her gait and posture to be evaluated. Assessments featured in this chapter are as follows:

- Observation
- Palpation
- Posture
- Gait
- Range of motion

Before assessment begins, explain briefly what you are planning to do, why you are doing it, how long it will take, what position changes it will require, and what equipment you will use. Eliminate as many distractions and disruptions as possible. Wash your hands before and after the assessment, preferably in the client's presence. Warm your hands and any equipment before touching the client, and be aware of your nonverbal communication and possible negative reactions from the client.

Observation

The initial component of all clinical assessments is observation. The therapist gains much information regarding the client when watching facial expressions while conversing. Palpation, posture, gait, and range of motion all involve observation. This assessment includes noting swelling, redness, bruising, lacerations, deformity, and the client's general demeanor.

Palpation

Palpation is touching with purpose and intent. In massage, the primary purpose of palpation is to locate treatment areas such as taut bands, spasms, and trigger points. However, palpation can also reveal other aspects of the client's health (e.g., swollen lymph nodes), which affect treatment (i.e., local or absolute contraindications). Palpation requires you to touch the client with different parts of your hands using varying degrees of pressure. The therapist looks for the following:

- **Anomalies:** Do any superficial or deep masses exist, such as lipomas or swollen lymph nodes? These masses represent a local contraindication. Swollen lymph nodes accompanied with fever represent an absolute contraindication.
- **Client reaction:** Does pressing the area produce pain or discomfort? Is it localized, or does it refer to other areas? These areas often represent a massage indication. Does the client report lack of sensation? This circumstance necessitates light pressure during massage until the cause is determined.
- **Edema:** Does the area feel swollen, mushy, or congested? Does any pitting edema exist (prolonged existence of pits produced by applying pressure)? The cause needs to be ascertained because edema from heart or kidney conditions denotes an absolute contraindication.
- **Twitching:** Is a muscle firing involuntarily or twitching when pressure is applied, indicating a trigger point? This circumstance often represents a massage indication.

- **Moisture:** Is the skin overly moist or dry? Dry skin suggests excessive stress (sympathetic nervous system activation). Dry skin may also indicate use of an emollient lubricant along with a stress-reduction element to the massage. Moist skin may also indicate excessive stress because the oil and sweat glands become activated under stress. Moist skin needs less lubricant than dry skin.
- **Temperature:** Is the skin overly warm, suggesting inflammation, or cool, indicating ischemia? Localized heat represents a local contraindication, and systemic heat represents an absolute contraindication.
- **Superficial fascia:** Does the skin glide easily or with difficulty when moved over the underlying structures? Most fascial restrictions can be addressed with massage

Posture

The body's position in space, such as sitting, standing, lying supine, and lying prone, is regarded as **posture.** Standing is the baseline measure of balance and alignment because posture is maintained through strength and tone of muscles against gravity. Misalignment of the body is frequently the source of chronic pain. Abnormal posture produces spasms and triggers points and vice versa. Improved posture reduces spasms and trigger points.

> **evolve** An anterior and a posterior view of the human body featuring major postural muscles are located on the Evolve website. Access your student account and choose course materials for this chapter. ■

Train your eyes to evaluate the structure by taking baseline measurements in several planes of the body. A plumb line, poster grid, or other aids may be used, but deviations may be determined without these items if you possess keen observational skill. Some therapists find that taking Polaroid photographs of the client is helpful in assessing posture.

Look for excess tension or atrophy in major muscle groups, comparing them bilaterally. Look for muscular imbalances between anterior and posterior musculature. Survey major postural signs of imbalance, such as a pelvic bowl, which spills the abdominal contents and signifies an anterior pelvic tilt; knees locked back, contributing to a posterior pelvic tilt, or overly bent; shoulders rolled forward and in; forward head posture; abnormal spinal curvatures (e.g., scoliosis, kyphosis, lordosis); long leg–short leg faulty base of support from collapsed arches or feet rotating out or in; high or low ear position on one side; and uneven facial features. Abnormal spinal curvatures require bolstering to increase client comfort while on the massage table (see Chapter 10). Chart any deviations. Use the following landmarks for posture assessment:

Horizontal landmarks are divided into two groups, and each landmark should appear relatively symmetrical left and right, as well as equidistant from the ground, on each side (Figure 26-4). Deviations should be noted.

Anterior
- Ears
- Eyes
- Top of the acromioclavicular joints
- Anterior superior iliac spines
- Top of the greater trochanters
- Top of the patellas
- Top of the fibular heads
- Top of the medial malleoli

Posterior
- Ears
- Occiput
- Scapulas
- Posterior superior iliac spines
- Top of the greater trochanters
- Calcaneus

Vertical landmarks are divided into two groups and should be in a vertical line that is perpendicular to the ground in respect to one of the following planes (Figure 26-5). Deviations to the left or right of the respective plane should be noted.

Midsagittal Plane
- Nasal septum
- Manubrium
- Umbilicus
- Pubic symphysis

Coronal Plane
- External auditory meatus
- Humeral head
- Femoral head
- Lateral epicondyle of femur
- Lateral malleolus

> ### TABLE TALK
> According to Andrew Taylor Still, because our body structure governs its function, tension in muscles and misaligned bones cause unnecessary strain on the body as a whole. This theory proposed in 1874 still holds true today.

> **evolve** Images of anterior and posterior pelvic tilts, as well as how a difference in leg length can affect pelvic alignment, are found in the course materials for Chapter 26. Log on to the Evolve website to access these important images. ■

Gait

A person's walking pattern is his or her **gait.** A normal gait pattern is smooth, coordinated, and rhythmic. A person's posture can be described as erect, with eyes looking forward and the arms extended to the sides and swinging forward in opposition to the legs. The thumb and forefinger of the hand should face forward. The toes point forward, with the feet positioned slightly apart.

HORIZONTAL LANDMARKS

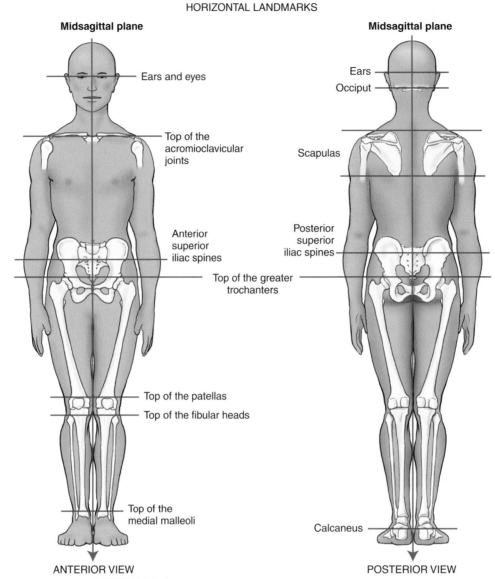

FIGURE 26-4 Horizontal landmarks—anterior and posterior views.

In describing the biomechanics of gait, two phases of gait are commonly used: (1) stance and (2) swing. The *stance phase* begins when the heel of one foot strikes the ground and ends when the toe of the same leg lifts off. The *swing phase* represents the period between a toe off on one foot and heel contact on the same foot. Perry states that the stance phase accounts for approximately 60% of one cycle, whereas the swing phase accounts for the remaining 40% at ordinary speeds. Keep in mind that assessing gait will be difficult unless the client is able to walk away from and toward the therapist.

MINI-LAB

Split the class into two groups: One group will observe while the other classmates walk. The observers will assess posture and gait. Hold a group discussion to identify structures and the muscle groups used. Have the two groups trade roles and repeat.

Range of Motion

Range of motion (ROM) is the movement around a joint or set of joints. Often called flexibility, ROM is used to determine which muscles, tendons, and ligaments to target during the massage. You can also use ROM to provide instant feedback to the client (e.g., whether treatment improved motion). Both passive and active movements are important.

When performing ROM, either move or have clients move the unaffected side first, if the condition is not bilateral. This factor establishes a baseline for the client's *normal* range. Next, address the affected side, stopping or asking clients to stop at the point of discomfort. Note when the client encounters pain by watching for facial grimaces, muscle guarding, apprehension, or the use of accessory muscles.

Active ROM measures the client's movement using voluntary muscles. Passive ROM measures movement by the therapist while the client relaxes. Note the **end-feel**; this is what is felt at the end of passive ROM and indicates limitation from

VERTICAL LANDMARKS

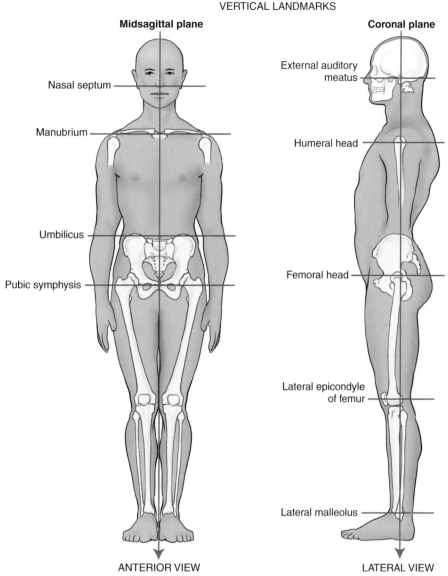

FIGURE 26-5 Vertical landmarks—anterior and lateral.

bone or muscle. *Hard end-feel* has an abrupt end of motion and is produced by an anatomical stop such as bone, which is what is felt at the end of elbow and knee extension. *Soft end-feel* has springy, spongy end of motion, such as the end of finger, shoulder, and hip movement. If a hard end-feel is felt at a joint that normally has a soft end-feel, then the presence of abnormal muscle contraction such as a contracture may be noted. If a soft end-feel is felt at a joint that normally has a hard end-feel, then a tight muscle crossing that joint may be noted.

Now that we have a better understanding of assessment protocols, let us examine which techniques may be used to address problems indicated by assessments.

TECHNIQUES

In this section, you will learn about techniques associated with a clinical practice. These techniques are needed to address pain at its source, such as a tight calf or trigger points

in the traps. Realize that the therapist has the flexibility to use any massage technique at any time. For example, flushing effleurage is used to warm up an area before deeper work begins and between clinical massage techniques. Swedish gymnastics such as joint mobilizations and stretching are used to reset tone and stretch muscles after sustained pressure and friction. Swedish gymnastics is discussed in Chapter 7. Dr. David Simons states that stretching is essential to the treatment of a muscle after releasing spasm and trigger points so as to rebalance the tissues surrounding an affected joint. Specific techniques include the following:

- Compression
- Sustained pressure
- Friction
- Myofascial release

Before discussing technique, we must first address pressure. Pressure applied in clinical applications of massage is slightly more aggressive than a relaxation massage. Some level of mild discomfort is usually associated with clinical massage—for example, a pressure that produces a discomfort level of a 6 to 7 on a 10-point scale. Do not exceed an 8 on a 10-point scale.

Compression

Description

Compression is rhythmic pumping on the muscle. With compression, blood is pushed out of the areas followed by a flush of blood when compression is released. This technique broadens the muscle, which will usually induce muscles to relax. Compressions are used on muscled areas such as the arms, thighs, back, hips, and posterior leg.

Technique

During compression, pressure is applied perpendicular to the muscle belly. The therapist shifts his or her weight forward, thereby transferring pressure down into the muscle belly and then releasing the pressure without breaking contact with the client's skin. Compression strokes are done rhythmically and may resemble a bounce. The therapist's wrist should be above a 90-degree angle (180 degrees is applying pressure with a fist) with the elbows slightly bent to prevent elbow joint strain. The client may be clothed or unclothed, with compression applied through a drape, if necessary. Lubricants are not required for most compression strokes.

Variations

One-handed compression. This variation implies that one hand is used to apply pumping pressure. When the palm is used, it is called *palmar compression*. The therapist may elect to place one hand over the other; this procedure is often referred to as *hand-over-hand compression*. The hand may be shaped as a fist, with the proximal phalanxes making contact with the client's skin and is called *fist compression*.

Two-handed compression. Two-handed compressions are executed using both hands simultaneously, usually side-by-side. The hands can also slide away from each other on the downward pressure and lift the tissue while moving toward the first position, called *fulling*. Because fulling effectively broadens the muscle, it is often referred to as *broadening*.

Twist compression. This compression is applied similar to one-handed compression except that the downward pressure ends with a twist. This twist is usually accomplished with an external rotation of the shoulder instead of a forearm supination to reduce wear and tear on the elbow. Because it is reminiscent of opening a jar of baby food, this move is often referred to as *baby jar lids*.

Sustained Pressure

Description

Sustained pressure is held pressure applied to trigger points and spasms for a 3- to 7-second time frame. This technique relieves pain and discomfort. It is referred to as *ischemic*

compression because the skin tends to blanch under the pressure as a result of compression of the capillaries and brief loss of blood flow to the area.

Technique

Apply pressure with thumb, forefinger, knuckle, or elbow. Generally the pressure is exerted perpendicular to the body's surface, but a diagonal angle may be needed to compress the tender area against a bone (Figure 26-6). Some tender areas, such as those found in sternocleidomastoid, require the tender area to be compressed between two fingers of the therapist's hand in a pincer grip fashion. This technique is done dry, using little or no lubricant.

Some muscles have a tendency to *roll* under pressure, such as the biceps brachii or muscles of the erector spinae. The therapist may have to stabilize the muscle with one hand while treating with the opposite hand to prevent rolling.

The pressure is sustained for 3 to 7 seconds. Release pressure (for 3 to 7 seconds), and reapply pressure for another 3 to 7 seconds. If the pressure produces a local twitch response, then pressure may be maintained until this muscle firing stops, even if it exceeds the 3- to 7-second recommendation. Continue pressure application, and release until (1) softening of the tissue is perceived or (2) the therapist realizes that other methods are needed to assist tissue release such as compression, friction, effleurage, or hydrotherapy.

When pressure is sustained, keep in mind that the tissue is not receiving nourishment. Consequently, less time spent over each trigger point and then repeated is preferred over a longer sustention.

Friction

Description

Friction is performed by rubbing one surface over another. Friction, specifically deep friction, is an excellent technique for reducing adhesions between tissue layers. Deep friction can also minimize the size of keloids, often in just a few sessions. Massage can aid scar maturation by further increasing scar pliability.

Technique

Friction, specifically deep friction may be applied with the palm of one or two hands, or specific work may be done with the tips of the thumb, fingers, knuckles or elbow (see Figures 7-34 and 7-35). The therapist's hands do not slide over the skin but move the skin (and superficial fascia) across tissue layers beneath the skin. Friction may be circular, pressing down and around an area, or you can use linear reciprocating movements. Frictioning techniques are done dry, using little or no lubricant.

Unlike sustained pressure, friction is applied for 12 to 15 seconds. Similar to sustained pressure, the pressure is released (for 3 to 7 seconds) and reapplied for another 12 to 15 seconds. Continue pressure application and release until (1) softening of the tissue is perceived or (2) the therapist

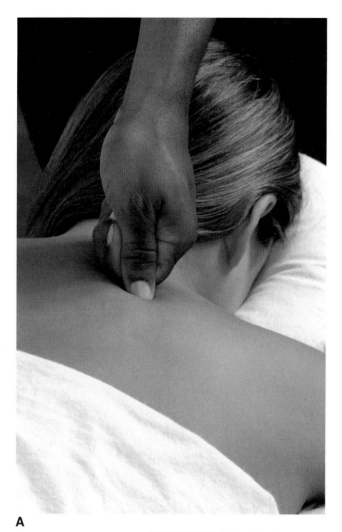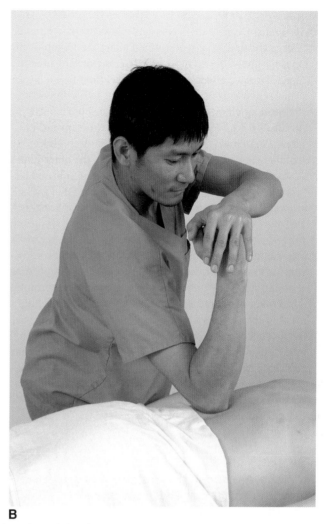

A   **B**

FIGURE 26-6 Sustained pressure. **A**, Using a braced thumb. **B**, Using an elbow.

realizes that other methods are needed to assist tissue release such as compression or hydrotherapy.

Variations

Cross-fiber friction. Also known as *deep-transverse friction,* cross-fiber friction is a precise and penetrating form of friction popularized by Dr. James Cyriax, who called it the most rehabilitative massage stroke. The direction of movement should be perpendicular to the pattern of muscle (see Figures 7-34 and 7-35).

Chucking friction. Chucking, or *parallel friction,* refers to deep friction applied in the same direction as muscle, tendon, or ligaments. The therapist uses his or her thumb or fingers to rub up and down forth, moving the superficial tissue over the underlying structure. Chucking is usually performed one handed while the other hand is supporting the limb that is being massaged (see Figure 7-36).

Circular friction. Circular friction uses small, circular movements that glide the superficial tissue layer over underlying tissue in several different directions using the fingers or palm of hand (see Figure 7-37). This move-

ment is particularly useful around joints and in bony areas (see Figure 7-38). Palmar circular friction applied using quick, circular movements is used to warm and prepare an area for skin rolling and myofascial release.

Myofascial Release

Description

Myofascial release (MFR) refers to a group of manual techniques used to reduce fascial restrictions. Several variations for achieving this result can be used, including *deep gliding, torquing,* and *skin rolling*.

Technique

Most techniques use a mild to moderate stretching pressure with specific directions into the fascia. This action is done to release the fascia from surrounding tissue to which it may have become adhered. The stretch to release this connective tissue can be created by pressure on a fascial plane or by tractioning a body part when held in a certain position.

Variations

Deep glide. Deep glides consist of slow, deep, controlled glides and are usually performed along the length of the muscle fibers. To be most effective, downward pressure creates a wave effect, separating muscle and fascia layers. This action can be done with thumb, index finger, fist, forearm, or elbow. The therapist may use both hands, one to direct the glide and the other to exert downward pressure. *Pin and stretch* is a variation of the deep glide. One hand anchors the tissue with pressure as the other glides away from it, stretching and releasing the muscle and fascia (Figure 26-7).

Torquing. Torquing is used for extremities and involves grasping the skin with both hands and rotating the tissues in one direction held around the bone's axis (Figure 26-8). As the fascia and muscular layers release, the tissues begin to loosen and unwind. This technique can be time consuming but is more practical for treating extremities than other methods of myofascial release. Massage lubricant is not necessary.

Skin rolling. Skin rolling involves lifting and compressing the skin and superficial fascia. Skin rolling is a technique essential to *Bindegewebsmassage* (connective tissue massage). Because no downward force is used, skin rolling is one of the few massage techniques that may be applied over bony areas.

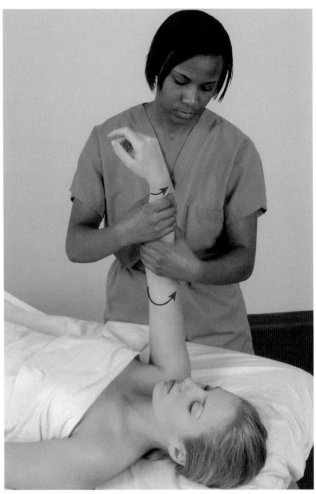

FIGURE 26-8 Torquing.

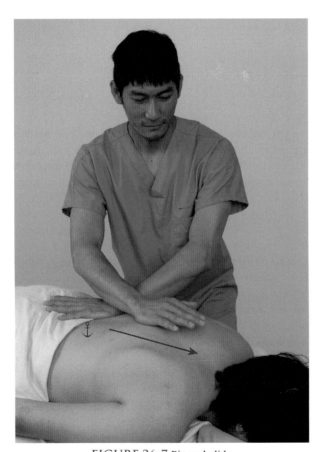

FIGURE 26-7 Pin and glide.

Skin rolling may be initially uncomfortable for the client; therefore move gently and respect the client's pain threshold. Some areas are vascular and sensitive; thus overworking an area may leave the client bruised and sore.

Remove any excess lubricant. Grasp and lift the skin between the fingers and thumbs, compressing the tissue. Roll the skin as though you were rolling a pencil, using your fingers to scoop up the skin as you move across the area (see Figure 7-26).

Continue the rolling technique until the designated area has been treated. Tissue may be lifted using the sides of two hands (see Figure 7-27). The skin may also be lifted between the thumb web of one hand and the fingers of the other hand (see Figure 7-28). Both thumbs may also be used with the thumbs apart and moving in opposite directions, called an S-curve (Figure 26-9). Because the superficial fascia lies in several planes, lift and roll the skin in several directions. If the skin is not lifting, then do not force the tissue into this position. You should address the area two or three times in a session, allowing time between each application.

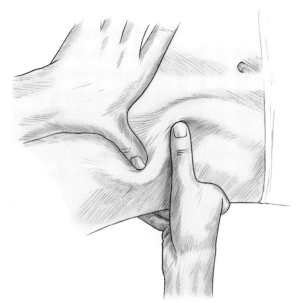

FIGURE 26-9 S-curve technique.

Lymphatic Drainage

Lymphatic drainage techniques enhance fluid movement in the treated area, thereby improving oxygenation, nutrient supply, and waste removal. Practitioners trained in lymphatic drainage are reminded to apply proper techniques before and after treatment. This method involves light pressure (i.e., less than an ounce per 2 cm^2) usually toward the node cluster draining a particular area. Light pressure is needed to encourage lymph flow without increasing blood filtration, as does deep gliding pressure, which creates a shearing force, and can temporarily inhibit lymph flow.

Practitioners who are not trained in lymphatic techniques may prepare and flush the treatment area using light effleurage applied centripetally (toward the heart) before and after treatment.

TREATMENT

The prudent therapist allows 72 hours to pass before beginning treatment. Given that reducing muscle spasm is the first priority, locate any tender spot, whether a spasm or trigger point. The premassage interview is needed to gather information about where to look for trigger points. The client may report persistent localized pain—areas in the body where pain comes and goes. A map of trigger points can assist in locating them (Figure 26-10). When using the trigger point map, locate tender areas. These areas will most likely be within the hollow circles, at 1-inch intervals along the serrated lines, and along the lines of the grids. Concentrate on the client's area of complaint.

When located, use a combination of effective techniques (e.g., sustained pressure, compression, direct pressure, friction) to reduce pain and discomfort. Remember that pressure should be approximately 6 to 7 on a 10-point scale. These spots are usually bilateral, with one side being more symptomatic than the other. Both sides need to be treated. Give central trigger points priority over attachment trigger points. Avoid even stretching the muscle before releasing its central trigger points, then its attachment trigger points, to avoid further inflaming the muscle's attachments.

When deciding when to release the muscle tension in an area, consider its purpose and usefulness. If the tension is caused by use of poor body mechanics to perform an activity, such as raking leaves, then this technique is appropriate; if it is caused by an intervertebral disc, then it should be left alone, at least until the problem has been assessed and corrected.

Treatment Tools

The most commonly used treatment tools of clinical massage therapists are pressure bars. These tools are used to help prevent overuse injuries to the thumb, as well as hard-to-reach or hard-to-treat areas such as the area between the ribs.

Caution is needed over any endangerment sites or areas near bony protuberances. Hard tissue, such as bone, can be felt with these instruments just as rock or even a grain of sand can be located with a small wooden stick.

Make sure all tools used are washed with soap and water or sterilized in the top tray of a dishwasher run on a hot water cycle. A bag or sheet of plastic can be used to wrap the treatment tool and discarded after use to exercise sterile technique or any other procedures recommended by their manufacturers.

COMMON MISTAKES

Overworking the tissue, especially injured tissue, is the most common mistake novice therapists make. The two types of overworking mistakes that can negatively affect any given treatment area are (1) working too deep and (2) working too long. Experience is the best teacher. Until you progress to a point at which you are comfortable judging pressure, tissue density, and tissue resistance, limit your pressure and duration of treatment. For the beginning therapist, the general rule for deep pressure is no more than 5 minutes of treatment to any given region. The best course of action is to treat the area for a short time and then move to another muscle for a while before returning to the original treatment site. In other words, three 2-minute treatments to the rhomboids are better than one 5-minute treatment.

With experience, the therapist gains skill and confidence. Using the following factors, the clinical therapist can properly judge how to modify treatment times:
1. **Client's massage experience.** Someone who has had weekly massages for the last 5 years is going to be more comfortable receiving deep pressure than a client who has never received a massage or who has had few massages. An experienced client will be better able to give direction and feedback to the therapist, even if it is their first session with the therapist. You can increase treatment time at the request of an experienced massage receiver.

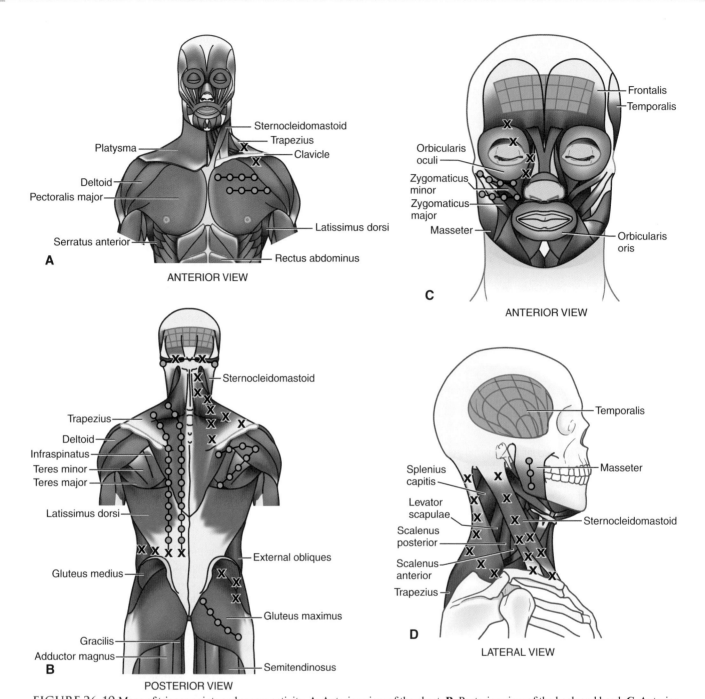

FIGURE 26-10 Maps of trigger points and spasm activity. **A,** Anterior view of the chest. **B,** Posterior view of the back and head. **C,** Anterior view of the head. **D,** Lateral view of the head. **E,** Anterior view of the right upper extremity. **F,** Posterior view of right upper extremity. **G,** Anterior view of right lower extremity. **H,** Posterior view of right lower extremity.

2. **Experience of the therapist.** A therapist with 5 or more years of full-time massage experience can better use his or her own judgment when exceeding the recommended guidelines.

3. **The level of familiarity between the client and the therapist.** If you are just starting to use clinical techniques but have done 20 to 50 massages on one certain client, then the established rapport and familiarity with the client's body are reason enough to exceed the treatment time for that client.

4. **Physical condition of the client.** Clients who are physically fit, such as athletes, are more conditioned, more

body aware, and can handle deeper pressure than the average client.

AFTERCARE

When working with injuries, treatment may increase the local sensation of discomfort and the referred pain patterns. Educating clients about expectations regarding their pain level following injury and treatment will be necessary. First of all, they should be taught that some increase in soreness is common and may be expected. This circumstance is true for almost any new therapeutic modality (chiropractic

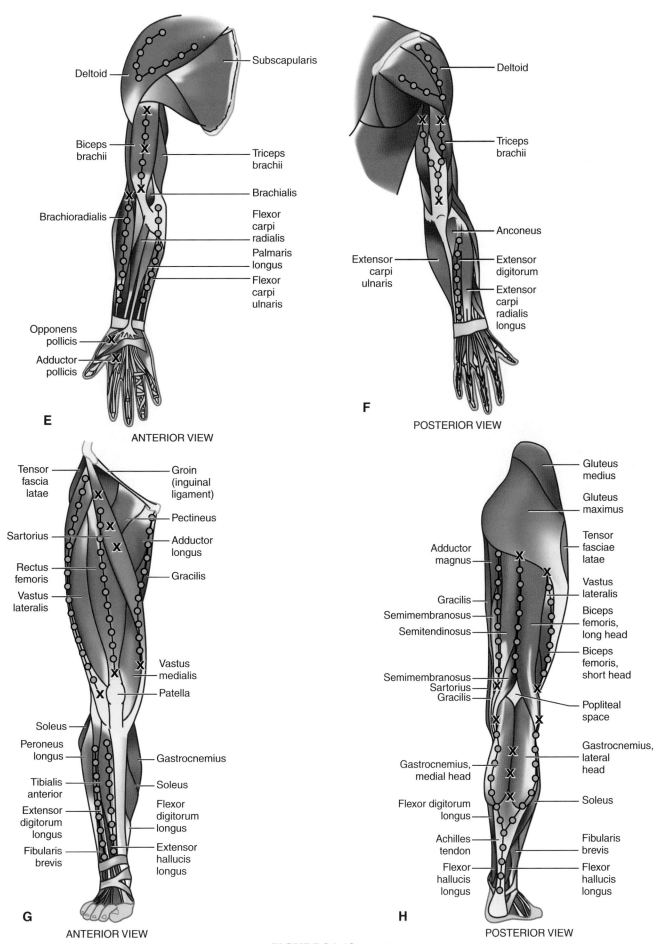

E
ANTERIOR VIEW

F
POSTERIOR VIEW

G
ANTERIOR VIEW

H
POSTERIOR VIEW

FIGURE 26-10, cont'd

adjustments, electrostimulation, acupuncture, exercise, yoga stretching, and so forth) but is especially applicable when the client has been injured. The body perceives the treatment as increased sensory input. While the occasional miracle client will feel better after just one session, in most instances, between four and six sessions are needed before the body becomes acclimated to the new treatment and begins to respond. Some recommended aftercare suggestions for clients are the following:

- Stretches
- Self-massage with or without tennis balls
- Stress-reduction techniques such as meditation, guided imagery, breathing exercises, and strolling outdoors
- Changing sleeping with proper support
- Nutrition such as increasing intake of fiber and water
- Ergonomics such as computer monitor height, keyboarding, or telephone headset
- Regular exercise
- Salt and soda bath (1 cup each; soak for 20 minutes)
- Ice and heat

---

evolve *Log onto your student account on Evolve for a detailed list of pain managing techniques.* ■

SPORTS MASSAGE

The goals of sports massage are similar to those of regular massage, with one big difference: Sports massage focuses on increasing human performance in an activity or sport. Sports massage is divided into three categories: (1) *event,* (2) *maintenance,* and (3) *rehabilitative* massage.

Event Massage

Event sports massage encompasses treatments given around a sports event and can be further divided into three subcategories: pre-event, inter-event, and post-event massage.

Pre-Event Massage
Pre-event sports massage focuses on increasing the circulation to muscles and increasing flexibility. Massages given before a sports event are quick and moderate in pressure, leaving the athlete's muscles relaxed yet ready for action. The most effective massage techniques to accomplish these goals are compression, fulling, tapotement, jostling, and nonspecific friction. Sports massage can enhance performance potential by reducing apprehension before the competition. Avoid using headrests or bolsters at events because time is a major consideration, and accessories slow treatment time. Begin with the client prone and the client's shoes left on with toes off the end of the table. The time frame is from 10 to 20 minutes.

Inter-Event Massage
Inter-event massage is given between games or events and within a 1- or 2-day period. This type of massage will be short and light; problem areas are addressed generally and

receive attention after assessment (rehabilitative massage). The goal of therapy is to assist the rapid return of the body to a state of homeostasis. Apply the same techniques used in pre-event massage, minus tapotement.

Post-Event Massage
Post-event sports massage occurs 30 minutes to 6 hours after the athletic event. During the post-event treatment, the therapist focuses on moving wastes out of the muscles, as well as spreading muscle fibers. This massage promotes rest and recovery by relaxing the muscle and increasing blood flow. Faster recovery time means that athletes can return to their sport promptly. Naturally, techniques that increase circulation and relieve muscle spasms and soreness are preferred (e.g., effleurage, compression, jostling, fulling, pétrissage). Avoid tapotement or deep, specific techniques because the athlete's muscles may spasm easily in their hypersensitive physical state. Avoid causing pain as a result of the aforementioned reason. For soreness, gentle movements in a pool or use of hydrotherapy (see Chapter 24) are also recommended.

Maintenance Massage

Maintenance massage encompasses the full picture of the client's subjective needs and emphasizes prevention. Sports massage not only enhances performance but also promotes healthy tissue by addressing common tension patterns, spasms, adhesions, and trigger points. The routine is essentially a modified Swedish massage that addresses tender areas with clinical techniques. This time is also good to implement self-care programs that facilitate independence and support the athlete's goals.

Rehabilitative Massage

Rehabilitative massage takes into consideration presentation of soft-tissue injuries. Enhanced recovery after injury is another benefit of sports massage. This goal is achieved through increased circulation, which brings much-needed oxygen and nutrients to the injured area. Review the section on rehabilitation earlier in the chapter for treatment recommendations.

"Everyone is ignorant, only in different subjects."
Will Rogers

TARGET AREAS IN THE ATHLETE

To develop a treatment plan for the athlete, several questions should be asked to gain insights (listed in Box 26-1). The following list will give you some ideas regarding specific areas to treat:

- **Running athletes,** including joggers, sprinters, hurdlers, and marathon runners, may have pain in the joints and muscles of the entire lower extremity.
- **Racquet sports,** which include tennis, squash, and racquetball, involve areas of the ankle and calf, lower back, shoulders, elbows and knees.

BOX 26-1

Questions to Ask Athletes at Every Session

Were you sore after the last massage? If so, for how long? Did it negatively affect your performance?

Was the blend of general and specific work a good combination for you?

Do you have any suggestions for this session?

- **Cycling sports,** which include mountain biking, may frequently involve the neck, shoulders, forearms, hands, the low back, and the entire lower extremity.
- **Swimming sports** typically involve tightening of the neck, shoulders, upper arms, and the entire lower extremity.
- **Contact sports** (football and rugby) involve the hands and shoulders, the low back, and entire lower extremity.
- **Jumping sports** (basketball, volleyball) involve the shoulders and entire lower extremity.
- **Baseball and softball** are sports that frequently tighten the neck, shoulders, chest, upper and lower back, and abdomen.
- **Golf** can involve the wrists, elbows, neck, shoulders, chest, upper and lower back, and knees.

COMMON TREATMENT AREAS

The following areas of the body are common treatment areas for a variety of pathological conditions. Each area has a list of muscles that should be on the therapist's *must treat* list for a given area. Use the trigger-points maps (see Figure 26-10) to locate important tender areas and the recommended techniques to address them.

Neck and Head

Suboccipitalis (rectus capitis major and minor, capitis oblique superior and inferior)
Temporalis
Sternocleidomastoid
Frontalis
Trapezius
Levator scapulae
Paraspinals (transversospinalis and erector spinae)
Splenii (capitis and cervicis)
Scalenes (anterior, medius, posterior) (Figure 26-11)

Shoulders

Rotator cuff (supraspinatus, infraspinatus, teres minor, subscapularis)
Deltoid
Trapezius
Pectoralis (major and minor)
Rhomboids (major and minor)
Serratus anterior (Figure 26-12)

Low Back and Hip

Quadratus lumborum
Paraspinals (transversospinalis and erector spinae)
Iliopsoas (iliacus and psoas major)
Gluteus maximus, medius, and minimus
Piriformis
Quadriceps femoris (rectus femoris, and vastus intermedius, medialis, and lateralis)
Hamstrings (semitendinous, semimembranosus, biceps femoris)

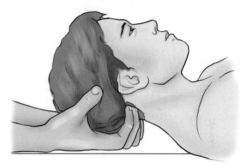

FIGURE 26-11 Cranial base release (suboccipitals and attachment sites of neck and shoulder muscles).

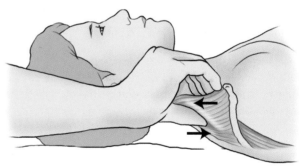

FIGURE 26-12 Unrolling upper traps

SUMMARY

Massage therapists are called on to work on clients who present various injuries and conditions. Having knowledge and skill in locating muscles, spasms, trigger points, and fascia is important. The therapist must also understand injury types, tissue healing, rehabilitation, clinical massage techniques, and treatment for specific areas of the body.

This chapter presents this information, and the student therapist is responsible for gaining as much experience as possible. Many people who seek massage services have aches and pains and need more than a relaxation massage. Therapists who possess knowledge and skills in both Swedish and clinical massage can address these needs. This knowledge includes working with athletes as well. Knowing the types of sports massage and which is appropriate for what setting, as well as technique skill, goes a long way toward meeting an athlete's unique needs.

evolve

Go to *Chapter Extras* on Evolve for additional illustrations and resources for this chapter. *Extras* for this chapter include:

1. Crossword puzzle (downloadable form)
2. Injury dynamics (flowchart)
3. Two-handed compression used in sports massage (photograph)
4. Fulling used in sports massage (photo series)
5. Treatment modalities (flowchart)
6. Clinical application protocol of massage therapy (flowchart)
7. Neurological laws: presentation and discussion (essay)
8. Overloading versus overtraining (essay)
9. Injury management: PRICE (essay)
10. Tissue healing rates (essay)

MATCHING I

Place the letter of the answer next to the term or phrase that best describes it.

A. Acute	E. End-feel	I. Lesion
B. Athlete	F. Fibrosis	J. Muscle fatigue
C. Chronic	G. Inflammation	K. Regeneration
D. Delayed-onset muscle soreness	H. Injury	L. Trigger point

_____ 1. Any noticeable or measurable deviation from normal healthy tissue

_____ 2. Someone who possesses natural or acquired abilities such as strength, endurance, or agility required for participating in sports

_____ 3. Soreness felt 8 to 14 hours after activity resulting from torn tissue, connective tissue damage, and inflammation

_____ 4. Hyperirritable knot found in muscle, tendon, ligament, fascia, or periosteum that is not mediated by the nervous system

_____ 5. State of exhaustion or a loss of strength or endurance felt after strenuous physical activity

_____ 6. Occurrence causing tissue damage resulting from violence or accident

_____ 7. Injuries that begin abruptly, usually have a recognizable cause, and are characterized by severe symptoms such as pain, swelling, and loss of function

_____ 8. Injuries that develop slowly and persist for long periods, sometimes for the remainder of the individual's lifetime

_____ 9. Protective mechanism that occurs in response to tissue disturbance from trauma, lacerations, or infection

_____ 10. Repair of damaged tissue with same tissue type

_____ 11. Repair of damaged tissue with a different tissue type, forming a scar

_____ 12. Feeling at the end of passive ROM indicating limitation caused by bone or muscle

MATCHING II

Place the letter of the answer next to the term or phrase that best describes it.

A. Active
B. Attachment
C. Central
D. Key

E. Latent
F. Local twitch response
G. Referred pain

H. Satellite
I. Spasm
J. Rigid zone or knot

_____ 1. Localized contraction caused by a lowered neurological threshold, often as a result of stress or injury

_____ 2. Common characteristic of a spasm and trigger point

_____ 3. Trigger points that cause pain even at rest

_____ 4. Trigger points that go unnoticed by client until pressure is applied

_____ 5. Trigger points that develop in center of muscle, often at the neuromuscular junction

_____ 6. Trigger points located at musculotendinous junctions, at the muscle's bony attachment, or both

_____ 7. Trigger points responsible for activating one or more satellite trigger points

_____ 8. Trigger point created by key trigger-point activity often arising in pain referral zones of the key trigger point

_____ 9. Tendency of trigger points to produce sensations (e.g., pain, tingling, numbness, burning, aching, itching) distal from that of the trigger point

_____ 10. Reflexive impulse that causes the affected muscle or an adjacent muscle to fire or twitch spontaneously

INTERNET ACTIVITIES

Visit http://www.sportsinjuryclinic.net and click on Sports Massage. After reading the link to Professionalism and Ethics, write a one-page report on the subject.

Visit http://www.fitness.gov and click on Resources. Choose Physical Activity Facts, and after reading, list four facts from memory.

Visit http://www.presidentschallenge.org and choose a category according to your age. Take the president's challenge and work toward earning the Presidential Active Lifestyle Award.

Bibliography

Abraham WM: Exercise-induced muscle soreness, *Physic Sports Med* 7:57-60, Oct 1979.

Applegate EJ: *The anatomy and physiology learning system,* ed 3, Philadelphia, 2006, Saunders.

Beers MH, Berkow R: *The Merck manual of diagnosis and therapy,* Whitehouse Station, NJ, 2006, Merck Research Laboratories.

Dominguez R, Gajda R: *Total body training,* New York, 1984, Warnerbooks.

Chaitow L: *Modern neuromuscular techniques,* ed 2, St Louis, 2003, Churchill Livingstone, Elsevier.

Chaitow L, Walker DeLany J: *Clinical application of neuromuscular techniques,* vol I, St Louis, 2000, Churchill Livingstone, Elsevier.

Chaitow L, Walker DeLany J: *Clinical application of neuromuscular techniques,* vol II, St Louis, 2000, Churchill Livingstone, Elsevier.

Como D, editor: *Mosby's medical, nursing, and allied health dictionary,* ed 6, St Louis, 2002, Mosby.

Crawley J, Van De Graaff KM: *A photographic atlas for anatomy and physiology,* Englewood, Colo, 2002, Morton.

Damjanov I: *Pathophysiology for the health-related professions,* ed 3, Philadelphia, 2006, Saunders.

Fernandez F : *Deep-tissue massage treatment : a handbook of neuromuscular therapy.* St Louis, 2006, Elsevier Mosby.

Foldi M, StroBenreuther R: *Foundations of manual lymph drainage,* ed 3, St Louis, 2005, Mosby.

Fritz S: *Sports and exercise massage: comprehensive care in athletics, fitness, and rehabilitation,* St Louis, 2005, Elsevier.

Frazier MS, Drzymkowski JW: *Essentials of human diseases and conditions,* ed 3, Philadelphia, 2004, Saunders.

Gehlsen GM, Ganion LR, Helfst R: Fibroblast responses to variation in soft tissue mobilization pressure, *Med Sci Sports Exerc* 31(4):531-535, 1999.

Gould BE: *Pathophysiology for the health professions,* ed 3, Philadelphia, 2006, Saunders.

Gray H, Pick TP, Howden R: *Gray's anatomy,* ed 29, Philadelphia, 1974, Running Press.

Haubrich WS: *Medical meanings: a glossary of word origins,* New York, 1984, Harcourt Brace Jovanovich.

Jacob S, Francone C: *Elements of anatomy and physiology,* Philadelphia, 1989, Saunders.

Juhan D: *Job's body, a handbook for bodyworkers,* ed 3, Barrington, NY, 2003, Station Hill Press.

Kalat JW: *Biological psychology,* ed 8, Belmont, Calif, 2003, Wadsworth.

Kapit W, Elson LM: *The anatomy coloring book,* ed 3, New York, 2002, Benjamin Cummings.

Klafs D, Arnheim DD: *Modern principles of athletic training,* ed 8, St Louis, 1992, Mosby.

Kordish M, Dickson S: *Introduction to basic human anatomy,* Lake Charles, La, 1995, McNeese State University.

Lowe WW: *Orthopedic massage: theory and technique,* St Louis, 2003, Mosby.

Marieb EN: *Essentials of human anatomy and physiology,* ed 8, New York, 2005, Benjamin Cummings.

Mattes AL: *Flexibility—active and assisted stretching,* Sarasota, Fla, 1995, self-published.

McAleer N: *The body almanac,* Garden City, NY, 1985, Doubleday.

McAtee R: *Facilitated stretching,* ed 2, Colorado Springs, Colo, 1999, Human Kinetics.

Merck manual, ed 17, Whitehouse Station, NJ, 1998, Merck and Company.

Moore KL: *Clinically oriented anatomy,* ed 5, Baltimore, 2005, Lippincott Williams & Wilkins.

Newton D: *Pathology for massage therapists,* ed 2, Portland, Ore, 1995, Simran.

Perry J: *Gait analysis: normal and pathological function,* New York, 1992, McGraw-Hill.

Platzer W: *Color atlas and textbook of human anatomy: locomotor system,* vol I, ed 5, New York, 2003, Thieme.

Premkumar K: *Pathology A to Z, a handbook for massage therapists,* Baltimore, 1999, Lippincott Williams & Wilkins.

Salvo S: *Massage therapy: principles and practice,* ed 1, Philadelphia, 1999, Saunders.

Salvo SG, Anderson SK: *Mosby's pathology for massage therapists,* St Louis, 2004, Mosby.

Solomon EP, Phillips GA: *Understanding human anatomy and physiology,* Philadelphia, 1987, Saunders.

Stanton P, Purdam C: Hamstring injuries in sprinting—the role of eccentric exercise, *J Orthopaed Sports Physic Ther* 10:343-348, March 1989.

Synder GE: Fascia—applied anatomy and physiology, *J Am Osteop Assoc* 68:675-685, March 1969.

Thibodeau G, Patton K: *Anatomy and physiology,* ed 6, St Louis, 2006, Mosby.

Thibodeau G, Patton K: *Structure and function of the body,* ed 12, St Louis, 2004, Mosby.

Tortora GJ: *Introduction to the human body: the essentials of anatomy and physiology,* ed 5, Hoboken, NJ, 2000, John Wiley & Sons.

Tortora GJ, Grabowksi SR: *Principles of anatomy and physiology,* ed 11, New York, 2005, John Wiley & Sons.

Venes D, Thomas CL, Taber CW: *Taber's cyclopedic medical dictionary,* ed 20, Philadelphia, 2005, FA Davis.

Walter JB, Israel MS: *General pathology,* ed 4, New York, 1974, Churchill Livingston.

Weineck J: *Functional anatomy in sports,* Chicago, 1986, Year Book Medical Publishers.

Wilmore JH, Costill DL: *Physiology of sport and exercise,* Leeds, UK, 2006, Human Kinetics.

Wilmore JH, Costill DL: Cardiovascular regulation. In: *Training for sport and activity: the physiological basis of the conditioning process,* ed 3, Dubuque, Iowa, 1988, William C Brown, pp 61-81.

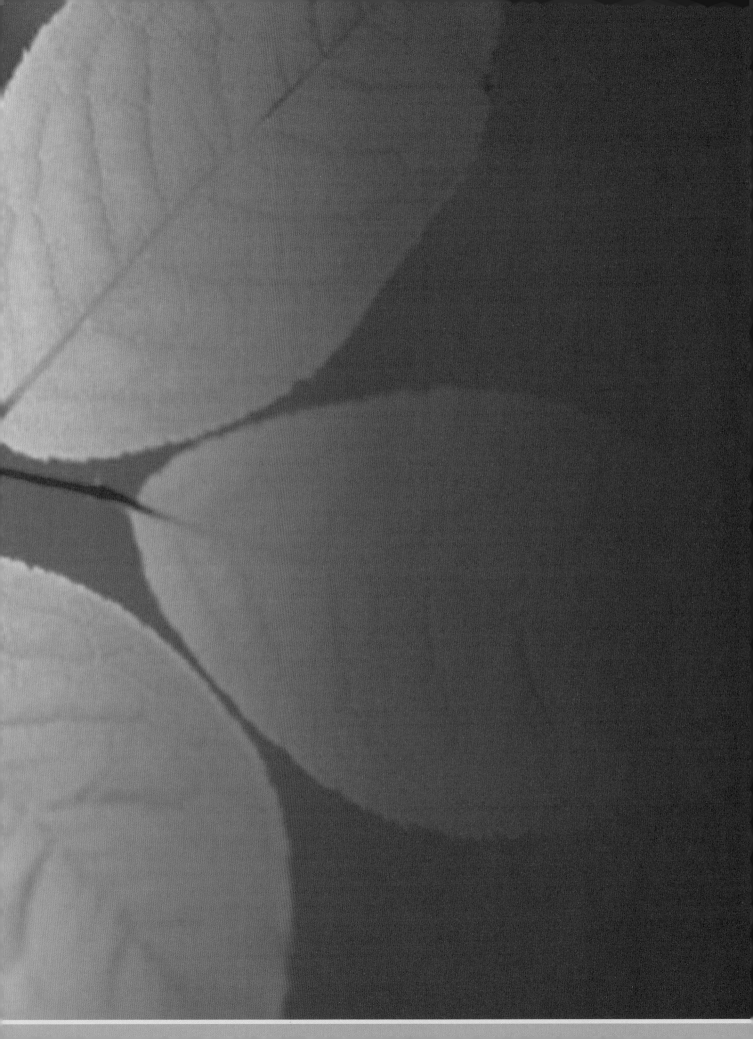

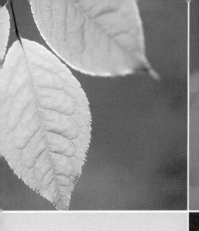

CHAPTER 27

"We can be knowledgeable with another man's knowledge, but we cannot be wise with another man's wisdom."

—Michel De Montaigne

Seated Massage

Ralph R. Stephens, BSEd, LMT, NCTMB

STUDENT OBJECTIVES

After completing this chapter, the student should be able to:

- List major considerations when purchasing a massage chair
- Describe types of seated massage equipment
- State reasons that a massage therapist might choose to massage a client in the seated position
- Explain and demonstrate procedures of sanitation and hygiene unique to seated massage
- Properly adjust the massage chair for the client
- Describe proper body mechanics and safety considerations for the massage therapist who uses a massage chair
- Use adaptive professional communication to communicate effectively with the client before and during the massage
- Perform a basic seated massage routine

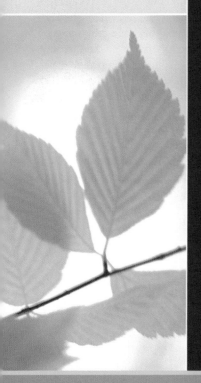

INTRODUCTION

Rubbing a person's shoulders while he or she is sitting in a chair is often instinctive. It is a natural and therapeutic urge. **Seated massage** is often referred to as *chair massage* and came to prominence through the efforts of David Palmer, whose vision was to make massage therapy safe, convenient, and affordable for anyone, anywhere, anytime. He introduced seated massage in the workplace in the early 1980s. Working at corporations such as Apple, Inc. and Pacific Bell, he developed the idea for a chair to complement the massage. In 1986, Palmer introduced the first special massage chair and coined the term *on-site massage.* Palmer adapted the traditional Japanese system of massage, called amma, to create massage routines performed on the client in a special portable chair (see Chapter 1). **Amma** routines use acupressure techniques, stretching, and percussion (tapotement).

Seated techniques have made massage more accessible to the mainstream public by making it as convenient and affordable as a haircut. Enterprising therapists have expanded this concept to every imaginable venue. Some of the opportunities to use seated massage are airports, beauty salons, large and small businesses, concerts (public and backstage), chiropractic offices, day spas, numerous events such as fairs and festivals, golf courses, health food stores, hospitals, hospices, institutions, locker rooms, nursing homes, offices, private practices, retail stores, schools, shopping malls, sporting events, and even street corners. The Massage Emergency Response Team (MERT) also uses seated massage.

TABLE TALK

The Massage Emergency Response Team (MERT), sponsored by the American Massage Therapy Association, was deployed during the rescue efforts after the September 11, 2001, terrorist attacks on the World Trade Center, Pennsylvania, and the Pentagon. MERT teams primarily used massage chairs to treat rescue workers and others at the disaster sites. The volunteer MERT therapists gave hundreds of seated massages to grateful emergency personnel. Seated massage skills were a vital part of the service that rescue workers provided.

Sessions are typically short (5 to 15 minutes), although they can last as long as 30 minutes. The cost is usually $10 to $20, averaging approximately $1 per minute. Some individuals who are not familiar with massage find seated massage more acceptable than table massage. Disrobing is unnecessary. Lubricants are not used. People generally feel less vulnerable seated in a chair than lying on a table, and the time commitment is considerably less, especially when the therapist goes to the client's place of business or on site.

TABLE TALK

How to Select a Massage Chair

Many different massage chairs are available on the market today. Just as with a massage table, different features appeal to different people. The following factors should be kept in mind when purchasing a massage chair:

• The massage chair should be lightweight because you may be moving it from location to location.
• It should be quick and simple to set up and take down.
• It should have enough adjustments to fit a variety of body styles but not so many that you spend a lot of time adjusting the chair. Avoid massage chairs requiring a series of smaller adjustments after making a major adjustment. Simple is better; simple and quick is best.
• It should be sturdy and strong. A creaky or wobbly chair makes the person sitting in it feel insecure and unsafe.
• Be sure that the armrest is strong enough to withstand deep compression and deep frictioning techniques performed on the client's arm.
• Face support adjustments on massage chairs should be completely enclosed. Exposed latches and locking mechanisms can pinch the therapist's fingers and catch the client's hair. Exposed latches and locking mechanisms can also come loose if bumped by the client or therapist and are difficult to keep clean and to sanitize.
• The chair manufacturer should offer a trial period during which the chair can be returned for a full refund if the therapist is not completely satisfied. The chair should come with a 5-year or longer warranty.
• Buying from a manufacturer that is well established is generally best. Such a manufacturer usually provides better customer service, and recognized brands typically have a better resale value should you decide to sell your chair at any time.

Several varieties of seated massage, equipment, and ways to accommodate clients who want a massage in a seated position are known. A massage chair (Figure 27-1) is made by most manufacturers of professional massage tables and offer a desktop face support, which is typically the face support from a massage chair designed to be clamped to or balanced on the edge of a counter, table, or desk. Many of these items have chest pads that hang vertically over the edge of the desk. A system of specially designed cushions can hang over the back of an armless chair, which are often the same cushion system used for positioning and support on a massage tabletop. If none of the previously mentioned options are available to you, then you can use a stack of pillows on a massage table, a regular table, or chair. As a last resort, the therapist may use a stool or chair, but this option provides no support for the head, upper body, or arms.

REASONS FOR USING THE CHAIR

Reasons for using the massage chair are as follows:
• Massage therapists may use seated massage techniques as their primary modality and source of revenue.

Seated massage is most often used for stress reduction and relaxation, as a *stress-buster break;* however, routines can be adapted to address specific complaints such as low back pain, headaches, neck and shoulder tension, and arm and wrist overuse injury. Combining clinical massage techniques with amma techniques gives the therapist the option of doing clinical massage in the seated position in either an on-site or a private office setting. Individuals are more likely to participate in a program of seated massage if it provides reduction of painful complaints and injuries. Employers are more likely to allow employees to participate if they believe it will prevent injuries, improve morale, and enhance productivity in the workplace.

In research published in 1996, Dr. Tiffany Field of the Touch Research Institute in Miami found that individuals who received a 15-minute seated massage twice a week showed increased cognitive ability, performed better on math tests, and completed problems with increased accuracy and speed. These individuals also experienced a significant decrease in tension compared with individuals who practiced traditional relaxation techniques while seated in a chair without receiving massage. Hence massage does not cost; it pays.

A massage chair takes up less room than a table, making it more adaptable to space limitations. This and the through-clothes technique has brought the chair into therapy areas, athletic training rooms, chiropractic offices, and many massage therapists' treatment rooms as an adjunct to their tables for specific work. Acquiring a massage chair and learning how to use it effectively are well worth the massage therapist's financial investment and time.

SANITIZATION AND HYGIENE CONSIDERATIONS

The need for hygiene for the massage therapist and sanitization of the massage chair cannot be overemphasized. The public is aware of the importance of cleanliness, and your clients will notice and appreciate that you keep your equipment sanitary and your work environment clean (see Chapter 4).

When conducting table massage in an office setting, the massage therapist must wash his or her hands before and after each client. However, with the shorter treatment protocols, taking time between clients to wash the hands twice is not economically feasible. When working on site, washroom facilities may be inaccessible. Seated massage therapy procedures must be self-contained, including hygiene.

Seated massage therapists can purchase **antimicrobial disposable towelettes** from a medical or massage supply business. These disposable towels sanitize your hands, face support, armrest, and chest pad of the chair between client sessions. Sanitize the leg rests if the client was wearing shorts or a skirt. These wipes are specially treated to destroy microscopic organisms that can cause diseases, such as staphylococci, streptococci, common cold and influenza viruses, herpes virus, human immunodeficiency virus, and tuberculosis. As a rule, if a disinfecting agent destroys tuberculosis

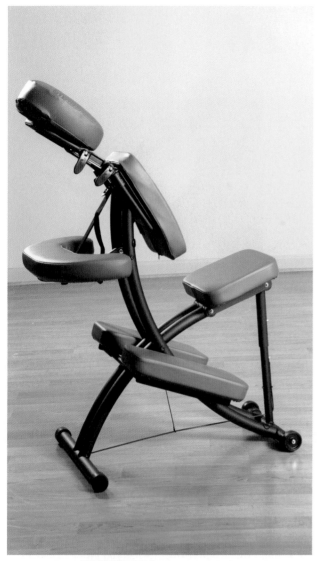

FIGURE 27-1 A massage chair.

- Massage therapists may use a massage chair as their secondary modality and supplemental source of revenue.
- Seated massage can be used as a promotional tool to introduce the public to massage therapy in a safe, nonthreatening way, thus promoting the therapist's practice in particular and the profession in general.
- Seated massage may be done on site or in the therapist's office.
- Massage chairs are often used at sporting events.
- Other opportunities include fundraisers, concerts, conventions, airports, beauty salons, and spas.
- On-site massage services may be used at professional offices and other workplaces for stress reduction, pain relief, and injury prevention.
- Seated massage is used by therapists in their offices for short treatments of the upper body.
- The massage chair is ideal for clients who have difficulty getting on and off a massage table.
- The chair is as versatile as your imagination.

bacteria, then all other microbes are also destroyed. These cleansers help protect the therapist and the client by preventing the spread of contagious pathogens.

Keeping your hands clean is important. The most common way to spread germs is by touching the eyes, ears, and nose. Keep your fingernails short and clean. Using an antimicrobial skin barrier, sometimes called a *skin protectorant,* further protects your hands. These products come in creams or foams that when rubbed onto the skin dry to form a barrier. Protect yourself and your clients.

Use a cover on the face cradle to make your clients feel more comfortable and to facilitate keeping the face support cushion clean. These covers help keep makeup off the vinyl. Face cradle covers feel more comfortable on the face than does vinyl fabric. One type of cover is a *nurse bouffant cap,* available through medical or massage supply businesses. Other types of covers are paper towels and specially designed paper covers, with the latter available through massage supply sources.

SAFETY CONSIDERATIONS AND BODY MECHANICS FOR THE SEATED MASSAGE THERAPIST

To prevent repetitive motion injuries, using proper body mechanics at all times is essential. Before you set up your massage chair, select an area that allows you to move completely around the chair during the massage. If you use a massage chair carrying case, then place it out of the way. Provide a clear, unobstructed pathway for your clients to and from the chair.

Work in the lunge (bow) stance, keeping the feet and body pointed in the direction of the force you are applying. Keep your back straight and your head erect. Your movement and pressure will be generated from the pelvis as you shift your weight from back leg to front leg (Figure 27-2). As you massage, the front knee is flexed and the arms are stretched in front, elbows only slightly flexed. For the majority of seated massage techniques, the wrists should not be extended more than 45 degrees.

When using the thumbs, maintain proper thumb alignment by *stacking the bones.* This technique means that the bones of the thumb are in relatively straight alignment with the bones of the wrist and arm. If you look straight down your arm, the thumb is then pointing straight ahead. As you use your thumb, the fingers of the working hand may be open or loosely closed. You may also use your fingertips, palm of the hand, or elbow to apply massage techniques. This method gives your thumbs a needed break and varies the quality of touch for the client. However, be sure to maintain proper body mechanics at all times. Spread your feet farther apart as you work closer to the floor. Avoid bending the back and neck.

> *"Ultimately, your only source of
> funding is satisfied clients."*
> Tim Mullen

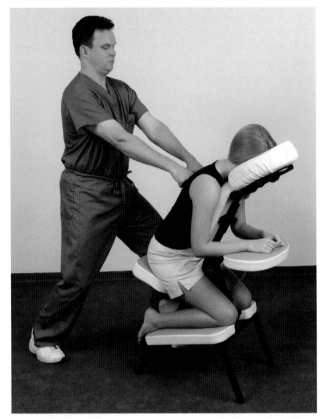

FIGURE 27-2 Seated massage with therapist in lunge position.

BEFORE THE SEATED MASSAGE BEGINS

If this session is your client's first time to sit in the massage chair, physically demonstrate how to do it properly. As you are sitting in the chair, explain what you are doing. For example, "I am sitting in the chair placing my knees and lower legs on these cushions while my forearms rest on this shelf and my face is supported by this crescent-shaped pillow." You will be amazed how many positions your clients will assume without directions. Some sit on the chair backward, whereas others climb onto it as if it were a motorcycle. Although this is entertaining, the client might upset the chair and be injured. Be specific with your directions and actions.

Most massage chairs have adjustments so they can properly support any body size or type (Figure 27-3). Before the seated massage session, adjust the chair to each client; do not expect the client to conform to the chair. The primary adjustments are the seat height, chest pad height, face support height and angle (tilt), and armrest height. A client will typically arch his or her back or slump if the chair is improperly adjusted to his or her body. *Be sure the client's back is straight and that the armrest is low enough so that the client's shoulders are not raised.* The proximal end of the forearm is just slightly off the armrest. For most clients, the most comfortable position of the face cradle is when the neck is slightly flexed forward. Once the chair is completely adjusted to the client, ask him or her if any adjustments should be made. Then ask whether the client is comfortable; most clients who do not know how the chair should feel will say *yes*. However, if given the option to make it better, they will point out any area of discomfort. This simple question takes a few seconds and has a significant impact on the session.

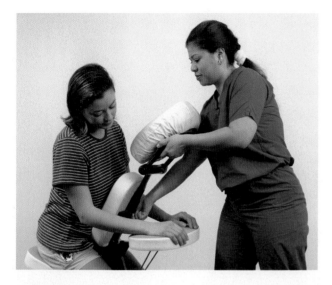

FIGURE 27-3 Therapist making adjustments on chair while client is seated.

MASSAGE STROKES USED FOR SEATED MASSAGE

Seated massage routines use East Asian and Swedish massage strokes (without oil) and ancillary massage strokes. These strokes include compression, sustained pressure (acupressure), stretching, deep and superficial friction, pétrissage, effleurage, nerve stroke, and tapotement. The strokes used vary according to the training of the therapist.

Compression

Compression is effective on the muscles of the forearm and back. Apply firm pressure primarily from the heel of the hand or loosely clenched fists. During compression of the forearm, face the client with your relaxed fingers and pointed toward the client's elbow. Apply pressure straight down while maintaining contact. Instruct the client to exhale as you apply pressure to the back and to inhale as you release. Avoid applying excessive pressure on the floating ribs and the lumbar region below the kidneys, as well as any previous injuries.

Sustained Pressure

Also known as *ischemic compression* or *acupressure,* sustained pressure is usually applied with a finger or thumb, elbow, or a handheld tool. Direct sustained pressure displaces fluids in the tissues being compressed, spreads muscle fibers, and relieves muscle spasms. It is primarily used to relieve trigger and tender points. In East Asian techniques, pressure is applied to points in a pattern to improve or balance energy flow in the meridians.

Deep Friction

Deep friction is applied with the thumb, finger, elbow, loosely clenched fist, palm, or heel of the hand. During friction, engage the skin through the client's clothes and move the skin over the underlying structures. Avoid sliding on the client's skin or clothes. The term *deep* does not denote hard pressure but rather the effect of shifting the skin over deeper structures.

Superficial Friction

A warming, stimulating stroke, superficial friction is applied with the palms of one or both hands in a rapid back-and-forth movement on the superficial tissues. A variation is to use the ulnar sides of the hands in a sawing motion. This variation is effective for reducing muscular tension around the shoulder joint on either side of the spine and across the top of the upper trapezius.

Pétrissage

Pétrissage involves grasping, lifting, and kneading the tissues or rolling the tissues between the thumb and fingers. This massage movement is used primarily in the neck and upper trapezius.

Effleurage

Effleurage, or light stroking, is applied over the client's clothing for relaxation and sedation. Nerve strokes can also be used.

Tapotement

Toward the end of the seated massage, tapotement can be used on the back, head, arms, and hips. Hacking, pounding, and rapping are best for the torso, hips, and arms, whereas tapping and pincement with the fingertips is best on the scalp. Do not use tapotement over areas where trigger points were found and treated because it can cause them to reform.

ADAPTIVE PROFESSIONAL COMMUNICATION

Because eye contact is impossible when the client is in the face cradle, a method of communication must be established in the initial interview before beginning the treatment. The following guideline is recommended for establishing communication:

When it hurts. Explain that you will be examining the tissues of the back, neck, and arms, looking for areas that are tight and contracted. When these areas are located, they will be tender. You should suggest, "Be sure to tell me whenever I find a tender area. Will you do that for me?" Not only does this give the client permission to tell you that something is tender, but he or she also agrees to do so.

When it gets better. Continue by saying, "When I find these tender places, I will stop and maintain the pressure. This sustained pressure will cause the nervous system to respond by relaxing the tender area. It may feel to you like I am letting up on the pressure, or it is beginning to feel better. Will you let me know when it gets better?"

If it refers. You should then add, "When I am examining or maintaining pressure on an area of tissue, you may experience some sensation somewhere else. It could be a pain, tingling, numbness, aching, or some other sensation somewhere besides right where I am massaging. These are trigger points. Will you tell me if you feel any sensation radiating anywhere other than where I am working?"

If it is too hard. Say, "If at any time I am working too hard, be sure and tell me right away. Will you do that?" This request is important because it gives the client permission to tell you that you are working too hard. In many instances, the client will not tell you because he or she thinks you are the professional and you must be doing it right. The client may think it is supposed to hurt. Some clients will endure anything if they believe it may make them better. You can also say, "Let me know if what I am doing feels good or if it hurts, especially if it hurts, because this work should not be painful."

During on-site massage, the massage area may be noisy, which makes hearing the client difficult. In this case, ask the client to communicate by raising his or her hand if pain is felt. If more specific information is needed regarding pain, then establish a pain-measuring system on a scale from 1 (no pain) through 5 (excruciating pain). You will know, by the number of fingers raised, how the client is responding to the pressure (Figure 27-4). This system also may be used in quiet places.

Some people will not tell you that something hurts. They may be accustomed to denying pain. However, the body never lies. You can tell that you are working too hard when the client begins to pull away from you or unconsciously

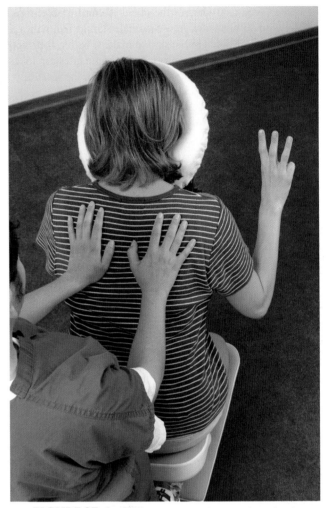

FIGURE 27-4 Client raising three fingers of one hand.

contracts muscles to limit your access into the tissues. If he or she is tensing up, squirming, or pulling away, then *you are using too much pressure.*

RECORD KEEPING

Have your clients fill out an intake form, and obtain informed consent. The initial interview with your client may be brief, but the form should ask questions regarding eye conditions that might be affected by the face cradle (e.g., contacts), and any medical conditions for which they are being treated. Establish your client's primary and secondary complaints and screen for possible contraindications using the PPALM assessment and planning method outlined in Chapter 8.

Clinical seated massage treatments require keeping additional detailed notes. Treatment notes document progress and remind the therapist of what procedures were performed and which treatments were helpful. In legal situations, proper documentation is helpful for you and your clients. Additionally, unless you give each client a receipt, it may not be considered a legal transaction by taxation authorities. To save time, receipts may be prepared in advance, with a place to fill in the client's name, date, and amount.

DAVID PALMER

Born: November 27, 1948.

"My vision is to make touch a positive social value in our culture."

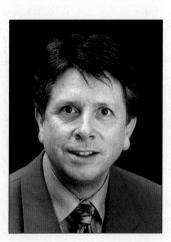

The topic of chair massage can hardly be discussed without the name David Palmer surfacing at least once. Read any article on the subject, and you will soon discover that he is the father of chair massage.

Palmer's career in massage began in 1980. Considering his previous profession of 10 years as an administrator of social service programs for nonprofit agencies in Chicago and San Francisco, it seemed only natural that he would focus on a field in which he could have a great effect on the well-being of people through the art of touch. He first encountered massage in his early 20s during a *rolfing* session. He had been experiencing chronic shoulder pain, and the rolfing combined with tai chi and stretching gave him a feeling of being back inside his body. This experience led him to explore massage.

After Palmer received a massage in a spa in San Francisco, a series of events over a 3-year period led to his position as director of a massage institute specializing in the Japanese art of *amma.* After only a short period of teaching, he realized that a serious gap existed between the people who wanted to give and receive professional massage. After a little investigating, he came to the conclusion that a significant packaging problem existed in the massage industry.

"The package that the mainstream massage community was selling to the general public was a package that the general public was not interested in buying," Palmer says. Convincing most people to accept an idea that required going into a private room, removing clothing, lying on a table, and being rubbed with oils by a stranger for a costly fee on a regular basis was difficult. The whole idea was just too frightening for the average individual. It was then that Palmer gave massage a hard look from a marketing point of view. He says, "They [mainstream massage community] were selling a graduate-level understanding of the field of touch to a population who had not even begun kindergarten regarding touch."

Palmer's solution to this problem was to make massage less frightening and more affordable. The result was his legacy of the seated chair massage. Although this type of massage had been done for thousands of years, as can been seen in ancient Japanese and Chinese woodcuts, Palmer's contribution was to revive its visibility and identity. Perceiving it as *strange* would be more difficult if the massage is given with the client fully clothed on an open sidewalk in a chair.

At the time, the chair massage was being done on a drummer's stool, but in 1983, Palmer decided to create a special chair. He had seen one of the Scandinavian computer chairs called *Balance* with slanted leg rests and thought it would be perfect, if only it had some sort of head rest and chest support. He hired a French cabinetmaker named Serge Bouyssou to be his design partner, and after 2 years the chair was introduced to the national market. The year was 1986, and chair massage was now viewed as being significant enough to have its own physical product.

Vision has clearly been an important factor in David Palmer's career. From the beginning, he saw a challenge and immediately acted on it. Chair massage has given so many people the opportunity to experience the wonderful benefits of massage. It allows the client to experience the much-needed sense of touch safely. "We're so touch phobic that you can't grow up in this culture without having some serious issues about touch," says Palmer. "Parents are afraid to touch their kids; teachers can't touch their students; it's crazy out there. My feeling is that we need to shift that around, and massage is a vehicle for doing that because it provides structured touch." Although he fully appreciates the many wonderful benefits of massage, it is not his main interest. He states, "My vision is to make touch a positive social value in our culture." He admits that this vision is what primarily motivates his professional life.

The most important thing Palmer believes that students can do in their massage therapy program is first learn how to touch and second learn how to be touched. He confesses, "I'm one of those unreformed 1960s brats who think it's still possible to change the world." If his previous record is any reflection on his future, he just might succeed.

SAMPLE SEATED MASSAGE ROUTINE

The following basic routine is a suggested protocol that you can accomplish in 15 minutes. Use it as a guide, but remain creative and intuitive. Accomplish as much as you can for each client within the time allowed. Concentrate the majority of time on the client's primary area of complaint, which is usually the low back, neck, or shoulders. However, in the workplace, quite common complaints involve the forearm, wrist, and hand. Start with some general strokes to acquaint clients with your touch and to establish their individual sensitivity in receiving; gradually become more specific as you go on. You cannot resolve everything from which a client has been suffering for years in one treatment. Even recent injuries usually require multiple treatments (see Chapter 26). One 15-minute session can reduce the main complaint and accomplish some general relaxation; therefore you have accomplished a great service for the client in that amount of time. Complete the seated massage treatment with general techniques. Work from general to specific, then back to general.

Upper Back and Neck

Begin the treatment with compression strokes to the paraspinal muscles. Use the heels of the hands or loosely clenched fists. Having the client breathe in rhythm with the compression is important. Ask your client to take a deep breath and exhale. As he or she exhales, apply firm pressure to the tissues on either side of the spine (ideally, the therapist breathes in the same pattern as the client). Begin between the scapulas and move inferiorly a hand width at a time until the ilium bones are reached. Then move back superiorly a hand width at a time until the starting point is reached. This technique establishes contact with the client, introduces relaxation, and gets him or her into a regular deep-breathing pattern.

You should be standing directly behind the center of the client's back. Keep your arms outstretched with just a slight bend in the elbows, back straight, head erect, moving from the pelvis in a lunge position. If you are using the heels of the hands, the wrists will be significantly extended. If pressure applied with the heels of the hands creates discomfort in your wrists, then switch to a loosely clenched fist. Using a loose fist to apply compression keeps the wrist straight as you apply pressure with the proximal phalanges.

Repeat this pattern using loosely clenched fists but with a circular deep frictioning stroke. Make four to eight circles with each hand, working simultaneously down and up the sides of the spine. If massaging in circles with both hands at the same time is too difficult or tiresome, then you may choose to switch to cross-fiber or chucking friction. Apply four friction strokes medially to laterally over the paraspinal muscles, then four friction strokes superiorly to inferiorly, and then move a hand width and repeat.

Every few minutes, ask the client how he or she perceives the pressure, using the guidelines discussed in the section Adaptive Professional Communication in this chapter.

Grasp the upper trapezius muscle with one or both hands, using a pincerlike grip. Begin just lateral to the base of the neck, in approximately the center of the upper trapezius muscle (Figure 27-5), and pétrissage the muscle between the thumb and fingers. Work laterally to the acromion process, then work medially to the base of the neck, and continue as far superior on the neck as you can while still isolating the trapezius fibers. The trapezius fibers will typically become too small to grasp at the third cervical (C3) level. When tender areas or trigger points are encountered, stop and maintain the pressure for 8 to 12 seconds. If your pressure is appropriate for the person, then the client will feel it relax within 12 seconds; if he or she does not, then you are applying too much pressure. Slowly release the pressure and move to another area, returning to the tender area in approximately 1 minute. Trigger points in the upper fibers of the trapezius commonly refer to the back of the head and up to the temple area.

You may now move to the side of the client in the chair and grasp and pétrissage the back of his or her neck in the lamina groove. Work all the way up to the occipital bone and back down to the shoulder. Because the thumb is more sensitive and powerful, you may choose to go to the other side and repeat this step. This decision is based on the sensitivity found in the tissues the first time over them and the client's main complaint. If the main complaint is the neck and shoulders, then you will want to be thorough in this area. If the main complaint is in the lower back, then less time will be spent in the posterior cervical region.

Tilt the face cradle forward to place the head and neck in 45 degrees of flexion. While standing at the side of the client, use the thumb and second finger of one hand to apply deep frictioning to the tissues between the occiput and C2. Work from lateral to medial and back. These tissues can be tender and ischemic; therefore be sure to check with the client about appropriate pressures when working this area.

Using the heel of the hand or fingertips, examine the rhomboid muscles and the posterior surface of the scapula with deep circular friction. When massaging the posterior region of the scapula, support the anterior aspect of the shoulder with the other hand. If this area is the client's primary complaint, a more specific examination of these tissues can then be done with the thumbs or a guided elbow (Figure 27-6). When this area is complete, move lateral to the shoulder joint and treat the rotator cuff tendons with circular friction.

Apply circular friction to the area below the scapulas using the heels of the hands, working both sides of the spine at once. This action addresses the latissimus dorsi muscle and paraspinal muscles in the midback.

Lower Back

Moving your hand inferiorly, use circular friction to relax the lower back. The quadratus lumborum muscle can be examined and treated effectively in the seated position. This muscle is responsible for many complaints of low back pain.

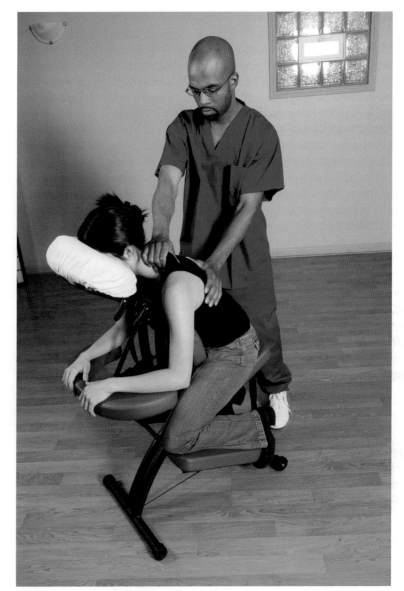

FIGURE 27-5 Therapist massaging upper trapezius.

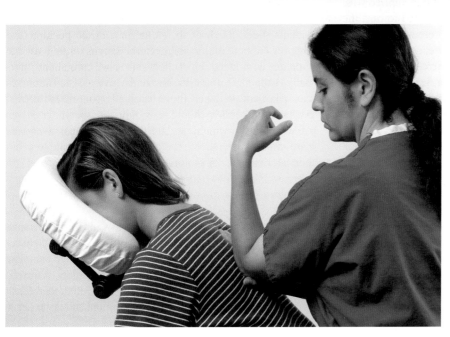

FIGURE 27-6 Guided elbow technique.

Trigger points in the quadratus lumborum often mimic hip and sciatic nerve pain. Palpate the client's waistline, being careful not to elicit a tickle response. After locating the lateral end of the twelfth rib, apply deep friction with your thumbs in a lateral to medial direction along its inferior surface. As you move medially, you will encounter a hard structure; this is the spine and is often more lateral than expected. Change directions of pressure to 45 degrees medial anterior. Using circular friction, examine the edge of the lumbar spine in the area of the transverse processes. Using deep circular friction, massage this area in thumb-width increments from the first lumbar region to the ilium bone. Change the direction of pressure to inferior anterior, and treat the superior surface of the ilium laterally to the midline of the body.

The lower portion of the paraspinal muscles can now be examined more thoroughly using fingertips, thumbs, or a guided elbow. Treat one side at a time with deep circular or cross-fiber friction, using sustained pressure on tender areas and trigger points. Apply friction on this area from medial to lateral, allowing the client to rock slightly in the chair. This technique is effective and relaxing.

Arm

Because no surface is available against which to compress the biceps and triceps during seated massage, the therapist is limited to pétrissage, rolling, jostling, nerve strokes, or squeezing the tissues of the upper arm with one or two hands.

Facing the front of the chair, slightly to one side, place the forearm with the palm down on the armrest to treat the forearm muscles. Apply compression to the extensor muscle group using the heel of the hand, working from wrist to elbow (Figure 27-7). Repeat this sequence three times, then rotate the arm, palm up, and apply three sets of compression to the flexor muscles.

Roll the hand over, palm down, and instead of compression, repeat this pattern using circular friction applied with the heel of the hand, with your fingers pointed toward the elbow of the client. Work from wrist to elbow in 1- or 2-inch intervals, making 5 to 10 circles on each spot. Repeat this sequence three times. Rotate the arm, palm up, and repeat the circular friction moves on the flexor muscles of the forearm.

Using the thumbs, apply circular friction to all sides of the wrist. Grasp the client's hand, shake out the arm, and return it to the armrest. Repeat this sequence on the other arm.

Face and Scalp

Facial and scalp massage feels great while in a chair; however, many people do not want their hair or makeup messed up, so always ask first. Using the pads of the fingers, apply circular friction to the temples, jaw, face, and forehead. During scalp massage, the tissue can be shifted back and forth across the cranium using deep friction in any direction. Gentle tapping or pincement tapotement also works well on the scalp, especially

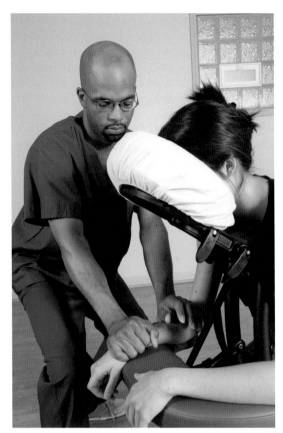

FIGURE 27-7 Therapist using palm to apply circular friction.

as part of the general finishing strokes. Tapotement on the cranium is not appropriate with someone who has a headache.

evolve Log on to the Evolve website to view a demonstration of scalp massage. ∎

Stretches

Stretches are useful in seated massage. Because most individuals spend much of their time in a flexed position, the anterior cervical region and pectoral regions of the body are typically contracted. Most clients also have chronically internally rotated shoulders. Passive and active-assisted stretches can relax and lengthen these habitually contracted tissues. Massage therapists should use only the specific systems of stretching in which they are trained and must always be careful not to overstretch the client's soft tissue and to avoid bouncy (ballistic) or prolonged stretching.

Final Procedure

As the seated massage session draws to a close, the therapist returns to general strokes. If the goal is to leave the client relaxed and sedated, then finish with some effleurage and slow downward nerve strokes on the back and shoulders. If the client is returning to work and needs to be more alert, then finish with tapotement, superficial (palmar) friction, and faster nerve strokes. Tapping or pincement tapotement on the head, hacking or quacking on the shoulders and back, and pounding or rapping on the hips is a stimulating way to finish the massage.

When the treatment is complete, tell the client, and ask him or her to get off the chair slowly. Remain close by because many people, especially older adults, may feel unsteady for a few moments. Some people actually doze off during the seated massage and may need time to become fully oriented. Be prepared to assist your client as needed.

Always have your appointment calendar handy to reschedule appointments and business cards to distribute. As you collect your fee from the client or just thank them and say good-bye, suggest that the client book another appointment. Also appropriate is to mention that, if the client liked your work, he or she should recommend it to others.

On completion of all transactions with the client, clean your hands, disinfect the chair, write your case notes, take a few deep breaths, and get ready for the next client.

SUMMARY

Seated massage is an important specialty area in the profession of massage therapy. It allows the therapist to reach a different group of clients who may not be available for traditional table massage. Usually done in a special portable chair, seated techniques can be used on site at the client's location or the therapist's office. Seated massage sessions tend to be shorter than table sessions, ranging from 5 to 30 minutes. The work is done through the clothes without lubricants. Seated massage is used for promoting the therapist's private practice or as a complete practice in itself. The portable massage chair has made massage as accessible to the general public as a haircut and has become a valuable adjunct to any therapist's practice.

evolve

Go to *Chapter Extras* on Evolve for additional illustrations and resources for this chapter. *Extras* for this chapter include:

1. Crossword puzzle (downloadable form)

MATCHING

Place the letter of the answer next to the term or phrase that best describes it.

A. *Amma*
B. An alternative method of communication
C. Antimicrobial disposable towelettes
D. Client begins to pull away from you or tense up

E. David Palmer
F. Explain and demonstrate how to sit in the chair properly
G. "Are you comfortable?"
H. Lubricated effleurage

I. Lunge position
J. Massage lubricants
K. Raise a hand
L. Select an area allowing the therapist to move around the chair during the massage

_____ 1. The father of seated massage

_____ 2. The traditional Japanese system of massage from which Palmer's techniques were derived

_____ 3. Media not used in seated massage

_____ 4. Item that replaces traditional hand washing at on-site massage locations

_____ 5. What the massage therapist must do before setting up the massage chair

_____ 6. Position most commonly used by therapists performing seated massage

_____ 7. System that must be established with the client because eye contact is not possible

_____ 8. Observation made by the therapist to determine whether he or she is working too hard or too deeply

_____ 9. Question verbalized to the client once the chair is completely adjusted to fit

_____ 10. Activities done if the client is experiencing seated massage for the first time

_____ 11. Method for obtaining the therapist's attention in a noisy treatment area

_____ 12. The stroke not used in seated massage

INTERNET ACTIVITIES

Visit http://www.massagemag.com/Magazine/2006/issue120/Chair.php and read the article Buying a Massage Chair. Using the Internet, look up all the chair manufacturers listed at the bottom of the article and choose the best chair for you.

Visit http://www.touchpro.org/about_touchpro/chair_massage_history.html and read the article about Chair Massage History. When did the phrase *on-site massage* originate?

Using the Internet, locate a reflexologist in your area. Place a telephone call and ask him or her three prepared questions regarding his or her practice.

Bibliography

Benjamin P, Tappan F: *Tappan's handbook of healing massage technique,* ed 4, Upper Saddle River, NJ, 2004, Prentice Hall.

Benjamin PJ: Seated massage in history, *Massage Ther J* 42(1):144, 2003.

Field T: Massage therapy reduces anxiety and enhances EEG pattern of alertness and math computations, *Int J Neurosci* 86:197-205, 1996.

Fritz S: *Fundamentals of therapeutic massage,* ed 3, St Louis, 2003, Elsevier.

Ironson G et al: Massage therapy is associated with enhancement of the immune system's cytotoxic capacity, *Int J Neurosci* 84:205-218, 1996.

Mattes A: *Active isolated stretching,* Sarasota, Fla, 1995, self-published.

Palmer D: *How to market on site massage,* Santa Rosa, Calif, 1986, Living Earth Crafts.

Palmer D: *The bodywork entrepreneur,* San Francisco, Calif, 1990, Thumb Press.

Parfitt A: *Seated acupressure bodywork: a practical handbook for therapists,* Berkeley, Calif, 2006, North Atlantic Books.

Stephens R: *Seated therapeutic massage,* vols I-III [video seminars], Cedar Rapids, Iowa, 1996.

Stephens R: *Therapeutic chair massage,* Baltimore, 2005, Lippincott Williams & Wilkins.

Travell JG, Simons D: *Myofascial pain and dysfunction, the trigger point manual,* Baltimore, 1992, Lippincott Williams & Wilkins.

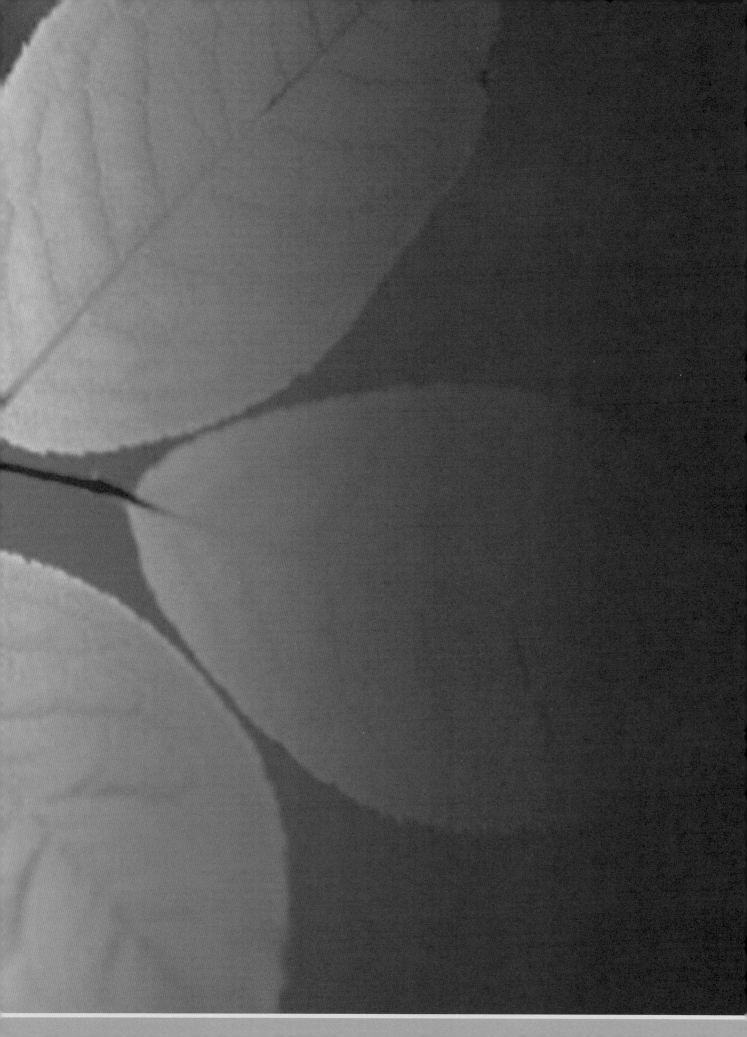

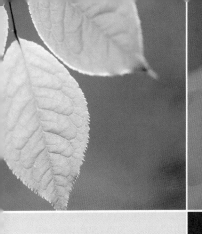

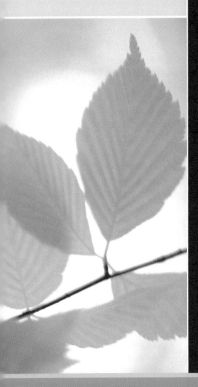

CHAPTER 28

"Experience is the hardest kind of teacher. It gives you the test first and the lesson afterward."
—Anonymous

Energy-Based Bodywork Therapy: Shiatsu and Ayurveda

Diego Sanchez, Dipl ABT (NCCAOM), CP (AOBTA), LMT
Kenneth G. Zysk, PhD, DPhil
Georgia Tetlow
Susan G. Salvo, BEd, LMT, NTS, CI, NCTMB

STUDENT OBJECTIVES

After completing this chapter, the student should be able to:

- Describe the unifying concept in shiatsu and Ayurveda
- Contrast and compare Asian and Western medicine
- Define Asian bodywork therapy
- State the definition of shiatsu
- Describe the theory of Yin and Yang and their major correspondences
- Name the twelve Regular Meridians, and delineate their path in the human body
- Define tsubo and their role in shiatsu
- Contrast and compare Zang organs to Fu organs
- State and describe the Five Element theory and its major correspondences
- Contrast and compare Creation Cycles with Control Cycles
- Discuss the concepts of Kyo and Jitsu and how they are used in treatment
- Apply appropriate techniques according to Ki (Qi) deficiency/Yin and/or excess/Yang conditions in the meridians while using proper body mechanics
- Incorporate the Zen shiatsu principles of touch during a session
- Demonstrate the techniques of thumbing and palming
- Explain Hara evaluation, and define its purpose
- Describe the three doshas
- State the Hindu meaning of prakriti
- Outline the seven chakras and their characteristics
- Contrast and compare traditional Chinese medicine and Ayurveda

INTRODUCTION TO ASIAN BODYWORK THERAPY

This chapter is designed to give the student an overview of Asian Bodywork Therapy, with a focus on shiatsu, a Japanese bodywork therapy. The chapter also examines Ayurveda, a Hindu science of health. Both systems are rooted in the philosophy of Traditional Asian Medicine.

The approach of Asian bodywork therapy is radically different from that of European massage. The Asian bodywork therapy principles are simple to understand and practice at a basic level; this chapter provides this basis. However, the professional practice of Asian bodywork therapy requires training and guidance of an instructor who is experienced in traditional Asian medicine. Should the material presented stimulate your curiosity, seek further training to expand the information provided in these pages. Asian bodywork therapy is a profession in itself, with nationally recognized standards of education.

TRADITIONAL ASIAN MEDICINE MODEL OF HEALTH

The central idea that runs through traditional Asian medicine is the concept of *energy*. Imagine a tree; the concept of energy is that the trunk and the branches are formed by the different ways of organizing energy for assessment and therapeutic purposes such as those taught in Chinese and Ayurvedic medicines (Figure 28-1). Traditional Asian medicine provides a basic model illustrating this concept. The

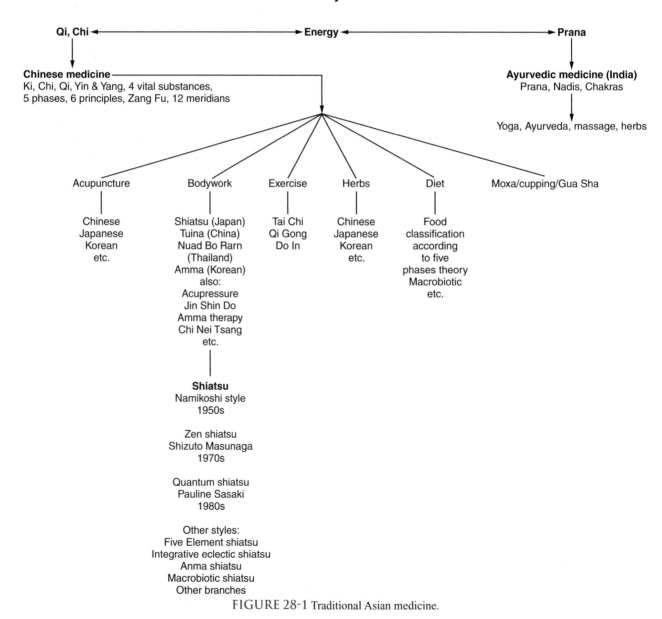

FIGURE 28-1 Traditional Asian medicine.

concept further branches out, following different styles that have originated in separate Asian regions (e.g., China, Japan, India) and have developed under the influence of many great teachers.

ENERGY

Energy, or **Ki** (in Japanese), *Qi* (sometimes spelled *Ch'i,* or *Chi*—all variations pronounced *chee*—in Chinese), or **Prana** (in India), also known as Life Force, is the element that creates and binds together all things and phenomena existing in the Universe (Figure 28-2). This composite includes everything that exhibits physically in Nature and in the human body, as well as the emotions, thoughts, and spirit.

Energy demonstrates itself as *movement* and *vibration.* Solid material and seemingly inanimate objects also have vibration that can be scientifically observed at a microscopic level in the vibration and movement of the atoms that form all things. Electrons spin around protons, and they constantly collide against each other and other atoms, releasing energy. The force of attraction and rejection between the protons and electrons and the space between them are also manifestations of energy in the form of a magnetic field that binds them. The human body also generates a magnetic field that can be measured around it.

Scientific studies done on particles of light determined that any given particle can be observed as a particle of matter or a wave of energy at the same time. This interchangeability between matter and wave (nonmatter) introduces the *concept of relativity* on which it is further expanded in the field of quantum physics. This concept coincides with the theories of Asian medicine.

Pauline Sasaki, a disciple of the renowned teacher Shizuto Masunaga and the creator of Quantum shiatsu, describes the observable energetic phenomena as variations in the speed of vibration in which the material aspects have the slowest speed of vibration (therefore easier to see to the naked eye), and the spiritual aspects have the fastest. The faster the vibration is, the harder it is to observe its manifestations, although by increasing the development of our sensory system, we are able to sense them. In any case, we can observe the effects of these faster vibrations the same as in the case of electricity,

in which we cannot see electricity itself, but we can see how a light turns on as we flip the switch.

> ### TABLE TALK
>
> #### Differences Between Asian and Western Medicine
>
> Allopathic or Western medicine is practiced by qualified physicians. Its model is *reductionist* in that using the scientific method strives to break down and separate the elements to find the smallest unit that can be modified to treat disease—for example, going to the molecular level and changing the chemical elements that interact in a symptom such as pain, using synthesized chemical compounds (drugs), or modifying or removing body parts with surgery. The emphasis is in the body parts and symptoms of disease. This system is the reason that you have a different specialist for the different organs, body parts or groups of diseases—cardiologist (heart), nephrologist (kidneys), oncologist (cancer), and so forth—thus each physician can narrow down his or her field of expertise to a smaller part of the body or a disease in particular. This process sometimes ends in having different physicians treating the same person for different things, in some cases prescribing conflicting treatment options. The circumstance that certain drugs used to improve one symptom caused harm to another function or organ of the body has occurred, such as a brand of pain medicine that had to be removed from the market because it caused increased rates of heart problems.
>
> Traditional Asian medicine is a system that includes all parts of the body, mind, and spirit, as well as the harmonious interaction of the individual with his or her surroundings (nature and the cosmos) in one indivisible continuum or unit. Any change in the parts of the system will affect the system as a whole; therefore any intervention is done having the whole system in consideration, not just the part being manipulated. Doing bodywork from the perspective of the traditional Asian medicine model of health, you will have the chance to create changes that will affect the person at many different levels, maybe changing how the person feels emotionally or even modifying patterns of behavior based on belief systems, such as how the person sees him or herself in the world. Any type of massage can have this effect, but knowing the theory of Asian bodywork therapy, you will have a method to evaluate and understand changes that occur beyond the purely physical aspects.
>
> The main difference between Eastern and Western European massage resides in the fact that the Eastern approach uses physical touch to balance the energetic system that includes, but is not solely defined by, the physical body.

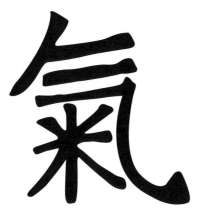

FIGURE 28-2 Symbol of Ki (Qi).

WHAT IS ASIAN BODYWORK THERAPY?

The American Organization for Bodywork Therapies of Asia (AOBTA) defines **Asian bodywork therapy (ABT)** as *the treatment of the human body/mind/spirit, including the electromagnetic or energetic field, which surrounds, infuses, and brings that body to life by pressure and/or manipulation.* Asian bodywork is based on traditional Chinese medicine (TCM) for assessing and evaluating the energetic system. It uses traditional Asian techniques and treatment strategies to affect and balance primarily the energetic system for the purpose of treating the human body, emotions, mind, energy field, and spirit for the promotion, maintenance, and restoration of health.

Many different bodywork therapies share the Asian origins and the definition mentioned previously—for example, shiatsu from Japan, Nuad Bo Rarn (Thai massage) from Thailand, Amma from Korea, Tuina from China, and other styles such as acupressure, Chi Nei Tsang, Jin Shin Do, Jin Shin Jyutsu, and so forth from different countries in Asia. Many of these styles developed further in countries such as the United States but keep referring to the same principles and philosophy originated in Asia more than 2500 years ago.

ABT is one of the three branches of traditional Asian medicine, as recognized by the National Certification Commission on Acupuncture and Oriental Medicine (NCCAOM). The other two branches are acupuncture and Oriental herbology. We might say that bodywork, acupuncture, and herbs are tools that can be used to apply the principles of traditional Asian medicine to regain and maintain health. The same principles of traditional Asian medicine can be applied through other means such as exercise (e.g., Tai Chi, Qi Gong), traditional Asian medicine dietary principles, **moxibustion** (stimulation of **acupoints** [see discussion in next section] with heat from burning an herb called mugwort or moxa above or on the acupoints), and other techniques such as **Gua-Sha** (a skin-scraping technique to help expel excess heat or remove energy stagnation) and **cupping** (a method in which a warmed cup is placed upside down directly on the skin, creating a vacuum that suctions the skin to relieve energy stagnation). Additionally, liniments, compresses, herbal baths, and essential oils on acupoints are used.

Herbs, foods, and essential oils have their own particular energetic qualities that have affinity for particular organs and functions of the body. They can be used to strengthen certain physiological functions and help resolve symptoms of disease. Only a qualified and experienced practitioner should use herbs.

SHIATSU

A Japanese bodywork therapy, **shiatsu,** uses pressure on the surface of the skin along energy channels called *meridians* to regain and maintain a harmonic flow of energy throughout the body-mind-spirit. The term *shiatsu* literally means "finger (*shi*) pressure (*atsu*)," but hands, elbows, knees and feet are also used and, when appropriate, joint mobilizations and stretches. Along the meridians are points called *tsubos,* also known as *acupoints* (although the term *acupoints* is more of an acupuncture term), which are energetic vortices on the surface of the skin where the energy of the meridian can be accessed.

From this perspective, health is a state of harmonious flow of the body-mind-spirit's energy (Ki) along the meridians. Symptoms of poor health can be interpreted as an imbalance of Ki flow. According to a person's state of health, his or her symptoms, and, depending on constitution and general energy levels, the shiatsu practitioner should use a variety of techniques to improve the energy flow. As the quality of Ki changes with the application of shiatsu, the symptoms associated with lack of Ki flow will gradually improve, facilitating pain relief; improved digestion, breathing, elimination, and sleep patterns; increased mobility; and reduced anxiety and depression. Following a treatment, a feeling of increased vitality can be felt, and the person may feel invigorated yet relaxed.

Traditional shiatsu is done on a floor mat; it can also be done on a massage table or with the person seated. Given that the client is fully clothed and no oils or ointments are used, shiatsu is extremely versatile for almost any environment and situation. It is popular not just for relaxation and well-being but also in pregnancy, during labor, in critical care of patients in hospitals, emergency relief support and in corporate, military, and other settings.

Based in TCM, shiatsu had been used in Japan for centuries until it was banned, alongside other folk medicine methods, during the U.S. occupation of Japan after World War II. In the 1950s, Tokujiro Namikoshi created a style of shiatsu that used Western anatomy references instead of traditional nomenclature. Thanks to this effort, the Ministry of Health in Japan approved his style of shiatsu as medical treatment. The Namikoshi Shiatsu School is still open today, and this style of shiatsu is very popular in Japan.

Shizuto Masunaga, creator of Zen Shiatsu, studied with Namikoshi but took a different turn with his work. He trained at the university as a psychologist but also studied the ancient Chinese medicine texts in which more mind-spirit references to clinical practice were commonplace. After meticulous research, Masunaga came up with an expanded model of health in which emotional and mental aspects of the person were taken more in consideration and blended into the physical touch technique of Zen Shiatsu. He created a new chart of meridians that had extensions of the meridian pathways and also contributed to the field with Hara diagnosis technique, which is widely used in shiatsu schools throughout the world today. Both the classical and Zen Shiatsu meridians are featured in some of the figures in this text. Hara diagnostic areas are also featured for each of the 12 sets of meridians.

YIN AND YANG

How is energy generated? The theory of Yin and Yang mentioned in the *Yellow Emperor's Inner Classic* (*Huang Di Nei Jing* in Chinese), a text that dates as far back as 300 to 100 BC and is still used today, provides a model to explain the creation of Ki. The widely reproduced symbol of the **Tai Ji,** which represents Yin and Yang, is formed by a complete circle (the One, completeness), divided in two sides (symbolizing Duality, struggle between opposites), one black, one white, each containing a smaller circle of the opposite color (symbolizing the nonabsolute quality of all things) within itself (Figure 28-3). Hence yin contains a speck of Yang within itself and vice versa.

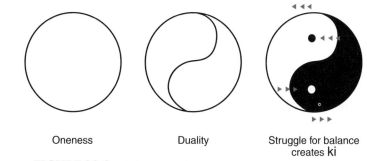

| Void | Oneness | Duality | Struggle for balance creates ki |

FIGURE 28-3 Tai Ji or symbol of Yin and Yang.

The two sides are constantly moving toward each other in a *circular* way, the same as during the day (Yang); the light of the sun decreases to make way to the darkness of the night (Yin), and dawn comes to end the night by bringing light (Yang) into the darkness (Yin). The constant movement of one thing into its opposite is what generates Ki. In this example, keep in mind that a moment of the day exists, after sunset or before sunrise, that is difficult to tell whether it is day or night. Day and night are relative to each other and also relative to the point where the observer is placed.

Yin and Yang literally mean in Chinese "the light (sunny) side of the hill and the dark (shadow) side of the hill." It poetically describes a dynamic that can be observed not only in the duality of the day-night or lightness-darkness cycle, but also in all aspects of Nature. Male/female, up/down, inside/outside, slow/fast, matter/energy, passive/active, and contraction/expansion are just some of the possible Yin/Yang pairs. An illustration of the sunny and dark sides of a hill can be seen on the Evolve website accompanying this text.

On the sunny side of the hill, more light, warmth, activity, and movement exist. Plants grow easily and have foliage and seeds that attract insects and birds. On the shadow side of the hill, it is darker, the temperature is cooler, plants grow more slowly, more dampness can be found, and less activity overall exists compared with the sunny side.

When comparing a list of Yin and Yang qualities, remember that one is not *better* than the other and that one is not necessarily *right* and the other is *wrong*. They are simply different aspects of the same thing: Ki (Table 28-1). They mutually create and balance each other; thus they are both necessary for the other one to exist. For example, in the West, we ascribe cultural value to *being on top* as better than *being down*, but *up* would not exist without a *down*. From the ABT perspective, both sides are necessary for everything in between to exist. They have equal value, being relative to each other. Health is a dynamic equilibrium between Yin and Yang.

Given that energy is movement, to experientially get in contact with the movement of Yin energy, we can focus on the contractive phase (movement from the periphery to the center and from the top to bottom). To get in contact with Yang energy, we can focus on the expansive phase of energy (movement from the center to the periphery and from be-

low to above). As an illustration, air expands and rises when heated, and it contracts and moves downward when cooled. These phases exhibit as *tendencies,* always in movement, not absolute.

The concept of direction of energy movement between Yin and Yang is often best understood with a picture, just as *a picture is worth a thousand words*. Log on to the Evolve web site using your student account to see this image and more.

In ABT, a symptom such as pain, for example, can be assessed energetically as being either predominantly Yin or predominantly Yang in nature and treated accordingly. Pain, as a manifestation of a Yang imbalance, is a feeling of heat,

TABLE 28-1   **Some Relative Correspondences of Yin and Yang**

YIN	YANG
Feminine	Masculine
Dark	Light
Cold (numb)	Hot (inflamed)
Moist	Dry
Interior	Exterior
Chronic	Acute
Anterior	Posterior
Medial	Lateral
Inferior	Superior
Community	Competition
Earth	Heaven
Water	Fire
Moon	Sun
Slow (still, lethargic)	Fast (restless, energetic)
Static, storing, conserving	Transforming, changing
Substantial	Nonsubstantial
Matter	Energy
Soft, mushy tissue	Hard, congested tissue
Concave	Convex
Passive (inhibited)	Active (excited)
Pale tongue	Red tongue
Thin pulse	Full pulse
Contraction	Expansion
Deficiency	Excess
Pain is dull, achy, stiff	Pain is sharp or moving
Deep	Shallow (on the surface)
Client says "Mm-mm-mm."	Client says "Ow!"

agitation, and restlessness; the area appears red, is warm to touch, feels hard, and is inflamed; symptoms are in the upper part of the body, and the pain is sharp and moves around. The person may feel additional pain if you touch the area directly.

Pain as a manifestation of a Yin imbalance is a feeling of cold, weakness, weight, and lethargy; the pain is dull rather than sharp, and it feels deep; if in the lower part of the body, the area can be soft (if hard, then it feels empty underneath), the skin is discolored or dark, and it feels good if the area is touched directly. Yang-type of pain can be observed in acute phases of injury. Yin-type of pain can be observed in chronic and prolonged phases of disease.

Therapeutically, you would address a Yang condition with soothing (Yin) techniques that would help *disperse the excess energy*. In the case of a Yin imbalance, you want to bring in a bit more movement (Yang) to break up the stagnation of energy or *tonify* or *strengthen the deficiency or weaknesses*. Using a bit of the opposite quality as needed, you are helping to restore the movement between Yin and Yang, and this action, in itself, will help the person regain balance at all levels. If a person is living with persistent physical pain, over time he or she will become impatient, angry, or depressed (emotional aspects). The person's perception of himself or herself and his or her ability to succeed in whatever aim the person has, his or her outlook on life (mental aspects), and even the person's relationship with others and the Universe (spiritual aspects) will be affected. The same happens the other way around; for example, a depressed person tends to develop certain types of physical imbalances or disease. ABT offers a coherent theory to understand and work with all these aspects of the person, using just our hands as tools to manipulate the body.

MERIDIANS

Energy circulates in the body through **meridians** (pathways of energy) and vessels, helping to move the *vital substances* (Ki, essence, blood, body fluids, and Spirit) to the *Zang/Fu* (Organ Systems that include the internal organs and functions associated to them and discussed in a later section). The meridians are the connections of the material body to the nonmaterial part of the body (energy field surrounding the body). They are systems of subtle channels of energy that distribute, balance, and connect the Ki of the interior organs with the surface and exterior of the body.

Meridians help "move the Ki and blood, regulate the Yin and the Yang, moisten the tendons and the bones, and benefit the joints...." *(Yellow Emperor's Classic)*. Ki circulates through the meridians in a fixed direction, one meridian ending where the following one starts, making one continuous interconnected channel.

Meridians meet at the distal ends of the extremities. The order of the flow follows the *Chinese Clock,* a system based in the circadian or biological cycle in which each organ has a time of the day when its energy is at its peak of activity, starting with the lung and ending with the liver (Figure 28-4).

Names of Organ Systems and meridians are depicted in capital letters (e.g., *heart*) to differentiate from the anatomi-

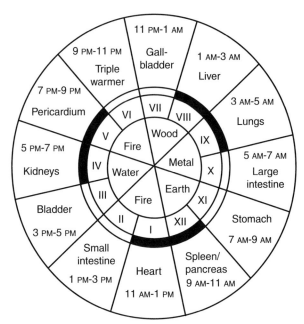

FIGURE 28-4 Chinese Clock.

BOX 28-1

Enrichment: Eastern Anatomical Position

In the Eastern anatomic position, the arms are raised above the head, with palms facing forward. The Yang channels descend from the ceiling downward along the backside of the body, and the Yin channels ascend from the feet upwards to the hands along the front and trunk of the body.

---

cal organs, such as the heart. If you find that a client has a heart meridian imbalance, then be careful with your language, and avoid making statements such as "You have a problem with your heart." This statement may cause unnecessary anxiety in your client about a possible medical condition of his or her heart, and it clearly falls outside our scope of practice.

The most important ones are the 12 Regular Meridians, which are bilateral and symmetric, and the eight Extraordinary Vessels. The twelve Regular Meridians (six Yang and six Yin) are named after the Organ Systems associated with them.

1. Lung (LU): 3 to 5 AM (Figure 26-5)
2. Large intestine (LI): 5 to 7 AM (Figure 26-6)
3. Stomach (ST): 7 to 9 AM (Figure 26-7)
4. Spleen (SP): 9 to 11 AM (Figure 26-8)
5. Heart (HT): 11 AM to 1 PM (Figure 26-9)
6. Small intestine (SI): 1 to 3 PM (Figure 26-10)
7. Bladder (BL): 3 to 5 PM (Figure 26-11)
8. Kidney (KID): 5 to 7 PM (Figure 26-12)
9. Heart protector (HP) or pericardium (P): 7 to 9 PM (Figure 26-13)
10. Triple heater (TH): 9 to 11 PM (Figure 26-14)
11. Gallbladder (GB): 11 PM to 1 AM (Figure 26-15)
12. Liver (LIV): 1 to 3 AM (Figure 26-16)

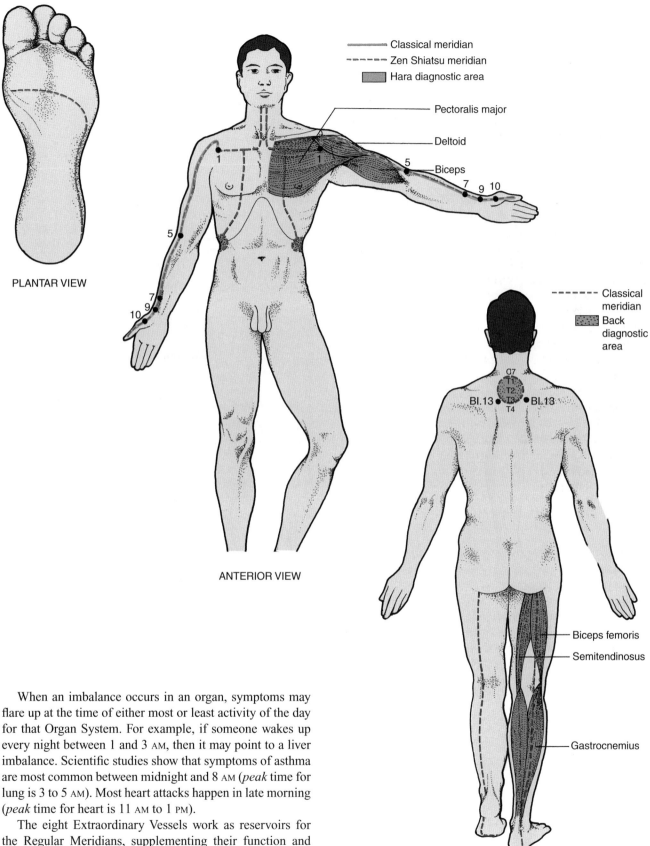

PLANTAR VIEW

ANTERIOR VIEW

POSTERIOR VIEW

FIGURE 28-5 The lung meridian. (From Beresford-Cooke C: *Shiatsu theory and practice,* Edinburgh, 1999, Churchill Livingstone.)

When an imbalance occurs in an organ, symptoms may flare up at the time of either most or least activity of the day for that Organ System. For example, if someone wakes up every night between 1 and 3 AM, then it may point to a liver imbalance. Scientific studies show that symptoms of asthma are most common between midnight and 8 AM (*peak* time for lung is 3 to 5 AM). Most heart attacks happen in late morning (*peak* time for heart is 11 AM to 1 PM).

The eight Extraordinary Vessels work as reservoirs for the Regular Meridians, supplementing their function and pooling and storing Ki as needed to preserve balance in the whole system. The Conception (ren), Governing (du). Penetrating (chong), and Belt (dai) Vessels are particularly important in the formation and support of the embryo.

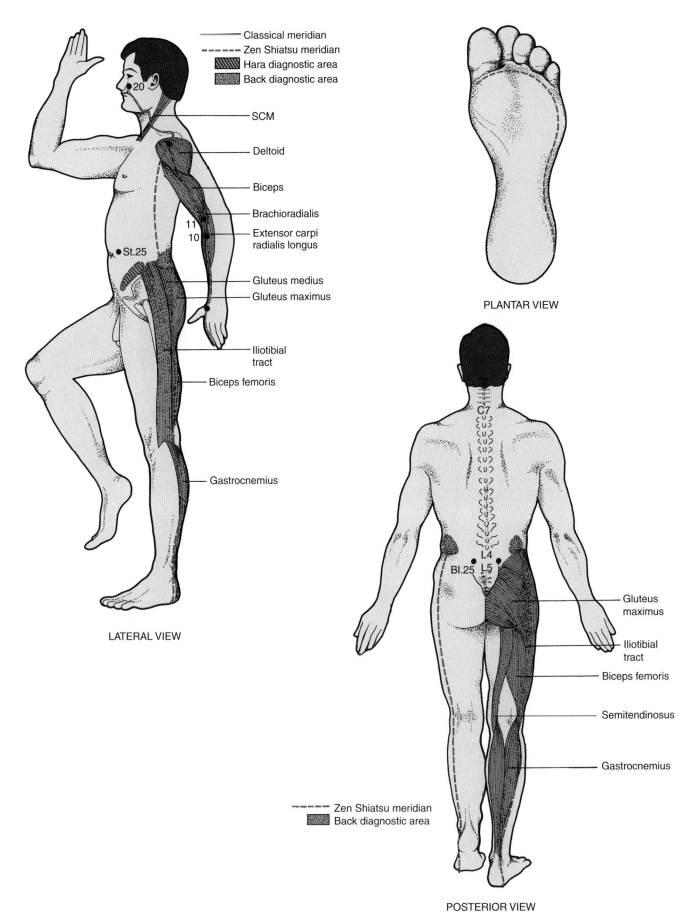

FIGURE 28-6 The large intestine meridian. (From Beresford-Cooke C: *Shiatsu theory and practice,* Edinburgh, 1999, Churchill Livingstone.)

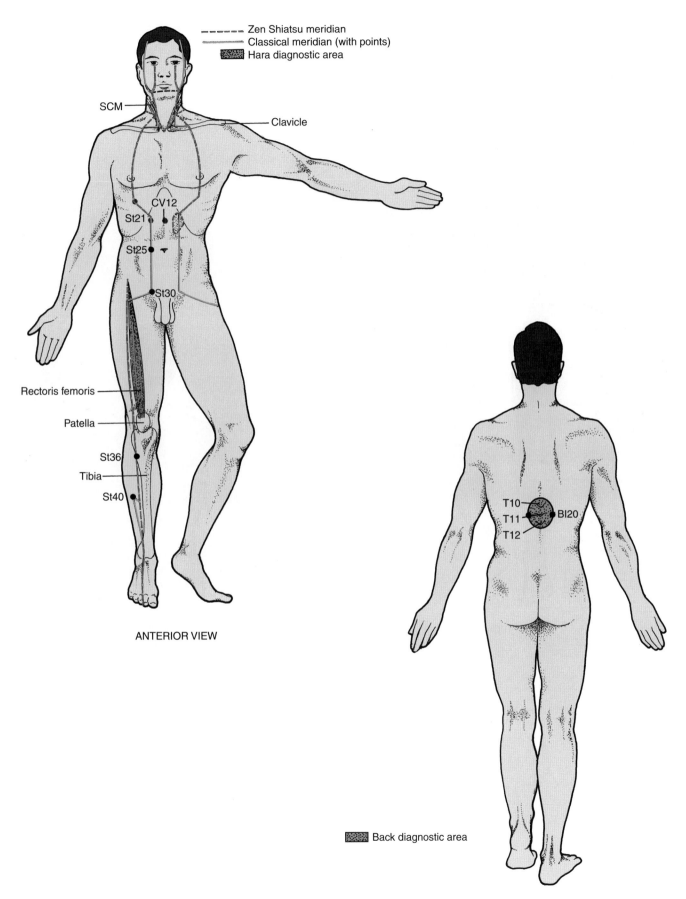

FIGURE 28-7 The stomach meridian. (From Beresford-Cooke C: *Shiatsu theory and practice,* Edinburgh, 1999, Churchill Livingstone.)

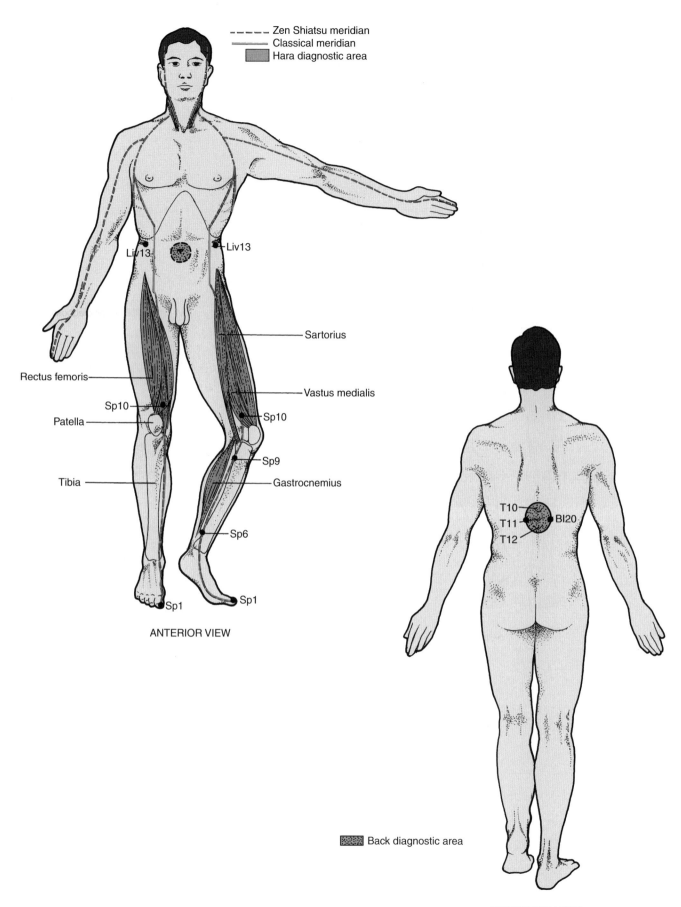

FIGURE 28-8 The spleen meridian. (From Beresford-Cooke C: *Shiatsu theory and practice,* Edinburgh, 1999, Churchill Livingstone.)

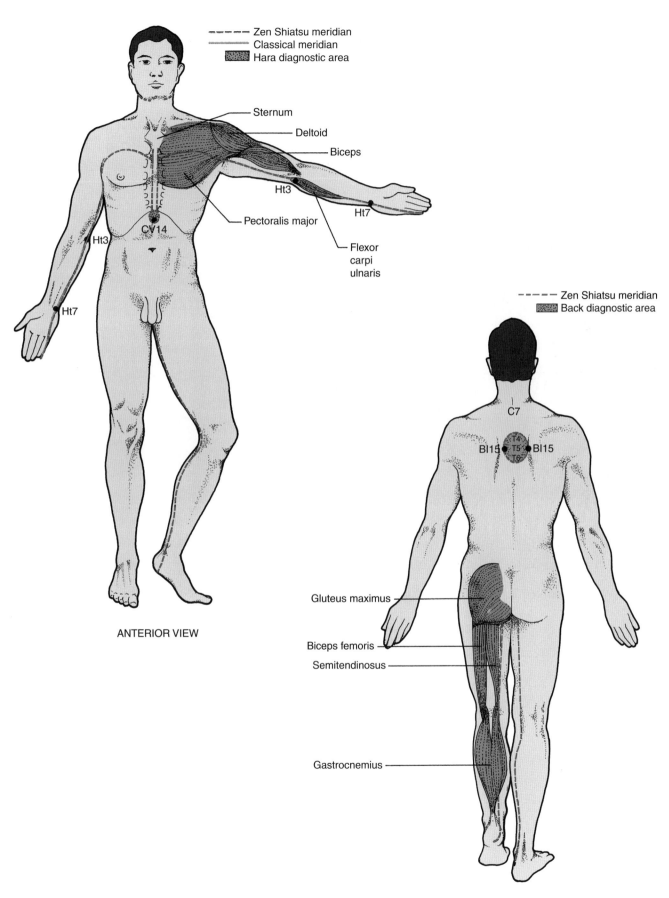

FIGURE 28-9 The heart meridian. (From Beresford-Cooke C: *Shiatsu theory and practice,* Edinburgh, 1999, Churchill Livingstone.)

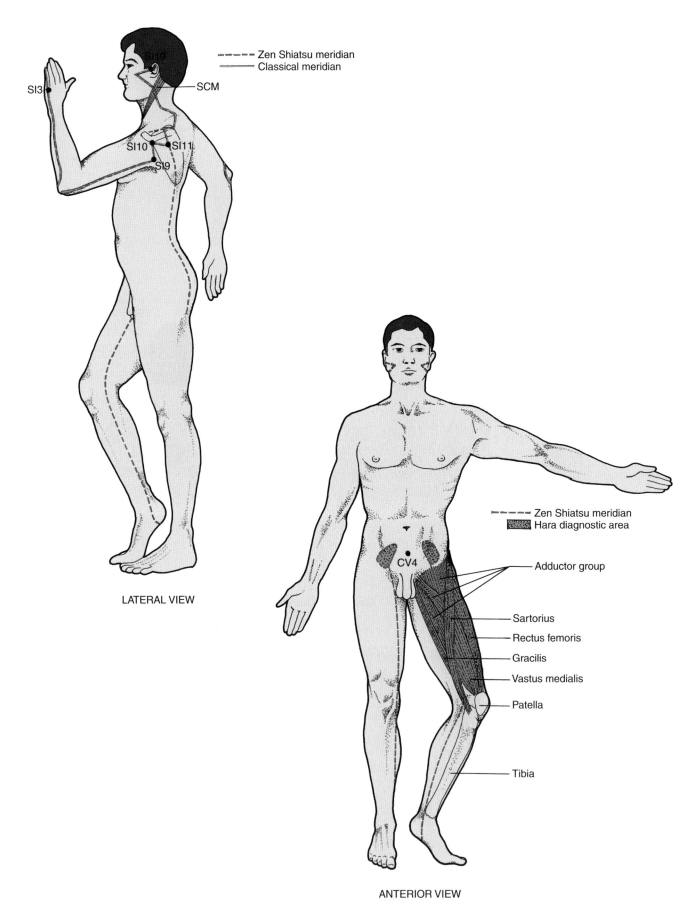

FIGURE 28-10 The small intestine meridian. (From Beresford-Cooke C: *Shiatsu theory and practice,* Edinburgh, 1999, Churchill Livingstone.) *(continued)*

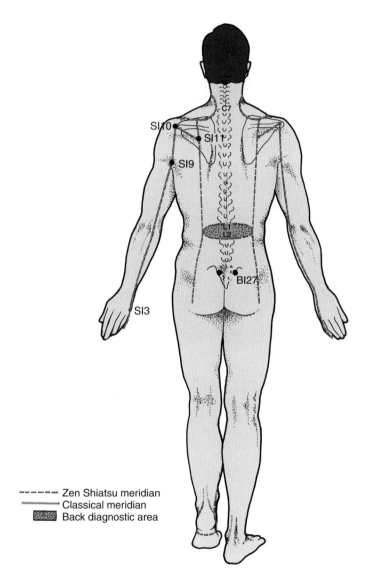

POSTERIOR VIEW

FIGURE 28-10, cont'd

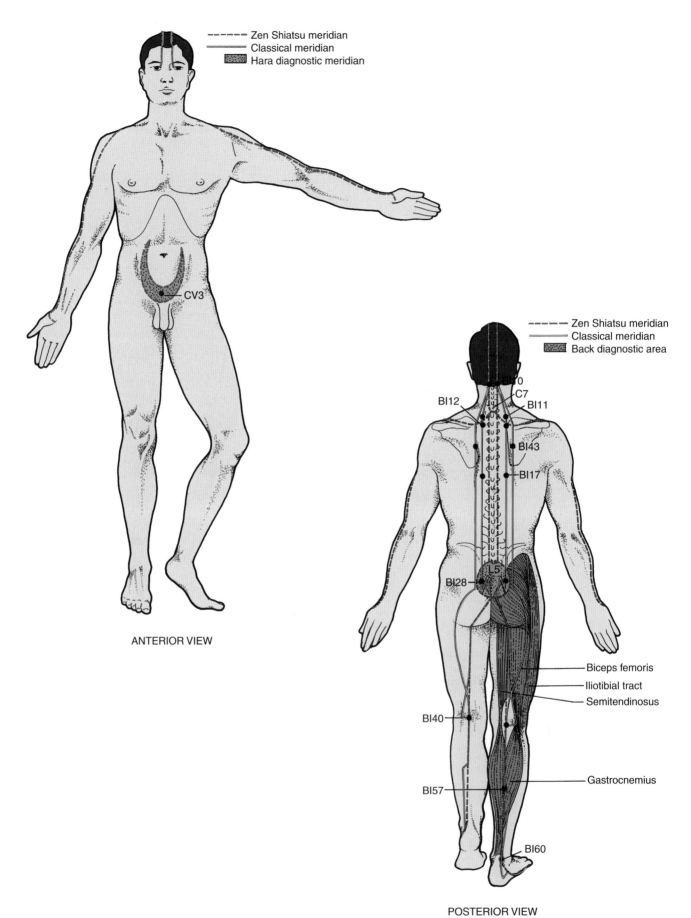

ANTERIOR VIEW

POSTERIOR VIEW

FIGURE 28-11 The bladder meridian. (From Beresford-Cooke C: *Shiatsu theory and practice,* Edinburgh, 1999, Churchill Livingstone.)

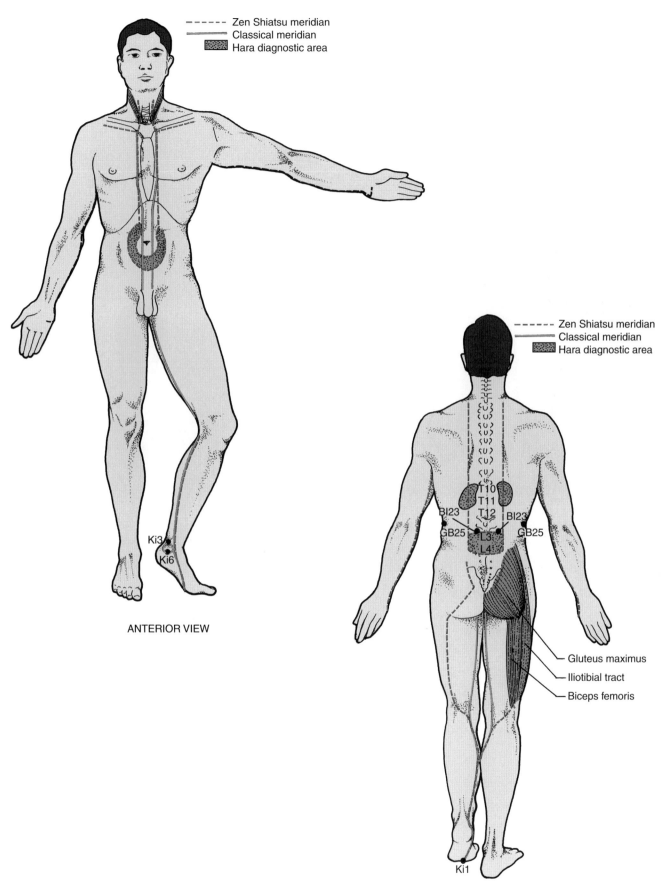

FIGURE 28-12 The kidney meridian. (From Beresford-Cooke C: *Shiatsu theory and practice,* Edinburgh, 1999, Churchill Livingstone.)

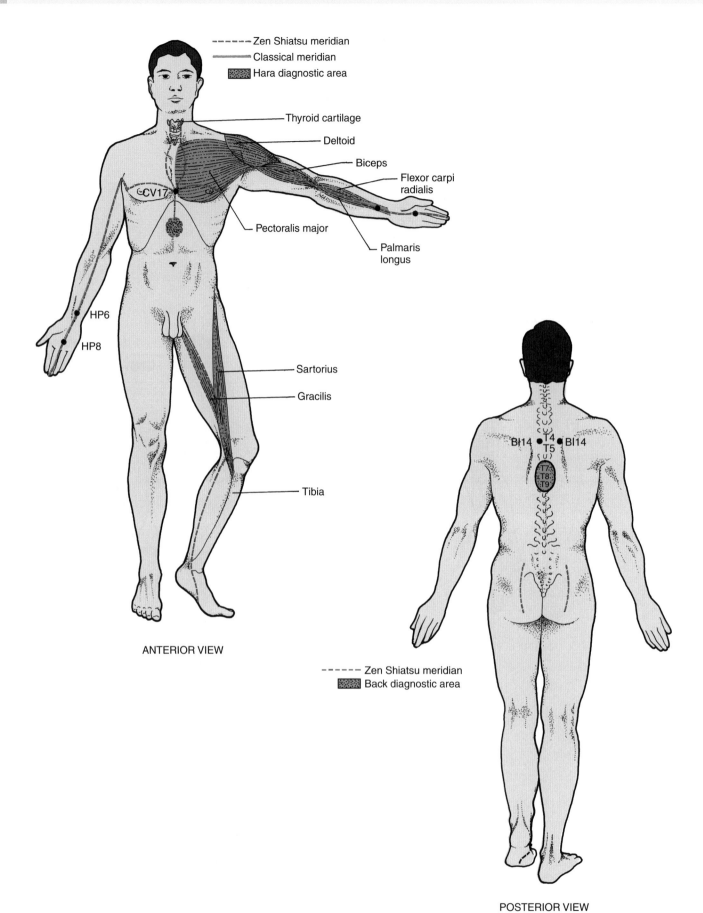

FIGURE 28-13 The heart protector or pericardium meridian. (From Beresford-Cooke C: *Shiatsu theory and practice,* Edinburgh, 1999, Churchill Livingstone.)

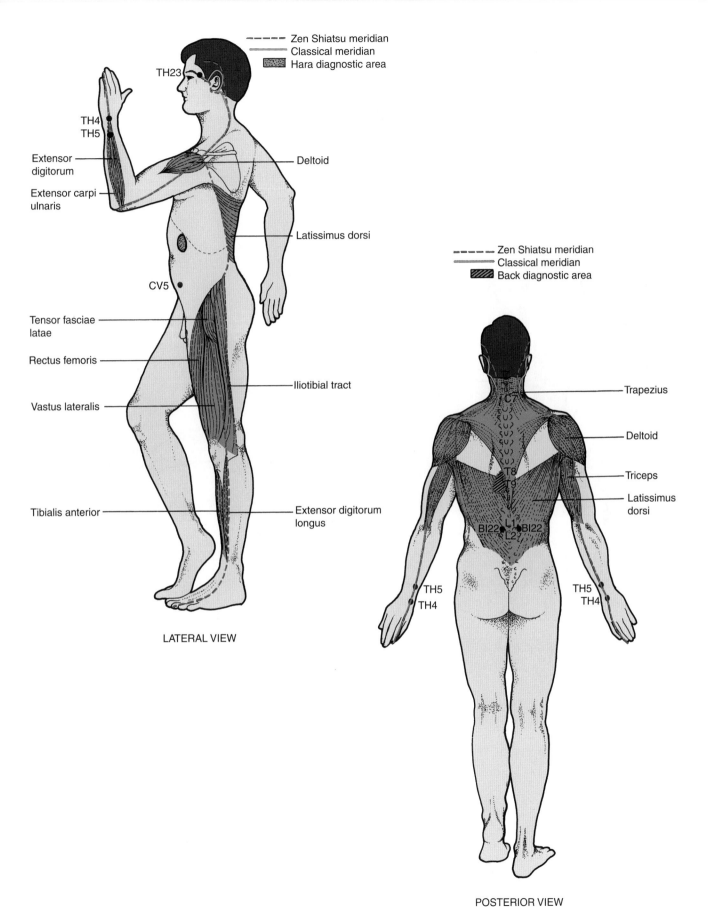

LATERAL VIEW

POSTERIOR VIEW

FIGURE 28-14 The triple heater meridian. (From Beresford-Cooke C: *Shiatsu theory and practice,* Edinburgh, 1999, Churchill Livingstone.)

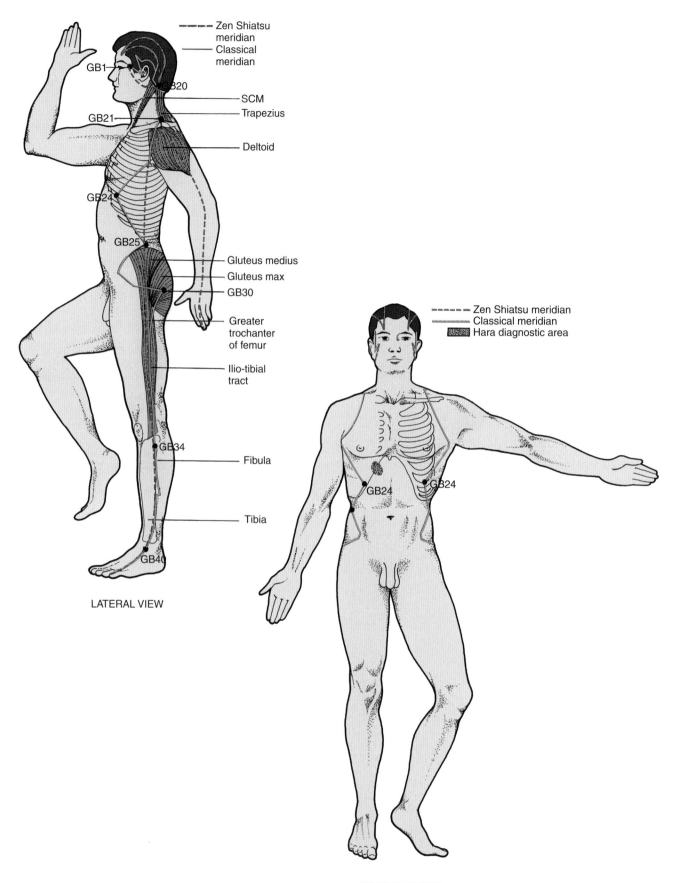

LATERAL VIEW

ANTERIOR VIEW

FIGURE 28-15 The gallbladder meridian. (From Beresford-Cooke C: *Shiatsu theory and practice,* Edinburgh, 1999, Churchill Livingstone.)

(continued)

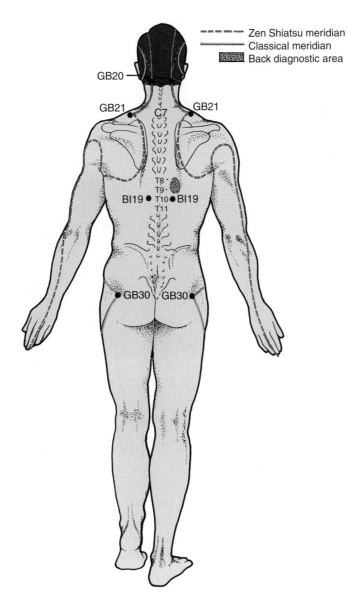

POSTERIOR VIEW
FIGURE 28-15, cont'd

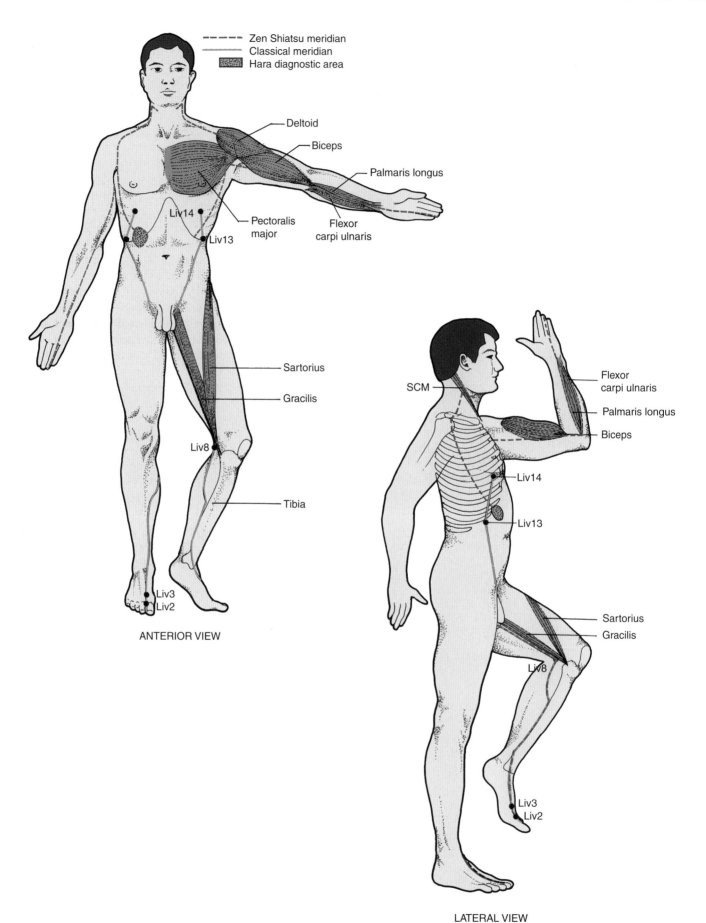

FIGURE 28-16 The liver meridian. (From Beresford-Cooke C: *Shiatsu theory and practice,* Edinburgh, 1999, Churchill Livingstone.)

TSUBOS

Along the meridians are points at which the energy concentrates and surfaces as vortices of Ki. These points are called **tsubos** (Japanese for *container* or *vase*). Meridian charts map the location of the tsubos related to each channel. The tsubos have specific actions when stimulated with pressure (shiatsu, acupressure), the insertion of needles (acupuncture), heat (moxibustion), essential oils, and even the vibration of tuning forks placed on them. They are identified with the name of the meridian plus numbers that increase in order from the origin to the end of the meridian pathway (SP1, SP2, SP3, and so forth). They also have Chinese names that sometimes evoke geographical features such as Kid1 *(Bubbling Spring),* LI4 *(Union Valley),* and HP7 *(Great Mound).* Knowing the indications for these points, you can include them in your treatment plan, according to the symptoms presented by your client. You can obtain reference guides with the names, locations, indications and actions of the 361 tsubos of the body.

TABLE TALK

To find the location of the tsubos, distance is measured in cun (pronounced *soon*), which is the body inch unit (Figure 28-17). For example, ST36 *(Leg Three Miles)* is located *3 cun below the lower edge of the patella, 1 cun lateral to the crest of the tibia.* Each cun is measured by the width of the client's own thumb knuckle.

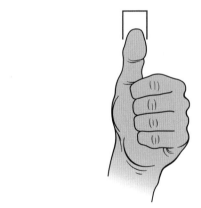

FIGURE 28-17 Cun illustration.

Kyo and Jitsu

When you palpate or lean on a tsubo, it will feel neutral, full, or empty. Kyo and Jitsu are terms used to describe the quantity of energy or the activity in a tsubo. **Kyo** means empty, Yin, depleted and not enough Ki. **Jitsu** means full, Yang, excess and too much Ki. Jitsu also means the quality of the Ki such as responsive, sluggish, soft, hard, expansive, or contractive.

In most instances, when you lean on a Kyo tsubo or area of the body, it feels as though you can go deep; it can feel

soft, cooler, nonresponsive, or sluggish. Energy in the tsubo is lacking; thus the Ki you are projecting in the form of pressure through your hand is welcome. While focusing on it, you are calling Ki to that particular tsubo, helping to draw energy towards it. This technique is called *tonification.* The Ki that pours into the tsubo comes from other places within the system of the client (where it is not needed or an excess exists) and the Universe. When you feel something start to stir or move, you move on to another point.

By bringing the attention to the tsubo, your Ki initiates a process, a process of transformation. This concept does not imply that you are pouring your own Ki into the tsubo, as in a gasoline filling station. By respecting the Zen shiatsu principles of touch (see later discussion), your own energy field will be expanded. Because of this expansion, the therapist should not feel drained at the end of a session.

A Jitsu tsubo feels full of energy. The point may feel hard, warm, and superficial. Your pressure feels *pushed out* or resisted to the extent that it feels as if you cannot stay there long. Your intention in this case should be to *disperse* or *sedate* the excess Ki in the tsubo. This technique is called *sedation.*

As with Yin and Yang, Kyo and Jitsu are relative to each other.

This entire system is designed to be self-regulating. Every Jitsu has a corresponding Kyo somewhere down the line, the depletion of which is bankrolling the excess; and every Kyo has a Jitsu that needs to overwork to balance the deficiency. You sometimes find Ko and Jitsu points next to each other on the same meridian. In fact, you will find meridians that are predominantly Kyo or predominantly Jitsu.

Through tonification and sedation, you want to even out the Ki in the whole channel. This process will balance the Ki in the whole system. The treatment strategy is to

1. Identify Kyo and Jitsu
2. Tonify the Kyo
3. If necessary, disperse the Jitsu
4. Check for changes until Ki evens out throughout the whole meridian or system.

You must first *address the need* (Kyo) wherever you find it because this action will start getting the whole system moving. Homeostasis, the natural tendency of the body to balance itself, will tend to move the system toward balance and equilibrium on its own. Probably by the time you go back to the first identified Jitsu area or tsubo, it would have already started to change before you touch it again.

If you push the Ki away from a Jitsu area or tsubo, without identifying and tonifying the Kyo first, it may feel temporarily better, but the results will not be long lasting. The difference between tonification and sedation techniques is your *intention* because you will always be applying relaxed, perpendicular, stationary projection of Ki on each tsubo.

---

evolve Technique tips for Eastern practitioners, as well as Hara diagnostic tips, are located on the Evolve web site for this chapter. ∎

ZANG/FU

The **Zang/Fu** are the Organ Systems, both Yin and Yang, the definition of which includes the internal organs and the meridians. The functions of the Organ Systems are not only physical (e.g., digestion, or transformation of foods for nourishment in the case of the stomach and the spleen) but also refer to the emotional, mental, and spiritual levels. Continuing with the example of stomach and spleen Organ Systems, emotional nourishment is as important for the full development of a child as food is. Mental stimulation and nourishment (learning) is vital for the development of intellectual capabilities, the same as nourishing your relationships with yourself, others, and the Universe can help you have a spiritually rich life. The same applies for all the other functions of the body (e.g., respiration, elimination, detoxification, assimilation). Organ Systems such as triple heater, also known as triple warmer, do not have a similar performing organ in Western anatomy.

Zang are the Yin organs: heart, liver, lungs, kidney, pericardium, and spleen. They tend to be *solid* organs. **Fu** are the Yang organs: small intestine, gallbladder, large intestine, bladder, triple heater, and stomach, which tend to be *hollow* organs. As Organ Systems, the Zang/Fu also have correspondences and associations to other organs (they associate in pairs, one Yin the other Yang, for example, liver/gallbladder, or lung/large intestine, and so forth), elemental forces in Nature (Wind, Fire, Earth, Metal, and Wood), climatic conditions (dampness, heat, cold, dryness), colors, sounds, flavors, smells, times of the day, seasons, and other characteristics.

A good flow of energy through the meridians and vessels to the whole system keeps the Zang/Fu and the body nourished, which is the foundation for health. An imbalance anywhere in the system—or an interruption, blockage, or depletion of the flow of energy—will affect not only the area, but also the system as a whole. ABT can be used as a preventive medicine by identifying the imbalances and helping to restore this flow. When an ABT practitioner works with this system, you must remember that the aim is not to fix the particular problem or symptom that might be calling our immediate attention but rather to restore a smooth flow of energy overall. This action, in itself, will help ensure that the functions of the Zang/Fu are performed properly, and, in turn, any imbalances or symptoms will tend to be resolved.

THEORY OF THE FIVE PHASES (OR FIVE ELEMENTS)

Another way to classify the information observed from natural phenomena is using the theory of Five Phases (also translated from Chinese as *Five Elements*), which has been compiled through centuries of careful observation of life cycles and Nature. The term *phases* is used here because it best describes a dynamic of the energy rather than a fixed state.

Of later appearance in history than the theory of Yin and Yang, another metaphor, or image, can help you understand what is going on with a person. Each phase describes a particular dynamic and resonance that a group of things and phenomena have in common. Health is the balanced expression of all these phases in harmony with each other.

The Five Phases, or Elements, are *Earth, Wood, Fire, Metal,* and *Water*. They can be correlated, for example, with the different stages in the biological cycle of birth, growth, climax, decay, and death. Another example can be the seasons of the year (the fifth season being what is called *Indian summer,* or late summer, or the transition between seasons) and how the seasons have particular qualities. The phases refer mainly to the process, or how the energy behaves, at these different stages.

Each phase has influence over, and is influenced by, its associated body organs, sense organs, body secretion, color, flavor, smell, sound, season of the year, time of the day, emotion, and by its general body-mind-spiritual function.

Wood

The Wood phase is associated with the exuberance and fast growth you can observe in the Spring as the seeds sprout, new and flexible shoots appear on the branches of the trees, and the activity that had decreased during the Winter suddenly picks up. Green, the color of foliage at its peak, is the color associated with the Wood phase. People also react to the influence of the Spring, and the Wood phase is observed in the renewed hope and bursts of energy you get with the first sunny days after a long Winter. Strong winds are common in Spring. Wind is associated with the Wood phase and is recognized as an element of influence. In a person, this dynamic can be observed as the emotional irritation we can develop when exposed to a draft of air for a long time. In addition, a burst of anger has a similar behavior to a burst of wind that pushes and breaks things for a few moments to suddenly disappear. The same as anger calms down once it has been vented (from Latin *ventus,* meaning "wind"). Anger and frustration, which can be repressed anger, are emotions associated with the Wood phase. These emotions are associated with the liver and gallbladder Organ Systems. The connection between emotions and physical health is starting to be understood by modern allopathic medicine. In TCM, this connection has been firmly and accurately established for many centuries. In common language, when a person talks with *bile* (a substance actually secreted by the liver and stored in gallbladder) or when someone is *green with envy,* you can recognize the connection between the liver *(Liv)* and gallbladder *(GB)* Organ Systems and the associations of the Wood phase such as the color green and the emotion of anger. By working liver or gallbladder meridians or their corresponding points on the surface of the skin, you might be able to help someone with chronic anger to change or moderate his or her behavior.

Liver stocks or stores Ki for decisive action, distributes Ki where it needed (the *general of the troops*), and is involved in the functions of planning and detoxification. Gallbladder together with liver is involved in decision making (deciding which way to turn) and affects the sides of the body and eyes. Sour flavor, craving for oils and fats, are also related to Wood.

Fire

The Fire Phase rules the heart, small intestine, heart protector (or pericardium), and triple heater (also known as triple warmer) Organ Systems; it also provides light, warmth, and *spark,* a lively and colorful dynamic. The Fire Phase is associated with the color red, summer, heat, bitter flavor, the tongue, the circulatory system and blood vessels, the emotion of joy, speech, sweat, meditation, insight, and inspiration. When imbalanced, a craving for alcohol may exist.

Main functions of these Organ Systems are (1) heart, *emotional stability,* (2) small intestine, *assimilation,* (3) heart protector, *circulation,* and (4) triple heater, *protection.* Together they are the *interpreters of experience.*

Earth

Being *down to earth* is an expression that sums up the centering, stable quality of this phase. Between all the other phases, a moment of transition exists that is ruled by the Earth.

All foods come from the soil and therefore are associated with Earth. Particularly grains and the act of eating have a calming, satisfying, and comforting effect. People eat *comfort foods* when sick or depressed. These foods are those that remind us of home, with its warmth, safety, sweet smells, and the figure of the mother. *Mother Earth* in its bountiful generosity, fertility, receptivity, and patience provides everything we need.

The yellow color associated with Earth comes from the color of the soil in the region of northern China, where the theory of Five Phases was reputedly born (Huang He, Yellow River). Carefully observing a person's face, you can sometimes distinguish a yellow hue or coloring that can point to an Earth Phase imbalance, probably affecting the spleen or stomach, the Organ Systems associated to Earth.

The main functions of stomach and spleen are digestion and transformation for nourishment. They are associated with fertility, reproductive organs, moisture, singing, sweet flavor, the flesh, lips, and saliva. Craving sugar is a sign of imbalance, pointing to these Organ Systems.

Metal

From the soil deep in the Earth, minerals are extracted to make strong and valuable metals. During our history as human beings, the metal blade of swords and other weapons has shaped much of our civilization structure. The borders of countries have been determined by wars fought with metal weapons or by the influence of commerce done with precious metals. Gold is the agreed measure of material worth in our society. Value, worth, structure, shape, and border are some of the words associated to the Metal phase. The border of our body, the skin, and keeping healthy psychological boundaries are necessary to protect ourselves from unwanted outside influences. A sense of self-worth (Metal), for example, is gained and supported from the grounded (Earth) knowledge of ourselves.

The lung and the large intestine Organ Systems are also associated with Metal. In TCM, lung gathers Ki from the air and creates Wei (protective) Ki, which circulates along the surface of the body as a barrier of defense. Our *first breath* and *last breath* mark the beginning and end boundaries of our life in physical form. The large intestine function of elimination or *letting go* is what helps us get rid of unwanted body waste. It also applies to unwanted emotional or mental structures we do not need anymore.

The nose, pungent and spicy flavors, color white, autumn, grief, mucus, dry climate, and imbalanced craving for protein are also associations with Metal phase. The figure of the father is traditionally associated to this element also. The main functions of the Organ Systems are (1) lung, *intake of Ki* and (2) large intestine, *elimination.*

Water

Water takes the shape of whichever vessel contains it, be it a river or a glass, but at the same time keeps its very unique characteristics. It always moves toward the lowest point in a smooth downward direction. Fluidity and adaptability are some of its defining characteristics.

This characteristic is what gives water its power and energy, as a stream coming down the mountain. If the mountain slopes are gentle, then water will move smoothly and easily in a continuous stream. If rocks and branches interrupt the stream, then water will go around, jump over, or carve into the obstacles until it finds its way through. *Willpower* is a trait associated to the Water phase.

Water rules the functioning of the kidney and bladder, the function of which is to provide the impetus (*get up and go* energy) for life. A precious and essential element for survival (our bodies are mostly water), water is sensitive to the pressures of stress in modern life. The adrenal glands that provide adrenalin for the *fight-or-flight* response when we are frightened are also part of this Organ System.

Kidney and bladder are in charge of the purification process and the balance of water in the body. The bones, bone marrow, teeth, central nervous system, ears, hearing, the emotion of fear, Winter, black or dark blue color, urine, groaning sound, and craving for stimulants are all correspondences to the Water phase.

Please see Table 28-2 for a list of the different associations and correspondences to the Five Phases.

Creative and Control Cycles

Many ways can be used to organize the information through the Five Phases theory. The process requires your input and interpretation; therefore finding apparent contradictions is possible. As you evolve in recognizing the different signs and associations to the Five Phases, you will feel more comfortable in their dynamic and flexible nature, when one thing can be interpreted in many ways according to who is observing and the particular circumstances of the moment in time.

Using these organizational patterns, you can expand your frame of reference to include another phase that might be

TABLE 28-2   Five Phases (Elements) Correspondences

ELEMENT	ORGAN SYSTEMS	SEASON	COLOR	SENSE ORGAN	FUNCTION	EMOTION
Fire	Ht/SI P/TH	Summer	Red	Tongue	Emotional stability Assimilation Circulation Protection	Excess joy
Earth	SP/ST	Late summer	Yellow	Mouth	Digestion Nourishment Support	Overthinking Pensiveness
Metal	Lu/LI	Autumn	White	Nose	Respiration Intake of Ki Letting go (LI)	Grief
Water	K/BL	Winter	Black/dark blue	Ears	Purification Impetus	Fear
Wood	Liv/GB	Spring	Green	Eyes	Gather Ki for decisive action	Anger

Ht/SI, Heart, small intestine; *P/TH*, pericardium, triple heater; *SP/ST*, spleen-pancreas, stomach; *Lu/LI*, lung, large intestine; *K/BL*, kidney, bladder; *Liv/GB*, liver, gallbladder.

underneath the one creating an apparent imbalance. The Creative (or Generative) Cycle describes the previous phase that as a *mother* generates or creates the *child* phase (Figure 28-18) The Creative Cycle feeds, nourishes, or generates the next in line.

The Control Cycle is a system of check and balances to keep any phase from overacting.

The Overacting Cycle is a stronger version of the Creative Cycle; excessive control weakens or suppresses the phase being controlled.

The Counteracting, or Insulting, Cycle inverts or goes in the opposite order of the Creative Cycle.

Table 28-3 list details of Creative and Control Cycles. Here are some examples of how you can use the cycles.

Wood Creates Fire

In a case in which you have a client who has a lot of Fire-associated symptoms, such as redness in the face, agitation, and inappropriate emotional responses, you can check not only the Fire meridians but also the Wood meridians.

In this case, Wood is the *mother* that creates or generates Fire, which is described as the *child*. Too much Wood can generate too much Fire. In this case, for example, the Fire Phase might be tamed by controlling the amount of *fuel* (Wood) that stokes the flame.

The inverse situation might also happen: a person without *sparkle*, pale face, constantly feeling cold, and showing other signs of lack of Fire might be treated by strengthening the *mother* phase, in this case Wood.

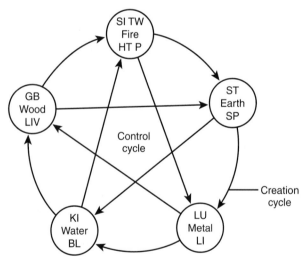

FIGURE 28-18 The Five Phases or Elements with Control Cycles and associated meridians.

TABLE 28-3   Five Element Correspondences

ELEMENT	ORGAN SYSTEMS	SEASON	COLOR	SENSE ORGAN	JOINTS OF THE BODY	EMOTION
Fire	Ht/SI P/TW	Summer	Red	Tongue	Elbows	Excess joy
Earth	SP/ST	Late summer	Yellow	Mouth	Hips	Overthinking
Metal	Lu/LI	Autumn	White	Nose	Wrists	Grief
Water	K/BL	Winter	Black/navy	Ears	Knees, ankles	Fear
Wood	Liv/GB	Spring	Green	Eyes	Shoulders	Anger

Ht/SI, Heart, small intestine; *P/TW*, pericardium, triple heater; *SP/ST*, spleen-pancreas, stomach; *Lu/LI*, lung, large intestine; *K/BL*, kidney, bladder; *Liv/GB*, liver, gallbladder.

Earth Controls *Water*

From the time of ancient Egypt, farmers along the Nile's riverbank knew that when the river flooded its banks, it could have dire consequences for their crops and livelihood. A strong Earth element will keep Water under control, just as a dam or riverbank does. If the Water phase (ruling the bladder, kidney, and the water balance in the body) overacts, then it can *swamp* the Earth-ruled function of the stomach and spleen, also dampening stomach fire. This action can cause slowed down digestion and increase bloating, tiredness, and edema, during which fluids get backed up in the interstitial space between the cells. A strong Earth phase helps *keep everything in its place* (one of the spleen functions). A person with this kind of imbalance would do well in exercising; eating cooked foods such as stews, grains, and soups; and receiving shiatsu to strengthen the stomach and spleen Organ Systems.

Ways to Evaluate an Energetic Imbalance

You have different tools that, used together, can help you guide your intuition to form an idea of what might be happening with your client. Clients might be having a particular leaning toward functioning at a more physical level, or emotional level, an affinity or aversion that can point to one of the Five Phases or Elements. They might tend to have more Yin- or Yang-type of responses. They may have a particular weakness or excess in a meridian. All these ideas put together, plus the valuable addition of your *hunches* or *gut feeling* about what is going on, can help you tailor your session for the specific needs of your client.

> **evolve** *An illustration, entitled* What Is Balance?, *of how the authors depict balance is found on the Evolve web site under course materials for this edition.* ∎

• **Look:** By observing how the person looks and behaves, his or her physical constitution, body proportions, posture, gait, mannerisms, level of activity, and strength in his or her movement, you can tell a lot about his or her state of health and personality.

  You can check the face color (hue), circles under eyes, condition of hair and nails, redness or discoloring of the skin, and *sparkle* in the eyes. Looking at the tongue, or tongue diagnosis, is an art regularly used by Chinese medicine practitioners to determine internal conditions of the body. Redness on the tip of the tongue, for example, points to heat in the heart. A thick white coating or fur at the back of the tongue might point to coldness in the kidney or bladder. Deep cracks at the center might point to stomach or spleen deficiency.

  When looking at a person, be discreetly discerning as you observe details. Keeping your gaze relaxed is important, which increases peripheric vision; thus you can have a *one-shot* look and impression of the whole person, instead of parts or details. The details will later fit into the big picture. Another way is to look at a figure larger than the physical body of your client, which contains the physical body and the energy field around it in one unit.

• **Listen/smell:** *Listening* refers not only to what the person is saying but also to how it is being said, what is not being said, and the tone of the voice. Is a complaining, angry, sad tone heard? Is the person talking in a hushed voice, growling, or shouting? Does it sound as though he or she is holding the breath? Does he or she have a dry mouth? You can sometimes distinguish a particular smell associated to the person such as sweet (relating to Earth), burnt (relating to Fire), damp (relating to Earth and Water), rancid (relating to Wood), metallic (relating to Metal), and urinelike (relating to Water).

• **Palpate:** You can check specific reflex areas in the abdomen (or Hara) and compare energetic states of different Organ Systems (see section Hara Evaluation). Many TCM practitioners rely on feeling the pulses at three different places on each wrist. This skill can give you information on the Ki, Zang/Fu, and meridians. As you work, check skin texture and firmness, temperature changes, areas of pain (or *Ah shi* points). *Ah shi*, which means "that's it," elicits a reaction from a client when touched. Other points are Shu/Yu (transporting) points and Bo or Mu (alarm) points.

• **Ask:** You can specifically inquire about symptoms, sleep patterns, elimination, digestion, appetite, diet, exercise, menstruation patterns, and health history, as well as climate likes or dislikes. For example, a person might strongly dislike cold, heat, or drafts of air, or a symptom might worsen on damp or rainy days.

ZEN SHIATSU PRINCIPLES OF TOUCH

The *Zen* part of Zen Shiatsu does not have a religious connotation, as in Zen Buddhism. The word *Zen* means "meditation" or "contemplation," and it is the state of mind in which the Zen shiatsu practitioner should be to perceive and be in contact with Ki, Ki of both the client and himself or herself.

The emphasis of Zen shiatsu techniques is to have an *in-the-moment* understanding of the quality and movement of Ki. Although the functions and actions of the individual tsubos are essential to learn and use in practice, the more inclusive concept of the meridian is what guides the Zen shiatsu practitioner during a session.

The principles of touch are designed to provide a way for the practitioner to be relaxed and present throughout the session. One of the ways to help the practitioner and client stay centered is to be present and paying attention to the process as it unfolds moment to moment. Your hands will be getting feedback and reactions from the client as you work. You should be able to interpret this information so as to adapt your technique to what is going on and what is appropriate for that person in that precise moment in time. Although you will be following a certain routine, especially at the beginning of your training, no two sessions will be the same because you will be tailoring your shiatsu for the unique circumstances of your client. The principles are the following:

I. Relax
II. Use your body weight, not your force
III. Move from the Hara
IV. Use two-handed connection
V. Stationary perpendicular penetration
VI. Project your Ki
VII. Continuity

I. Relax

Some bodywork styles emphasize the practitioner's muscular strength as a way to perform techniques and are vigorous and very physical. To have muscular strength, your muscles have to be contracted. As you know, muscle contraction, once it reaches a threshold, cannot be sustained for prolonged periods. You can push the threshold to sustain more and more contraction with practice (as weight lifters do), but a point always comes when the muscles need to relax before they can contract again. As a practitioner keeping high levels of contraction throughout the hour or more that a bodywork session takes is difficult. Never mind doing many sessions in a day! In addition, if your effectiveness is tied to your muscular strength, then it puts a lot of pressure on you to always be contracted to do your job properly.

Zen shiatsu is based on the opposite principle that you are relaxed so as to be effective. Relaxed does not mean that you will collapse in a heap of flaccid flesh and bone or that your touch will be too soft or ineffective. You can perform any task that demands physical power while keeping a sense of openness and relaxation. Think of the grace of a top-class dancer or skater, whose muscular effort is guided by a prevailing sense of calm and groundedness even in the midst of a challenging performance.

Being aware of your body, consciously releasing areas of tension, breathing fully, having a comfortable posture, and adjusting it to keep relaxed and open as you work are some of the ways to ensure that you are not using your muscular force in a purely contractive way. Besides, helping your client relax is difficult if you are not relaxed yourself.

As you relax, your own energy field expands, and immediately you start being aware of the space around you. Your perception of yourself and your client increases, and figuring out what is going on and what to do becomes relatively easy. The expansion of your field happens in all directions (not only up) at the same time. As you expand downward, you increase your connection to the Earth, further relaxing and stabilizing you and your client. As you expand forward, you increase the connection with your client, and your Ki travels further along the meridians, affecting the person beyond the local point of contact. As you expand upward, you get in contact with Cosmic Ki that might help as inspiration to guide your session.

Given that the meridians vibrate at a higher speed than the physical body, they resonate more with the expansive phase of movement rather than the contracting phase. When you relax and expand your field, being in contact with the Ki in the meridians is relatively easy.

II. Use Your Body Weight, Not Your Force

Using the relaxed weight of your body to lean on the area of work not only is the most effective way to ensure a supportive and effective touch but will also help you better perceive the reaction of the client to your touch.

Proper body mechanics include having your spine aligned; a good connection of your legs, knees, and feet to the floor; and having your arms extended rather than flexed.

III. Move from the Hara

The **Hara,** a Japanese word to describe the lower abdomen, is the geographic center of balance of your body. More precisely, a point in the Hara called the **Dan Tien** (three fingerwidths distance below the navel), also called the *Sea of Ki,* is traditionally described as the center of focused power and action, where all movement of the body originates. In Japan, a person is said to *have a good Hara* when he or she enjoys good health, stability, and strength. Several Qi Gong and Tai Chi exercises and meditations can be used to develop the Dan Tien because it is the center of power for the practice of martial arts. It is the point at which you physically embody the Ki of the Earth into your being, allowing it to permeate every action you do.

Moving from the Hara means to have the connection of your body to the ground activated as you are working. Simple exercises such as bringing your breathing down to the Hara can help you center yourself and feel grounded very quickly. A practical thing to check is to have your Hara relaxed and facing the area of work.

IV. Use Two-Handed Connection

Having both hands in contact with your client as you work is a good way to give stability, support, and continuous connection. You will also benefit yourself from having the support of the Earth through the body of your client as you move around him or her.

Your hands will intermittently become more Yin (receptive, listening, slower, supportive) or more Yang (active, faster, directive), respectively, throughout the whole session. A more Yin *mother hand* is the one that stays stable in one place, supporting and listening to the reaction to the work you are doing at the same time with the *child hand,* the more Yang and active hand that moves along the meridian. Ideally, both hands are on the same meridian, or pathway. If you have to move around, keeping a hand on your client would be a good idea, when possible.

Feeling the reaction underneath the mother hand is relatively easy if both hand and wrist are relaxed. Your hands connect through your client's meridian, forming a closed circuit that includes your Hara, your mother hand, your child hand, and your client's meridian or area you are contacting. You can increase your perception of subtle reactions as you work by visualizing a sphere of Ki within this closed circuit.

V. Stationary Perpendicular Penetration

Probably the most defining principle in Zen shiatsu technique, approaching the area of work *perpendicularly* allows you to connect energetically with Ki in the meridians. Touch that approaches the surface of the skin nonperpendicularly creates tissue resistance, bringing up the dense, slow vibrations of Ki. This approach restricts your work to the physical range of Ki only. It can be effective but it is *hit and miss,* and the effect will be localized. When leaning with your body weight perpendicularly into a tsubo, you reach the full range of vibrations of the meridian (emotional, mental, and spiritual but *including* the physical), stimulating the whole meridian at once.

You need to adjust the angle of pressure as you go, adapting to the different curvatures of the body.

Lean perpendicularly into the tsubo until you feel you have contacted the Ki in the meridian, and then release the pressure and move on to the next tsubo. Circling, rubbing, or moving your thumb or palm on the tsubo restricts your work to the physical and local aspects of the area you are working instead of the more inclusive quality you would get by contacting the Ki in the meridian in a *stationary* way.

You should time yourself so you do not spend too much or not enough time in each tsubo. Getting a stable rhythm (for example, moving on at the count of five or ten, as appropriate for you and the client) helps give continuity to your session and is reassuring for your client. You may want to go back to the tsubos that felt particularly depleted or Kyo.

VI. Project Your Ki

By relaxing your body weight perpendicularly into a tsubo, you allow your Ki to project itself beyond the point of contact with the surface of your client's skin, allowing a better contact with his or her Ki. You can visualize the area you are working as a sphere, and you project your Ki toward the center of the sphere.

VII. Continuity

Follow along the same meridian, instead of jumping back and forth from different meridians or areas of the body. Continue along the whole pathway of the meridian. A Zen shiatsu session normally involves treating the whole body, irrespective of where symptoms are. You can pay specific attention to the troublesome areas but always within the context of the whole.

TECHNIQUES: PALMING AND THUMBING

Palming, a Yin technique, is done with relaxed hands placed on the body of your client. Extend your arms and bring your body weight forward so you feel the pressure under your hands. Without moving your hands, as you move your body weight backwards, the pressure is relieved from underneath them. Palming is a good way to *listen* and evaluate the quality of the Ki in the meridian, comparing the different sensations on each tsubo as you work. You will have a *mother* hand and a *child* hand that can switch positions as needed.

Thumbing should be done with extended arms and thumbs, with fingers relaxed. The extended thumb should continue a line projected from the extended arm. In other words, the thumb should be aligned with the wrist, elbow, and shoulder. Have the elbows extended and the shoulders relaxed. Be mindful of not flexing the distal phalanx of the thumb, keeping the distal interphalangeal joint extended. The point of contact of the thumb with the tsubo should be midway between the pad of the thumb and the nail of the thumb, with care taken to be not too close to the nail. Thumbing can be done effectively only if your nails are short.

When thumbing, use the *child* hand, and keep the *mother* hand in the palming position, stabilizing and supporting yourself and the client.

Palming and thumbing should be done rhythmically while following the direction of the flow along the meridian. You should work each meridian in the following direction of the flow:

Supine
- From the Hara down the legs to the feet
- From the chest out to the arms
- From the chest up the throat, neck and face, to the head

Prone
- From the base of the neck, laterally to shoulders and arms
- From the base of the neck down along the back toward the sacrum
- From the sacrum down each leg to the feet

HARA EVALUATION

Palpating the different reflex areas of the meridians on the Hara, you can compare the overall energetic state of the person and a clear picture of where the imbalance may be. The aim is to find the Kyo-Jitsu pair of meridians that will be the focus of your treatment. By working the Kyo and Jitsu meridians you have found through this method, you will have the fastest and most direct way to balance the whole system (Figure 28-19).

- Sit in a comfortable position by your client's Hara so you can reach all the diagnostic (meridian) reflex areas evenly.
- Align your spine and center yourself by bringing your attention to the connection of your legs to the Earth, and bring your breathing down to the lower abdomen.
- Place your *mother* hand by the side of your client's trunk.
- With the other hand relaxed, *land* gently and perpendicularly with your relaxed fingertips on each of the Hara diagnostic areas. The pressure should be light and comfortable for the client but still deep enough to be present and make contact with the Ki.
- Feel for the most Kyo diagnostic area, comparing all the areas with even pressure and for an equal amount of time.

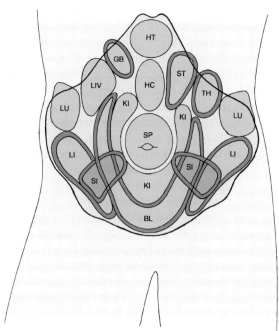

FIGURE 28-19 Hara diagnostic area map.

- Feel for the most Jitsu diagnostic area, comparing all the areas with even pressure and for an equal amount of time.
- Look for the Kyo/Jitsu reaction:
  - Place your *mother* hand's fingertips on the most Kyo area, making contact with the Ki.
  - Then place the *child* hand on the most Jitsu area and feel for a reaction in the most Kyo area, underneath your *mother* hand. You may feel a subtle movement or change under your fingertips.

If you do not get a reaction of any kind with the most Jitsu area, then leave your mother hand on the most Kyo area, and with the other hand make another round of the remaining diagnostic areas, this time going in gently but a bit deeper than before until you find the area that reacts. That will be the Jitsu meridian that you will use in your treatment.

Some guidelines for Hara diagnosis:

- Meridians such as kidney, bladder, large intestine, small intestine, and lung have either broad or bilateral diagnostic areas in the Hara. Make sure you palpate them evenly. If one side feels Jitsu and the other side of the same meridian diagnostic area feels Kyo, then you discard them and look for an alternative one that has a consistent Kyo or Jitsu feeling throughout the whole diagnostic area.
- You cannot have one meridian of a Yin-Yang pair (Liv/GB, Lu/LI, Ht/SI, and so forth) being most Kyo and the other one being most Jitsu.

INTRODUCTION TO TRADITIONAL AYURVEDA

As health care professionals become better acquainted with the various forms of complementary, alternative, and integrative medical treatments, they often discover that India's traditional healing modality of Ayurveda is one of the world's oldest healing systems currently practiced. It is based on Hinduism with some ideas that have evolved from ancient Persia. More specifically, **Ayurveda** is a science of health and medicine designed to maintain or improve health through the use of dietary modification, massage, yoga, herbal preparations, and other measures. Health care practitioners who find themselves drawn to Ayurveda deserve the most reliable and up-to-date information about it. Therefore this section discusses the fundamental principles and practices of traditional Ayurveda as understood from their original Sanskrit sources and traditional practitioners.

The four phases of Indian medical history provide a chronological grid that is necessary to understand the development of this traditional system of medicine and are as follows.

Based on available literary sources, the history of Indian medicine occurred in four main phases. The first, or *Vedic*, phase dates from approximately 1200 to 800 BC. Information about medicine during this period is obtained from numerous curative incantations and references to healing that are found in the *Atharvaveda* and the *Rigveda*, two religious scriptures that reveal a *magico-religious* approach to healing.

The second, or *classical*, phase is marked by the advent of the first complete Sanskrit medical treatises, the *Caraka* and *Sushruta Samhitas*, which probably date from a few centuries before to several centuries after the start of the Common Era. This period includes all subsequent medical treatises dating from before the Muslim invasions of India at the beginning of the eleventh century, given that these works tend to follow the earlier classical compilations closely and provide the basis of traditional Ayurveda.

The third, or *syncretic*, phase is marked by clear influences on the classical paradigm from Islamic or Unani, South Indian Siddha, and other nonclassical medical systems. Bhavamishra's sixteenth-century *Bhavaprakasha* is one text that reveals the results of these influences, which includes diagnosis by examination of pulse and urine. This phase extends from the Muslim incursions to the present era.

This author would term the final or current phase as *New Age Ayurveda*, wherein the classical paradigm is being adapted to the world of modern science and technology, including quantum physics, mind-body science, and advanced biomedical science. This recent manifestation of Ayurveda is most visible in the Western world, although much of New Age Ayurveda is filtering back to India.

From its beginnings during the Vedic era, Indian medicine has always adhered closely to the principle of a fundamental connection between the microcosm and macrocosm. Humans are minute representations of the universe, and contained within them is everything that makes up the surrounding world. The interconnectedness of humans and their world makes understanding one completely without the other impossible.

HUMAN BODY

According to Ayurveda, the cosmos consists of five basic elements: earth, air, fire, water, and space or ether. Certain forces cause these elements to interact, giving rise to all that exists. In humans, these five elements combine in such a way as to produce the three *doshas*, psychophysical elements and forces that, along with the seven *dhatus* (tissues) and three *malas* (waste products), make up the human body.

Three Doshas

Doshas, a word that means *that which changes,* are constantly moving in dynamic balance, one with the others. Recall that the five elements combine and give rise to the **doshas.** In Ayurveda, dosha is also known as the governing principles such that every living thing in nature is characterized by the dosha. The three active doshas, or **tri-doshas,** are called Vata, Pitta, and Kapha.

The three doshas occur in varying amounts in every human body, and the proportion that is appropriate to an individual's body is called the person's innate, natural state, or *prakriti,* which is different for each person. When in equilibrium in the human body, the three doshas maintain health, but when an imbalance occurs among them, they defile the normal functioning of the body, leading to the manifestation of disease. An imbalance indicates an increase or decrease in one, two, or all three of the doshas.

Vata

Vata, or Vayu, meaning *wind,* is composed of the elements air and space. It is the principle of kinetic energy and is responsible for all bodily movement, evacuation, and nervous functions. Vata is located below the navel and in the bladder, large intestines, nervous system, pelvic region, thighs, bone marrow, and legs; its principal seat is the colon. When disrupted, its primary manifestation is gas and muscular or nervous energy, leading to pain.

Pitta

Pitta, or bile, is made up of the elements fire and water. It governs enzymes and hormones and is responsible for digestion, pigmentation, body temperature, hunger, thirst, sight, courage, and mental activity. Pitta is located between the navel and the chest and in the stomach, small intestines, liver, spleen, skin, and blood; its principal seat is the stomach. When disrupted, its primary manifestation is acid and bile, leading to inflammation.

Kapha

Kapha, or Shleshman, meaning *phlegm,* is made up of the elements of earth and water. It connotes the principle of cohesion and stability. Kapha regulates Vata and Pitta and is responsible for keeping the body lubricated and maintaining its solid nature, tissues, sexual power, and strength. It also controls patience. The normal locations of Kapha are the upper part of the body, the thorax, head, neck, upper portion of the stomach, pleural cavity, fat tissues, and areas between joints; its principal seat is the lung. When it is disrupted, its primary manifestation is fluids and mucus, leading to swelling, with or without discharge.

The attributes of each dosha help determine the individual's basic bodily and mental makeup and to isolate which dosha or combination of doshas is responsible for a disease. The qualities of Vata are dryness, cold, light, irregularity, mobility, roughness,

and abundance. Dryness occurs when Vata is disturbed and is a side effect of motion. Too much dryness produces irregularity in the body and mind. Pitta is hot, light, intense, fluid, liquid, putrid, pungent, and sour. Heat appears when Pitta is disturbed, resulting from change caused by Pitta. The intensity of excessive heat produces irritability in the body and mind. Kapha is heavy, unctuous, cold, stable, dense, soft, and smooth. Heaviness occurs when Kapha is disturbed and results from firmness caused by Kapha. The viscosity of excessive heaviness and stability produces slowness in body and mind.

Nadis

Similar to the Chinese meridians, the **nadis** are channels in which Prana energy flows. Nadis are sometimes viewed as extending only to the skin of the body but are often thought to extend to the boundary of the aura. The three main nadis include *Shushumna, Ida,* and *Pingala,* but a total of 72,000 nadis exist. Nadis all start from the central channel of the chakras (see later section) to the periphery where they gradually become thinner.

The nadis are stimulated through the practice of Pranayama, which involves alternate breathing through left and right nostrils, which alternately stimulate, respectively, the left and right sides of the brain.

Seven Dhatus

The seven dhatus, or tissues, are responsible for sustaining the body. Each dhatu is responsible for the one that comes next in the following order:

1. Rasa, meaning "sap" or "juice," includes the tissue fluids, chyle, lymph, and plasma. It functions as nourishment and comes from digested food.
2. Blood includes the red blood cells and functions to invigorate the body.
3. Flesh includes muscle tissue and functions as stabilization.
4. Fat includes adipose tissue and functions as lubrication.
5. Bone includes bone and cartilage and functions as support.
6. Marrow includes red and yellow bone marrow and functions as filling for the bones.
7. Shukra includes male and female sexual fluids and functions in reproduction and immunity.

Three Malas

The malas are the waste products of digested and processed food and drink. Ayurveda delineates three principal malas: *urine, feces,* and *sweat.* A fourth category of other waste products includes fatty excretions from the skin and intestines, ear wax, mucus of the nose, saliva, tears, hair, and nails. According to Ayurveda, an individual should evacuate the bowels once a day and eliminate urine six times a day.

Ayurveda considers digestion to be the most important function that takes place in the human body. It provides all that is required to sustain the organism and is the principal cause for all maladies from which an individual may suffer. The process of digestion and assimilation of nutrients is discussed under the topics of the Agnis (enzymes), Ama (improperly digested food and drink), and the Srotas (channels of circulation).

Three Agnis

The *Agnis,* or enzymes, assist in the digestion and assimilation of food and are divided into three types, as follows:

Jatharagni is active in the mouth, stomach, and gastrointestinal tract and helps break down food. The waste product of feces results from this activity.

Bhutagnis are five enzymes located in the liver. They adapt the broken-down food into a homologous chyle according to the five elements and assist the chyle to assimilate with the corresponding five elements in the body. The homologous chyle circulates in the blood channels as rasa, nourishing the body and supplying the seven dhatus.

Dhatvagnis are seven enzymes that synthesize the seven dhatus from the assimilated chyle homologized with the five elements. The remaining waste products result from this activity.

AMA

Ama, the chief cause of disease, is formed when a decrease in enzyme activity occurs. A product of improperly digested food and drink, it takes the form of a liquid sludge that travels through the same channels as the chyle. Because of its density, however, it lodges in different parts of the body, blocking the channels. Ama often mixes with the doshas that circulate through the same pathways and usually gravitates to a weak or stressed organ or to a site of a disease manifestation. Because all diseases invariably come from Ama, the word *Amaya,* meaning "coming from Ama," is a synonym for disease. Internal diseases begin with Ama, and external diseases produce Ama. In general, Ama can be detected by a coating on the tongue, turbid urine with foul odor, and feces that are passed with undigested food, an offensive odor, or abundant gas. The principal course of treatment in Ayurveda involves the elimination of Ama and the restoration of the balance of the doshas.

SROTAS

The Srotas are the vessels or channels of the body through which all substances circulate. They are either large, such as the large and small intestines, uterus, arteries, and veins, or small, such as the capillaries. A healthy body has open and free-flowing channels. Blockage of the channels, usually by Ama, results in disease. The 13 Srotas are as follows:

1. Pranavahisrotas convey vitality and vital wind or breath (Prana) and originate in the heart and alimentary tract.
2. Udakavahisrotas convey water and fluids and originate in the palate and pancreas.
3. Annavahisrotas convey food from the outside and originate in the stomach.
4. Rasavahisrotas convey chyle, lymph, and plasma and originate in the heart and in the 10 vessels connected with the heart. Ama primarily accumulates within them.
5. Raktavahisrotas convey red blood cells and originate in the liver and spleen.
6. Mamsavahisrotas convey ingredients for muscle tissue and originate in the tendons, ligaments, and skin.
7. Medovahisrotas convey ingredients for fat tissue and originate in the kidneys and fat tissues of the abdomen.
8. Asthavahisrotas convey ingredients for bone tissue and originate in hipbone.
9. Majjavahisrotas convey ingredients for marrow and originate in the bones and joints.
10. Shukravahisrotas convey ingredients for the male and female reproductive tissues and originate in the testicles and ovary, respectively.
11. Mutravahisrotas convey urine and originate in the kidney and bladder.
12. Purishavahisrotas convey feces and originate in the colon and rectum.
13. Svedavahisrotas convey sweat and originate in the fat tissues and hair follicles.

This broad outline shows that Ayurveda understands that the human body's anatomical parts are composed of the five basic elements, which have undergone a process of metabolism and assimilation in the body. Humans differ, depending on their normal bodily constitution, or prakriti, which is determined at the moment of conception and remains until death. The four factors that influence constitutional type are (1) the father, (2) the mother (particularly her food intake), (3) the womb, and (4) the season of the year. A large imbalance of the doshas in the mother will affect the growth of the embryo and fetus, and a moderate excess of one or two of the doshas will affect the constitution of the child.

PRAKRITI

A person's constitution is called the **prakriti.** Seven normal body constitutions exist and are based on the three doshas: Vata, Pitta, Kapha, Vata-Pitta, Pitta-Kapha, Vata-Kapha, and Sama. The last is a state in which all three occur in equal proportions. It is the best condition but is extremely rare. Most people are a combination of doshas, in which one dosha predominates. In general, Vata-type people tend to be anxious and fearful, exhibit light and *airy* characteristics, and are prone to Vata-diseases. Pitta-type people are aggressive and impatient, exhibit fiery and hotheaded characteristics, and are prone to Pitta-diseases. Kapha-type people are stable and entrenched, if not sluggish at times; they exhibit heavy, wet, and earthy characteristics and are prone to Kapha-diseases.

These concepts are the principal factors that help the Ayurvedic physician determine the correct course of treatment to be administered to a patient for a particular ailment.

CHAKRA SYSTEM

The word **chakra** comes from a Sanskrit word meaning "wheel" or "circle," referring to the seven energy centers in the body. The functions of the chakras are to receive, process, and distribute energy and to keep the spiritual, mental, emotional and physical health of the body in balance. Some traditional sources describe five chakras; others describe eight.

The earliest mentions of chakras are found in the *Vedas,* the oldest written tradition in India, dating from 2000 to 600 BC, and the *Yoga Upanishads* (circa 600 AD). The chakra system came to be an integral part of the yoga philosophy.

The main text about chakras came to the West in a translation by the Englishman, Sir John Woodroffe, alias Arthur Avalon, in a book entitled *The Serpent Power,* published in 1919. The book lists seven basic chakras, and they all exist within the subtle body, overlaying the physical body.

Chakras are described as being located in ascending order from the base of the spine to the top of the head (Figure 28-20), even though they may express themselves externally at points along the front of the body (navel, heart, throat, and so forth). Chakras are associated with a color, an element, a sound, a symbol (a different number of lotus petals in each chakra), and many other distinguishing characteristics.

Characteristics of Chakras

Although some discrepancies exist, here are the more traditional chakra characteristics.

The Root Chakra (First Chakra)
Location: in the perineum at base of spine
Sanskrit name: Muladhara
Gland: adrenal medulla
Symbol: four-petaled lotus
Color: red

Element: earth
Qualities: grounding, patience, structure, stability, security, survival
Essential oils: cinnamon, garlic, sandalwood
Gem: ruby
Herb: mugwort
Musical note: C

The Sacral Chakra (Second Chakra)
Location: sacrum, 2 inches below the navel and 2 inches into the pelvis
Sanskrit name: Svadhisthana
Gland: gonads
Symbol: six-petaled lotus
Color: orange
Element: water
Qualities: well-being, sexuality, sensuality, pleasure, abundance, seat of the emotions
Essential oils: jasmine, neroli, orange blossom
Gem: moonstone
Herb: cedar
Musical note: D

The Solar Plexus Chakra (Third Chakra)
Location: directly below the sternum and just above the navel
Sanskrit name: Manipura
Gland: pancreas

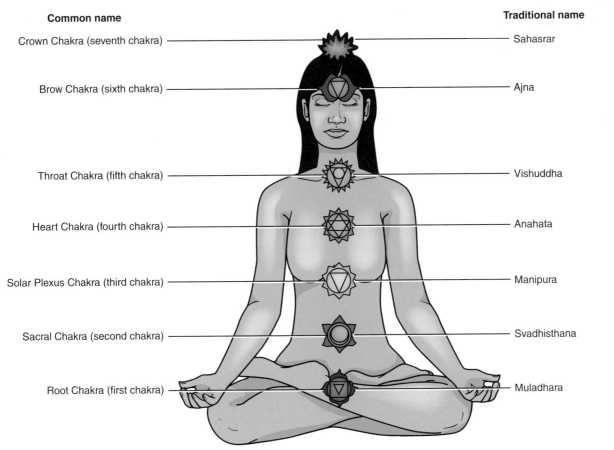

Common name		Traditional name
Crown Chakra (seventh chakra)		Sahasrar
Brow Chakra (sixth chakra)		Ajna
Throat Chakra (fifth chakra)		Vishuddha
Heart Chakra (fourth chakra)		Anahata
Solar Plexus Chakra (third chakra)		Manipura
Sacral Chakra (second chakra)		Svadhisthana
Root Chakra (first chakra)		Muladhara

FIGURE 28-20 The Chakra system.

Symbol: 10-petaled lotus
Color: yellow
Element: fire
Qualities: self-worth, self-esteem, confidence, personal
  power, mentality
Essential oils: lemon, grapefruit, juniper
Gem: yellow sapphire, topaz, citrine
Herb: rosemary
Musical note: E

The Heart Chakra (Fourth Chakra)
Location: middle of chest
Sanskrit name: Anahata
Gland: thymus
Symbol: 12-petaled lotus
Color: green
Element: air
Qualities: unity, love, peace, purity, and innocence
Essential oils: rose, carnation, lily of the valley
Gem: emerald, rose quartz
Herb: lavender
Musical note: F

The Throat Chakra (Fifth Chakra)
Location: throat
Sanskrit name: Vishuddha
Gland: thyroid
Symbol: 16-petaled lotus, circle
Color: blue or turquoise
Element: ether (contains all elements)
Qualities: communication, will, creativity, truthfulness,
  integrity
Essential oils: blue chamomile, gardenia, ylang-ylang
Gem: blue sapphire, blue pearl
Herb: wintergreen
Musical note: G

The Brow Chakra (Sixth Chakra)
Location: between the eyebrows (third eye or eye of psy-
  chic vision)
Sanskrit name: Ajna
Gland: pineal
Symbol: two-petaled lotus
Color: indigo
Element: the cosmos
Qualities: intuition, discernment, wisdom, imagination,
  knowledge

Essential oils: camphor, sweet pea
Gem: amethyst
Herb: sage
Musical note: A

The Crown Chakra (Seventh Chakra)
Location: top of skull (some say just above the skull)
Sanskrit name: Sahasrar
Gland: pituitary
Symbol: 1000-petaled lotus
Color: white (sometimes purple) or white streaked with
  purple
Element: the cosmos
Qualities: enlightenment, grace, beauty, serenity, oneness
  with all that is
Essential oils: violet, lavender, lotus
Gem: alexandrite
Herbs: frankincense and myrrh
Musical note: B

TABLE TALK

Differences and Similarities Between Traditional Chinese Medicine and Ayurveda

Although the concept of energy is the same in India and China, the Ayurvedic and TCM models of reference differ in how this energy can be observed and organized for therapeutic uses.

In India, the Ayurvedic tradition of the deities Shiva (contracting, manifesting, downward stream of Prana) and Shakti (expansive, liberating, upward stream of Prana) have a similar dynamic as the Chinese theory of Yin and Yang (see later discussion). The same as the nadis, subtle energy pathways in Ayurveda, have a resemblance with the meridian system in TCM.

The chakras are centers of energy of pivotal importance in Ayurveda. They receive, process, and distribute energy in the body. They have their own system of correspondences that are the point of reference for some types of bodywork and energy healing systems, even beyond Ayurveda. Seven major chakras exist along the centerline of the body (Shushumna). Three doshas (grosser forms of Prana in the body) and their various combinations help detect tendencies toward disease or weaknesses. Each chakra and dosha has its own correspondence with sounds, colors, elements, body organs, foods, and psychological and physiological functions, among other things. Ayurvedic massage, yoga, meditation, diet, and herbology are used to prevent and treat imbalances and to support the good functioning of the body.

Within both Chinese medicine and Ayurveda are *Five Elements* and *Vital Substances* theories, but they differ consistently.

SUMMARY

For *energy-based* bodywork therapies such as shiatsu, the physical body is only one aspect of the person set within a larger frame of reference that also includes the emotional, mental, and spiritual aspects of the human being. The concept of energy (Ki in Japanese, Qi or Chi in Chinese, Prana in India) is the central element that is common to all the aspects of the person. Specific techniques are used to evaluate and treat according to the flow and cycles of energy. Steeped in traditions originated in Asia 2500 to 4000 years ago, two major branches, one from India (Ayurvedic medicine) and one from China (TCM), still remain and are being practiced with increasing relevance.

In this chapter, we discuss the central concepts of Ayurveda and particularly of TCM that lays the background and are the origin of the so-called ABTs. Among these concepts we find the theories of Yin and Yang, the Five Phases or Elements, meridians, Zang/Fu, and tsubos. We go into detail and discuss the principles of touch of a particular ABT originated in Japan, called Zen Shiatsu.

Traditional Ayurveda is a sophisticated system of medicine that has been practiced in one form or another in India for the last 2500 years. It includes the chakra system. As with other forms of alternative, complementary, and integrative medicine, Ayurveda focuses on the whole organism and its relationship to the external world to reestablish and maintain the harmonious balance that exists within the body and between the body and its environment.

evolve

Go to *Chapter Extras* on Evolve for additional illustrations and resources for this chapter. *Extras* for this chapter include:

1. Crossword puzzle (downloadable form)
2. Speed of vibrations and their manifestations (illustration)
3. Governing vessel (illustration)
4. Conception vessel (illustration)
5. Tonifying touch (illustration)
6. Dispersing touch (illustration)
7. Two-handed connectedness (illustration)
8. Perpendicular penetration (illustration)
9. Internal and external causes of disease in traditional Chinese medicine (essay)
10. Classification of disease according to the eight principles (essay)

MATCHING I

Place the letter of the answer next to the term or phrase that best describes it.

A. Ashi points
B. Asian Bodywork Therapy
C. Chi or Qi
D. Dan Tien

E. Hara
F. Jitsu
G. Ki
H. Kyo

I. Meridians
J. Shiatsu
K. Tai Ji
L. Tsubo

_____ 1. In Chinese medicine, points on the body that get a reaction from the client when touched and means "that's it!"

_____ 2. Japanese bodywork therapy that uses pressure on the surface of the skin along energy channels called *meridians* to regain and maintain a harmonic flow of energy throughout the body-mind-spirit

_____ 3. Japanese term to describe a quality of energy in a tsubo that feels full or excessive, Yang, hard, warm, and where your pressure is *pushed out* or resisted

_____ 4. Japanese term to describe a quality of energy in a tsubo that feels empty or depleted, Yin, soft, cold, and where your pressure is *welcome* or accepted

_____ 5. Treatment of the body-mind-spirit by pressure and/or manipulation and includes the body's energetic field

_____ 6. In China, the energy of the body-mind-spirit

_____ 7. In Japan, the energy of the body-mind-spirit

_____ 8. In Chinese Medicine, channels or pathways through which Ki flows

_____ 9. Japanese term used to describe energetic vortices on the surface of the skin where the energy of the meridian can be accessed

_____ 10. In Japan, the geographic center of gravity and the energetic center in the body located in the lower abdomen

_____ 11. In Japan, a point in the Hara located three finger-widths' distance below the navel that is the center of focused power and action and where all movement of the body originates

_____ 12. In ABT, the familiar black and white icon that symbolizes the interaction of Yin and Yang

MATCHING II

Place the letter of the answer next to the term or phrase that best describes it.

A. Chakras	E. Moxibustion	I. Prana
B. Cun	F. Nadis	J. Tri-doshas
C. Doshas	G. Pitta	K. Vata
D. Kapha	H. Prakriti	L. Zang/Fu

_____ 1. In Chinese medicine, the Organ Systems, both Yin and Yang, the definition of which includes the internal organs and the meridians

_____ 2. Technique to stimulate the tsubos with heat by burning the herb mugwort above them

_____ 3. The body inch in Chinese medicine; the width of the client's own thumb knuckle

_____ 4. In Ayurveda, term used to describe the three active doshas, or Vata, Pitta, and Kapha

_____ 5. In Ayurveda, a person's unique constitution or the innate, natural state

_____ 6. In Ayurveda, the governing principles is produced as the five elements combine

_____ 7. The dosha composed of the elements Air and Space

_____ 8. The dosha made up of the elements Fire and Water

_____ 9. The dosha made up of the elements of Earth and Water

_____ 10. In India, the energy of the body-mind-spirit

_____ 11. In Ayurveda, the seven energy centers in the body that receive, process, and distribute energy and keep the spiritual, mental, emotional, and physical health of the body in balance

_____ 12. In Ayurveda, channels in which Prana energy flows

INTERNET ACTIVITIES

Log on to http://www.shiatsuassociation.com, the official web site for the Shiatsu Therapy Association of Ontario, and choose the link for FAQs. Write down three questions and their answers. Be sure to paraphrase the answers in your own words.

Visit the web site for the National Center for Complimentary and Alternative Heath and read about Ayurvedic medicine at http://nccam.nih.gov/health/ayurveda/. Share this information with your classmates.

To learn more about chakras, visit http://www.chakraenergy.com/seven.html. Note how each charka has a lesson associated with it.

Bibliography

American Organization for Bodywork Therapies of Asia (AOBTA), 2006, *http://www.aobta.org/*

Beinfeld H, Korngold E: *Between heaven and earth: a guide to Chinese medicine,* New York, 1992, Random House.

Beresford-Cooke C: *Shiatsu theory and practice: a comprehensive text for the student and professional,* St Louis, 2002, Elsevier Health Sciences, Churchill Livingstone.

Brennan BA: *Light emerging: the journey of personal healing,* New York, 1993, Bantam Books.

Connelly D: *Traditional acupuncture: the law of the five elements,* Laurel, Md, 1994, Tai Sophia Institute.

Dash BD, Lalitesh K: *Basic principles of Ayurveda,* New Delhi, 1980, Asia Book Corporation of America, New Delhi, Concept Publishing.

Dash VB: *Fundamentals of Ayurvedic medicine,* Twin Lakes, Wis, 1990, Lotus Press.

Dubitsky C: *Bodywork shiatsu; bringing the art of finger pressure to the massage table,* Rochester, Vt, 1997, Inner Traditions International, Ltd.

Ellis A: *Fundamentals of Chinese acupuncture,* Brookline, Mass, 1994, Paradigm Publications.

Ferguson P: *Take five: the five elements guide to health and harmony,* Dublin, Ireland, 2000, Gill & MacMillan, Ltd.

Holland A: *Voices of Qi: an introductory guide to traditional Chinese medicine,* ed 2, Berkeley, Calif, 1999, North Atlantic Books.

Jolly J: *Indian medicine,* New Delhi, 1977, Munshiram Manoharial Publishers Private, Ltd.

Judith A, Ravenwolf S: *Wheels of life: a journey through the chakras,* Woodbury, Minn, 1999, Llewellyn Worldwide, Ltd.

Kaptchuk TJ: *The web that has no weaver: understanding Chinese medicine,* Lincolnwood, Ill, 2000, NTC Publishing Group.

Lad V: *Ayurveda: the science of self-healing,* Twin Lakes, Wis, 1990, Lotus Press.

Leggett D: *Recipes for self-healing,* London, 1999, Meridian Press.

Leslie CM, Young AH: *Paths to Asian medical knowledge,* Berkeley, Calif, 1992, University of California Press.

Lundberg P: *The book of shiatsu: a complete guide to using hand pressure and gentle manipulation to improve your health, vitality, and stamina,* New York, 2003, Simon & Schuster.

Maciocia G: *Tongue diagnosis in Chinese medicine,* Vista, Calif, 1995, Eastland Press.

Maciocia G: *Foundations of Chinese medicine: a comprehensive text,* St Louis, 2005, Elsevier Health Sciences, Churchill Livingstone.

Masunaga S, Ohashi W: *Zen shiatsu: how to harmonize yin and yang for better health,* Tokyo, 1997, Japan Publications.

Matsumoto K: *Extraordinary vessels,* Brookline, Mass, 1983, Paradigm Publications.

Meulenbeld G, Wujastyk JM, Wujastyk D: *Studies on Indian medical history,* Amsterdam, 2001, Egbert Forsten Publishers.

Nadkarni AK: *Indian materia medica,* New Delhi, 1989, Popular Prakashan.

Namikoshi T: *Complete book of shiatsu therapy: health and vitality at your fingertips,* Tokyo, 1981, Japan Publications.

Pitman V: *On the nature of the whole, Indian medical tradition series,* vol 7, New Delhi, 2004, Motilal Banarsidass.

Sasaki P: Personal Communication, Connecticut Center for Massage Therapy, Westport, Conn, Fall 1989.

Sharma HM, Clark C: *Contemporary Ayur-Veda: medicine and research in Maharishi Ayur-Veda,* St Louis, 2002, Elsevier Health Sciences.

Sharma PV: *Essentials of Ayurveda Soasangahrdayam,* New Delhi, 1999, Motilal Banarsidass Publishers.

Svoboda RE, Lade A: *Tao and dharma: Chinese medicine and Ayurveda,* Twin Lakes, Wis, 1995, Lotus Press.

Svoboda R: *Prakriti: your AyurVedic constitution,* Twin Lakes, Wis, 1998, Lotus Press.

Tsu L: *Tao Te Ching,* New York, 1989, Knopf Publishing Group, [translation by Gia Fu Feng and Jane English].

Upadhyay SD: *Nadivijana (ancient pulse science),* Delhi, India, 1986, Chaukhamba Sanskrit Pratisthan.

Xinnong C: *Chinese acupuncture and moxibustion,* Beijing, 2002, Beijing Foreign Languages Press.

Zimmermann F: *Jungle and the aroma of meats: an ecological theme in Hindu medicine,* New Delhi, 1999, Motilal Banarsidass.

Zysk KG: *Asceticism and healing in ancient India: medicine in the Buddhist monastery,* New Delhi, 1998, Motilal Banarsidass.

Zysk KG: *Conjugal love in India: Ratisastra and Ratiramana: text, translation and notes,* New York, 2000, Kegan Paul International, Ltd.

Zysk KG: *Medicine in the Veda: religious healing in the Veda,* Ottawa, 1998, Laurier Books, Ltd.

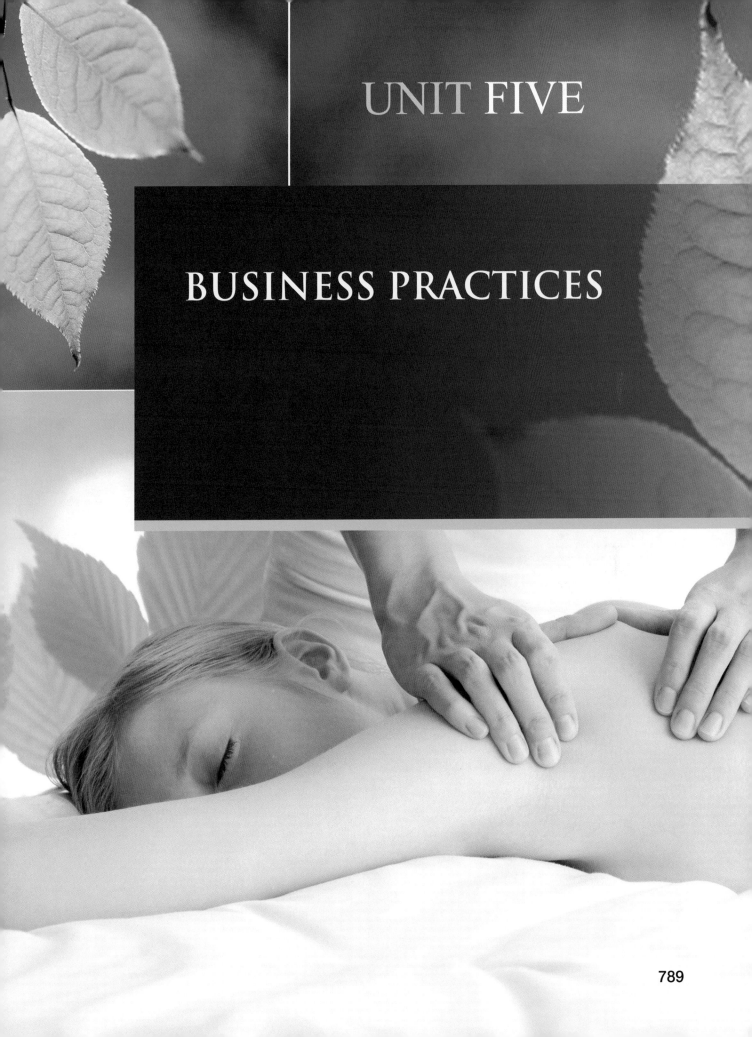

UNIT FIVE

BUSINESS PRACTICES

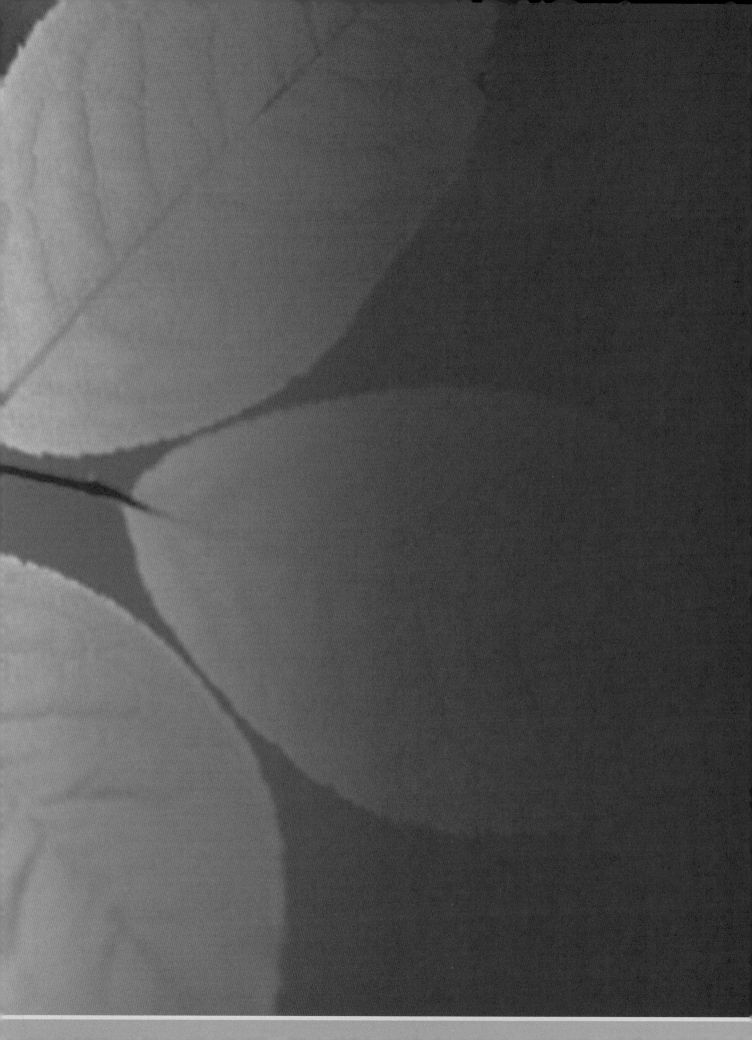

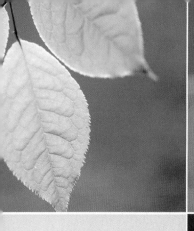

CHAPTER 29

The Business of Massage

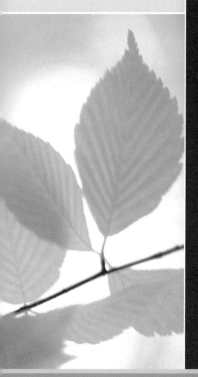

"To accomplish great things, we must not only act, but also dream; not only plan, but also believe."
—Anatole France

STUDENT OBJECTIVES
After completing this chapter, the student should be able to:

- Identify primary values
- Write a vision and a mission statement
- Choose a business entity that is appropriate for your future business vision
- Develop a business plan
- Outline all pertinent licenses and permits required by law to operate a massage business
- List all types of insurance required by law to operate a massage business
- Determine initial costs for beginning your massage career
- Create a curriculum vitae
- Describe various promotional activities such as advertising
- Design a business logo, letterhead, business card, brochure, and web site
- Write three sample business advertisements
- Use proper telephone etiquette for business-related calls
- Compare and contrast contracts and proposals
- List ways of using business resources
- Describe a typical day for a massage therapist
- Discuss insurance reimbursement for massage therapy
- Identify taxes you are responsible for paying and tax deductions
- Compare and contrast an employee versus an independent contractor
- Create a plan for avoiding burnout
- Devise a plan for building a cash reserve and investing toward retirement using securities and retirement accounts

INTRODUCTION

Achieving gratification from a career in massage therapy can happen in many ways: from monetary compensation to personal satisfaction. Many students enter this profession because they felt *drawn* or *called* to become a massage therapist. For some, the attraction is simply a matter of the personal success achieved as a massage client. What does a career in massage mean to you?

- Financial reward of a part- or full-time job
- Supplemental income of a part-time job
- More free time without loss of income
- Personal recognition
- Travel opportunities
- Being your own boss
- Personal fulfillment of helping others
- Flexible hours
- A retirement career

The world of massage is evolving. In the May 2000 issue of *Consumer Reports,* deep massage was reported as the most effective treatment for fibromyalgia, the second most effective treatment for back pain (chiropractic care is first), and the second most effective treatment for headaches (prescription drugs are first). Furthermore, in the 1994 September/October issue of *Money Magazine,* being a massage therapist is listed as the Best Business for Enjoying Life While You Work.

Many people go into business for themselves without ever really knowing the first thing about it. They love their craft, and they are good at it, but being unable to give a great massage is rarely the cause of a failed business. It is rather the lack of business acumen and insufficient capital. The purpose of this chapter is to provide the new therapist with basic business knowledge to build a prosperous practice, from surveying the site and laying the foundation (planning and development) to erecting the framework (employment, promotion, and support) to the finishing touches, regular maintenance, and eventual remodeling (diversifying your income, tracking your finances, avoiding burnout, and planning for retirement). This chapter is both a tool kit and a survival kit.

Whether you work for yourself or someone else, your practice is a business. If your practice is going to thrive, you must become a proficient businessperson. A successful massage practice will require scheduling, purchasing, accounting, and so forth. The massage therapist needs to be well organized to handle these responsibilities (or have them handled), as well as being able to perform massage itself. Having a mentor who is successful can be a major help with business issues.

The first section of this chapter identifies your hopes, dreams, and aspirations. You will map your approach by beginning a business plan, followed by acquiring business permits, obtaining the proper insurance, and determining startup costs. Once these essential elements have been established, you need to market yourself and your services, advertise and promote your business, write contracts and proposals, locate resources, plan career advancement, diversify your income, and return something to the community through volunteering. Finally, you will learn how to manage discouragement, avoid burnout, and plan for retirement.

SURVEYING THE SITE AND LAYING THE FOUNDATION: BUSINESS PLANNING AND DEVELOPMENT

Massage therapists have two main choices of employment: (1) they can work for someone else or (2) they can become self-employed. The majority of therapists, even those who start out working for someone else, eventually become self-employed. Starting your own business can be a daunting project, but broken down into steps and taken one step at a time, it can be accomplished by anyone.

Why do businesses fail? Dun and Bradstreet, the world's largest business database manager, claims that 90% of all businesses fail because of lack of business planning (not lack of professional skills). This section assists the student therapist in business planning and development. First, conduct a survey of your personal values by listing your dreams and desires and stating the purpose of your business. Building a practice requires a vision, a mission, and a working plan. Having a vision, mission, and business plan helps keep your attention and business focused. This plan will help you map your course so as to get where you want your business to go. After developing a business plan, we will then explore business entities, obtaining the necessary licenses and insurance to lay the foundation of your practice.

What Do You Value?

Your massage practice will reflect who you are. Who you are (your character) and how you behave (your personality) naturally come from your needs, desires, attitudes, and beliefs about life. A big part of your success is, and will be, embedded in your personal, business, and spiritual philosophies. If your work is not an extension of your self—that is, if your inner life and outer life are not congruent—then you will experience a mental and emotional tug of war.

Identifying what you value is often difficult because values themselves are abstract concepts. However, as experience teaches us and scientific research tells us, we spend time and energy on things we value or on acquiring things we value. Using a backdoor approach, the following activity may help you identify important elements about yourself.

On a sheet of paper, list 15 to 20 things you like or want to do. These activities can range from cooking to hiking to reading to your kids to watching television or to getting *or* receiving massages. After reading over your list, assign a *value* to the right of each activity. For example, cooking may be linked to spending time with family, creative expression, or nurturing. This evaluation may take some time, but the underlying motivation of each activity should emerge. During this exercise, you will be shifting the focus from things you like or want to do to things you value.

Next, create a new list from the values you have identified in the previous section. From the most important to the least important, number each value. Although it may feel as though you are soul searching, this exercise is often liberating because it helps you identify your most important values, making it easier to make decisions involving your energy and your time—two of your most valuable assets! This list will change to reflect your changing needs.

Copy the new list on several sheets of paper, and tape them where you can see them, such as on the bathroom mirror, on the refrigerator door, and on the dashboard of your car. This exercise is also a beneficial activity to teach clients about stress reduction. If your clients feel overwhelmed, ask them to go through this process and help them identify what is important to them.

"Things which matter most must never be at the mercy of the things which matter least."
Goethe

Vision Statement

Every business follows a path. Several signs indicate what type of path you will take or are currently taking. Some indicators are profit (or loss), décor, services offered, clientele, referral base, and your own level of satisfaction. Any type of business should be guided by a vision instead of the therapist's worries, anxieties, or fears. The harsh truth is that if you do not consciously design your business vision, circumstances will. Unless you give thought to it and create your vision, you will be trying to navigate your business without an idea about where you are and where you are headed.

A vision statement embraces what you want—the desires for your business. Built from your value list, your business vision should both create excitement and energize you. This vision is not necessarily a preview of the future but is rather a glimpse of how things might be if certain obstacles were removed, such as time, money, training, experience, confidence, and so on. Embark on a *vision quest,* and describe on paper what you see. Wake up the following morning and move about as if you are living this vision—a vision of how busy you are, the kind of work environment in which you are located, the kind of modalities you are practicing, and so forth. Continue building this vision until it is complete. When talking about your business with others, speak of it affectionately and not with impatience. As you create your vision, notice how it makes you feel. If it does not feel right, then alter the vision until it makes you smile and stirs you into action. Note if you must make any changes within yourself to fulfill your business vision. Once your vision is clear, move on to writing your mission statement and then on to the business plan. The business plan will help you turn your dreams into a reality.

"Argue for your limitations and they're yours."
Richard Bach

Mission Statement

A **mission statement**, or statement of purpose, briefly and succinctly defines your type of business and its objective. Mission statements give businesses direction. The U.S. Constitution can be viewed as a mission statement. When writing your mission statement, you might say that you are in the massage industry, and your mission is to help people relax or feel better. This textbook has a mission, too; its mission is to assist in the educational process of individuals who wish to become knowledgeable, well-informed, and competent massage therapists.

A few guidelines are available for writing a mission statement. First, it must be short. If not, you are probably not going to remember it or read it often; being able to recite it by memory is a good idea. Next, it must focus on meeting the needs of other people while not conflicting with your own. Every successful massage therapist will tell you the same thing: When your focus is serving humanity, opportunities are never in short supply. Last, your mission statement must be totally compatible with your most important values; it will evolve as you evolve; therefore it must be flexible and revised as needed. Your birthday or New Year's Day may be a good time to reevaluate your mission statement on an annual basis.

"A true definition of an entrepreneur comes closer to: a poet, visionary, or packager of social change."
Robert Schwartz

Business Evaluation and Planning

Once you know more about your values, dreams, and mission, the time has come for evaluation and planning. The following is a list of questions; it is the beginning of your business map. Remember, no single *right way* exists to construct a successful business; the trick is to find your own way, one that fits who you are and what your business represents.

Answering the following questions to the best of your ability will help you (1) identify your business parameters and (2) develop a better understanding of what areas need attention. Beginning to respond to these questions now rather than later is best. Put them down on paper, and go back to them after graduation for completion, refinement, and implementation. The components of basic business and marketing plans are personal information; general description of your business; services, fees and pricing; competition; your location and operations; and your management and personnel. A complete list of questions for the business plan is located at the end of the chapter for you to read or answer.

"The only place where success comes before work is in the dictionary."
Vidal Sassoon

Choice of Business Entity

Business enterprises may take many forms. Common choices in for-profit entities include *proprietorships, limited liability companies, partnerships,* and *corporations.* The choice of format has compliance, tax, and liability consequences that call for consultation with lawyers, accountants, and other experts; however, some insight into these matters can make these consultations more efficient and beneficial.

Proprietorship

Proprietorship, or *sole proprietorship,* involves a single owner. It is the simplest and least-expensive type of business to open. The owner provides all the capital and receives all the profits. Legally, no distinction exists between the business and the owner. Creditors of the proprietorship may look to both the owner's personal assets and the business assets to satisfy their claims. Additionally, people injured by an employee of the proprietorship during the course of employment may pursue a claim against the owner of the proprietorship. In the case of a proprietorship that uses a different name than that of the owner, the proprietor often must make a filing under local statutes to protect the use of the assumed name, which is referred to as *doing business as* (DBA). The profits or losses of the business are reported on the owner's personal tax return, which in most cases is on Schedule C of Form 1040 federal individual tax return. A sole proprietorship is recommended for the small-business person who is just getting started. Other benefits of sole proprietorship are that the owner has complete control and that the business may be easily terminated.

Advantages
- It is easy to start.
- You own it, and you control it.
- Profit and loss are reported on Schedule C on your individual Form 1040 tax return.

Disadvantages
- You are personally liable; any court judgment may affect your personal assets.
- If you decide to expand, locating financial resources (loan or credit) depends on your personal credit history and net worth.

What You Will Need to Do
- Obtain an occupational license, which is issued by the city, county, or parish in which you operate.
- Acquire liability insurance.

Limited Liability Company

Limited liability company (LLC) has appeared fairly recently as an organizational choice. As a consequence of the check-the-box regulations, the owner of a single-member company can treat the business as a corporation for tax purposes or report any income and expense on the owner's Schedule C of Form 1040. An LLC with two or more members may elect corporate or partnership taxation. Members can generally limit their liability to their equity in the company. However, as a practical matter, banks, landlords, and other significant

creditors may require the members to personally guarantee some of the company's obligations. LLCs contrast with limited partnerships in that a member can retain protection against the company's general creditors while actively participating in the business. The laws of most jurisdictions permit the owners of LLCs to conduct most of their affairs in private.

Advantages
- It is easy to start.
- It is the same as proprietorship or partnership (LLC can be either).
- Members retain protection against the company's creditors while actively participating in business activities.

Disadvantages
- Banks, landlords, and other significant creditors may require the members to personally guarantee some of the company's financial obligations.
- If more than one member exists, then each member is required to file a separate tax return.
- If you decide to expand, locating financial resources (loan or credit) may depend on the personal credit history and net worth of the LLC members.

What You Will Need to Do
- Contact an attorney to discuss creating an LLC.
- Obtain an occupational license, which is issued by the city, county, or parish in which you operate.
- If the LLC has more than one member, then acquire federal and state identification employee numbers.
- Acquire liability insurance.

Partnerships

Partnerships have flow-through taxation. Each partner files his or her own individual tax return (Form 1040), and the partnership accounts for its income and losses on Form 1065. Business partnerships are similar to domestic partnerships in that both parties agree to share both the responsibilities and the rewards of the business. Similar to domestic partnerships, it helps if business partners have good personal chemistry (similar to domestic partnerships, business partnerships have approximately a 50% mortality rate). Additionally, as with domestic partners who choose not to formally marry, two people can enter the business relationship without a formal written agreement. However, having a written agreement drawn up and reviewed by an attorney is advisable. Investment expense is usually shared among the partners, whereas authority is divided. Partnerships can have *general partners* who have shared responsibility for decisions, share in the profits, and share in personal liability. *Limited partners,* referred to as *silent partners,* do not actively participate in the management of the partnership but still receive a profit and are only liable up to the amount of their personal investment. Most small business partnerships are general partnerships that have no limited partners.

Advantages
- It is easy to start.
- Startup costs are divided between two or more people.
- It provides a broader base of skills and interest (two heads are better than one).

Disadvantages

- Decision making must be shared with one or more partner.
- If one partner dies, then the other is left with the business debts.
- As with sole proprietorship, the partners are liable for business-related mistakes.
- Unlike a sole proprietorship, you can be personally liable for suits against your partner (the exception to this would be a limited liability partnership, which is a separate legal structure with limiting liability).
- Although a partnership is only a tax-reporting rather than a tax-paying entity, it must still file a tax return.
- Think carefully about entering into a partnership with your best friend; many business partnerships end in dispute.

What You Will Need to Do

- Obtain an occupational license, which is issued by the city, county, or parish in which you operate.
- Acquire liability insurance.
- Consider drawing up a partnership agreement.
- Acquire federal and state identification employee numbers.

Corporations

For Internal Revenue Service (IRS) purposes, a small business may be either an S corporation or a C corporation. A C corporation pays federal taxes on its taxable income. Subject to exceptions, the income or loss of an S corporation flows to its shareholders in proportion to share ownership. A properly organized and operated corporation of either type limits the owner's liability. Limiting liability is the principal reason most small-business owners organize in the corporate format. After the corporation is organized by the articles of incorporation with the secretary of state or other appropriate state (and, if applicable, local) officers, shares of stock are issued to the stockholders. The shareholders must elect a board of directors annually, which oversees business operations. Corporate officers who run the daily affairs of the company can be elected or appointed by the board. Apart from filing tax returns, corporations must pay fees annually and give certain notices to state government periodically. Questions that organizers may wish to discuss with their attorneys include the following:

1. What happens if the shareholders disagree on a fundamental issue?
2. If a death or divorce changes share ownership, will the remaining shareholders then have a right to purchase and, if so, at what price?
3. What happens if a shareholder working in the business becomes disabled?

Advantages

- You are not liable to third parties.
- Your personal assets cannot be attached in a lawsuit against the business.
- The practice can continue in the event an owner leaves or dies.

- Because of its limited liability and accounting requirements, the corporate structure is attractive to a broader range of financial resources; over time, a profitable corporation is an attractive risk to banks and investors.
- Your financial risk is generally limited to the amount you pay for your stock.

Disadvantages

- A corporation is the most legally complicated business structure, and creating a corporate entity requires the assistance of an attorney.
- C corporations pay taxes separately from its shareholders (Form 1120); if the corporation pays dividends to its shareholders, then such payments are not tax deductible to the corporation, but the shareholders are required to pay tax on the dividend distribution.
- Most states charge a corporate franchise tax each year.

What You Will Need to Do

- Employ an attorney to help draw up articles of incorporation.
- File the articles of incorporation with the state where you wish to be incorporated (usually the secretary of state); you may ask the attorney you hire to take care of this task.
- Obtain an occupational license, which is issued by the city, county, or parish in which you operate.
- Acquire federal and state employee tax identification numbers.
- Acquire liability insurance.

Licenses, Permits, and Registrations

The following is a list of licenses and permits that may be required before starting your massage therapy business. Each state, county, and municipality differs in issuing these licenses and permits. Please contact your local city hall for the proper procedure. The local Small Business Administration (SBA) also may be of assistance.

If you do not know whether your state has a massage licensing board, then contact your state attorney's office or the secretary of state. If no massage board or a state licensing program is available for massage, then contact the National Certification Board for Therapeutic Massage and Bodywork at 800-296-0664 or visit *http://www.ncbtmb.org* and request an application for certification. Although not required, you may want to do this for the recognition of being nationally certified.

If your state does have a licensing board, then request by mail or telephone an information packet, application, and list of upcoming testing dates. Carefully read the state requirements, and ensure that the educational program you choose meets or exceeds the state standards. Preparation for certification may include successfully completing an approved course of study and an internship program. Some states require not only a minimum number of hours but also a number of hours in specific subject areas. Obtaining a copy of your state's massage therapy laws may also be helpful. Many massage therapy boards will not provide these laws for you; therefore you may have to check at your local library or download the laws off the Internet.

Provisional License

In most states, a massage therapist must obtain a state license before he or she is allowed to practice. However, because of lag time between graduation and state testing, many states grant a provisional license to therapists who have completed their pre-licensing coursework. Although not mandatory, a provisional license allows the therapist to practice legally for a specified period. This time frame may be for a fixed period such as 1 month, or it may be flexible, being valid until the next scheduled state testing date. The provisional license assumes that the therapist is fully trained and will be able to pass the state examination. In some states, the required provision may be that a licensed therapist must be willing to supervise the unlicensed therapist. In other words, the provisionally licensed therapist must not do any massages unless the supervising therapist is on the premises. In this way, if problem situation arises, the provisional therapist can ask for advice from the licensed therapist. Other restrictions are also made, such as with advertising. Some states may require that provisionally licensed therapists declare in all advertisements that they are provisionally licensed and that they must list the name and license number of their supervising therapist. Check with your own state or regional law for specifics. An extra form and fee often must be submitted to the state to apply for a provisional license.

State License

Once you have graduated from a massage therapy program, the time comes to take the state or national examination. Obtain an application form from the state or national board and fill it out completely; an incomplete application may delay or void your testing date and may cost you a resubmission fee. If your application is approved, you may then be able to apply for a provisional or temporary license while you are waiting for the examination date and your test scores. If not, then do not practice massage for compensation until you have received verification that you have successfully passed your state examination. In some states, you may have passed your examination, but you cannot legally practice until you receive your state license. This procedure varies from state to state; therefore obtain specific licensing instructions from your state board.

Your state board of massage therapy exists to protect the public. Informing you of proposed or current changes in the law is not its responsibility. Each massage therapist must keep abreast of changes in the state law by attending open board meetings or local massage therapy association meetings or by notices posted on the state board's website.

Occupational License

In most cities, you must acquire a business or occupational license to operate any kind of business. Contact the clerk of court, city planning department, or appropriate public office in your area. Typically, part of the procedure of obtaining your business license is to have your business location approved through the city zoning department and the fire marshal. This process includes a home, or cottage business. All business licenses and permits should be displayed in a public place.

Sales Tax Permit

If you sell any product to a client, you may then be required to obtain a sales tax permit through state, county, or parish taxing authorities. You will receive a taxpayer identification number and instructions on how to pay your sales tax, which usually involves monthly, quarterly, or twice-yearly tax payments. You are usually allowed to choose a payment schedule when you apply for your sales tax number. Some municipalities tax services such as massage, whereas others do not.

Registration of a Business Name

If you have a business name other than your name, also known as a *trade name,* or a *DBA* name, then it should be registered with the city or county clerk's office. The statement filed with the clerk's office protects you from other businesses using your name and ensures that you are not using a name currently registered by someone else in your area.

Federal Tax Identification Number

Also known as an *employer identification number* (EIN), a federal tax identification number is issued to a business if you have employees or are incorporated. If your business falls into either of these categories, then apply for an EIN by filling out Form SS-4, available at your local IRS office. Your EIN will usually begin with the prefix *72-*. All other businesses can operate using an individual social security number.

Insurance Needs

What types of insurance do you have? What types of insurance will you need to operate your business? Insurance needs vary from person to person and from time to time. Find out which type of insurance is required by law for your business to operate. Additionally, an insurance agent should be contacted to discuss your individual insurance needs. Some of your commercial and personal insurance needs can be obtained through professional massage organizations. The following sections should help you understand the different types of insurance that affect your business.

Professional Liability

Also referred to as *malpractice insurance* and *errors and omission insurance,* professional liability covers liability costs arising from your professional activities. Massage therapists are accountable for their actions and may be held liable for any mistakes made while performing their service, such as soft-tissue damage. Most affordable professional liability policies are available through the major massage and bodywork professional associations. This type of insurance can also be purchased while you are a student. If you operate a home-based practice, then your homeowner's policy does not cover your professional activities. Professional liability is required in most states.

General Liability

Also referred to as *premise liability,* general liability takes care of liability costs that are a result of bodily injury, property damage, and personal injury incurred when the client is on your premises. An example would be if your client slips and falls on your property or if a tree limb falls and damages a client's parked car.

Business Personal Property

This type of insurance covers the cost of business property such as a desk, massage table, chairs, and stereo equipment in your business location. Again, your homeowner's policy probably does not cover the costs of your business property if you operate a home-based business. An inexpensive rider can usually be purchased under your homeowner's policy to cover these costs in the event of flood, fire, or theft.

Automobile Insurance

Some states require that you have an automobile policy that is rated for business use if you travel to and from a client's home or office.

Health Insurance

Expenses such as physician visits and hospitalization are covered with health insurance. If you are self-employed, then this type of insurance can be purchased through the *National Association for the Self-Employed* (NASE; available online at http://www.nase.org).

Life Insurance

If you have dependents, then this type of insurance provides your loved ones with financial support in the event of your death. *Term life* is the least expensive choice and is the insurance policy most frequently purchased.

Disability Insurance

If you need income protection, you may then want to obtain disability insurance. This type of insurance provides you with disability income in the event that you cannot work as a result of a disability such as an illness or injury.

Determining Startup Costs

Startup costs vary from person to person and from one geographical region to the next. Take a realistic look at how much money you will need to open your doors. This section assumes that you will be working for yourself. Once you have made your initial calculations, you can make adjustments before purchases are made if you find that the figures are high. For example, you may decide that asking another therapist to share certain expenses with you will be advantageous financially. High overhead and an office are risky when you are just starting out and do not have any clients. Some of these items, such as advertising and printing costs, must eventually be repeated. Box 29-1 is a worksheet that helps clarify startup costs.

FRAMEWORK: EMPLOYMENT, PROMOTIONAL STRATEGIES, AND SUPPORT

Great diversity exists within the categories of the self-employed and employee massage therapist. This section explores various employment opportunities and strategies for promoting massage through the use of advertising, marketing, business cards, brochures, and Internet web sites. It focuses on the importance of curriculum vitae and how to develop contracts and proposals, get publicity, and write press releases. Last, this section examines the advantages of support services that can be gained by networking with other therapists, business owners, and health care professionals.

"Luck is talent meeting opportunity."
Monica Reno

Employment Opportunities

A career in massage therapy offers many employment opportunities for working with people in the health and fitness industry, beauty and spa industry, travel and recreation industry, and health care industry. A variety of settings are available for massage therapists, including the following:

- Acupuncturists
- Airports
- Athletic teams and dance companies
- Casinos
- Chiropractic clinics
- Corporate wellness programs
- Cruise lines
- Day spas
- Facial, nail, and beauty salons
- Golf, tennis, and country clubs
- Gyms and health clubs
- Hospitals
- Hotels
- Nursing homes
- On-site massage in offices
- Pain management clinics
- Physical therapy and sports medicine clinics
- Private practice (in office or out-call)
- Psychiatric treatment centers
- Resorts
- Shopping malls
- Upscale grocery stores
- Veterinarians and race tracks (animal massage)

Marketing

Marketing involves moving goods and services from the provider to the consumer. This process involves promoting business with image, purpose, and direction. Ideas include the following:

- Paid advertising and publicity
- Passing out business cards at a local country club

BOX 29-1

Determining Startup Costs

Opening a business checking account: _____

Equipment and machinery (massage tables, stereo, telephone):   _____

Room furnishings and fixtures (shelves, lamp, chair):   _____

Office rent (first and last month's rent plus security deposit):   _____

Telephone deposit and installation costs: _____

Utility deposits and installation costs: _____

Legal and professional services (accountant, attorney):   _____

Personnel: _____

Insurance (auto, general liability, malpractice, property):   _____

Professional society membership (may be an insurance payment):   _____

Initial licenses and permits: _____

Remodeling: _____

Initial office supplies (appointment book, stapler, pens):   _____

Initial massage supplies (linens, massage lubricants):   _____

Advertising and promotion: _____

Printing cost (business cards, gift certificates, stationery, forms):   _____

Petty cash: _____

Miscellaneous: _____

Total: _____

- Giving gift certificates to potential referral sources
- Sending a proposal to a hospital for massage services
- Setting up a booth at a local heath fair
- Sending a résumé to a prospective employer

In developing a marketing strategy, consider the competition. Asking direct questions and answering honestly about competitors help develop and evaluate marketing ideas.

> *"Doing business without advertising is like winking at a beautiful girl in the dark. You know what you're doing but nobody else does."*
> Stuart H. Britt

Advertising

Making a business noticeable to the public by purchasing print space or broadcast media time is **advertising**. Airtime or space can be purchased from the **media** (systems of mass communication). Massage therapists often use media in the form of phone book advertising, newspaper and newsletter advertising (display or classified), radio or television commercials, direct mailing, or even the Internet by setting up a website. Most media sell advertising and offer prospective customers a media kit. Media kits include things such as the coverage area and market information, including total population statistics by groups (women, men, teens and children);

information about households with televisions, cable, DVD players, and videocassette recorders; and demographics about household income, education level, and occupation. Also included is a price sheet, which lays out the deadlines and pricing structure; history of the company; its mission statement, owners, and stock listing; and any advantages regarding buying this particular media over other media. Last, your advertising should include a website address so that people can go online to learn more about the company or business or obtain a telephone number, address, and contact person. Polish your telephone skills before such calls come in.

When choosing the right advertising for your business, consider not only the price but also the amount of return, its target audience, circulation, and when it is released. For example, more people read Sunday papers than weekday papers, but only a certain sector of the population reads the travel section of the newspaper. People who are working are not likely to watch soap operas, and only approximately 5% of people who get your direct-mail piece actually read it, with even fewer actually calling for an appointment. Advertising also influences your business image in the client's mind. The appearance of the advertisement is just as important as when it comes out and what it says. Soliciting the help of advertising specialists would be helpful. Some therapists employ an advertising agency, which helps make decisions about how, when, and where to advertise.

Advertising lets people know who you are and what services you provide. *General advertising* announces or reminds the current or potential clients about your business. *Specific advertising* targets an objective such as gift certificate sales or increasing the purchase of a new or existent service, such as body wraps or reflexology. By determining your target group, you can decide what advertising and promotional strategies are most effective because the most effective advertisements target a specific population. Keep in mind that a lag time always exists between action and results, and you cannot always predict the results.

Business Cards

Business cards should let people know who you are, what services you provide, and how to contact you; they should also project a favorable image. Having a business card also says that you are serious about our work. Be generous and hand your business cards out often. They serve no purpose in a box on the shelf. As you give them to people, introduce yourself and clearly state what business you practice. People will often remember what you do rather than your name, which is another reason why business cards are important.

Business cards may also be used for appointment cards. You may even use your business card as part of an incentive program by writing something on the back, such as "$10 off next massage." Be creative and have fun, but remember, this is your *business face*.

Your card should be well spaced and not crowded with words or graphics; beauty lies in simplicity. If you have a logo, then use it on your business card and on every other piece of printed material. Make sure the type style or font is easy to read and the telephone number with area code is easily located by a large and bold type. If you have an office in your home, then you may choose to specify your geographic area (e.g., the Garden District) but not your home address. Be sure to proofread all information before it goes to print.

MINI-LAB

Design your own business card, letting it reflect your area of specialty.

Brochures

The purpose of a brochure is to explain to prospective clients in some detail about you and your services. Professionally printed brochures are more expensive than business cards, but because of space, they can be effective in promoting your business. If you have an adequate computer, printer, and computer program, you can print your own. The most popular format is a trifold, which is printed double-sided on an 8.5" × 11" sheet of paper. This size can also be used as a mailer.

Begin your brochure with an attention grabber that conveys some benefit of massage, such as "Feel comfortable in your body again." Then describe the benefits people often experience (in your clients' words). Next, describe what you actually do and give a short autobiography. In your autobiography, state a brief description of your qualifications and, if appropriate, your years of experience. Your telephone number should be large and readable at the end of the brochure. Close with a statement that may provoke action, such as "Call now." Use vivid language, appealing to vision, hearing, and emotion—for example, "One part therapy, one part luxury" or "Visit the tranquil place." Note that you do not have to say things directly, as with "Feel comfortable in your body again" or "Must be experienced to be fully understood." What are the mental images that come to mind when you read those words? A brochure is easier to read if you use bullet points and attractive graphics instead of paragraphs of text.

If you include your fees and menu of services, then print them on a separate sheet of paper that slips into your brochure as an insert. Avoid dating your flyer; put "practicing since 1994" instead of "13 years of experience." Use facsimile machines and electronic mail to send out your brochure when someone calls you with an inquiry.

Once you have a rough draft, give it to three trusted friends and ask for feedback. Revise it as often as needed. Ensure that after reading your brochure, a potential client then knows what needs you fulfill and how you are different from others providing a similar service.

Internet Websites

Although radio and television advertising are occasionally cost prohibitive for people with small practices, an Internet website can be an inexpensive way to reach large numbers of clients. The exposure can range from a free listing on established massage sites to creating and publishing your own web site. Six guidelines and standards for designing your web site are as follows:

1. Select a color scheme. If have a logo or preferred colors on business cards and stationery, then that is a good start. If not, then choose two or three complementary colors and stay with them—do not change colors on every page. If you are unsure, then surf the Net and find a website that you like. The most common color schemes are as follows:
   - Red, yellow, and white
   - Blue and white
   - Red, grey, and white
   - Blue, orange, and white
   - Yellow, grey, and white
2. Use a template. Most website-design software (such as FrontPage) includes some templates, or you can check out some websites that specialize in designing templates. Visit:
   - *http://www.templatesbox.com*
   - *http://www.templatemonster.com*

- *http://freesitetemplates.com*
- *http://www.freelayouts.com*

3. Provide an easy-to-use navigation system. This aspect is one of the most important considerations. Make sure that visitors can find information easily. Most websites display their navigation bar on the left or at the top. Do the same because most people are used to this type of navigation. Include a navigation bar at the bottom of each page to save your visitors from having to scroll back to the top.

4. Do not go overboard on special effects. Although including one or two special effects to spice up a website is nice, avoid rotating graphics because they serve to distract from the site's content and consume download time. Visitors may move off your site even before your spinning logo finishes loading.

5. Backgrounds. Make sure that your visitors can read the text on the background (avoid dark blue writing on a black background or yellow on white). The default for links in most programs is blue (before being visited) and burgundy (after being visited). If you have a dark background, then the make sure your links are light.

6. Content is king. Although your website should looks clean and professional, a far more important aspect is that you concentrate your efforts on the content and promotion. If you want a professional website, then avoid the following:
   - Flashy intros, revolving globes, beveled line separators, animated mail boxes
   - Busy backgrounds
   - Loads of pop-up or pop-under boxes
   - Autoplay music (allow your customer to play music only if desired)
   - Hit counters of the free variety, which say "you are 27th visitor"
   - Date and time stamps, unless your website is updated daily or weekly

Telephone Etiquette

The telephone is the second contact between the client and the therapist. The first is promotional advertising such as a business card, brochure, or word of mouth. Because of the importance of *telephone communication*, spending time learning how to manage incoming calls and telephone communications makes good sense. This aspect is known as *telephone etiquette*—the behavior observed and used by people on the telephone when communicating for social or professional activities. The following tips are for communicating with your current and prospective clients by telephone:

General telephone standards
- Always answer between the second and third ring.
- Speak slowly and use a pleasant, expressive tone of voice; smile at the person on the other end of the telephone.
- Give the caller or person you are calling your undivided attention; do not carry on two conversations at once.
- Say "please," "thank you," and "you're welcome."
- Do not chew while on the telephone. This action is considered impolite.
- End each call with a sincere closing remark.
- Keep your promises, and follow up on the call.
- Return calls within 24 hours; this is known as the *sundown rule*.

Placing a call
- Identify yourself by name and business or title (if applicable).
- Be cordial, and explain the purpose of the call.
- Have all necessary information handy before placing the call.

Answering a call
- Begin with "Good morning," "Good afternoon," or "Good evening," followed by your name, the name of your establishment, and an inquiry. For example, "Good afternoon. This is Jane at the Downtown Spa. How may I help you?"
- Find out the caller's name, and use it as you speak to him or her.
- Be a good listener; find out what the caller wants first.
- Let the caller end the conversation, allowing him or her to hang up first.

Putting a caller on hold
- If you must place the caller on hold, ask permission and wait for a reply. For example, "May I put you on hold?"
- If the caller says no, get his or her name and number and say that you will return the call shortly. Keep this promise.
- If the caller concurs, then do not leave him or her on hold for more than 30 seconds. If the caller must be on hold longer than that, offer to return the call. The caller may choose to continue holding.
- Always thank the caller for holding.

Taking messages
- Clearly write down the date, time the call was received, who called, why the person called, and a return telephone number and extension (if applicable).
- Make sure you understand the message.
- Repeat all the information to the caller, and check for accuracy before hanging up.
- Give the message to the proper person as soon as possible.

Massage inquires by telephone
- Inform the caller of available services and fees.
- State appointments that are available. Avoid telling the caller when massages are not available.
- If the caller schedules an appointment, recommend that he or she avoid eating or eat only lightly 1 hour before the scheduled session.
- If he or she comes directly from his or her work, suggest that the person bring alternate clothing to wear after the massage session.
- If you require that the client bring special items such as shorts, a swimsuit, or a towel, inform him or her at this time.

- Suggest that the client schedule *downtime,* or time to relax, after the session.
- If you have a cancellation or late policy, then let him or her know about it at this time.
- Verify the appointment day and time.
- Give the client directions to your establishment and any other information that you deem necessary.
- Finally, ask if he or she has any questions.

> *"Every artist was an amateur."*
> Ralph Waldo Emerson

Curriculum Vitae

Curriculum vitae (CV), also known as a *résumé,* is an autobiographical sketch that documents all your achievements, including occupational, avocational, academic, and personal information that you wish to disclose to a prospective employer or business contact. Even if you are self-employed, your CV can help you in business meetings, with developing business relationships, and in acquiring a referral base. A well-written CV lets your business contacts know who you are and what you can offer their employers, members, clients, or patients. A well-written and properly distributed CV can help you advance your practice.

Before you sit down to write your CV, take time to reflect on your life. What are the accomplishments of which you are proud? What are the things that have brought you the most joy? Your list of accomplishments may include acting in a community play or assisting with a political campaign. Now, study the list. You might notice a pattern of personal strengths or interests emerging. You may find that you are a natural leader or that you work best with groups of people. This information can help you write your personal data section.

Begin organizing and writing your CV. The most widely used format is the *reverse chronological format,* which emphasizes your education and work experience from most to least recent. Begin by posting your name, address, telephone number, and e-mail address at the top center of the page at a larger font the rest of the text.

> *evolve* I keep my résumé as a Word document and update it annually. A sample résumé is on the Evolve website under course materials for Chapter 29. Research other formats and choose the one that works best for you. ■

Education: List all of your academic achievements in reverse chronological order. If you did not attend college, then list your high school; if you did attend college, then omit your high school in this section. Your education section should include the name of the educational institution, any college degrees, postgraduate degrees, certificates, and any awards or honors. Also include the schools you attended and any major and minor courses that have helped you as a massage therapist (e.g., psychology, anatomy and physiology, kinesiology). If you have attended any postgradu-

ate workshops, then list them after your formal educational achievements.

Work experience: Starting with the most recent, list all the jobs held within the last 10 years. Include the names of your employers, titles or positions held, job descriptions, and starting and termination dates. Focus on your field experience while you were at school. Did you provide sports massage for athletes? Did you massage residents in a nursing home? Select the activities that enhance your qualifications, such as hobbies, sports, and professional affiliations.

Personal data: Although not necessary, this section is your opportunity for the reader to know about you. List your marital status, number and ages of your children, your general health status, and whether you are a nonsmoker. Use only the personal information that will help you project the positive image that you began to formulate in the preceding sections. You might even mention that you like to coach baseball or that you enjoy playing chess. These activities may create a pleasant image to the reader.

Once your CV is organized, type it on 8.5" × 11" white bond paper. Keep your writing style simple. After you have proofread it once, let three other people proofread it for you. This exercise is a good system for reducing grammar and spelling errors. Typos in a professional CV are taboo.

If you have a specific employer in mind, then send him or her your CV along with a well-written cover letter addressed to a specific person in the company or organization. Avoid phrases such as "Dear Madam," "Dear Sir," or "To Whom It May Concern." Spell his or her full name correctly. If you are invited to an interview or a business meeting, then call the day before to confirm. Arrive 15 minutes before the meeting begins. Within a week, send him or her a thank-you note, and mention how much you enjoyed the opportunity to share ideas.

Contracts and Proposals

When embarking on a new business venture, you may be asked to write a business contract or a proposal. Writing down these ideas and formal agreements does many things. It outlines and details your ideas, helps avoid communication problems, states specifically how problems will be handled and who will handle them when they do arise, and helps keep both parties focused.

A **contract** is a written voluntary agreement between two or more parties that communicates expectations, duties, and responsibilities. A signed and dated contract is enforceable by law. Ideally, all parties should draw up an informal contract, or draft, outlining what they perceive as a reasonable agreement. Make sure your draft (1) clarifies the business relationship of each party (e.g., lessor, lessee, employer, employee, partner, independent contractor); (2) states the duration of the contract (e.g., 6 months, 1 year); and (3) predetermines on what grounds the contract can be terminated, if before the previously agreed time. Write down any other ideas you have concerning the proposed business arrangement. Regardless of which party prepares the final draft of the contract, have your attorney look it over to point out possible problems. Everything is negotiable, but do negotiate *before* signing.

A **proposal** is a written idea put forward for consideration, discussion, or adoption. Many massage therapists entering the field have the opportunity to approach businesses that do not offer massage therapy and create a position for themselves or for other therapists. The following sections are elements that should be included when writing a proposal to a sports group, nursing home, or any other business endeavor where you wish to be hired or volunteer your services.

Cover Letter

The cover letter of the proposal is actually your *letter of introduction* and should include your name (or name of person submitting the proposal), title, and all contact information such as your mailing address, e-mail address, telephone number, cellular telephone number, and pager number. This page should also include the title of the project and a 25-word summary introducing your concept of the proposed massage therapy services.

Objective

A broad statement should embody the aim, expected results of the project, or both—for example, "by providing stress-reduction services to the employees of said corporation to enhance employee productivity and reduce absenteeism." Next, the objective describes whom the project will serve and the geographic location. Then discuss the significance and need for this project; compare your project with other projects in the same field and geographic locations (when applicable). Last, state the anticipated outcomes and a method of evaluating and reporting these outcomes.

Logistics

Logistics are the managing details of the operation—that is, the what, when, and where section of the proposal. If you are familiar with the facility, then you may recommend a specific location where massage services will be provided. Briefly discuss physical arrangements such as room dimensions, bathroom location, lighting, equipment, and supplies. Mention which of these items you are willing to provide. Are you proposing full-time or part-time work? Will massage services be available during the day, evenings, or weekends? One idea is to propose a part-time availability and to increase your hours as demand increases. Within what time frame would you conduct the proposed massage services? What hours of the day will massage services be offered, and who will pay for them? Also include who should be contacted as ideas are developed and problems arise. State which person in the company will be responsible for managing the project, and define your organization's contact person, if different from the person negotiating the proposal. Specify how you can be reached. Also include a mutually agreed on mediator (or third party) to help settle disputes if irreconcilable problems arise.

Qualifications

An effective qualification section introduces you as a health care professional. Include a brief CV of your training and experience. If you do not have postgraduate experience, then focus on the field experience you acquired while you were in school. Introduce other people (e.g., staff, volunteers) who are key to the project, and provide their backgrounds. Mention any professional affiliations such as the American Massage Therapy Association (AMTA), National Certification Board for Therapeutic Massage and Bodywork (NCBTMB), and Associated Bodywork and Massage Professionals (ABMP) and whether the participating massage therapists are insured.

Funding

This important section outlines the projected budget for the project and includes the amount you are contributing, if any; the names and amounts of funds received from other participants; and the amount you are requesting from the agency or corporation. If needed, suggest plans for additional fundraising. The budget should include both expenses and revenues for the entire proposed project. If revenue is to be generated by this project, then outline who will benefit financially. This section should also include payment schedules and payment method.

Summary

The summary, or closing remarks, should recap your proposal and convey a sense of warmth, camaraderie, confidence, and willingness to be of service in this project. Also helpful is to include a brief synopsis on a separate sheet of paper listing or bulleting all the elements in your proposal, outlining their contents, which can be used during the meeting in which your proposal is presented before the board members. Do not use complete sentences but rather a rough description of what each element entails, which is similar to using note cards for a speech; it will keep you on track and allow others to follow your presentation easily.

MINI-LAB

Using the guidelines outlined in this chapter, write a proposal and a contract.

Publicity

Publicity is free media exposure. You can attract attention for your business in many ways. One way is to *become the expert*. After you have some initial experience in massage therapy, write a column for a local paper or magazine. Write about anything with which you are experienced and tie it back into massage. Stress and stress reduction are always good topics. If you like sports, then write about ways to manage common sports injuries. Submit this information for publication to newspapers, magazines, or newsletters as an article. Contact these resources ahead of time and request a copy of their writers' guidelines. Use this information when preparing your final draft. If accepted, then you may even be paid for your work. Take advantage of the release date, and run a display advertisement in the same publication, or if you have the time and resources, publish your own newsletter.

Use this same information and dispense it by speaking publicly; give talks, speeches, or lectures. You may be asked to appear on a television or radio show. You can also begin teaching classes or workshops in massage or a related topic. Promoting massage instead of your practice is an effective way of increasing clientele. This tactic is called a *soft sell*. Tell people about massage, and teach them how to use it to take care of themselves. Pass out informational material that includes your name and contact information. Prospective clients can contact you if they have any questions or need to schedule an appointment.

Another way to use publicity is to participate in *community service* or to *volunteer*. A volunteer is someone who renders aid or performs a service without direct monetary gain. Volunteering is done of your own free will, usually with a sense of charity, but virtually every known religion or philosophy is concerned with some form of volunteerism or charity. Volunteerism is also a way to give back to the community that supports your practice. Through donations of time and talent, massage can touch lives. Many ideas exist for volunteering, such as doing postevent sports massage at local athletic events or donating gift certificates to civic and church groups as door prizes or auction items for fundraisers. Get a group of therapists together, and support your local police and fire departments by offering free foot rubs or massages to each officer or firefighter. Donate time at retirement homes or with hospice programs. When donating time, wear professional attire with a nametag or monogrammed shirt. Not only will you be promoting massage, personal recognition will also come as more and more people recognize your name. Donate gift certificates to schools for teacher appreciation week. The possibilities are limited only by your imagination.

Press Releases

Part of your promotional strategy might include publicity writing and submitting press releases to newspapers as a way of letting people know what you are doing. Each workshop you attend, each office you hold, and each lecture you give should be announced in the newspaper as a noteworthy event. This tactic provides a subtle reminder of who you are and gives the message that you are active in your community and your profession. A press release is not an advertisement. If yours has the sound of an advertisement, then the editor of the newspaper will not print it.

evolve Learning how to write and submit a press release is a simple, quick, and inexpensive way to get your name out in the public eye. Log on to the Evolve website to view a sample press release. ■

Begin your press release with something that a newspaper normally considers interesting and newsworthy. Keep it simple, and use a writing style that is direct and delivers a clear, concise message.

MINI-LAB

Using the guidelines outlined in this chapter, write a press release.

When writing your press release, use short words, sentences, and paragraphs, and write in the present tense as much as possible. Make sure your press release answers the who, what, where, when, why, and how of your event. Use the inverted pyramid style of journalistic writing—that is, place the most important information in the beginning of the press release and less important information in each subsequent paragraph. This way, if the editor has to cut the size of the release, then important information located at the beginning of it will not be eliminated (most editors cut from the bottom of the release). Last, and most important, proofread your work and ask at least three other objective people to proofread it. The following guidelines are helpful in putting together your press release:

- Type on 8.5" × 11" white bond paper.
- Leave a 2-inch margin on the top and bottom of the press release; side margins are 1.5 inches.
- Date it and identify it as a press release by typing the words PRESS RELEASE at the top center of the page, followed by the phrase *For Immediate Release.* A specific date can be substituted if the release should be delayed.
- At the upper left-hand corner of the page, identify yourself (or the appropriate person) as the *contact person* and include an address and daytime telephone number.
- Type only the lead sentence in capital letters; it should be action oriented.
- Double-space the text if the press release is for print, and triple space the release if it is for broadcast. Confine the release to one page (if possible), and type on only one side of the paper. If the press release is more than one page, then write MORE at the bottom of the first page. End the press release with either *-30-* or consecutive number symbols (#) tabbed consecutively across the page.

Preceptors, Resources, and Networking

Building a support structure is vital for the health of any business. This process involves reaching out to others and asking for help. Several methods are available for accomplishing this task. First, locate an established therapist and ask him or her to become your preceptor. Your massage instructor can often arrange these meetings. Participating in a preceptorship can be rewarding for both the novice and the preceptor. During class time, instructors are available to teach you the knowledge and skills of your trade. A **preceptor** is someone who guides you during your postgraduate clinical practice; this person is similar to a mentor. He or she may be physically on the premises while you engage in your professional activities, or he or she may be available to be contacted as you have questions about how to handle certain situations. This person may be one of your instructors but most often is a veteran massage therapist who has agreed to help you get started. Someone who was once a massage student and new graduate can better understand your concerns.

You can also locate a *business coach,* which is a cross between a consultant and a teacher and not necessarily in the massage business. This person helps you bridge the gap between where you are and where you want to be. A business coach may offer honest, direct feedback and professional advice. Your business coach may be a chiropractor, physical or occupational therapist, banker, or experienced self-employed person. Do not be afraid to approach people from whom you would like to learn. These individuals are often flattered that you are asking them for their guidance and can act as a sounding board if you need help in making decisions. The following is a list of keys to finding and keeping a business coach relationship:

1. Find someone you admire.
2. Find someone who is successful.
3. Find someone who is willing to be a coach.
4. Be willing to learn from his or her mistakes.
5. Give something back to him or her. Money is probably not appropriate in this circumstance, but find a service that he or she needs such as cooking or baby-sitting, or give a gift such as flowers, a book, or even a massage. Show the person how much he or she is appreciated.
6. Remember that, regardless of what advice is offered, the decision and responsibility are ultimately your own.

Another important aspect of support is using established business *resources.* These resources include a variety of business and civic organizations such as your public library, the Small Business Administration (SBA, http://www.sba.org), and the Service Corps of Retired Executives (SCORE, http://www.score.org). Most major hospitals have medical librarians who can help you locate important information. In many instances, your secretary of state's office can put you in touch with these resource organizations. Membership in a professional massage organization is also am important resource tool. Belonging to a massage association helps you keep up with current trends, exchange ideas with the only people who truly understand your problems, and actively support your industry as a whole. Attend massage conferences and conventions often. Nothing is quite as inspiring as thousands of people gathered together who share a common experience.

If you are fortunate to live in the vicinity of a college or university, most colleges and universities have business and marketing departments. Volunteer your business as a project for graduate students who must analyze and prepare business proposals. The college library, which typically has scientific resources available, is also a wealth of information and generally includes large periodical indexes such as *Index Medicus.*

> *"It isn't what you know when you start, but what you learn when you get out there."*
> Carol Kresge

The next support method involves *networking,* which is essentially a referral system. During this process, you are reaching out and developing business relationships with vast groups of people who are looking for the same thing you are—promoting their businesses. You may network informally by referring your clients to people you know or with whom you do business. Formal networking involves joining a networking group, local chamber of commerce, or other civic or social group to begin meeting people. When you meet someone who is a potential networking associate, exchange business cards and clearly state your line of work. People often remember what you do rather than your name, which is why business cards are important. At your next opportunity, write down where and when you met these people and who introduced you. Keep track of all the business cards you collect in a rotary file, a computer program, or a special card folder.

As your base of support widens, you will have a large number of people you can call when you have a question, need guidance, or want a sounding board for your concerns. At the same time, the process is also reciprocal; be there for your network friends. So much of this business comes by word of mouth; it makes sense to network.

SAMPLE DAY OF A MASSAGE THERAPIST

This section examines the massage routine in its various segments and discusses the therapist's responsibilities during each segment. The sections of the massage are (1) before the client arrives, (2) when the client arrives, (3) before the massage session, (4) during the massage session, and (5) after the massage session.

Hands-on experience is your best and final teacher. By palpating, questioning, listening, and treating, you develop a sense of what is familiar, which, in turn, breeds knowledge, enhances skill, and promotes confidence. You will learn that mastery comes not only in the doing but also in the deciding. Many small decisions are made in the course of a workday. Let this section serve as a guide.

Before the Client Arrives

This section is concerned with the time frame beginning when you report to work until the client arrives. If possible, arrive at least 60 minutes before your first appointment. Check your answering machine or answering service and take care of any calls. You may want to call each person the day before the scheduled massage to verify the appointment, which reduces any confusion and minimizes absenteeism. Look over your schedule; pull and review client intake forms and past notes for any clients scheduled that day. If you are expecting a first-time client, then have a blank intake form and pertinent literature ready.

Check the table for safety and security. Are the knobs that connect the table legs to the tabletop loose? If so, then tighten them. If you massage on a portable table, then make sure the latches that keep the table closed are now flat and not protruding. Check and correct the extension of the table legs, and make sure any table cords are straight and taut.

Dress the treatment table and ready the massage room. If you have prepared your massage room the day before, then inspect the room for any unexpected items (e.g., dead insects). When your client enters the massage room, have the music playing, the lighting dim and indirect, and the room warm. Having the massage area visually appealing and ready to go (i.e., bolsters, linens, lubricant) is a mark of professionalism. If you do not allow enough time between massages for this preparation, then have a place (e.g., waiting room, office) where your client can wait while you prepare the massage room.

Using a mirror, critique your own appearance. Is your hair in place? Are your nails trimmed, neat, and clean? Are your pockets empty of keys and change? Have you removed your jewelry and watch?

MINI-LAB

Visit a massage therapist's office. What is the initial impression you have approaching the door? List the words that describe how you feel. Is the mood serene, business-like, busy, chaotic, impersonal, or cluttered? What do you hear or smell?

When the Client Arrives: Room Orientation and Preparation for Massage

This period is the time frame between the client's arrival and when he or she undresses for the massage. Greet your client with a smile, making eye contact and calling him or her by name whenever possible. Introduce yourself (if this is your first time as his or her therapist), and escort the client to the area where the massage consultation will take place. Be calm, confident, friendly, and courteous while in the presence of your client. The therapeutic relationship, which is an ongoing process, is built on a foundation of trust and good communication skills, which builds rapport (see Chapter 2). To show respect for the client and the relationship, avoid using tobacco in any form while in the company of a client. The smell of tobacco is often offensive to nonsmoking clients. Although many smoking therapists are unaware of their tobacco odor, it can be detected on their clothes, hair, and linens.

Ask the client to fill out an intake form (see Chapter 8), and review the informed consent section with him or her. If the person is a previous client, then go over the health history information and record any changes. Perform any assessments related to treatment, and prioritize the client's needs based on the consultation. Explain to the client what will be done during the session and why. Ask the client if he or she has any questions, and answer them to the best of your ability.

If any special considerations need to be addressed, then discuss how the massage will be adapted to suit the client's special needs (see Chapter 10). The client may be overwhelmed by all the information that is needed to prepare for a safe and well-tailored massage session. Asking the client to show up 15 minutes early for his or her first appointment may be helpful, or you may want to mail out in advance all the forms that you require (e.g., initial intake, consent, brochure of your practice, policies and procedures). This packet may be titled *What to Expect* or *What a Massage is Like.* The purpose of this procedure is to decrease the client's stress and anxiety and to save you time.

You may wish to direct your client to the music selection, telling him or her what is currently playing and asking the client to make a selection if he or she prefers a different kind of music. Next, direct the client to your massage lubricant selection, and ask him or her to make a choice (see Chapter 3). Point out the most popular lubricant so as to make the selection process easier. Take into consideration any skin sensitivities and allergies. You may need to get an ingredient list in large type so the client can read the ingredients. The use of aromatherapy can also help the client to unwind (see Chapter 24).

Even though draping is discussed in the premassage consultation, many emotions are often associated with disrobing and touch that distort the new client's perspective, making directions and instructions difficult to hear. Simple and concise instructions assist the client in the transition from the mental focus of the consultation to the physical and emotional focus of a massage session. Be sure to allow the client time to settle into the space provided for him or her before giving directions on the use of linens, positioning himself or herself on the table, indicating when you will return to begin the massage (see Chapter 6). Every precaution should be taken to ensure the client's comfort, physical and emotional safety, and privacy.

Before you exit the room, address any comfort needs your client may have. Offer the client a glass of water, and suggest a trip to the restroom. Show the client where to place his or her clothes and personal items, and explain to the client any special procedures you use to handle these items. Tell the client how to lie on the table (either to get underneath the top sheet or to drape towels over her body). Tell him or her that you are going to leave the room so he or she may disrobe in privacy and that, when you reenter the room, you will knock before you open the door. This precaution alleviates any apprehension he or she may have about your unannounced return.

TABLE TALK

Client empathy is one of the reasons that you, as the therapist, must receive massages from other therapists. By getting back in touch with how it feels to be a client, you will be a more attentive and sensitive therapist.

Clients often wear a watch or jewelry and may bring a purse, wallet, or other valuables to the massage office. Because most jewelry and watches are removed before the massage begins, care must be taken to safeguard these items. Large articles, such as purses, should not leave the client's

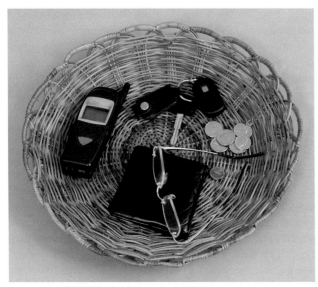

FIGURE 29-1 A basket for personal items.

sight. For smaller items, use a large envelope, small basket, or small bowl to accommodate the client's belongings (Figure 29-1). A portable container allows these items to remain with the client if he or she must move from one room to another. A locker or locked box may also be used to store these items safely during the massage.

MINI-LAB

Once you have learned a basic massage routine, perform a massage blindfolded. The recipient on the table may have to assist with the draping and turning aspects of the massage because these tasks may be too difficult for you without your sense of sight. This activity will help you get out of your head and intellect and into your hands and feeling skills.

Before the Massage Session

This section deals with the period when you leave the massage room until you return to begin the massage. Wash and dry your hands and forearms (see Chapter 4). Because your hands may become cool from the hand washing, warm them by rubbing them together before the massage begins. Rubbing your hands together helps warm the massage lubricant, too.

You have spent much time and energy learning a craft and preparing your massage room; spend a little time preparing your mind, body, and spirit. Grounding and centering yourself before the massage is an integral part of your therapy session. If you feel distracted and not present with your client, then you will not be able to give the best massage possible. Learning how to clear your thoughts, how to prepare your body, and how to ground and center yourself will help you be a more skilled and sensitive therapist (see Chapter 6).

Breathing and performing body movements are some techniques you can use to prepare yourself before the massage begins. No matter what style of massage you practice,

you will expend energy. Before you enter the massage room, move and stretch your body while practicing deep breathing. If all you have is a few seconds, then simply squat down to stretch your low back (only if your knees can do this comfortably) and stand up to shake out your entire body. Stretch your upper body (Figure 29-2). Relaxation allows a calm to exist. A therapist who is calm will easily project professionalism, confidence, and peace to the client with her presence and touch.

Some massage therapists choose to incorporate elements of their own spirituality into the massage. Some therapists choose to turn their skills and the direction of the massage over to the care of God (or a higher power). A simple prayer, verbal or silent, of gratitude for the opportunity to work with this client helps create the atmosphere for healing to occur (most massage therapists prefer to pray in silence). If you decide to pray in the massage room, ask permission from the client. Some clients will be fine with prayer; others will consider it too personal an issue and may be uncomfortable.

> *"No one is useless in this world who lightens the burdens of another."*
> Charles Dickens

Many clients will ask you how many massages you have done today and if you are tired, or after noting the physical

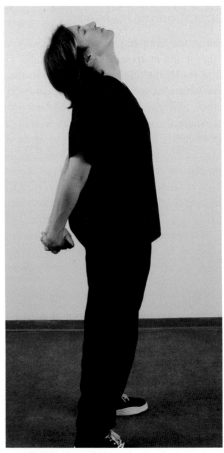

FIGURE 29-2 Massage therapist stretching before entering massage room.

nature of your work, they will ask if your hands become tired. What they may really be asking is "Do you have enough energy for me?" Assure them that you have stamina and endurance built up from frequently doing massage and that when your hands do feel tired you massage them back to happiness. At this point, they seem to be less fearful and greatly relieved.

During the Massage Session

This section of the chapter addresses the time frame that begins when the massage therapist reenters the room and ends when the massage therapist leaves the room after the massage is complete.

Before you begin the massage, address the client's care and comfort needs one more time. Ask your client if the room temperature is comfortable. Relaxing is difficult if you feel chilled. Encourage your client's proper body alignment with the placement of bolsters or pillows underneath the areas of the body that require support (e.g., neck, knees, ankles; see Chapter 6). Remind the client about the importance of being relaxed and offering feedback during the massage. If the client is uncomfortable in any way, then he or she may not become or stay engaged with the massage.

Begin by making physical contact with the client, perhaps with quiet, motionless touch (Figure 29-3). Help your client relax by asking him or her to take a few deep breaths. Once you and the client are ready, proceed with the massage routine. The dozens of methods for massaging the body, each effective in its own way, are best learned in the classroom under a skilled and caring instructor.

The length of treatment is offered by the therapist but determined by the client. The client schedules the session, often in 30- to 90-minute increments. If the client is undecided about the length of the session, tell him or her that you will schedule a half-hour session but will block out a full hour. When 30 minutes is up, let the client know, and he or she can then decide if the massage will continue.

Focus on the client's areas of complaint during the session while working out areas that you find during the massage through palpation. Although the therapist is confined to a specific length of time, try not to let the massage feel hurried. Address the client's concerns first (e.g., back, neck, shoulder) so as to avoid accidentally running out of time.

In some instances, as you massage, the client's body may tense. Silently, you may decide to respond by changing your pressure or rhythm. If the client remains tense, then ask for feedback. Reiterate how important communication is during the massage. You may discover that the client is ticklish or is in pain and is therefore splinting, or contracting, his or her muscles. The client may also have to use the restroom. Address his or her needs, and then continue with the massage. Be patient and caring; enhance your client's ability to relax.

Regarding conversation during the massage, take your cues from the client. If he or she is there for stress reduction,

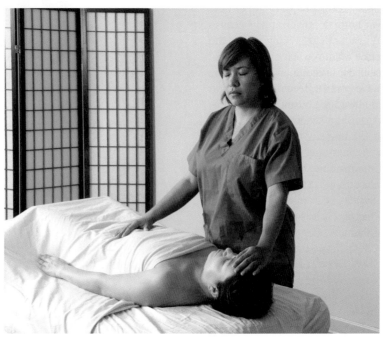

FIGURE 29-3 Therapist making physical contact with client before massage.

then avoid becoming too talkative because doing so may distract from his or her overall relaxation. One guideline is to talk only when answering the client's questions and when addressing the client's comfort needs. Otherwise, stay silent and follow the client's lead.

Designing and tailoring the session to the client's individual needs is the hallmark of a proficient massage therapist. Everybody responds differently to massage. The more you learn and practice, the greater are the number of massage styles you can offer your clients. Know all your options and honor your limits. As your experience increases, you can incorporate new moves into your routine. As with any art, mastery is a lifelong process.

The following few general guidelines can be considered as you are applying massage:

- Practice good hygiene with hand washing before and after each massage.
- Protect yourself by using good body mechanics.
- Promote client comfort through a restful environment and bolstering devices.
- Screen your client for local and absolute contraindications.
- Stroke lightly over bony prominences and endangerment sites.
- Address client needs regarding work on a specific area.
- Be thorough and complete. Always connect body parts to themselves and to one another.
- Work deeply enough to contact and release tension but not so deep that you cause tension and pain.
- Stay relaxed and present; be focused and respect the client.

> *"A ship in harbor is safe—but that*
> *is not what ships are for."*
> John A. Shedd

Providing communication and direction during the massage is a little different than normal conversation because eye contact is infrequent. When a client is lying prone, the head is to one side or in a face cradle; when a client is supine, either the eyes are closed or a client must strain his or her neck muscles to obtain eye contact. Establish a method of communication in the premassage consultation, and reinforce your instructions during the session when needed. The most important feedback a massage therapist needs is how the client is receiving the massage. More specifically, the therapist must know if the massage causes any pain or discomfort. Massage therapist Ralph Stephens developed the following abbreviated system of communication. This system is also featured in Chapter 27; it is particularly helpful in establishing and maintaining communication and in building rapport with your client during the session.

When it Hurts or if the Pressure is Too Hard

Tell the client, "Be sure to tell me whenever I find a tender area. Will you do that for me?" or "If at any time I am working too hard, be sure to tell me right away. Will you

do that?" Quantitative measuring scales you can use are as follows:

- Ask the client to simply raise a hand if pain is felt.
- Use the 1-to-5 scale: 1 represents *no pain* and 5 represents *excruciating pain*. You will know, by the number vocalized or the number of fingers raised, how he or she is responding to the pressure. A 1-to-5 scale is necessary to allow easy one-handed response.
- Establish a thumbs up-thumbs down-okay gesture system. Thumbs up means that the pressure is too great (Figure 29-4). Thumbs down means that more pressure is requested. An okay symbol (index finger touching thumb with other fingers extended) means the pressure is perfect.

When it Gets Better

Tell the client, "When I find these tender places, I will stop and maintain the pressure. This sustained pressure will cause the nervous system to respond by relaxing the tender area. It may feel to you like I am letting up on the pressure or that it is beginning to feel better. Will you let me know when it gets better?"

If it Refers

Tell the client, "When I am examining or maintaining pressure on an area of tissue, you may experience some sensation somewhere else. It might be a pain, tingling, numbness, aching, or some other sensation, somewhere besides right where I am massaging. These may be trigger points that also

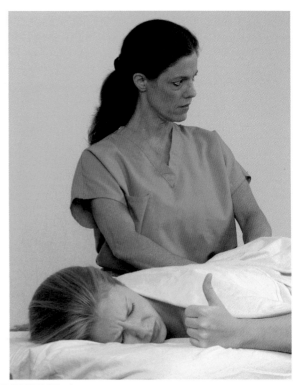

FIGURE 29-4 Prone client giving *thumbs up* for pressure during massage.

need to be massaged. Will you tell me if you feel anything other than pressure where I am working?"

Regardless of which system of feedback you use for assessing pain and pressure, use your peripheral vision and look for physical signs of discomfort (Figure 29-5). Some clients do not volunteer feedback about pain. They may be accustomed to denying pain and discomfort, or they may have a different sensation and perception assigned to pain. However, the body rarely lies. Body gestures that may indicate you are working too hard include (1) the client pulling away from you or contracting muscles to limit your access into the tissues, (2) general squirming, (3) raising eyebrows or frowning, (4) holding the breath, (5) white knuckles, and (6) raising the head or foot up off the table.

Another helpful tool to use when giving directions is to use tactile cues and gestures. For example, as you ask the client to scoot over to the edge of the table, gently touch his or her shoulder or tap the tabletop on the side toward which you want him or her to move. This method can be used when you need the client to move up or down the table and also when to turn the head to one side or another. When asking a client to turn over, if eye contact is possible, supinate or pronate your hand to indicate the direction he or she should roll. When giving directions in which a client should place his or her arms or other body part a certain way, demonstrate it, too. If you need the client to raise his or her head, feet, or knees to accommodate a bolster, then use a gentle lifting motion with your hand. Your client may be so relaxed that verbal directions are processed slowly. Kinetic cues help the client understand what you need him or her to do.

When you are finished with the massage, avoid hurrying the client off the massage table. In fact, invite the client to rest a few minutes. Because the client has been in one position for an extended period, asking him or her to roll over on his or her side and bend the knees to his or her chest is often helpful. Place a soft pillow under the client's head, and ask

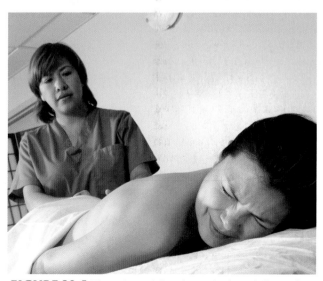

FIGURE 29-5 Therapist noticing signs of pain and discomfort.

him or her to lie in this position for a few minutes before getting up to dress. If the client is afraid of falling asleep and losing track of time, then tell him or her that you will be back in 10 minutes to remind him or her to get up. This short rest period allows the client some quiet time devoid of stimuli to integrate the physical and emotional aspects of the massage. It also allows transition time to move from internal focus to external focus before rescheduling an appointment, leaving your facility, and driving away. Before you leave the room, remove the bolsters and wipe off any excess lubricant from the soles of your client's feet.

You may need to instruct the client on how to get up off the table. Once lying on his or her side, suggest that the client allow the lower legs to fall off the edge of the table. The client can then use the arm that is not lying against the massage table to push the upper body up into a seated position. Avoid letting the client sit straight up from a supine position because he or she may strain the back or neck. Remind the client that the best way to get off the massage table is also the best way to get out of bed in the morning. If your client requires assistance getting off the table, refer to Chapter 6.

A small portion of the population (approximately 10%) finds difficulty in standing up after lying down for an extended period. This circumstance is the result of insufficient cerebral circulation and a sudden drop in blood pressure that often occurs when moving into an upright position. Symptoms of this condition may include dizziness, impaired vision, and buzzing in the ears. In severe cases, fainting may occur. With this fact in mind, performing one of the following exercises after the massage is helpful: (1) remind your client to sit up for a few moments before standing, or (2) assist him or her into a standing position, pausing for a few moments to make sure he or she is oriented in the upright position.

If you remove a client's eyeglasses while he or she is on the massage table, or if a client gives you his or her eyeglasses before the massage, hand them back to the client before he or she gets off the massage table and before you leave the massage room to allow time to redress. If you neglect this important procedure, then you may be liable if your client trips or falls in your massage room and incurs injuries because he or she was unable to see clearly.

As you leave the massage room, let the client know if he or she is to wait in the room for you to return or if he or she needs to exit the room to find you in another area.

After the Massage Session

This last section concerns the therapist's activities from the time he or she exits the massage room after the massage until the client leaves the premises. While your client is dressing, wash your hands and write any case notes. Make sure the lighting in the postmassage area is not too bright or too noisy because this type of environment is not relaxing. Provide a transitional space. Take a few deep breaths, and prepare to greet the client with a smile.

Have ready any parting information that you wish to give the client. Information sheets can be anything from tips on how to use ice, self-massage, relaxation techniques, and theories about muscle soreness and how to preserve and prolong the effects of the massage (Box 29-2). Without the educational element of massage therapy, the massage session may be no more than an expensive aspirin or bandage. Avoid just putting out fires; show clients how to prevent them. Clients really appreciate this added service of information on items such as how to alter sleeping positions to reduce muscle strain or how to sit in a chair comfortably. Be familiar with your scope of practice to make sure client education is legal for a massage therapist in your state.

If the therapist removes jewelry or wristwatches for the client, part of the therapist's responsibility is to make sure the client leaves with these items. The therapist may simply indicate where the items have been placed before leaving the room for the client to dress. In the case of a client who is physically unable to put the jewelry back on himself or herself, the therapist should offer assistance.

Clients may be disoriented after a massage and may accidentally forget some of their belongings. If you do discover personal articles in a room after a massage, then you should place them inside an envelope and seal it. Write the date, the item, and the owner of the item. If you do not know who owns the item, then call the clients who were there that day and ask them if they left anything in your studio. Letting them tell you what they are missing and give you a complete description before returning the item is generally best.

Some clients report becoming *sore* after a massage because it may produce a mild inflammatory response that is usually resolved within 48 hours. Some reasons for this reaction are the amount of pressure used during the massage, the length of time spent massaging an area, the health of the client's tissues, lack of client hydration, client inactivity, exposure to environmental toxins, and lack of postmassage care. If you worked an area deeply or for an extended period, or if you suspect a client may be sore, then recommend that the client drink lots of fresh water (at least 0.5 oz of water per 1 lb of body weight) and ice the area for 20 minutes.

How often a client schedules a massage can be influenced by the therapist but, once again, is determined by the client. Massage rarely can resolve everything that has been bothering the client for years in one session. Typically, clients schedule (1) once a week, (2) once a month, (3) only when they are in a crisis, such as a headache or stiff shoulder. A client who is in the crisis management category may become a regular client if he or she begins to experience that massage is keeping crises from occurring. If a client asks you to decide when you think he or she should come back, politely tell him or her that only when everything you have shown him or her (e.g., stretching, self-massage, cold and hot packs) fails to work. This approach builds trust and confidence between the client and therapist by empowering the client.

Collect fees if you have not already done so, and ask the client if he or she would like to reschedule. Offer the client another glass of water before he or she departs. After the client has gone, ready your room for your next client, take a few deep breaths, and stretch out your muscles.

Some clients may want to stay and talk after the massage. If the conversation is related to the massage and the client's health and progress, then the therapist should make some time to address the client's concerns. If, on the other hand, the conversation is just a friendly chat, then the therapist may have other priorities. The massage therapist may often need to tend to telephone messages, wash linens, ready the massage room for the next client, or break for lunch. Usually, simply walking the client to the door, perhaps even stepping outside with him or her, saying thank you and good-bye, and walking back in the office is enough. You may have to say something such as, "I really enjoy talking with you, but I have a few things to take care of." Setting a boundary is necessary to take care of yourself and to serve the other clients you have scheduled for the rest of the day.

FINISHING TOUCHES, REGULAR MAINTENANCE, AND REMODELING: HOW TO STAY IN BUSINESS

Now that your business is started and you have learned some ways to nurture and promote it, you need to know the long-term strategies for *staying* in business. The economics of private practice move in a spiral, not linear, pattern. This section explores ideas for diversifying your income, adding insurance billing and reimbursement to your practice, and monitoring the pulse of your business through basic accounting and financial reports. This section also discusses taxes and tax deductions, hiring employees and independent contractors, handling insufficient funds checks, preventing professional burnout, and investing in your future.

BOX 29-2

Ten Daily Steps for Preserving and Prolonging the Effects of Your Massage

- Drink at least 0.5 oz of fresh water per 1 lb of body weight.
- Maintain a neutral sleeping posture by using pillows to bolster the extremities to keep the spine straight.
- Stretch.
- Apply ice packs on painful areas (20 minutes).
- Be aware of your posture during the day.
- Decrease the intake of caffeine and sugar as much as possible (these neurostimulants can increase pain perception and dehydrate the body).
- Breathe slowly, extending the exhale.
- Develop a positive attitude.
- Simplify and prioritize, and take stress breaks.
- Love yourself.

Diversifying Your Income

The business world is a jungle, and the law of the jungle is survival of the fittest. One way for massage therapists to survive in the ever-changing business environment is by diversifying their income. Diversification helps minimize the effects of fluctuation in the market (the consumer market or the stock market); diversification helps reduce financial stress while you are building a clientele. The idea of diversity follows the same idea as in financial investments: Do not put all your eggs in one basket. Finding 10 places to scrape up $1000 each year is easier than finding one place that provides $10,000. Diversify your income by using different strategies for producing revenue. Here are a few ideas to protect you from extinction.

Retail sales can bring in extra money. Clients may choose to buy individual containers of massage cream; massage tools; relaxation music; aromatherapy oils, candles, or bath salts; and eye, neck, and back pillows. If you are going to sell retail goods, then make sure that you have the proper license requirements. You must also collect and pay sales tax regularly. The following should be considered when engaging in retail sales:

- Make sure that the items are affordable. Many clients will buy a $5 item, but only a few will buy a $100 item.
- Have a significant markup. Common markups are between 50% and 100% above the wholesale price.
- The items should be related to massage or relaxation. Do not sell candy and cigarettes.
- Do not tie up your money in a large inventory.
- Sell what you use yourself or what you would recommend.

Assess this last option carefully because conflicts of interest may arise and may be considered unethical in some situations. See Chapter 2 for a complete discussion.

Expand your services by offering clients a variety of treatment options. Some therapists offer whirlpool baths, steam rooms, saunas, salt scrubs, facials, and other services. Make sure that the services offered do not detract from the atmosphere of the massage environment. The sound of hair dryers and the smell of nail polish and acetone are usually not conducive to relaxation.

Specialized training is a good way to attract new business and expand your client base. Most states and the NCBTMB require massage therapists to earn continuing education units (CEUs) each year. Taking additional training for developing a new area of expertise may be worthwhile. Learn an approach or technique that is unique to your community—something that will fill a gap in the existing market. For example, if you practice relaxation massage, then you might want to attend a workshop in hydrotherapy, get some experience in the field, and develop a day spa facility.

Work in more than one location. This factor is especially true if you are self-employed. Locate part-time work a couple of afternoons a week for a chiropractor. Offer chair massage at the local health food store, a busy office building, or anywhere else with high traffic. Practice foot reflexology treatments at shoeshine booths, and split the proceeds with the owner. Take a new technique you learned and teach an introductory version at the local massage school. Offer a low-cost class in massage or relaxation techniques at your local college or university or community center for people who want to learn massage.

Insurance Billing and Reimbursement

Insurance billing is another aspect of expanding your practice and increasing your income. As clients learn that insurance coverage is available for massage services, therapists will be contacted regarding insurance billing and reimbursements. Massage has been proven effective in treating musculoskeletal and myofascial pain, and physicians are referring patients to massage therapists. Physical therapists are hiring massage therapists to work in their offices. When the time-consuming work of massage is handled by massage therapists, the physical therapist becomes free to perform the more technically demanding tasks of evaluations, assigning exercise protocols, and so on. Chiropractors also are taking advantage of the success of massage therapy by employing therapists within their practices and billing insurance for massage services.

Many rewards and frustrations exist related to insurance reimbursement. The therapist must be willing and able to prepare and submit all required documents related to client care and wait for reimbursement, which may take months or even years, at which time the therapist's bill may be reduced or even denied.

> *"If I had really wanted to do all this damned*
> *secretarial work, I'd have gone to secretarial school."*
> S. Devillier

Health maintenance organizations (HMOs) and preferred-provider organizations (PPOs) will cover services provided only by therapists who are on their approved list. At this time (2007), Medicare and Medicaid do not cover massage in most states. Most major medical policies issued by insurance companies do not include massage therapy. The types of cases most likely to cover the cost of massage therapy are personal injury (PI) cases, automobile medical insurance and automobile liability, and workers' compensation.

When accepting a client who has these special needs, additional signed documents are needed—not only a completed client intake form but a medical release form (see Chapter 8) as well. These forms allow the therapist to communicate legally with the client's health care providers, as well as agents of the insurance company, about the client's injuries. Also obtain the physician's prescription.

When submitting a claim, include a receipt for services. This receipt should include the client's name, date of services, fees for services, payments and adjustments, previous and current balance due, Current Procedural Terminology (CPT) codes, the therapist's contact information and provider number (if applicable), the therapist's tax identification number, and the client's next appointment. Avoid using a social security number as a tax identification number because of identification theft issues.

Accurate documentation is essential when expecting reimbursement from an insurance company. Progress notes of each session document the course and progress of treatments and are required because they establish the validity of massage and help determine whether to approve current and future treatments because insurance companies pay only for services that are deemed medically necessary.

HCFA 1500 Form

The Health Care Financing Administration created the *HCFA 1500 form* as a method of standardizing claims, eliminating the confusion of different forms for different insurance companies. Medicare and Medicaid use the Centers for Medicare & Medicaid Services (CMS) form, which is identical to the HCFA 1500 form and therefore interchangeable. Both forms are designed to be read by an optical character-recognition program to assist in the processing of insurance claims.

When filing a claim, insurance companies require a diagnosis code, or *ICD-9* code, identifying the attending physician's diagnosis. The United States Health Services and Health Care Financing Administration publish these codes. ICD-9 is an acronym for *Internal Classification of Disease,* ninth edition. Only a physician can provide a medical diagnosis and its corresponding ICD-9 code.

Also required is a procedural code, or *CPT code*, identifying services provided to the client. The American Medical Association developed the CPT code and publishes it annually. These codes establish a common language for everyone involved with the client's care. CPT codes list allowable fees associated with each service. These codes are arranged according to their specialty; massage is classified as physical medicine. These codes change. Stay informed of changes by referring to the most current CPT code manual or by consulting the attending physician's office or the insurance agent. A few current codes are:

97010—Hot and Cold Packs
97124—Soft Tissue
97140—Myofascial Release
97139—Therapeutic Procedure

Once the claim is submitted, the insurance company has 30 days to respond to the request. If 6 weeks have lapsed and the insurance company has not contacted you, then you should contact the insurance company. Document the inquiry by stating the time and date of the telephone call. Include the names of the person or persons to whom you spoke and what was said. If no reasonable action has been taken after the second inquiry, then contact the client's attorney (if one is available) or file a compliant with your state insurance commissioner. If the claim was denied, then contact the client and inform him or her of the insurance company's decision and that he or she is now responsible for the balance due. A signed agreement stating this before treatment begins is standard protocol.

Prioritizing Insurance Claims

The first rule of insurance filing is to *never compromise your cash flow*. In other words, do not take insurance cases over cash-paying clients. Insurance cases should be used to fill in dead time in your practice. Realize that insurance clients may be seen as often as three times a week; therefore one client will take up a lot of your time. The second rule is to *avoid cases that involve attorneys whenever possible*. These claims are the most risky insurance claims regarding payment. By the very nature of litigation, it slows down the payment process. Occasionally, a case is lost; therefore, in such an instance, you may not be paid. When an attorney is not involved, the therapist can often bill the insurance company weekly or monthly for long treatment periods. With an attorney involved, you may not get payment until the case is settled, which can sometimes take years. If an attorney is involved, then request that the attorney or the client pay your bill (or at least 50% of it) during treatment to increase your cash flow or, in the event that your client's attorney loses the case, to protect yourself from a significant loss. If the attorney is unwilling to negotiate, then you do have the right to refuse to accept the case. Paperwork for insurance claims is time consuming and runs up costs because it takes away from time with your regular clientele. You can also hire a medical billing company to take care of treatment authorization and filing for you.

Accounting

Accounting can be defined as the art of interpreting, measuring, and describing economic activity. Whether you are preparing a household budget, balancing a checkbook, preparing an income tax return, or running your massage practice or a major corporation, you are working with accounting concepts (Box 29-3). Accounting has often been called the *language of business*. Begin by opening up a business checking account. Use this account when depositing all money earned as a result of your business and paying business expenses. If possible, use checks to pay for all business-related expenses because this method provides the best documentation of payment. If you are sharing expenses with another therapist, then avoid co-mingling funds to maintain your separate business entity.

Petty Cash

Establish a petty-cash account by writing yourself a check and cashing it. Keep this money in a separate envelope or small lock box. This fund is for small incidental business expenses you pay in cash. Do not put cash received from clients in this account. Write *petty cash* on any cash receipts and file them in the lock box. When the fund is running low, total the receipts and write another check to cash for the amount of the receipts. This exchange will replenish the fund to its original balance. Most businesses keep $100 to $200 in this fund. At any given time, you should be able to count the money and receipts and balance back to the originally established total.

BOX 29-3

Accounting Terminology

Accounting: process of interpreting, measuring, and describing economic activity.

Accounts payable: money you owe to suppliers.

Accounts receivable: money owed to you or your business.

Accrual-basis accounting: charging the income and expense to the period in which they were incurred or recognized.

Assets: things that offer value to the company. Current assets are cash on hand; fixed assets are hard goods such as machines, equipment, furniture, vehicles, property, and buildings that are owned by the company.

Balance sheet: summary of the company's *assets, liabilities,* and owner's *equity* at an exact point in time.

Cash-based accounting: record transactions, both monies collected and expenses, at the time they are received or paid.

Cash flow: amounts and sources of money coming into and going out of the company.

Credits: entries made on the *right side* of an account. Credits reduce assets and expense accounts and increase liability, capital, and income accounts.

Debits: entries made on the *left side* of an account. Debits increase assets and expense accounts and reduce liability, capital, and income accounts.

Depreciation: process of spreading out the deduction for the cost of an asset over time.

Equity: difference between total assets and liabilities; also called *net worth.*

Gross income: money earned or accumulated before taxes.

Inventory: unsold retail items on hand.

Liabilities: what the business owes, both current and long-term liabilities.

Net income: money left after taxes.

Petty cash: cash used to pay for incidental expenses, usually set up and treated as a separate account.

Profit and loss statement: statement of income that outlines revenues and expenses over a fixed period, indicating whether your business made a *profit* or a *loss.*

Accountant Versus Accounting Software

Acquiring an accountant or a bookkeeper can help you with record keeping, financial statements, and preparation of tax forms. A good accountant can help you save money and evaluate tax consequences of tax deductions and major purchases. Software packages that help with all your accounting needs can be purchased for less than $200. If you have an accountant or plan to get one, then ask him or her which software program he or she recommends because you will be giving him or her copies of files on disks periodically throughout the year. Your records should outline some basic information such as *cash flow, inventory and purchases, payroll* (if applicable), *assets,* and some financial reports such as *cash flow statements, profit and loss statements,* and *balance sheets.*

Cash Flow

Record all monies received from clients and collected from other sources such as retail sales. Deposit this money in the proper account, and balance this account when your statement arrives. The two ways to track cash flow are the cash-based method and the accrual-based method. *Cash-based accounting* requires you to record the transaction, both monies collected and expenses, at the time they are received or paid. *Accrual-based accounting* involves charging the income and expense to the period in which they were incurred or recognized. For example, if you gave a massage last month and you will not be collecting payment until this month, record the transaction in last month's financial statement with an accounts receivable for the money due this month.

Inventory and Purchases

Document all your purchases of business supplies. If you are involved with the retail sales of massage products such as lubricants, music, or books and periodicals, then record when these items were purchased, how much you paid for them, and how much they sold. Your **inventory** is the unsold retail items you have on hand.

Payroll

If you have employees, then you need to keep track of their wages, federal income taxes, and social security taxes withheld, as well as any taxes and social security paid to local and state governments.

Assets

Keep a record of your fixed assets such as equipment, machines, furniture, computer and computer peripherals, vehicles, and other business-related property. The value of these items will be depreciated at tax time. **Depreciation** is the process of spreading out the deduction for the cost of an asset over time. Some fixed assets can be deducted in one fiscal year. Check with your accountant to see whether it is tax advantageous for you to take the deduction in one or multiple years.

Financial Reports

All of the financial information you gather (cash flow, inventory, purchases, payroll, and assets) is vital in preparing three key financial reports (cash flow statement, profit and loss statement, balance sheet). The accuracy of these financial reports reflects the accuracy of the financial information you collect and record throughout the year. These reports will help you track business and financial trends and spot potential problem areas that may need attention. If you are trying to get a business loan or have another financial need, then you will probably need to produce these reports.

Cash flow statements – Cash flow statements provide an overview of the amounts and sources of money coming into and going out of the company. Because cash flow is regarded as the *life-giving blood of a business,* keeping track of these amounts and having the opportunity to regulate these amounts may make the difference between whether your business thrives.

Profit and loss statements – Profit and loss (P & L) statements are essentially statements of income that outline revenues and expenses over a fixed period, indicating whether your business made a *profit* or sustained a *loss*. Most businesses prepare these statements monthly, quarterly, or annually.

Balance sheets – Balance sheets summarize all of the company's *assets* and *liabilities* and the owner's *equity* at an exact point in time, usually at the end of a quarter or a fiscal year. Here are some important terms and their definitions:

- **Assets.** Business assets are things that offer value to the company. Assets are divided into current and fixed assets. *Current assets* are cash on hand, including petty cash; money in checking and savings accounts; accounts receivable (money owed to you or your business); prepaid expenses such as deposits on rent, utilities, and insurance; and the value of your inventory. *Fixed assets* include machinery, equipment, and furniture such as a massage table, computer, telephone, answering machine, wet room spa, and steam cabinet. Vehicles, property, and buildings that are owned by the company are also considered fixed assets.
- **Liabilities.** Debts that the business owes are its liabilities, which can be classified as current and long-term liabilities. Examples of *current liabilities* are **accounts payable** (what you owe to suppliers); payments you owe on business loans within 1 year; accrued expenses such as salaries, wages, and commissions that you owe but have not yet paid; and taxes that you owe but have not paid. Examples of taxes are payroll, sales, income, property, and self-employment taxes. *Long-term liabilities* are mortgage payments for your business location and promissory notes taken out on the business's behalf for major purchases. Long-term liabilities are expenses that extend beyond one calendar year.
- **Equity.** Also called *net worth*, equity is the difference between your total assets and your liabilities.

Taxes

All businesses and individuals pay tax on their income. *Gross income* is the money a person or company earns or accumulates before taxes. The amount you have left or the money you pocket after taxes is your *net income.* Expenses and taxes, which are part of running and keeping a business, include sales tax, income tax, and self-employment tax. Not all of these taxes will apply to your situation, but having some understanding of what each type of business tax entails is always a good idea. Tax laws change periodically; consult with your accountant about current tax information.

Sales Tax
If you sell any product to a client, then you may be required to collect sales tax. These collected taxes are paid to state and local governments on a regular basis, usually once a month. Some municipalities tax services, whereas others do not. You will also need a sales tax number. Contact your local department of revenue and taxation for more information.

Income Tax
Federal and state taxes must be paid on profits gained by your business operations. These profits are derived from your revenues minus your expenses. The percentage paid to the federal government relates to the amount of your bottom line (how much you actually made). The amount paid to state and local governments varies from region to region. Contact your state and local department of revenue for more information. Track how much profit (or loss) you are generating throughout the year. If you notice a large profit during the year, then begin preparing for a sizable income tax payment by saving money or by making quarterly estimated tax payments.

Self-Employment Tax
Most self-employed people pay a quarterly self-employment tax of 15.3% (both the employer's and the employee's portion of Social Security and Medicare taxes), in addition to income tax, to the federal government on their business net income. You may also be required to pay an amount to your state and local governments on a quarterly basis. Ask your accountant or contact the your state's department of revenue and taxation for more information. Some localities also tax equipment used in business. Your local city hall is a good place to check for information as this percentage changes.

Tax Deductions
Anyone who is regarded as self-employed (files a Schedule C on Form 1040) or operates as a corporate business can deduct business-related expenses. The IRS says that you may deduct any ordinary and necessary items from your business; therefore you may deduct needed items that may not be common in other businesses but that make your business function efficiently. For tax purposes, keep all your business receipts, past income tax returns, and documents related to your tax returns for 7 years. Be sure to consult with your accountant to help you make timely decisions when purchasing assets (from a tax liability perspective). Examples of tax deductions are as follows:
- Accounting and bookkeeping fees
- Accounting or computer courses (may be deductible as continuing education)
- Advertising and promotion
- Bank service charges and card merchant fees
- Books and periodicals
- Business-related insurance
- Continuing education and professional development
- Conventions and conferences of business and trade organizations
- Depreciation on major purchases
- Gifts to and entertaining current or prospective clients (IRS limits apply)
- Health insurance

- Interest on business and investment loans; business bank card interest and annual fees incurred
- Laundry and cleaning services
- Legal, consulting, and professional services
- License fees
- Mileage (IRS mileage cost per mile or deduct actual cost), excluding travel to and from work; keep a mileage log
- Office supplies (including lubricants)
- Postage and shipping charges and supplies
- Printing and duplication
- Rent (home office; use a ratio of office space to total square footage)
- Repairs to office or equipment
- Uniforms and protective clothing
- Utilities and telephone service (home office; unless you have a business-dedicated meter, use a percentage of utilities; should be the same percentage used to determine rent amount; cannot deduct personal telephone line but can deduct business-related long distance calls or get a separate business line)

Employees and Independent Contractors

When your business has grown to the point at which you are turning down clients because of heavy workload, you may have to recruit another therapist. Massage therapists often associate with one another and other businesses as common law employees or independent contractors. These classifications have extensive legal and tax consequences.

An employer usually sets the hours and place for employee massage services. Employers generally provide employees with the tools and materials required to perform the work and exercise at least a measure of control and supervision over how the employees go about their tasks. The employment relationship typically involves a single employer and continues for an indefinite period (i.e., term of employment).

Independent contractors, in most cases, receive a fee based on completion of the task. They usually have special skills, training, or licensure that allows operation without detailed supervision by others. Independent contractors often provide their own tools and equipment. They generally determine the precise time for performing services and work for more than one party.

Contracting parties occasionally attempt to characterize employees as independent contractors. This temptation may arise from an employer's responsibility to withhold income taxes on wages, contribute to social security, pay unemployment compensation insurance, and obtain workers' compensation coverage. These costs are significant compliance and financial burdens, particularly when the employer lacks bookkeepers and other associates who are adept at handling the necessary paperwork.

However, a mischaracterization can expose an employer to interest and penalties for missing tax payments. A common law employee treated as an independent contractor may take legal action for gaps in social security and unemployment compensation coverage. Even worse, if the employee has failed to pay income taxes due, the employer may have to pay the employee's taxes to the extent of the tax-withholding shortfall. A massage therapist who is considering an independent contractor relationship should obtain tax advice from a lawyer or accountant to confirm that a proper characterization of the relationship exists.

MINI-LAB

In your own words, define *success* and *security*.

Insufficient Funds Checks

When you receive an insufficient funds check, call the client and politely explain the situation. Tell the client that you are mailing him or her a letter to serve as official notification, and ask him or her for a specific time and date when he or she can deliver or mail payment. Write this information down. Send two copies of the letter—one by certified mail with return receipt requested and one by regular mail. Receiving payment in a certified check, cash, or money order is best. Be sure to collect any insufficient funds check fees.

If you have not received payment within 10 days after receiving verification that the certified letter was claimed, or if your certified letter was unclaimed or refused, then contact your local district attorney's office. Do not open the certified letter if it is returned to you. The district attorney's office may require a copy of the certified letter, your returned receipt card, or the unopened returned certified letter before collection can be pursued.

If you accepted a postdated check and it was returned, then you have accepted a check knowing the person did not have money in his or her bank account. In this case, the district attorney's office may not be able to help you.

In any case, be pleasant, patient, understanding, and persistent. See Box 29-4 for a sample letter to be used in these circumstances.

How to Prevent Burnout

Burnout is the condition of being tired of or unhappy with one's work. It does not discriminate against any race, gender, religion, or age and is not specific to one type of profession. Burnout affects everyone from teachers to neurosurgeons. Symptoms of burnout can include simple disinterest in the job, dreading your next client, boredom, restlessness, inability to remain focused, fatigue, and outright hatred of a job or associates. Burnout can include depression, lack of productivity, increased tardiness, increased absenteeism, decline of social skills, workaholism, and a decline in professional boundaries. The added stress can also affect your health.

Burnout affects people for different reasons. Many massage therapists are entrepreneurs and are highly motivated, hardworking people. Many self-employed people have difficulty

---

BOX 29-4

Sample Letter to Client Regarding Insufficient Funds

NOTE: Personalize the terms in bold type to fit your specific situation.

Your letterhead with name, logo, address, and telephone and facsimile numbers here.
Name
Address
City, State, Zip
Date
Dear **Name,**

The check we received from you in the amount of **fifty dollars ($50.00)** dated **August 15, 2006,** was returned.

We understand that occasionally these mishaps occur as a result of mathematical errors, mistakes on the bank's behalf, or a deposit not being credited to your account. These situations are often embarrassing, but please be assured that we are willing to work with you.

Please bring the above-mentioned amount plus a **twenty-dollar ($20.00)** insufficient funds check charge for a total amount of **seventy dollars ($70.00)** to our offices as soon as possible. This payment must be made in cash, money order, or certified check. If you cannot come by our office, you have 10 days from receipt of this letter to mail your payment to us at the above address. Please do not send cash through the mail.

We are happy to provide you with massage therapy services and try to keep all collection attempts inside our office.

Please note the following office policies:

1. Payment is due at the time of service.
2. Should a check or credit card fail to clear, a notice (this letter) is sent to the client.
3. Failure to comply with making payment of the original amount plus insufficient funds fees within the designated time frame will result in filing collections with the district attorney's office.
4. We reserve the right to place any client whose check or credit card has failed to clear on a cash-only basis.

Please contact us so that we can take care of this matter.

Sincerely,
Terry White, L.M.T.

cc: certified mail, regular mail, file

---

setting limits on their professional time. Because delineating a 40-hour week can be difficult, self-employed people may overwork.

Not setting and maintaining limits for yourself or your time is maintaining poor boundaries and overscheduling, which may lead to early burnout. We can prevent *professional burnout* by taking steps to ensure our own wellness. Achieve harmony in our own lives first, and then assist others who are struggling to do the same.

If burnout is the result of overwork, then the therapist may be mad at himself or herself for not maintaining good boundaries. The inherent danger with this type of burnout is that this anger can, at times, be directed toward the client. The strategies for dealing with burnout are varied and depend on the type of problem. A few suggestions for managing burnout follow.

Nurture Yourself

Eat right, get enough rest, and exercise. Spend time with people you enjoy, read a book, or take a photography class. Rediscover things you like to do, or try new things that you might enjoy. Write down 10 things you currently like to do and how long it has been since you have done them. This activity may be quite revealing. List each activity on a separate strip of paper and place the strips in a jar. When you feel excessively stressed or on the verge of burnout, pick one of the activities from the jar and do it. This exercise is also a great stress-reduction activity for your clients.

Sojourn

Scheduling a certain amount of time off is extremely important for massage professionals. Schedule some time away from work on a *daily* and *weekly* basis. Be flexible; if your massage days are Monday through Friday, then take off Saturday and Sunday; or if everyone wants Saturday massages, then take off Sunday and Monday. Remember that you cannot give away what you do not have and that recharging your own batteries is necessary. Do not forget to vacation at least once a year. Get away from the office, especially if you work out of your home. Better yet, get out of town. If you feel the need, then take a break from massage altogether. Shift gears and take a sabbatical. Use this time not only to recharge your batteries but also to reevaluate important decisions or situations.

Stimulate Yourself

Some therapists burn out from the boredom of repetitious routines and lack of challenge. Use CEUs for this purpose. Take a class in something interesting and outrageous, not just massage technique and anatomy. Workshops also bring you together with your colleagues.

Relax

Get massages yourself! Regular massages are a necessity because of the tremendous physical requirements of this job. The recommended minimum is one massage per month. No maximum number of massages you can receive exists.

"I am indeed rich, since my income is superior to my expense, and my expense is equal to my wishes."
Edward Gibson

Building a Cash Reserve and Investing in Your Future

A business plan will help you chart your business course (Box 29-5). Also important is putting away money for a rainy day because of the influx of clients; thus cash flow fluctuates from day to day. You need to build a cash reserve to get you through tough times when more money is going out than coming in, when you are unemployed, or when any other financial disaster occurs. Because you

---

BOX 29-5

Business Plan

Introduction
1. Cover letter
2. Table of contents

Personal Information
1. What is my experience in this business, if any?
2. What do I love about my work?
3. What are my weaknesses and shortcomings?
4. What are my strengths and talents?
5. What is special and distinct about me as a massage therapist? Why will these attributes appeal to clients?
6. What are my values?
7. What have I learned about this business from fellow therapists, teachers, trade journals, and trade suppliers?

General Description of Business
1. What is my vision statement?
2. What is my mission statement?
3. What services do I or will I offer? (Describe these services and the benefits of these services.)
4. For what purpose will people buy my services?
5. Am I willing to change what I offer, to some extent, to meet my clients' changing needs?

Operating Procedures
1. What types of licenses are required for me to operate my business?
2. What will be the opening date of my business? What hours of the day and days of the week will I be in operation?
3. What will my office policies be for late clients, cancellations, out-of-date gift certificate redemption, insufficient funds checks, and credit card sales?

Management and Personnel
1. What is my management experience?
2. What do I predict my legal structure will be?
3. Who will be the other key figures in my business? (Include an organizational chart, list of duties and backgrounds of key individuals, outside consultants or advisers, and board of directors.)
4. How will services be provided? Will I do all the work, or will I use employees or contract labor?

5. What are the types of support that my business may require? (Include childcare, janitorial service, lawn and garden care, and bookkeeping and accounting.)
6. What are the wages and benefits I can offer each type of employee and support person?

Insurance Needs
1. What are my insurance needs? (These may include professional and general liability, business personal property, automotive, life and health insurance, and disability insurance.)
2. Have I contacted an agent to discuss what types of policies they offer and the cost and benefit of each?

Marketing and Competition
1. What do I want my business identity to be? (Describe the image you want to project. *You never get a second chance to make a first impression.*)
2. What do I want people to say to others about my services?
3. Who is my target market? Who will want to buy my services? (Identify important characteristics such as age, gender, occupation, income, and so on.)
4. Who else provides a similar service? (In order of their strength in the market, list your five closest competitors by name and address. Next, describe each competitor's strengths and weaknesses.) What have I learned from my competitors, operations and from their advertising?
5. What will my fee schedule look like? How have I determined these fees? Will this price cover my material costs, labor costs, and overhead?
6. What are my competitors charging?
7. How am I different from my competitors in ways that matter to potential clients? (Refer to the previous business plan section on personal information.)

Advertising, Promotion, and Location
1. How can I get the attention of the people I want to reach? Which advertising media are appropriate for my business and targeted clients?
2. What other channels such as networking, referrals, and publicity will I use to reach clients?
3. How can I discover whether a promotion is working?

(continued)

BOX 29-5, cont'd

Business Plan, cont'd

Advertising, Promotion, and Location, cont'd

4. What is my advertising budget for 6 months? (Include specific media you will use and the cost of each.)
5. What type of location does my business require? (Describe the type of building your business needs, including office and studio space, parking, exterior lighting, security needs, and proximity to other businesses for added exposure.)
6. Where do I plan to locate my business? Is this location right for my business and me?
7. In what geographic area will my business serve? Are sufficient numbers of potential clients located there?
8. What type of physical layout is needed for my business? (Include layout for reception area, restroom, hydrotherapy and spa room [if applicable], retail and inventory areas, and gift certificate sales.)

Financial Projections

1. How much money do I have to begin this business?
2. What is the cost of my capital equipment, supply list, and other startup items?
3. If money is to be borrowed, do I have a bank and loan officer in mind?
4. How will my business be profitable? (Produce an income projection [profit and loss statements], balance sheet, cash flow statement, and break-even analysis. The projection should cover 3 years—that is, the first year projects monthly and the next 2 years project quarterly.)
5. Based on these documents, how much money will I need to make to stay in business?
6. What are the growth opportunities?

Supporting Documents

1. Tax returns for the last 3 years
2. Personal financial statements
3. Copy of proposed lease for building space
4. Copy of licenses and other legal documents
5. Copy of your curriculum vitae

---

will always have bills to pay, do not wait until you have extra money to begin saving. Instead, consider yourself a creditor. Once a month, pay yourself 10% of what you gross. Put this money in a liquid account (e.g., savings account, interest-bearing checking account) so you can access it quickly and easily. When you have enough money saved to pay for 1 to 6 months of living expenses, you have reached your goal of an adequate cash reserve to be used in emergencies and when you are ready to begin your next financial goal, investing.

Do not wait until you have a goal (college for children, retirement) to start investing in your future. Continue with the 10% rule (pay yourself 10% of your gross income). This money will be invested so it can grow over time. If you work for a company that makes regular contributions to a retirement account or offers incentive for you to put money in a retirement account, then you are among the few. Most therapists are self-employed or work for small companies that do not participate in employee retirement plans. Therefore massage therapists must become motivated and disciplined enough to invest for themselves to meet future financial goals. The following investment guidelines can help you with market investing.

Invest for the Long Term

The market does not move in one direction all year, but historically the stock market moves up over time, even with relatively sharp downturns. Investing for the long term allows you to weather the inevitable storms. This strategy is not unlike a marriage commitment. However, if you cannot sleep at night worrying about your investments, then you probably should not be investing in the market or you are in the wrong area of the market.

Invest Systematically

Buying stocks when they are at their lowest price is almost impossible (unless you have a crystal ball). If you invest the same dollar amount and buy the same stock or fund regularly and systematically, then you will naturally buy it at different prices. Over time, your average cost will be lower than the average price of the stock or fund. This strategy is called *dollar-cost averaging*.

Diversify

Do not put all your eggs in one basket. If you allocate your money among several different sectors of the market (energy, consumer goods, pharmaceuticals), or different types of securities (stocks, bonds, mutual funds), your portfolio performs better. A **financial portfolio** is all of the various investments held by an individual investor. What you choose to buy will depend on your need for income, your personality (whether you can handle it when the stock, bond, or fund price fluctuates), and your risk tolerance. Many investors use the *diversity by five* strategy, which means carefully selecting five quality stocks (names you know such as Coca Cola, Wal-Mart, or Exxon Mobil). Odds are that three of these will perform well, one will offer a stellar performance, and one will be disappointing.

Use Professional Advice

Finding a good financial advisor is tricky. Brokers make their living whether you make money or not; they get a commission if you buy or sell. Many horror stories have been told about unscrupulous financial advisors who recommend purchasing something for an exorbitant fee that only later you discover never performed even though you were charged. Ask around for someone who gives you the pros and cons of an investment and lets you make the decision. It is important that you like and trust him or her. Ask him or her for references, too.

Securities

Securities are the vehicles in which you put your money to optimize your return. Types of securities are stocks and bonds. A mutual fund contains many types of securities. The securities listed in the following sections will help you decide where to invest. Unless your money is invested in a retirement account or other tax shelter, you will owe tax on your investment income.

Stocks

Buying stock establishes your proportionate ownership in that company represented by shares. As a stockholder, you reap rewards of the company's profits but also suffer the company's losses. Most stocks pay their stockholders dividends. A **dividend** is part of a company's earnings that is distributed at regular intervals to its shareholders; dividends can be reinvested to buy more shares or can be paid to you in cash.

Bonds

A bond is basically a loan. Examples of bonds are corporate bonds (loan to a corporation), municipal bonds (loan to a municipality or revenue district), and government bonds and types of government bonds called *treasury bills* (loan to Uncle Sam). When you purchase a bond, most agencies pay you interest on a biannual basis. Interest on municipal and government bonds is usually tax free. When the bond matures (ranging from 1 to 40 years), the agency returns your initial investment. Most people who buy bonds need to receive a regular income from their investments, such as individuals who are already retired.

Funds

A *mutual fund* is established by an investment company that pools money from its shareholders and invests it in a variety of securities. Each individual mutual fund has varying degrees of investment objectives and accompanying risks. Some mutual funds charge a fee to join and to withdraw; other funds are no-load funds, which means no fee is charged when shares are bought or sold. *Index funds* are unmanaged mutual funds that seek to replicate the performance of established market indices. Some well-known indexes include the Dow Jones Industrial Average, Standard & Poor's 500 Index, the NASDAQ Composite Index, Russell 2000, and the Consumer Price Index.

Retirement Accounts

The federal government wants you to save for your own retirement, too. In fact, they help you by allowing you to treat contributions to your retirement account as a tax deduction. Some restrictions include how much you can claim as a deduction.

If you withdraw funds from a retirement account before you qualify, then you have 90 days to replace it or you may pay income tax on the amount withdrawn plus a penalty. The income you earn from your investment is tax-deferred income; therefore taxes are not due until you begin withdrawing the money at retirement. At this future time, you will probably be in a lower tax bracket (the exception is the Roth IRA). You can sometimes borrow against retirement accounts; thus it can be regarded as an asset and therefore loan collateral. The most common retirement accounts are an individual retirement account (IRA), simplified employee pension (SEPP), savings incentive match plan for employees (SIMPLE), and annuities. You have until April 15 to make contributions for the previous year, and rules and restrictions change annually. Please consult your accountant or your financial advisor for current information.

Individual Retirement Account

Money in an individual retirement account (IRA) can be invested in a wide variety of ways (certificates of deposit, stocks, bonds, or mutual funds). Traditional IRAs are tax-deferred retirement accounts in which some or all contributions may be deductible from current taxes, depending on the individual's adjusted gross income and coverage by an employer-sponsored retirement plan. Through 2007, the maximum deductible contribution is $4000. This amount will increase to $5000 in 2008 and be subject to annual adjustments thereafter. The federal government does allow you to withdraw the money under certain hardships (college education and down payment on a house, among other reasons). Under these conditions, you are taxed on the distribution but not penalized. For individuals over 50 years of age, an additional $1000 can be contributed; this is known as a *catch-up* contribution. A Roth IRA, which was created through the Taxpayer Relief Act of 1997, does not allow you to write off contributions, but income derived as a result of distributions during retirement is tax free.

Simplified Employee Pension Plan

In many ways, a SEPP plan is similar to an IRA, except that the SEPP plan allows an employer to make tax-deductible contributions to the employees retirement account while they are also contributing.

Savings Incentive Match Plan for Employees

A SIMPLE IRA is a company-sponsored retirement plan that allows employees to contribute through deductions from their paycheck. The company must match the employee contribution or contribute 2% of the employee's annual gross income to any employee who earns $5000 or more during the year.

Annuities

Often used as a retirement account, an annuity is a type of investment in which the policyholder makes a lump sum or installment payments to an insurance company. The income is tax deferred, and distributions are made at retirement. This type of account is expensive to open and maintain because of many hidden costs.

SUMMARY

Basic business consists of three phases: preparatory work, actual business operation, and long-term strategies for the future operation of your business. The preparatory work includes the development of a business plan, which should be built around your personal values, goals, visions, and professional mission. Your business plan will include details of all phases of your future business, such as services offered, hours, fees, marketing, insurance needs, startup costs, and necessary licenses and permits. Once this task is accomplished, you can open your doors.

People say that anyone can open a business, but keeping it open is the hard part. Business growth depends on how we relate to the public, both individually as clients and collectively as a target market for our advertising and promotional strategies. This aspect applies to the use of media and networking with other professionals.

Finally, proof of true business success is defined in terms of longevity. You can go the distance by diversifying your income, managing your finances with basic accounting and financial reports, planning tax strategies, avoiding professional burnout, and investing wisely for retirement.

If you find all this business thinking helpful, then you should realize that this information is just the tip of the iceberg. You can learn more about business in many ways. Your public library contains a wealth of books about promotion, publicity, advertising, marketing, and selling. Your local massage schools, universities, and many professional organizations also offer continuing education courses in business.

evolve

Go to *Chapter Extras* on Evolve for additional illustrations and resources for this chapter. *Extras* for this chapter include:

1. Crossword puzzle (downloadable form)

MATCHING I

Place the letter of the answer next to the term or phrase that best describes it.

A. Advertising
B. Contract
C. Curriculum vitae
D. Marketing
E. Media
F. Mission statement
G. Preceptor
H. Professional liability
I. Publicity
J. Sole proprietorship

_____   1. Making your business noticeable to the public by purchasing print space or broadcast media time

_____   2. Systems of mass communication

_____   3. Promoting your business with image, purpose, and direction

_____   4. A written agreement between two or more parties that communicates expectations, duties, and responsibilities and is enforceable by law

_____   5. Business of a single owner

_____   6. Free media exposure

_____   7. Malpractice insurance

_____   8. Someone who guides you during your postgraduate clinical practice

_____   9. An autobiographical sketch that documents all your achievements: occupational, avocational, and academic

_____ 10. Statement of purpose

MATCHING II

Place the letter of the answer next to the term or phrase that best describes it. Some answers are used more than once.

A. Accounts receivable
B. Balance sheet
C. Cash-based accounting
D. Depreciation

E. Dividend
F. Equity or net worth
G. Gross income
H. Individual retirement account

I. Inventory
J. Financial portfolio
K. Profit and loss statement
L. Securities

_____   1. Unsold retail items you have on hand

_____   2. Money owed to you or your business

_____   3. All the various investments held by an individual investor

_____   4. The process of spreading the deduction for the cost of an asset over time

_____   5. Statement of income that outlines revenues and expenses over a fixed period, indicating whether your business earned a profit or a loss

_____   6. Tax-deferred retirement account in which some or all contributions may be deductible from current taxes, depending on the individual's adjusted gross income and coverage by an employer-sponsored retirement plan

_____   7. The difference between your total assets and your liabilities

_____   8. Part of a company's earnings distributed at regular intervals to its shareholders

_____   9. The money one earns or accumulates before deductions

_____   10. Vehicles in which you put your money to optimize your return

_____   11. A financial statement that summarizes all of the company's assets, liabilities, and owner's equity at an exact point in time, usually at the end of a quarter or a fiscal year

_____   12. Accounting method whereby you record the transaction, monies collected, and expenses at the time they are received or paid

INTERNET ACTIVITIES

Visit http://www.sba.gov and under Small Business Planner, choose Plan your Business. After reading al the material in this section, prepare your own business plan.

Visit http://www.score.org and choose How To. Locate Create Market Plan on the web page and read the information when it pops up. Write a short summary and present it to your instructor.

Visit http://www.sohnen-moe.com and click on Business Tips. List 10 suggestions from the section on marketing tips.

Bibliography

Ashley M: *Massage: a career at your fingertips,* ed 2, Mahopac Falls, NY, 2005, Enterprise.

Associated Bodywork and Massage Professionals: *Successful business handbook,* Evergreen, Colo, 2001, ABMP.

Barnhart T: *The five rituals of wealth: proven strategies for turning the little you have into more than enough,* New York, 1996, HarperCollins.

Beck MF: *Theory and practice of therapeutic massage,* ed 4, Clifton Park, NY, 2006, Thomson Delmar Learning.

Boldt LG: *Zen and the art of making a living: a practical guide to creative career design,* New York, 1999, Penguin Books USA.

Charles Schwab: Individual Retirement Accounts, 2006. Available at: *http://www.schwab.com/*

Denning E: Massage therapy medical codes for 2002, *Massage Bodywork: Nurture Body, Mind, Spirit,* Feb/Mar 2002, pp 144-145.

Downes J, Goodman JE: *Barron's dictionary of finance and investment terms,* ed 5, Hauppauge, NY, 1995, Barron's Educational Services.

Edward Jones: Retirement Planning, 2006. Available at: *http://www.edwardjones.com/*

Fritz S: *Fundamental of therapeutic massage,* ed 3, St Louis, 2003, Elsevier.

Gaedeke R, Tootelian D: *Small business management,* ed 3, Needham Heights, Mass, 1991, Simon and Schuster.

Grodzki L: *Building your ideal private practice: how to love what you do and be highly profitable too!* New York, 2000, WW Norton.

Harrison BJ: *Business practices: a guide to starting your massage therapy practice in New Mexico,* Albuquerque, NM, 1994.

Mainstreaming of alternative medicine, *Consumer Reports,* May 2000, pp 17-25.

Meigs WB, Roberts F: *Accounting: the basis for business decisions,* ed 13, New York, 2004, McGraw-Hill.

Money Magazine, Sept/Oct 1994, p 56.

Palmer DA: *The bodywork entrepreneur,* San Francisco, 1990, Thumb Press.

Sohnen-Moe C: *Business mastery: a guide for creating a fulfilling, thriving business and keeping it successful,* ed 3, Tucson, Ariz, 1997, Sohnen-Moe Associates.

The National Certification Board for Therapeutic Massage and Bodywork Code of Ethics

The Code of Ethics of the National Certification Board for Therapeutic Massage and Bodywork (NCBTMB) specifies professional standards that allow for the proper discharge of the massage therapist's and/or bodyworker's responsibilities to those served, that protect the integrity of the profession, and that safeguard the interest of individual clients.

Those practitioners nationally certified in therapeutic massage and bodywork in the exercise of professional accountability will conduct themselves as follows:

1. Have a sincere commitment to provide the highest quality of care to those who seek their professional services.
2. Represent their qualifications honestly, including education and professional affiliations, and provide only those services that they are qualified to perform.
3. Accurately inform clients, other health care practitioners, and the public of the scope and limitations of their discipline.
4. Acknowledge the limitations of and contraindications for massage therapy and bodywork, and refer clients to appropriate health professionals.
5. Provide treatment only when there is reasonable expectation that it will be advantageous to the client.
6. Consistently maintain and improve professional knowledge and competence, striving for professional excellence through regular assessment of personal and professional strengths and weaknesses and through continued educational training.
7. Conduct their business and professional activities with honesty and integrity, and respect the inherent worth of all people.
8. Refuse to unjustly discriminate against clients or other ethical health professionals.
9. Safeguard the confidentiality of all client information, unless disclosure is required by law, court order, or absolutely necessary for the protection of the public.
10. Respect the client's right to treatment with informed and voluntary consent. The NCTMB practitioner will obtain and record the informed consent of the client, or client's advocate, before providing treatment. This consent may be written or verbal.
11. Respect the client's right to refuse, modify, or terminate treatment regardless of prior consent given.
12. Provide draping and treatment in a way that ensures the safety, comfort, and privacy of the client.
13. Exercise the right to refuse to treat any person or part of the body for just and reasonable cause.
14. Refrain, under all circumstances, from initiating or engaging in any sexual conduct, sexual activities, or sexualizing behavior involving a client, even if the client attempts to sexualize the relationship.
15. Avoid any interest, activity, or influence that might be in conflict with the practitioner's obligation to act in the best interests of the client or the profession.
16. Respect the client's boundaries with regard to privacy, disclosure, exposure, emotional expression, beliefs, and the client's reasonable expectations of professional behavior. Practitioners will respect the client's autonomy.
17. Refuse any gifts or benefits that are intended to influence a referral, decision, or treatment and that are purely for personal gain and not for the good of the client.
18. Follow all policies, procedures, guidelines, regulations, codes, and requirements promulgated by the National Certification Board for Therapeutic Massage and Bodywork.

From National Certification Board for Therapeutic Massage and Bodywork: *Code of ethics (adopted 2/17/95),* McLean, Va, The Board.

The National Certification Board for Therapeutic Massage and Bodywork Standards of Practice

STANDARD I: PROFESSIONALISM

The certificant must provide optimal levels of professional massage and bodywork services and demonstrate excellence in practice by promoting healing and well-being through responsible, compassionate, and respectful touch. In his or her professional role the certificant shall commit to the following:

1. Adhere to the NCBTMB Code of Ethics, Standards of Practice, policies, and procedures.
2. Comply with the peer review process conducted by the NCBTMB Ethics and Standards Committee regarding any alleged violations against the NCBTMB Code of Ethics and Standards of Practice.
3. Conduct themselves in a manner in all settings meriting the respect of the public and other professionals.
4. Treat each client with respect, dignity, and worth.
5. Use professional verbal, nonverbal, and written communications.
6. Provide an environment that is safe and comfortable for the client and which, at a minimum, meets all legal requirements for health and safety.
7. Use standard precautions to ensure professional hygienic practices and maintain a level of personal hygiene appropriate for practitioners in the therapeutic setting.
8. Wear clothing that is clean, modest, and professional.
9. Obtain voluntary and informed consent from the client before initiating the session.
10. If applicable, conduct an accurate needs assessment, develop a plan of care with the client, and update the plan as needed.
11. Use appropriate draping to protect the client's physical and emotional privacy.
12. Be knowledgeable of their scope of practice and practice only within these limitations.
13. Refer to other professionals when in the best interest of the client and/or practitioner.
14. Seek other professional advice when needed.
15. Respect the traditions and practices of other professionals and foster collegial relationships.
16. Not falsely impugn the reputation of any colleague.
17. Use the initials NCTMB to designate his or her professional ability and competency to practice therapeutic massage and bodywork only.
18. Remain in good standing with and maintain NCBTMB certification.
19. Understand that the NCBTMB certificate may be displayed prominently in the certificant's principal place of practice.
20. When using the NCBTMB logo and certification number on business cards, brochures, advertisements, and stationery, do so only in a manner that is within established NCBTMB guidelines.
21. Not duplicate the NCBTMB certificate for purposes other than verification of the practitioner's credentials.
22. Immediately return the certificate to NCBTMB if it is revoked or suspended.

STANDARD II: LEGAL AND ETHICAL REQUIREMENTS

The certificant must comply with all the legal requirements in applicable jurisdictions regulating the profession of massage therapy and bodywork. In his or her professional role the certificant shall commit to the following:

1. Obey all applicable local, state, and federal laws.
2. Refrain from any behavior that results in illegal, discriminatory, or unethical actions.
3. Accept responsibility for his or her own actions.
4. Report to the proper authorities any alleged violations of the law by other certificants.
5. Maintain accurate and truthful records.
6. Report to the NCBTMB any criminal convictions regarding himself or herself and other certificants.
7. Report to NCBTMB any pending litigation and resulting resolution related to his or her professional practice and the professional practice of other certificants.
8. Respect existing publishing rights and copyright laws.

STANDARD III: CONFIDENTIALITY

The certificant shall respect the confidentiality of client information and safeguard all records. In his or her professional role the certificant shall commit to the following:

1. Protect the client's identity in social conversations, all advertisements, and any and all other manners unless requested by the client in writing, medically necessary, or required by law.
2. Protect the interests of clients who are minors or who are unable to give voluntary consent by securing permission from an appropriate third party or guardian.

3. Solicit only information that is relevant to the professional client/therapist relationship.
4. Share pertinent information about the client with third parties when required by law.
5. Maintain the client files for a minimum period of four years.
6. Store and dispose of client files in a secure manner.

STANDARD IV: BUSINESS PRACTICES

The certificant shall practice with honesty, integrity, and lawfulness in the business of massage and bodywork. In his or her professional role the certificant shall commit to the following:

1. Provide a physical setting that is safe and meets all applicable legal requirements for health and safety.
2. Maintain adequate and customary liability insurance.
3. Maintain adequate progress notes for each client session, if applicable.
4. Accurately and truthfully inform the public of services provided.
5. Honestly represent all professional qualifications and affiliations.
6. Promote his or her business with integrity and avoid potential and actual conflicts of interest.
7. Advertise in a manner that is honest, dignified, and representative of services that can be delivered and remains consistent with the NCBTMB Code of Ethics.
8. Advertise in a manner that is not misleading to the public by, among other things, the use of sensational, sexual, or provocative language and/or pictures to promote business.
9. Comply with all laws regarding sexual harassment.
10. Not exploit the trust and dependency of others, including clients and employees or co-workers.
11. Display or discuss schedule of fees in advance of the session that are clearly understood by the client or potential client.
12. Make financial arrangements in advance that are clearly understood by and safeguard the best interests of the client or consumer.
13. Follow acceptable accounting practices.
14. File all applicable municipal, state and federal taxes.
15. Maintain accurate financial records, contracts and legal obligations, appointment records, tax reports, and receipts for at least 4 years.

STANDARD V: ROLES AND BOUNDARIES

The certificant shall adhere to ethical boundaries and perform the professional roles designed to protect the client and practitioner and safeguard the therapeutic value of the relationship. In his or her professional role the certificant shall commit to the following:

1. Recognize his or her personal limitations and practice only within these limitations.

2. Recognize his or her influential position with the client and shall not exploit the relationship for personal or other gain.
3. Recognize and limit the impact of transference and countertransference between the client and the certificant.
4. Avoid dual or multidimensional relationships that could impair professional judgment or result in exploitation of the client or employees and/or co-workers.
5. Not engage in any sexual activity with a client.
6. Acknowledge and respect the client's freedom of choice in the therapeutic session.
7. Respect the client's right to refuse the therapeutic session.
8. Refrain from practicing under the influence of alcohol, drugs, or any illegal substances (with the exception of prescribed dosage of prescription medication, which does not significantly impair the certificant).
9. Have the right to refuse and/or terminate the service to a client who is abusive or under the influence of alcohol, drugs, or any illegal substance.

STANDARD VI: PREVENTION OF SEXUAL MISCONDUCT

The certificant shall refrain from any behavior that sexualizes, or appears to sexualize, the client/therapist relationship. The certificant recognizes that the intimacy of the therapeutic relationship may activate practitioner and/or client needs and/or desires that weaken objectivity and may lead to sexualizing the therapeutic relationship. In his or her professional role the certificant shall commit to the following:

1. Refrain from participating in a sexual relationship or sexual conduct with the client, whether consensual or otherwise, from the beginning of the client/therapist relationship and for a minimum of 6 months after the termination of the client/therapist relationship.
2. In the event that the client initiates sexual behavior, clarify the purpose of the therapeutic session, and if such conduct does not cease, terminate or refuse the session.
3. Recognize that sexual activity with clients, students, employees, supervisors, or trainees is prohibited even if consensual.
4. Not touch the genitalia.
5. Only perform therapeutic treatments beyond the normal narrowing of the ear canal and normal narrowing of the nasal passages as indicated in the plan of care and only after receiving informed voluntary written consent.
6. Only perform therapeutic treatments in the oropharynx as indicated in the plan of care and only after receiving informed voluntary consent.
7. Only perform therapeutic treatments into the anal canal as indicated in the plan of care and only after receiving informed voluntary written consent.
8. Only provide therapeutic breast massage as indicated in the plan of care and only after receiving informed voluntary consent from the client.

From National Certification Board for Therapeutic Massage and Bodywork: *Code of ethics (adopted 2/17/95) and standards of practice (adopted 2/9/00),* McLean, Va, The Board.

Common Abbreviations, Symbols, Prescriptive Directions, Medical Terminology, Pathologies, Modalities, and Findings

ABBREVIATION OR SYMBOL	MEANING	ABBREVIATION OR SYMBOL	MEANING
General			
Abd; ABD	abduction	stat	immediately
Add; ADD	adduction	↑	increase, above
p; post	after	INF	inferior
ANT	anterior	INT	internal
≈	approximately	int. rot.	internal rotation
ASAP	as soon as possible	inver	inversion
PRN	as needed	LAT	lateral, left anterior thigh
@	at	L	left
hs	at bedtime	<	less than, minus, negative, absent
a; pre	before	LTG	long-term goal
BIL	bilateral	LN	lymph node
CAUD	caudal	#	number
CEPH	cephalic	qwk	once a week
c/o	complains of	OTC	over-the-counter
CSTx	continue same treatment	pt	patient
CNT	could not test	+	positive, plus, present, and
CSR	craniosacral rhythm	Rx	prescription, drug, or medication
DOB	date of birth	Px	prognosis, physical examination
DOI	date of injury	PROX	proximal
↓	decrease, below	0—<	recumbent
Dx	diagnosis	ROS	review of symptoms/systems
DNK	did not keep	R	right
dist.	distal	2°	secondary, due to, as a result of
Eval	evaluate	STG	short-term goal
ever	eversion	SUP	superior, supination
qd	every day	per, /	through, by
qod	every other day	×	times, time
EXT	external, extension	Tx	treatment, therapy
ext. rot.	external rotation	b.i.d.	twice a day
FLEX	flexion	c; w/	with
>	greater than	WNL	within normal limits
Hx	history	s; w/o	without
Symptoms			
Abr	abrasion	INFLAM	inflammation
ASP	abnormal spine posture	max	maximum
AI	accidental injury	min	minimum
Adh	adhesion, fibrosis	MAEW	moves all extremities well
AOB	alcohol on breath	P & B	pain and burning
BA	backache	POM	pain on motion
CON	congested	SFLE	stress from life experience
crep	crepitus	SOB	shortness of breath
Flat	flatulence	SOBOE	shortness of breath on exercise

Continued

ABBREVIATION OR SYMBOL	MEANING	ABBREVIATION OR SYMBOL	MEANING	—cont'd

Symptoms—cont'd

FOOSH	fell on outstretched hand	SP	spasm
HA	headache	st	stiffness
HOH	hard of hearing	STI	soft-tissue injury
HT	hypertonus, tension, tight muscles	TP	trigger point

Pathological Conditions

CTS	carpal tunnel syndrome	lord	lordosis
CVA	cerebral vascular accident	LBP	low back pain
CFS	chronic fatigue syndrome	OA	osteoarthritis
CHF	congested heart failure	PTSD	posttraumatic stress disorder
DDD	degenerative disk disease	RA	rheumatoid arthritis
DJD	degenerative joint disease	RTC	rotator cuff
DEV	deviation	spr.	sprain
ed	edema	str.	strain
FT	fibrous tissue	TMJD	temporomandibular joint dysfunction
Fl up	flare up	TeP	tender point
FX	fracture	TOS	thoracic outlet syndrome
HBP	high blood pressure	TP	trigger point
HTR	hypertrophy	V V	varicose vein
kyph	kyphosis		

Massage Techniques and Modalities

AAS	active-assisted stretching	NMT	neuromuscular therapy
AROM	active range of motion	PB	paraffin bath
aroma	aromatherapy	PAROM	passive-assisted range of motion
CST	craniosacral therapy	Pas Ex	passive exercise
XFF	cross-fiber friction	PNF	proprioceptive neuromuscular facilitation
DP	direct pressure	PROM	passive range of motion
MLD	manual lymphatic drainage	PT	physical therapy
M	massage	ROM	range of motion
MET	muscle energy technique	SFT	soft-tissue mobilization
MFR	myofascial release	SCS	strain, counterstrain
MFW	myofascial web, continuous fascial planes	SwM	Swedish massage
		Ther-X	therapeutic exercise or procedure

Muscles and Landmarks

abs	abdominal	LEV	levator scapulae
AC	acromioclavicular	L1-L5	lumbar vertebrae, spine
ACL	anterior cruciate ligament	M	major
ASIS	anterior superior iliac spine	m	minor
bi	biceps	Ms	muscle, musculoskeletal
C1-C7	cervical vertebrae, spine	pecs	pectoralis
DH	dominant hand	QL	quadratus lumborum
ES	erector spinae group	S1-S5	sacral vertebrae, sacrum
gastroc	gastrocnemius	SI	sacroiliac
IF	iliofemoral	SCM	sternocleidomastoid
IP	iliopsoas	TMJ	temporal mandibular joint
ITB	iliotibial band	TFL	tensor fascia latae
IT	ischial tuberosity	T1-T12	thoracic vertebrae, spine
lats	latissimus dorsi	traps	trapezius

INTRODUCTION

We live in a society inundated with misconceptions about health, and no area has more misconceptions than nutrition. Although the term is familiar, the concept is often unclear; nutrition is often used in place of the word *diet*. More accurately, **nutrition** is the sum of the processes involved in the taking in of nutrients and using them for proper function, growth, and health. **Diet** is the food consumed to supply the process of nutrition. Diet directly affects a body's nutrition, which has an impact on one's general health.

Individual nutritional needs vary. Factors such as age, gender, activity levels, and disease are important considerations when calculating proper diet. Determining what and how much to eat is the first step in obtaining health through nutrition. In the pages to follow, we will examine general and specific nutritional needs and develop a dietary plan to supply those needs. Let's begin with essential nutrients.

ESSENTIAL NUTRIENTS

A **nutrient** is a substance that provides nourishment and affects metabolic processes such as cell growth and repair. The body produces some nutrients such as cholesterol in adequate amounts, making dietary supplements unnecessary. There are some nutrients, **essential nutrients**, that are either produced by the body in insufficient amounts or not produced at all. Examples of essential nutrients are carbohydrates, proteins, fats, minerals, and vitamins, which are obtained by the foods we eat.

Essential nutrients can be subdivided into micronutrients and macronutrients.

Micronutrients are required in minute amounts. Vitamins, minerals, and water fall into this category. Because micronutrients lack caloric value, they are referred to as the "no-calorie group." Despite the low levels required for health, micronutrient deficiency is fairly common, affecting one in three people.

Macronutrients are required in relatively large quantities. Examples of macronutrients are proteins, carbohydrates, and fats. These provide the majority of the body's energy through calories and are referred to as the "calorie group."

Nutrients are combinations of chemicals made available by the process of digestion. Based on its chemical makeup, each nutrient provides for different biological functions.

Next we will examine the most common essential nutrients, including their basic functions and dietary sources.

PROTEIN

Description—Proteins are composed of chains of amino acids. The body uses about 24 amino acids; 8 are essential. These are the main building blocks of the body. Chromosomes, hormones, enzymes, and cell membranes are all composed of proteins.

Function—Proteins assist in the body's growth and energy needs. They also help build and repair tissues and blood and form antibodies to fight infection.

Source—Good sources of proteins are both animal and plant sources such as meat, fish, poultry, eggs, milk, cheese, dried beans, peas, and nuts.

Commentary—It is important to realize there are two distinct types of proteins: complete and incomplete. Complete proteins contain all eight essential amino acids and are found in animal sources. Plant proteins are often deficient in one or more amino acids; however, combining multiple plant proteins can provide all of the essential amino acids. Legumes and grains together can make a complete protein. It is not by chance that numerous cultures consume dishes combining beans and rice. This knowledge is especially important for vegetarian or vegan diets.

CARBOHYDRATES

Description—Carbohydrates are also known as saccharides, or sugar. All carbohydrates are composed of carbon, hydrogen, and oxygen (CHO); the different types are distinguished by their complexity. The hierarchy from simple to complex is monosaccharides, disaccharides, and polysaccharides. Monosaccharides, *simple sugars*, are glucose (blood sugar), fructose (fruit sugar), and galactose (milk sugar). Disaccharides, the union of two monosaccharides, are sucrose (table sugar), lactose (milk sugar), and maltose (malt sugar). Polysaccharides, trisaccharides (carbohydrates containing three or more simple sugar molecules) are dextrins, glycogen (stored glucose), cellulose, and gums.

Function—Carbohydrates are the most common source of energy for the body. They require the least amount of water to digest, so they can be broken down more readily.

Carbohydrates also help generate adenosine triphosphate (ATP), provide roughage, and satisfy hunger.

Source—Good sources of carbohydrates are plant sources, such as bread, cereals, potatoes, corn, dried beans and peas, fresh fruits, sugar, syrup, jelly, jam, and honey.

Commentary—It is a common misconception to associate the term *carbohydrate* with bread instead of sugar because most sources consumed will be some form of grain. The end result, however, produces sugar in the body. Therefore, honey and toast are both forms of carbohydrates. Carbohydrates were once dubbed *simple* or *complex*. The now antiquated terms, first used in 1977, merely deemed mono- and disaccharides as simple carbohydrates, and polysaccharides as complex carbohydrates. The terms were designed to help distinguish the recommended types of carbohydrates to be consumed. Their distinction was dispensed by the United States Department of Agriculture (USDA) in 2005, in favor of recommending fiber-rich or whole grain foods.

FATS

Description—Fats are a subgroup of lipids called *triglycerides*. They are composed of three fatty acids and a glycerol molecule. Fats can be unsaturated or saturated. The distinction is simple; at room temperature unsaturated fats are liquid, whereas saturated fats are solid.

Function—Fats can be an energy source, but they act more as the body's reserve fuel. Fats also protect and insulate the body.

Source—Good sources of fats are animal and plant sources, such as nuts, seeds, oils, butter, cream, fatty meats, olives, avocados, and other fatty foods.

Commentary—Trans fats are a type of unsaturated fat that occur naturally only in very small quantities but are produced industrially on a large scale. Created by a chemical process of partial hydrogenation of plant oils, trans fats provide a longer shelf life, cheaper production costs, and often adhere to vegetarian standards. However, trans fats have been linked frequently to an increased risk of coronary artery disease. At the time of this writing, many countries have banned the use of trans fats and legislation is being proposed to ban or limit the use of trans fats in the United States.

VITAMINS

Description—Vitamins are an important group of micronutrients, essential for metabolic reactions in the body. They are either soluble by water or fat. Water-soluble vitamins are absorbed easily and excreted within hours. Examples of water-soluble vitamins are the B vitamins and vitamin C. Fat-soluble vitamins are absorbed slowly and often reside in the liver and fat cells. Examples of fat-soluble vitamins are A, D, E, and K.

Function—Vitamins regulate metabolic processes by acting as catalysts in chemical reactions and coenzymes (transporters) that carry chemical groups in the cell.

Source—Good sources for vitamins can be both plant and animal, such as vegetables, fruits, and fish.

Commentary—In the following, we will discuss in detail a few specific examples of vitamins. The following is intended to be a brief look at vitamins. Although there are numerous vitamins in existence, food labels often cite information only for the more prominent vitamins: A, the B complex, C, D, and E. Recommended daily values (RDVs) will be included for both the adult male and the adult female (e.g., 10 mg/6 mg).

Vitamin A (retinol)

Function—Vitamin A acts as an antioxidant, supports immune system function, promotes healthy eyes, helps maintain skin smoothness and clarity, and helps control bone growth. A deficiency in retinol can cause night blindness.

Source—Good sources for retinol include liver, spinach, sweet potatoes, pumpkin, collard greens, and milk.

RDV—900 μg/700 μg

The vitamin B complex

Once considered a single vitamin, there are now more than 20 types of B vitamin. The B complex refers to eight B vitamins: B_1, B_2, B_3, B_5, B_6, B_7, B_9, and B_{12}.

B_1 (thiamine)

Function—Thiamine promotes proper heart function and helps convert carbohydrates and fat into energy. A deficiency in this vitamin can cause beriberi.

Source—Good sources for thiamine include pork, whole grains, spinach, wheat germ, and fortified cereals.

RDV—1.2 mg/1.1 mg

B_2 (riboflavin)

Function—Riboflavin promotes red blood cell formation and helps prevent cataracts. Riboflavin deficiency can cause ariboflavinosis.

Source—Good sources for riboflavin include asparagus, organ meats, milk, yogurt, almonds, soybeans, and fortified cereals. Riboflavin is so delicate it can be destroyed by heat or light. Many dairy companies switched from glass bottles to cartons to protect the riboflavin content.

RDV—1.3 mg/1.1 mg

B_3 (niacin)

Function—Niacin promotes adrenal gland production, assisting in expelling toxins, and helps maintain muscle tone. A niacin deficiency can cause pellagra.

Source—Good sources for niacin include beets, chicken, turkey, veal, salmon, tuna, sunflower seeds, and peanuts.

RDV—16 mg/14 mg

B_5 (pantothenic acid)

Function—Pantothenic acid promotes red blood cell production, aids in the breakdown of fats and carbohydrates for energy, and helps maintain a healthy digestive tract. Pantothenic acid is found in all living cells, so a deficiency is rare. Deficiency symptoms may include fatigue, insomnia, stomach pains, and upper respiratory tract infections.

Source—Good sources for pantothenic acid include brewer's yeast, corn, tomatoes, egg yolks, beef, duck, sweet potatoes, whole grains, and lobster.

RDV—5 mg/5 mg

B_6 (pyridoxine)

Function—Vitamin B_6 promotes healthy nerve and brain function, aids in the production of DNA and RNA, and helps the proper absorption of vitamin B_{12}. A deficiency in this vitamin creates symptoms such as muscle weakness, depression, nervousness, and short-term memory loss.

Source—Good sources for pyridoxine include brown rice, whole grain flour, bran, shrimp, lentils, fish, and nuts.

RDV—1.3 mg/1.3 mg

B_7 (biotin, vitamin H)

Function—Biotin aids in the metabolism of carbohydrates, fats, and amino acids. Deficiency is rare; symptoms may include hair loss, dry scaly skin, cracking in the corners of the mouth and a swollen tongue.

Source—Good sources of biotin include brewer's yeast, organ meats, nut butters, soybeans, legumes, and cooked eggs (raw egg white can interfere with biotin absorption).

RDV—30 µg/30 µg

B_9 (folic acid)

Function—Folic acid aids in the production of DNA and RNA and is crucial for proper brain development and function. Folic acid is the most common B vitamin deficiency; it can cause poor growth and gingivitis. Deficiency during pregnancy can cause birth defects including spina bifida, cleft palate, and brain damage.

Source—Good sources for folic acid include spinach, whole grains, orange juice, wheat germ, asparagus, salmon, avocado, root vegetables (carrots, potatoes), and milk.

RDV—400 µg/400 µg (600 µg during pregnancy)

B_{12} (cobalamin)

Function—Cobalamin promotes proper iron function and regulates red blood cell formation. Deficiency may cause anemia and cognitive decline. Vegetarians are often at a higher risk for this deficiency.

Source—Good sources for cobalamin include fish, dairy, organ meats (liver, kidney) eggs, beef, and pork.

RDV—2.4 µg/2.4 µg

Vitamin C (ascorbic acid)

Function—Vitamin C acts as an antioxidant, helps the body resist infection, promotes adrenal gland function, aids in collagen production, and can reduce high blood pressure and cholesterol. A deficiency can cause scurvy.

Source—Good sources for ascorbic acid are citrus fruits (oranges, limes), strawberries, broccoli, and sweet red peppers.

RDV—90 mg/75 mg

Vitamin D (cholecalciferol)

Function—Vitamin D promotes bone development, helps absorb and metabolize calcium, and aids the immune system. A deficiency can cause rickets and lead to osteoporosis.

Source—Good sources for this vitamin include fortified milk, fish liver oils, and sun exposure (sunlight helps skin to synthesize vitamin D).

RDV—5 µg/5 µg

Vitamin E (tocopherol)

Function—Vitamin E acts as a powerful antioxidant, repairs tissue, reduces blood pressure, promotes sperm development, helps prevent cataracts, and increases maternal circulation during pregnancy. Deficiency symptoms include muscle weakness, impaired vision, and unsteady gait.

Source—Good sources for vitamin E include almonds, peanuts, sunflower seeds, spinach, avocado, oils (wheat germ, safflower), and carrot juice.

RDV—15 mg/15 mg

Vitamin K

Function—Vitamin K aids in blood clotting and maintains bone health. Bacteria found in the intestines produce this vitamin. Deficiency is rare and may lead to hemorrhaging.

Source—Good sources of vitamin K include beef liver, green tea, spinach, dark green lettuce, asparagus, broccoli, and kale.

RDV—120 µg/90 µg

MINERALS

Description—Minerals are chemical elements required by living organisms. They are all nonorganic compounds found in nature. Minerals divide into two categories: macro (bulk) minerals such as calcium and micro (trace) minerals such as iron.

Function—Minerals are vital in regulating many body functions. They act as coenzymes (iron can transport oxygen), support organs (potassium supports kidney function), build bone (calcium), and aid healthy growth and development (zinc). Minerals often work with vitamins to perform bodily functions.

Source—Good sources can be found in both plant and animal products, such as vegetables, meats, dairy, and soy.

Commentary—Like the description of vitamins, a detailed examination of minerals will be limited to a few examples. Each mineral will be followed with its atomic letters as designated by the periodic table. RDVs will present the needs of the adult male followed by the adult female.

Calcium (Ca)

Function—Calcium supports the development and maintenance of strong bones and teeth and promotes heart, nerve, and muscle function. To properly function, calcium requires other nutrients, such as vitamin D. Calcium is the most abundant bulk mineral in the body. A deficiency of this mineral can contribute to osteoporosis, hair loss, and seizures.

Source—Good sources of calcium include cheese, ice cream, yogurt, broccoli, almonds, Swiss chard, and milk (however, heavy caffeine use can diminish calcium levels; adding cream in your coffee does not count).

RDV—1,000 mg/1,000 mg

Potassium (K)

Function—Potassium is essential for proper kidney function. It also supports normal heart function and aids digestive function. Potassium is a relatively delicate bulk mineral, because it relies on the balance of many other nutrients to maintain proper levels. Excessive amounts of sodium, coffee, or alcohol may deplete the body's stores of potassium. Potassium deficiency, or hypokalemia, can cause weakness and lack of energy.

Source—Good sources of potassium include unprocessed foods, including meat, fish, vegetables (especially potatoes), fruit (especially avocados, bananas, and orange juice), dairy, and whole grains.

RDV—2,000 mg/2,000 mg

Iron (Fe)

Function—Iron attaches to the hemoglobin in red blood cells, thereby delivering oxygen to the tissues. Iron is the most abundant trace mineral in the body. A deficiency can lead to anemia, causing weakness and fatigue. Excessive iron may lead to iron toxicity, which can cause diabetes and liver damage.

Source—Good sources of iron include liver, lean red meat, fish, poultry, oysters, whole grains, dried beans, legumes, fortified breads, and cereals.

RDV—18 mg/18 mg (27 mg during pregnancy)

Zinc (Zn)

Function—Zinc acts as an antioxidant, promotes immune system function, and helps regulate appetite, taste, and smell. It is essential for normal growth and development and supports most aspects of reproduction. Zinc, the second most abundant trace mineral, is stored primarily in muscle tissue, although high concentrations exist in the blood and the male prostate gland. Proteins help absorb zinc; hence animal sources are best to attain an adequate amount of zinc. A deficiency may cause skin abnormalities such as psoriasis, impaired taste or smell, poor growth, hypogonadism, and amenorrhea (lack of a menstrual period).

Source—Good sources of zinc include oysters, red meats, poultry, cheese, shellfish, legumes, whole grains, and mushrooms.

RDV—11 mg/8 mg

WATER

Function—Water, the most important nutrient, regulates body temperature and transports all the other nutrients. The body is roughly 70% water. This statistic is often varied, because it breaks down further: the brain is 70% water, the lungs are 90%, the blood is 83%, and so on.

Source—Although all water comes essentially from the same source, the important factor is purity. The Environmental Protection Agency (EPA) governs tap water standards. The Food and Drug Administration (FDA) sets the standards for bottled water based on the EPA's recommendations. Tap water quality will vary by location but must adhere to the EPA's standards. Every region of the United States produces annual reports on tap water quality, available online. Bottled waters offer a consistent product and are often chosen for taste reasons.

Commentary—The standard calculation for daily water intake is simply a half ounce per pound of body weight. However soda, coffee, sports drinks, and tea do not count toward this total. Fortunately, bottled water has become the fastest growing beverage market. There are many brands now in five categories: artesian (water from well tapping), mineral (water with natural minerals), purified (water produced by distillation or other suitable processes), sparkling (water with higher CO_2 levels), and spring (water from an underground source that naturally flows to the surface).

DIETARY FIBER

Fiber, or roughage, is found in the walls of plant cells. It is essential to human health, despite the fact that enzymes in the digestive tract cannot break it down. There are two types of fiber: soluble and insoluble.

Fiber helps maintain intestinal tract health. Soluble fiber mixes with water to form a gel that slows digestion in the stomach and intestine, resulting in a lower absorption rate of starches and sugars. It also reduces cholesterol levels. Insoluble fiber acts as a laxative and gives stool its bulk, helping it move quickly through the digestive tract.

All plant foods are sources of fiber. Good sources of soluble fiber include dried beans and peas, oats, barley, and fruits. Good sources of insoluble fiber include fruits, vegetables, and whole grains.

It was once thought that a high-fiber diet lowers the risk of colon cancer; however, studies have been conflicting. In 2002 the FDA allowed food labels to state that a high-fiber diet may reduce the risk of some cancers, recalling that the development of cancer was dependent upon many factors.

DETERMINING DIETARY NEEDS

All the nutrients we have listed can be found on most food nutrition labels. Understanding how to read and utilize the information on a nutrition label is vital for healthy diet planning. In this section, we will discuss how to read nutrition labels and what to look for when planning a limited calorie diet.

A **calorie** is a unit of measure for the energy you receive when you eat a food. In the United States, a calorie is equal to the heat energy needed to raise the temperature of 1 kg of water by 1° C. It is also referred to as a kilocalorie (kcal). Macronutrients each have set caloric values: fat has 9 kcal, and protein and carbohydrates both have 4 kcal. As stated earlier, micronutrients such as vitamins and water do not have any caloric value.

The General Guide to Calories, developed by the FDA, determines an individual's daily caloric needs to be 2,000 kcal. This number is the basis for percentages found on nutrition labels. This means on average, an adult requires 2,000 calories to provide the energy needed to accomplish their daily activities. Many factors will determine a specific individual's daily caloric needs: age, gender, weight, height, lifestyle, and exercise. This is also true for determining an individual's basal metabolic rate (BMR). This number represents the energy you expend completely at rest or the calories you burn just lying in bed all day. Although it may to fun to know your BMR, it will be of little help in diet planning. Calculators are available online to determine the caloric needs and BMR of a specific individual (http://nutritiondata.com/calories-burned.html and http://health.discovery.com/tools/calculators/basal/basal.html). These equations are based on the average healthy adult. They do not take into consideration special needs, conditions, or disorders.

WEIGHT LOSS

Once an individual's base caloric need is established, his or her current weight can be maintained with a diet based on that number. By reading nutrition labels and paying close attention to serving size, you can plan a healthy diet without gaining weight. To lose weight, one needs simply to consume less than his or her base caloric need. One pound is equal to 3,500 calories, so to lose one pound per week, a person can cut back 500 calories per day.

Although we live in a society overwhelmed with fad diets, "miracle" pills, and radical surgeries, weight loss comes down to a simple math equation: expend more energy than you take in. This can be accomplished by taking in fewer calories (dieting) or expending more energy (exercising), or a combination of both. Once again, this is true for the average healthy adult. Always consult your physician before beginning any diet or exercise regimen.

HOW TO READ A NUTRITION LABEL

It is important to remember that when limiting your caloric intake, the body must still obtain the proper amount of nutrients. Although there are supplements available, balancing your diet with foods rich in vitamins and minerals is recommended. It is possible to overdo vitamin intake with the use of supplements. Consult the nutrition label to ensure you are selecting the best food for your needs; items are often not as healthy as one might think.

Sample Label of Peanut Butter

The first thing on the label is serving size. Portion control is vital. Most canned foods contain at least 2 servings but are often eaten by one person in one sitting.

Calories are listed next. Peanut butter is considered a moderate calorie. The general rule: 40 kcal is low, 100 kcal, is moderate and 400 kcal are high.

Macronutrients are the next section. Most Americans consume adequate amounts of these. Limit yourself by making well-balanced choices. One serving of this peanut butter, only two tablespoons, would count for a quarter of your daily fat allowance. To balance this, your next meal may need to include leaner options.

Micronutrients come next on the label. Most Americans will need to increase their daily intake of the items found here. Plan your diet to be high in fiber, vitamins, and minerals. Take a supplement if necessary.

The bottom portion is a standard footnote that must be on all labels. It simply serves as a reference.

Nutrition Facts

Serving Size 2 Tbsp (31g)
Servings Per About 16

Amount Per Serving

Calories 190   Calories from Fat 130

	% Daily Value*
Total Fat 17g	25%
Saturated Fat 3g	16%
Trans Fat 0g	
Cholesterol 0mg	0%
Sodium 70mg	3%
Total Carbohydrate 31g	2%
Dietary Fiber 2g	9%
Sugars 3g	
Protein 8g	
Vitamin E	15%
Riboflavin	2%
Niacin	20%
Iron	4%

* Percent Daily Values are based on a 2,000 calorie diet. Your Daily Values may be higher or lower depending on your calorie needs.

	Calories:	2,000	2,500
Total Fat	Less than	65g	80g
Sat Fat	Less than	20g	25g
Cholesterol	Less than	300mg	300mg
Sodium	Less than	2,400mg	2,400mg
Total Carbohydrate		300g	375g
Dietary Fiber		25g	30g

THE NEW FOOD PYRAMID

Another useful tool in diet planning is the Food Pyramid. It was developed by the USDA in 1992 to illustrate the five major food groups and identify the number of servings from each group that are needed daily to provide a healthy, well-balanced diet. In 2005 the USDA unveiled MyPyramid, the pyramid's new look. It was redesigned to include an emphasis on physical activity as well as a new customizable edge, offering 12 different versions of MyPyramid.

The five major groups have remained consistent, but serving suggestions are more tailored for each of the 12 options. The look now includes color coding for each group and a slogan. The bottom width of the colored bands denotes the comparative amount required daily. The figure climbing the steps represents the importance of daily physical activity. Visit www.MyPyramid.gov for more resources, including videos and games.

SPECIAL CONSIDERATIONS

Vegetarianism

Vegetarians can meet all the nutritional recommendations by consuming a variety of foods to meet their daily caloric needs. Vegetarianism can be a very healthy choice; grains, vegetables and fruits tend to represent the majority of the food consumed, which is exactly what MyPyramid suggests. A vegetarian diet usually results in higher than average amounts of most nutrients, with a few exceptions. Meat can be a primary source of protein, iron, calcium, zinc and

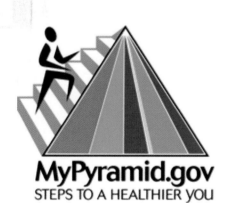

MyPyramid.gov
STEPS TO A HEALTHIER YOU

Grains – Make half your grains whole
Vegetables – Vary your veggies
Fruits – Focus on fruits
Oils – Know your fats
Milk – Get your calcium-rich foods
Meats & Beans – Go lean on protein

vitamin B_{12}, so vegetarians may need to focus on finding other foods to give them these nutrients. All of these *can* be obtained through adherence to a vegetarian diet, mostly by eating beans, nuts, vegetables, and fortified foods.

The food industry has never been more accommodating to the vegetarian diet. For nearly every meat and dairy product, there is a soy or vegetable equivalent. Technology has advanced so that many vegetarian products look and even taste like their counterparts. Most restaurants have vegetarian options or can make the necessary modifications to provide one. Asian and Indian restaurants especially tend to offer such options.

Pregnancy and Breastfeeding

Studies have shown that diet can weigh considerably in the outcome of a pregnancy. The standard MyPyramid recommendations are a good foundation for healthy diet planning during pregnancy, allowing consideration for the changing caloric needs of the mother. Consulting a physician is vital for any pregnant woman concerned about a proper dietary plan.

Although macronutrient needs may generally remain consistent, nearly all micronutrients will require a higher RDV for a pregnant woman. It is often hard to achieve this nutrition through diet alone. Iron and folic acid intake are especially important; the increase of both is considerable (RDVs for pregnancy are 27 mg of iron compared with the standard 18 mg, and 600 μg of folic acid compared with the standard 400 μg). Prenatal vitamins are routinely recommended to supply the additional needs of pregnancy and nursing.

NUTRITION AND THE MASSAGE THERAPIST

Nutrition is a valuable component to overall health, and as massage therapists, it is our duty to recognize that relationship. We are health care practitioners, and our clients will often seek our advice on health topics outside our field of expertise. Although we must be careful not to overstep the boundaries of our practice, any suggestions made must be with an understanding of nutrition and its role in bodily health.

This knowledge is vital not only for the benefit of our clients but for ourselves. The body is our primary tool. Comprehension about how to care for the body is massage therapists' best form of insurance. Your career longevity depends on self-care. Recall that our occupation is rated in the strenuous category on Bonnie Prudden's scale. It is on par with a professional athlete or dancer, two occupations that obviously require special attention to nutritional needs. Education is the first step to proper nutrition, and there are a multitude of resources available. Remember, you cannot give what you do not have. Managing your nutritional health is the best gift you can give yourself.

SUMMARY

The body requires essential nutrients to carry out its physiological process. These nutrients are obtained through diet. Determining your nutritional needs is the first step to diet management. The calorie, or *energy*, needs of an individual can be calculated based on a number of factors, such as age or gender. Weight loss can be planned around the caloric needs of an individual. Resources such as nutritional labels and the food pyramid are available to assist with beneficial diet planning. Special issues such as pregnancy should always be taken into consideration for proper nutritional health. Nutrition is intrinsically linked to massage therapy, for the benefit of the therapist and client. It is our duty to be informed on the subject and to lead by example.

Bibliography

CNPP. 2005 Food Pyramid Guideline. Available at: http://www.mypyramid.gov/. Retrieved November 21, 2006.

Environmental Protection Agency: Drinking water and health, 2005. Available at: http://www.epa.gov/safewater/faq/pdfs/fs_healthseries _bottlewater.pdf. Retrieved November 26, 2006.

Gallaher D: Present knowledge in nutrition. Available at: http://www.umm.edu/altmed/ConsSupplements/Fibercs.html. Retrieved November 25, 2006.

Hart J: Supplements. Available at: http://www.umm.edu/altmed/ConsLookups/ Supplements.html. Retrieved November 23, 2006.

Mardis A: A look at the diet of pregnant women, 2000. Available at: http://www.cnpp.usda.gov/Publications/NutritionInsights/ Insight17.pdf. Retrieved November 26, 2006.

Posnick L et al: Bottled water regulation and the FDA. Available at: http://www.cfsan.fda.gov/~dms/botwatr.html. Retrieved November 25, 2006.

USDA: Dietary guidelines for Americans 2005. Available at: http://www.health.gov/dietaryguidelines/dga2005/document /pdf/DGA2005.pdf. Retrieved November 20, 2006

USFDA: How to understand and use nutritional facts labels. Available at: http://www.cfsan.fda.gov/~dms/foodlab.html. Retrieved November 20, 2006.

Links to Nutritional Calculators

Nutrition Data. Nutrition facts and calorie counter. Available at: http://nutritiondata.com/calories-burned.html. © 2006 Condé-Net Inc.

Discovery Health. Basal metabolic rate calculator. Available at: http://health.discovery.com/tools/calculators/basal/basal.html. © 2006 Discovery Communications Inc.

Pharmacology

Unless a massage therapist has training in pharmacology, the world of medications is potentially bewildering. Most massage therapist do not have this training. They need to rely on information given to them by their clients. Sometimes, clients either do not know what medications they are taking or they do not know why they are taking them.

Because the effects and side effects of medications have a bearing on how a massage needs to be performed, the massage therapist needs to be as knowledgeable as possible about clients' conditions. The massage therapist needs to elicit client information before, during, and after the massage to make the most informed decisions about treatment. A strategy to obtain this crucial information could be the following:

1. During the client interview, determine the client's use of medications.
2. Ask if the client is experiencing any side effects from the medications, including any sensory deprivation such as a decrease in the ability to sense pressure.
   a. If not, proceed with the massage as usual.
   b. If so, modify the massage to accommodate the side effect. If the client has not informed his or her physician as to the side effects, then recommend that he or she do so.
3. Re-evaluate the client during subsequent sessions.
4. Modify the treatment plan as needed.

A different strategy is needed for clients taking anticoagulants or blood thinners, which are medications that prevent coagulation or blood clotting. People taking anticoagulants are particularly prone to bruising. This strategy could be the following:

1. Ask if the client is prone to bruising.
   a. If so, then do not apply above a medium or moderate pressure.
   b. If not or the client does not know, examine the skin from the elbows down.
      i. If the skin looks healthy and unblemished, then proceed with the massage as usual.
      ii. If the skin looks blemished or bruised, then do not apply above a medium or moderate pressure.
2. Re-evaluate the client during subsequent sessions.
3. Modify the treatment plan as needed.

The following glossary includes pharmacological terminology.

TERMINOLOGY

Analgesic   Pain reliever that does not cause the loss of consciousness.

Angina pectoris   Also called *angina*, angina pectoris is chest pain that occurs when the blood flow to cardiac muscle is reduced, such as through atherosclerosis, arteriosclerosis, a blood clot, and spasm of cardiac blood vessels.

Antibiotic   Medication that kills or prevents the growth of bacteria.

Anticoagulant   Substance that prevents coagulation or blood clotting.

Anticonvulsant   Medication used in the prevention of epileptic seizures.

Antidepressant   Medication designed to treat or alleviate the symptoms of clinical depression.

Antidiabetic   Medication used to treat diabetes mellitus by decreasing blood glucose levels. This medication is also known as a *hypoglycemic substance*.

Antifungal   Medication used to treat fungal infections.

Antihistamine   Medication used to reduce or eliminate the effects of histamine, a chemical released by the body during allergic reactions. Histamine is partially responsible for inflammation.

Antiviral   Medication used to treat viral infections.

Arteriosclerosis   Hardening of the arteries from a variety of causes, one of which is atherosclerosis.

Arrhythmia   Any of a number of conditions in which cardiac muscle contraction is irregular or is faster or slower than normal (e.g., tachycardia, bradycardia).

Atherosclerosis   Hardening of the arteries as a result of the formation of plaques in the walls of the arteries. The plaques, or lesions, are made of cholesterol and white blood cells. Older lesions can become calcified.

Beta blockers   Group of medications that decrease blood pressure and affect heart rate and the strength of the heart's contraction. These medications are used to treat angina pectoris, hypertension, hypertrophic cardiomyopathy, irregular heartbeat, migraine headaches, anxiety, tremors, overproduction of thyroid hormones, and glaucoma.

Blood thinner   Anticoagulant substance that prevents coagulation or blood clotting.

Bronchodilator   Opens the bronchial tubes of the lungs.

Cardiomyopathy Diseased heart muscle that can develop as a result of a variety of causes. It results in the loss of cardiac muscle function. People with cardiomyopathy are often at risk for arrhythmia or sudden cardiac death or both.

Congestive heart failure (CHF) Also known as *heart failure*, CHF is a condition in which the heart is a slowly failing pump. If the right side of the heart fails first, then blood will back up in peripheral veins and edema will result. If the left side of the heart fails first, then blood will back up in the pulmonary veins and pulmonary edema will result.

Corticosteroids Natural substances made by the body. In pharmacological terms, corticosteroids are synthetic forms of what the body makes. They are groups of medications that suppress the immune system and reduce inflammation and are commonly used in organ transplants to prevent organ rejection. Corticosteroids are also used in the treatment of autoimmune and inflammatory diseases such as Crohn's disease, asthma, and poison ivy. Taking these medications, especially over 30 days, results in a loss of integrity of various body tissues. Muscles may atrophy; connective tissues of the skin, ligaments, joints, bones, and tendons may weaken. Massage that stresses these structures, such as joint mobilizations, ribcage compressions, stretching, heavy percussion, skin rolling, wringing, and deep friction (e.g., cross-fiber, chucking, circular), should be monitored or avoided. This is particularly true for women who have or are at risk for osteoporosis (e.g., postmenopausal women or older adults).

Cushing's syndrome Disorder that results from excessive corticosteroids, either from the overproduction by the body or from ingesting them. Signs and symptoms include rapid weight gain, a "moon face," excess sweating, thinning of the skin, easy bruising, muscle weakness, excess growth of fat along the collar bone and back of the neck (known as a "buffalo hump"), depression, anxiety, hypertension, hyperglycemia, and, if left untreated, heart disease and death.

Edema Swelling of any organ or tissue from an excessive accumulation of interstitial fluid.

Glaucoma Group of diseases of the optic nerve. If left untreated, then glaucoma can result in permanent damage of the optic nerve and partial or total loss of vision.

Hypertension High blood pressure.

Hypertrophic cardiomyopathy Diseased heart muscle that results in an enlarged heart that cannot be traced to a definite cause.

Hypoglycemia Low level of blood glucose (sugar) with symptoms that include anxiety, sweating, tremors, increased heart rate, hunger, and weakness. Severe hypoglycemia leads to mental disorientation, convulsions, unconsciousness, and shock.

Hypotension Low blood pressure.

Hypothyroidism Condition in which the thyroid gland is producing extremely low levels of or no thyroid hormones.

IM (intramuscular) Injection of a substance directly into muscle.

Inhaler Medical device used to deliver medication into the lungs. An inhaler is often used in the treatment of asthma. It is also known as a *puffer*.

Injection Method of putting liquid into the body with a syringe and hollow needle that punctures the skin.

Muscle relaxers Muscle relaxants that decrease muscle tone.

Myocardial infarction Heart attack.

Narcotic Medication derived from opium that reduces pain, induces sleep, and may alter mood or behavior. Narcotics are addictive drugs.

NSAIDs (nonsteroidal antiinflammatory drugs) Medications that reduce pain, fever, and inflammation. *Nonsteroidal* differentiates these medications from steroids (corticosteroids), which are also antiinflammatory medications. NSAIDS are nonnarcotic. The most common NSAIDs are aspirin, ibuprofen, and naproxen.

Orthostatic hypotension Excessive decrease in blood pressure that occurs with standing from a sitting or lying position. Symptoms include light-headedness and dizziness, which can lead, in some cases, to fainting.

Over-the-counter (OTC) Medications that may be sold without a prescription and without a visit to a medical professional.

Prescription Written order by a qualified health care professional to a pharmacist or other therapist for treatment.

SubQ (subcutaneous) Injection of a substance into the subcutaneous layer just below the epidermis.

Topical Applied to the surface of the body.

Transdermal patch Adhesive skin patch that contains medication that passes through the skin and into the blood vessels in the dermis. These patches are often used to administer nitroglycerin, birth control, antinausea medication, and medication used to stop smoking or to reduce pain.

Urinary incontinence Lack of voluntary control over urination.

Urinary retention Lack of the ability to urinate.

MEDICATIONS LISTED ALPHABETICALLY

The following list includes the most commonly prescribed medications. The common name (if generic) or trade name is listed first in **bold**. The chemical name, if it is different from the common name, is listed second in parentheses. After the name of the medication is the method by which it is usually taken or administered. Common side effects and massage considerations are also included. If the client is not experiencing any side effects or the side effects are mild, then modification of the treatment plan may be unnecessary. These descriptions are meant to be taken as general guidelines only.

Every person reacts differently to medications. It is important to ask the client what effects and side effects he or she is experiencing and perform the massage accordingly.

Acetaminophen Oral medication used to reduce pain and fever. This medication is administered orally. No side effects occur that will affect how massage should be performed.

Actifed (triprolidine, usually in combination with pseudoephedrine) Antihistamine used to treat allergies. This medication is administered orally. Side effects include dizziness, fatigue, and sometimes hypotension. If the client is experiencing these symptoms, then the client should be asked if he or she needs assistance with positional changes such as getting on the table or sitting up and getting off the table after treatment.

Advil (ibuprofen) NSAID used to reduce inflammation, relieve pain, and reduce fever. Side effects include dizziness and drowsiness. The client should be asked if he or she needs assistance with positional changes such as getting on the table or sitting up and getting off the table after treatment.

Aleve (naproxen sodium) NSAID used to reduce inflammation, relieve pain, and reduce fever. Side effects include dizziness and drowsiness. The client should be asked if he or she needs assistance with positional changes such as getting on the table or sitting up and getting off the table after treatment.

Allegra (fexofenadine), **Allegra-D** Antihistamine used to treat allergies. This medication is administered orally. Side effects include dizziness, fatigue, and sometimes hypotension. If the client is experiencing these symptoms, then the client should be asked if he or she needs assistance with positional changes such as getting on the table or sitting up and getting off the table after treatment.

Amoxicillin Oral antibiotic that is administered orally. Generally, clients who have been taking antibiotics for at least 3 days are no longer considered contagious. However, if the question remains as to whether a client is contagious, then his or her physician should be consulted. If the client is contagious, then massage is contraindicated. The main side effects of amoxicillin are digestive tract upset and diarrhea. If the client is experiencing discomfort from these side effects, then abdominal massage may be contraindicated.

Ampicillin Oral antibiotic that is administered by injection. Generally, clients who have been taking antibiotics for at least 3 days are no longer considered contagious. However, if a question remains as to whether a client is contagious, then his or her physician should be consulted. If the client is contagious, then massage is contraindicated. If a client received an injection of ampicillin, then massage over the injection site is contraindicated for at least 10 days after the last injection because it may increase the medication's absorption rate. The main side effects of ampicillin are digestive tract upset and diarrhea.

If the client is experiencing discomfort from these side effects symptoms, then abdominal massage may be contraindicated.

Aricept (donepezil) Used to treat mild-to-moderate Alzheimer's disease. Although usually administered orally, Aricept may be administered by injection if rapid action is desired. Side effects can include hypotension, orthostatic hypotension, and dizziness. If a client has received an injection of Aricept, massage over the injection site is contraindicated for at least 10 days after the last injection because it may increase the medication's absorption rate. Clients who are taking Aricept are subject to orthostatic hypotension. The client should be asked if he or she needs assistance with positional changes such as getting on the table or sitting up and getting off the table after treatment.

Armour Thyroid (thyroid extract) Synthetic thyroid hormone used to treat hypothyroidism, goiters, and thyroid cancer. This medication is administered orally. The main side effects include anxiety and insomnia. A gentle, relaxing massage is indicated.

Aspirin (acetylsalicylic acid) Oral medication used to relieve pain and fever and to prevent blood clot formation. Aspirin is prescribed for people who are at risk for conditions that can result from blood clots such as myocardial infarction (MI) or heart attack, angina pectoris, stroke, and peripheral vascular disease. This medication is administered orally. Side effects include heartburn, constipation, and easy bruising. If a client who is taking aspirin is subject to these side effects, then he or she may need to be propped in a semireclining position to enable gravity to help keep stomach acid from refluxing into the client's esophagus. Abdominal massage that includes gliding and kneading strokes should be performed clockwise around the client's abdomen to alleviate constipation.

Ativan (lorazepam) Medication used to treat insomnia, anxiety, and tension, including muscle tension. This medication is usually administered orally, but it may be given by injection if rapid action is desired. If a client has received an injection of Ativan, then massage over the injection site is contraindicated for at least 10 days after the last injection because it may increase the medication's absorption rate. Side effects include fatigue, dizziness, drowsiness, and hypotension. The client should be asked if he or she needs assistance with positional changes such as getting on the table or sitting up and getting off the table after treatment.

Atrovent (ipratropium bromide) Bronchodilator designed to open the bronchial tubes during an asthma attack. This medication is usually administered through an inhaler. Side effects can include restlessness, anxiety, dizziness, headache, insomnia, weakness, tremors, and heart palpitations. If a client is experiencing any of these effects, then a gentle massage with long, gliding strokes may help the client relax and possibly alleviate the side effects.

Betapace, Betapace AF (sotalol)   Beta blocker used to treat angina pectoris, hypertension, hypertrophic cardiomyopathy, irregular heartbeat, migraine headaches, anxiety, tremors, overproduction of thyroid hormones, and glaucoma. This medication is administered orally. A gentle, relaxing treatment, possibly of shorter duration, is indicated for any client who has a cardiac disorder. Clearance from the client's health care practitioner is necessary before the client can receive massage. Hypotension is the main side effect. Clients who are taking Betapace or Betapace AF are subject to orthostatic hypotension. The client should be asked if he or she needs assistance with positional changes such as getting on the table or sitting up and getting off the table after treatment.

Birth control pills   Combination of estrogens and progesterone that is administered orally. Side effects include headache, breast swelling and tenderness, nausea, and leg cramps. Face and scalp massage may help alleviate headache. Propping with a soft pillow under the chest when prone may be more comfortable for the client. If the client is experiencing leg cramps, then propping the legs up when supine may help. Lighter pressure over the legs is indicated. A serious side effect is an increased chance of blood clots and phlebitis, most often in the legs. Signs and symptoms include redness, heat, swelling, and pain. If these effects are present, then the client needs to be referred to her health care provider. Phlebitis is a local contraindication for massage. For blood clots, deep, vigorous massage in the area is contraindicated because of the danger of dislodging the clot.

Celebrex (celecoxib)   NSAID used to reduce inflammation, relieve pain, and reduce fever. Side effects include dizziness and drowsiness. The client should be asked if he or she needs assistance with positional changes such as getting on the table or sitting up and getting off the table after treatment.

Claritin (loratadine)   Antihistamine used to treat allergies. This medication is administered orally. Side effects include dizziness, fatigue, and sometimes hypotension. If the client is experiencing any of these effects, then the client should be asked if he or she needs assistance with positional changes such as getting on the table or sitting up and getting off the table after treatment.

Climara (estradiol patches)   Synthetic estrogens used in hormone replacement therapy for menopausal symptoms, osteoporosis treatment and prevention, and sometimes breast cancer. No side effects occur that affect massage.

Codeine   Narcotic used to relieve severe acute and chronic pain and pain associated with terminal illness. Codeine can also be used to treat diarrhea and to suppress coughing. This medication is usually administered orally. Narcotic pain relievers affect the brain and the perception of pain. Many side effects are associated with narcotic pain relievers. The most common are drowsiness, constipation, hypotension, and euphoria. The euphoria is part of the altered perception of pain. Therefore the massage therapist should closely monitor the client's verbal and nonverbal responses to the pressure being applied during the massage treatment and adjust the pressure accordingly. Abdominal massage that includes gliding and kneading strokes performed clockwise around the client's abdomen may help alleviate constipation. The client should be asked if he or she needs assistance with positional changes such as getting on the table or sitting up and getting off the table after treatment.

Coreg (carvedilol)   Beta blocker used to treat angina pectoris, hypertension, hypertrophic cardiomyopathy, irregular heartbeat, migraine headaches, anxiety, tremors, overproduction of thyroid hormones, and glaucoma. This medication is administered orally. A gentle, relaxing treatment, possibly of shorter duration, is indicated for any client who has a cardiac disorder. Clearance from the client's health care practitioner is necessary before the client can receive massage. The main side effect is hypotension. Clients who are taking Coreg are subject to orthostatic hypotension. The client should be asked if he or she needs assistance with positional changes such as getting on the table or sitting up and getting off the table after treatment.

Corgard (nadolol)   Beta blocker used to treat angina pectoris, hypertension, hypertrophic cardiomyopathy, irregular heartbeat, migraine headaches, anxiety, tremors, overproduction of thyroid hormones, and glaucoma. The medication is administered orally. A gentle, relaxing treatment, possibly of shorter duration, is indicated for any client who has a cardiac disorder. Clearance from the client's health care practitioner is necessary before the client can receive massage. The main side effect of Corgard is hypotension. Clients who are taking Corgard are subject to orthostatic hypotension. The client should be asked if he or she needs assistance with positional changes such as getting on the table or sitting up and getting off the table after treatment.

Cortef (hydrocortisone tablets)   Corticosteroid used to treat inflammation such as that occurring with allergies, asthma, and certain types of arthritis. It is also used to suppress immune responses. This medication is administered orally. If used for a short periods, such as for acute conditions, then usually serious side effects do not occur. If, however, Cortef is being taken for chronic conditions, then severe effects such as osteoporosis, slow wound healing, easy bruising, muscle wasting, and possibly Cushing's syndrome can develop. If any of these effects are present, then massage is contraindicated and the client needs to be referred to his or her health care practitioner. Clearance from the client's health care practitioner is necessary before the client can receive massage. If clearance is given, then a lighter massage, possibly of shorter duration, is indicated.

Coumadin (warfarin sodium)   Anticoagulant used to prevent blood clot formation. This medication is administered orally. The most common side effect is easy bruising.

For a client taking Coumadin, clearance from the client's health care practitioner is necessary before the client can receive massage. If clearance is given, then a lighter massage, possibly of shorter duration, is indicated. The client should be asked if he or she needs assistance with positional changes such as getting on the table or sitting up and getting off the table after treatment.

Crestor (rosuvastatin calcium)   Medication used to lower blood cholesterol levels. This medication is administered orally. A rare side effect is muscle pain. If a client taking Crestor is experiencing this side effect, then clearance from the client's health care practitioner is necessary before the client can receive massage. If the client is cleared for massage, then a lighter pressure is indicated.

Darvocet (propoxyphene hydrochloride and acetaminophen)   Narcotic used to relieve severe acute and chronic pain. This medication is usually administered orally. Narcotic pain relievers affect the brain and the perception of pain. Many side effects are associated with narcotic pain relievers. The most common effects are drowsiness, hypotension, constipation, and euphoria. The euphoria is part of the altered perception of pain. Therefore the massage therapist should closely monitor the client's verbal and nonverbal responses to the pressure being applied during the massage treatment and adjust the pressure accordingly. Abdominal massage that includes gliding and kneading strokes performed clockwise around the client's abdomen may help alleviate constipation. The client should be asked if he or she needs assistance with positional changes such as getting on the table or sitting up and getting off the table after treatment.

Detrol, **Detrol LA** (tolterodine)   Medication used to treat urinary frequency, urgency, and incontinence. This medication is administered orally. The most common side effects are dizziness, drowsiness, constipation or diarrhea, nausea, joint pain, and headache. Abdominal massage that includes gliding and kneading strokes performed clockwise around the client's abdomen may help alleviate constipation. Face and scalp massage may help reduce headache. If the client is experiencing joint pain, then joint mobilization techniques are contraindicated.

Diflucan (fluconazole)   Antibiotic is administered orally. Generally, clients who have been taking antibiotics for at least 3 days are no longer considered contagious. However, if a question remains as to whether a client is contagious, then his or her physician should be consulted. If the client is contagious, then massage is contraindicated. The main side effect of Diflucan is headache, which face and scalp massage may help alleviate.

Digitalis   Medication used to treat congestive heart failure and abnormally high heart rate. This medication is administered orally. A gentle, relaxing treatment, possibly of shorter duration, is indicated for any client who has a cardiac disorder. Clearance from the client's health care practitioner is necessary before the client can receive massage. However, massage is contraindicated for a client with congestive heart failure. The main side effect of digitalis is hypotension. Clients who are taking digitalis are subject to orthostatic hypotension. The client should be asked if he or she needs assistance with positional changes such as getting on the table or sitting up and getting off the table after treatment.

Digoxin (digitalis)   Medication used to treat congestive heart failure and abnormally high heart rate. This medication is administered orally. A gentle, relaxing treatment, possibly of shorter duration, is indicated for any client who has a cardiac disorder. Clearance from the client's health care practitioner is necessary before the client can receive massage. However, massage is contraindicated for a client with congestive heart failure. The main side effect of Digoxin is hypotension. Clients who are taking Digoxin are subject to orthostatic hypotension. The client should be asked if he or she needs assistance with positional changes such as getting on the table or sitting up and getting off the table after treatment.

Dilantin (phenytoin)   Anticonvulsant used to treat seizures. Administered orally or by injection. Side effects include drowsiness, dizziness, restlessness, and irritability. Gentle, relaxing massage with light pressure is indicated. If the client has had an injection of Dilantin, then massage over the site is contraindicated for at least 10 days after the last injection because it may increase the medication's absorption rate. The client should be asked if he or she needs assistance with positional changes such as getting on the table or sitting up and getting off the table after treatment.

Ditropan XL (oxybutynin)   Medication used to treat urinary frequency, urgency, and incontinence. This medication is administered orally. The most common side effects are dizziness, drowsiness, constipation or diarrhea, nausea, joint pain, and headache. Abdominal massage that includes gliding and kneading strokes performed clockwise around the client's abdomen may help alleviate constipation. Face and scalp massage may help headache. If the client is experiencing joint pain, then joint mobilization techniques are contraindicated.

Estrace (estradiol tablets)   Synthetic estrogens used in hormone replacement therapy for menopausal symptoms, osteoporosis treatment and prevention, and sometimes breast cancer. No side effects occur that affect massage.

Estraderm (estradiol)   Synthetic estrogens used in hormone replacement therapy for menopausal symptoms, osteoporosis treatment and prevention, and sometimes breast cancer. No side effects occur that affect massage.

Flomax (tamsulosin)   Medication used to treat urinary retention and enlarged prostate; should be taken only by men. This medication is administered orally. The most common side effects include dizziness, orthostatic hypotension, and vasodilation of skin blood vessels (flushing). The client should be asked if he or she needs assistance with positional changes such as getting on the table or sitting up and getting off the table after treatment.

Glucophage (metformin)   Antidiabetic medication used to treat type 2 (non–insulin-dependent) diabetes. This medication is administered orally. If the client is experiencing neuropathy as a side effect from diabetes, then lighter massage is indicated over the affected areas. A side effect could be hypoglycemia. The client should have a sugar source, such as candy or juice, within easy reach should hypoglycemia occur during the massage.

Glucotrol (glipizide), **Glucotrol XL** (glipizide extended-release)   Antidiabetic medication used to treat type 2 (non–insulin-dependent) diabetes. This medication is administered orally. If the client is experiencing neuropathy as a side effect from diabetes, then lighter massage is indicated over the affected areas. A side effect could be hypoglycemia. The client should have a sugar source, such as candy or juice, within easy reach should hypoglycemia occur during the massage.

Humulin (insulin)   Antidiabetic medication used to treat type 1 (insulin-dependent) diabetes; also often prescribed for people with type 2 (non–insulin-dependent) diabetes. This medication is administered by injection. Massage over the injection site is contraindicated because it may increase the medication's absorption rate. A major side effect of insulin injection could be hypoglycemia. The client should have a sugar source, such as candy or juice, within easy reach should hypoglycemia occur during the massage.

Ibuprofen   NSAID used to reduce inflammation, relieve pain, and reduce fever. Side effects include dizziness and drowsiness. A gentle, relaxing massage is indicated. The client should be asked if he or she needs assistance with positional changes such as getting on the table or sitting up and getting off the table after treatment.

Inderal (propranolol)   Beta blocker used to treat angina pectoris, hypertension, hypertrophic cardiomyopathy, irregular heartbeat, migraine headaches, anxiety, tremors, overproduction of thyroid hormones, and glaucoma. This medication is administered orally. A gentle, relaxing treatment, possibly of shorter duration, is indicated for any client who has a cardiac disorder. Clearance from the client's health care practitioner is necessary before the client can receive massage. The main side effect of Inderal is hypotension. Clients who are taking Inderal are subject to orthostatic hypotension. The client should be asked if he or she needs assistance with positional changes such as getting on the table or sitting up and getting off the table after treatment.

Insulin   Antidiabetic medication used to treat type 1 (insulin-dependent) diabetes; often also prescribed for people with type 2 (non–insulin-dependent) diabetes. Medication is administered by injection. Massage over the injection site is contraindicated because it may increase the medication's absorption rate. A major side effect of insulin injection could be hypoglycemia. The client should have a sugar source, such as candy or juice, within easy reach should hypoglycemia occur during the massage.

Keflex (cephalexin)   Antibiotic is administered orally. Generally, clients who have been taking antibiotics for at least 3 days are no longer considered contagious. However, if a question remains as to whether a client is contagious, then his or her physician should be consulted. If the client is contagious, then massage is contraindicated. The main side effects of Keflex are digestive tract upset and diarrhea. If the client is experiencing discomfort from these side effects, then abdominal massage may be contraindicated.

Keppra (levetiracetam)   Anticonvulsant used to treat seizures. This medication is administered orally. Side effects include drowsiness, dizziness, restlessness, and irritability. Gentle, relaxing massage with light pressure is indicated. The client should be asked if he or she needs assistance with positional changes such as getting on the table or sitting up and getting off the table after treatment.

Lamisil (terbinafine hydrochloride)   Antifungal medication is administered orally. The main side effects are nausea, heartburn, diarrhea, and headache. If the client is experiencing heartburn and acid reflux, then he or she may need to be propped in a semireclining position to enable gravity to help keep stomach acid from refluxing into his or her esophagus. Face and scalp massage may help alleviate headache.

Lanoxin (digoxin)   Medication used to treat congestive heart failure and abnormally high heart rate. This medication is administered orally. A gentle, relaxing treatment, possibly of shorter duration, is indicated for any client who has a cardiac disorder. Clearance from the client's health care practitioner is necessary before the client can receive massage. However, massage is contraindicated for a client with congestive heart failure. The main side effect of Lanoxin is hypotension. Clients who are taking Lanoxin are subject to orthostatic hypotension. The client should be asked if he or she needs assistance with positional changes such as getting on the table or sitting up and getting off the table after treatment.

Lantus (insulin)   Antidiabetic medication used to treat type 1 (insulin-dependent) diabetes; occasionally prescribed for people with type 2 (non–insulin-dependent) diabetes. This medication is administered by injection. Massage over the injection site is contraindicated because it may increase the medication's absorption rate. A major side effect of insulin injection could be hypoglycemia. The client should have a sugar source, such as candy or juice, within easy reach should hypoglycemia occur during the massage.

Lasix (furosemide)   Diuretic used to treat high blood pressure and edema that results from congestive heart failure. This medication is administered orally. A gentle, relaxing treatment, possibly of shorter duration, is indicated for any client who has a cardiac disorder. Clearance from the client's health care practitioner is necessary before the client can receive massage. However, massage is contraindicated for a client with congestive heart failure. The main side effects of Lasix are muscle cramps because of a loss of electrolytes and orthostatic hypotension. The client may require careful positioning, such as a bolster or pillow under the knees in supine position and under the ankles in prone position, to prevent muscle cramping during the treatment. In addition, because deep pressure can sometimes cause muscle cramping, it should be avoided for this reason and because it is contraindicated for those with congestive heart failure. The client should be asked if he or she needs assistance with positional changes such as getting on the table or sitting up and getting off the table after treatment. Because diuretics cause an increase in urine production, the client taking Lasix may need to use the bathroom frequently during the massage.

Levoxyl (levothyroxine sodium) Synthetic thyroid hormone used to treat hypothyroidism, goiters, and thyroid cancer. This medication is administered orally. The main side effects are anxiety and insomnia. A gentle, relaxing massage is indicated.

Lipitor (atorvastatin) Medication used to lower blood cholesterol levels. This medication is administered orally. The main side effects are nausea and heartburn. If a client taking Lipitor is subject to these side effects, then he or she may need to be propped in a semireclining position to enable gravity to help keep stomach acid from refluxing into the client's esophagus.

Lithium (lithium carbonate, lithium citrate) Medication used as a mood stabilizer in the treatment of bipolar disorder, mania, and depression. Can also be prescribed along with other antidepressant medications. Lithium is also sometimes prescribed for migraine and cluster headaches. This medication is administered orally. A host of side effects may result from taking lithium. The most common are dizziness, drowsiness, slow reactions, hypotension, and rash. A rash is a local contraindication for massage. A gentle, relaxing massage is indicated. The client should be asked if he or she needs assistance with positional changes such as getting on the table or sitting up and getting off the table after treatment.

Lopid (gemfibrozil) Medication used to lower blood cholesterol levels. This medication is administered orally. The main side effect is constipation, which may be alleviated by abdominal massage that includes gliding and kneading strokes performed clockwise around the client's abdomen.

Lopressor (metoprolol) Beta blocker used to treat angina pectoris, hypertension, hypertrophic cardiomyopathy, irregular heartbeat, migraine headaches, anxiety, tremors, overproduction of thyroid hormones, and glaucoma. This medication is administered orally. A gentle, relaxing treatment, possibly of shorter duration, is indicated for any client who has a cardiac disorder. Clearance from the client's health care practitioner is necessary before the client can receive massage. The main side effect of a beta blocker is hypotension. Clients who are taking Lopressor are subject to orthostatic hypotension. The client should be asked if he or she needs assistance with positional

changes such as getting on the table or sitting up and getting off the table after treatment.

Lotensin (benazepril hydrochloride) Medication used to treat hypertension. This medication is administered orally. The main side effect is hypotension. Clients who are taking Lotensin are subject to orthostatic hypotension. The client should be asked if he or she needs assistance with positional changes such as getting on the table or sitting up and getting off the table after treatment.

Micronase (glyburide) Antidiabetic medication used to treat type 2 (non–insulin-dependent) diabetes. This medication is administered orally. If the client is experiencing neuropathy as a side effect from diabetes, then lighter massage is indicated over the affected areas. A side effect could be hypoglycemia. The client should have a sugar source, such as candy or juice, within easy reach should hypoglycemia occur during the massage.

Morphine (morphine sulfate) Narcotic used to relieve severe acute and chronic pain and pain associated with terminal illness. Morphine can also be used to treat shortness of breath from pulmonary edema and congestive heart failure. Usually administered orally or by injection. Narcotic pain relievers affect the brain and the perception of pain. Many side effects are associated with narcotic pain relievers. The most common are drowsiness, hypotension, constipation, and euphoria. The euphoria is part of the altered perception of pain. For a client taking morphine, clearance from the client's health care practitioner is necessary before the client can receive massage. The massage therapist should closely monitor the client's verbal and nonverbal responses to the pressure being applied during the massage treatment and adjust the pressure accordingly. For a terminally ill client taking morphine, the massage treatment should be dictated by whatever the client wants and needs. If the client has had an injection of morphine, then massage over the site is contraindicated for at least 10 days after the last injection. Massage over a recent injection site may increase the medication's absorption rate. Abdominal massage that includes gliding and kneading strokes performed clockwise around the client's abdomen may help alleviate constipation. The client should be asked if he or she needs assistance with positional changes such as getting on the table or sitting up and getting off the table after treatment.

Motrin (ibuprofen) NSAID used to reduce inflammation, relieve pain, and reduce fever. Side effects include dizziness and drowsiness. The client should be asked if he or she needs assistance with positional changes such as getting on the table or sitting up and getting off the table after treatment.

Naprosyn (naproxen sodium) NSAID used to reduce inflammation, relieve pain, and reduce fever. Side effects include dizziness and drowsiness. The client should be asked if he or she needs assistance with positional changes such as getting on the table or sitting up and getting off the table after treatment.

Nexium (esomeprazole) Medication used to relieve heartburn and acid reflux. This medication is administered orally. If the client is experiencing heartburn and acid reflux, then he or she may need to be propped in a semireclining position to enable gravity to help keep stomach acid from refluxing into his or her esophagus. The main side effect is constipation, which abdominal massage that includes gliding and kneading strokes performed clockwise around the client's abdomen may help alleviate.

Nitro-Dur (nitroglycerin) Medication used to relieve and prevent angina pectoris. Can be administered orally, or the medication can be delivered through the skin through the use of ointments or transdermal patches. A gentle, relaxing treatment, possibly of shorter duration, is indicated for any client who has a cardiac disorder. Clearance from the client's health care practitioner is necessary before the client can receive massage. If the client uses a nitroglycerin ointment or transdermal patch, then massage over or near the application site or patch is contraindicated. The main side effects of nitroglycerin are orthostatic hypotension, dizziness, weakness, and vasodilation of skin blood vessels (flushing). The client should be asked if he or she needs assistance with positional changes such as getting on the table or sitting up and getting off the table after treatment.

Nitrogard (nitroglycerin) Medication used to relieve and prevent angina pectoris. This medication is administered orally. A gentle, relaxing treatment, possibly of shorter duration, is indicated for any client who has a cardiac disorder. Clearance from the client's health care practitioner is necessary before the client can receive massage. The main side effects of nitroglycerin are orthostatic hypotension, dizziness, weakness, and vasodilation of skin blood vessels (flushing). The client should be asked if he or she needs assistance with positional changes such as getting on the table or sitting up and getting off the table after treatment.

Nitroglycerin Medication used to relieve and prevent angina pectoris. Can be administered orally, or the medication can be delivered through the skin through the use of ointments or transdermal patches. A gentle, relaxing treatment, possibly of shorter duration, is indicated for any client who has a cardiac disorder. Clearance from the client's health care practitioner is necessary before the client can receive massage. If the client uses a nitroglycerin ointment or transdermal patch, then massage over or near the application site or patch is contraindicated. The main side effects of nitroglycerin are orthostatic hypotension, dizziness, weakness, and vasodilation of skin blood vessels (flushing). The client should be asked if he or she needs assistance with positional changes such as getting on the table or sitting up and getting off the table after treatment.

Nitrostat (nitroglycerin) Medication used to relieve and prevent angina pectoris. This medication can be administered orally or delivered through the skin through the use of ointments or transdermal patches. A gentle, relaxing treatment, possibly of shorter duration, is indicated for any client who has a cardiac disorder. Clearance from the client's health care practitioner is necessary before the client can receive massage. If the client uses a nitroglycerin ointment or transdermal patch, then massage over or near the application site or patch is contraindicated. The main side effects of nitroglycerin are orthostatic hypotension, dizziness, weakness, and vasodilation of skin blood vessels (flushing). The client should be asked if he or she needs assistance with positional changes such as getting on the table or sitting up and getting off the table after treatment.

Novolin (insulin) Antidiabetic medication used to treat type 1 (insulin-dependent) diabetes; often also prescribed for people with type 2 (non–insulin-dependent) diabetes. This medication is administered by injection. Massage over the injection site is contraindicated for at least 10 days after the last injection. Massage over a recent injection site may increase the medication's absorption rate. A major side effect of insulin injection could be hypoglycemia. The client should have a sugar source, such as candy or juice, within easy reach should hypoglycemia occur during the massage.

Orapred (prednisolone) Corticosteroid used to treat inflammation, which can occur with allergies, asthma, and certain types of arthritis. This corticosteroid is also prescribed to suppress immune responses. This medication is administered orally. If used for a short period, such as for acute conditions, then serious side effects do not usually occur. If, however, it is being administered for chronic conditions, then severe effects such as osteoporosis, slow wound healing, easy bruising, muscle wasting, and possibly Cushing's syndrome may occur. If any of these effects are present, then massage is contraindicated; the client needs to be referred to his or her health care practitioner. Clearance from the client's health care practitioner is necessary before the client can receive massage. If clearance is given, then a lighter massage, possibly of shorter duration, is indicated.

Ortho Evra (norelgestromin/ethinyl estradiol transdermal system) Combination of estrogens and progesterone used for birth control. This medication is administered through a transdermal patch. Massage over or near the patch is contraindicated. Side effects can include headache, breast swelling and tenderness, nausea, and leg cramps. Face and scalp massage may help alleviate headache. Propping with a soft pillow under the chest when prone may be more comfortable for the client. If the client is experiencing leg cramps, then propping the legs up when supine may help. A serious side effect of Ortho Evra is an increased chance of blood clots and phlebitis, most often in the legs. Signs and symptoms include redness, heat, swelling, and pain. If any of these signs are present, then the client needs to be referred to her health care practitioner. Phlebitis is a local contraindication for massage. For blood clots, deep, vigorous massage in the area is contraindicated because of the danger of dislodging the clot.

Ortho Tri-Cyclen (norgestimate/ethinyl estradiol) Combination of estrogens and progesterone used for birth control. This medication is administered orally. Side effects can include headache, breast swelling and tenderness, nausea, and leg cramps. Face and scalp massage may help alleviate headache. Propping with a soft pillow under the chest when prone may be more comfortable for the client. If the client is experiencing leg cramps, then propping the legs up when supine may help. A serious side effect is an increased chance of blood clots and phlebitis, most often in the legs. Signs and symptoms include redness, heat, swelling, and pain. If any of these signs are present, then the client needs to be referred to her health care practitioner. Phlebitis is a local contraindication for massage. For blood clots, deep, vigorous massage in the area is contraindicated because of the danger of dislodging the clot.

OxyContin (oxycodone hydrochloride) Narcotic used to relieve severe acute and chronic pain. This medication is usually administered orally. Narcotic pain relievers affect the brain and the perception of pain. Many side effects are associated with narcotic pain relievers. The most common are drowsiness, hypotension, constipation, and euphoria. The euphoria is part of the altered perception of pain. Therefore the massage therapist should closely monitor the client's verbal and nonverbal responses to the pressure being applied during the massage treatment and adjust the pressure accordingly. Abdominal massage that includes gliding and kneading strokes performed clockwise around the client's abdomen may help alleviate constipation. The client should be asked if he or she needs assistance with positional changes such as getting on the table or sitting up and getting off the table after treatment.

Paxil (paroxetine HCl) Medication used to treat depression. This medication is administered orally. Side effects include drowsiness, anxiety, insomnia, and orthostatic hypotension. The client should be asked if he or she needs assistance with positional changes such as getting on the table or sitting up and getting off the table after treatment.

Penicillin Oral antibiotic, but it can be administered by injection. Generally, clients who have been taking antibiotics for at least 3 days are no longer considered contagious. However, if a question as to whether a client is contagious remains, then his or her physician should be consulted. If the client is contagious, then massage is contraindicated. If a client received an injection of penicillin, then massage over the injection site is contraindicated for at least 10 days after the last injection because it may increase the medication's absorption rate. The main side effects are digestive tract upset and diarrhea. If the client is experiencing discomfort from these side effects, then abdominal massage may be contraindicated.

Pepcid (famotidine) Medication used to relieve heartburn and acid reflux. This medication is administered orally. If the client is experiencing heartburn and acid reflux, then he or she may need to be propped in a semireclining position to enable gravity to help keep stomach acid from refluxing into his or her esophagus. The main side effect is constipation, which abdominal massage that includes gliding and kneading strokes performed clockwise around the client's abdomen may help alleviate.

Percocet (oxycodone and acetaminophen) Narcotic used to relieve severe acute and chronic pain. This medication is usually administered orally. Narcotic pain relievers affect the brain and the perception of pain. Many side effects are associated with narcotic pain relievers. The most common effects are drowsiness, hypotension, constipation, and euphoria. The euphoria is part of the altered perception of pain. Therefore the massage therapist should closely monitor the client's verbal and nonverbal responses to the pressure being applied during the massage treatment and adjust the pressure accordingly. Abdominal massage that includes gliding and kneading strokes performed clockwise around the client's abdomen may help alleviate constipation. The client should be asked if he or she needs assistance with positional changes such as getting on the table or sitting up and getting off the table after treatment.

Plavix (clopidogrel) Anticoagulant used to prevent blood clot formation. This medication is prescribed for people who are at risk for conditions that can result from blood clots such as myocardial infarction (MI) or heart attack, angina pectoris, stroke, and peripheral vascular disease. This medication is administered orally. Side effects include heartburn, constipation, and easy bruising. If the client taking Plavix is subject to these, then he or she may need to be propped in a semireclining position to enable gravity to help keep stomach acid from refluxing into the client's esophagus, and lighter pressure during the massage is indicated. Abdominal massage that includes gliding and kneading strokes performed clockwise around the client's abdomen may help alleviate constipation.

Prednisone Corticosteroid used to treat inflammation that may occur with allergies, asthma, and certain types of arthritis. It is also used to suppress immune responses. This medication is administered orally or by injection. If a client has received an injection of prednisone, then massage over the injection site is contraindicated for at least 10 days after the last injection because it may increase the medication's absorption rate. If used for a short period for acute conditions, then serious side effects do not usually occur. If, however, it is being taken for chronic conditions, then severe effects, such as osteoporosis, slow wound healing, easy bruising, muscle wasting, and possibly Cushing's syndrome, may develop. If any of these effects are present, then massage is contraindicated, and the client needs to be referred to his or her health care practitioner. Clearance from the client's health care practitioner is necessary before the client can receive massage.

If clearance is given, then a lighter massage, possibly of shorter duration, is indicated.

Premarin (conjugated estrogens)   Synthetic estrogens used in hormone replacement therapy for menopausal symptoms, osteoporosis treatment and prevention, and sometimes for breast cancer. This medication is administered orally or as a vaginal cream. Side effects can include headache, breast swelling and tenderness, nausea, and leg cramps. Face and scalp massage may help alleviate headache. Propping with a soft pillow under the chest when prone may be more comfortable for the client. If the client is experiencing leg cramps, then propping the legs up when supine may help. Lighter pressure over the legs is indicated. A serious side effect is an increased chance of blood clots and phlebitis, most often in the legs. Signs and symptoms include redness, heat, swelling, and pain. If any of these effects are present, then the client needs to be referred to her health care practitioner. Phlebitis is a local contraindication for massage. For blood clots, deep, vigorous massage in the area is contraindicated because of the danger of dislodging the clot.

Prempro (medroxyprogesterone with conjugated equine estrogens)   Synthetic progesterone used to treat perimenopausal and menopausal symptoms and premenstrual syndrome (PMS). This medication is administered orally. Side effects can include headache, breast swelling and tenderness, nausea, and leg cramps. Face and scalp massage may help alleviate headache. Propping with a soft pillow under the chest when prone may be more comfortable for the client. If the client is experiencing leg cramps, then propping the legs up when supine may also help. A serious side effect is an increased chance of blood clots and phlebitis, most often in the legs. Signs and symptoms include redness, heat, swelling, and pain. If any of these effects are present, then the client needs to be referred to her health care practitioner. Phlebitis is a local contraindication for massage. For blood clots, deep, vigorous massage in the area is contraindicated because of the danger of dislodging the clot.

Prevacid (lansoprazole)   Medication used to relieve heartburn and acid reflux. This medication is administered orally. If the client is experiencing heartburn and acid reflux, then he or she may need to be propped in a semireclining position to enable gravity to help keep stomach acid from refluxing into his or her esophagus.

Prilosec (omeprazole delayed-release)   Medication used to relieve heartburn and acid reflux. This medication is administered orally. If the client is experiencing heartburn and acid reflux, then he or she may need to be propped in a semireclining position to enable gravity to help keep stomach acid from refluxing into his or her esophagus. The main side effect is constipation, which abdominal massage with gliding and kneading strokes performed clockwise around the client's abdomen may help alleviate.

Primatene Mist (epinephrine)   Bronchodilator used to treat an asthma attack. This medication is administered through an inhaler. Side effects can include restlessness, anxiety, dizziness, headache, insomnia, weakness, tremors, and heart palpitations. If a client is experiencing these effects, then a gentle massage with long, gliding strokes may help the client relax and possibly alleviate the side effects.

Procrit (epoetin alfa)   Medication stimulates red blood cell formation and is used to treat anemia caused by renal failure, certain types of leukemia, and anemia that occurs with certain medications for human immunodeficiency viral (HIV) infection. This medication is administered by injection. Side effects include fatigue, weakness, muscle pain, and weakness. For a client taking Procrit, clearance from the client's health care practitioner is necessary before the client can receive massage. If clearance is given, then a lighter massage, possibly of shorter duration, is indicated. Massage over the injection site is contraindicated for at least 10 days after the last injection because it may increase the medication's absorption rate. The client should be asked if he or she needs assistance with positional changes such as getting on the table or sitting up and getting off the table after treatment.

Prometrium (micronized progesterone)   Synthetic progesterone used to treat perimenopausal and menopausal symptoms and PMS. This medication is administered orally. Side effects can include headache, breast swelling and tenderness, nausea, and leg cramps. Face and scalp massage may help alleviate headache. Propping with a soft pillow under the chest when prone may be more comfortable for the client. If the client is experiencing leg cramps, then propping the legs up when supine may help. A serious side effect is an increased chance of blood clots and phlebitis, most often in the legs. Signs and symptoms include redness, heat, swelling, and pain. If any of these effects are present, then the client needs to be referred to her health care practitioner. Phlebitis is a local contraindication for massage. For blood clots, deep, vigorous massage in the area is contraindicated because of the danger of dislodging the clot.

Proventil (albuterol inhaler)   Bronchodilator used to treat an asthma attack. This medication is administered orally or through an inhaler. Side effects can include restlessness, anxiety, dizziness, headache, insomnia, weakness, tremors, and heart palpitations. If a client is experiencing these signs, then a gentle massage with long, gliding strokes may help the client relax and possibly alleviate the side effects.

Provera (medroxyprogesterone acetate)   Synthetic progesterone used to treat perimenopausal and menopausal symptoms and PMS. This medication is administered orally. Side effects can include headache, breast swelling and tenderness, nausea, and leg cramps. Face and scalp massage may help alleviate headache. Propping with a soft pillow under the chest when prone may be more comfortable for the client. If the client is experiencing leg cramps, then propping the legs up when supine may help. A serious side effect is an increased chance of blood clots and phlebitis, most often in the legs. Signs and symptoms include redness, heat, swelling, and pain. If any of these effects are present, then the client needs to be referred to her health care practitioner. Phlebitis is a local contraindication for massage. For blood clots, deep, vigorous massage in the area is contraindicated because of the danger of dislodging the clot.

Prozac (fluoxetine) Medication used to treat depression. This medication is administered orally. Side effects include drowsiness, anxiety, insomnia, and orthostatic hypotension. The client should be asked if he or she needs assistance with positional changes such as getting on the table or sitting up and getting off the table after treatment.

Restoril (temazepam) Medication used to treat insomnia, anxiety, and tension, including muscle tension. Although usually administered orally, this medication may be administered by injection if rapid action is desired. If a client has received an injection of Restoril, then massage over the injection site is contraindicated for at least 10 days after the last injection because it may increase the medication's absorption rate. Side effects include fatigue, dizziness, drowsiness, and hypotension. The client should be asked if he or she needs assistance with positional changes, such as getting on the table or sitting up and getting off the table after treatment.

Ritalin (methylphenidate) Medication used to treat attention deficit disorder (ADD), attention deficit hyperactivity disorder (ADHD), and narcolepsy. This medication is administered orally. Side effects include drowsiness, dizziness, blurred vision, and impaired concentration. The client should be asked if he or she needs assistance with positional changes such as getting on the table or sitting up and getting off the table after treatment.

Starlix (nateglinide) Antidiabetic medication used to treat type 2 (non–insulin-dependent) diabetes. This medication is administered orally. If the client is experiencing neuropathy as a side effect from diabetes, then a lighter massage is indicated over the affected areas. A side effect could be hypoglycemia. The client should have a sugar source, such as candy or juice, within easy reach should hypoglycemia occur during the massage.

Synthroid (levothyroxine sodium) Synthetic thyroid hormone used to treat hypothyroidism, goiters, and thyroid cancer. This medication is administered orally. The main side effects are anxiety and insomnia. A gentle, relaxing massage may be indicated.

Tagamet (cimetidine) Medication used to relieve heartburn and acid reflux. This medication is administered orally. If the client is experiencing heartburn and acid reflux, then he or she may need to be propped in a semireclining position to enable gravity to help keep stomach acid from refluxing into his or her esophagus. The main side effect is constipation, which abdominal massage that includes gliding and kneading strokes

performed clockwise around the client's abdomen may help alleviate.

Tegretol (carbamazepine) Anticonvulsant used to treat seizures. This medication is administered orally. Side effects include drowsiness, dizziness, fatigue, hypotension, and dry mouth. The client may need to drink water during the massage. The client should be asked if he or she needs assistance with positional changes such as getting on the table or sitting up and getting off the table after treatment.

Tetracycline Antibiotic is administered orally. Generally, clients who have been taking antibiotics for at least 3 days are no longer considered contagious. However, if a question remains as whether a client is contagious, then his or her physician should be consulted. If the client is contagious, then massage is contraindicated. The main side effects of tetracycline are digestive tract upset and diarrhea. If the client is experiencing discomfort from these side effects, then abdominal massage may be contraindicated.

Transderm-Nitro (nitroglycerin) Medication used to relieve and prevent angina pectoris. This medication is administered through a transdermal patch. A gentle, relaxing treatment, possibly of shorter duration, is indicated for any client who has a cardiac disorder. Clearance from the client's health care practitioner is necessary before the client can receive massage. Massage over or near the patch is contraindicated. The main side effects of nitroglycerin are orthostatic hypotension, dizziness, weakness, and vasodilation of skin blood vessels (flushing). The client should be asked if he or she needs assistance with positional changes such as getting on the table or sitting up and getting off the table after treatment.

Tricor (fenofibrate) Medication used to lower blood cholesterol levels. This medication is administered orally. The main side effect is constipation, which abdominal massage that includes gliding and kneading strokes performed clockwise around the client's abdomen may help alleviate.

Tylenol (acetaminophen) Medication used to reduce pain and fever. This medication is administered orally. No side effects occur that affect massage.

Valium (diazepam) Medication used to treat insomnia, anxiety, and tension, including muscle tension. Usually an oral medication, but Valium may be also be administered by injection if rapid action is desired. If a client has received an injection of Valium, then massage over the injection site is contraindicated for at least 10 days after the last injection because it may increase the medication's absorption rate. Side effects include fatigue, dizziness, drowsiness, and hypotension. The client should be asked if he or she needs assistance with positional changes such as getting on the table or sitting up and getting off the table after treatment.

Valtrex (valacyclovir) Antiviral medication administered orally. The main side effect is headache, which face and scalp massage may help alleviate.

Vasotec (enalapril) Medication used to treat high blood pressure. This medication is administered orally. The main side effects are dizziness and hypotension. Clients who are taking Vasotec are subject to orthostatic hypotension. The client should be asked if he or she needs assistance with positional changes such as getting on the table or sitting up and getting off the table after treatment.

Vicodin (hydrocodone and acetaminophen) Narcotic used to relieve severe acute and chronic pain. This medication is usually administered orally. Narcotic pain relievers affect the brain and the perception of pain. Many side effects are associated with narcotic pain relievers. The most common are drowsiness, hypotension, constipation, and euphoria. The euphoria is part of the altered perception of pain. Therefore the massage therapist should closely monitor the client's verbal and nonverbal responses to the pressure being applied during the massage treatment and adjust the pressure accordingly. Abdominal massage that includes gliding and kneading strokes performed clockwise around the client's abdomen may help alleviate constipation. The client should be asked if he or she needs assistance with positional changes such as getting on the table or sitting up and getting off the table after treatment.

Wellbutrin and **Wellbutrin SR** (bupropion, bupropion extended-release) Medication used to treat depression. This medication is administered orally. Side effects include dizziness, drowsiness, constipation, and orthostatic hypotension. Abdominal massage that includes gliding and kneading strokes performed clockwise around the client's abdomen may help alleviate constipation. The client should be asked if he or she needs assistance with positional changes such as getting on the table or sitting up and getting off the table after treatment.

Xanax (alprazolam) Medication used to treat insomnia, anxiety, and tension, including muscle tension. This medi-cation is administered orally. Side effects include fatigue, dizziness, drowsiness, and hypotension. The client should be asked if he or she needs assistance with positional changes such as getting on the table or sitting up and getting off the table after treatment.

Zantac (ranitidine) Medication used to relieve heartburn and acid reflux. This medication is administered orally. If the client is experiencing heartburn and acid reflux, then he or she may need to be propped in a semireclining position to enable gravity to help keep stomach acid from refluxing into his or her esophagus. The main side effect is constipation, which abdominal massage that includes gliding and kneading strokes performed clockwise around the client's abdomen may help alleviate.

Zocor (simvastatin) Medication used to lower blood cholesterol levels. This medication is administered orally. The main side effects are nausea and heartburn. If a client taking Zocor is subject to these, then he or she may need to be propped in a semireclining position to enable gravity to help keep stomach acid from refluxing into the client's esophagus.

Zoloft (sertraline) Medication used to treat depression. This medication is administered orally. Side effects include drowsiness, anxiety, insomnia, and orthostatic hypotension. The client should be asked if he or she needs assistance with positional changes such as getting on the table or sitting up and getting off the table after treatment.

Zyrtec, **Zyrtec-D** (cetirizine) Antihistamine used to treat allergies. This medication is administered orally. Side effects include dizziness, fatigue, and sometimes hypotension. If the client is experiencing these symptoms, then the client should be asked if he or she needs assistance with positional changes such as getting on the table or sitting up and getting off the table after treatment.

Glossary

Abdominal Relating to the anterior trunk or area between the thorax and the pelvis

Abduction Movement away from the median plane

Absolute contraindication Condition in which massage is inappropriate, not advised, and may be harmful to the client

Absorption Process by which products of digestion move into the bloodstream or lymph vessels and then into the body's cells

Accounting Art of interpreting, measuring, and describing economic activity

Acetabulum Hip socket with the ilium, ischium, and pubic bones contributing equally to its makeup

Acetylcholine Neurotransmitter involved in muscle contraction

Acquired immunity Diverse but specific response to invading pathogens involving lymphocytes

Acromial Relating to the top of the shoulder

Active-assisted movements Movements that the client performs while the therapist assists

Active movements Movements that the therapist describes or demonstrates while the client actively performs the movement; types are *active-assisted* and *active-resisted* movements

Active-resisted movements Movements whereby the therapist applies gentle resistance while the client is actively engaged in the movement

Active transport Movement of atoms and molecules such as ions against the concentration gradient from low levels to high levels, the mechanism of which is both chemical and physical

Active trigger point Trigger point that causes pain even at rest

Acupoint See *Tsubo*

Acute disease Disease with abrupt onset of severe symptoms that run a brief course (less than 6 months) and then resolve or, in some cases, bring death

Acute injury Injury that begins abruptly, usually having a recognizable cause and characterized by severe symptoms such as pain, swelling, and loss of function

Adaptation Decrease in sensitivity to a prolonged stimulus

Adduction Movement toward the median plane

Adenosine triphosphate Molecule involved in muscle contraction

Adipose tissue Connective tissue specialized for fat storage that includes yellow bone marrow; also insulates the body against heat loss, provides fuel reserves for energy, and provides a cushion around certain structures (e.g., heart, kidneys, some joints)

Adrenal cortex Outer region of the adrenals

Adrenal gland Gland located superior to each kidney

Adrenal medulla Inner region of the adrenals

Adrenocorticotropic hormone Pituitary hormone regulating endocrine activity of the adrenal cortex

Advertising Making your business noticeable to the public by purchasing print space or broadcast media time

Agonist Muscle most responsible for causing a specific or desired action

Aldosterone Adrenal hormone that stimulates kidneys to conserve sodium, which triggers the release of antidiuretic hormone and results in water retention, helps maintain proper mineral balance, and monitors blood volume

Alimentary canal Muscular passageway leading from the mouth to the anus

All-or-none response Physiological response whereby each individual muscle fiber, when sufficiently stimulated, contracts to its fullest extent or not at all

Alveoli Tiny sacs attached to alveolar ducts within the lungs

Amino acids Building blocks of protein

Amma Precursor to all other therapies, manual and energetic—the grandparent of all massage techniques

Amphiarthrosis (cartilaginous) joint Joint that is slightly movable

Anal canal Canal leading from the rectum to the anus

Analgesics Agents that reduce pain

Anatomic position Standard body position used in Western medicine, with the body erect and facing forward, arms to the side, palms facing forward, thumbs to the side, feet approximately hip distance apart, and with toes pointing forward

Anatomy Study of the structures of the human body and their positional relationship to one another

Antagonist Muscle that must relax and stretch or eccentrically contract to allow actions of the agonist to occur

Antebrachial Relating to the forearm area between wrist and elbow

Antecubital   Relating to the space in front of elbow or at the bend of the elbow

Anterior   Pertaining to the front side of a structure

Anterior fontanel   Diamond-shaped membrane located where the coronal suture and sagittal sutures meet and will completely ossify by 18 to 24 months of age

Antidiuretic hormone (vasopressin)   Pituitary hormone that promotes water retention by the kidneys

Antimicrobial disposable wipes   Special wipes that destroy microscopic organisms that can cause diseases, such as staphylococci, streptococci, common cold and influenza viruses, herpesvirus, human immunodeficiency virus (HIV), and tuberculosis

Anus   Terminal end of the gastrointestinal tract

Aortic semilunar valve   Valve between the left ventricle and the aorta

Aponeurosis   Broad, flat tendon

Arachnoid   Middle meningeal layer

Archer stance   See *Bow stance*

Areolar connective tissue   Connective tissue that is widely distributed and possesses little tensile strength forming the subcutaneous layer

Aromatherapy   Use of plant-derived essential oils for therapeutic purposes

Arrhythmia   Any deviation from a normal heart rate pattern

Arteriole   Small-sized arteries

Artery   Vessel that moves blood away from the heart

Articular cartilage   Hyaline cartilage covering an epiphysis

Articulation (arthrosis)   Two bones joined together

Asclepiades   Founder of the group of ancient Greek physicians known as the Methodists

Asclepius   Greek physician who was believed to have evolved into a god and whose holy snake and staff are the symbol of the medical profession

Asian bodywork therapy   Treatment of the body, mind, and spirit by pressure and/or manipulation and includes the body's energetic field

Assessment   Process involved in appraising a client's condition based on subjective reporting and objective findings

Astrocyte   Neuroglia cell used for structural support of central nervous system's neurons; part of the blood-brain barrier

Athlete   Someone who possesses natural or acquired abilities such as strength, endurance, or agility required for participating in a sport

Atrial natriuretic hormone   Hormone that decreases blood volume and blood pressure

Atrium   Superior heart chamber

Attachment trigger point   Trigger point located at a musculotendinous junction caused by unrelieved tension of a central trigger point

Autoimmune disease   Disease marked by inappropriate or excessive response of the body's immune functions

Autonomic nervous system   Division of peripheral nervous system supplying impulses to smooth muscle, cardiac muscle, and glands

Avicenna (980-1037)   Name by which Persian physician Abu-Ali al-Husayn ibn-Sina was known in the West; authored over 100 books that compiled all the theoretical and practical medical knowledge of his time and was thus greatly influenced by the works of Galen of Pergamon

Axillary   Armpit region

Axon   Neural extension that carries nerve impulses away from the neuron toward another neuron, a muscle cell, or gland

Ayurveda   Hindu science of health and medicine designed to maintain or improve health through the use of dietary modification, massage, yoga, herbal preparations, and other measures

Ball-and-socket (triaxial) joint   Joint permitting all movements

Bath   Category of hydrotherapy encompassing partial or full immersion in (most often) water or heated air

Benign tumor   Noncancerous tumor

Biarticular   Term used to describe muscles that cross two joints

Bicuspid valve   See *Mitral valve*

Bile   Emulsifier of fat produced in the liver and stored in the gallbladder

Biogenic amine   Hormones that function as neurotransmitters and help regulate blood pressure, waste elimination, and body temperature

Birth canal   See *Vagina*

Blood   Fluid medium of plasma containing erythrocytes, leukocytes, and platelets

Blood pressure   Pressure exerted by blood on arterial walls during contraction of the left ventricle

Blood-brain barrier   Selective semipermeable wall of tissue that prevents or slows down the passage of some chemical compounds and disease-causing organisms from traveling from the blood into the central nervous system

Body mask   Application of mud or other products to most of the body

Body mechanics   Component of massage addressing issues of how the therapist stands and moves during the session to enhance treatment effectiveness and reduce injury risks

Body polish   Method of exfoliation using a fine grainy substance

Body scrub   Method of exfoliation using a dry natural bristle brush (or loofah) or grainy product

Body shampoo   Method of gently scrubbing the skin using a brush dipped in warm, soapy water

Bonding   A reciprocal relationship from the caregiver to the infant and from the infant to the caregiver

Bone marrow   Hollow center of bone

Bone   Connective tissue that consists of compact bone, spongy bone, collagenous fibers, and mineral salts

Bony marking   Place on bones where muscles, tendons, and ligaments attach and where nerve and blood vessels pass

Borelli, Giovanni Alfonso (1608-1679)   Italian anatomist who carried out extensive anatomic dissections and analyzed the phenomenon of muscular contraction

Boundary, professional   Differences between a client and therapists, creating a sense of separateness

Bow stance   Stance used when the therapist proceeds from one point to the next along the client's body with the therapist's feet placed on the floor in a 30- to 50-degree angle, one pointing straight forward *(lead foot—pointing in the direction of movement)* and the other pointing toward the side *(trailing foot)*

Bowman's capsule   Hollow cup-shaped mouth of a nephron

Brachial   Upper arm or area between the shoulder and the elbow

Bradycardia   Slow heart rate (≤50 beats per minute)

Brain   Organ that contains an estimated 100 billion neurons and is divided into four major regions: cerebrum, diencephalon, cerebellum, and brainstem

Brainstem   Structure that is continuous with the spinal cord and possesses three main divisions: midbrain, pons, and medulla oblongata

Breast   Gland consisting of a duct system for the passage of milk to the nipple

Breathing   Two-phase process consisting of inspiration and expiration

Bright, Timothy (c. 1551-1615)   British Renaissance–era physician who taught and published on the use of baths, exercise, and massage to restore health

Bronchi   Passageways from the trachea to each lung

Brunner's gland   Duodenal gland that secrete alkaline mucus

Buccal   Relating to the cheek area

Bulbourethral (Cowper's) gland   Gland located on either side of the prostate that secretes an alkaline substance, making up approximately 5% of semen volume

Bursa   Collapsed saclike structure with an interior lining of synovial membrane; contains synovial fluid

Calcaneal   Relating to the heel of the foot

Calcitonin   Thyroid hormone that increases calcium storage in bones by stimulating osteoblasts, lowering blood calcium levels

Calf (sural)   Posterior leg

Calorie (kilocalorie)   A unit of measure for the energy from a food; it is equal to the heat energy needed to raise the temperature of 1 kg of water by 1° C

Calyx   Cuplike structure protruding from the renal papilla; minor calyces join to form a major calyx that leads to the renal pelvis

Cancerous disease   Disease characterized by uncontrollable growth of abnormal cells most often with the development of a *neoplasm* or *tumor*

Capillary   Vessel between an arteriole and a venule that possess a thin, permeable membrane for efficient gas exchange

Carbohydrate   Also known as starches and sugars and are classified according to molecular structure as mono-, di-, and polysaccharides

Cardioesophageal sphincter   Sphincter located between the esophagus and stomach

Carpal   Relating to the wrist

Carrier oil   Fatty material used to *carry* one or more essential oil

Cartilage   Connective tissue found chiefly in the thorax, joints, and some rigid tubes of the body (trachea, larynx) that is tough and protective

Catecholamines   Chemical family containing norepinephrine, epinephrine, and dopamine that has a direct effect on the sympathetic nervous system

Caudal   See *Inferior*

Cecum   A small saclike structure that is the first section of the large intestine

Cell   Fundamental unit or building blocks of all living organisms and the simplest form of life that can exist as a self-sustaining unit

Cell body   Main region of the neuron containing the nucleus, ribosomes, and other organelles

Cell membrane   Membrane that separates cytoplasm from the surrounding external environment

Celsus, Aulus   Roman writer, considered to be the first important medical historian

Central   Pertaining to the center of the body

Central nervous system   Body system that includes the brain, meninges, cerebrospinal fluid, and spinal cord

Central trigger point   Trigger point that develops almost directly in the center of the muscle, often where the motor end plate innervates it at the neuromuscular junction

Centripetally   Toward the center

Cephalic   Pertaining to the head area

Cerebellum   Structure located posterior and inferior to the cerebrum concerned with muscle tone, coordinates skeletal muscles and balance, and controls fine and gross motor movements

Cerebrospinal fluid   Fluid circulating around the brain and spinal cord within the subarachnoid space that supplies tissues with oxygen and nutrients, carries away wastes, and acts as a shock absorber

Cerebrum   Largest part of the brain where vision, smell, taste, and body movements are consciously perceived, where skeletal muscle movements are initiated, and where emotional and intellectual processes occur

Cervical   Relating to the neck area

Chakra   In Ayurveda, one of seven energy centers in the body that receives, processes, and distributes energy and to keep the spiritual, mental, emotional, and physical health of the body in balance

Chi   In China, the energy of the body, mind, and spirit

Chief cell   Stomach's exocrine cell that produces pepsinogen, a precursor to pepsin

Cholecystokinin   Hormone produced by the intestinal mucosa that stimulates the gallbladder to release bile and the pancreas to secrete enzymes

Chronic disease (illness)   Disease that develops slowly and lasts 6 months or longer, in some cases, a lifetime; no cure is known

Chronic illness   See *Chronic disease*

Chronic injury   Injury that develops slowly and persists for long periods, sometimes the remainder of the individual's lifetime

Circumduction   Cone-shaped range of motion that occurs when the distal end moves in a circle and the proximal end is fixed

Class-1 lever   Lever in which the fulcrum is positioned between the effort and the resistance, similar to a seesaw

Class-2 lever   Lever in which the fulcrum is at one end, the resistance is in the middle, and the effort is at the opposite end, similar to a wheelbarrow

Class-3 lever   Lever in which the fulcrum is at one end, the effort is located in the center, and the resistance is at the opposite end, similar to sweeping with a broom

Client web   Diagram used to arrange information gathered in the assessment process

Clitoris   Small cylindrical mass of erectile tissue and nerves located at the anterior junction of the labia minora

Coccygeal   Relating to the bottom of the spine

Cocoa butter   Butter obtained from the cacao seed; also known as theobroma oil

Code of ethics   Set of guiding moral principles that members of particular professions are expected to follow

Cold mitten friction   See *Cold towel friction*

Cold towel friction   Ice application through towels dipped in icy water and applied to the body with friction movements

Collecting duct   Structure made up of the distal tubules of several nephrons that join several larger ducts to become the renal papilla

Communication   Act of exchanging information through words, actions, behaviors, body language, and feelings

Compact bone   Forms the periphery of bones providing protection, support, and resistance to stress of weight and movement

Compress   Cloth that has had water wrung from it and is applied to the skin's surface

Compression   Rhythmic pumping on the muscle

Concentric contraction   Type of isotonic contraction when contraction results in shortening of a muscle

Conduction   Exchange of thermal energy while the body's surface is in direct contact with the thermal agent or conductor

Confidentiality   Safekeeping or nondisclosure of privileged information

Congenital disorder   Disorder that is present at birth

Connective tissue   Tissue that makes up most of the body and helps transport nutrients, defends the body against disease, assists in blood clotting, and acts as a supportive framework

Contamination   Infectious agent residing on an organism

Contract   Written agreement between two or more parties that is enforceable by law and communicates expectations, duties, and responsibilities

Contraindication   Presence of a disease or physical condition making the act of treating a particular client in the usual manner impossible or undesirable

Contralateral   Related to opposite sides of the body

Contrast method   Combining heat and cold in the same treatment

Convection   Transfer of heat energy through movement of air or liquid

Conversion   One energy source changing (or converting) into a heat energy source as it passes into the body

Coronal plane   See *Frontal plane*

Coronal suture   Suture that separates the frontal bone from the parietal bones

Corpus callosum   Transverse fibers that connect and provide a communicative pathway between the two cerebral hemispheres

Cortisol (hydrocortisone)   Adrenal hormone that affects carbohydrate, protein, and fat metabolism; in large amounts, produces an antiinflammatory response

Costal   Relating to the ribs

Coughing   Sudden expulsion of air to clear the lungs and lower respiratory passageways of irritants or foreign materials

Coulter, John S.   American physician who, in 1926, became the first full-time academic physician in the field of physical medicine, which became known as physiatry or physical therapy

Countertransference   When the therapist brings his or her own unresolved issues or personal needs into the therapeutic relationship

Coxal   Relating to the hip region

Cranial (skull)   Relating to the head

Cranial nerve   Nerve originating from the brain

Cranial   See *Superior*

Cross-contamination   Passing of microorganisms from one person to another

Crural   Relating to the leg between the knee and ankle

Crying   Response to emotions involving a sudden inspiration followed by the release of air in short breaths

Cryokinetics   Application of a cold pack, ice immersion, or ice massage with or followed by full joint range of motion

Cryotherapy   External, therapeutic application of cold

Cubital   Relating to the elbow

Cun   Body inch in traditional Chinese medicine; the width of the client's own thumb knuckle

Cupping   In shiatsu, a method in which a warmed cup is placed upside down directly on the skin creating a vacuum that suctions the skin to relieve energy stagnation

Curriculum vitae   Autobiographical sketch that documents all your achievements: occupational, avocational, and academic

Cutaneous membrane   Membrane that covers the entire surface of the body

Cuticle (eponychium)   Tough ridge of skin that grows out over the nail from its base

Cytoplasm   Gel-like fluid within the cell membrane cradling cellular structures called organelles

Dan Tien   In Japan, a point in the Hara located three finger-widths' distance below the navel that is the center of focused power and action and where all movement of the body originates

Day spa   Spa providing beauty, health, and therapeutic treatments on a day-use basis with no overnight accommodations

Decoction   Tea made from boiling parts of a plant, usually bark, roots, or seeds

Defecation   Process of eliminating indigestible or unabsorbed material from the body

Deficiency disease   Disease caused by a lack of an essential vitamin, mineral, or nutrient in the individual's diet or caused by the individual's inability to properly digest and absorb a particular nutrient

Degenerative disease   Disease in which tissue breakdown occurs caused by an overuse syndrome or the aging process

Deglutition   Swallowing

Delayed-onset muscle soreness   Soreness felt 8 to 14 hours after activity, reaching a peak 48 hours after activity resulting from either inflammation or connective tissue damage

Deltoid   Curve of the shoulder and upper arm formed by the deltoid muscle

Dendrite   Short, narrow, neural extensions that receive and transmit stimuli toward the neuron's cell body

Dense irregular connective tissue   Connective tissue that resists pulling forces generally in more than two directions, such as deep fascia

Dense regular connective tissue   Connective tissue that resists pulling forces generally in two directions, such as ligaments, tendons, retinacula, and aponeuroses

Deoxyribonucleic acid   Chemical within chromosomes that resembles a small, coiled string

Depreciation   Process of spreading the deduction for the cost of an asset over time

Depression   Lowering or dropping a body part, moving inferiorly

Dermatome   Area of skin served by a specific sensory nerve root

Dermis   True skin lying under the epidermis possessing a network of nerves and vessels

Destination spa   Spa offering on-site accommodations, professionally administered spa services, physical fitness and wellness elements, educational programming, and spa cuisine

Diagnosing   Science and skill of distinguishing diseases or disorders from each other

Diaphysis   Cylindrical shaft of a long bone

Diarthrosis (synovial) joint   Freely movable joints

Diastole   Bottom number in the blood pressure equation that represents pressure against arterial walls during the pause between ventricular contractions

Diencephalon   Part of the brain that houses the thalamus and the hypothalamus

Diet   Food consumed to supply the process of nutrition

Diffusion   Movement of molecules, or other particles, from an area of high concentration to an area of low concentration, a process that will continue until the distribution of particulate is equal in all areas

Digestion   Process that occurs as food is mixed with digestive enzymes and converted into an absorbable state

Digital (phalangeal)   Relating to fingers or toes

Disability   Loss, absence, or impairment of physical or mental fitness

Disassociation   Coping mechanism in which the client *leaves his or her body* or believes his or her own past abuse has happened to someone else

Disease   Illness characterized by signs and symptoms

Disorder   Functional abnormality

Distal   Farther from the point of reference and term used when referencing the extremities

Distal convoluted tubule   Last section of the renal tubule

Diureses   Urine production

Diuretic   Substance promoting the formation and excretion of urine

Dividend   Part of a company's earnings distributed at regular intervals to its shareholders

Documentation   Process of providing written information of client care

Dopamine   Neurotransmitter involved in emotions, moods, regulating motor control, attention, and learning

Dorsal   See *Posterior*

Dorsal cavity   Cavity located on the posterior aspect of the body that can be further divided into the cranial and spinal cavities

Dorsiflexion   Flexing the ankle dorsally so that the toes are moving toward the shin

Dorsum   Top of the foot

Doshas   In Ayurveda, the governing principles and that which is produced as the five elements combine

Draping   Covering the body with cloth to provide a professional atmosphere, support the client's need for emotional privacy (modesty), offer warmth, and provide access to individual parts of the client's body

Dual relationships   Having more than one relationship with a client

Ductus deferens   See *Vas deferens*

Duodenum   First section of the small intestine

Dura mater   Outermost meningeal layer

Eccentric contraction   Type of isotonic contraction occurring when contraction results in lengthening of a muscle

Ectoderm   Embryonic cell layer giving rise to structures of the nervous system, including the special senses, the mucosa of the mouth and anus, the epidermis, and epidermal tissues

Edema   Swelling; occurs when lymph pools in an area

Effleurage   Application of unbroken gliding movements that are repeated and follow the contour of the client's body

Eicosanoid   Tissue hormones that alter smooth muscle contractions, blood flow, nerve impulse transmission, and immune responses

Ejaculatory duct   Tube that transports sperm from the vas deferens to the urethra during ejaculation

Elastic cartilage   Type of cartilage that is soft and pliable and gives shape to the external nose and ears and internal structures such as the epiglottis, part of the larynx, and the auditory tubes

Electrocardiogram   Graphic tracing of variations in electrical potential caused by the heart's contraction

Elevation   Raising or lifting a body part, moving superiorly

Ellipsoidal (biaxial) joint   Joint with movement limited to flexion, extension, abduction, and adduction

Empirical   Information that is measurable and verifiable via the senses

Endangerment site   Area of the body meriting caution during massage because it contains superficial delicate structures that are relatively unprotected and are therefore prone to injury

End-feel   What is felt at the end of passive range of motion such as a hard or soft

Endocrine gland   Ductless gland that produces hormones

Endocytosis   Process such as phagocytosis and pinocytosis that moves large particles across the cell membrane into the cell

Endoderm   Embryonic cell layer giving rise to the lining of the body's passages and the covering for most of the internal organs

Endoplasmic reticulum   Complex network of membranous channels within the cytoplasm to aid in the synthesis of protein and lipids and to assist in the transportation of these materials from one part of the cell to another

Endorphin   Neurotransmitter that functions as opiates to block pain

Enkephalin   Similar to endorphin (see *Endorphin*)

Ependymocyte   Neuroglia cell that lines cranial ventricles and the central canal of the spinal cord that assists in the circulation of cerebrospinal fluid

Epidermis   Outer layer of skin that contains pigment cells called melanocytes, as well as pores, to allow passage for hair and specialized glands

Epididymis   Tightly coiled duct located on the posterior border of the testes and is the site for final sperm maturation

Epidural space   Space between the dura mater and the vertebral canal filled with connective tissue and blood vessels

Epiglottis   One of the laryngeal cartilages that closes the trachea during swallowing to prevent food from entering the inferior respiratory passageways

Epinephrine (adrenaline)   Neurotransmitter located in several areas of the central nervous system and in the sympathetic division of the autonomic nervous system; can be excitatory or inhibitory; also a hormone

Epiphyseal line   Replaces the epiphyseal plate when bone growth is complete in mature bone

Epiphyseal plate   Thin layer of cartilage between epiphysis and diaphysis where new bone is formed in immature bone; also known as growth plate

Epiphysis   End of a long bone

Epithelial tissue   Tissue that lines or covers internal and external (skin) organs of the body; blood vessels and body cavities; and digestive, respiratory, urinary, and reproductive tracts

Erythrocyte   Red blood cell that transport oxygen and carbon dioxide

Esophagus   Muscular tube that connects the pharynx to the stomach

Essential nutrient   A nutrient that is either produced by the body in insufficient amounts or not at all and which must be obtained by the diet

Essential oil   Concentrated essence of one or more aromatic plants

Essential oil therapy   See *Aromatherapy*

Estrogen   Hormone responsible for female secondary sex characteristics and menstrual cycles; triggers the preparation of the female organs for fertilization and implantation of the early embryo

Eversion   Elevation of the lateral edge of the foot so that the sole is turned outward (or laterally)

Exacerbation   Period of full-blown symptoms occurring with the disease process

Exfoliation   Removal of dead skin by products, loofah, or body brush

Exocrine gland   Gland that secretes products into ducts that may empty into body cavities, hollow center of organs, or the body's surface

Expiration (exhalation)   Process of expelling air from the lungs

Extension   Straightening or increasing the angle of a joint

External   Nearest the outside of a body cavity

External (pulmonary) respiration   Gas exchange in the lungs, between blood and air in the alveoli

Exteroceptor   Receptor located in the skin, mucous membranes, and sense organs, responding to stimuli originating from outside of the body

Facial   Relating to the face

Fallopian tube   Tube extending laterally from the uterus that serves as a passage for an ovum; site of fertilization

Fasciculi   Groups of muscle fibers

Father Sebastian Kneipp (1821-1897)   Father of hydrotherapy

Fats   Lipids or fatty acids that can range in consistency from a solid to a liquid and are classified as saturated or unsaturated

Femoral   Relating to the thigh or area between the hip and the knee

Fertilization   Process of uniting sperm with an egg

Fibrocartilage   Cartilage that has the greatest tensile strength of all cartilage types and is found between the vertebrae, in knee joints, and between the pubic bones

Filtrate   Fluids filtered from the kidney

Filtration   Movement of particles across the cellular membrane as a result of pressure

Financial portfolio   All the various investments held by an individual investor

Fixator   Specialized synergists that act as stabilizers

Flexion   Bending or decreasing the angle of a joint

Follicle-stimulating hormone   Pituitary hormone that stimulates estrogen production and ovarian follicle development in women and sperm production in men

Foot reflexology   Modality asserting that our entire body has reflex points located on the feet and, through applied pressure, releases blocked energy in corresponding zones

Free nail edge   Most distal portion of the nail, the part that is trimmed as a result of nail growth

Friction   Massage movement applied by rubbing one surface over another

Frictions   In hydrotherapy, any treatment in which the client skin is rubbed or frictioned, with exfoliation being one of the benefits

Frontal   Relating to the forehead

Frontal lobe   Cerebral lobe regulating motor output, cognition, and speech production (Broca's area; typically left lobe)

Frontal plane   Plane passing through the body from side to side, creating anterior and posterior sections

Fu   In shiatsu, organs that are the Yang and more hollow organs such as the small intestine, gallbladder, large intestine, bladder, triple heater, and stomach

G cell   Stomach's endocrine cells that secrete the hormone gastrin

Gait   Person's walking pattern

Galen of Pergamon (c. 130-200 AD)   Roman physician who synthesized and unified Greek medical knowledge and whose works dominated Western medicine for over 1500 years

Gallbladder   Hollow organ located on the inferior surface of the liver that stores bile

Gamete   Male and female sex cell

Ganglion   Cluster of nerve cell bodies located in the peripheral nervous system

Gastrin   Hormone initiating the production and secretion of gastric juices and stimulating bile and pancreatic enzyme emissions into the small intestines

Gene   Section of deoxyribonucleic acid on a chromosome that codes for a specific enzyme

Genetic disease   Disease caused by an abnormal genetic code

Genetics   Study of inheritance

Geriatric   Refers to someone who is 70 years of age or older

Gliding (triaxial) joint   Joints permit all movements but limited to gliding

Glomerulus   Tuftlike network of fine capillaries within the Bowman's capsule formed by the afferent arteriole

Glucagon   Pancreatic hormone that increases blood glucose levels

Gluteal (buttock)   Curve of the buttocks formed by the gluteal muscles

Golgi body   Series of four to six horizontal membranous sacs that packs and stores proteins and lipids until needed

Golgi tendon organ   Receptor located at musculotendinous junctions that becomes activated by both tension and excessive stretch and responds by inhibiting motor neurons

Gonads   Primary reproductive organ that is testes in men and ovaries in women

Graham, Douglas O.   American physician and Swedish massage practitioner who authored several works on the history of massage

Greater omentum   Part of the mesentery that connects to the greater curvature of the stomach and duodenum and attaches to the transverse colon

Groin (inguinal)   Area where the thigh meets the abdomen

Growth hormone (somatotropin)   Pituitary hormone that stimulates protein synthesis for muscle and bone growth and maintenance

Gua-Sha   In shiatsu, a skin scraping technique to help expel excess heat or remove energy stagnation

Gustatory organ   Taste bud located on the superior and lateral surfaces of the tongue

Hair root plexus (hair follicle receptor)   Nerve receptor that responds to light touch and hair movement

Hallux   Great toe

Handicap   Congenital or acquired mental or physical defect that interferes with normal functioning of the body system or the ability to be self-sufficient in modern society

Hara   In Japan, the geographic center of gravity and the energetic center in the body located in the lower abdomen

Harvey, William (1578-1657)   British anatomist who demonstrated that blood circulation in animals is caused by the beat of the heart

Haustra   Series of pouches in the large intestine

Haversian canal   Minute vascular canal that runs longitudinally through the bone

Health   Condition of physical, mental, and social well-being and the absence of disease or other abnormal condition

Hemoglobin   Red respiratory pigment on an erythrocyte

Hepatic portal system   Circuit that collects blood from the digestive organs and delivers this blood to the liver for processing and storage

Hiccup (hiccough)   Intermittent contractions of the diaphragm followed by a spasmodic closure of the vocal cords

High-risk pregnancies   Pregnancies that put the mother, the developing fetus, or both at higher-than-normal risk for complications during or after the pregnancy and birth

Hilum   Indentation in the medially concave region of the kidney

Hinge (monoaxial) joint   Joint limited to flexion and extension

Hippocrates of Cos (c. 460-375 BC)   Greek physician; considered the father of modern Western medicine

Histamine   Neurotransmitter involved in emotions and regulation of body temperature, water balance, and stimulation of inflammatory responses

Homeostasis   Constancy of the body's internal environment representing a relatively stable condition within a very limited range

Homolateral   Related to the same side of the body

Horizontal plane   See *Transverse plane*

Hormonal control system   Mechanism in which a hormone stimulates or inhibits the release of other hormones

Hormone   Glandular secretions that act as catalysts in biochemical reactions and regulate the physiological activity of other cells

Horse stance   See *Warrior stance*

Host   Organisms in which disease-causing agents reside

Hot tub   Wooden barrel of hot or cool water used for soaking or dipping

Hotel spa   See *Resort spa*

Human chorionic gonadotropin   Placental hormone excreted in urine used to detect pregnancy

Hunting response   Cycles of vasodilation and vasoconstriction associated with cold application

Hyaline cartilage   Type of cartilage that is elastic, rubbery, and smooth and covers articulating ends of bones; connects ribs to the sternum; and supports the nose, trachea, and part of the larynx

Hydrotherapy   Therapeutic use of water

Hygiene   Collective principles of health preservation

Hyperemia   Increased local blood flow

Hypodermis   See *Subcutaneous layer*

Hypothalamus   Part of the diencephalon that governs and regulates the autonomic nervous system and pituitary gland and controls hunger, thirst, temperature, anger and aggression, release of hormones, sexual behavior, sleep patterns, and consciousness

Ice massage   Ice applied using circular friction

Ileocecal sphincter   Sphincter located between the small and large intestine

Ileum   Final division of the small intestine

Immunity   Anatomical and physiological defense reactions to invading microorganisms

Infectious disease   Communicable disease caused by biological agents such as viruses, bacteria, fungi, protozoa, or parasites

Inferior   Situated below or toward the tail end

Inflammation   Protective mechanism that is a response to tissue damage from trauma and serves to stabilize the area, contain infection, and prepare the damaged tissue for repair

Informed consent   Client's authorization for professional services based on information provided by the massage therapist; permission for treatment

Infusion   Tea made from steeping the parts of a plant, usually stems and leaves

Ingestion   Process of orally taking materials into the body

Inheritance   Expression of genetic material

Insertion   Tendinous muscle attachment on the more movable bone

Inspiration (inhalation)   Process of drawing air into the lungs

Insula (island of Reil)   Structure hidden by parts of the frontal, parietal, and temporal lobes that is sometimes considered a fifth cerebral lobe

Insulin   Pancreatic hormone that decreases blood glucose levels

Integrity   Being whole with undivided integrating thoughts, values, intention, and actions

Internal   Nearest the inside (within) of a body cavity

Internal (tissue) respiration   Gas exchange between blood and body's tissues

Interneuron (association nerve)   Nerve connecting sensory nerve to motor nerve and vice versa

Interoceptor   Receptor located in the viscera that detects stimuli originating from within the body regarding the function of the internal organs, such as digestion, excretion, and blood pressure

Interosseous ligament   Membrane that interconnects select bones by attaching to their periosteum; also provides muscle attachment

Interstitial cells of Leydig   Endocrine cells located in the testes that produce testosterone

Intracartilaginous ossification   Bone formation from cartilage found in extremities

Intramembranous ossification   Bone formation from membranes found on the roof and sides of the skull

Inventory   Unsold retail items that a business has on hand

Inversion   Elevation of the medial edge of the foot so that the sole is turned inward (or medially)

Ipsilateral   See *Homolateral*

Ischemia   Local decrease in blood flow

Islets of Langerhans (pancreatic islets)   Islands of endocrine cells located on the pancreas

Isometric contraction   Contraction in which muscle length remains the same while muscle tension increases

Isotonic contraction   Contraction in which muscle tone or tension remains the same as the length of the muscle changes

Jejunum   Intermediate portion of the small intestine

Jitsu   Japanese term to describe the quality of energy in a tsubo that feels full or excessive, Yang, hard, warm, and when your pressure is *pushed out* or resisted

Joint capsule   Sleevelike structure around a synovial joint

Joint cavity   Inner region of a joint capsule and is lined with a synovial membrane and filled with synovial fluid

Joint mobilizations   Movements of a joint through its normal range of motion

Jojoba   An almost liquid wax taken from a desert shrub's seeds; chemically similar to the skin's oil

Jump sign   Spontaneous reaction of pain or discomfort that causes a client to wince, jump, or verbalize on application of pressure

Juxtaglomerular apparatus   Structure located where the afferent arteriole touches part of the distal convoluted tubule and consists of the juxtaglomerular cells and the macula densa

Juxtaglomerular cell   Structure located in the afferent arteriole that acts as a mechanoreceptor stimulating the secretion of renin

Kapha   In Ayurveda, dosha made up of the elements of earth and water

Kellogg, John Harvey (1852-1943)   American who popularized health concerns; wrote numerous articles and books on massage that brought the issue to the general populace

Keratinocyte   Epidermal cell filled with a tough, fibrous protein called keratin that provides protection by waterproofing the skin's surface

Key trigger point   Trigger point, either active or latent, responsible for activating one or more satellite trigger points

Ki   In Japan, the energy of the body, mind, and spirit

Kidney   Principal organs of the urinary system located in the upper lumbar region

Kinesiology   Study of human motion

Krause end bulb   Nerve receptor involved in discriminatory touch and low-frequency vibration with some references calling it a cold receptor because it can detect temperatures below 65° F

Kyo   Japanese term to describe the quality of energy in a tsubo that feels empty or depleted, Yin, soft, cold, and when your pressure is *welcome* or accepted

Labia majora   Two folds of skin extending inferiorly and posteriorly from the mons pubis; covered with pubic hair in adult women

Labia minora   Two folds of skin inside the labia majora containing numerous oil glands

Labor   Process the body undergoes to expel a fetus; includes dilation, expulsion, and placental stage

Lacteal   Lymph capillary located within a villus of the small intestines

Lambdoidal suture   Suture that separates the parietal bones from the occipital bone

Langerhans cell   Epidermal cell thought to play a limited role in immunologic reactions

Large intestine (colon)   Final section of the gastrointestinal tract that undigested and unabsorbed food takes before the body eliminates it

Larynx   Triangle-shaped structured housing the vocal cords; also known as the voice box

Latent trigger point   Trigger point that goes unnoticed by the client until pressure is applied

Lateral   Oriented farther away from the midline of the body

Lateral deviation   Movements to the side often used when discussing mandibular movements

Laughing   See *Crying*

Lesion   Any noticeable or measurable deviation from normal healthy tissue

Lesser omentum   Part of the mesentery that attaches from the right side of stomach and first section of the duodenum to the liver

Leukocyte   White blood cell that serves as part of the body's immune system

Ling, Pehr Henrik (1776-1839)   Swedish physiologist and gymnastics instructor; considered the father of Swedish massage; developed his own system of medical gymnastics and exercise, known by several different names—the Ling System, Swedish Movements, and the Swedish Movement Cure; important part of the Ling System was a particular style of massage, known today as Swedish massage

Liniments   Alcoholic, oily, or soapy agents used as analgesics to create the sensation of heat

Liquid connective tissue   Connective tissue that consists of blood, lymph, and interstitial fluid

Liver   Organ located in the upper right quadrant of the abdominal cavity

Lobe   Region of the cerebrum named for the bone it lies beneath; frontal, parietal, temporal, and occipital lobes

Local contraindication   Area avoided during massage caused by local infection or other reason

Local disease   Disease affecting only one area of the body, such as a foot fungus

Local twitch response   Reflexive impulse that causes the affected muscle or an adjacent muscle to fire or twitch spontaneously

Loop of Henle   Section of the renal tubule just past the proximal convoluted tubule that consists of a descending limb, a hairpin turn, and an ascending limb

Loose connective tissue   Connective tissue that attaches skin to underlying structures, wraps and supports body cells, fills in spaces between structures, and helps keep them in their proper place

Lucas-Championniere, Just (1843-1913)   French physician who advocated the use of massage and passive-motion exercises after certain injuries

Lumbar   Relating to the back region between the ribs and the hips

Lung   Organ of respiration that extends from the diaphragm to just above the clavicles

Lunge position   See *Bow stance*

Luteinizing hormone   Pituitary hormone that triggers ovulation in women and testosterone production in men

Lymph   Fluid of the lymphatic system

Lymph capillary   Small lymph vessels

Lymph node   Bean-shaped structures located along lymph vessels that collect and filter lymph

Lymphatic trunk   Large vessels where lymph collects

Lymphocyte   Type of white blood cell of which can be a B cell or T cell

Lysosome   Organelle containing digestive enzymes to engulf and digest pathogens and cellular debris

Macula densa   Structure located in the distal convoluted tubule of Henle's that acts as chemoreceptors stimulating the secretion of renin

Major duodenal papilla   Site of entry for secretions from the pancreas, liver, and gallbladder into the duodenum

Malignant tumor   Cancerous tumor

Mammary gland   See *Breast*

Mandibular   Lower jaw

Marketing   Promoting your business with image, purpose, and direction

Massage   Systematic and scientific manipulation of the soft tissues of the body for the purpose of obtaining or maintaining health

Mastication   Chewing

Mechanical response   Response of the body to massage that occurs as a result of pressure, force, or range of motion

Mechanoreceptor   Receptor found in the skin, blood vessels, ears, muscles, tendons, joints, and fascia that detects sensations such as pressure, blood pressure, vibration, stretching, muscular contraction, proprioception, sound, and equilibrium

Media   Systems of mass communication

Medial   Oriented toward the midline of the body

Median plane   See *Midsagittal plane*

Mediastinal   Pertaining to the portion of the thoracic cavity occupying the area between the lungs

Medical spa   Spa providing medical and wellness care of both conventional and complimentary therapies

Medulla oblongata   Part of the brainstem that conducts sensory and motor impulses between other parts of the brain and the spinal cord

Medullary cavity   Hollow space within the center of the bone's shaft

Medullary pyramid   Structure made by numerous collecting tubules that appear as a distant triangular wedge in the kidney

Meissner (tactile) corpuscle   Nerve ending that mediates sensations of discriminative touch such as light versus deep pressure, as well as low-frequency vibration

Melanocyte   Epidermal cells that contribute to the skin's color; also found in hair and eye's iris

Melanocyte-stimulating hormone   Pituitary hormone that increases skin pigmentation by stimulating distribution of melanin granules

Melatonin   Pineal gland hormone involved in circadian rhythms (the body's 24-hour cycle) and the growth and development of sexual organs

Membrane   Thin, soft, pliable sheets of tissue that cover the body, line tubes or body cavities, cover organs, and separate one part of a cavity from another

Meninges   Connective tissue coverings surrounding the brain and spinal cord

Mental   In anatomy, relating to the chin

Mercuriale, Girolamo (1530-1606)   Italian Renaissance–era physician who synthesized ancient medical writings; wrote *De Arte Gymnastica,* considered to be the first book written in the field of sports medicine

Meridian   In traditional Chinese medicine, a channel or pathway through which Ki flows

Merkel disk   Nerve receptor that responds to light touch and discriminative touch

Mesentery   Section of the peritoneum consisting of the two omentums

Mesoderm   Embryonic cell layer giving rise to muscles and connective tissues of the body

Metabolic disease   Disease that disrupts the body's metabolism

Metabolism   Total of all physical and chemical processes that occur in an organism such as growth, digestion, and waste elimination

Metaphysis   Growth portion of a bone; where the diaphysis and epiphysis converge

Metastasize   Spreading of cancerous cells

Mezger, Johann (1817-1983)   Dutch physician who is generally given credit for making massage a fundamental component of physical rehabilitation; also credited for the introduction of French terminology into the massage profession

Microglia   Neuroglia cell protecting the central nervous system by destroying pathogens and removing dead neural tissue

Micturition   Urination

Midbrain   Part of the brainstem that conducts nerve impulses from the cerebrum to the pons and conducts sensory impulses from the spinal cord to the thalamus

Midsagittal plane   Plane that runs longitudinally or vertically down the body, anterior to posterior, dividing the body into right and left sections

Minerals   Essential nonorganic compounds found in nature that play a vital role in regulating many body functions

Mission statement   Statement of purpose that briefly and succinctly defines your type of business and its objective

Mitochondrion   Site of cellular respiration providing most of a cell's adenosine triphosphate

Mitral valve (bicuspid)   Left atrioventricular valve

Mons pubis   Mound of adipose tissue covered by skin and pubic hair cushioning the pubic symphysis

Motor (efferent) nerve   Nerve that carries impulses from the brain or spinal cord to activate or inhibit a muscle or gland

Motor neuron   Neuron sending the impulse to the muscle cell

Motor unit   Single motor neuron plus all the muscle fibers to which it innervates

Moxibustion   In Asian bodywork therapy, a technique to stimulate the tsubos with heat by burning the herb mugwort above them

Mucosal-associated lymphoid tissue   Collection of lymphoid cells in the mucosa or submucosa of the digestive tract and includes the tonsils, Peyer's patches, and vermiform appendix

Mucous membrane   Membrane that lines openings to the outside of the body

Multiarticular   Term used to describe muscles that cross more than two joints

Muscle fatigue   State of exhaustion or a loss of strength or endurance such as that felt after strenuous physical activity caused by the muscle's use of glucose without adequate oxygen, resulting in a buildup of lactic acid

Muscle fiber   Threadlike muscle cell

Muscle soreness   See *Delayed-onset muscle soreness*

Muscle spindle   Receptor wrapped around muscle fibers that are stretch-sensitive and respond by causing reflexive contraction

Muscle tissue   Tissue that has the ability to shorten (contract) and elongate (stretch) to produce movement and includes types such as smooth, cardiac, and skeletal tissue

Mutation   Mistakes in the gene coding system

Myelin sheath   Sheath surrounding axons that electrically insulates the neuron and increases nerve impulse speed

Myofascial   Pertaining to skeletal muscles and their related fascia

Myofascial release   Group of manual techniques used to reduce fascial restrictions

Myofibril   Structure in muscle fibers containing myofilaments

Myotome   Group of skeletal muscles innervated by a single spinal segment

Nadis   In Ayurveda, channels in which Prana energy flows

Nail   Heavily keratinized, nonliving tissue forming the thin hard plates found on the distal surfaces of the fingers and toes

Nail bed   Area beneath the nail

Nail body   Main and most visible part of the nail

Nail root   Place where nail production takes place

Narrative report   Summarization of client progress stretching through numerous sessions and prescriptive periods

Nasal   Relating to the nose

Nasal cavity   Cavity just behind the nose

Natural immunity   Nonspecific response to invading pathogens

Negative feedback system   Mechanism that triggers the negative, or opposite, response

Nephron   Kidney's filtering unit that contains three main parts: glomerulus, Bowman's capsule, and renal tubule

Nerve   Bundle of neurons held together by several layers of connective tissue

Nerve impulse (action potential)   Electrical fluctuation traveling along the surface of a neural cell membrane

Nervous tissue   Tissue that has the ability to detect and transmit electrical signals by converting stimuli into nerve impulses

Neural control system   Mechanism in which hormones are secreted by nerve stimulation

Neuroglia   Connective tissue that supports, nourishes, protects, insulates, and organizes neurons

Neuromuscular junction   Junction between the motor neuron and the motor end plate

Neuron   Impulse-conducting cells possessing excitability and conductibility

Neurotransmitter   Collective term for chemical messengers involved in nerve impulse transmission; it is how neurons talk to one another.

Nissen, Hartvig   Prominent early practitioner of Swedish massage (created by Pehr Ling) in the United States; helped popularize Ling's methods with his numerous publications

Nociceptor   Receptor that detects pain

Node of Ranvier   Gap along myelinated axons

Norepinephrine (noradrenaline)   See *Epinephrine*

Nose   Port of entry for air and beginning of the air conduction pathway of the respiratory system

Nuchal   Relating to the posterior neck region

Nucleus   Control center of the cell, directing nearly all metabolic activities

Nutrient   A substance that provides nourishment and affects metabolic processes such as growth and repair

Nutrition   Taking in nutrients and using them for proper function, growth, and health

Objective data   Information the therapist obtains that is measurable and quantitative

Occipital   Relating to the posterior and inferior surface of the head

Occipital lobe   Cerebral lobe that contains a center for visual input

Oligodendrocyte   Neuroglia cell forming a myelin sheath around some axons in the central nervous system

Oocyte   Female sex cell

Opposition   Movement in which the tip of the thumb comes into contact with the tip of any other digit on the same hand

Oral   Related to the mouth

Oral cavity   Port of entry for food and drink in the gastrointestinal tract

Orbital (ophthalmic)   Relating to the eye

Organelle   Cellular structures that possess distinct structure and function and include the nucleus, ribosomes, endoplasmic reticulum, Golgi body, mitochondria, and lysosomes

Origin   Tendinous muscle attachment on the less movable bone

Osmosis   Movement of a pure solvent such as water from an area of low concentration (most dilute) to an area of high concentration (least dilute); movement will continue until the two concentrations equalize

Ossification   Process of bone development that begins between the sixth and seventh week of embryonic life and continues throughout adulthood

Osteoblast   Bone-forming cells found in the periosteum

Osteoclast   Cells in bone that break down bone tissue to maintain homeostasis of calcium and phosphates and to repair bone

Osteocyte   Bone cell

Otic (auricular)   Related to the ear

Ovary   Gland located in the superior part of the pelvic cavity, lateral to the uterus that house developing follicles and produces the hormones progesterone and estrogen

Oviduct   See *Fallopian tube*

Ovum   Female oocyte that has been released by the ovary

Oxytocin   Pituitary hormone that stimulates uterine contractions and milk expression in women

Pacinian corpuscle   Nerve ending that responds to crude and deep pressure, vibration, and stretch and perceives proprioceptive information about joint position

Pack   Device for the application of heat, cold, or nutrients. It can refer to the actual item (i.e., hot stones, fabrics), a pouch (i.e., canvas or vinyl bag filled with substances such as silica or gel), or the products themselves (i.e., clay, seaweed)

Palliative care   Care that is directed toward reducing or relieving the intensity of uncomfortable symptoms but that cannot affect a cure; in some cases, represents pain management or comfort care

Palmar (volar)   Pertaining to the anterior surface of the hand

Palpation   Touching with purpose and intent

Pancreas   Organ located inferior and posterior to the greater curvature of the stomach

Pancreatic islets   See *Islets of Langerhans*

Paracelsus (1493-1541)   Name by which Philippus Aureolus Theophrastus Bombastus von Hohenheim was generally known; Swiss physician and chemist who promoted chemically prepared medicines instead of herbal remedies

Paraffin bath   Dipped bath in a heated waxy mixture

Parasite   Organism living in or on a host organism and relying on that host for nourishment

Parasympathetic   Part of the autonomic nervous system that conserves body's energy resources

Parathyroid   Gland located on the posterolateral surface of the thyroid; usually four in number

Parathyroid hormone   Hormone that decreases calcium storage in bones by stimulating osteoclasts and increases calcium reabsorption from urine and the intestines back into the blood, all to raise blood calcium levels

Paré, Ambroise (c. 1510-1590)   French military surgeon who, in addition to inventing several surgical instruments, was among the earliest modern physicians to discuss the therapeutic effects of massage, especially in orthopedic surgery cases

Parietal cell   Stomach's exocrine cell that produces intrinsic factor and hydrochloric acid

Parietal lobe   Cerebral lobe that governs somatosensory input (namely the skin and muscles) and taste

Passive movements   Movements applied by the therapist while the client remains relaxed (or passive)

Patellar   Relating to the kneecap area

Pathogen   Biological agent capable of causing disease

Pathology   Study of disease

Pectoral (mammary)   Related to the upper anterior thorax or chest area

Pedal   Related to a foot or feet

Pediatric   Refers to young people between 3 and 18 years of age

Pelvic   Related to the inferior region of the abdominopelvic cavity

Pelvic girdle   Pairing of the ilium, ischium, and pubis

Pelvic obliquity   One side of the pelvis positioned higher than the other side in the horizontal plane

Pelvic rotation   One side of the pelvis placed further forward, or more anteriorly, than the other around a central axis

Pelvic tilt   Anterior or posterior tilting of the entire pelvis in the frontal plane

Penis   Structure that introduces sperm into the vagina

Peptide hormone   Hormone that introduces a series of chemical reactions to alter metabolism

Perineal   Related to the region between the pubis and coccyx; inferior pelvic cavity

Periosteum   Fibrous sheath surrounding the bone's shaft containing blood and lymphatic vessels, nerves, and bone-forming cells for growth and fracture healing

Peripheral   See *Superficial*

Peripheral nervous system   Composed of the cranial and spinal nerves emerging from the central nervous system

Peristalsis   Wavelike contractions that mix and propel materials in the gastrointestinal tract

Peritoneum   Serous membrane that envelops the entire abdominal wall

Pétrissage   Application of cycles of rhythmic lifting, squeezing, and releasing of tissue, often working parallel to the muscle fibers

Peyer's patches (intestinal tonsils)   Groups of lymphatic nodules found in the mucous membrane of the small intestine

Phagocytosis   Process by which specialized cells ingest harmful microorganisms and cellular debris, break them down, and expel the harmless remains back into the body

Pharynx   Muscular tube shared by respiratory and digestive systems; also known as the throat

Photoreceptor   Receptor that is sensitive to light; two types: rods and cones

Physiology   Study of how the body and its individual parts function in normal body processes

Physiopathological reflex arc   Reflex caused by increased stimuli or an increase in the amount of afferent impulses

Pia mater   Innermost meningeal layer

Pineal gland   Gland located on the posterior aspect of the brain's diencephalon

Pinocytosis   Process by which specialized cells engulf harmful liquid microorganisms and cellular debris, break them down, and expel the harmless remains back into the body

Pitta   In Ayurveda, dosha made up of the elements fire and water

Pituitary   Bilobed gland that extends from the hypothalamus

Pivot (monoaxial) joint   Joint with movement limited to rotation

Placenta   Organ formed against the uterine lining that serves to bring blood and oxygen and remove waste from the developing child

Planning   Therapist's strategy to help the client achieve his or her goals

Plantar (volar)   Related to the bottom surface or sole of the foot

Plantar flexion   Extension of the ankle such that the toes are pointing downward, increasing the ankle angle anteriorly

Plasma   Liquid portion of blood

Plasma membrane   See *Cell membrane*

Platelet   See *Thrombocyte*

Plexus   Network of intersecting nerves in the peripheral nervous system

Plicae circulares   Circular folds located in the lumen of the small intestine

Pollex   Thumb

Pons   Part of the brainstem that relays nerve impulses from one side of the cerebellum to another

Popliteal   Relating to the posterior aspect of the knee

Posterior   Pertaining to the back of a structure

Posterior fontanel   Membrane located where the sagittal and lambdoidal sutures meet that will ossify by 2 months of age

Posture   Body's position in space, such as sitting, standing, lying supine, and lying prone

Prakriti   In Ayurveda, a person's unique constitution or the innate, natural state

Prana   In India, the energy of the body, mind, and spirit

Preceptor   Someone who guides you during your postgraduate clinical practice

Pregnancy   Also known as the gestational process, the sequence of events including implantation and embryonic and fetal growth that ends in birth; normal pregnancy is divided into three trimesters

Progesterone   Hormone that prepares the endometrium for pregnancy and helps maintain the corpus luteum once conception and implantation occurs

Progress report   Summarization of client progress over a period, usually 30 days or the length of a prescriptive period, whichever comes first

Prolactin   Pituitary hormone that stimulates milk production

Pronation   Medial (inward) rotation of the forearm so that the palm is turned down

Proprioceptor   Receptor located in the skin, ears, muscles, tendons, joints, and fascia; responds to movement and position

Prostate   Gland located inferior to the urinary bladder that produces an alkaline secretion, making up approximately 25% of semen volume

Protein   Naturally occurring organic compounds that contain large combinations of amino acids

Protraction   Movement forward or anteriorly

Proximal   Nearer to the point of reference; term used when referring to the extremities

Proximal convoluted tubule   First section of the renal tubule

Pubic   Related to the region of the pubic symphysis or genital area

Publicity   Free media exposure

Pulmonary circuit   Circuit that brings deoxygenated blood from right ventricle to the lungs to release carbon dioxide and reacquire oxygen

Pulmonary semilunar valve   Valve between the right ventricle and the pulmonary trunk

Pulse   Expansion effect of arteries that occurs when the left ventricle contracts and produces a wave of blood

Pyloric sphincter   Sphincter located between the stomach and small intestine

Qi   See *Ki*

Radiation   Transfer of heat energy in rays

Range of motion   Movement around a joint or set of joints

Recidivism   Relapse into a previous condition such as substance abuse

Recruitment   Process of motor unit activation based on need

Rectum   Section of the large intestine between the sigmoid colon and the anal canal

Referred pain phenomena   Tendency of a trigger point to produce sensations (e.g., pain, tingling, numbness, burning, aching, itching) distal from that of the trigger point when subjected to compression

Reflex   Instantaneous, automatic response to a stimulus from either inside or outside the body

Reflex arc   Functional unit of nervous system consisting of an afferent, inter, and efferent neuron

Reflexive response   Response of the body to massage that occurs as nerves are stimulated, activating a reflex arc

Rehabilitation   Process of restoration of a person who has had an illness or injury so as to regain maximum self-sufficiency and function in a normal or as near normal manner as possible

Relaxin   Hormone facilitating implantation of fertilized ovum and softening of connective tissue in pregnant women

Remission   Period of partial or complete disappearance of symptoms occurring with the disease process

Renaissance (c. 1250-1550)   Intellectual and artistic movement (a *rebirth*) beginning in northern Italy in the fourteenth century and extending throughout much of Europe by the seventeenth century

Renal pelvis   Upper region of a ureter

Renal tubule   Structure within the nephron subdivided into the proximal and distal tubule and the loop of Henle

Renin   Substance secreted by the juxtaglomerular cells that increases blood volume and blood pressure

Repetitive motion injuries   Self-inflicted injuries related to poor biomechanics, including general posture, sporting movements, and work habits; also known as repetitive strain injuries

Reservoir   Source of infection that may lead to disease

Resort spa   Spa owned by and located within a resort or hotel that provides professionally administered spa services, fitness and wellness components, and spa cuisine

Respiratory diaphragm   Dome-shaped muscle of respiration that separates the thoracic cavity from the abdominal cavity

Reticular connective tissue   Connective tissue that forms a supportive framework for bones and certain organs such as liver and spleen

Retina   Nervous tissue membrane of the eye continuous with the optic nerve where rods and cones are located

Retinacula   Bandagelike retaining strips of connective tissue

Retraction   Movement backward or posteriorly

Retroperitoneal   Behind the abdominal peritoneum

Rhazes (c. 850-932)   Name by which Persian physician Abu Bakr Muhammad ibn-Zakariya al-Razi was known in the West; noted physician of his time and the first important Arab medical writer

Ribosome   Small granules of ribonucleic acid and protein in the cytoplasm that synthesize protein for use within the cell and produce other proteins that are exported outside the cell

Right lymphatic duct   Lymphatic trunk that drains the right arm and the right side of the head and the right half of the thorax into the right subclavian vein

Rotation   Circular movement when a bone moves around its own central axis

Rubefacient   Agents that redden the skin as the ingredients cause irritation

Ruffini's corpuscle   Nerve ending that mediates deep or continuous pressure, with some references calling it a heat receptor because it can also detect rising temperatures

Sacral   Relating to the sacrum

Sacroiliac   Between the sacrum and the pelvic bone

Saddle (biaxial) joint   Joints possessing movements of flexion, extension, abduction, adduction, opposition, reposition, and circumduction

Sagittal plane   Plane passing through the body parallel to the median plane

Sagittal suture   Suture that joins the two parietal bones

Saliva   Fluid secreted by salivary and mucous glands in the mouth

Sanitation   Application of measures to promote a healthy, disease-free environment

Sarcolemma   Muscle cell membrane

Sarcomere   Muscle's contractile unit

Sarcoplasm   Muscle cell cytoplasm

Sarcoplasmic reticulum   A fluid-filled system of cavities that contain sarcomeres

Satellite cell   Neuroglia cell used for structural support of neurons in the peripheral nervous system; found only surrounding neuron cell bodies within ganglia

Satellite trigger point   Trigger point created by key trigger point activity often arising in pain referral zones of the key trigger point

Sauna   Dry heat treatment in a wood-lined room with temperatures ranging from 160° to 210° F with 10% to 20% humidity

Scapular   Relating to the shoulder blade

Schwann cell   Neuroglia cell forming a myelin sheath around axons in the peripheral nervous system

Scope of practice   Profession's working parameters

Scrotum   Pouch that supports the testes

Seated massage   Type of massage developed by David Palmer, whose vision was to make massage therapy safe, convenient, and affordable for anyone, anywhere, anytime

Sebaceous (oil) gland   Skin gland that secretes sebum that lubricates both the hair and the epidermis

Secretin   Hormone produced by the intestinal mucosa that stimulates the pancreas to secrete an alkaline liquid that neutralizes the acid chyme and facilitates the action of intestinal enzymes

Securities   Vehicles into which you put your money to optimize your return

Self-disclosure   Honest and open sharing of emotions, ideas, and insights

Semen   Thick, milky alkaline fluid that is a mixture of sperm (10%) and seminal fluid (90%)

Seminal vesicle   Saclike pouch located posterior to the base of the urinary bladder that secretes a thick alkaline fluid that makes up 60% of semen volume

Seminiferous tubule   Tightly coiled tubes within the testes that produce sperm

Sensory (afferent) nerve   Nerve or receptor that carries impulses to the brain or spinal cord

Serotonin   Neurotransmitter important for sensory perception, mood regulation, and normal sleep

Serous membrane   Membrane that lines closed body cavities that do not open to the outside of the body

Sexual misconduct   Sexual contact between a therapist and a client or any sexualizing of therapeutic relationship

Sexual reproduction   Process by which male and female sex cells unite to produce offspring

Shea butter   Butter extracted from the nut or fruit of the African Shea tree

Shiatsu   Japanese bodywork therapy that uses pressure on the surface of the skin along energy channels called meridians to regain and maintain a harmonic flow of energy throughout the body-mind-spirit

Shoulder girdle   Pairing of the clavicle and scapula

Shower   Water sprayed in fine streams from a showerhead under low to medium pressure

Sign   Objective changes in the body that can be observed and measured such as swelling, rashes, fever, high blood pressure, and paralysis

Sliding filament theory   Theory of muscle contraction in which thin filaments sliding toward the sarcomeres center shorten the muscle fiber

Small intestine   Longest section of the alimentary canal situated in the central abdomen

Sneezing   Forceful involuntary expulsion of air through the nose and mouth to clear upper respiratory passageways

Snoring   Audible breathing during sleep

Sodium-potassium pump   Mechanism used to maintain the resting potential of a neural cell membrane

Somatic nervous system   Division of peripheral nervous system that carries information from bones, muscles, joints, skin, and special senses of vision, hearing, taste, and smell

Somatic reflex   Reflex that is responsible for contraction of skeletal muscles

Spa   Place where water therapies are administered

Spa therapy   Service administered in a spa

Spa tub   Heated pool using high-pressure jets to agitate and circulate chemically treated water

Spasm   Local contraction caused by the stress of an injury that lowers the neural threshold (strength of stimuli required to generate a nerve impulse)

Spermatic duct   Duct system in the male reproductive system that includes the epididymis, vas deferens, ejaculatory duct, and urethra

Spermatozoon   Male sex cell

Sphincter Ring of muscle fibers that regulate movement of materials from one compartment of the gastrointestinal tract to another

Sphincter of Oddi Sphincter regulating the flow of secretions from the pancreas, liver, and gallbladder into the duodenum

Spinal cord Structure that exits the skull through the foramen magnum and extends to approximately the second lumbar region and functions as an integrating center and an information highway

Spinal nerve Nerve originating from the spinal cord

Spleen Largest lymphatic organ located within the left lateral rib cage just posterior to the stomach

Spongy bone Latticelike network found in the center of long bones, typically filled with red and yellow bone marrow, and where blood cells are made

Squamosal suture Suture located where the parietal bones and temporal bones meet

Standards of practice Guiding principles by which members of a particular organization conduct their day-to-day professional responsibilities

State-dependent memory Type of memory triggered by duplicating the original position, location, or amount of pressure, body movements, and emotions at the time of an abusive or traumatic event

Steam bath Heat treatment in a ceramic-tiled room filled with steam at 105° to 120° F with 100% humidity

Steroid hormone Hormones that alter cell activity by turning genes on or off

Stomach Organ that is an enlargement of the gastrointestinal tract bound at both ends by sphincters

Stretching Movements of a muscle (and its synergist) being drawn out to its fullest length

Stroke volume Amount of blood ejected from the left ventricle during each contraction

Subacute Condition in which the client appears to be well with regard to an absence of measurable signs but is still experiencing symptoms

Subarachnoid space Space between the pia mater and the arachnoid filled with cerebrospinal fluid

Subcutaneous layer Layer beneath the dermis; it is rich in fat and areolar connective tissue

Subdural space Space between the arachnoid and the dura mater filled with serous fluid

Subjective data Information learned from the client or the client's family and friends; includes most written information obtained on the intake form and information gathered during conversation

Sudoriferous (sweat) gland Skin gland that secretes sweat in response to excess heat or emotional arousal

Superficial Pertaining to the outside surface or surrounding the external area of a structure

Superficial fascia See *Subcutaneous layer*

Superior Situated above or toward the head end

Supination Lateral (outward) rotation of the forearm so that the palm is turned up

Sustained pressure Held applied pressure usually on trigger points and spasms for a 3- to 7-second time frame

Swedish gymnastics Part of the Ling system and includes movements of joints (range of motion) or muscles (stretching) to reduce pain, restore mobility, and maintain health

Swedish massage Systematic and scientific manipulation of the body's soft tissues for the purpose of establishing or maintaining good health

Sympathetic Part of the autonomic nervous system that that spends the body's energy resources

Symptom Subjective changes in the body of which only the person experiencing them is aware, such as headaches, nausea, and anxiety

Synapse Junction between two neurons or between a neuron and a muscle or gland, where transmission of nerve impulses takes place; not actually touching other neurons, muscles, or glands

Synaptic bulb Small budlike structure on the ends of axons containing synaptic vesicles

Synaptic vesicle Saclike structure located within the synaptic bulbs that produce and store neurotransmitters

Synarthrosis (fibrous) joint Joint with movement that is absent or extremely limited

Syndrome Group of signs and symptoms that occur to present a pattern defining a particular disease or abnormality

Synergist Muscle that aids movement by contracting at the same time as prime movers so they can produce more effective movement

Synovial fluid Viscous fluid secreted by synovial membranes

Synovial membrane Membrane that line cavities of freely moving joints

Synovial sheath Tubelike structure lined with synovial membranes surrounding long tendons

Systemic circuit Circuit that brings oxygenated blood from the left ventricle through numerous arteries into the capillaries, then moves it back to the heart

Systemic disease Disease affecting large parts of the body or the entire body

Systole Top number in the blood pressure equation that represents pressure exerted on the arterial wall during ventricular contraction

Table mechanics Component of massage addressing issues surrounding the massage table, such as table height and positioning, bolstering, and draping

Tachycardia Rapid heart rate ($\geq$100 beats per minute)

Taenia coli Thick, longitudinal bands located in the muscularis tunic of the large intestine

Tai Ji In Asian bodywork therapy, the familiar black and white icon, which symbolizes the interaction of Yin and Yang

Tapotement Application of repetitive staccato striking movements of the hands, moving either simultaneously or alternately

Target cell   Type of cell containing receptor sites that are chemically compatible with their corresponding hormone

Tarsal   Related to the ankle

Taylor, Charles Fayette   American physician who, along with his brother, George Henry Taylor, introduced the Swedish movement system into the United States; helped popularize Ling's methods

Taylor, George Henry   American physician who, along with his brother, Charles Fayette Taylor, introduced the Swedish movement system into the United States; helped popularize Ling's methods

Telodendria   Clusters of short fine filaments located at the end of each axon

Temporal lobe   Cerebral lobe that houses auditory and olfactory areas and Wernicke's area

Tendon   Cordlike structure anchoring the end of a muscle to a bone

Terminal illness   Condition in which the person is expected to die within a time frame, usually 6 months

Testicle   Gland that is the site of sperm production

Testosterone   Hormone that promotes secondary male sex characteristics, libido, and sperm production

Thalamus   Part of the diencephalon that relays sensory information (except olfaction) to appropriate parts of the cerebrum

Thermoreceptor   Receptor that detects temperature changes

Thermotherapy   External application of heat for therapeutic purposes

Thixotropism   Ability of fascia to change the physical state of its ground substance from a gel to a sol state and vice versa

Thoracic   Relating to the area between the neck and the respiratory diaphragm

Thoracic duct   Lymphatic trunk that drains most of the body's lymph into the left subclavian vein

Thrombocyte (platelet)   Fragmented cell that helps repair blood vessels through clotting mechanisms

Thymopoietin   See *Thymosin*

Thymosin   Thymus hormone that stimulates the production of T cells

Thymus   Bilobed gland posterior to the sternum

Thyroid   Bilobed gland located at base of the throat, posterior and inferior to the larynx

Thyroid-stimulating hormone   Pituitary hormone that stimulates thyroid activity

Thyroxine (tetraiodothyronine or T4)   See *Triiodothyronine*

Tissot, Simon André (1728-1797)   French hygienist who was an important figure in physical therapy; published several works on gymnastics and massage

Tissue   Group of similar cells that act together to perform a specific function and include epithelial, connective, muscle, and nerve

Tonsils   Group of large specialized lymph tissues embedded in the mucous membranes around the throat

Trachea   Tube from the larynx to the upper chest just anterior to the esophagus; also known as the windpipe

Transference   Client *transfers* feelings, thoughts, and behaviors related to a significant person in the client's early life (e.g., parents) onto the therapist

Transverse plane   Plane passing through the body creating superior and inferior sections

Traumatic disorder   Disorder that disrupts homeostasis

Treatment plan   Plan that outlines steps the therapist will follow to provide a tailor-made session for each client

Tricuspid valve   Right atrioventricular valve

Tri-doshas   In Ayurveda, term used to describe the three active doshas: Vata, Pitta, and Kapha

Trigger point   Rigid zone or knot found in muscle, tendons, fascia, ligaments, and periosteum caused by a neurochemical event that cause fibers to stick together; pressure applied on the point may refer pain

Triiodothyronine (T3)   Thyroid hormone that increases metabolism

Tsubo   Japanese term used to describe energetic vortices on the surface of the skin where the energy of the meridian can be accessed

Umbilical   Related to the midabdomen or navel area

Uniarticular   Term used to describe muscles that cross one joint

Universal donor   Person who has blood type O whose blood can be donated to all of the blood types

Universal recipient   Person who has blood type AB and can receive all other blood types

Ureter   Slender hollow tube transporting urine formed by the kidneys to the urinary bladder

Urethra   Small tubular structure transporting urine from the urinary bladder out of the body during urination

Urinary bladder   Storage reservoir for urine; located in the pelvis behind the symphysis pubis

Urine   Concentrated filtrate from the kidneys that is slightly acidic and amber in color

Uterus   Hollow, pear-shaped organ in which the fertilized ovum implants, the fetus develops, and from which menses flows

Vagina   Canal extending from the uterine cervix to outside the body that is the passageway for menstrual flow and childbirth and the receptacle for the penis during sexual intercourse

Vas deferens   Also known as the seminal duct; carries sperm from the epididymis to the ejaculatory duct

Vasoconstriction   Narrowing of the vascular lumen's diameter

Vasodilation   Enlargement of the vascular lumen's diameter

Vata   In Ayurveda, the dosha composed of the elements air and space

Vein   Vessel that moves blood toward the heart

Venous pump   Mechanisms that assists blood flow in the veins

Ventral cavity   Body cavity located on the anterior aspect of the body and can be further divided into the thoracic and abdominopelvic cavities

Ventral   See *Anterior*

Ventricle   Inferior heart chamber

Venule   Small-sized veins

Vermiform appendix   Lymphoid tissue located inferior to the cecum

Vertebral   Relating to vertebrae

Vesalius, Andreas (1514-1564)   Flemish physician who wrote *De Humani Corporis Fabrica* (1543), considered one of the most important studies in the history of medicine

Vibration   Application of rapid shaking, quivering, trembling, or rocking movements

Villus   Fingerlike projection on the plicae circulares in the small intestine

Visceral (autonomic) reflex   Reflex responsible for maintaining homeostasis through coughing, sneezing, and blinking and correcting the heart rate, respiratory rate, and blood pressure

Vitamins   Organic compounds that are essential for normal physiological and metabolical functioning of the body

Vocal cords   Cords located in the larynx used for voice production

Volkmann's canal   Minute vascular canal that runs horizontally through the bone, connecting Haversian canals

Vulva   Female external genitalia that include the mons pubis, labia majora and minora, and the clitoris

Warrior stance   Stance used when the therapist applies strokes that traverse relatively short distances with both of the therapist's feet placed on the floor a little more than hip-width distance apart, with toes pointing forward

Whirlpool   Tub filled with water just before use and drained after each use

Womb   See *Uterus*

Yawn   Very deep breath initiated by opening the mouth wide

Zang/Fu   In traditional Chinese medicine, the Organ Systems, both Yin and Yang, the definition of which includes the internal organs and the meridians but mostly refers to the functions of the body that are necessary for life

Zang   In shiatsu, organs that are the Yin, more solid organs such as the heart, liver, lungs, kidney, pericardium, and spleen

Zone   Mapping used in foot reflexology

Illustration Credits

Chapter 1

Figure 1-2, 1-3 Courtesy U.S. National Library of Medicine, Bethesda, Maryland
Figure 1-4 Courtesy Stadt Archives, Schaffhaussen, Germany

Chapter 2

Biography figure Courtesy Feldenkrais Institute, Tel Aviv, Israel

Chapter 3

Figure 3-4 Courtesy Oakworks, Shrewsbury, Pennsylvania

Chapter 5

Figure 5-2 Courtesy Harlow Primate Laboratory, University of Wisconsin, Madison, Wisconsin
Figure 5-3 Courtesy Courbis, Inc.
Figure 5-4 Courtesy Kathy Wilmering, 2005
Figure 5-5 Courtesy Tiffany Field

Chapter 8

Figure 8-6 Hockenberry MJ: *Wong's nursing care of infants and children*, ed 7, St Louis, 2003, Mosby (Reprinted with permission)
Biography figure Courtesy Trager Institute, Mill Valley, California

Chapter 10

Figure 10-2A,B Courtesy Oakworks, Shrewsbury, Pennsylvania
Biography figure Courtesy Tiffany Field

Chapter 11

Figures 11-9, 11-10 Herlihy B, Maebuis NK: *The human body in health and illness*, ed 2, Philadelphia, 2003, Saunders
Figures 11-11A Courtesy Phototake, New York, New York
Figures 11-12A, 11-13A Courtesy Ed Reschke, Muskegon, Michigan
Figures 11-11B, 11-12B, 11-13B, 11-14B Thibodeau GA, Patton KT: *Anatomy and physiology*, ed 6, St Louis, 2006, Mosby

Figure 11-14A Courtesy Robert L. Calentine, River Falls, Wisconsin
Figure 11-21A,B Muscolino J: *Kinesiology: the skeletal system and muscle function*, St. Louis, 2006, Mosby

Chapter 12

Figure 12-2 Jarvis C: *Physical examination and health assessment*, ed 4, Philadelphia, 2004, Saunders

Chapter 13

Figure 13-4A,B Herlihy B, Maebuis NK: *The human body in health and illness*, ed 2, Philadelphia, 2003, Saunders
Biography figure Courtesy Rolf Institute, Boulder, Colorado (photo by David Kirk Campbell)

Chapter 14

Figures 14-1, 14-3A,B, 14-4A,B, 14-5A,B, 14-7A,B, 14-8A,B, 14-9A,B, 14-13A-C, 14-15A,B, 14-20A,B Muscolino J: *Muscular system manual: the skeletal muscles of the human body*, ed 2, St. Louis, 2005, Mosby
Figure 14-3C Thibodeau GA, Patton KT: *Anatomy and physiology*, ed 5, St Louis, 2003, Mosby
Figure 14-6 Courtesy Charles Eaton, MD, Jupiter, Florida

Chapter 15

Figures 15-3A-C, 15-5B Thibodeau GA, Patton KT: *Anatomy and physiology*, ed 6, St Louis, 2006

Chapter 16

All figures (excluding 16-1A,B and 16-55) Muscolino J: *Muscular system manual: the skeletal muscles of the human body*, ed 2, St. Louis, 2005, Mosby
Figure 16-1A,B Herlihy B, Maebuis NK: *The human body in health and illness*, ed 2, Philadelphia, 2003, Saunders

Chapter 17

Figures 17-2, 17-7, 17-18 Applegate E: *The anatomy and physiology learning system*, ed 3, St Louis, 2006, Saunders
Figure 17-8 Vidic B, Suarez FR: *Photographic atlas of the human body*, St. Louis, 1984, Mosby

Figures 17-13, 17-19, 17-21 Herlihy B, Maebuis NK: *The human body in health and illness*, ed 2, Philadelphia, 2003, Saunders

Figure 17-17 Thibodeau GA, Patton KT: *Anatomy and physiology*, ed 6, St Louis, 2006, Mosby

Chapter 18

Figures 18-4, 18-5, 18-6 Herlihy B, Maebuis NK: *The human body in health and illness*, ed 2, Philadelphia, 2003, Saunders

Chapter 19

Figure 19-1 Applegate E: *The anatomy and physiology learning system*, ed 3, St Louis, 2006, Saunders

Figures 19-2, 19-5 Solomon EP: *Introduction to human anatomy and physiology*, ed 2, St Louis, 2003, Saunders

Figure 19-3 Bevelander G, Ramaley JA: *Essentials of histology*, ed 8, St Louis, 1979, Mosby

Figure 19-4 Thibodeau GA, Patton KT: *Anatomy and physiology*, ed 6, St Louis, 2006, Mosby; © Dennis Kunkel

Figures 19-7, 19-18 Thibodeau GA, Patton KT: *Anatomy and physiology*, ed 6, St Louis, 2006, Mosby

Figures 19-6, 19-8, 19-10, 19-11, 19-12, 19-14, 19-15, 19-16, 19-17, Table 19-1 Herlihy B, Maebuis NK: *The human body in health and illness*, ed 2, Philadelphia, 2003, Saunders

Chapter 20

Figures 20-3, 20-4, 20-6 Herlihy B, Maebuis NK: *The human body in health and illness*, ed 2, Philadelphia, 2003, Saunders

Figure 20-5 Thibodeau GA, Patton KT: *Anatomy and physiology*, ed 6, St Louis, 2006, Mosby

Figure 20-7A McMinn RMH, Hutchings RT: *Color atlas of human anatomy*, ed 2, Chicago, 1988, Year Book Medical Publishers

Figure 20-7B Vidic B, Suarez FR: *Photographic atlas of the human body*, St Louis, 1984, Mosby

Chapter 21

Figures 21-2, 21-3A-C, 21-7 Thibodeau GA, Patton KT: *Anatomy and physiology*, ed 6, St Louis, 2006, Mosby

Figures 21-4A-C Herlihy B, Maebuis NK: *The human body in health and illness*, ed 2, Philadelphia, 2003, Saunders

Figure 21-9 Abrahams P, Hutchings RT, Marks SC: *McMinn's color atlas of human anatomy*, ed 4, St Louis, 1999, Mosby

Chapter 22

Figures 22-1A, 22-4 Applegate E: *The anatomy and physiology learning system*, ed 3, St Louis, 2006, Saunders

Figures 22-1B, 22-2B Abrahams P, Hutchings RT, Marks SC: *McMinn's color atlas of human anatomy*, ed 4, St Louis, 1999, Mosby

Figure 22-2A Brundage DJ: *Renal disorders*, St Louis, 1992, Mosby

Figures 22-3A,B, 22-5 Herlihy B, Maebuis NK: *The human body in health and illness*, ed 2, Philadelphia, 2003, Saunders

Chapter 23

Figure 23-1 McCance KL, Huether SE: *Pathophysiology: the biologic basis for disease in adults and children*, ed 5, St Louis, 2006, Mosby

Figure 23-5 Stevens A, Lowe J: *Human histology*, ed 3, Philadelphia, 2005, Mosby

Figures 23-2, 23-6, 23-9 Applegate E: *The anatomy and physiology learning system*, ed 3, St Louis, 2006, Saunders

Figures 23-4, 23-7 Herlihy B, Maebuis NK: *The human body in health and illness*, ed 2, Philadelphia, 2003, Saunders

Figures 23-3, 23-12 Thibodeau GA, Patton KT: *Anatomy and physiology*, ed 6, St Louis, 2006, Mosby

Figure 23-8 Solomon EP: *Introduction to human anatomy and physiology*, ed 2, St Louis, 2003, Saunders

Chapter 24

Figure 24-1 Courtesy Lancaster City Museum, part of Lancashire County Museum Service, Lancaster, Pennsylvania

Figures 24-3, 24-14, 24-15 Courtesy TouchAmerica, Hillsborough, North Carolina

Figures 24-7B, 24-13 Courtesy Golden Ratio, Emigrant, Montana

Figure 24-11 Courtesy Brook Slezak/Taxi/Getty Images

Chapter 25

Figure 25-1 Courtesy International Institute of Reflexology

Chapter 26

Figure 26-3 Damjanov I: *Pathology for the health professions*, ed 3, St. Louis, 2006, Mosby

Figure 26-9 Chaitow L: *Modern neuromuscular techniques*, ed 2, Edinburgh, 2003, Churchill Livingstone

Chapter 28

Figure 28-4 Modified from Hass EM: *Staying healthy with seasons*, Milbrae, CA, 1981, Celestial Art

Figures 28-5, 28-6, 28-7, 28-8, 28-9, 28-10, 28-11, 28-12, 28-13, 28-14, 28-15, 28-16, 28-19 Beresford-Cook C: *Shiatsu theory and practice*, ed 2, Edinburgh, 2003, Churchill Livingstone

Index

A

AAMM. *See* American Association of Masseurs and Masseuses
A-band, 381
Abbreviations, 828–829
ABCDEF. *See* Asymmetry Border Color Diameter Elevated Fast growing
Abdomen
  alternate-hand circular effleurage, usage. *See* Supine client
  diffused tapotement. *See* Supine client
  endangerment site, 97–98
Abdominal, definition, 849
Abdominal area, treatment suggestions, 706
Abdominal cavity, 281f
Abdominal (celiac) area, 283
Abdominal massage. *See* Pregnancy massage; Self-applied abdominal massage
Abdominal muscles
  anterior/posterior view, 485f
  lateral view, 485f
Abdominopelvic cavity, 281f
Abdominopelvic quadrants, 280
Abducens nerve, 521f
Abduction, 321. *See also* Horizontal abduction
  definition, 849
Abductor digiti minimi
  action, 428f
  nerve, 428f
  origin/insertion, 428f
Abductor pollicis brevis
  action, 427f
  nerve, 427f
  origins/insertions, 427f
Abductor pollicis longus
  action, 427f
  nerve, 427
  origins/insertions, 427f
ABMP. *See* Associated Bodywork and Massage Professionals
ABO blood groups, 563t
Aborth, 656
Absolute contraindications, 96
  definition, 849
  treatment, 97b, 207b
Absorption, 610
  definition, 849
ABT. *See* Asian bodywork therapy
Abu-Ali al-Husayn ibn-Sina. *See* Avicenna
Abu Bakr Muhammad ibn Zakariya al-Razi. *See* Rhazes
Academic performance, increase, 93
Accessory digestive organs, 618–619
  illustration, 618f
Accessory flexor. *See* Ulnar nerve
Accessory ligaments, 321
Accessory male sex glands, 648
Accessory nerve, 519, 521f
Accountants, accounting software (contrast), 813

Accounting
  definition, 849
  description, 812
  terminology, 813b
  usage, 812–815
Accounts payable, 814
  description, 813b
Accounts receivable, 814
  description, 813b
Acetabulum, 347
  definition, 849
Acetaminophen. *See* Darvocet; Percocet; Tylenol; Vicodin
  definition, 839
Acetylcholine (ACh), 512–513
  definition, 849
  release, stimulation, 89, 583b
Acetylsalicylic acid. *See* Aspirin
Acne, 303
Acne vulgaris, 295
Acoustic nerve, 519
Acquired immunity, 579
  definition, 849
Acquired immunodeficiency syndrome (AIDS), 66, 582
  guidelines, 246
  massage, impact, 245–247
  precautions, 246
Acromegaly, 548
Acromial, definition, 849
Acromial area, 282
Acromion process, 340f, 341f
ACTH. *See* Adrenocorticotropic hormone
Actifed, definition, 839
Actin, 380
Action, 402b
  potentials, 510. *See also* Nerve impulses
  terminology, 321–327
Active-assisted movements
  definition, 849
  performing, 172
Active cell processes, 267–270
Active movements, 8
  therapist involvement, 172
Active occupations, 111b
  (physical activity category), 110
Active-resisted movements, therapist involvement, 172
Active transport, 268–269
  definition, 849
  illustration, 269f
Active trigger points, 714
  definition, 849
Acupoints. *See* Tsubo
Acupressure, 743
Acupuncture, illustration, 754f
Acute disease, definition, 849
Acute injury, definition, 849
Adaptation, 525
  definition, 849

Adaptive massage
  bibliography, 257
  case study, 255
  Internet activities, 257
  introduction, 240–244
  self test, 256
  student objectives, 239
  summary, 254
Adaptive professional communication, 744
Addison's disease, 549
Adduction, 321. *See also* Horizontal adduction
  definition, 849
Adductor brevis, 445f
  actions, 447f
  nerve, 447f
  origin/insertion, 447f
Adductor longus, 445f
  actions, 447f
  nerve, 447f
  origin/insertion, 447
Adductor magnus, 445f
  actions, 446f
  nerve, 446f
  origins/insertions, 446f
Adductors, 445f
Adenohypophysis, 544
Adenosine triphosphate (ATP), 267
  availability, 91
  breakdown, 268
  definition, 849
  depletion, 388
ADH. *See* Antidiurectic hormone
ADHD. *See* Attention deficit hyperactivity disorder
Adhesions, 720
  breakdown/freeing, 162
  formation, decrease, 92, 331b
Adipose connective tissue, 273
  illustration, 272f
Adipose tissue, 650f
  definition, 849
  interaction, 249
Adolescent boys, massage (caution), 248
Adrenal androgen, 548t
Adrenal cortex, 546
  definition, 849
Adrenal estrogens, 548t
Adrenal glands, 546
  definition, 849
  hormones, inclusion, 548t
  illustration, 547f
Adrenaline. *See* Epinephrine
Adrenal medulla, 546
  definition, 849
  hormones, memorization, 546
Adrenocorticotropic hormone (ACTH), 545t
  definition, 849
Adrenohypophysis, 545f
Adult massage, infant massage (contrast), 227

Advertising. *See* Massage business
  definition, 849
  description, 798
Advil (ibuprofen), definition, 839
Aerobic stage, 384
Aesclepius (Asclepius)
  evolvement, 5
  explanation, 850
Afferent arteriole, 635f
  positional relationship, 636f
Afferent nerves. *See* Sensory nerves
Afferent neuron, 509f
Affusion showers. *See* Vichy showers
Aftercare. *See* Sports/rehabilitation
Agnis, 782
Agonists (prime movers), 386
  definition, 849
Agranular endoplasmic reticulum. *See* Smooth
  endoplasmic reticulum
Agranular leukocytes, 561f
AIDS. *See* Acquired immunodeficiency
  syndrome
Air-conditioning chambers, 591
Air movements. *See* Modified respiratory air
  movements
Airways, guardian, 593
Akin
  absorption, properties, 294
Albinism, 296
Albuterol inhaler. *See* Proventil
Alcohol, influence. *See* Massage
Aldosterone, 548t, 639
  definition, 849
Ale, H. Fred, 505
Aleve (naproxen sodium), definition, 839
Alimentary canal
  definition, 849
  divisions, 611–618
Allegra (fexofenadine), definition, 839
Allen, Gracie, 229
Allergies, 205, 582. *See also* Purpose Pain Al-
  lergies Lifestyle Medical
  discomfort, 221
All-or-none response, 383, 511
  definition, 849
Alpha cells, 546
Alpha state, 516
Alpha waves, increase, 90, 535b
Alprazolam. *See* Xanax
Alter, Lisa, 514
Alternate finger raking, 148
Alternate-hand circle effleurage, usage. *See*
  Shoulders
Alternate-hand circular effleurage, 148
  usage. *See* Supine client
Alternate-hand effleurage, 145, 148
  usage. *See* Prone client
Alternate-hand pétrissage, 154–155. *See also*
  Quadriceps
Alternate hand superficial friction. *See* Prone
  client
Alveolar duct, 591f, 594f
Alveolar sac, 591f, 593, 594f
Alveoli, 593–594
  definition, 849
  illustration, 591f, 594f
Alzheimer's disease, 529
  massage, usage, 93
Ama, 782
  impact. *See* Disease
Amblyopia, 250
Amenorrhea, 656
American Association of Masseurs and Mas-
  seuses (AAMM), creation, 10

American Massage and Therapy Association
  (AMTA), 802
  name change, 10
American Organization for Bodywork Therapies
  of Asia (AOBTA), 755
American Society of Physical Therapy Physi-
  cians, formation, 9
Amino acids
  classification, 621t
  definition, 849
  description, 620
Amma (amna // anmo) (therapy precursor), 5, 756
  definition, 849
Amoxicillin, definition, 839
Amphiarthroses, 319
  examples, 320f
Amphiarthrosis joint (cartilaginous joint),
  definition, 849
Ampicillin, definition, 839
Amputations, 251
  massage, impact, 240
AMTA. *See* American Massage and Therapy
  Association
Anabolism, 263
Anaerobic stage, 384
Anal canal, 617
  definition, 849
Analgesia, production, 156
Analgesic, 51
  definition, 837
  use, reduction, 90
Anatomical neck, 341f
Anatomical position, 280
Anatomic position, definition, 849
Anatomic snuffbox. *See* Hypothenar eminence
Anatomy. *See* Applied anatomy; Comparative
  anatomy; Gross anatomy; Microscopic
  anatomy; Surface anatomy
  definition, 262, 849
  introduction, 262–263
  physiology, connection, 262
  regional approach, 262
  relationship. *See* Body systems
  systemic approach, 262
  terminology, introduction, 263–265
Anchoring. *See* Towel
Ancient Roman public bath, 666f
Ancient world, 5–6
Anconeus
  actions, 418f
  nerve, 418f
  origin/insertion, 418f
Anemia, 580
  discomfort, 220
  massage, usage, 93
Aneurysm, 580
Anger, feelings (decrease), 93
Angina pectoris, 580
  definition, 837
Angle, bony marking, 317t
ANH. *See* Atrial natriuretic hormone
Ankles
  anterior view, 460f
  bolstered area, 121
  bolster placement, 130f
  bones, 349–350
  flop, illustration, 701f
  gymnastics, 185t
  movements, 180
    muscles, 452f–461f
    muscles, list, 459
  posterior view, 461f
Ankylosing spondylitis, 328
Annuities, investment, 818

Annulus fibrosus, 360
Anomalies, observation, 722
Anorexia nervosa, 622
Anothomia (dei Luzzi), 7
Anoxia, 595
ANS. *See* Autonomic nervous system
Antagonists, 386
  definition, 849
Antebrachial, definition, 849
Antebrachial area, 282
Antecubital, definition, 849
Antecubital area, 282
Anterior, definition, 849
Anterior cervical triangle, endangerment sites, 98
Anterior deviations, 723
Anterior fontanel, 356
  definition, 850
Anterior horizontal landmarks, 724
Anterior lobe, 544
Anterior nares, 590
Anterior pituitary, hormones
  inclusion, 545t
  memorization, 544
Anterior reference (ventral reference), 280, 282f
Anterior rotation, 326
Anterior scalene, 472f
Anterior thigh, ocean waves (usage), 155f
Anterior tilt, 326
Anterior torso, regional terms, 283–284
Antibiotic, definition, 837
Antibody testing, 245
Anticoagulants
  definition, 837
  impact, 207b
Anticonvulsant, definition, 837
Antidepressants
  definition, 837
  impact, 207b
Antidiabetic, definition, 837
Antidiuretic hormone (vasopressin // ADH), 572
  definition, 850
Antifungal, definition, 837
Antigens, 563
Antihistamine, definition, 837
Antipsychotics, impact, 207b
Antiviral, definition, 837
Anus, 617
  definition, 850
Anxiety
  disorders, 529
  massage, usage, 96
  reduction, 90, 219, 535b
AOBTA. *See* American Organization for Body-
  work Therapies of Asia
Aorta, 573
Aortic semilunar (SL) valve, 566
  definition, 850
APIE. *See* Assessment Plan Implementation and
  Evaluation
Apnea, 595, 600
Apocrine skin glands, 301f
Apocrine sweat glands, 301
Aponeurosis, definition, 850
Appendicitis, 622
Appendicular skeleton, 315, 317
  muscles, 404f–461f
Appendix. *See* Vermiform appendix
Applied anatomy, 262
Appointments, handling, 27–28
Appropriateness, 26
Arachnoid, definition, 850
Arachnoid mater, 513f
  description, 513f
Archer stances. *See* Bow stances

Arches. *See* Feet
  imprint. *See* Feet; High arches
Archimedes, 668–669
Area circumference, decrease (edema, impact), 584b
Areolar connective tissue, 273
  definition, 850
  illustration, 272f
Aricept (donepezil), definition, 839
Armour thyroid (thyroid extract), definition, 839
Arms
  bones, 341–342
  extended
    rolling friction. *See* Supine client
    wringing friction. *See* Supine client
  massage, 133f
  positioning, 118
  seated massage routine, 748
  swelling, inquiry, 221
  two-handed effleurage, usage. *See* Prone client
Arm shelf, addition. *See* Prone client
Arndt's Law, 530b
Aromatherapy (essential oil therapy), 685–688
  definition, 850
  description, 686
  impact. *See* Hydrotherapy; Spa
  olfaction, relationship, 686–687
  usage. *See* Massage; Spa
Arrector pili, 300
Arrhythmia, 568
  definition, 837, 850
Arterial pulse, 569–570
Arteries, 569. *See also* Major arteries
  definition, 850
  memorization, 569
Arterioles. *See* Afferent arteriole; Efferent arteriole
  definition, 850
  description, 569
  illustration, 577f
Arteriosclerosis, 580
  definition, 837
Arthritis. *See* Gouty arthritis; Osteoarthritis; Rheumatoid arthritis
Arthrosis. *See* Articulation
Articular cartilage, 313, 313f, 319
  definition, 850
Articular facet, 361f
Articulated skeleton, obtaining, 362
Articulation (arthrosis), definition, 850
Articulations (joints), 319–321, 362
  list, 366t
  types, 319
Ascending limb, 635f, 636f
Ascending tracts, 514
Asclepiades, 6
  definition, 850
Asclepius. *See* Aesclepius
Ascorbic acid. *See* Vitamin C
Asian bodywork therapy (ABT)
  definition, 850
  description, 755–756
  introduction, 754
Asian medicine
  illustration, 754f
  model. *See* Health
  Western medicine, contrast, 755
Asking, evaluation technique, 777
Aspirin (acetylsalicylic acid), definition, 839
Assessment. *See* Initial assessments
  definition, 192, 850
  domains, 203
  methods. *See* Reassessment methods
  session, purpose, 205

Assessment Plan Implementation and Evaluation (APIE), 744
  notes, 194
    contrast. *See* Subjective Objective Assessment Plan notes
    format, 196b
Assessment/planning
  bibliography, 215
  case study, 213
  importance, 192
  Internet activities, 215
  introduction, 192
  self test, 214
  sessions, 208
  student objectives, 191
  summary, 213
Assets
  description, 813b
  recording, 813
  usage, 814
Associated Bodywork and Massage Professionals (ABMP), 11, 802
Association nerves. *See* Interneurons
Asthma, 600–601
  attacks, decrease, 92, 602b
  massage, usage, 93
Astigmatism, 524
Astrocytes, 508
  definition, 850
Asymmetry, term (usage), 303
Asymmetry Border Color Diameter Elevated Fast growing (ABCDEF), 303
Atharvaveda, 780
Atherosclerosis, 580–581
  definition, 837
Athletes
  assessment, 722–725
  definition, 850
  description, 712
  interaction, 718, 722
  rehabilitation, 722
  target areas, 733
Athlete's foot, 303
Athletics, questions, 733b
Ativan (lorazepam), definition, 839
Atlas
  atlantoaxial joint, 362f
  lateral view, 363f
  superior view, 363f
Atorvastatin. *See* Lipitor
ATP. *See* Adenosine triphosphate
Atria, 565
Atrial conduction fibers, 568f
Atrial natriuretic hormone (ANH), 548, 639
  definition, 850
Atrioventricular (AV) node, 241, 567, 568f
Atrioventricular (AV) valves, 566, 567f
Atrium. *See* Left atrium; Right atrium
  definition, 850
Atrophy, 390
Atrovent (ipratropium bromide), definition, 839
Attachment trigger points, 714–715
  definition, 850
Attention deficit hyperactivity disorder (ADHD), massage (usage), 93
Atwood, Margaret, 252
Atypical vertebrae, 360–361
Auditory association area, 515f
Auditory nerve, 519
Aulus Celsus (medical historian), 6. *See also* De Medicina
Auricular area. *See* Otic area
Autoimmune diseases, 65
  definition, 850
Automobile insurance, 797

Autonomic nervous system (ANS), 507, 520–523
  divisions, 522f
  reactions, 523t
  regulation, 517
Autonomic reflexes. *See* Visceral reflexes
AV. *See* Atrioventricular
Avicenna (Abu-Ali al-Husayn ibn-Sina) (Persian physician), 7
  explanation, 850
Awareness/clarity, 26
Axial skeleton, 315
Axilla, endangerment sites, 98
Axillary, definition, 850
Axillary artery, 573
  description, 569
Axillary border, 341f
Axillary nerve, 519
Axillary nodes, 578
Axillary vein, 574
Axis
  atlantoaxial joint, 362f
  lateral view, 262f
  superior view, 363f
Axons, 275, 508–509. *See also* Transmitting neuron
  definition, 850
  illustration, 508f, 510f
  terminal, 512f
Ayurveda
  bibliography, 788
  contrast/comparison. *See* Traditional Chinese medicine
  definition, 850
  description, 780
  Internet activities, 788
  introduction, 780
  self test, 786–787
  student objectives, 753
  summary, 785
Ayur-Veda (code of life), sacred practice, 5
Ayurvedic medicine, illustration, 754f

B
Bach, Richard, 793
Back
  alternate hand superficial friction. *See* Prone client
  cupping tapotement, 166f
  gymnastics, 181t
  massage, 133f
  movements, 175
  mud, application, 677f
  pain, massage (usage). *See* Low back
  pincement tapotement, 164f
  posterior view, 730f
  sides, massage, 149f
  skin rolling pétrissage, 157f
  tapping tapotement, 163f
Backaches, discomfort, 220
Bacteria, agent, 66
Baker's cyst, 328
Balance
  improvement, 392b
  requirement, 115
  struggle, 757f
Balance sheet
  description, 813b
  usage, 814
Ball, therapist squeeze, 109f
Ball-and-socket articulations, 366t
Ball-and-socket joints (triaxial joints), 326f, 327f, 328
  definition, 850
Ballistic movements, avoidance, 173
Ball squeeze, 110

Balneology, 679
Barnes, John F., 94–95
Baroreceptor, 527
Bartholin's gland, 649f
Basal metabolic rate (BMR), 834
Basophils, 561f
Bass, Ellen, 254
Baths, 679–683. *See also* Ancient Roman public
    bath; Herbal bath; Hot air bath; Immersion
    baths; Milk bath
  definition, 850
  hydrotherapeutic applications, 674b
  usage, 672. *See also* Contrast baths; Paraffin
    baths; Steam bath
B cells, 579–580
  development, 578f
Beginning prone position, 123–124
Beginning supine position, 124–125
Behavior, consequences, 38
Bell's palsy, 529
Belly. *See* Muscles
Benazepril hydrochloride. *See* Lotensin
Benign prostatic hypertrophy, 656
Benign tumor, 245
  definition, 850
Berlioz, Hector, 5
Beta blockers, definition, 837
Beta cells, 546
Betapace (solatol), definition, 840
Beta state, 516
Beta wave activity, decrease, 90, 535b
Bhavaprakasha, 780
Biarticular, definition, 850
Biarticular muscles, 385
Biaxial joints. *See* Ellipsoidal joints; Saddle joints
Biceps brachii
  actions, 416f
  nerve, 416f
  origins/insertion, 416f
Biceps femoris (long head), 443f
  actions, 445f
  nerve, 445f
  origins/insertion, 445f
Biceps femoris (short head), 443f
Bicipital groove, 340f
Bicuspid valve. *See* Mitral valve
Big shoulder circle movement, 175, 178t
  illustration, 179f
Bile. *See* Pitta
  definition, 850
  duct. *See* Common bile duct
  entry, 618
  impact, 614t
Bindegewebsmassage (connective tissue mas-
    sage), 155–156
Biogenic amine, definition, 850
Biologic prefixes/suffixes, 263–264
Biomechanics, 110
Biotin. *See* Vitamin B₇
Bipennate muscle fiber, 385f
Bipolar disorder, 529
Birch wood, usage, 682
Birth canal. *See* Vagina
Birth control pills, definition, 840
Birth (parturition), 655
  expulsion, 655
Bladder
  epithelium, location, 271f
  infection, 639
  meridian, 758
    anterior view, 766f
    posterior view, 766f
Blastocyst
  illustration, 653f
  stages, 653f

Blood
  cells, 561–563
    types, 561f
    characteristics, 561
    chemical composition, regulation,
      632
    circulation
  illustration, 570f
  improvement, 89, 219
  paths, 572–574
  components, 561–563
  composition, 561f
  creatine kinase activity, reduction, 91,
    392b
  definition, 850
  description, 560–563
  groups. *See* ABO blood groups
  inclusion, 781
  oxygen saturation, increase, 89, 583b
  pH, regulation, 632
  plasma, 577
  supply, passage, 636
  thinner, definition, 838
  types, 563–564
  volume, 572
    regulation, 632
Blood-brain barrier, 517
  definition, 850
Blood flow. *See* Contracted muscle; Relaxed
    muscle
  increase, 156. *See also* Local blood flow
  muscle tensions, relationship, 91f
  promotion. *See* Venous blood flow
Blood pressure, 571–572
  control, assistance, 219
  decrease, 89, 583b
  definition, 850
  massage, usage. *See* High blood pressure
  regulation, 632
Blood vessels, 568–571
  diameter, 572
  dilation, 89, 583b
  endangerment sites, 97
  illustration, 314f, 566f
  wall layers, 569f
BMR. *See* Basal metabolic rate
Body
  aging, effects, 247
  alignment/posture, improvement, 180
  bibliography, 290
  cavities, 280, 281f
  coordination. *See* Movements
  diarthrosis joints (synovial joints)
    anterior view, 365f
    posterior view, 365f
  disease, relationship, 65
  examination, 780–782
  hair, lubricants (addition), 50
  image, improvement, 93
  Internet activities, 290
  introduction, 262
  language, 20
    usage, 249
  major joints, 362–368
  major muscles
    anterior view, 400f
    posterior view, 401f
  map, 698
  mask
    definition, 850
    usage, 676–677
  mechanics. *See* Seated massage
  membranes, 277–278
  placement. *See* Work
  planes, 281f

Body (*Continued*)
  polish
    definition, 850
    usage, 684
  regions, 283f
  scrubs
    definition, 850
    usage, 684
  self test, 285–289
  shampoo, definition, 850
  student objectives, 261
  summary, 284
  temperature
    impact, 668b
    ranges, 668b
    regulation, 294
  tissues, 270–277
  trauma, leaving, 253
  water balance, control, 639
  weight, usage, 778
  wrap, 677–679
    setup. *See* Massage tables
    usage. *See* Supine client
Body compass, 278–284
  bibliography, 290
  Internet activities, 290
  introduction, 262
  self test, 285–289
  student objectives, 261
  summary, 284
Body mechanics, 110–113
  attire, wearing, 117
  definition, 850
  foot stances, relationship, 115–117
  guidelines, 117–120
  inclusion, 108
  initiation, decisions, 123–125
  principles, 113–115
  quick check, 120b
Body mechanics, science
  bibliography, 139
  case study, 137
  Internet activities, 139
  introduction, 108
  objectives, 107
  self test, 138
  summary, 137
Body systems, 279t
  anatomy, relationship, 279t
  overview, 278
  physiology, relationship, 279t
Bodywork, 4
  illustration, 754f
Bodywork therapy. *See* Energy-based bodywork
    therapy
  introduction. *See* Asian bodywork therapy
Boils, 303
  term, usage, 295
Bolsters
  placement, 134f. *See also* Ankles
  usage. *See* Prone client; Supine client
Bolus, approach, 611
Bonding, importance. *See* Infant massage
Bonds, investment, 817–818
Bone marrow
  definition, 850
  description, 577–578
  illustration, 272f
Bones (osseous tissue), 271–272. *See also* Flat
    bones; Irregular bones; Long bones; Lower
    extremity; Sesamoid bones; Short bones;
    Spongy bone; Upper extremity
  aging, 314–315
  classification, 312
  connective tissue, 272f

Bones (*Continued*)
  definition, 850
  development, 314
  examples, 313f
  exercise, 314–315
  health, 314–315
  inclusion, 781
  mineral retention, increase, 92, 331b
Bony landmarks, 317
Bony markings, 317
  anterior view, 339f
  definition, 850
  lateral view, 339f
  locations, 339f
  posterior view, 339f
  types, list, 317t
Bony structures, endangerment sites, 97
Border
  bony marking, 317t
  term, usage, 303
Borelli, Giovanni Alfonso, 7
  explanation, 850
Bottom leg, massage, 133f
Bounce test, 47
Boundaries, 25–31. *See also* Professional
    boundaries
  characteristics. *See* Healthy boundaries
  clarification, 25
  crossing, mistakes, 29–31
  management, 29
  violation, 30
Boundaries, standard, 827
Bowman's capsule
  definition, 851
  description, 634
  illustration, 635f
Bow stances (archer stances), 115–116
  definition, 850
  usage, 116–117. *See also* Massage
    therapists
Braced finger technique, 119f
Braced thumb
  technique, 119f
  usage. *See* Sustained pressure
Brachial, definition, 851
Brachial area, 282
Brachial artery, 573
  description, 570
  illustration, 569f
Brachialis
  action, 416f
  nerve, 416f
  origin/insertion, 416f
Brachial plexus (C5-T1), 518, 519
Brachial vein, 574
Brachiocephalic artery, 573
Brachiocephalic vein, 574
Brachioradialis
  action, 417f
  nerves, 417f
  origin/insertion, 417f
Bradycardia, 568
  definition, 851
Brain, 515–517
  definition, 851
  hippocampal region, development (increase),
    90, 535b
  parts, 515f
Brainstem
  definition, 851
  description, 517
  illustration, 514f, 517f, 518f
Breast feeding
  nutrition considerations, 835
  oils/scents, avoidance, 223b

Breasts (mammary glands), 650. *See also*
    Female breast
  comfort system, massage table padding
    (usage), 242f
  definition, 851
  disease. *See* Fibrocystic breast disease
  glandular tissue, 545f
  implants, massage (impact), 241
  massage, impact. *See* Large breasts
  soreness, inquiry, 221
  tenderness, discomfort, 220
  tissue retraction, hands (usage), 243f
Breathing (pulmonary ventilation), 595
  definition, 851
  description, 595
  importance, 113–114
  massage therapy, relationship, 600
  mechanisms, 595–599
  usage, 120, 221
Bright, Timothy, 7. *See also* Hygienina on Re-
    storing Health; Therapeutica on Restoring
    Health
  explanation, 851
Bright's disease, 639
British Chartered Society of Massage and
    Medical Gymnastics (name
    change), 10
Britt, Stuart H., 798
Broad ligament, 649f
Broca's area (motor speech area), 515f
Brochures, purpose, 799
Broken skin, infection route, 68
Bronchi, 591f. *See also* Primary bronchi;
    Secondary bronchi
  definition, 851
Bronchioles, 591f, 593
Bronchitis, 601
Bronchodilator, definition, 838
Brow chakra (sixth chakra), 784
Brueton, Diana, 673
Bruise, 303–304
  term, usage, 295
Brunner's glands (duodenal glands), 616
  definition, 851
Buccal, definition, 851
Buccal area, 282
Buccinator
  actions, 466f
  nerve, 466f
  origins/insertion, 466f
Bulbourethral glands (Cowper's glands),
    648
  definition, 851
Bulimia, 622
Bundle of His, 567, 568f
Bunions, 328
Bupropion. *See* Wellbutrin
Burnout, prevention, 815–817
Burns, 304
Burn victims, massage (usage), 93
Burroughs, William S., 377
Bursae, 321
  definition, 851
Bursitis, 328
Business. *See* Massage business
Business cards, purpose, 799
Busy waves, 516
Butters, lubricant, 51
Buttock area. *See* Gluteal area
Byers, Dwight, 703–704

C
Café au lait spots, 305
Calcaneal, definition, 851
Calcitonin, definition, 851

Calcium (Ca)
  function, 832
  source, 832–833
Calf, two-handed pétrissage. *See* Prone client
Calf (sural), definition, 851
Calligraphy, communication (depiction), 202f
Calluses, 304
Calorie, description, 833
Calyx, 634
  definition, 851
Campbell, Joseph, 191
Cancer. *See* Skin
  massage, usage, 93, 244–245
  viewpoint, 245
Cancerous diseases, 65
  definition, 851
Candida albicans infection, 66, 245
Canon of Medicine (Avicenna), 7
Cantor, Robert, 523
Capillaries. *See* Peritubular capillaries
  definition, 851
  description, 570
  dilation, 162
  exchange, 570
  illustration, 577f
Capitate, 342
Capitulum, 340f
Carbamazepine. *See* Tegretol
Carbohydrates
  classification, 621t
  definition, 851
  description, 620–621, 830–831
  functions, 620t, 831
  source, 831
Carboxypeptidase, impact, 614t
Carcinogens, definition, 245
Cardiac cycle, 567
Cardiac muscle, 274
  pictomicrograph, 275f
  line drawing, 275f
Cardiac notch, 594
Cardiac output, 572
Cardioesophageal sphincter, 613
  definition, 851
Cardiomyopathy, definition, 838
Cardiovascular system, 560
  massage, impact, 89, 583b
  pathologic conditions, 580–582
Care, quality (principle), 24
Care plan, 192, 210b
  formulation, 206–208
Carotid artery, 573. *See also* Common carotid
    artery
Carpal, definition, 851
Carpal area, 283
Carpals, 342
  bony marking, 347t
Carpal tunnel, 346f
  syndrome, 529–530
Carradine, David, 93
Carrier oils, 687
  definition, 851
Cartilage, 272
  connective tissue, 272f
  definition, 851
Cartilaginous joint. *See* Amphiarthrosis joint
Cartilaginous tissue, 272–273
Carvedilol. *See* Coreg
Cash-based accounting, description, 813b
Cash flow
  description, 813b
  recording, 813
  statements, 813–814
Cash reserve, building, 817
Catabolism, 263

Cataract, 530
Catecholamines, 513
    definition, 851
Cauda equina, 514
Caudal reference. *See* Inferior reference
CD4/CD8 ratio, increase, 89, 584b
CD4 cells
    decline, 245
    number/function, increase, 89, 584b
CDC. *See* Centers for Disease Control and
    Prevention
Cecum, 617
    definition, 851
Celebrex (celecoxib), definition, 840
Celiac, definition, 849
Celiac area. *See* Abdominal area
Cells, 265–267
    bibliography, 290
    body, 275, 508f
        definition, 851
        description, 508
    death, 267
    definition, 851
    drinking. *See* Pinocytosis
    eating. *See* Phagocytosis
    elements, 265
    illustration, 266f
    Internet activities, 290
    introduction, 262
    membrane, 266
        definition, 851
    organization, levels, 265
    self test, 285–289
    student objectives, 261
    summary, 284
    types, 296
Cellular level, operation, 265
Cellular nutrition, improvement, 156
Cellular organization, level, 265t
Cellulite, surface dimpling (reduction), 92, 331b
Cellulitis, 304
Celsius-to-Fahrenheit conversion, 667b
Celsus, Aulus (definition), 851
Centeredness, requirement, 115
Centers for Disease Control and Prevention
    (CDC)
    establishment. *See* Universal precaution
    HIV/AIDS estimate, 245–246
Central, definition, 851
Central canal, 514
Central nervous system (CNS), 507
    definition, 851
    supporting cells, 508
Central reference (deep reference), 282
Central sulcus (central sulci), 515f, 516
Central trigger points, 714–715
    definition, 851
Central venous catheter, massage (impact), 241
Centripetally, definition, 851
Centripetal pressure, application, 146
Cephalexin. *See* Keflex
Cephalic, definition, 851
Cephalic area, 282
Cerebellar cortex, illustration, 517f
Cerebellum
    definition, 851
    description, 517
    illustration, 514f, 516f
Cerebral aqueduct, 517
Cerebral cortex, 513f, 515
Cerebral hemispheres, 515
    specialization, 516
Cerebral palsy (CP), 530–531
    massage, usage, 93
    Cerebrospinal fluid (CSF), 514

Cerebral palsy (CP) (*Continued*)
    definition, 851
    Cerebrum
    definition, 851
    description, 515–516
    illustration, 514f, 517f
Certification, explanation, 30b
Ceruminous glands, 300
Cervical, definition, 851
Cervical anterior curve, 364f
Cervical area, 282
Cervical dilation, 655
Cervical nodes, 578
Cervical pillow, bath-size towel (rolling), 123f
Cervical plexus (C1-C5), 518
Cervix, illustration, 648f, 649f
Cesarean section (C-section), usage, 225, 226
Cetirizine. *See* Zyrtec
CFS. *See* Chronic fatigue syndrome
Chain of trust. *See* Trust
Chair. *See* Massage chair
Chakra. *See* Brow chakra; Crown chakra; Heart;
    Root chakra; Sacral chakra; Solar plexus;
    Throat
    characteristics, 783–784
    definition, 851
    system, 782–784
        illustration, 783f
    term origin, 782
Charity, 74
Charley horse. *See* Legs
Chartered Society of Massage and Medical
    Gymnastics (formation), 9
Chartered Society of Physiotherapy (name
    change), 10
Chemical barrier, 579
Chemical synapses, 311
Chemoreceptors, 525
Chen-chiu ta-ch'eng (Chinese massage
    writings), 7
Cherkin, Daniel, 88
Cherry hemangiomas, 305
Chest
    anterior view, 730f
    gymnastics, 180t
    movements, 175
    treatment suggestions, 706
CHF. *See* Congestive heart failure
Chi. *See* Energy
    definition, 851
    illustration, 754f
    symbol, 755f
Chief cells, 614
    definition, 851
Chief Sealth, 590
Chi Nei Tsang, 756
Chinese clock, 758b
Chinese medicine. *See* Traditional Chinese
    medicine
    illustration, 754f
Chlamydia, 656
Chloasma (mask of pregnancy), 296
Choice, element, 35
Cholecalciferol. *See* Vitamin D
Cholecystitis, 622
Cholecystokinin, 548
    definition, 851
    impact, 614t
Chondroblast, 270
Chordae tendineae, 566
Chromosomal diseases, 655
Chronic diarrhea, 245
Chronic disease, definition, 851
Chronic fatigue syndrome (CFS), 582
    massage, usage, 93–94

Chronic illnesses
    definition, 244, 851
    equipment, caring, 246t
    massage, impact, 244–252
Chronic injury, definition, 851
Chronic obstructive pulmonary disease (COPD),
    601
Chronic pain, massage (usage), 96
Chucking friction, 160, 727. *See also* Supine
    client
Churchill, Winston, 63
Chymosin, impact, 614t
Cigarette smoking, impact, 600
Cilia, 266, 266f, 591
Cimetidine. *See* Tagamet
Circular friction, 160, 727. *See also* Forearms
    palm, application, 748f
Circular muscle, 614, 615f
    fiber, 385, 385f
Circular one-handed effleurage, 147–148
Circular two-handed effleurage, 148
Circulation
    importance, 720
    increase, 162, 171, 180
    massage, usage, 96
Circulatory system, 279t
    anatomy, 560
    bibliography, 587
    Internet activities, 587
    introduction, 560
    physiology, 560
    self test, 585–586
    student objectives, 559
    summary, 584
    terms/meanings, 560
Circumduct fingers, 175t
    traction, involvement, 177f
Circumduction, 323. *See also* Fingers; Shoulders
    definition, 851
Circumduct toes movement, 185t
    illustration, 186f
Cirrhosis. *See* Liver
Cisterna chyli, 577
Clapping tapotement, 167
Clarifying, involvement, 20
Claritin (loratadine), definition, 840
Clark, Frank A., 226
Class-1 levers, 328
    definition, 851
Class-2 levers, 328
    definition, 851
Class-3 levers, 328
    definition, 851
Clavicle, 340, 340f, 341
    bony marking, 341t
Cleavage
    lines
        Langer's lines, 298f
        map. *See* Langer's cleavage line map
    stage, 653
Client-centered care. *See* Therapeutic relationship
Client interview, 200–206
    conducting, 203–206
    control, loss, 202
    interests, signaling, 203
    orientation, initiation, 202
    setting, 202
    silence, usage, 202
    time, necessity, 202
Clients
    abuse, 30–31
    appearance, comments (avoidance), 30
    arrival
        procedure, 805–806
        therapist preparation, 28, 804–805

Clients (*Continued*)
  assistance. *See* Massage tables
  background/education, consideration, 202
  contraindications, interaction (avoidance), 30
  counseling, usage, 253–254
  dating, 36
  dissatisfaction, therapist handling, 28
  draping. *See* Massage session
  dual relationships, occurrence, 34–36
  empathy, 805
  fingers, raising, 744f
  friendship, 35
    boundary violation, 30
  harm, extreme hot/cold (impact), 672
  illness, massage (avoidance), 70
  information, collection/documentation
      (reasons), 192–193
  initial session. *See* New clients
  insufficient funds, letter (usage), 816b
  intake form
    preparation, 197
    sample, 198f
  intimacy, 35
  legs, towel draping, 130f
  listening, 19–20
  massage experience, examination, 730, 732
  mid-turn position, 131f, 132f
  neglect, 30–31
  oil recommendations. *See* Pregnant clients
  personal items, basket (usage), 806f
  physical condition, 732
  positioning. *See* Massage table mechanics
  progress, summary, 210b
  prone position, 132f
  prone to supine turning. *See* Sheet draping;
      Towel draping
  questions. *See* Hydrotherapy; Spa
  reaction, 722
  records
    no show/cancellation/no reschedule, 201
    ownership/retention, 193
  referrals, 208
  refusal right, 199
  rolling over, 129f, 130f
  rotation, 136f
  seduction, 34
  semireclining position, 602f
  side-lying to supine turning. *See* Sheet draping
  speaking, 19
  stance, 135f
  supine position, 131f, 147f
  supine to prone turning. *See* Sheet draping;
      Towel draping
  supine to side-lying turning. *See* Sheet draping
  therapist
    communication. *See* Lip-reading clients
    familiarity level, 732
    physical contact, 807f
  therapist shoulder, grasping, 135f
  towel draping, 126f
  web, 192
    definition, 852
  wheelchairs. *See* Wheelchair-bound clients
Climara (estrodiol patches), definition, 840
Clinical assessments, 722–725
Clinical massage. *See* Sports/rehabilitation
  tolerance, 726
Clitoris
  definition, 852
  description, 650
  illustration, 648f
Clopidogrel. *See* Plavix
Closed-ended questions, usage, 19, 202
Clot creation, fibrin threads (impact), 562f
Cluster headaches, 581

CNS. *See* Central nervous system
Coagulation, 562
Coarse vibration, 168. *See also* Supine client
Cobalamin. *See* Vitamin B$_{12}$
Coccygeal, definition, 852
Coccygeal area, 283
Cochlea, 525
Codeine, definition, 840
Code of ethics, 24, 36
  definition, 852
Cold. *See* Common cold
Cold compress, 673–674
Cold gel pack, 675f
Cold mitten friction. *See* Cold towel friction
Cold packs, 675
Cold stones, usage, 676
Cold (temperature)
  applications, 667
    impact, 671
  comparative effects, 680b
  contraindications, 671
Cold towel friction (cold mitten friction), 685
  definition, 852
  photograph, 686f
Colic, relief, 226
Colic gas, relief, 93, 625b
Colitis, 622. *See also* Ulcerative colitis
Collagenblast, 270
Collagen fibers, formation, 719
Collateral branch, 508f
Colleagues, sexual misconduct, 38–39
Collecting duct
  definition, 852
  description, 634
  illustration, 626f, 635f
Collegial relationships. *See* Therapeutic
    relationship
Colon
  definition, 857
  evacuation, promotion, 93, 625b
Color, term (usage), 303
Colostomy, massage (impact), 241, 243–244
Columns, 514
Common bile duct, 618, 619f
Common carotid artery
  description, 569
Common cold, 601
Common peroneal artery, 573
Common peroneal nerve, 519
Communication. *See* Adaptive professional
    communication; Nonverbal communica-
    tion; Therapeutic relationship
  definition, 19, 852
  establishment, guidelines, 744
  improvement, 93
  skills, 19–20
Compact bone, 313f, 314, 314f
  definition, 852
Comparative anatomy, 262
Comparative physiology, 262
Compassion. *See* Therapeutic relationship
Complement proteins, 579
Compliance, 595
Compress, 672–673. *See also* Cold compress;
    Hot compress
  definition, 852
Compression. *See* One-handed compression;
    Twist compression; Two-handed
    compression
  definition, 852
  description, 726
  technique, 726
  usage, 725, 726, 743
  variations, 726
Compression wraps, 677

Compress ribcage movement, 175, 180t
  illustration, 180f
Concentric contraction, 388–389
  definition, 852
  illustration, 389f
Conditioning stage. *See* Rehabilitation
Conductibility, 508
Conduction
  description, 669
  example, 669f
  system. *See* Heart
Condyle, bony marking, 317t
Cones. *See* Retina
  description, 527–528
Confidentiality, 23
  definition, 852
  principle, 24
  standard, 826–827
Conflict/conflict resolution, 21–22
  strategies. *See* Healthy conflict resolution
      strategies; Unhealthy conflict resolution
      strategies
Conflict of interest. *See* Interest conflict
Congenital disorders, 66
  definition, 852
Congestive heart failure (CHF), definition, 838
Congruency, 26
Conjugated equine estrogens, inclusion. *See*
    Prempro
Conjugated estrogens. *See* Premarin
Connective tissues, 270–274. *See also* Bones;
    Liquid connective tissue
  damage theory. *See* Muscle soreness
  definition, 852
  healing, improvement, 92, 331b
  massage. *See* Bindegewebsmassage
    impact, 92, 331b, 368b
  membranes, 277
  structures. *See* Knees
  types/locations, 272f, 273t
  vascularization, 270
Consciousness
  emotional state, 115
  mental state, 115
  physical state, 115
  states, 516
Consent form, review, 203
Constipation
  description, 623
  massage, usage, 94
  relief, 93, 625b
Contact dermatitis, 304
Contact lens users, massage (impact), 251
Contaminated linens, method, 69
Contamination. *See* Cross-contamination
  definition, 852
Continuing education
  principle, 24
  providing, 31
Continuity
  application, 144
  concept, 144
  usage, 779
Contracted muscle, blood flow, 91f
Contractility, 381, 569
Contraction. *See* Concentric contraction; Ec-
    centric contraction; Isometric contractions;
    Isotonic contractions
  energy sources, 383–384
  illustration. *See* Muscles
  mechanism, 381–383
  review, 382
  strength, 383
  thresholds, 383
Contractors, usage. *See* Independent contractors

Contracts
  definition, 852
  description, 802
  funding, 802
  logistics, 802
  proposal, 802
  qualifications, 802
  summary, 802
  usage, 801–802
Contracture, 390
Contraindications. *See* Absolute contraindications; Infant massage; Local contraindications; Massage; Pregnancy
  definition, 96, 206, 852
  ruling out, 206
Contralateral, definition, 852
Contralateral reference, 282
Contrast bath, usage, 683
Contrast method, 679. *See also* Simultaneous contrast method
  definition, 852
Contrast pack, usage, 679
Control cycles, 775–777
  inclusion. *See* Five phases
Controlled experiments, 83
Convection
  definition, 852
  description, 669
  examples, 669f
Convergent muscle fiber, 385, 385f
Conversion. *See* Energy
  definition, 852
Convoluted tubule. *See* Distal convoluted tubule; Proximal convoluted tubule
Coolidge, Calvin, 20
COPD. *See* Chronic obstructive pulmonary disease
Coracobrachialis
  actions, 415f
  nerve, 415f
  origin/insertion, 415f
Coracoid process, 340f, 341f
Coreg (carvedilol), definition, 840
Corgard (nadolol), definition, 840
Corium (hide), 297
  term, usage, 295
Corns, 304
Coronal plane. *See* Frontal plane
Coronal suture, 355
  definition, 852
Coronary artery, 573
  disease, 581
Coronoid process, 340f
Corporations, advantages/disadvantages, 795
Corpus albicans, 652f
Corpus callosum, 514f, 516f
  definition, 852
Corpus Hippocraticum (Hippocratic writings), 6
Corpus luteum, 651f
Correlational research, 83
Cortef (hydrocortisone tablets), 840
Cortex, 514f, 633
  urine manufacturing, 637
Cortical hormones, 545f
Corticosteroids
  definition, 838
  impact, 207
Cortisol (hydrocortisone), 548t
  definition, 852
  levels, reduction, 90, 535b, 552
Costal, definition, 852
Costal area, 283
Costochondral joint, 320f
Cotton sheet, usage, 678f
Cotton thermal blanket, usage, 678f

Coughing, 599
  definition, 852
Coulter, John S., 9
  explanation, 852
Coumadin (warfarin sodium), definition, 840–841
Countertransference, 32–34
  definition, 852
  red flags, 33–34
Courage (martial arts principle), 110
Cover letter, usage, 802
Cover wraps, 677
Cowper's glands. *See* Bulbourethral glands
Coxal, definition, 852
Coxal bones, 347
CP. *See* Cerebral palsy
Cranial, definition, 852
Cranial area, 282
Cranial base release, 733b
Cranial bones, 354–356
  anterior view, 356f
  bony marking, 357t
  inferior view, 358f
  posterior view, 357f
Cranial meninges, 513f
Cranial nerves, 507, 519
  definition, 852
  illustration, 521f
Cranial reference. *See* Superior reference
Cranial (skull), definition, 852
Craniosacral outflow, 521
Cream, lubricant, 50–51
Creatine kinase activity, reduction. *See* Blood
Creative cycles, 775–777
Credits, description, 813b
Crest, bony marking, 317t
Crestor (rosuvastatin calcium), definition, 841
Cretinism, 549
Crohn's disease, 623
Cross-bridge effect, 382
Cross-contamination, definition, 852
Cross-fiber friction, 159–160, 727
  fingertips, usage. *See* Paraspinals
  mini-lab, 162
Crown chakra (seventh chakra), 784
Crural, definition, 852
Crying, 599
  acceptance, 254
  definition, 852
  response. *See* Infant massage
  therapist comfort, 253f
Cryokinetics
  definition, 852
  usage, 675–676
Cryotherapy, 670–671
  definition, 852
C-section. *See* Cesarean section
CSF. *See* Cerebrospinal fluid
Cubital, definition, 852
Cubital area, 283
Cun, definition, 852
Cupping, 756
  definition, 852
Cupping tapotement, 164. *See also* Prone client
Current assets, 814
Current liabilities, 814
Curriculum vitae (CV), 801
  definition, 852
  educational achievements, 801
  organization, 801
  personal data, 801
  work experience, 801
Cushing's disease, 549
Cushing's syndrome, definition, 838
Cutaneous, term (usage), 295

Cutaneous membranes, 277
  definition, 852
  types/locations, 278f
Cuticle (eponychium), 301, 301f
  definition, 852
  term, usage, 295
CV. *See* Curriculum vitae
Cyanotic appearance. *See* Nails
Cyriax, James Henry, 159, 169
Cystitis, 639
Cytoplasm (cytosol), 266
  illustration, 646f
Cytotoxicity, 584b
Cytotoxic T cells, 580

D

Dan Tien, 778
  definition, 852
Dantien (center of gravity), 114
Darvocet (propoxyphene hydrochloride // acetaminophen), definition, 841
da Vinci, Leonardo, 54
Davis, Laura, 254
Davis's Law, 530b
Day spa, 667
  definition, 852
DDT. *See* Dichlorodiphenyltrichloroethane
De Arte Gymnastica (Mercuriale), 7
Debits, description, 813b
Decoction, 678
  definition, 852
Decubitus, term (usage), 295
Decubitus ulcers, 304
Deep fascia, 270f, 378
Deep friction, 726
  usage, 743
Deep glide, usage, 728
Deep hip outward rotators, medial/lateral view, 433f
Deep pressure massage, 712
Deep reference. *See* Central reference
Deep tissue massage, 712
Deep transverse friction, 159
Defecation, 610
  definition, 852
Deficiency diseases, 65
  definition, 852
Degenerative diseases, 65
  definition, 852
Deglutition, 611
  definition, 853
De Humani Corporis Fabrica (Vesalius), 7
dei Luzzi, Mondino, 7. *See also* Anothomia
Delayed-onset muscle soreness (DOMS), 715–718
  definition, 853
Delight, 35
Delta state, 516
Delta wave activity, increase, 90, 535b
Deltoid
  actions, 414f
  area, 283
  definition, 853
  nerve, 414f
  origins/insertion, 414f
Deltoid tuberosity, 340f, 341f
De Medicina (Celsus), 6, 7
Dementia, 531–532
De Montaigne, Michel, 739
Dendrites, 275, 508f
  definition, 853
Dennis, Wayne (touch studies), 85
Dense connective tissue, 273
  illustration, 273t
  types, 273

Dense fibrous connective tissue, 272f
Dense irregular (unorganized) connective tissue,
    273
    definition, 853
Dense regular (organized) connective tissue, 273
    definition, 853
Density, 668–669
    principle. *See* Relative density
Denvillier, S., 811
Deoxyribonucleic acid (DNA), 267, 655
    definition, 853
Depreciation, definition, 853
Depression, 251, 532
    definition, 853
    feelings, reduction, 90, 535b, 552
    relief, 219
Depression (body), 324. *See also* Mandibular
    depression; Scapular depression
Depth, application, 143–144
De Quervain's tendonitis, 390
Dermal-epidermal junction, 297
Dermal growth/repair, 298
Dermatitis. *See* Contact dermatitis; Seborrheic
    dermatitis
Dermatomes, 518
    definition, 853
    map, 518, 519f
Dermis, 295, 297–298
    definition, 853
    term, usage, 295
    true skin, 297–298
de Saint-Exupéry, Antoine, 239
De Sanitae Tuenda (Galen), 6
Descending limb, 635f, 636f
Descending tracts, 514
Descriptive research, 83
Deserts, illustration, 701f
Deshimaru, Taisen, 278
Destination spa, 667
    definition, 853
Detrol (Detrol LA // tolterodine), definition, 841
Developmental physiology, 262
Deviations. *See* Anterior deviations; Posterior
    deviations
Devillier, S., 811
Dhatus, 781
DHT. *See* Dihydrotestosterone
Diabetes, massage (usage), 94
Diabetes insipidus, 549
Diabetes mellitus, 549
Diagnosing, definition, 853
Diameter, term (usage), 303
Diaphragm
    action, 493f
    illustration, 591f
    line, 698
        horizontal landmark, 698f
    nerve, 493f
    origins/insertion, 493f
    relaxation, 599f
Diaphysis, 313, 313f
    definition, 853
Diarrhea, 233, 623
Diarthroses, 319
    examples, 320f
Diarthrosis joint (synovial joint), 319, 321
    anterior/posterior view. *See* Body
    definition, 853
    structures, 320f
    types, 326f, 327–328
Diastole, 571–572
    definition, 853
Diazepam. *See* Valium
Dichlorodiphenyltrichloroethane (DDT), 618
Dickens, Charles, 806

Dickinson, Emily, 399
Diencephalon
    definition, 853
    description, 516–517
    illustration, 514f, 517f, 518f
Diet, description, 831
Dietary fiber, 833
Dietary needs, determination, 833–834
Diffused tapotement, 167. *See also* Supine client
Diffusion, 267–268, 597. *See also* Liquid
    definition, 853
    illustration. *See* Facilitated diffusion; Passive
        diffusion
Diflucan (fluconazole), definition, 841
Digestion, 610
    definition, 853
    promotion, 226
    stimulation, 93, 625b
    substances, impact, 614t
Digestive organs. *See* Accessory digestive
    organs
Digestive system, 279t
    bibliography, 628
    illustration, 610f
    impact. *See* Waste elimination
    Internet activities, 628
    introduction, 610
    massage, impact, 93, 625b
    physiology, 610–611
    self test, 627
    student objectives, 609
    summary, 626
    terms/meanings, 625
Digestive tract
    absorption sites, 616f
    epithelium, location, 271f
Digital abduction, 321
Digital adduction, 321
Digital extension, 321
Digital flexion, 321
Digitalis. *See* Digoxin
    definition, 841
Digital (phalangeal), definition, 853
Digital (phalangeal) area, 283
Digits, 350
    hyperextension, avoidance, 118
Digoxin (digitalis). *See* Lanoxin
    definition, 841
Dihydrotestosterone (DHT), 647
Dilantin (phenytoin), definition, 841
Dilation. *See* Cervical dilation
Dinesen, Isak, 685
Direction, application. *See* Massage
Directional references, 280–282
Direct nerve stimulation, 569
Direct physical contact. *See* Pathogens; Toxic
    agents
Direct questioning, 203
Direct trauma, impact, 713
Disability
    definition, 853
    insurance, 797
Disaccharides, 620
Disarticulated skeleton, obtaining, 362
Disassociation, 253
    definition, 853
Discomfort, observation, 809f
Discrimination, principle, 24
Disease. *See* Acute disease; Chronic disease;
    Local disease; Vascular disease
    agents, 66–67
    ama, impact, 782
    awareness, 64–68
    definition, 853
    impact, 713

Disease (*Continued*)
    relationship. *See* Body; Organism/pathogen
    types, 65–66
Dislocation, 328–329
Disorders
    definition, 853
    impact, 713
Disposable gloves, removal, 71f
Distal, definition, 853
Distal convoluted tubule
    definition, 853
    description, 634
    illustration, 626f, 635f
Distal reference, 282, 282f
Distal tubule, positional relationship, 636f
Ditropan XL (oxybutynin), definition, 841
Diureses, definition, 853
Diuretic, definition, 853
Diverticulitis, 623
Diverticulosis, 623
Dividend, definition, 853
DNA. *See* Deoxyribonucleic acid
Doctorow, E.L., 244
Documentation
    definition, 192, 853
    formats, 194–196
    reasons. *See* Clients
    tips, 201–202
DOMS. *See* Delayed-onset muscle soreness
Donepezil. *See* Aricept
Dopamine, 513
    definition, 853
    levels, increase, 90, 535b, 552
Dorsal. *See* Posterior
Dorsal cavity, 280
    definition, 853
Dorsalis pedis artery, 573
    description, 570
    illustration, 569f
    Dorsal reference. *See* Posterior reference
Dorsal root ganglion, 518
    Dorsiflex ankle movement, 185t
    illustration, 185f
Dorsiflexion, 323
    definition, 853
    illustration, 324f, 701f
Dorsum, definition, 853
Doshas, 781. *See also* Tri-doshas
    definition, 853
Down syndrome (trisomy 21), 655
Downward rotation, 323–324
Drape
    adjustment, 135f
    maintenance, 136f
Draping, 125. *See also* Massage; Sheet draping;
    Towel
    definition, 853
    rules, 125–126
Drop, 326
Drowsy waves, 516
Drug addiction, issues, 252
Dry brush massage, usage, 684
Dry natural bristle brush, usage. *See* Feet
Duality, 757f
Dual licensure/roles. *See* Licensed massage
    therapist
Dual relationships
    definition, 853
    occurrence. *See* Clients
    type, 35
Duchamp, Marcel, 541
Ductless glands. *See* Endocrine glands
Ductus deferens. *See* Vas deferens
Dull, Harold, 673
Duodenal glands. *See* Brunner's glands

Duodenal papilla. *See* Major duodenal papilla
Duodenum
    definition, 853
    description, 616
    illustration, 618f
Duplicated movements, 8
Dura mater, 513f
    definition, 853
    description, 513
Durant, Will, 350
Duration, application, 145
Dynamic contractions. *See* Isotonic contractions
Dysmenorrhea, 656
Dyspnea, 595
    sensation, decrease, 92, 602b
    Dystrophy. *See* Reflex sympathetic dystrophy

E
Ear, structures, 526f
Earth
    control. *See* Water
    correspondences, 776t
    phase, 775
Eastern anatomical position, 758b
Eating disorders, massage (usage), 94
Eccentric contraction, 389
    definition, 853
    illustration, 389f
Eccrine skin glands, 301f
Eccrine sweat glands, 300
ECG. *See* Electrocardiogram
Ectoderm, 653
    definition, 853
Eczema, 305
    term, usage, 295
Edema, 577, 582–583. *See also* Lymphedema
    definition, 838, 853
    discomfort, 220
    impact. *See* Area circumference
    massage, usage, 94
    observation, 722
    patients, weight decrease, 584b
    reduction, 89, 584b
Educated Heart (McIntosh), 35
Educational achievements. *See* Curriculum vitae
Efferent arteriole, 635f
Efferent nerves. *See* Motor nerves
Efferent neuron. *See* First efferent neuron;
        Second efferent neuron
Effleurage (gliding strokes), 142, 145–152. *See
        also* Heart; Ironing effleurage; Metatarsals;
        Upper trapezius
    benefits, 152
    definition, 145, 853
    description, 145–146
    technique, 146
    usage, 743
    variations, 146t, 147–151
Eicosanoid, definition, 853
Einstein, Albert, 47
Ejaculatory duct, 647
    definition, 853
Elastic cartilage, 273
    definition, 853
Elasticity, 381, 569
Elastic layer, 569f
Elastic recoil, 595
Elbows
    endangerment sites, 98
    extension, 321, 322f
    flexion, 321, 322f
    gymnastics, 178t
    joints, 327f, 341f
    movements, 175
        muscles, 416f–418f, 418t

Elbows (*Continued*)
    technique. *See* Guided elbow technique
    usage. *See* Sustained pressure
    wetting. *See* Hand washing
Elderly people
    blood pressure, sudden drop, 247
    massaging, care, 247
Electrical brain waves, 516
Electrical synapses, 511
Electrocardiogram (ECG)
    definition, 853
    description, 568
Electromyography (EMG) readings, decrease,
        92, 392b
Elements. *See* Five elements
Elevated, term (usage), 303
Elevation, 324. *See also* Mandibular elevation;
        Scapular elevation
    definition, 853
Elimination problems, discomfort, 220
Eliot, George, 38
Ellipsoidal articulations, 366t
Ellipsoidal joints (biaxial joints), 326f,
        327f, 328
    definition, 853
Embolism, 581
Embryo, time, 653
Embryonic development, 653–654
Emerson, Ralph Waldo, 645, 801
EMG. *See* Electromyography
Emmetropia, 524
Emollientcy, 50
Emotional baggage, 33
Emotional expression, acceptance, 253
Emotional needs, satisfaction, 93
Emotional release
    discomfort, 254
    massage, impact, 253–254
    response, 254
Emotional responsiveness, 507
Empathy. *See* Clients
Emphysema, 601
Empirical, definition, 853
Empirical means, usage. *See* Objective data
Employees, usage, 815
Employment. *See* Massage business
Enalapril. *See* Vasotec
Encephalitis, 532
Endangerment sites, 97–99. *See also* Popliteal
    anterior view, map, 98f
    definition, 853
    posterior view, map, 99f
End-feel. *See* Hard end-feel; Soft end-feel
    definition, 854
    notation, 724–725
Ending prone position, 124–125
Ending supine position, 123–124
Endocardium, 566f
Endocrine glands (ductless glands)
    anatomy, 542
    bibliography, 556
    definition, 854
    description, 542
    Internet activities, 556
    introduction, 542
    list, 543–548
    location. *See* Major endocrine glands
    physiology, 542
    self test, 554–555
    student objectives, 541
Endocrine hormones
    anatomy, 542
    bibliography, 556
    Internet activities, 556
    introduction, 542

Endocrine hormones (*Continued*)
    physiology, 542
    self test, 554–555
    student objectives, 541
    summary, 552
Endocrine system, 279t
    massage, impact, 90–91, 552
    pathological conditions, 548–552
    terms/meanings, 543
Endocytosis, 269
    definition, 854
Endoderm, 654
    definition, 854
End-of-life massage, 244
Endometrial changes. *See* Uterine cycle
Endometriosis, 656
Endometrium, 649f
Endomysium, 378
Endoneurium, illustration, 510f
Endoplasmic reticulum, 267. *See also* Rough
        endoplasmic reticulum; Smooth endoplas-
        mic reticulum
    definition, 854
Endorphins, 513
    definition, 854
    release, stimulation, 156
Energetic imbalance, evaluation process, 777
Energy
    conversion, 669--670
    generation, explanation, 756–758
    illustration, 754f
    snack. *See* Sixty-second energy snack
    sources. *See* Contraction
Energy-based bodywork therapy
    bibliography, 788
    Internet activities, 788
    self test, 786–787
    student objectives, 753
    summary, 785
    techniques, 779
Energy (ki/qi/chi), 755
Energy points (tsubo), 5, 773
Engulfing microbe, 269f
Enkephalins, 513
    definition, 854
Enlightenment, 7–8
Enterocrinin, impact, 614t
Enunciation, 249
Enveloping microbe, 269f
Enzyme, 611
Eosinophils, 561f
Ependymocytes, 508
    definition, 854
Epicardium, 565, 566f
Epicondyle, bony marking, 317t
Epidermal growth, 297
Epidermal layer, 296–297
Epidermis, 295–298
    definition, 854
    term, usage, 295
Epididymis, 647
    definition, 854
Epidural space, 513
    definition, 854
Epiglottis, definition, 854
Epimysium, 378
Epinephrine (adrenaline), 513, 548t. *See also*
        Primatene Mist
    definition, 854
    levels, reduction, 90, 535b, 552
Epineurium, illustration, 510f
Epiphyseal line, 313f, 314
    definition, 854
Epiphyseal plate, 314
    definition, 854

Epiphysis (epiphyses), 313–314, 313f
    definition, 854
Epistaxis, 591
Epithelial membranes, composition, 277
Epithelial tissue (epithelium), 270
    composition, 295
    definition, 854
    location. *See* Bladder
    locations, 271f
Epoetin alfa. *See* Procrit
Eponychium. *See* Cuticle
Epsom salts, usage, 680
Equipment, unsuitability, 718
Equity, 814
    description, 813b
Erb's palsy, 532
Erection. *See* Female erection; Male
    erection
Erector spinae, 491
Ernst, Edzard, 88
Errors and omission insurance, 797
Erwin, Joey, 619
Erythrocytes, 561–562
    definition, 854
    illustration, 562f
Esomeprazole. *See* Nexium
Esophagus, 612
    definition, 854
Essential nutrients, 830
    types, 830
Essential oils, 687
    definition, 854
    examples, 687
    storage, 687
    therapy. *See* Aromatherapy
Estrace (estradiol tablets), definition, 841
Estraderm (estradiol), definition, 841
Estradiol
    patches. *See* Climara
    tablets. *See* Estrace
Estrogen, 545f, 549t
    definition, 854
    levels, 651f
Ethical decisions, making, 24–25
Ethical requirements, standard, 826
Ethical responsibility, 199
Ethics
    code. *See* Code of ethics
    committee, consultation, 25
Ethinyl estradiol. *See* Ortho Tri-Cyclen
    transdermal system. *See* Ortho Evra
Ethmoidal sinus, 356, 591
Ethmoid sinus, 358f
Ethnographic research, 84
Eucalyptus, 688
European Renaissance, 7–8
    definition, 861
Evaluation stage. *See* Rehabilitation
Eversion, 323
    definition, 854
    illustration, 324f, 701f
Exacerbation, definition, 854
Excitability, 381, 508
Excitation, 382. *See also* Sarcolemma
Excitatory neurotransmitters, 512
Excursion, application, 144
Exercise
    combination. *See* Water
    illustration, 754f
Exfoliation, definition, 854
Exhalation. *See* Expiration
Exocrine glands, 542
    definition, 854
Experimental research, 83
Experiments, definition, 83

Expiration (exhalation), 595
    definition, 854
    illustration, 599f
Exploring, usage, 20
Expression, improvement, 93
Expulsion. *See* Birth
Extended arm
    rolling friction. *See* Supine client
    wringing friction. *See* Supine client
Extensibility, 381
Extension, 321. *See also* Fingers; Hyperexten-
    sion; Lateral extension; Myosin head; Toes
    definition, 854
Extensor carpi radialis brevis
    actions, 423f
    nerve, 423f
    origins/insertions, 423f
Extensor carpi radialis longus
    actions, 423f
    nerve, 423f
    origins/insertions, 423f
Extensor carpi ulnaris
    actions, 424f
    nerve, 424f
    origin/insertion, 424f
Extensor digiti minimi
    action, 425f
    nerve, 425f
    origin/insertion, 425f
Extensor digitorum
    actions, 424f
    nerve, 424f
    origin/insertions, 424f
Extensor digitorum brevis
    actions, 453f
    nerve, 453f
    origins/insertions, 453f
Extensor digitorum longus
    actions, 453f
    nerve, 453f
    origins/insertions, 453f
Extensor hallucis longus
    actions, 453f
    nerve, 453f
    origins/insertion, 453f
Extensor indicis
    action, 425f
    nerve, 425f
    origin/insertion, 425f
Extensor pollicis brevis
    action, 426f
    nerve, 426f
    origins/insertions, 426f
Extensor pollicis longus
    action, 426f
    nerve, 426f
    origins/insertions, 426f
External, definition, 854
External intercostal
    actions, 494f
    nerve, 494f
    origin/insertion, 494f
External obliques
    actions, 486f
    nerve, 486f
    origins/insertions, 486f
External reference, 282
External respiration (pulmonary respiration),
    597, 599
    definition, 854
    muscles, 493–495
    list, 496
Exteroceptors, 525
    definition, 854
Extracellular fluid, 577

Extrafusal muscle, 528f
Extreme behavior, 252–253
Extremities, 317
Eyes
    conditions, 251
    martial arts principle, 110
    orbits, 354

F
Face
    bolstered area, 121
    cradle, usage, 746
    endangerment sites, 98
    great sensory nerve, 519
    raindrops tapotement. *See* Supine client
    rest, usage. *See* Prone client
    seated massage routine, 748
Face rest, usage. *See* Massage tables
Facet, bony marking, 317t
Facial, definition, 854
Facial area, 282
Facial artery
    description, 569
    illustration, 569f
Facial bones, 359
    bony marking, 359t
Facial expressions
    communication, 20
    usage, 249
Facial nerve, 519, 521f
Facial tissues, offering, 253
Facilitated diffusion, 268
    illustration, 268f
Facilitation. *See* Law of Facilitation
Fallen arches, 350
Fallopian tube (oviducts)
    definition, 854
    description, 649
    illustration, 648f, 649f
False vocal cords, 593
Falx cerebelli, 513
Falx cerebri, 513
Famotidine. *See* Pepcid
Fanfolds, unfolding. *See* Towel
Fahrenheit-to-Celsius conversion, 667b
Fascia, ground substance, 274
Fascia connective tissue, 274
    information, 712
Fascial restrictions, release, 92, 331b
Fascia viscoelastic state, 274
Fascicle, illustration, 510f
Fasciculi, definition, 854
Fast growing, term (usage), 303
Fast twitch muscles (white muscles), 388
Father Sebastian Kneipp. *See* Kneipp
Fatigue
    discomfort, 220
    impact, 713
    reduction, 93
    relief, 156, 219
Fats
    classification, 621t
    definition, 854
    description, 621, 831
    function, 620t, 831
    inclusion, 781
    source, 831
Fat-soluble vitamins, 294
Fatty apron, 616
Fe. *See* Iron
Fear, acceptance, 254
Federal tax identification number, 796
Feedback systems. *See* Negative feedback sys-
    tem; Positive feedback system
    role, 64

Feelings, contact, 254
Feet
    anterior view, 460f
    arches, 350, 353
        imprint, 355f
    bones, 349–350
    flop, illustration, 701f
    ground, contact points, 355f
    gymnastics, 185t
    movements, 180
        muscles, 452f–461f
        muscles, list, 459
    placement, examination, 118
    posterior view, 461f
    stances, relationship. See Body
        mechanics
    stimulation, dry natural bristle brush (usage),
        702f
    stool, therapist usage, 119f
    support base, 116f
    swelling, inquiry, 221
    treatment areas, 705f
    winging out, 701f
Feldenkrais, Moshe (biography), 26–27
Female breast, 650f
Female clients
    abdominal area, access, 126–127
    back, exposure. See Side-lying female
        client
    towel draping, 126. See also Supine female
        client
Female erection, 652
Female lubrication, 652
Female orgasm, 652
Female reproductive cycle, 650–652
    first phase, 650–651
    fourth cycle, 652
    illustration, 651f
    second phase, 651–652
    third phase, 652
Female reproductive organs, 648–650
Femoral, definition, 854
Femoral artery, 573
    description, 570
    illustration, 569f
Femoral nerve, 519
Femoral triangle, endangerment sites, 98
Femoral vein, 574
Femur, 347, 448f
    anterior view, 348f
    bony marking, 350t
    posterior view, 349f
Fenofibrate. See Tricor
Fertilization
    definition, 854
    description, 646
    illustration, 646f, 653f
Fetal delivery, perineum (preparation), 219
Fetal development, 655
Fetal movement, reduction (inquiry), 221
Fever, 579. See also Hay fever
Fexofenadine. See Allegra
Fiber. See Dietary fiber
Fibrinogen, 561
Fibrin threads, impact. See Clot creation
Fibroblasts, 270
Fibrocartilage, 273
    definition, 854
Fibrocystic breast disease, 656
Fibromyalgia, 390
    massage, usage, 94
Fibrosis. See Tissue healing
Fibrous joint. See Synarthrosis joint
Fibula, 348–349
    bony marking, 353t

Fibularis brevis
    actions, 454f
    nerve, 454f
    origin/insertion, 454f
Fibularis longus
    actions, 454f
    nerve, 454f
    origins/insertions, 454f
Field, Tiffany, 87, 248, 741
    photograph, 87f
Fight-or-flight division, 522
Fight-or-flight response, 543, 775
Filtrate, 637
    definition, 854
Filtration, 268, 637
    definition, 854
    process, 636–637
Filum terminale, 514
Fimbriae, 649f
Financial portfolio, definition, 854
Financial projections. See Massage business
Financial reports, importance, 813–814
Findings, 828–829
Fine-motor movements, 713
Fine vibration, 167–168. See also Prone client;
        Supine client
Fingernails
    cleaning. See Hand washing
    cleanliness/length, 69
    polish, absence, 69
Finger pressure. See Shiatsu
Fingers
    abduction, 323f
    adduction, 323f
    circumduction, 324f
    flexion/extension, 321f
    interlacing, 175t
    movements, muscles, 429t
    pads, usage. See Supine client
    positioning, 118
    usage. See Rubber band; Skin
Finger stretch, 110
Fingertips, usage. See Paraspinals
Finger-walking technique, 700f
Fire
    correspondences, 776t
    phase, 774–775
    wood control, 776
First cervical vertebrae, second cervical verte-
        brae (joints), 327f
First-class levers, 329f
First-degree strain, 392
First efferent neuron, 509f
Fist effleurage. See Upper trapezius
Fitzgerald, William, 696
Five elements (phases), correspondences, 776t
Five phases (elements)
    control cycles, inclusion, 776t
    correspondences, 776t
    meridians, inclusion, 776t
    theory, 774–777
Fixators, 386
    definition, 854
Flaccid muscles, 390
    toning, 167
Flat bones, 312
    example, 313f
Flat feet (pes planus), 350
    imprint, 355f
Flesh, inclusion, 781
Flexibility
    absence, 718
    increase, 392b
    maintenance, 180
Flexibility/adaptability, 26

Flexion, 321. See also Fingers; Toes
    definition, 854
Flexor carpi radialis
    actions, 420f
    nerve, 420f
    origin/insertion, 420f
Flexor carpi ulnaris
    actions, 421f
    nerve, 421f
    origin/insertions, 421f
Flexor digiti minimi
    action, 428f
    nerve, 428f
    origin/insertion, 428f
Flexor digitorum longus
    actions, 458f
    nerve, 458f
    origin/insertions, 458f
Flexor digitorum profundus
    action, 422f
    nerve, 422f
    origins/insertions, 422f
Flexor digitorum superficialis
    actions, 422f
    nerve, 422f
    origins/insertions, 422f
Flexor hallucis longus
    actions, 458f
    nerve, 458f
    origin/insertion, 458f
Flexor pollicis brevis
    action, 426f
    nerve, 426f
    origins/insertions, 426f
Flexor pollicis longus
    action, 426f
    nerve, 426f
    origins/insertions, 426f
Flip wrist
    illustration, 176f
    movement, 175t
Flomax (tamsulosin), definition, 841
Flotation, 682
Fluconazole. See Diflucan
Fluid balance, regulation, 632
Fluoxetine. See Prozac
Folic acid. See Vitamin B$_9$
Follicle. See Primary follicles
    development, 651f
        stages. See Ovarian follicle development
    illustration, 652f
    term, usage, 295
Follicle-stimulating hormone (FSH), 545t, 652
    definition, 854
    levels, 651f
Follicular cells (granulosa), 646f
Follicular phase, 651f
Folliculitis, 305
Fomentation packs, 674
Fontanel. See Anterior fontanel; Posterior
        fontanel
Foods
    disassembly, 619–622
    pyramid. See New food pyramid
Footprint, skeletal overlay, 355f
Foot reflexology
    definition, 854
    description, 697
    introduction, 696
    map, 699f
    student objectives, 695
    techniques, 698–700
    treatment
        guidelines, 700–703
        suggestions, 704–707

Footwork (martial arts principle), 110
Foramen, bony marking, 317t
Force, nonusage, 778
Forced expiratory volume/flow, increase.
    See Lungs
Forced vital capacity, increase. See Lungs
Forearm iron effleurage, 148f
Forearms
    anterior view, 430f
    bones, 342
    muscles, 419f–431f
        list, 429t
    musculature
        circular friction, 162f
        one-thumb cross-fiber technique, 161f
    posterior view, 431f
    wetting. See Hand washing
Forebrain, turning in, 515
Foreign substances, elimination, 632
Form, function (relationship), 262
Fossa, bony marking, 317t
Foundation, laying, 792–797
Foundational touch research, 84–87
Fourth ventricle, 517f
Fractures, 329
    healing, promotion, 92, 331b
France, Anatole, 791
Free edge, 301f
Free nail edge, 301
    definition, 854
Free nerve endings, 296f, 528
Friction, 142, 156–162, 725. See also Chucking
        friction; Circular friction; Cold-towel fric-
        tion; Cross-fiber friction; Hydrotherapeutic
        friction; Towel
    benefits, 162
    definition, 854
    description, 156–158, 726
    hydrotherapeutic applications, 674b
    technique, 158–161, 726–727–727
    usage, 672, 683–685, 726–727. See also Deep
        friction; Superficial friction
    variations, 146t, 727
Frictions (hydro/spa treatment), definition,
    854
Friendship. See Clients
Frontal, definition, 854
Frontal area, 282
Frontal bone, 320f, 467f
Frontalis
    actions, 462f
    nerve, 462f
    origin/insertion, 462f
Frontal lobe, 515f
    definition, 854
    description, 515
Frontal plane (coronal plane), 280, 281f, 723
    definition, 855
Frontal sinus, 356, 591
    illustration, 358f
Frost, Robert (quotation), 15
FSH. See Follicle-stimulating hormone
Fu. See Zang/fu
Fuller, Buckminster, 82
Fulling pétrissage, 155. See also Quadriceps;
        Thighs
Function. See Muscles
Functional reversibility, 384
Funds, investment, 818. See also Index funds;
        Mutual funds
Fundus, 613, 649f
Fungi, agent, 66
Furosemide. See Lasix
Fusiform muscle fiber, 385f
Future, investment, 817

G
Gait
    consideration, 723–724
    definition, 855
Galea aponeurotica, 462f
Galen of Pergamon (Hippocratic follower), 6
    explanation, 855
Gallbladder
    definition, 855
    description, 618
    illustration, 618f
    meridian, 758
        anterior view, 770f
        lateral view, 770f
        posterior view, 771f
Gallstones, 623
Gametes, 646
    definition, 855
Ganglion cyst, 391
Ganglion (ganglia), 508
    definition, 855
    description, 518
    illustration, 509f
Garshana, 672
Gas discomfort, relief, 226
Gases, exchange, 590. See also Lungs
Gastric mucosa, 548t, 614
Gastrin
    definition, 855
    impact, 614t
Gastritis, 623
Gastrocnemius, 455f
    actions, 456f
    nerve, 456f
    origins/insertion, 456f
Gastroenteritis, 623
Gastroesophageal reflux disease (GERD)
    description, 623
    discomfort, 220–221
Gastrointestinal (GI) complaints, discomfort,
    220–221
Gastrointestinal (GI) tract, 610
    pathologic conditions, 622–625
Gate theory, 91
G cell, definition, 855
Gel pack. See Cold gel pack
Gels, lubricant, 51
Gel state, 712
Gemellus inferior
    action, 435f
    nerve, 435f
    origin/insertion, 435f
Gemellus superior
    action, 435f
    nerve, 435f
    origin/insertion, 435f
Gemfibrozil. See Lopid
Gene, 655
    definition, 855
General Guide to Calories (FDA), 833–834
Generalization. See Law of Generalization
General liability, 797
General sense organs, 523
Genetic diseases, 65
    definition, 855
Genetics, 655
    definition, 855
Genital herpes, 656
Genital warts, 656
GERD. See Gastroesophageal reflux disease
Geriatric
    definition, 855
    reference, 247
Geriatric clients, massage (impact), 247
Germ layers. See Primary germ layers

Gestures, communication, 20
GH. See Growth hormone
GI. See Gastrointestinal
Gibson, Edward, 817
Gide, Andre, 631
Glands. See Endocrine glands
    endangerment sites, 97
Glantz, Kalman, 16
Glaucoma, 532
    definition, 838
Glenohumeral joints. See Shoulders
Gliding articulations, 366f
Gliding joints (triaxial joints), 326f, 327f, 328
    definition, 855
Gliding strokes. See Effleurage
Glipizide. See Glucotrol
Glomerulonephritis, 639–640
Glomerulus, 636
    definition, 855
    description, 634
    illustration, 635f
Glossopharyngeal nerve, 519, 521f
Gloves, usage, 70
    guidelines, 70–72
Glucagon, 548t
    definition, 855
Glucophage (metformin), definition, 842
Glucose
    requirement, 383–384
    utilization, 383
Glucotrol (glipizide), definition, 842
Gluteal (buttock), definition, 855
Gluteal (buttock) area, 283
Gluteals (buttocks), 437f
Gluteus maximus, 437f
    actions, 438f
    nerve, 438f
    origins/insertion, 438f
Gluteus medius, 437f
    actions, 438f
    nerve, 438f
    origin/insertions, 438f
Gluteus minimus
    actions, 439f
    nerve, 439f
    origin/insertion, 439f
Glyburide. See Micronase
Goblet cells, 591
Goethe, 793
Goiter, 549, 553
Golgi body, 267
    definition, 855
    illustration, 266f
Golgi tendon organs, 388, 509
    definition, 855
    description, 527
    illustration, 529f
    mediation, 173
Gonads, 547, 646
    definition, 855
    hormones, inclusion, 549t
Gonorrhea, 656–657
Good Health (Kellogg), 9
Gout, 640
Gouty arthritis, 329
Gracilis, 445f, 448f
    actions, 446f
    nerver, 446f
    origin/insertion, 446f
Grad, Bernard (touch research), 85
Graham, Douglas O., 9. See also Treatise on
        Massage, Its History, Mode of Application
        and Effects
    explanation, 855

Graham, Martha, 208
Granular endoplasmic reticulum. *See* Rough endoplasmic reticulum
Granular leukocytes, 561f
Granulosa. *See* Follicular cells
Granulosum, term (usage), 295
Graves' disease, 551
Greater omentum
    definition, 855
    description, 616
    illustration, 612f
Greater tubercle, 340f, 341f
Great extensor. *See* Radial nerve
Great flexor. *See* Median nerve
Groin (inguinal), definition, 855
Groin (inguinal) area, 283
Groin stretch movement, 180, 182t
    illustration, 183f
Groove, bony marking, 317t
Groshong catheters, 241
Gross anatomy, 262
Gross income, description, 813b
Gross-motor movements, 713
Groundedness, requirement, 115
Grounded theory, 84
Growing child, massage (adaptation), 232–233
Growth hormone (somatropin) (GH // STH), 545t
    definition, 855
Gua-Sha, 756
    definition, 855
Guided elbow technique, 747f
Guillain-Barré syndrome, 532
Gustatory organs, 523, 611
    definition, 855
Gyri, 515

H
Hacking, 163–164
Haganah, 26
Hair
    cleanliness, 69
    follicles, 302
    lubricants, addition. *See* Body
    related structures, 298–301
    root plexus (hair follicle receptor), 302, 526
        definition, 855
Hairstyle, selection, 69
Hallux, definition, 855
Halpern, Steve, 55
Hamate, 342
Hammertoe, 329
Hamstrings, 443f
Handicap, definition, 855
Hands
    bones, 342–347
    C formation, usage. *See* Pétrissage
    gymnastics, 175t
    joints, 320f
    movements, 174–175
        muscles, 419f–431f
    position, demonstration. *See* Push hands
    swelling, inquiry, 221
    ulnar sides, usage. *See* Scapula
    usage. *See* Skin
Hand swishing, 110
    performing, 109f
Hand washing
    fingernails, cleaning, 72f
    forearms/elbows, wetting, 72f
    hands
        drying, 73f
        soaping, 72f
        wetting, 72f

Hand washing (*Continued*)
    importance, 72–73
    procedure, 72–73
    usage, 69
    rinsing, 73f
    water, usage, 72f, 73f
Hannigan, Mary, 676
Hara (lower abdomen), 114
    definition, 855
    diagnostic area map, 780f
    evaluation, 779–780
    movement, 778
Hard end-feel, 725
Harlow, Harry
    photograph, 86f
    touch research, 85
Harnate, 346f
Harvey, William, 7
Harvey, William (explanation), 855
    illustration, 8f
Haustra, definition, 855
Haversian canals, 313, 314f
    definition, 855
Hawthorne, Nathaniel, 6
Hay fever, 601
H-band, 381
HCFA. *See* Health Care Financing Administration
hCG. *See* Human chorionic gonadotropin
Head
    anterior view, 480f, 730f
    bolstered area, 121
    bony attachments, 482f–484f
        lateral view, 483f, 484f
        superior/inferior view, 483f, 484f
    bony marking, 317t
    great sensory nerve, 519
    lateral view, 730f
    movements, muscles, 462f–484f
        list, 479
    posterior view, 481f, 730f
    regional terms, 282
    stool, therapist usage, 119f
    treatment
        areas, 733
        suggestions, 706
Headaches, 391. *See also* Cluster headaches
    discomfort, 221
    massage, usage, 94
    reduction, 219
Head pillow, usage. *See* Supine female client
Healing, 718
    agent. *See* Spa
    magico-religious approach, 780
    process. *See* Tissue healing
Health. *See* Massage therapists
    Asian medicine model, 754–755
    bibliography, 79
    case study, 75
    definition, 74, 855
    homeostasis, relationship, 64
    information, 206
    insurance, 797
    Internet activities, 79
    introduction, 64
    self test, 76–78
    student objectives, 63
Health Care Financing Administration (HCFA)
    1500 Form, 812
Health care team members, networking, 209–212
Health Insurance Portability and Accountability Act of 1996 (HIPAA), 192, 211–212
    confidentiality notice, 212b
    guidelines. *See* Massage therapists
Healthy boundaries, characteristics, 26

Healthy conflict resolution strategies, 21t
Hearing, sense organs, 524–525
Hearing-impaired clients
    massage, impact, 249–250
    premassage interview, time (allowance), 249
Heart, 548, 565–568
    beats, number, 565
    chakra (fourth chakra), 784
    chambers, 565–566
        illustration, 567f
    conduction system, 567–568
        illustration, 568f
    coverings, 565
    cross-section, 565f
    description, 565
    effleurage, 148
        usage. *See* Prone client
    meridian, 758
        anterior view, 763f
        posterior view, 763f
    murmur, 581
    protector, meridian, 758
        anterior view, 768f
        posterior view, 768f
    rates, 567–568
        reduction, 89, 583b
    valves, 566
        illustration, 567f
    wall, 565
        cross-section, 566f
Heartburn, complaints, 220
Heat
    applications, 667
        impact, 670
    comparative effects, 680b
    conservation (vasoconstriction), 295f
    contraindications, 670
    generation, 162
    loss, increase (vasodilation), 295f
Heel, praying hands two-handed pétrissage. *See* Prone client
Heel to hip movement, 180, 182t
    illustration, 184f
Hefty, Brenda, 120
Helper T cells, 580
Hemangiomas. *See* Cherry hemangiomas; Strawberry hemangiomas
Hematoma, 581
Hemiplegia, 251
Hemispheres. *See* Left hemisphere; Right hemisphere
    specialization. *See* Cerebral hemispheres
Hemoglobin
    definition, 855
    description, 562
Hendricks, Gay, 29, 253. *See also Year of Living Consciously*
Hendricks, Kathlyn, 253
Hepatic duct, 618f. *See also* Left hepatic duct; Right hepatic duct
Hepatic portal circulation, 574f
Hepatic portal system, 573
    definition, 855
Hepatitis, 623
Heraclitus, 669
Herbal bath, 680
Herbal wraps, 677–678
Hernia, 624
Herniated disk, 329–330
Herodicus (Hippocrates teacher), 8
Herophilies, 275
Herpes simplex, 305
Hiccups, 599
    definition, 855
Hickman catheters, 241

High arches, imprint, 355f
High blood pressure, massage (usage), 94
High-risk pregnancy, 222
Hike, 326
Hilton's Law, 530b
Hilum, 633
    definition, 855
Hinge articulations, 366t
Hinge joint (monoaxial joint), 326f, 327, 327f
    definition, 855
HIPAA. See Health Insurance Portability and
    Accountability Act of 1996
Hip circle movement, 180, 182t
    illustration, 183f
Hip clock stretch movement, 180, 182t
    illustration, 183f
Hip hyperextension movement, 180, 182t
    illustration, 184f
Hippocampal region, development. See Brain
Hippocrates of Cos, 8, 666, 682. See also On
        Joints
    emphasis, 5–6
    explanation, 855
    image, 6f
Hip rotation movement, 180, 182t
    illustration, 184f
Hip rotators, access, 167, 171
Hips
    abduction, 321, 323f
    adduction, 321, 323f
    anterior view, 450f
    bones, 347
    extension, 321, 322f
    flexion, 321, 322f
    gymnastics, 182t
    joint jostling vibration. See Prone client
    joints, 327f
    movements, 175, 180
        muscles, 432f–451f
        muscles, list, 449f
    placement, examination, 118
    posterior view, 451f
    rotation, 325f
    treatment areas, 733
Histamine, 513
    definition, 855
    release, stimulation, 89, 583b
Histology, 270. See also Skeletal system
Historical research, 84
HIV. See Human immunodeficiency virus
Hives, 305
Homeostasis, 64, 590
    definition, 262, 855
    maintenance, 632, 667
    relationship. See Health
Homeostatic regulation, 572
Homolateral, definition, 855
Homolateral reference (ipsilateral reference),
        282, 282f
Homunculus, illustration, 302f
Honesty, principle, 24
Hooke, Robert, 265
Horizontal abduction, 321
Horizontal adduction, 321
Horizontal landmarks, 698f, 723. See also
        Anterior horizontal landmarks; Posterior
        horizontal landmarks
Horizontal plane. See Transverse plane
Hormonal control systems, 543
    definition, 855
Hormonal functions, 553t
Hormones. See Endocrine hormones; Steroid
        hormone
    definition, 855
    description, 542–543

Hormones (Continued)
    inclusion. See Adrenal glands; Anterior
        pituitary; Gonads; Pancreatic islets;
        Parathyroid gland; Thyroid gland
    types, 543
Horns, 514
Horse stances. See Warrior stances
Hose shower, 683
Hospice patients, massage (usage), 95
Hospitalized patients, massage (usage), 95
Host, definition, 855
Host-pathogen relationship, 68
Hot air baths, 682
Hot compress, 673
Hotel spa, 667
    definition. See Resort spa
Hot pack, terrycloth pouch (usage), 674f
Hot tubs
    definition, 855
    usage, 681
Housekeeping system, 521
HPV. See Human papillomavirus
HSV2. See Type 2 herpes simplex virus
Huang-ti nei-ching (Chinese medicine), 5
    recognition, 5
Hubbard, Carl, 680
Hubbard tank, 680
Human body. See Body
Human chorionic gonadotropin (hCG), 548
    definition, 855
    secretion, 654
Human development, 652–655
Human genetics, 655
Human immunodeficiency virus (HIV)
    guidelines, 246–247
        HIV-positive clients, massage (impact),
            245–247
    infections, 246
    massage, usage, 94–95
    precautions, 246
Human needs, hierarchy, 86b
Human papillomavirus (HPV), impact, 245
Human skeleton, relationships, 338f
Humeral head, 341f
Humerus, 340f, 341–342, 341f
    bony marking, 342t
Humulin (insulin), definition, 842
Hunchback, 330
Hunger, cause, 615
Hunting response, 671
    definition, 855
Huxley, Hugh, 378
Hyaline cartilage (tracheal ring), 272–273
    definition, 855
    illustration, 594f
Hydrochloric acid, impact, 614t
Hydrocodone. See Vicodin
Hydrocollator, 674
    unit, 674f
Hydrocortisone. See Cortisol
    tablets. See Cortef
Hydrogenated oils, 621
Hydrostatic pressure, 669
Hydrotherapeutic applications, 674b
Hydrotherapeutic friction, 672
Hydrotherapy
    application methods, 672
    bibliography, 692
    clients, questions, 672b
    definition, 856
    description, 666
    effectiveness (enhancement), aromatherapy
        (impact), 686
    Internet activities, 692
    introduction, 666

Hydrotherapy (Continued)
    self test, 690
    student objectives, 665
    summary, 689
    treatment guidelines, 671–685
Hygiene. See Massage therapists
    bibliography, 79
    case study, 75
    considerations. See Massage chair
    definition, 74, 856
    Internet activities, 79
    introduction, 64
    self test, 76–78
    student objectives, 63
Hygienina on Restoring Health (Bright), 7
Hyoid bone, 356
Hyperemia, 572
    creation, 89, 583b
    definition, 856
Hyperextension, 321
    avoidance. See Digits
Hyperkyphosis, 330
Hyperopia, 524
Hyperparathyroidism, 551
Hyperpituitarism, 551
Hyperplasia, softening, 162
Hypersensitive area, desensitization, 167
Hypertension, 581
    definition, 838
Hyperthyroidism, 551–552
Hypertrophic cardiomyopathy, definition,
        838
Hypoglossal nerve, 519
Hypoglycemia, 552
    definition, 838
Hypoparathyroidism, 552
Hypopituitarism, 552
Hypotension, definition, 838
Hypothalamus, 544f
    definition, 856
    description, 517
    illustration, 514f, 518f
Hypothenar eminence
    anatomic snuffbox, 429
Hypothyroidism, 552
    definition, 838
Hypoxia, 595

I
I-band, 381
Ibuprofen. See Advil; Motrin
    definition, 842
ICD. See Implantable cardioverter defibrillator
Ice massage, 685
    definition, 856
    hydrotherapeutic applications, 674b
    photograph, 685f
Ice pack, usage. See Prone client
Ida, 781
Ileocecal sphincter, 615
    definition, 856
Ileostomy, massage (impact), 241, 243–244
Ileum, definition, 856
Iliac artery, 573
Iliacus
    actions, 433f
    nerve, 433f
    origins/insertion, 433f
Iliac vein, 574
Iliocostalis, 488b, 491f
    actions, 492f
    nerve, 492f
    origins/insertions, 492f
Iliolumbar ligament, 361
Iliopsoas, 432f

Iliotibial band
  knee flexion/hip outward rotation, palmar circular effleurage, 148f
  palmar circular friction, 162f
Ilium, 347
  bony marking, 350t
IM. *See* Intramuscular
Imbalance, evaluation process. *See* Energetic imbalance
Immersion baths, 680–681
Immune system, massage (impact), 89
Immunity, 579–580. *See also* Acquired immunity; Natural immunity
  definition, 856
  skin, role, 294
Impetigo, 305
Implantable cardioverter defibrillator (ICD), massage (impact), 241
Implantation
  description, 653
  illustration, 653f
Implanted devices, massage, 241
Impulses. *See* Nerve impulses
Inactivity
  impact, 251
  periods, impact, 713
Incident reports, 31–32
  form, 32f
Income
  diversification, 811
  tax, 814
Incompetent cervix, inquiry, 221
Incontinence. *See* Urinary incontinence
Independent contractors, usage, 815
Inderal (propranolol), definition, 842
Index funds, investment, 818
Indigestion, complaints, 220
Individual Retirement Accounts (IRAs), usage, 818
Infant massage
  avoidance, 228
  baby, reading, 229–230
  background music, usage, 232
  benefits, 226. *See also* Parents
  bibliography, 236
  bonding, importance, 227
  case study, 234
  contraindications, 233
  contrast. *See* Adult massage
  crying, response, 228–229
  environment, organization, 232
  infant behavior, guide, 228
  initiation, 227–228
  instructor, becoming, 233
  Internet activities, 236
  introduction, 218, 226–227
  lighting, usage, 232
  noise, control, 232
  parent instruction, dolls (usage), 231–232
  personnel, identification, 232
  positioning, importance, 232
  precautions, 233
  self test, 235
  strokes, usage, 229–232
  student objectives, 217
  summary, 233
  usage, 95
Infants
  comfort positioning, 229
  cues, 229–230
  sleep stages, 228
Infection
  relationship. *See* Organism/pathogen
  route. *See* Broken skin; Ingestion; Inhalation; Intact skin; Mucous membranes
  transmission, modes, 67–68

Infection control. *See* Massage therapists
  bibliography, 79
  case study, 75
  Internet activities, 79
  introduction, 64
  self test, 76–78
  student objectives, 63
Infectious diseases, 65–66
  definition, 856
Inferior, definition, 856
Inferior angle, 341f
Inferior reference (caudal reference), 282
Inflammation, 579, 713
  cardinal signs, 719f
  definition, 856
  theory. *See* Muscle soreness
Influenza, 601
Information
  nondisclosure. *See* Privileged information
  usage, 199
Informed consent, 199–200
  definition, 856
  mini-lab, 199
  principle, 24
Infraglenoid tubercle, 340f, 341f
Infraspinatus
  action, 412f
  nerve, 412f
  origin/insertion, 412f
Infraspinous fossa, 341f
Infundibulum, 516f, 649f
Infusion (tea)
  definition, 856
  usage, 678
Ingestion, 610
  definition, 856
  infection route, 68
Ingham, Eunice, 696f
Inguinal area. *See* Groin area
Inguinal nodes, 578
Inhalation. *See* Inspiration
Inhaler, definition, 838
Inheritance, 655
  definition, 856
Inhibin, 6478
Inhibitory neurotransmitters, 512
Initial assessments, 210b
Injected medications, impact, 207b
Injection, definition, 838
Injuries, 718
  causes. *See* Sports injuries
  massage, usage, 95
  type (importance). *See* Tissue
Innominate bones, 347
Inorganic phosphorus, excretion (promotion), 93, 641b
Insects, extermination, 70
Insertion. *See* Muscles
  definition, 856
Insomnia
  massage, usage, 95
  reduction, 219
Inspiration (inhalation), 595
  definition, 856
  illustration, 599f
  ingestion route, 68
Institute of Massage and Remedial Exercise, merger, 9
Insufficient funds
  checks, receiving, 815
  letter, usage. *See* Clients
Insula (island of Reil), 515f, 516
  definition, 856
  description, 516
  illustration, 515f

Insulin, 548t. *See also* Humulin; Novolin
  definition, 842, 856
Insurance. *See* Automobile insurance; Disability; Health; Life insurance
  billing/reimbursement, 811–812
  claims, prioritization, 812
  needs, 796–797. *See also* Massage business
Intact skin, infection route, 68
Intake form
  briefness/convenience, 197
  preparation. *See* Clients
  presentation, 197
  readability/organization, 197
  review, 203
  sample. *See* Clients
Integrity, 29
  definition, 856
Integument, term (usage), 295
Integumentary system, 279t
  anatomy, 294
  bibliography, 309
  impact. *See* Waste elimination
  Internet activities, 309
  introduction, 294
  physiology, 294–295
  self test, 308
  student objectives, 293
  summary, 307
Intensity. *See* Law of Intensity
Intention, 142–143
Interatrial septum, 565
Interest conflict, 31
Inter-event sports massage, 732
Interlace fingers movement, 175
  illustration, 176f
Intermediate muscle fibers, 388
Internal, definition, 856
Internal intercostal
  actions, 494f
  nerve, 494f
  origin/insertion, 494f
Internal obliques
  actions, 487f
  nerve, 487f
  origins/insertions, 487f
Internal reference, 282
Internal respiration (tissue respiration), 597, 599
  definition, 856
International Institute of Reflexology, 696
Internet websites
  backgrounds, control, 800
  color scheme, selection, 799–800
  content, importance, 800
  navigation system, providing, 800
  purpose, 799–800
  special effects, limitation, 800
  template, usage, 800
Interneurons (association nerves), 509
  definition, 856
  illustration, 509f
Interoceptors, 525
  definition, 856
Interosseous ligament, 270f, 313
  definition, 856
Interpretive functions, 507
Interstitial cells of Leydig, 547
  definition, 856
  description, 647
  illustration, 647f
Interstitial fluid, 577
Interventricular septum, 565
Intervertebral disk, 360
  location, 361f
Intervertebral foramen, 360
Intervertebral joint, 320f

Interview. *See* Client interview
Interviewing skills, 202–203
Intestinal gas, relief, 93, 625b
Intestinal mucosa, 548
Intestinal tonsils. *See* Peyer's patches
Intimacy. *See* Clients
Intimate relationships, therapeutic relationships
    (contrast), 29f
Intracartilaginous ossification, 314
    definition, 856
Intrafusal muscle, 528f
Intramembranous ossification, 314
    definition, 856
Intramuscular (IM), definition, 838
Intrinsic factor, impact, 614t
Inventory
    definition, 856
    description, 813b
    documentation, 813b
Inverse stretch reflex, 173
Inversion, 323
    definition, 856
    illustration, 324f, 701f
Investing. *See* Long-term investing
    diversification, 817
    professional advice, usage, 817
    system, 817
Involuntary system, 507
Ions, concentration, 269f
Ipratropium bromide. *See* Atrovent
Ipsilateral reference. *See* Homolateral reference
IRA. *See* Individual Retirement Accounts
Iron (Fe)
    function, 833
    source, 833
Ironing effleurage, 147
Iron oxide, mineral water, 668
Irregular bones, 312
    example, 313f
Irritable bowel syndrome, 624
Ischemia, 572
    definition, 856
    reduction, 89, 583b
Ischemic compression, 743
Ischium, 347
    bony marking, 350t
Island of Reil. *See* Insula
Islets of Langerhans (pancreatic islets),
    546–547
    definition, 856
    description, 546
    hormones, inclusion, 548t
Isometric contractions, 389–390
    definition, 856
    illustration, 389f
Isometrics, usage, 390
Isotonic contractions (dynamic contractions),
    388–389
    definition, 856
    illustration, 389f
Isthmus, 545

J

Jaundice, 233
Jejunum, 616
    definition, 856
    etymology, 616
Jet blitz/douche, 683
Jin Shin Do, 756
Jin Shin Jyutsu, 756
Jitsu, 773
    definition, 856
Job-related stress, reduction, 93
Joint capsule, 319, 321
    definition, 856

Joint cavity, 319
    definition, 856
Joint mobilizations, 172
    definition, 856
    involvement, 173
Joint movements
    anatomy, 312
    bibliography, 335
    Internet activities, 335
    introduction, 312
    physiology, 312
    self test, 333–334
    student objectives, 311
    summary, 332
Joints. *See* Articulations; Body; Synovial joints
    classification, 320f
    mobility, increase, 180
    ranges of motion, checking, 729
Jojoba, 51
Jostling vibration, 168. *See also* Supine client
Jugular vein, 574
Juhan, Deane, 276–277, 293
Jump sign, 715
    definition, 856
Jung, C.G., 171
Juxtaglomerular apparatus
    definition, 856
    description, 634
    illustration, 636f
Juxtaglomerular cells
    definition, 856
    description, 634
    illustration, 636f

K

K. *See* Potassium
Kapha (Shleshman), 781, 782
    definition, 856
Kaposi's sarcoma, 245
Keflex (cephalexin), definition, 842
Kegels (pubococcygeus exercise), recommenda-
    tion, 222
Kellogg, John Harvey, 9. *See also* Good Health
    explanation, 856
Keloids, 720
    formation, reduction, 92, 331b
Keppra (levetiracetam), definition, 842
Keratin, production, 296
Keratinocytes, 296
    definition, 856
Key trigger points, 715
    definition, 856
Ki. *See* Energy
    creation, 757f
    definition, 856
    projection, 779
    symbol, 755f
Kidneys
    blood flow, 634–636
    blood sequence, 636
    blood vessels, 634–636
    cross-section, 633f
    definition, 856
    description, 632–633
    meridian, 758
        anterior view, 767f
        posterior view, 767f
    posterior location, 633f
    urine formation, 637
    water reabsorption, 545f
Kidney stones, 640
Kinesiology
    bibliography, 502
    definition, 401, 856
    Internet activities, 502

Kinesiology (*Continued*)
    introduction, 400–403
    self test, 497–501
    student objectives, 399
    summary, 496
Kinesthetic awareness, increase, 180
King, Jr., Martin Luther, 43
Kitabu'l Hawi Fi't-Tibb (Rhazes), 6–7
Klinefelter's syndrome. *See* XXY male
Kneading stroke. *See* Pétrissage
Knee-jerk reflex, 509
Knees
    bolstered area, 121
    connective tissue structures, 368t
    extension, 321, 322f
    flexion, 321, 322f
    gymnastics, 182t
    joints, 320f, 367
        anterior view, 367f
        ligaments, inclusion, 367f
        posterior view, 367f
    movements, 175, 180
        muscles, 432f–451f
        muscles, list, 450
    placement, examination, 118
    rotation, 325f
    therapist reaching, 136f
Kneipp, Sebastian, 666
    explanation, 854
Knuckles, usage. *See* Supine client
Kool-Aid experiment, 268
Korzbyski, Alfred, 337
Krause, term (usage), 295
Krause end bulb, 302
    definition, 856
Kresge, Carol, 804
Krieger, Delores, 86–87
    photograph, 87f
Kübler-Ross, Elisabeth, 244
Kupffer's cells, 618
Kyo, 773. *See also* Energy points
    definition, 857
Kyphosis, 330. *See also* Hyperkyphosis
    massage, impact, 251

L

Labia majora
    definition, 857
    description, 650
    illustration, 648f
Labia minora
    definition, 857
    description, 650
    illustration, 648f
Labor, 218
    assistance, 219
    massage, usage, 225
Lacrimal, term (usage), 295
Lactase, impact, 614t
Lactation
    description, 655
    illustration, 545f
Lacteal, 615
    definition, 857
Lamboidal suture, 355
    definition, 857
Lamina groove, 360
Lamisil (terbinafine hydrochloride), definition, 842
Lamott, Annie, 247
Landmarks, 698. *See also* Horizontal landmarks;
    Vertical landmarks
    abbreviations, 829
    illustration. *See* Reflexology
Langerhans cells, 294, 296
    definition, 857

Langer's cleavage line map, 298f
Langer's lines. *See* Cleavage
Lanoxin (digoxin), definition, 842
Lansoprazole. *See* Prevacid
Lao Tsu, 28, 665
Large-breasted women
    prone position, cylindrical pillows (positioning), 242f
    upper arm, holding. *See* Side-lying large-breasted women
Large breasts, massage (impact), 241
Large clients
    floor massage, 249f
    massage, impact, 249
    therapist body/mechanics, considerations, 249
Large intestine, 616–618
    definition, 857
    illustration, 617f
    meridian, 758
        lateral view, 760f
        plantar view, 760f
        posterior view, 760f
    peristalsis, stimulation, 171
Laryngeal tension, reduction, 92, 602b
Laryngitis, 601
Larynogpharynx, 591f
Larynx, 593
    definition, 857
    illustration, 593f
Lasix (furosemide), definition, 842–843
La stone therapy, 676
Latent trigger points, 714
    definition, 857
Lateral, definition, 857
Lateral border, 340f, 341f
Lateral deviation, 325. *See also* Mandible
    definition, 857
Lateral epicondyle, 340f
Lateral extension, 321
Lateral fissure, 515f
Lateral flexion, 321
Lateral longitudinal arch, 350, 355f
Lateral nail fold, 301f
Lateral pterygoid, 467f
    actions, 469f
    nerve, 469f
    origins/insertions, 469f
Lateral reference, 281f, 282
Lateral rotation, 323–324
Lateral supracondylar ridge, 340f
Latex gloves, assets/liabilities, 71
Latissimus dorsi
    actions, 410f
    alternate hand pétrissage. *See* Prone client
    nerve, 410f
    origins/insertion, 410f
Laughing, 599
Lavender, 688
Lavoisier, Antonie, 667
Law of Facilitation, 531b
Law of Generalization, 531b
Law of Intensity, 531b
Law of Pascal, 669
Law of Radiation, 531b
Law of Symmetry, 530b-531b
Law of Unilaterality, 530b
Laws/legislation, principle, 24
Leading foot, placement, 116
Lean-and-drag technique, 146
Lean (position), examination, 118
Left atrium
    description, 566
    illustration, 565f
Left hemisphere, 516
Left hepatic duct, 618

Left obliquity, 326
Left rotation, 323
Left ventricle
    description, 566
    illustration, 565f
Legal issues, ethical issues (contrast), 22-23
Legal requirements, standard, 826
Leg pull movement, 180, 182t
    illustration, 182f
Leg rock movement, 180, 182t
    illustration, 182f
Legs
    alternate-hand effleurage, usage. *See* Prone client
    bones, 348–349
    circulation problems, inquiry, 221
    cramps (Charley cramps)
        discomfort, 220
        reduction, 219
    massage. *See* Bottom leg; Pregnant women; Top leg
    nerve stroke, usage. *See* Supine client
    rotations, 185t
        illustration, 186f
    swelling, inquiry, 221
    two-handed effleurage, usage. *See* Supine client
Lemon, 688
Lesions
    definition, 857
    description, 718
Lesser omentum, definition, 857
Leukemia, 245
Leukocytes
    definition, 857
    description, 562
    illustration, 561f
Levator scapulae
    actions, 405f
    nerves, 405f
    origins/insertion, 405f
Levers. *See* Class-1 levers; Class-2 levers; Class-3 levers; First-class levers; Second-class levers; Third-class levers
    classification, 327f, 328
Levetiracetam. *See* Keppra
Levine, Stephen, 244
Levothyroxine sodium. *See* Synthroid
Levoxyl (levothyroxine sodium), definition, 843
LH. *See* Luteinizing hormone
Liabilities, description, 813b
Liability. *See* General liability; Professional liability
Lice, 305
Licensed massage therapist, dual licensure/roles, 36
Licenses. *See* Occupational icense; State license requirements, 795–796
Licensure, explanation, 30b
Life insurance, 797
Life ribcage movement, 175
Lifestyle. *See* Purpose Pain Allergies Lifestyle Medical
    habits, improvement, 93
    vocation, 205
Lift ribcage movement, 180t
    illustration, 180f
Lift technique, 120
Ligaments, 272f
Limbs. *See* Lower limbs; Upper limbs
Limited liability company (LLC), advantages/disadvantages, 794
Line, bony marking, 317t
Linear diagramming, sample. *See* Purpose Pain Allergies Lifestyle Medical

Linens
    care. *See* Massage
    cleanliness, 69
    handling. *See* Contaminated linens
    laundering, 69
    massage media, impact, 50
Ling, Pehr Henrik, 8. *See also* Swedish Movement Cure
    biography, 10
    explanation, 857
Ling System, Swedish Movements (Ling), 8
Lingual lipase, impact, 614t
Liniments, lubricants, 51
Lipitor (atorvastatin), definition, 843
Lippman, Walter, 8
Lip-reading clients, therapist communication, 249–250
Liquid, diffusion, 268f
Liquid connective tissue (vascular tissue), 270–271, 273t
    definition, 857
Listening
    effectiveness, 20
    evaluation technique, 777
Lithium (lithium carbonate // lithium citrate), definition, 843
Little shoulder circle movement, 175, 178t
    illustration, 179f
Liver, 618
    cirrhosis, 622
    definition, 857
    meridian, 758
        anterior view, 772f
        lateral view, 772f
LLC. *See* Limited liability company
Lobe. *See* Anterior lobe; Frontal lobe; Occipital lobe; Parietal lobe, Posterior lobe; Temporal lobe
    definition, 857
Local blood flow, increase, 167f
Local contraindications, 96
    definition, 857
    treatment, 97b, 207b
Local disease, definition, 857
Local reflex response, 569
Local swelling, reduction, 156
Local twitch response, 715
    definition, 857
Long bones, 312
    anatomy, 313–314, 313f
    example, 313f
Long head. *See* Biceps femoris
Longissimus, 488b, 491f
    actions, 492f
    nerve, 492f
    origins/insertions, 492f
Longitudinal muscle, 614, 615f
Long-term investing, 817
Longus capitis, 470f
    actions, 470f
    nerve, 470f
    origins/insertion, 470f
Longus colli, 470f
    actions, 471f
    nerve, 471f
    origins/insertions, 471f
Longus colli inferior oblique, 470f
Longus colli superior oblique, 470f
Longus colli vertical, 470f
Looking, evaluation technique, 777
Loop of Henle
    definition, 857
    description, 634
    illustration, 635f

Loose connective tissue, 273, 273t
  definition, 857
  illustration, 272f
Lopid (gemfibrozil), definition, 843
Lopressor (metoprolol), definition, 843
Loratidine. *See* Claritin
Lorazepam, definition, 839
Lordosis, 330
  massage, impact, 251
Loren, Sophia, 217
Lotensin (benazepril hydrochloride), definition, 843
Lotion, lubricant, 51
Lou Gehrig's disease, 532
Low back
  endangerment sites, 98
  ocean waves, usage, 156f
  pain, massage (usage), 95
  posture, examination, 118
  treatment areas, 733
Lower back, seated massage routine, 748
Lower extremity
  anterior/posterior views. *See* Right lower extremity
  bones, 347–353
  regional terms, 284
Lower gastrointestinal tract, gas movement, 171
Lower limbs, 317
Lower respiratory tract, 593–595
  illustration, 591f
Lubricants
  addition. *See* Body
  dispenser, 51
  emollientcy, 50
  impact. *See* Skin
  pump dispenser, usage, 70
  selection, 50
  single-use dish, usage, 70
  storage/shelf life, 51-52
  texture, 50
  types, 50-52
Lubrication. *See* Female lubrication; Male lubrication
Lucas-Championniere, Just, 9
  explanation, 857
Lucidum, term (usage), 295
Lumbar, definition, 857
Lumbar anterior curve, 364f
Lumbar area, 283
Lumbar plexus (L1-L4), 518, 519
Lumbar vertebrae
  lateral view, 363f
  superior view, 363f
Lumen, 569
Lunate, 342
Lunge position, 116. *See also* Massage chair
Lungs, 594
  air sacs, epithelium (location), 271f
  air space, 598f
  buds, 654f
  definition, 857
  disease, massage (usage), 95
  fluid discharge, increase, 92, 602b
  forced expiratory flow/volume, increase, 92
  forced vital capacity, increase, 92
  gas exchange, 600f
  meridian, 758
    anterior view, 759f
    plantar view, 759f
    posterior view, 759f
  peak expiratory flow, improvement, 92
  photograph, 598f
  vital capacity, increase, 92
Lunula, 301f
Lupus erythematosus, 583

Luteal phase, 651f
Luteinizing hormone (LH), 545t, 652
  definition, 857
  levels, 651f
Lyme disease (Lyme arthritis), 330
Lymph, 577
  capillary, definition, 857
  circulation
    paths, 579
    promotion, 89, 584b
  definition, 857
  description, 575
  one-way circulation, 577f
  organs, 577–579
  vessels, 577
Lymphatic capillaries, 577f
Lymphatic circulation, improvement, 219
Lymphatic drainage techniques, 729
Lymphatic-immune system
  massage, impact, 584b
  pathologic conditions, 582–584
Lymphatic system, 575
  anatomy, 576
  illustration, 578f
  massage, impact, 89
  physiology, 576–577
Lymphatic trunks, 577
  definition, 857
Lymphatic vessel, 577f
Lymphedema, 577
Lymph nodes, 578
  definition, 857
  swelling, 722
    lymphadenopathy, 245
Lymphocytes
  count, increase, 89, 584b
  definition, 857
  description, 562, 577–578
  illustration, 561f
Lymphoma, definition, 245
Lymph space, illustration, 510f
Lysosome, 267
  definition, 857
  illustration, 266f

M

Macronutrients, 830
Macula densa, 634
  definition, 857
Macular degeneration, 532
Maintenance, 810–818
Maintenance massage, 732
Maintenance stage. *See* Rehabilitation
Majno, Guido, 565
Major arteries, 574f
Major duodenal papilla, 616
  definition, 857
  illustration, 618f
Major endocrine glands, location, 544f
Major joints. *See* Body
Major muscles. *See* Body
Major pituitary hormones, target organs, 545f
Major systemic arteries, 573–574
Major systemic veins, 574
Major veins, 576f
Malas, 781–782
Male clients
  feet, uncovered. *See* Supine male client
  towel draping, 126
Male erection, 652
Male lubrication, 652
Male orgasm, 652
Male reproductive organs, 646–648
  illustration, 647f
Male sex glands. *See* Accessory male sex glands

Malignant tumor, 244
  definition, 857
Malpractice insurance, 797
MALT. *See* Mucosal-associated lymphoid tissue
Maltase, impact, 614t
Mammary area. *See* Pectoral area
Mammary glands. *See* Breasts
Manav Dharma Shastra, 5
Mandible
  angle, 467f
  lateral deviations, 326f
Mandibular, definition, 857
Mandibular area, 282
Mandibular depression, 325f
Mandibular elevation, 325f
Mandibular movement, muscles, 479
Mandibular protraction, 325f
Mandibular retraction, 325f
Marketing. *See* Massage business
  definition, 857
  description, 798
Marley, Bob, 81
Marrow. *See* Bone marrow
  inclusion, 781
Martial arts, principles, 110
Mashesh, 4
Mask, usage. *See* Body
Mask of pregnancy. *See* Chloasma
Maslow, Abraham, 86
  photograph, 86f
  quote, 68
Massa, 4
Massage. *See* Ice massage; Maintenance massage; Postpartum massage; Rehabilitative massage; Sports massage; Swedish massage; Therapeutic massage
  adaptation. *See* Growing child
  aromatherapy, usage, 688
  avoidance
    alcohol, impact, 70
    cold-like symptoms, impact, 70
  blankets, 49
  contraindication, 82
  definition, 4, 857
  direction, application, 144
  discontinuation, 253
  effects, 88-93
  experience, examination. *See* Clients
  foundation, 114
  goal, 383
  impact. *See* Pain
    preservation/prolongation, 810b
  indications, 93-96
  linens, 49
    care, 49
  masterful application, 142
  mechanical responses, 88
  media, 49-50
    cost, 50
  media, impact. *See* Skin
  modalities, abbreviations, 829
  negative perception, 37
  pain cycle, relationship, 90
  parlor, 37
  practice
    commonness, 668
    value, assessment, 792–793
  preparation, 109–110, 805–806
    warm-up, 109
  principles, 24
  reflexive responses, 88
  refusal, timing (learning), 28
  risks, 199
  safety

Massage (*Continued*)
    discussion, 87-88
    guidelines, 70-73
  scientific application, 142
  sheets, 49
  side effects, 199
  supplies, 52
    checklist, 52
  techniques, abbreviations, 829
  timeline, 4f
  tools, handling, 69
  towels, 49
  treatment guidelines, 97b
  type, 50
  usage. *See* Dry brush massage; Labor; Nursing mothers; Underwater massage
  warmup, 118
Massage, historical perspective
  bibliography, 13
  introduction, 1-2
  self test, 12
  summary, 11
Massage business
  advertising, 819b-820b
    usage, 798–803
  bibliography, 823
  competition, 819b
  description, 819b
  employment, 797–804
    opportunities, 797–798
  evaluation/planning, 793
  financial projections, 820b
  framework, 797–804
  insurance needs, 819b
  Internet activities, 823
  introduction, 792
  location, 819b-820b
  maintenance, 810–818
  management/personnel, 819b
  marketing, 798, 819b
  name, registration, 796
  operating procedures, 819b
  plan, 819b-820b
    business description, 794–795
    personal information, 793–794
  planning/development, 792–797
  practices, standard, 827
  promotion, 819b-820b
  promotional strategies, 797–804
  self test, 821–822
  startup costs, determination, 797
    illustration, 798b
  student objectives, 791
  summary, 819–820
  support, 797–804
  supporting documents, 820b
Massage chair, 49
  adjustments, 743
  photograph, 741f
  selection process, 740
  therapist adjustments, 743f
  usage, 125f
    reasons, 740–741
Massage Emergency Response Team (MERT), 740
Massage environment
  case study, 57
  information resources, 59
  Internet activities, 59
  introduction, 44
  objectives, 43
  self test, 58
  summary, 57
Massage objectives
  bibliography, 102–105
  case study, 100

Massage objectives (*Continued*)
  Internet activities, 102
  introduction, 82
  objectives, 81
  scientific method, 83-84
  self test, 101
  summary, 99
Massage room
  ambiance, 53
  chairs/stools, placement, 53
  client personal items, placement, 53
  clocks, usage, 52-53
  color, impact, 56
  environment, 54, 56
  flooring, impact, 54
  furnishing, 52-54
  light, impact, 54
  mirrors, usage, 52
  music, usage, 54, 56
  orientation, 805–806
  soundproofing, impact, 54
  supply cabinet, usage, 53
  temperature, 56
  wall hangings, 53
  wastebasket, usage, 53
  water dispenser, usage, 53
  window treatments, 53-54
Massage session
  clients, draping, 125–131
  completion, 809–810
  preparation, 806–807
  procedure, 807–809
Massage strokes
  application, elements, 142–145
  types, 142
  usage/variety, 118
  variations, 146t
Massage table mechanics, 120–131
  client positioning, 120–123
  definition, 863
  inclusion, 108
  initiation, decisions, 123–125
Massage table mechanics, science
  bibliography, 139
  case study, 137
  Internet activities, 139
  introduction, 108
  objectives, 107
  self test, 138
  summary, 137
Massage table padding, 46. *See also* Breasts
  density, 46
  durability, 46
  layering systems, 46
  loft, 46
Massage tables, 44-49
  accessories, 47-49
  arm shelf, 48
  arm support side extension, 47f
  arrival, 45
  body wrap setup, 678f
  bolsters, 48-49
    usage, 48f
  carrying case, 48
  carts, 48
  clients, assistance, 131–132
  fabric, 46-47
  face rest, 47f
    usage, 47-48
  features, 45-47
  feet, dangling, 136f
  footrest, 48
  frames, 46
  height, 45-46. *See also* Pregnancy massage
    determination, 45f, 117

Massage tables (*Continued*)
  illustration, 44f
  length, 46
  manufacturer, selection, 44-45
  multiple-layer systems, usage, 46
  ready set go test, 47
  rock test, 47
  side extensions, 48
  single layer, usage, 46
  tests, 47
  vinyl fabric care, 47
  widening accessory, 123f
  width, 45. *See also* Pregnancy massage
Massage therapists, 10
  arm support, usage, 136f
  bow stance, usage, 116f
  client, therapeutic relationship (illustration), 20f
  conditions/situations, relevance, 197
  credentials, 199
  dual licensure/roles. *See* Licensed massage therapist
  health/hygiene, 74
  HIPAA guidelines, 212
  infection control, 68-70
  intent, 50
  law, obligation, 23
  nutrition, 835
  position, 135f
  professional image, 22
  professionalism, illustration, 16f
  professional standards, 23-25
  qualities. *See* Professional massage therapist
  sales activity, conflict of interest, 31
  sample day, 804–810
  self-assessment guide, 145b
  shoulder, grasping. *See* Clients
  stretching, example, 806f
  warrior stance, usage, 117f
Massage therapy
  application, 243f
  contraindications, 96-97
  medications, impact, 207b
  relationship. *See* Breathing
Massage Therapy Research Agenda, development, 82
Masseter, 467f
  actions, 468f
  nerve, 468f
  origin/insertions, 468f
Masso (massin), 4
Masterful application. *See* Massage
Master gland, 544
Mastication, 611
  definition, 857
  muscles, 467f
Mastitis, 657
Mathias, Wayne, 233
Maxilla, 467f
Maxillary sinus, 356, 591
  illustration, 358f
Mayland, Elaine, 194
McClure, Vimala Schneider, 230–231
McIntosh, Nina, 35
Meagher, Jack, 564, 720
Meatus (meatuses), 591
  bony marking, 317t
Mechanical effect, 668–669
Mechanical response, 88. *See also* Massage
  definition, 857
Mechanical vibration, usage, 170–171
Mechanoreceptors, 526–527
  definition, 857
Media
  definition, 857
  description, 798

Medial, definition, 857
Medial border, 340f
    sawing superficial friction, hands (ulnar
        sides), usage. *See* Scapula
Medial epicondyle, 340f
Medial longitudinal arch, 350, 355f
Medial pterygoid, 467f
    actions, 469f
    nerve, 469f
    origin/insertions, 469f
Medial reference, 281f, 282, 282f
Medial rotation, 323–324
Medial thigh
    endangerment sites, 98
    pregnancy massage, 224
Median cubital vein, 574
Median nerve (great flexor), 519
Median plane, 280
Mediastinal, definition, 857
Mediastinal area, 283
Medical clearance, obtaining, 244
Medical history, disclosure (refusal), 96
Medical information, 206. *See also* Purpose
        Pain Allergies Lifestyle Medical
    release, 209f
Medical release form, 209f
Medical spa, 667
    definition, 857
Medical terminology, 828–829
    exposure, 265
Medications, list, 838–848
Medroxyprogesterone, conjugated equine estro-
        gens (inclusion). *See* Prempro
Medroxyprogesterone acetate. *See* Provera
Medulla, 633
    urine collection, 637
Medulla oblongata
    definition, 857
    description, 517
    illustration, 514f, 518f
Medullar cavity, 313, 313f
Medullary cavity, definition, 857
Medullary pyramids, 634
    definition, 858
Mehrabian, Albert, 21b
Meissner, term (usage), 295
Meissner corpuscle (tactile corpuscle), 302
    definition, 858
Melanin, 298
    production, 296
Melano, term (usage), 295
Melanocytes, 296
    definition, 858
Melanocyte-stimulating hormone (MSH), 545t
    definition, 858
Melanomas, definition, 245
Melatonin, definition, 858
Melzack, Patrick, 91
Membranes
    definition, 858
    types/locations, 278f
Memory T cells, 580
Meninges, 513. *See also* Cranial meninges
    definition, 858
Meningitis, 532
Menopause, 657
Menstruation (first phase), 650–651
    pathologic condition, 657
Mental, definition, 858
Mental alertness, increase, 93
Mental area, 282
Mental functioning, 507
Mentastics (mental gymnastics), 201
Mercuriale, Girolamo, 7. *See also* De Arte
        Gymnastica
    definition, 858

Meridians, 758–759
    definition, 858
    inclusion. *See* Five phases
    Kyo-Jitsu combination, 779
Merkel disk, 302, 526
    definition, 858
MERT. *See* Massage Emergency Response
        Team
Mesenteric artery, 573
Mesenteries
    definition, 858
    description, 616
    illustration, 612f
Mesoderm, 653
    definition, 858
Metabolic diseases, 66
    definition, 858
Metabolic wastes, excretion, 156
Metabolism, definition, 262–263, 858
Metacarpals, 347
Metacarpal scissors, 175t
    illustration, 176f
Metal
    correspondences, 776t
    phase, 775
Metaphysis, 314
    definition, 858
Metastasize, definition, 858
Metatarsal arch. *See* Transverse arch
    transverse, 355f
Metatarsals
    bones, 350
    chucking friction. *See* Supine client
    scissor movements, 185t
        illustration, 186f
    thumb effleurage, 147f
Metformin. *See* Glucophage
Methylphenidate. *See* Ritalin
Metoprolol. *See* Lopressor
Mezger, Johann (Dutch physician), 8-9
    explanation, 856
    illustration, 9f
MFR. *See* Myofascial release
Microglia, 508
    definition, 858
Micronase (glyburide), definition, 843
Micronized progesterone. *See* Prometrium
Micronutrients, 831
Microscopic anatomy, 262
Microvilli, 266, 266f, 615f
Micturition, definition, 858
Midbrain
    definition, 858
    description, 517
    illustration, 514f, 516f, 518f
Middle Ages, 6-7
Middle scalene, 472f
Midsagittal plane, 280, 723
    definition, 858
    illustration, 724f, 725f
Miesler, Deitrich W., 247
Migraines, 581
Migrating WBC, adhesion (enhancement),
        89, 583b
Milk bath, 680
Mindwork, 95
Minerals
    classification, 622
    content, 668
    definition, 858
    functions, 620t, 832–833
    retention, increase. *See* Bones
    source, 832–833
Mineral waters, types, 668
Minimalism (music), 56
Miscarriage, 656

Mission statement, 793
    definition, 858
Mitochondrion (mitochondria), 267
    definition, 858
    illustration, 266f
Mitral valve (bicuspid valve), 566
    definition, 850, 858
Mizner, Wilson, 11
Modalities, 828–829
    abbreviations. *See* Massage
    description, 199
    expectations/benefits, 199
    restrictions. *See* Pregnancy massage
Modern era, 8-11
Modified respiratory air movements, 599–600
Moisture, 668
    observation, 723
Moles
    ABCDEF assessment, 303
    changes, 303
Monoaxial joint. *See* Hinge joint; Pivot joint
Monocytes, 561f
Mononucleosis, 583
Monosaccharides, 620
Mons pubis
    definition, 858
    description, 650
    illustration, 648f
Montagu, Ashley, 299
Mood, improvement, 93
Moor mud, formation, 677
Morning sickness. *See* Nausea
Morphine (morphine sulfate), definition, 843
Morula, 653f
Mosby's Pathology for Massage Therapists
        (Salvo/Anderson), 97
Motility, 378
Motion, range. *See* Range of motion
Motor end plate, 381
Motor nerves (efferent nerves), 509, 528f
    definition, 858
Motor neuron, definition, 858
Motor output, 507
Motor units, 382f
    definition, 858
    electron microscope photograph, 382f
    neuromuscular junction, inclusion, 382f
Motrin (ibuprofen), definition, 843
Mouth, epithelium (location), 271f
Movements. *See* Active movements; Duplicated
        movements; Passive movements
    body coordination, 385–387
    smoothness, 120
    types, 142
Mowles, Sallie, 218
Moxibustion, 756
    definition, 858
MS. *See* Multiple sclerosis
MSH. *See* Melanocyte-stimulating hormone
Mucosa, 615f
Mucosal-associated lymphoid tissue (MALT),
        578–579
    definition, 858
Mucous coat, 594f
Mucous membranes, 277–278
    definition, 858
    infection route, 67-68
    types/locations, 278f
Mud, application. *See* Back
Mullen, Tim, 707, 742
Multiarticular, definition, 858
Multiarticular muscles, 385
Multifidus, 488b, 489f
    actions, 490f
    nerve, 490f
    origin/insertions, 490f

Multiple-layer systems, usage. *See* Massage tables
Multiple sclerosis (MS), 532–533
  massage, usage, 96
Muscle cells, 379–381
  illustration, 380f
  properties, 381
  transition, 378–379
Muscle fibers. *See* Bipennate muscle fiber; Circular muscle fiber; Convergent muscle fiber; Fusiform muscle fiber; Parallel muscle fiber; Pennate muscle fiber; Unipennate muscle fiber
  arrangement, 385
  finition, 858
  location/direction, 402b
  manual separation, 91, 392b
  types. *See* Skeletal muscle fibers
Muscles. *See* Cardiac muscle; Skeletal muscle; Smooth muscle
  abbreviations, 829
  attachment sites, 402b
  belly, 384
  broadening, mimicking, 162
  contraction, illustration, 383f
  fatigue, 715
    definition, 858
    reduction, 91, 392b
  flexibility, increase, 91
  function, 402b
  guarding, reduction, 180
  histological table, 274t
  information, 712
  insertion, 384–385, 402b
  labor/delivery, assistance, 219
  lengthening, 91, 392b
  massage, impact, 91-92, 392b
  mechanical relaxation/lengthening, 156
  naming, 402b
    combinations, 402b
  organs, 378–379
    structure, 379f
  origin, 384, 402b
    research, 403
  palpation, process, 403b
  performance, improvement, 91
  range of motion, increase, 91
  ranking, 403
  relative position, 402b
  relaxation, 91, 172, 392b
  relaxers
    definition, 838
    impact, 207
  spasms, 391
  stiffness, reduction, 156
  strengthening. *See* Respiratory muscles
  stretching, mimicking, 162
  tendinous attachments, 403
  tensions, relationship. *See* Blood flow
  tissues, 274
    definition, 858
  tone, relationship. *See* Posture
  toning. *See* Weak muscles
Muscle soreness, 715–718. *See also* Delayed-onset muscle soreness
  connective tissue damage theory, 716–717
  inflammation theory, 716
  reduction, 91, 156, 392b
  relief, 180
Muscle spindles, 526–527
  definition, 858
  illustration, 528f
  stimulation, 171
Muscular discomfort, reduction, 219
Muscular dystrophy, 391

Muscular nomenclature
  bibliography, 502
  Internet activities, 502
  introduction, 400–403
  self test, 497–501
  student objectives, 399
  summary, 496
Muscular spasm, release, 383
Muscular system, 279t
  anatomy, 378
  bibliography, 396
  Internet activities, 396
  introduction, 378
  pathological conditions, 390–392
  physiology, 378
  self test, 394–395
  student objectives, 377
  summary, 393
  terms/meanings, 393
Muscular tension, relief, 91, 392b
Muscular tone, reset, 180
Musculature, one-thumb cross-fiber technique. *See* Forearms
Musculocutaneous nerve, 519
Musculoskeletal component, 329f
Musculoskeletal problems, rehabilitative approach, 387
Musculotendinous cuff
  anterior view, 411f
  posterior view, 411f
Mutations, 655
  definition, 858
Mutual funds, investment, 818
Mutuality, 35
Myasthenia gravis, 533
Myelin, 508f
  sheath, 509
    definition, 858
Mylar foil sheet, usage, 678f
Myocardial infarction, definition, 838
Myocardium, 565, 566f
Myofascial, definition, 858
Myofascial release (MFR), 725, 727–729
  definition, 858
  description, 727
  practice, 95
  technique, 727–728
  variation, 728
Myofibril, definition, 858
Myofilaments, 380. *See also* Thick myofilament; Thin myofilament
  cross-section, 380f
Myometrium, 649f
Myopia, 524
Myosin, 380
Myosin head, 380
  extensions, 380f
Myotatic stretch reflex, 173
Myotomes, 518–519
  definition, 858
  map, 520f
My Water Cure (Kneipp), 666

N
Nadis, 781
  definition, 858
Nadolol. *See* Corgard
Nails, 300–301
  bed, 301f
    definition, 858
  body, 301f
    definition, 858
  cross section, 301f
  cyanotic appearance, 301
  definition, 858
  edge. *See* Free nail edge

Nails (*Continued*)
  fold. *See* Lateral nail fold
  root, 301f
    definition, 858
Name-dropping, impressiveness (absence), 23
Namikoshi, Tokujiro, 756
Naprosyn (naproxen sodium), definition, 843–844
Naproxen sodium. *See* Aleve
Narcotic, definition, 838
Narcotic analgesics, impact, 207b
Nares, 590. *See also* Anterior nares; Posterior nares
Narrative report, 210
  definition, 858
  letter format, 211b
  progress report, contrast, 210
Nasal, definition, 858
Nasal area, 282
Nasal cavity
  definition, 858
  description, 590–591
  illustration, 591f
Nasal conchae, 590–591
Nasal congestion, discomfort, 221
NASE. *See* National Association for the Self-Employed
Nasopharynx, 591f
Nateglinide. *See* Starlix
National Association for the Self-Employed (NASE), 797
National Certification Board for Therapeutic Massage and Bodywork (NCBTMB), 24, 796
  business practices, standard, 827
  code of ethics, 825
  confidentiality, standard, 826–827
  legal/ethical requirements, standard, 826
  professionalism, standard, 826
  recommentation, 31, 193
  roles/boundaries, standard, 827
  sexual misconduct, prevention (standard), 827
  standards of practice, 826–827
National Certification Commission on Acupuncture and Oriental Medicine (NCCAOM), 756
National Certification Test, development/administration, 23
Natural immunity, 579
  definition, 858
Natural killer cells, 579–580
  number/function, increase, 89, 584b
Nausea, feeling, 679
Nausea (morning sickness), 233
  discomfort, 221
  inquiry, 221
Navel, jaw (superiority), 282
NCBTMB. *See* National Certification Board for Therapeutic Massage and Bodywork
NCCAOM. *See* National Certification Commission on Acupuncture and Oriental Medicine
Neck
  bolstered area, 121
  circles, 174f, 174t
  extension, 321, 322f
  flexion, 321, 322f
  forward flexion, 174t, 175f
  gymnastics, 174t
  lateral extension, 321, 322f
  lateral flexion, 174f, 174t, 321
    rotation, involvement, 175f
  line, 698
    horizontal landmark, 698f
  movements, 174
    muscles, 462f-484f
    muscles, list, 479
  regional terms, 282
  rotation, 324f

Neck (*Continued*)
seated massage, 746
treatment areas, 733
Necrosis, 267
Negative feedback system, 64, 543
definition, 859
Nei Ching. *See* Huang-ti nei-ching
Neoplasm, 65, 244
Nephron, 633–634
definition, 859
fluid flow, 634
loop, 636f
tubular/vascular network, 635f
Nerve fascicles, 510
Nerve impulses (action potentials), 510–511
arrival, 512f
conduction, 510–511
illustration, 511f
definition, 859
propagation, 382
Nerves
compression, 533
definition, 859
description, 509–510
endangerment sites, 97
endings, stimulation, 167
entrapment, 533
massage, usage, 96
illustration, 510f
importance, massage therapists (impact), 519, 520f
plexuses, 518
Nerve stroke, 145 149
usage. *See* Supine client
Nervous system, 279t. *See also* Autonomic nervous system; Central nervous system; Peripheral nervous system; Somatic nervous system
anatomy, 506
bibliography, 539
cells, 507–509
divisions, 507f
Internet activities, 539
introduction, 506
massage, impact, 90-91, 535b
organization, 507
pathologic conditions, 529–535
physiology, 506–507
role. *See* Touch
self test, 537–538
student objectives, 505
summary, 536
terms/meanings, 506
Nervous tissue, 274–275
definition, 859
pictomicrograph, 276f
line drawing, 276f
Net income, description, 813b
Networking, usage, 803–804
Neural control system, 543
definition, 859
Neurilemma, 508f, 510
Neuroglia, 507–508
definition, 859
Neurohormones, 546
Neurohypophysis, 545
Neurologic laws
presentation/discussion, 530b-531b
principles, 721
Neuromuscular junction, 392f
definition, 859
Neuromuscular therapy, 712
Neurons, 508. *See also* Interneurons
definition, 859
illustration, 508f
nerves, connections, 510
parts, 275, 508–509

Neuropathy, 533
Neurotransmitters, 511–512
definition, 859
molecule, release, 512f
types, 512–513
Neutrophils, 561f
New Age Ayurveda, 780
New clients, initial session, 197–200
mini-lab, 197
New food pyramid, 834–835
Nexium (esomeprazole), definition, 844
Niacin. *See* Vitamin B$_3$
Nipple, 650f
Nissen, Hartvig, 9. *See also* Swedish Movement and Massage; Swedish Movement and Massage Treatment
definition, 859
Nitro-Dur (nitroglycerin), definition, 844
Nitrogard (nitroglycerin), definition, 844
Nitrogen, excretion (promotion), 93, 641b
Nitroglycerin. *See* Nitro-Dur; Nitrogard; Nitrostat; Transderm-Nitro
Nitrostat (nitroglycerin), definition, 844
Nociceptor, definition, 859
Node of Ranvier, 508f
definition, 859
description, 509
Nondisclosure. *See* Privileged information
Nonsteroidal antiinflammatory drugs (NSAIDs)
definition, 838
impact, 207b
Nonverbal communication, 20-21
Norelgestromin. *See* Ortho Evra
Norepinephrine (noradrenaline), 513
levels, reduction, 90, 535b, 552
Norgestimate. *See* Ortho Tri-Cyclen
Nose, 590
definition, 859
No shows, handling, 28
Nostrils, 590
Notch, bony marking, 317t
Notice of Privacy Policies, receipt, 212
Novolin (insulin), definition, 844
NSAIDs. *See* Nonsteroidal antiinflammatory drugs
Nuad Bo Rarn, 756
Nuchal, definition, 859
Nuchal ligament, 359
Nuclear membrane, 266f
Nucleolus, 266f, 508f
Nucleus, 267, 508f
definition, 859
illustration, 266f, 646f
Nucleus pulposus, 360
Nursing mothers, massage (usage), 226
Nutrients. *See* Essential nutrients; Macronutrients; Micronutrients
classification, 621t
functions, 620t
Nutrition
bibliography, 836
considerations, 835
importance, 720
introduction, 830
label, understanding, 834
summary, 836
Nutritive materials, replenishment, 89, 583b

O

Obesity, 624
consideration, 251
Objective data, 193–194
contrast/comparison. *See* Subjective data
definition, 859
empirical means, usage, 193

Oblique capitis inferior
action, 478f
nerve, 478f
origin/insertion, 478f
Oblique capitis superior
actions, 478f
nerve, 478f
origin/insertion, 478f
Oblique muscle, 614
Obliquities. *See* Pelvic obliquities
anterior view, 326f
Obliqus capitis inferior, 476f
Obliqus capitis superior, 476f
Observation, consideration, 722
Obsessive-compulsive disorder (OCD), 533
Obturator externus
action, 436f
nerve, 436f
origins/insertion, 436f
Obturator foramen, 347
Obturator internus
action, 436f
nerve, 436f
origin/insertion, 436f
Obturator nerve, 519
Occipital, definition, 859
Occipital area, 282
Occipital bone, 467f
Occipitalis, 462f
action, 463f
nerve, 463f
origin/insertion, 463f
Occipital lobe
definition, 859
description, 516
illustration, 515f
Occipitofrontalis, 462f
Occiput, 476f
Occupational license, 796
Occupational Safety and Health Administration (OSHA), blood-borne/fluid-borne pathogen exposure prevention, 68
Occupations
pain hazards, relationship, 111b
physical activity, requirement, 111b
OCD. *See* Obsessive-compulsive disorder
Ocean waves, usage. *See* Anterior thigh; Low back
Oculomotor nerve, 519, 521f
Office policies, 199
Oil glands. *See* Sebaceous glands
Oils. *See* Carrier oils; Essential oils
lubricant, 51
safety, 687–688
starter kit, 688
Olecranon fossa, 341f
Olecranon process, 338, 341f
Olfaction, 524, 590
illustration, 524f
relationship. *See* Aromatherapy
Olfactory nerve, 519, 521f
Oligodendrocytes, 508
definition, 859
Omentum. *See* Greater omentum; Lesser omentum
Omeprazole delayed-release. *See* Prilosec
Oncogenes, 245
Oncology, 244
Oncoviruses, 245
Oncoviruses, impact, 245
One-handed compression, 726
One-handed effleurage, 145, 147–148. *See also* Circular one-handed effleurage
One-handed hacking. *See* Prone client
One-handed pétrissage, 153. *See also* Triceps
finger pads, usage. *See* Supine client
thumbs, usage. *See* Supine client

One-knee test, 47
Oneness, 757f
One-thumb cross-fiber technique. *See*
　　Forearms
On Joints (Hippocrates), 6
Onset Provocative Palliative Quality Radiation
　　Site Timing (OPPQRST), 205
　usage. *See* Pain
Oocytes
　definition, 859
　description, 646
　development, 646f
　illustration, 646f, 652f
Open-ended questions, usage, 19, 202
Operative toilet, providing, 70
Ophthalmic area. *See* Orbital area
Opponens digiti minimi
　action, 429f
　nerve, 429f
　origin/insertion, 429f
Opponens pollicis
　actions, 427f
　nerve, 427f
　origins/insertion, 427f
Opposite shoulder, therapist hand (sliding),
　　135f
Opposition, 325. *See also* Thumbs
　definition, 859
OPPQRST. *See* Onset Provocative Palliative
　　Quality Radiation Site Timing
Optic chiasma, illustration, 518f
Optic nerve, 519, 521f
Oral, definition, 859
Oral area, 282
Oral cavity, 611–612
　definition, 859
Orapred (prednisolone), definition, 844
Orbicularis oculi
　actions, 463f
　nerve, 463f
　origin/insertion, 463f
Orbicularis oris
　actions, 464f
　nerve, 464f
　origins/insertions, 464f
Orbital (ophthalmic), definition, 859
Orbital (ophthalmic) area, 282
Organelles, 266–267
　definition, 859
Organism
　level, 265
　organization, levels, 265, 265t
Organism/pathogen
　infection/disease, relationship, 67t
　reservoir, relationship, 67t
Organization levels, 265t
Organs
　endangerment sites, 97
　organization, levels, 265t
　systems, organization (levels), 265t
Orgasm. *See* Female orgasm; Male orgasm
Origins. *See* Muscles
　definition, 859
　number, 402b
Ornate jewelry, wearing (avoidance), 69
Oropharynx, 591f
Ortho Evra (norelgestromin // ethinyl estradiol
　　transdermal system), definition, 844–845
Orthostatic hypotension, 247
　definition, 838
Ortho Tri-Cyclen (norgestimate // ethinyl estra-
　　diol), 845
Os coxa, 347
Osgood-Schlatter disease, 330
OSHA. *See* Occupational Safety and Health
　　Administration

Osmosis, 268
　definition, 859
　illustration, 269f
Osseous connective tissue, 273t
Osseous tissue. *See* Bones
Ossification. *See* Intracartilaginous ossification;
　　Intramembranous ossification
　definition, 859
Osteoarthritis, 330
Osteoblast, 270, 314
　definition, 859
Osteoclasts, 314
　definition, 859
Osteocyte (mature osteoblast), 314, 314f
　definition, 859
Osteoporosis, 330
OTC. *See* Over-the-counter
Otic (auricular), definition, 859
Otic (auricular) area, 282
Oval window, 525
Ovarian cycle, 651f
Ovarian cysts, 657
Ovarian follicles, 649
　development, stages, 652f
Ovaries, 547, 648–649
　definition, 859
　illustration, 648f, 649f, 653f
　menstruation, 651
　pre-ovulation, 652
Ovary surface, epithelium (location), 271f
Over-the-counter (OTC), definition, 838
Overtraining, problem, 718
Oviducts. *See* Fallopian tube
Ovulation (third phase), 652. *See also*
　　Post-ovulation; Pre-ovulation
　illustration, 651f
Ovum
　definition, 859
　discharge, 653f
　illustration, 646f
Oxybutynin. *See* Ditropan XL
Oxycodone. *See* Percocet
OxyContin (oxycodone hydrochloride), 845
Oxygen
　requirement, 383–384
　saturation, increase. *See* Blood
Oxytocin, 545f

P

Pacemaker, massage (impact), 241
Pacini, term (usage), 295
Pacinian corpuscle, 296f, 302
　definition, 859
Packs. *See* Cold packs
　definition, 859
　description, 672
　hydrotherapeutic applications, 674b
　pouch, usage, 674–675
　terrycloth pouch, usage. *See* Hot pack
　usage, 672–677
　usge. *See* Contrast pack
Padding. *See* Massage table padding
Pain. *See* Purpose Pain Allergies Lifestyle
　　Medical; Referred pain
　assessment, OPPQRST (usage), 205f
　cycle
　　interruption, massage (impact), 90f
　　relationship. *See* Massage
　decrease, 90, 180, 208, 535b
　discomfort, 205
　hazards, relationship. *See* Occupations
　massage, usage. *See* Chronic pain; Low back
　rating scale. *See* Wong-Baker FACES Pain
　　Rating Scale
　relief, 167, 171, 219

Pain (*Continued*)
　scale (10-point scale), 206f
　signs, observation, 809f
Pain Erasure: The Bonnie Prudden Way
　　(Prudden), 110
Pain-relieving substances, release (stimulation),
　　156
Palliative care, definition, 859
Palm, usage. *See* Circular friction
Palmar circular effleurage, 148f. *See also*
　　Iliotibial band
　usage. *See* Iliotibial band
Palmar friction, 727
Palmaris longus
　actions, 421f
　nerve, 421f
　origin/insertions, 421f
Palmar (volar), definition, 859
Palmar (volar) area, 283
Palmer, David, 740, 745
Palming, technique, 779
Palpate, term (usage), 295
Palpation, 194
　consideration, 722–723
　definition, 859
　importance/usage, 722–723
　usage, 777
Pancreas
　definition, 859
　description, 618–619
　illustration, 620f
Pancreatic amylase, impact, 614t
Pancreatic duct, 618f
Pancreatic islets. *See* Islets of Langerhans
Pancreatic lipase, impact, 614t
Pancreatitis, 624
Pantothenic acid. *See* Vitamin B_5
Paper office, 44
Papez, J.W., 687
Papillae, 523
Papillary muscles, 566
Paracelsus (Philippus von Hohenheim) (Swiss
　　physician), 7
　explanation, 859
Paraffin baths
　definition, 859
　usage, 682–683
Paraffin wraps, 678–679
Parahormone. *See* Parathyroid hormone
Parallel friction, 160
Parallel muscle fiber, 385, 385f
Paralysis, 533
Paranasal sinuses, 358f
Paraphrasing, involvement, 20
Paraplegia, 251
Parasite, definition, 859
Paraspinal muscles, posterior view, 488b
Paraspinals, 488
　cross-fiber friction, fingertips (usage), 161f
　raking, usage, 151f
　superficial warming friction, fingertips (us-
　　age), 159f
Parasympathetic, definition, 859
Parasympathetic nerve, 520–523
　system, 521–522
Parasympathetic nervous system, 520
Parathyroid, definition, 859
Parathyroid gland, 545
　definition, 859
　hormones, inclusion, 547t
Parathyroid hormone (parahormone), 547t
Paré, Ambroise (French military surgeon), 7
　explanation, 859–860
Parents
　back support, necessity, 232
　infant bonding, fostering, 226

Parents (*Continued*)
  infant massage
    benefits, 226
    instructor, interaction, 228f
    instruction, dolls (usage). *See* Infant massage
Parietal bone, 320f, 467f
Parietal cells, 614
  definition, 860
Parietal layer, 278
Parietal lobe, 515f
  definition, 860
  description, 515
Parietal pericardium, 278f
Parietal peritoneum, 278f
Parietal pleura, 278f
Parkinson's disease, 533–534
Paroxetine hydrochloride. *See* Paxil
Partially hydrogenated oils, 621
Participants, 84
Partnerships, 794–795
  advantages/disadvantages, 795
Parturition. *See* Birth
Pascal, law. *See* Law of Pascal
Passive cell processes, 267–270
Passive diffusion, illustration, 268f
Passive movements, 8
  application, 172
  definition, 860
Patella, 347, 448f
  anterior view, 348f
  posterior view, 349f
Patellar, definition, 860
Patellar reflex, 509
Pathogens
  definition, 860
  direct physical contact, 67-68
  indirect physical contact, 68
  relationship. *See* Host-pathogen relationship; Organism/pathogen
Pathological conditions, abbreviations, 829
Pathology, 828–829
  definition, 860
  introduction, 64-68
  terminology, introduction, 263–265
Pathophysiology, 262
Patient
  age, importance, 720
  health/habits, importance, 720
Paxil (paroxetine hydrochloride), 845
Payroll, tracking, 813
PDD. *See* Pervasive developmental disorder
Peak expiratory flow, improvement. *See* Lungs
Peanut butter, sample label, 834
Pearce, John, 16
Peck, M. Scott, 698
Pectineus, 445f
  actions, 448f
  nerve, 448f
  origin/insertion, 448f
Pectoralis major, 221, 414–415
  actions, 414f
  muscle, 650f
  nerves, 414f
  origins/insertion, 414f
  superficial warming friction, knuckles (usage). *See* Supine client
Pectoralis minor
  actions, 407f
  nerves, 407f
  origins/insertion, 407f
Pectoral (mammary), definition, 860
Pectoral (mammary) area, 283
Pedal, definition, 860
Pediatric, definition, 860
Pediatric clients, massage (impact), 248
Pedicle, 361f

Pelvic, definition, 860
Pelvic angles, 326–327
Pelvic area, 283
  treatment suggestions, 706
Pelvic cavity, 281f
Pelvic girdle, 317
  bones, 347
  definition, 860
Pelvic inflammatory disease (PID), 657
Pelvic inlet, 347
Pelvic line, 698
  horizontal landmark, 698f
Pelvic obliquities, 326f
  definition, 860
  movement, 326
Pelvic outlet, 347
Pelvic rotations, 326f
  definition, 860
  walking motion, 326f
Pelvic tilts, 326f
  definition, 860
Penetration, usage. *See* Stationary perpendicular penetration
Penicillin, definition, 845
Penis, 648
  definition, 860
Pennate muscle fiber, 385
Pepcid (famotidine), definition, 845
Peppermint, 688
Pepsinogen, impact, 614t
Peptide hormone, definition, 860
Percocet (oxycodone // acetaminophen), definition, 845
Percussion. *See* Tapotement
  receiving, 602
Performance, improvement, 392b
Pericardial space, 566f
Pericardium, 566f
Perimetrium, 649f
Perimysium, 378
Perineal, definition, 860
Perineal area, 283
Perineal massage, 219
Perineum
  area, 650
  preparation. *See* Fetal delivery
Perineurium, 510
Periosteum, 270f, 313, 313f, 314f
  definition, 860
Peripheral nervous system (PNS), 507, 517–520
  definition, 860
  supporting cells, 508
Peripheral reference. *See* Superficial reference
Peripheral vascular disease, 581
Peristalsis
  definition, 860
  description, 611
  illustration, 611
  stimulation. *See* Large intestine
Peritoneal. *See* Retroperitoneal
Peritoneum
  definition, 860
  description, 611
  illustration, 612f
  Peritonitis, 624
Peritubular capillaries, 635f
Permits. *See* Sales tax
  requirements, 795–796
Peroneal artery. *See* Common peroneal artery
Peroneal nerve. *See* Common peroneal nerve
Perpendicular penetration, usage. *See* Stationary perpendicular penetration
Personal information. *See* Massage business
Pervasive developmental disorder (PDD), massage (usage), 96
Pes anserinus, lateral view, 448f

Pes planus. *See* Flat feet
Pétrissage (kneading stroke), 142, 153–156
  application, 153
  benefits, 156
  definition, 860
  description, 153
  hands, C formation (usage), 153f
  technique, 153
  usage, 743
  variations, 146t, 153–156
Petty cash, 812–813
  description, 813b
Peyer's patches (intestinal tonsils), 579
  definition, 860
Pfluger's Law, 530b
pH, regulation. *See* Blood
Phagocytes, 579
Phagocytosis (cell eating), 269, 562
  definition, 860
  illustration, 269f
Phalangeal area. *See* Digital area
Phalanges, 347, 350
Phantom limb sensation, 240
Pharmacology
  appendix, 837
  terminology, 837–848
Pharyngitis, 624
Pharynx, 612
  definition, 860
  description, 591
  illustration, 592f
Phases. *See* Five elements; Five phases
Phenomenological research, 84
Phenytoin. *See* Dilantin
Phlebitis, 581
Photoreceptors, 527–528
  definition, 860
Physical activities
  categories, 110
  relationship. *See* Occupations
Physical condition. *See* Clients
Physical contact, addressing, 28
Physical strength, requirement, 113
Physical therapy, 10
  modality, 683
Physical well-being, increase, 93
Physiology. *See* Comparative physiology; Developmental physiology; Pathophysiology
  connection. *See* Anatomy
  definition, 262, 860
  introduction, 262–263
  regional approach, 262
  relationship. *See* Body systems
  systemic approach, 262
  terminology, introduction, 263–265
Physiopathological reflex arc, definition, 860
Pia mater, 513f
  definition, 860
  description, 513
PID. *See* Pelvic inflammatory disease
Pigmentation. *See* Skin
Pillows
  bath-size towel, rolling. *See* Cervical pillow
  placement, 134f
  usage. *See* Side-lying clients
Pin and glide, illustration, 728f
Pincement tapotement, 163. *See also* Back
Pineal body, 514f, 545
Pineal gland, 545
  definition, 860
  description, 517
  hormone, 546t
  illustration, 516f, 518f
Pingala, 781
Pinkeye, 534

Pinocytosis (cell drinking), 269–270, 562
  definition, 860
  illustration, 269f
Piriformis
  actions, 434f
  nerve, 434f
  origin/insertion, 434f
Pisiform, 342, 346f
Pitch, 525
Pitta (bile), 781, 782
  definition, 860
Pituitary, definition, 860
Pituitary gland, 516f, 543–545
  location/structure, 544f
Pituitary hormone
  release, assistance, 226
  target organs. See Major pituitary hormones
Pituitary reflex, location, 706
Pivot articulations, 366t
Pivot joint (monoaxial joint), 326f, 327, 327f
  definition, 860
P&L. See Profit and loss
Placenta, 548
  definition, 860
  previa/abruptio, inquiry, 221
Placental stage, 655
Planes of reference. See Reference planes
Planning. See Assessment/planning
  definition, 192, 860
Plantar fascitis, 391
Plantar flex ankle movement, 185t
  illustration, 185f
Plantar flexion, 323
  definition, 860
  illustration, 324f, 701f
Plantaris
  actions, 456f
  nerve, 456f
  origin/insertion, 456f
Plantar (volar), definition, 860
Plasma, 271
  definition, 860
  description, 561
  membrane, 266
Plastic sheet, usage, 678f
Platelet. See Thrombocytes
  count, increase, 583b
  inhibitors, impact, 207b
  plug, 562
Platysma
  actions, 466f
  nerve, 466f
  origins/insertions, 466f
Plavix (clopidogrel), definition, 845
Pleurisy, 601
Plexus, definition, 860
Plicae circulares, 615
  definition, 860
Plural endings, usage, 263b
Pluripotent stem cell, 561, 577
PMS. See Premenstrual syndrome
Pneumocystis carinii pneumonia, 245
Pneumonia, 601
PNS. See Peripheral nervous system
Poliomyelitis, 534
Polish, usage. See Body
Pollex
  area, 283
  definition, 860
Pollicis, 347
Polyps, 624
Polysaccharides, 620
Pons
  definition, 860
  description, 517
  illustration, 514f, 518f

Pool plunge, 681
Pope John Paul II, 107
Popliteal
  definition, 860
  endangerment sites, 98
Popliteal artery, 573
  description, 570
  illustration, 569f
Popliteal vein, 574
Popliteus
  actions, 449f
  nerve, 449f
  origin/insertion, 449f
Port wine spots, 305
Positioning. See Massage table mechanics
  equipment, 121–123
Positive feedback system, 64
Postcentral gyrus, 301, 302f, 515f
Posterior, definition, 860
Posterior cervical triangle, endangerment sites, 98
Posterior deviations, 723
Posterior (dorsal), definition, 860
Posterior fontanel, 356
  definition, 860
Posterior horizontal landmarks, 724f
Posterior lobe, 545
Posterior nares, 591
Posterior pituitary, hormones, 546t
Posterior reference (dorsal reference), 280
Posterior root ganglion, 518
Posterior rotation, 326
Posterior scalene, 472f
Posterior tibial artery
  description, 570
  illustration, 569f
Posterior tilt, 326
Posterior torso, regional terms, 284
Post-event sports massage, 732
Post-ovulation, 652
Postpartum massage, 225–226
Postpartum pregnancy, massage (usage), 96
Postsynaptic neuron, plasma membrane, 511, 512f
Posttraumatic stress, reduction, 93
Posture
  communication, 20
  consideration, 723
  definition, 860
  impact, 713
  improvement, 392b
  muscle tone, relationship, 390
Potassium (K)
  function, 833
  source, 833
Pounding tapotement, 167. See also Prone client
Powder, lubricant, 51
Power differential. See Therapeutic relationship
Power stroke, 382, 390
PPALM. See Purpose Pain Allergies Lifestyle
    Medical
Practice
  scope. See Scope of practice
  standards, 25
  definition, 862
Prakriti, 782
  definition, 860
Prana, 755
  definition, 860
  illustration, 754f
Praying two-handed pétrissage. See Prone client
Precentral gyrus, 515f
Preceptors
  definition, 860
  description, 803
  usage, 803–804
Prednisolone. See Orapred
Prednisone, definition, 845–846

Pre-event sports massage, 732
Prefix, definition, 264
Prefrontal area, 515f
Pregnancy. See High-risk pregnancy
  contractions, relaxation, 219
  contraindications, 222
  discomforts, 219–221
  due date, inquiry, 221
  first trimester, 218
  high-risk factors, 222
  intake process, 221–222
  mask. See Chloasma
  nutrition considerations, 835
  oils, avoidance, 223b
  progression, 218–219
  scents, avoidance, 223b
  second trimester, 218
  singleton/multiples, 653
  third trimester, 218–219
Pregnancy massage. See Medial thigh
  abdominal massage, 223–224
  benefits, 219
  bibliography, 236
  case study, 234
  client comfort, 223
  comfort issues, 224
  draping, 222
  duration/frequency, 222–224
  Internet activities, 236
  introduction, 218
  massage table
    height, 222
    width, 223
  modality restrictions, 223
  prone position, avoidance, 223
  self test, 235
  sheet drape, towel usage, 223f
  student objectives, 217
  summary, 233
  supplies, 222b
  treatment guidelines, 222–224
  usage, 96
Pregnancy-related complications, 218
Pregnant clients
  oil recommendations, 223b
  positioning, 224–225
  seated position, 225
  semireclining position, pillow supports
      (usage), 225f
  side lying, 224–225
  supine position
    left tilt, 224
    right flank, wedge (usage), 224f
    semireclining, 224
Pregnant women, legs (massage), 222
Prehistoric world, 5
Premassage interview, 221
Premarin (conjugated estrogens), definition, 846
Premenstrual syndrome (PMS), 657
  massage, usage, 96
Premise liability, 797
Premotor area, 515f
Prempro (medroxyprogesterone, conjugated
    equine estrogens [inclusion]), definition, 846
Pre-ovulation (second phase), 651–652
Presbyopia, 524
Prescription
  definition, 838
  referral form, contrast, 193
Prescriptive directions, 828–829
Prescriptive directives, 193
Press releases, usage, 803
Pressure
  application, 109f, 143–144. See also Cen-
      tripetal pressure
  pain, inducement, 808

Pressure (*Continued*)
   receptors, 526
   release, 109f
Prevacid (lansoprazole), definition, 846
PRICE. *See* Protection rest ice compression and elevation
Prilosec (omeprazole delayed-release), definition, 846
Primary auditory area, 515f
Primary bronchi, 594f
Primary follicles, 652f
Primary germ layers, 654f
Primary reproductive organs, 646
Primary taste area, 515f
Primatene Mist (epinephrine), definition, 846
Prime movers. *See* Agonists
Privileged information, nondisclosure, 23
PRL. *See* Prolactin
Process, bony marking, 317t
Procrit (epoetin alfa), definition, 846
Professional attitude, development, 31
Professional boundaries
   definition, 850
   examples, 27-28
   principle, 24
   usage, 30
Professional distance, 28-29
Professional image. *See* Massage therapists
Professionalism, 22
   standard, 826
Professional liability, 797
Professional massage therapist, qualities, 22b
Professional responsibility, 199
Professional standards. *See* Massage therapists
Professional techniques, preformation, 28
Profit and loss (P&L) statement
   description, 813b
   usage, 814
Progesterone, 545f, 549t
   definition, 860
   levels, 651f
Progress report
   contrast. *See* Narrative report
   definition, 860
   usage, 209–210
Prolactin (PRL), 545t
   definition, 860
   release, assistance, 226
Prometrium (micronized progesterone), definition, 846
Promotional strategies. *See* Massage business
Pronation, 323, 324f
   definition, 860
Pronator quadratus
   action, 419f
   nerve, 419f
   origin/insertion, 419f
Pronator teres
   actions, 419f
   nerve, 419f
   origins/insertions, 419f
Prone client
   arm, two-handed effleurage (usage), 150f
   back
      alternate hand superficial friction, 158f
      cupping tapotement, 166f
      one-handed hacking, 164f
      pounding tapotement, 166f
      rapping tapotement, 166f
      slapping tapotement, 167f
   bolsters/face rest, usage, 122f
      arm shelf, addition, 122f
   calf, praying hands two-handed pétrissage, 155f
   heart effleurage, usage, 148f
   heel, praying hands two-handed pétrissage, 155f

Prone client (*Continued*)
   hip joint jostling vibration, 171f
   hips, rocking vibration, 172
   ice pack, usage, 675f
   latissimus dorsi muscle, alternate hand pétrissage, 156f
   leg
      alternate-hand effleurage, 151f
      fine vibration, 170f
   pressure, thumbs up indication, 808f
   rhomboids, quacking tapotement, 165f
   rocking vibration, hand-over-hand usage, 171f
   shoulder, two-handed circular effleurage (usage), 150f
   stones, arrangement, 676f
Prone female client
   lower towel rotation, 129f
   turning, preparation, 131f
Prone position, 121
Proposals
   description, 802
   funding, 802
   logistics, 802
   objective, 802
   qualifications, 802
   summary, 802
   usage, 801–802
Propoxyphene hydrochloride. *See* Darvocet
Propranolol. *See* Inderal
Proprietorship, advantages/disadvantages, 794
Proprioceptors, 525
   definition, 861
Prostate, 648
   definition, 861
Prostatitis, 657
Protection rest ice compression and elevation (PRICE), 718
Protectiveness, 26
Proteins. *See* Complement proteins
   definition, 861
   description, 830
   functions, 620t, 830
   source, 830
   usage, 620
Protozoa, agent, 66
Protraction, 325. *See also* Mandibular protraction; Scapular protraction
   definition, 861
Protuberance, bony marking, 317t
Proventil (albuterol inhaler), definition, 846
Provera (medroxyprogesterone acetate), definition, 846–847
Provisional licensure, 796
Proximal, definition, 861
Proximal convoluted tubule
   definition, 861
   description, 634
   illustration, 635f
Proximal reference, 282, 282f
Prozac (fluoxetine), definition, 847
Prudden, Bonnie, 110, 711, 716–718
Psoas major
   access, 618
   actions, 432f
   nerve, 432f
   origins/insertion, 432f
Psoriasis, 305
   term, usage, 295
Psychiatric patients, massage (usage), 96
Psychotherapist, playing (danger), 30
Ptyalin, impact, 614t
Pubic, definition, 861
Pubic area, 283
Pubic bone, 347
Pubis, bony marking, 350t
Public bath. *See* Ancient Roman public bath

Publicity
   definition, 861
   description, 802
   usage, 802–803
Pubococcygeus exercise. *See* Kegels
Pull abducted arm movement, 175, 178t
   illustration, 178f
Pull arm down side movement, 175, 178t
   illustration, 178f
Pull arm overhead movement, 175, 178t
   illustration, 178f
Pull fingers, 175t
   illustration, 177f
Pull toes movement, 185t
   illustration, 186f
Pulmonary circuit, 572
   definition, 861
   illustration, 573f
Pulmonary functions, improvement, 92, 602b
Pulmonary respiration. *See* External respiration
Pulmonary semilunar (SL) valve, 566
   definition, 861
Pulmonary ventilation. *See* Breathing
Pulse. *See* Arterial pulse
   definition, 861
   description, 569
   rates, reduction, 89, 583b
Pulsing tapotement, 163
Pump dispenser, usage. *See* Lubricants
Purchases, documentation, 813
Purkinje fibers, 567, 568f
Purpose Pain Allergies Lifestyle Medical (PPALM)
   assessment/planning method, 744
   domain, 203
   form, 199
   notation, linear diagramming (sample), 204f
Push adducted arm movement, 175, 178t
   illustration, 178f
Push hands, position (demonstration), 143
Pyloric sphincter, 613
   definition, 861
Pylorus, 613
Pyroxidine. *See* Vitamin B$_6$

Q
Qi. *See* Energy
   illustration, 754f
Quacking tapotement, 164. *See also* Prone client
Quadratus femoris
   action, 437f
   nerve, 437f
   origin/insertion, 437f
Quadratus lumborum, 489f
   actions, 488f
   nerves, 488f
   origin/insertion, 488f
Quadriceps
   alternate-hand pétrissage, 154f
   fine vibration. *See* Supine client
   fulling pétrissage, 157f
Quadriceps femoris, 440f
Quadriplegia, 251
Qualitative research, 84
Quality of care. *See* Care
Quantitative research, 83
Quasiexperimental research, 83
Questions. *See* Closed-ended questions; Open-ended questions
Quinton catheters, 241

R
RA. *See* Rheumatoid arthritis
Radial artery, 573
   description, 570
   illustration, 569f

Radial deviation, 321, 323
  ulnar deviation, contrast, 321
Radial flexion, 321
Radial fossa, 340f
Radial groove, 341f
Radial nerve (great extensor), 519
Radial tuberosity, 340f, 341f
Radial vein, 574
Radiation. *See* Law of Radiation
  definition, 861
  description, 669
  examples, 669f
Radius, 340f, 341f, 342
  bony marking, 345t
Raindrops tapotement, 163. *See also* Supine client
Raking, 147. *See also* Alternate finger raking
  usage. *See* Paraspinals
Ramus, bony marking, 317t
Range of motion (ROM)
  consideration, 724–725
  definition, 861
  increase, 180, 208, 392b
  movement, 173–174
Ranitidine. *See* Zantac
Rapping tapotement. *See* Prone client
Rasa, 781
Raynaud's syndrome, 581
RBC. *See* Red blood cell
RDVs. *See* Recommended daily values
Reabsorption, 637
Reach and pull, 110
Reassessment methods, 208
Receptor nerves, 538f
Receptor sites, 542
Recidivism, 252
  definition, 861
Reciprocity, 35
  granting, 30
Recommended daily values (RDVs), 831–832
Record keeping, 744, 746
Recovery time, factors, 720
Recruitment, definition, 861
Rectum
  definition, 861
  description, 617
  illustration, 616f, 648f
Rectus abdominis
  actions, 486f
  nerve, 486f
  origins/insertions, 486f
Rectus capitis posterior major, 476f
  actions, 477f
  nerve, 477f
  origin/insertion, 477f
Rectus capitis posterior minor, 476f
  action, 477f
  nerve, 477f
  origin/insertion, 477f
Rectus femoris
  actions, 440f
  nerve, 440f
  origin/insertion, 440f
Red blood cell (RBC)
  count, increase, 89, 583b
  function, 561
  surface, proteins, 562
Red muscles. *See* Slow twitch muscles
Reference planes, 280
Referral form, contrast. *See* Prescription
Referred pain phenomena, 715
  definition, 861
Reflective questions, asking, 202
Reflex
  arc, 509–510. *See also* Physiopathological
      reflex arc
    definition, 861

Reflex (*Continued*)
  definition, 861
  description, 509
  illustration, 509f
Reflexes, 698
Reflexive responses, 88. *See also* Massage
  definition, 861
Reflexology. *See* Foot reflexology
  foot map, 699f
  landmarks, illustration, 698f
  theories, 697–698
  treatment
    guidelines, 700–703
    suggestions, 704–707
  zone map, 697f
Reflex sympathetic dystrophy, 534
Reflux, 233
Refusal right. *See* Clients
Regeneration. *See* Tissue healing
Regional terms, 282–284
Registration. *See* Massage business
  explanation, 30b
  requirement, 795–796
Rehabilitation, 720–722. *See also* Athletes
  aid, 180
  clinical massage. *See* Sports/rehabilitation
  conditioning stage, 721
  definition, 861
  evaluation stage, 721
  maintenance stage, 721–722
  stages, 721–722
Rehabilitative massage, 732
Reimbursement. *See* Insurance
Relative density, principle, 668–669
Relativity, concept, 755
Relaxation, 383
  emphasis, 778
  enhancement, 171
  promotion, 90, 180, 535b
  response, 610
  strokes, interjection, 702
  usage, 817
Relaxed muscle, blood flow, 91f
Relaxed waves, 516
Relaxin, 549t
  definition, 861
Release form. *See* Medical release form
  usage, 209
Remen, Rachel Naomi, 589
Remission, definition, 861
Remodeling, 810–818
Renaissance. *See* European Renaissance
Renal papilla, 634
Renal pelvis, 634
  definition, 861
Renal tubule, 634
  definition, 861
Renin, definition, 861
Rennin, impact, 614t
Reno, Monica, 797
Repetitive motion injuries, 108–109
  definition, 861
Repetitive strain injuries (RSIs), 108, 391
Reproductive area, treatment suggestions,
    706
Reproductive organs, 646–655. *See also*
    Female reproductive organs; Male
    reproductive organs; Primary
    reproductive organs; Secondary
    reproductive organs
Reproductive system, 279t
  anatomy, 646
  bibliography, 661
  Internet activities, 661
  introduction, 646
  pathological conditions, 656–657

Reproductive system (*Continued*)
  physiology, 646
  self test, 659–660
  student objectives, 645
  summary, 658
  terms/meanings, 658
Reservoir, definition, 861
Resistance, 572
Resolution. *See* Tissue healing
Resort spa, 667
  definition, 861
Resources, usage, 803–804
Respect. *See* Therapeutic relationship
Respiration. *See* External respiration; Internal
    respiration
Respiration rate
  reduction, 92, 602b
  slowing/deepening, 226
Respiratory air movements. *See* Modified respi-
    ratory air movements
Respiratory airways, epithelium (location), 271f
Respiratory conditions, discomfort, 221
Respiratory diaphragm, 594–595
  definition, 861
Respiratory muscles, strengthening, 92, 602b
Respiratory system, 279t
  anatomy, 590
  bibliography, 606
  illustration, 591f
  impact. *See* Waste elimination
  Internet activities, 606
  introduction, 590
  massage, impact, 92, 602b
  pathological conditions, 600–602
  physiology, 590
  self test, 604–605
  student objectives, 589
  summary, 603
  terms/meanings, 590
Responsibility. *See* Therapeutic relationship
Rest and digest, 610
Resting potentials, 510
Restoril (temazepam), definition, 847
Reticular activating system, 517
Reticular connective tissue, 273
  definition, 861
  illustration, 272f
Retina
  definition, 861
  description, 527
  rods/cones, 525f
Retinacula, definition, 861
Retinol. *See* Vitamin A
Retirement accounts, usage, 818
Retraction, 325. *See also* Mandibular retraction;
    Scapular retraction
  definition, 861
Retroperitoneal, 632–633
  definition, 861
Rhazes (Abu Bakr Muhammad ibn Zakariya
    al-Razi) (Persian physician), 6-7
  explanation, 861
Rheumatoid arthritis (RA), 330
  massage, usage, 96
Rh factor, 563
Rhomboids
  actions, 405f
  major/minor, 405f
  nerve, 405f
  origins/insertion, 405f
  quacking tapotement. *See* Prone client
Rhythm, application, 144
Rhythmic contraction, 611
Riboflavin. *See* Vitamin B$_2$
Ribonucleic acid (RNA), 267. *See also* Deoxyri-
    bonucleic acid

Ribosome, 267
 definition, 861
 illustration, 266f
Ribs, 317, 359
 bony marking, 361t
Ridge, bony marking, 317t
Right atrium
 description, 565–566
 illustration, 565f
Right clavicle
 anterior view, 340f
 lateral view, 341f
 posterior view, 341f
Right fibula
 anterior view, 351f
 posterior view, 352f
Right foot
 anterior view, 351f
 arches, 355f
 dorsal view, 353f
 left foot, contralateral relationship, 282
 plantar view, 354f
 posterior view, 352f
Right hand
 anterior view, 343f, 345f
 posterior view, 344f, 346f
Right hemisphere, 516
Right hepatic duct, 618
Right humerus
 anterior view, 340f
 lateral view, 341f
 posterior view, 341f
Right lower extremity
 anterior view, 731f
 posterior view, 731f
Right lymphatic duct, 577
 definition, 861
Right obliquity, 326
Right pelvis
 anterior view, 348f
 posterior view, 349f
Right radius
 anterior view, 343f
 posterior view, 344f
Right rotation, 323
Right scapula
 anterior view, 340f, 411f
 lateral view, 341f, 411f
 medial view, 411f
 posterior view, 341f, 411f
Right scapula/arm
 anterior view, 408f
 posterior view, 408f
Right tibia
 anterior view, 351f
 posterior view, 352f
Right ulna
 anterior view, 343f
 posterior view, 344f
Right upper extermity
 anterior view, 731f
 posterior view, 731f
Right ventricle
 description, 566
 illustration, 565f
Rigveda, 780
Ringworm, 305
Ritalin (methylphenidate), definition, 847
RNA. See Ribonucleic acid
Rocking vibration, 168–170. See also Prone
 client
 hand-over-hand usage. See Prone client
Rodents, extermination, 70
Rods. See Retina
 description, 527
Rogers, Martha, 97

Rogers, Will, 733
Roles, standard, 827
Rolf, Ida Pauline, 318–319
Rolling friction, 158
ROM. See Range of motion
Romand public bath. See Ancient Roman public
 bath
Room. See Massage room
Root chakra (first chakra), 783
Rosacea, 305
Rose geranium, 688
Rosemary, 688
Rosuvastatin calcium. See Crestor
Rotation, 323–324. See also Hips; Knees; Neck;
 Pelvic rotations; Scapular rotation; Shoul-
 ders; Spinal rotation
 definition, 861
 movement, 326
 superior view, 326f
Rotatores, 488b, 489f
 actions, 490f
 nerve, 490f
 origin/insertion, 490f
Rott, definition, 263
Rough endoplasmic reticulum (granular endo-
 plasmic reticulum), 267
 illustration, 266f
Routine, application, 145
Royal Central Institute of Gymnastics, 8
RSIs. See Repetitive strain injuries
Rubber band
 stretch, 110
 stretching, fingers (usage), 109f
Rubefacient, 51
Rubenstein, Leonard, 311
Ruffini, term (usage), 295
Ruffini's corpuscle, 302
 definition, 861
Rugae, 637, 649f
Rumi, 559

S
SA. See Sinoatrial
Sacral, definition, 861
Sacral area, 283
Sacral chakra (second chakra), 783
Sacral plexus (L4-S4), 518
Sacrococcygeal posterior curve, 364f
Sacroiliac, definition, 861
Sacroiliac area, 283
Sacrotuberous ligament, 361
Saddle articulations, 366t
Saddle joints (biaxial joints), 327–328, 327f
 definition, 861
Safety. See Therapeutic relationship
 bibliography, 79
 case study, 75
 discussion. See Massage
 guidelines. See Massage
 Internet activities, 79
 introduction, 64
 self test, 76-78
 student objectives, 63
Safety of Massage Therapy, The (Ernst), 88
Sagittal plane, 280, 281f
 definition, 861
Sagittal suture, 355
 definition, 861
Sales tax, 814
 permit, 796
Saline, mineral water, 668
Saliva, 611
 definition, 861
Salivary amylase, impact, 614t
Saltatory conduction, 511

Salt glow, 684
Sama, 782
Samhitas, 5
Sandalwood, 688
Sanitation
 definition, 862
 guidelines, 69-70
Sanitization. See Massage chair
San-tsai-tou-hoei (Japanese massage
 writings), 7
Saphenous vein, 574
Sarcolemma
 definition, 862
 excitation, 381–382
Sarcomas, 245
Sarcomeres, 380–381
 definition, 862
Sarcoplasm, definition, 862
Sarcoplasmic reticulum, 382
 system, 388
Sartorius, 448f
 actions, 442
 nerve, 442f
 origin/insertion, 442f
Sasaki, Pauline, 755
Sassoon, Vidal, 794
Satellite cells, 508
 definition, 862
Satellite trigger points, 715
 definition, 862
Saunas
 definition, 862
 usage, 682
Savings Incentive Match Plan for Employees
 (SIMPLE) plan, usage, 818
Sawing, 158
 superficial friction, hands (ulnar sides) usage.
 See Scapula
SC. See Sternoclavicular
Scabies, 305
Scalenes, 221, 472f
Scalenus anterior
 actions, 473f
 nerve, 473f
 origins/insertion, 473f
Scalenus medius
 actions, 473f
 nerve, 473f
 origins/insertion, 473f
Scalenus posterior
 actions, 474f
 nerve, 474f
 origins/insertion, 474f
Scalp, seated massage routine, 748
Scaphoid, 342, 346f
Scapular, definition, 862
Scapular area, 283
Scapular depression, 325f
Scapular elevation, 325f
Scapular movement, muscles, 404f-409f
 list, 407
Scapular protraction, 325f
Scapular retraction, 325f
Scapular rotation, 325f
Scapular spine, 341f
Scapula (shoulder blade), 338, 340
 bony marking, 341t
 medial border, sawing superficial friction
 (hands [ulnar sides], usage), 160f
Scar formation
 promotion, 162
 reduction, 92, 331b
Scars, 305–306
 maturation. See Tissue healing
Schnabel, Arthur, 695
Schuyler, James, 96

Schwann cells, 508, 509
  definition, 862
  illustration, 510f
  nucelus, 508f
Schwartz, Jan, 640
Schwartz, Robert, 793
Sciatica, 534
Sciatic nerve, 519
Science, definition, 83
Scientific application. *See* Massage
Scientific method. *See* Massage objectives
  definition, 83
  illustration, 83f
Scleroderma, 306
  term, usage, 295
SCM. *See* Sternocleidomastoid
Scoliosis, 330
  massage, impact, 251
Scope of practice, 23-24
  definition, 862
  principle, 24
  statement, 199
  staying, 30
Scotoma, 250
Scrotum, 647
  definition, 862
Scrubs, usage. *See* Body
S-curve technique, 729f
Seated massage
  bibliography, 751
  hygiene considerations, 741–742
  Internet activities, 751
  introduction, 740
  massage strokes, usage, 743–744
  preparation, 742–743
  routine. *See* Arms; Face; Lower back; Neck;
    Scalp; Stretch; Upper back
    final procedure, 748–749
    massage, 746–749
  sanitization, 741–742
  self test, 750
  student objectives, 739
  summary, 749
  therapist
    lunge position, 742f
    safety considerations/body mechanics, 742
Seated position, 123
Seating massage, chair (usage), 125f
Sebaceous cysts, 306
Sebaceous glands (oil glands), 300
  definition, 862
  stimulation, 89
Seborrhea, term (usage), 295
Seborrheic dermatitis, 306
Sebum, term (usage), 295
Secondary bronchi, 594f
Secondary reproductive organs, 646
Second-class levers, 329f
Second-degree strain, 392
Second efferent neuron, 509f
Secretin, 548
  definition, 862
  impact, 614t
Securities
  definition, 862
  investment, 817–818
Seduction. *See* Clients
Seizure disorders, 534
Self-applied abdominal massage, 224
Self-disclosure
  action, 19
  definition, 23, 862
Self-employment tax, 814
Self-esteem, improvement, 93
Self-image, enhancement, 219
Self-nurturance, 816

Self-report forms, 212
Semen, 648
  definition, 862
Semicircular canals, 525
Semilunar (SL) valve, 566. *See also* Aortic semi-
    lunar valve; Pulmonary semilunar valve
    illustration, 567f
Semimembranosus, 443f
  actions, 444f
  nerve, 444f
  origin/insertion, 444f
Seminal vesicles, 648
  definition, 862
Seminiferous tubules, 647
  definition, 862
Semipermeable bounday, 266
Semireclining position. *See* Clients
Semispinalis, 488b
  actions, 489f
  nerve, 489f
  origin/insertions, 489f
Semitendinosus, 443f, 448f
  actions, 444f
  nerve, 444f
  origin/insertion, 444f
Sense organs, 523–529. *See also* General sense
    organs
Sensory input, 506–507
Sensory nerves (afferent nerves), 508, 528f
  definition, 862
Sensory receptors
  activation, 90, 535b
  illustration, 527f
  types, 525–529
SEP. *See* Simplified Employee Pension
Separation, 331
Septum, 565. *See* Interatrial septum; Interven-
    tricular septum
Sequence, application, 145
Serenity prayer, 115b
Serotonin, 513
  definition, 862
  levels, increase, 90, 535b, 552
Serous membranes, 277, 278
  definition, 862
  types/locations, 278f
Serratus anterior
  actions, 406f
  nerve, 406f
  origins/insertion, 406f
Serratus posterior inferior
  actions, 495f
  nerve, 495f
  origins/insertions, 495f
Serratus posterior superior
  actions, 495f
  nerve, 495f
  origins/insertions, 495f
Sertraline. *See* Zoloft
Sesamoid bones, 312
  example, 313f
Sex cells, 646
Sex glands. *See* Accessory male sex glands
Sexual abuse
  extreme behaviors, 252–253
  massage, relationship, 252–253
  trauma, reasons, 252
Sexual conduct, principle, 24
Sexual intercourse, 652
Sexually transmitted diseases (STDs)
  pathologic conditions, 656–657
  spreading process, 68
Sexual misconduct, 36-39. *See also* Colleagues
  definition, 862
  examples, 37
  prevention, standard, 827

Sexual reproduction, definition, 862
Sexual risk management, 37-38
Shaft, 340f, 341f
Shaking. *See* Vibration
  acceptance, 254
Shampoos, 684. *See also* Body
Shea butter, 51
Shedd, John A., 808
Sheet draping, 127–131
  prone to supine draping, 127–128
  side-lying to supine turning, 131
  supine to prone turning, 128
  supine to side-lying turning, 131
  usage. *See* Side-lying
Sherrington, Charles Scott, 531b
Sherrington's Law, 531b
Shiatsu (finger pressure), 5, 756
  bibliography, 788
  definition, 862
  Internet activities, 788
  Japanese modality, 5
  principles. *See* Touch
  self test, 786–787
  student objectives, 753
  summary, 785
Shingles, 306
Shin splints, 391
Shirodhara, 672, 679
  photograph, 679f
Shleshman. *See* Kapha
Short bones, 312
  example, 313f
Short head. *See* Biceps femoris
Shortness of breath (SOB), 201
  discomfort, 221
Short-term injuries, 251
Shoulders
  abduction, 321, 323f
  adduction, 321, 323f
  alternate-hand circle effleurage, usage, 152f
  circumduction, 324f
  extension, 321, 322f
  flexion, 321, 322f
  girdle, 317, 340
    definition, 862
  grasping, 135f
  gymnastics, 178t
  joints (glenohumeral joints), 340f, 341f
  line, 698
    horizontal landmark, 698f
  movements, 175
    muscles, 410f-415f, 415t
  positioning, 118
  rolling, 109f
  rotation, 324f
  therapist hand, sliding. *See* Opposite shoulder
  treatment areas, 733
  two-handed circular effleurage, usage. *See*
    Prone client
Showers. *See* Hose shower; Spray shower; Swiss
    showers; Vichy showers
  definition, 862
  facilities, maintenance, 70
  usage, 683
Shukra, inclusion, 781
Shushumna, 781
Sickle cell disease, 582
Side-lying, sheet draping (usage), 128, 131
Side-lying clients
  pillows, usage, 124f
  rolling over, 134f
Side-lying female client, back exposure, 133f
Side-lying large-breasted women, upper arm
    (holding), 243f
Side-lying position, 121–123
Siegel, Bernie, 244

Sight conditions, terms, 524
Sign, definition, 862
Silence, usage. *See* Client interview
SIMPLE. *See* Savings Incentive Match Plan for Employees
Simplified Employee Pension (SEP) plan, usage, 818
Simultaneous contrast method, 680f
    usage, 679
Simvastatin. *See* Zocor
Single-use dish, usage. *See* Lubricants
Sinoatrial (SA) node, 241, 567, 568f
Sinus congestion, relief, 171
Sinus discomfort, 221
Sinusitis, 602
Site, survey, 792–797
Sit (position), examination, 118
Sitting occupations, 111b
    (physical activity category), 110
Sitz bath, usage, 683
Sixty-second energy snack, 113b
Skeletal distribution, 315–317
Skeletal muscle, 270f, 274
    contractions, 388–390
    parts, 384–385
        illustration, 384f
    pictomicrograph, 275f
        line drawing, 275f
    pump, 571f
Skeletal muscle fibers, types, 387–388
Skeletal nomenclature
    bibliography, 374
    Internet activities, 374
    introduction, 338
    self test, 369–373
    student objectives, 337
    summary, 368
Skeletal system, 279t
    anatomy, 312
    anterior view, 315f
    appendicular divisions, 315f
    axial divisions, 315f
    bibliography, 335
    histology, 314
    Internet activities, 335
    introduction, 312
    pathological conditions, 328–331
    physiology, 312
    posterior view, 316f
    self test, 333–334
    student objectives, 311
    summary, 332
    terms/meanings, 312
Skeleton. *See* Appendicular skeleton; Axial skeleton
    anterior view, 283f
    posterior view, 283f
    terms/meanings, 339
Skin
    appearance, 294
    appendages, 298–301
    cancer, 304
    color, 298
    condition, 205
        improvement, 89–90
    coverage, 294
    dryness, lubricants (impact), 50
    epithelium, location, 271f
    glands, 300. *See also* Apocrine skin glands; Eccrine skin glands
    glandular action, improvement, 162
    hands, contact, 165f
    involvement. *See* Vitamin D synthesis
    lifting
        fingers/thumb web, usage, 158f
        hands, usage, 157f

Skin (*Continued*)
    massage, impact, 89–90
    membrane, classification, 294
    microscopic view, 296f
    nourishment, massage media (impact), 50
    pathological conditions, 303–306
    physiological data, 294
    pigmentation, 305
    protection, function, 294
    protectorant, 742
    regions, 295–298
    role. *See* Immunity
    rolling, 155–156
        pétrissage. *See* Back
        usage, 728
    sensation, role, 294
    sensory receptors, 297t
    suppleness, maintenance, 219
    tags, 306
    temperature, increase, 89
    terms/meanings, 295
    touch, significance, 82
    waste elimination, role, 294
Skull, 317
    bones, 353–359
    sacrum, relationship, 282
Slapin, Beverly, 219
Slapping tapotement, 167. *See also* Prone client
Sliding filament theory, 381f, 382
    definition, 862
Slow twitch muscles (red muscles), 387–388
Small intestine
    absorption sites, 616f
    definition, 862
    description, 615–616
    meridian, 758
        anterior view, 764f
        lateral view, 764f
        posterior view, 765f
    wall, illustration, 615f
Smelling, evaluation technique, 777
Smooth endoplasmic reticulum (agranular endoplasmic reticulum), 267
    illustration, 266f
Smooth muscle, 274
    illustration, 594f
    pictomicrograph, 275f
        line drawing, 275f
Sneezing, 599
    definition, 862
Snoring, 599
    definition, 862
SOAP. *See* Subjective Objective Assessment Plan
Society of Trained Masseuses, The
    formation, 9
    merger, 9
Sodium chloride, excretion (promotion). *See* Urine
Sodium-potassium pump, 510
    definition, 862
Soft end-feel, 725
Sojourns, usage, 816
Solar plexus
    chakra, 783–784
    points (holding), thumbs (usage), 706f
Solatol. *See* Betapace
Soleus, 455f
    action, 457f
    nerve, 457f
    origins/insertion, 457f
Sol state, 712
Somatic nervous system, definition, 862
Somatic reflexes, 509
    definition, 862
Somatic sensory association area, 515f
Somatropin. *See* Growth hormone

Soreness. *See* Muscle soreness
Spa, 666–667. *See also* Day spa; Destination spa; Hotel spa; Medical spa; Resort spa
    applications, 683. *See also* Hydrotherapy
    aromatherapy, usage, 688
    bibliography, 692
    clients, questions, 672b
    definition, 862
    effectiveness (enhancement), aromatherapy (impact), 686
    Internet activities, 692
    introduction, 666
    self test, 690
    student objectives, 665
    summary, 689
    therapies, 667
        definition, 862
    treatment guidelines, 671–685
    tubs
        definition, 862
        usage, 681
Spasms
    activity, maps, 730f
    definition, 862
    generation, explanation, 713–714
    information, 712–713
    location process, 714
    reduction, 219
Spasticity, 391–392
Spastic muscles, 390
Speech, 590
    difficulties, 250
Speed, application, 144
Spermatic duct, 647
    definition, 862
Spermatozoon (spermatozoa)
    definition, 862
    description, 646
    illustration, 646f, 653f
Sphenoidal sinus, 356
Sphenoid sinus, 591
    description, 358f
Sphincter, 611. *See also* Cardioesophageal sphincter; Ileocecal sphincter; Pyloric sphincter
    definition, 862
Sphincter of Oddi, 616, 618
    definition, 862
    illustration, 618f
Sphygmomanometer, 571
Spina bifida, 534
Spinal abnormalities, massage (impact), 251
Spinal accessory nerve, 519
Spinal area, treatment suggestions, 706–707
Spinal cavity, 281f
Spinal cord, 514
    definition, 862
    illustration, 509f
    injury, 251
Spinal extension, 321, 322f
Spinal flexion, 321, 322f
Spinalis, 488b
    actions, 491f
    nerve, 491f
    origins/insertions, 491f
Spinal lateral flexion/extension, 321, 322f
Spinal nerves, 518, 521f
    definition, 862
    exit, 507
Spinal rotation, 324f
Spinal twist, 175, 181t
    illustration, 181f
Spindles. *See* Muscle spindles
Spine
    alignment, 118, 120
    bony marking, 317t

Spine (*Continued*)
  massage, stoppage, 149f
  root, 341f
Spinous process, 361f
Spitz, Rene (touch studies), 85
Spleen
  definition, 862
  description, 578
  illustration, 618f
  meridian, 758
    anterior view, 762f
    posterior view, 762f
Splenius capitis
  actions, 474f
  nerve, 474f
  origins/insertions, 474f
Splenius cervicis
  actions, 475f
  nerve, 475f
  origins/insertions, 475f
Spondylolisthesis, 331
Spondylosis, 331
Spongy bone, 313f, 314, 314f
  definition, 862
Sports injuries, causes, 718
Sports massage, 732–733. *See also* Inter-event
    sports massage; Post-event sports massage;
    Pre-event sports massage
Sports/rehabilitation, clinical massage
  aftercare, 732
  assessments, 722–725
  bibliography, 737
  gait, consideration, 723–724
  information, 712–718
  Internet activities, 737
  introduction, 712
  mistakes, 730–732
  observation, 722
  palpation, 722–723
  posture, consideration, 273
  ROM, consideration, 724–725
  self test, 735–736
  student objectives, 711
  summary, 734
  techniques, 725–729
  treatment, 729
    areas, 733
    tools, 729
Sprain, 331
Spray shower, 683
Squamosal suture, definition, 862
Srotas, 782
St. John, Paul, 112–113
Stability, requirement, 114–115
Stabilizers, 386
Stamina, requirement, 113
Standards of practice. *See* Practice
Standing occupations, 111b
  (physical activity category), 110
Starlix (nateglinide), definition, 847
Startup costs, determination. *See* Massage
    business
State-dependent memory, 253
  definition, 862
State license, 796
Stationary perpendicular penetration, usage, 779
STDs. *See* Sexually transmitted diseases
Steam bath
  definition, 862
  usage, 682
Steam canopy, 682
Stent, massage (impact), 241
Sternoclavicular (SC) joint, 367
Sternocleidomastoid (SCM), 221
  actions, 471f
  muscles, 392

Sternocleidomastoid (SCM) (*Continued*)
  nerve, 471f
  origins/insertion, 471f
Sternum, 317, 359
  bony marking, 360t
Steroid hormone, definition, 862
STH. *See* Growth hormone
Stiffness, reducation, 219
Still, Andrew Taylor, 356, 723
Stimulation, 816
Stimuli, 506
Stirrup, 524–525
Stocks, investment, 817
Stoma, 243
Stomach, 613–615
  absorption sites, 616f
  definition, 863
  illustration, 613f
  lining, cross-section, 613f
  meridian, 758
    anterior view, 761f
    posterior view, 761f
  muscle layers, 613f
  structures, 613f
Stones
  arrangement. *See* Prone client
  placement. *See* Toes
  usage, 676
Stool, therapist usage. *See* Feet; Head
Strabismus, 250
Strain, 392. *See also* First-degree strain; Second-
    degree strain; Third-degree strain
Stratum, term (usage), 295
Stratum corneum, 296, 297
Stratum germinativum, 296–297
Stratum granulosum, 296, 297
Stratum lucidum, 296, 297
Stratum spinosum, 296, 297
Strawberry hemangiomas, 305
Strength
  martial arts principle, 110
  requirement. *See* Physical strength
Strenuous occupations, 111b
  (physical activity category), 110
Stress
  impact, 713
  massage, usage, 96
  reduction, 90, 219, 535b
  response, 543
Stretch
  breaks, usage, 120
  movement, 172
  receptors, 526
  reflex, 527. *See also* Inverse stretch reflex;
      Myotatic stretch reflex
  reflexes, 173b
  seated massage routine, 748
Stretching
  contraction, opposite, 388
  definition, 863
  involvement, 173
Stretch marks, 306
  discomfort, 221
  prevention, 219
Stroke, 534
Strokes. *See* Massage strokes
Stroke volume, 566
  definition, 863
  increase, 89, 583b
Structured time. *See* Therapeutic relationship
Subacute, definition, 863
Subarachnoid space, 513
  definition, 863
  description, 513
Subclavian artery, 573
Subclavian vein, 574

Subcutaneous layer, 298
  definition, 863
Subcutaneous (SubQ), definition, 838
Subdural space, 513
  definition, 863
Subjective data, 193
  definition, 863
  objective data
    comparision, 194
    contrast, 193–194
Subjective Objective Assessment Plan (SOAP)
  format, 195b
  notes, APIE notes (contrast), 194–196
  SOAPIER note, 194
  variations, 194
Subjects, 83
Submucosa, 615f
Suboccipitals, 476f
SubQ. *See* Subcutaneous
Subscapular fossa, 340f
Subscapularis
  actions, 413f
  nerve, 413f
  origin/insertion, 413f
Substance, treatment, 69
Substance abuse, 534–535
  issues, 252
Substantia nigra, 517
Sucrase, impact, 614t
Sudoriferous, term (usage), 295
Sudoriferous gland (sweat gland), 296f, 300
  definition, 863
Suffix, definition, 263
Sulci, 515. *See also* Central sulcus
Sulfur, mineral water, 668
Summation, 512l
Sun-moon effleurage, 148
Superficial, definition, 863
Superficial fascia, 270f, 274
  observation, 723
  softening, 156
Superficial friction, usage, 743
Superficial reference (peripheral reference), 282
Superficial warming friction, 158
  fingertips, usage. *See* Paraspinals
  knuckles, usage. *See* Supine client
Superior, definition, 863
Superior angle, 341f
Superior reference (cranial reference), 282
Supination, 323, 324f
  definition, 863
Supinator
  action, 420f
  nerve, 420f
  origins/insertion, 420f
Supine client
  abdomen
    alternate-hand circular effleurage, usage, 152f
    diffused tapotement, 168f
    fine vibration, 168f
  body wrap, usage, 677f
  bolsters, usage, 122f
  extended arm
    rolling friction, 160f
    wringing friction, 160f
  face, raindrops tapotement, 164f
  legs
    coarse vibration, 171f
    nerve stroke, usage, 153f
    two-handed effleurage, usage, 150f
  metatarsals, chucking friction, 161f
  pectoralis major, superficial warming friction
      (knuckles, usage), 159f
  quadriceps
    fine vibration, 170f
    jostling, 170f

Supine client (*Continued*)
    touch, 143f
    towel draping, T formation, 129f
    upper trapezius (one-handed pétrissage),
        finger pads/thumbs (usage), 154f
Supine female client
    head pillow, usage, 134f
    towel draping, 127f
        abdomen, exposure, 128f
Supine male client, feet (uncovered), 132f
Supine position, 121
Supraglenoid tubercle, 340f, 341f
Supraspinatus
    action, 412f
    nerve, 412f
    origin/insertion, 412f
Supraspinous fossa, 341f
Supraspinous ligament, 359
Sural. *See* Calf
Surface anatomy, 262
Surface dimpling, reduction. *See* Cellulite
Surface markings, 317
Surfactants, 593
Surgery, recovery, 251
Surgical neck, 341f
Survivors of Incest Anonymous, 254
Sustained pressure
    braced thumb, usage, 727f
    definition, 863
    description, 726
    elbow, usage, 727f
    technique, 726
    usage, 725, 726, 743
Sutherland, William, 356
Suture, 320f. *See also* Coronal suture; Lamb-
    doidal suture; Sagittal suture; Squamosal
    suture
Swanson, Rebecca, 206
Sweat glands. *See* Apocrine sweat glands;
    Eccrine sweat glands; Sudoriferous gland
    openings, 296f
Swedhana, 672
Swedish gymnastics, 8, 172–186
    benefits, 180–186
    bibliography, 189
    case study, 187
    definition, 863
    description, 172–173
    flow chart, 173f
    Internet activities, 189
    introduction, 142
    mini-lab, 173
    objectives, 141
    self test, 188
    summary, 186
    technique, 173–180
Swedish massage, 8, 88
    definition, 142, 863
Swedish massage movements
    bibliography, 189
    case study, 187
    classification, 145
    Internet activities, 189
    introduction, 142
    objectives, 141
    self test, 188
    summary, 186
Swedish milking, 229
Swedish Movement and Massage (Nissen), 9
Swedish Movement and Massage Treatment
    (Nissen), 9
Swedish Movement Cure (Ling), 8
Swiss showers, 683
Sydenham, Thomas, 7
Symbols, 828–829
Symmetry. *See* Law of Symmetry

Sympathetic, definition, 863
Sympathetic nerve, 520–523
    system, 522–523
Sympathetic nervous system, 520. *See also*
    Parasympathetic nervous system
Symphysis pubis, illustration, 648f
Symptoms
    abbreviations, 828
    definition, 863
Synapses, 381, 511–513
    definition, 863
    illustration, 512f
Synaptic bulb, 508f, 511
    definition, 863
    description, 508
    illustration, 512f
Synaptic cleft, 511
Synaptic transmission, 382, 511–513
Synaptic vesicles, 509
    definition, 863
Synarthroses, 319
    examples, 320f
Synarthrosis joint (fibrous joint), definition, 863
Syncretic phase, 780
Syndrome, definition, 863
Synergists, 386
    definition, 863
Synovial fluid, 321
    definition, 863
    production, stimulation, 180
Synovial joint. *See* Diarthrosis joint
Synovial membranes, 278, 319
    definition, 863
    types/locations, 278f
Synovial sheath, 321
    definition, 863
Synthroid (levothyroxine sodium), definition,
    847
Syphilis, 657
Systemic arteries. *See* Major systemic arteries
Systemic circuit, 572–573
    definition, 863
    illustration, 573f
Systemic disease, definition, 863
Systemic veins. *See* Major systemic veins
Systole, 571–572
    definition, 863

T
T3. *See* Triiodothyronine
T4. *See* Thyroxine
Tables. *See* Massage tables
    mechanics. *See* Massage table mechanics
    padding. *See* Massage table padding
Tachycardia, 568
    definition, 863
Tactile corpuscle. *See* Meissner corpuscle
Taenia coli, definition, 863
Tagamet (cimetidine), definition, 847
Tai Ji
    definition, 863
    illustration, 757f
Tamsulosin. *See* Flomax
Tangerine, 688
Tapotement. *See* Pulsing tapotement; Raindrops
    tapotement
    benefits, 167
    definition, 863
    description, 163
    percussion, 142
        variations, 146t
    percussive strokes, 163–167
    technique, 163
    usage, 743–744
    variations, 163–167
Tapping tapotement, 163. *See also* Back

Target cells, 542–543
    definition, 863
Tarsal, definition, 863
Tarsals, bones, 349–350, 354t
Taste
    hairs, 523
    pores, 523
    sense organ, 523–524
Taut band, palpation, 713f
Taxes. *See* Income; Sales tax; Self-employment
    tax
    deductions, 814–815
    impact, 814–815
Taylor, Charles Fayette, 9
    explanation, 863
Taylor, George Henry, 9
    explanation, 863
T cells, 579–580
    development, 578f
TCM. *See* Traditional Chinese medicine
Tea tree, 688
Techne Iatriche (healing science), 5
    development, 6
Teeth, root, 320f
Teething, discomfort (relief), 226
Tegretol (carbamazepine), definition, 847
Telangiectasia, 582
Telephone
    calls
        answering, 800
        placing, 800
    etiquette, importance, 800–801
    messages, taking, 800
    standards, 800
Telodendria, 508f
    definition, 863
    illustration, 508
Temazepam. *See* Restoril
Temperature, 667–668
    conversion, 667b
    observation, 723
    ranges. *See* Body
    regulation. *See* Body
Temporal artery
    description, 569
    illustration, 569f
Temporal bone, 467f, 476f
Temporalis, 467f
    actions, 468f
    nerve, 468f
    origin/insertion, 468f
Temporal lobe
    definition, 863
    description, 516
    illustration, 515f
Temporomandibular joint (TMJ), 367
    dysfunction, 331
        massage, usage, 96
Temporoparietal suture, 355
Tenderness, meaning, 703–704
Tender point activity, reduction, 162,
    171
Tender point formation, reduction,
    162
Tendinitis, 392
Tendonitis. *See* De Quervain's tendonitis
Tendons, 384f
    definition, 863
    reflex, 527
    sheaths, 379
Tension, addressing, 156
Tensor fascia lata
    actions, 439f
    nerve, 439f
    origins/insertion, 439f
Tentorium cerebelli, 513

Terbafine hydrochloride. *See* Lamisil
Teres major
    actions, 410f
    nerve, 410f
    origin/insertion, 410f
Teres minor
    actions, 413f
    nerve, 413f
    origin/insertion, 413f
Terminal illnesses
    definition, 244, 863
    equipment, caring, 246t
    massage, impact, 244–252
Termites, extermination, 70
Term life insurance, 797
Terrycloth pouch, usage. *See* Hot pack
Testes, 547
Testicles, 647
    definition, 863
Testosterone, 545f, 549t
    definition, 863
Tetracycline, definition, 847
Tetraiodothyronine. *See* Thyroxine
Texture, 50
T formation. *See* Supine client; Towel
Thalamus
    definition, 863
    description, 517
    illustration, 514f, 516f, 518f
Thalassotherapy, 668
Theca cells, development, 646f
Theisen, Kathleen Casey, 390
Thenar eminence, 427. *See also* Hypothenar
        eminence
Theory of Human Motivation (Maslow), 86
Theory of the five phases (elements). *See* Five
        phases
Therapeutica on Restoring Health (Bright), 7
Therapeutic exercise, 172
Therapeutic massage, 88
Therapeutic relationship, 16-19
    bibliography, 41
    case study, 39
    client-centered care, 17
    collegial relationships, 19
    communication, 17
    compassion, 17
    Internet activities, 41
    introduction, 16
    power differential, 19
    respect, 18
    responsibility, 18
    safety, 18
    self test, 40
    structured time, 18
    summary, 39
    trust, 17
Therapists. *See* Massage therapists
    experience, 732
    physical contact. *See* Clients
    rotation, direction, 127–128
Thermal-dynamic process, 667
Thermal mittens/booties, 676
Thermoreceptor, definition, 863
Thermotherapy, 669–670
    definition, 864
Theta state, 516
Thiamine. *See* Vitamin B₁
Thick myofilament, 380f
Thighs
    bones, 347
    endangerment sites. *See* Medial thigh
    sides, fulling pétrissage, 157f
    top, fulling pétrissage, 157f
Thin myofilament, 380f
Third-class levers, 329f

Third-degree strain, 392
Third ventricle, 516f, 518f
Thixotropism, 274
    definition, 864
Thixotropy, 274
Thomas, Lewis, 261
Thoracic, definition, 864
Thoracic area, 283
Thoracic cavity, 281f
Thoracic duct, 577
    definition, 864
Thoracic outlet syndrome, 535
Thoracic posterior curve, 364f
Thoracic vertebrae
    lateral view, 363f
    superior view, 363f
Thoracolumbar outflow, 523
Thorax, 359
    anterior view, 360f
    bones, 359–362
    posterior view, 361f
Thoreau, Henry David, 194
Thresholds, 512. *See also* Contraction
Throat
    chakra (fifth chakra), 784
    endangerment sites, 98
Thrombocytes (platelets)
    definition, 864
    description, 562
    illustration, 561f
Thrombophlebitis, 582
Thrush, 624
Thumbing, technique, 779
Thumb-over-thumb stroke, 229
Thumbs
    effleurage. *See* Metatarsals
    joints, 327f
    opposition, 325f
    spreading, 229
    usage. *See* Skin; Solar plexus; Supine
        client
Thumb walk, usage. *See* Zones
Thymopoietin, 548
Thymosin, 438
    definition, 864
Thymus, 548
    definition, 864
Thymus gland, 578
Thyroid, definition, 864
Thyroid extract. *See* Armour thyroid
Thyroid gland, 545
    hormones, inclusion, 547t
Thyroid hormones, 545f
Thyroid-stimulating hormone (TSH), 545t
    definition, 864
Thyroxine (tetraiodothyronine // T4), 547t
    definition, 864
TIA. *See* Transient ischemic attach
Tibia, 348, 448f
    bony marking, 353t
Tibial artery, 573
Tibialis anterior
    actions, 452f
    nerve, 452f
    origins/insertions, 452f
Tibialis posterior
    actions, 457f
    nerve, 457f
    origins/insertions, 457f
Tibial nerve, 519
Tibial vein, 574
Tibiofemoral joint, 367
Tilts. *See* Anterior tilt; Pelvic tilts; Posterior tilt
    right lateral view, 326f
Time of the embryo. *See* Embryo
Tisserand, Robert, 596–597

Tissot, Simon André, 8
    explanation, 864
Tissue
    assessment, therapist assistance, 180
    bibliography, 290
    cells, 577f
    definition, 270, 864
    hormones, 543
    injury, type (importance), 720
    Internet activities, 290
    introduction, 262
    level, composition, 265
    milking, 153
    organization, level, 265t
    oxygenation, increase, 219
    pushing, 146
    respiration. *See* Internal respiration
    self test, 285–289
    slurping, 153
    spaces, 577f
    student objective, 261
    summary, 284
Tissue healing
    fibrosis, 719–720
    process, 718–720
    regeneration, 719
    resolution, 719
    scar maturation, 720
TMJ. *See* Temporomandibular joint
Tocopherol. *See* Vitamin E
Toes
    abduction, 323f
    adduction, 323f
    extension, 321f
    flexion, 321f
    stone, placement, 676f
Tolterodine. *See* Detrol
Tones, communication, 20
Tongue, taste buds, 524f
Tonic contraction, 611
Tonification, 773
Tonsilitis, 624
Tonsils, 579. *See also* Peyer's patches
    definition, 864
Topical, definition, 838
Top leg, massage, 133f
Torquing
    illustration, 728f
    usage, 728
Torticollis (wryneck), 392
Touch
    application, 143
    aversion, reduction, 93
    nervous systems, role, 301–303
    receptors, 526
    research. *See* Foundational touch
        research
    sensitivity, reduction, 93
    significance. *See* Skin
    Zen shiatsu principles, 777–779
Touch-holds, 229
Touch Research Institute (TRI), 87, 248
Towel
    anchoring, 129f, 130f
    draping, 126–127
    fanfolds, unfolding, 128f
    friction, 158
    holding, 130f
    rolling. *See* Cervical pillow
    rotation, 130f
    T formation, 129f
Towel draping. *See* Clients; Female clients;
        Legs; Male clients
    client prone to supine turning, 127
    client supine to prone turning, 127
    T formation. *See* Supine client

Toxic agents
  direct physical contact, 67-68
  indirect physical contact, 68
Trachea
  definition, 864
  illustration, 591f, 594f
Tracheal ring. *See* Hyaline cartilage
Tracts, 514
Traditional Chinese medicine (TCM), 755–756
  ayurveda, contrast/comparison, 784
Trager, Milton, 200–201
Trailing foot, placement, 116
Transdermal patches
  definition, 838
  impact, 207b
  usage, 306
Transderm-Nitro (nitroglycerin), definition, 847
Transference, 32-34
  definition, 864
Transient ischemic attach (TIA), 582
Transmitting neuron, axon, 512f
Transverse abdominis
  action, 487f
  nerve, 487f
  origins/insertions, 487f
Transverse arch (metatarsal arch), 350
Transverse carpal ligament, 342, 346f
Transverse plane (horizontal plane), 280
  definition, 864
Transverse process, 361f
Trapezium, 342, 346f
Trapezius
  actions, 404f
  nerves, 404f
  origins/insertions, 404f
Trapezoid, 342
Trash, removal, 70
Trauma, impact. *See* Direct trauma
Traumatic disorders, 66
  definition, 864
Travell, Janet, 550–551, 568
*Treatise on Massage, Its History, Mode of
  Application and Effects* (Graham), 9
Treatment
  facility, safety guidelines, 56
  guidelines, 207
  plan, 192
    definition, 192, 864
  tools, 729
TRI. *See* Touch Research Institute
Triaxial joints. *See* Ball-and-socket joints;
  Gliding joints
Triceps, one-handed pétrissage, 154f
Triceps brachii
  actions, 417f
  nerve, 417f
  origins/insertion, 417f
Triceps surae, 455f
Trichomoniasis, 657
Tricor (fenofibrate), definition, 847
Tricuspid valve, 566
  definition, 864
Tri-doshas, 781
  definition, 864
Trigeminal nerve, 519, 521f
Trigeminal neuralgia, 535
Trigger points, 713. *See also* Active trigger
    points; Attachment trigger points; Central
    trigger points; Key trigger points; Latent
    trigger points; Satellite trigger points
  activity, reduction, 162, 171
  classification, 714–718
  definition, 864
  formation, reduction, 91, 162, 392b
  generation, explanation, 713–714

Trigger points (*Continued*)
  location process, 714
  maps, 730f
  palpation, 713f
  work, 712
Triglycerides, 831
Triiodothyronine (T3), 547t
  definition, 864
Triple heater, meridian, 758
  lateral view, 769f
  posterior view, 769f
Triquetrum, 342
Trisomy 21. *See* Down syndrome
Trochanter, bony marking, 317t
Trochlea, 340f
Trochlear nerve, 519, 521f
Tropomyosin, 380, 382
Troponin, 380
True ribs, 359
True vocal cords, 593
Trunk, muscles, 485f-496f
Trust, 35. *See also* Therapeutic relationship
  chain, 212
Trypsinogen (trypsin), impact, 614t
TSH. *See* Thyroid-stimulating hormone
Tsubo (acupoints). *See* Energy points
  definition, 864
  stimulation, 756
T-tubules, 382
  system, 388
Tubercle, bony marking, 317t
Tuberculosis, 602
Tuberosity, bony marking, 317t
Tubular secretion, 637
Tuina, 756
Tumor, 65, 244. *See also* Benign tumor; Malig-
    nant tumor
Tunica externa, 568, 569f
Tunica interna, 568
Tunica intima, 569f
Tunica media, 568, 569f
Turner's syndrome. *See* XO female
Twain, Mark, 3, 609
Twist compression, 726
Twitching, observation, 722
Twitch response. *See* Local twitch response
Two-handed circular effleurage, usage. *See*
    Prone client
Two-handed compression, 726
Two-handed connection, usage, 778–779
Two-handed effleurage, 145, 148. *See also*
    Circular two-handed effleurage
  usage. *See* Prone client; Supine client
Two-handed pétrissage, 154
Tylenol (acetaminophen), definition, 847
Tympanic membrane, 524
Type 2 herpes simplex virus (HSV2), 656
Typical vertebrae
  exploded view, 361f
  parts, 359–360, 361f

U

Udvartana, 672, 685
Ulcerative colitis, 624
Ulcers, 625. *See also* Decubitus ulcers
  attribution, 625
Ulna, 340f, 341f, 342
  bony marking, 343t
Ulnar artery, 573
Ulnar deviation, 323
  contrast. *See* Radial deviation
Ulnar nerve (accessory flexor), 519
Ulnar tuberosity, 340f
Ulnar vein, 574

Ultrasound
  acoustic mechanical vibration, 168b
  effect, manual creation, 167
Ultraviolet (UV) radiation
  amount, reduction, 296
  protection, 294
Umbilical, definition, 864
Umbilical area, 283
Underwater massage, usage, 681
Unhealthy conflict resolution strategies, 21t
Uniarticular, definition, 864
Uniarticular muscles, 385
Uniforms, cleanliness, 69-70
Unilaterality. *See* Law of Unilaterality
Unipennate muscle fiber, 385f
Universal donor, 563
  definition, 864
Universal precaution, 246
  CDC establishment, 69
Universal recipient, 563
  definition, 864
Upper back, seated massage, 746
Upper extremity
  anterior/posterior views. *See* Right upper
    extermity
  bones, 340–347
  regional terms, 282–283
Upper limbs, 317
Upper respiratory tract, 590–593
  illustration, 591f
Upper respiratory tract congestion, relief,
  171
Upper trapezius
  fist effleurage, 147f
  one-handed pétrissage, usage. *See* Supine
    client
  therapist massage, 747f
  unrolling, 733b
Upward rotation, 323–324
Ureters
  definition, 864
  description, 637
  illustration, 638f
Urethra
  definition, 864
  description, 639, 647
  illustration, 638f, 649f
Urinary bladder
  definition, 864
  description, 637, 639
  illustration, 509f, 638f, 648f
Urinary incontinence, 641
  definition, 838
Urinary retention, definition, 838
Urinary structures, 633f
Urinary system, 279t
  anatomy, 632
  illustration, 633f
  impact. *See* Waste elimination
  introduction, 632
  massage, impact, 93, 641b
  pathologic conditions, 639–641
  physiology, 632–639
  student objectives, 631
Urinary tract infection (UTI), 641
Urine, 639
  definition, 864
  elimination, 632
  formation. *See* Kidneys
  output, increase, 93, 641b
  sodium chloride, excretion (promotion),
    93, 641b
Uterine abnormalities, inquiry, 221
Uterine contraction, 545f
Uterine cycle, endometrial changes, 651f

Uterus (womb)
  definition, 864
  description, 649–650
  illustration, 648f, 649f
  menstruation, 650–651
  pre-ovulation, 651
UTI. See Urinary tract infection

V
Vagina (birth canal)
  definition, 864
  description, 650
  illustration, 648f
Vaginal births, 225–226
Vaginal bleeding/discharge, inquiry, 221
Vaginal candidiasis, 657
Vagus nerve, 519, 521f
Valacyclovir. See Valtrex
Valium (diazepam), definition, 847
Valtrex (valacyclovir), definition, 848
Value, assessment, 792–793. See also
    Massage
Variables, 83
Varicose veins, 582
Vasa vasorum, 568
Vascular disease, 572
Vascular problems, 221
Vascular spasm, 562
Vascular tissue. See Liquid connective tissue
Vas deferens (ductus deferens), 647
  definition, 864
Vasoconstriction, 569, 670. See also Heat
  definition, 864
Vasodilation, 569. See also Heat
  definition, 864
Vasopressin. See Antidiuretic hormone
Vasotec (enalapril), definition, 848
Vastus intermedius
  action, 441f
  nerve, 441f
  origins/insertion, 441f
Vastus lateralis, 440f
  action, 442f
  nerve, 442f
  origins/insertion, 442f
Vastus medialis, 440f
  action, 441f
  nerve, 441f
  origin/insertion, 441f
Vata (vayu), 781, 782
  definition, 864
Vegetarianism, 835
Veins, 570–571. See also Major veins; Varicose
    veins
  definition, 864
Vena cava, 574
Venereal warts, 656
Venous blood flow, promotion, 162
Venous portal systems, 573
Venous pump, 571
  definition, 864
Ventilation. See Pulmonary ventilation
Ventral cavity, 280
  definition, 864
Ventral reference. See Anterior reference
Ventricles. See Fourth ventricle; Left ventricle;
    Right ventricle; Third ventricle
  definition, 864
  description, 565
Venules
  definition, 864
  description, 570
  illustration, 577f
Vermiform appendix, 617
  definition, 864

Vertebrae, 359. See also Atypical vertebrae
  articular facets, joints, 327f
  parts. See Typical vertebrae
Vertebral, definition, 864
Vertebral arch, 360, 361f
Vertebral area, 283
Vertebral body, 361f
Vertebral canal, 360, 361f
Vertebral column, 317, 359–362
  anterior view, 364f
  bones, 359–362
  curves/divisions, 364f
  divisions, 361–362
  lateral view, 363f
  movement, muscles, 493
  muscles, 485f-496f
  posterior view, 364f
  regions/traits, 364t
  superior view, 363f
  vertebrae, components, 363f
Vertebral components, bony marking, 362t
Vertebral preminens
  lateral view, 363f
  superior view, 363f
Vertebra prominens, 361
Vertical landmarks, 723
Vesalius, Andreas, 7. See also De Humani
    Corporis Fabrica
  explanation, 864
Vesicle, 266f
Vessels of the vessels, 568
Vestibulocochlear nerve, 519
Vibration (shaking), 142, 167–172
  benefits, 171
  definition, 864
  description, 167
  mini-lab, 172
  technique, 167
  variations, 146t, 167–171
Vichy showers (affusion showers), 683
  photograph, 684f
Vicodin (hydrocodone // acetaminophen), 848
Vigor, increase, 93
Villus (villi)
  definition, 864
  description, 615
  epithelium, cells, 615f
  illustration, 615f
Vinyl gloves, assets/liabilities, 71
Viruses, agent, 66-67
Visceral layer, 278
Visceral pericardium, 278f
Visceral peritoneum, 278f
Visceral pleura, 278f
Visceral reflexes (autonomic reflexes), 509
  definition, 864
Viscosity, 572
Vision, sense organs, 524
Vision statement, 793
Visual association area, 515f
Visual cortex, 515f
Visually impaired clients, 250
  initial consultation, 250
Vital capacity, 596
  increase. See Lungs
Vitamin A (retinol), 831
Vitamin B_1 (thiamine), 831
Vitamin B_2 (riboflavin), 831
Vitamin B_3 (niacin), 831
Vitamin B_5 (pantothenic acid), 832
Vitamin B_6 (pyroxidine), 832
Vitamin B_7 (biotin // vitamin H), 832
Vitamin B_9 (folic acid), 832
Vitamin B_{12} (cobalamin), 832
Vitamin B complex, 831–832

Vitamin C (ascorbic acid), 832
Vitamin D (cholecalciferol), 832
  deficiency, 330
  synthesis, skin (involvement), 294
Vitamin E (tocopherol), 832
Vitamin H. See Vitamin B_7
Vitamin K, 832
Vitamins
  classification, 621t
  definition, 864
  description, 621–622, 831
  functions, 620t, 831–832
  source, 831–832
Vitiligo, 296
Vocal cords. See False vocal cords; True vocal
    cords
  definition, 864
  illustration, 593f
  sets, 593
Void, 757f
Volar. See Palmar; Plantar
Volkmann's canals, 313
  definition, 864
Volume, 525
Voluntary system, 507
Vomiting, 233
  inquiry, 221
von Hohenheim, Philippus. See Paracelsus
Vulva, 650
  definition, 864

W
Waistline, 698
  horizontal landmark, 698f
Walking occupations, 111b
    (physical activity category), 110
Wall, Ronald, 91
Warfarin sodium. See Coumadin
Warm-up, problems, 719
Warrior stances (horse stances), 115–117
  definition, 865
  usage, 117. See also Massage therapists
Warts, 306. See also Genital warts; Venereal
    warts
  term, usage, 295
Waste elimination
  digestive system, impact, 632
  integumentary system, impact, 632
  respiratory system, impact, 632
  role. See Skin
  urinary system, impact, 632
Waste products, removal (promotion), 89, 583b
Wasting away, 245
Water
  balance, control. See Body
  classification, 622
  correspondences, 776t
  Earth control, 776–777
  function, 620t, 833
  healing agent, 667–669
  immersion, exercise (combination), 680
  loss, 639
  phase, 775
  shiatsu. See Watsu
  source, 833
  usage. See Hand washing
Watsu (water shiatsu), 681
WBC. See White blood cell
Weak muscles, toning, 91, 392b
Websites. See Internet websites
Weekend workshop warrior syndrome, 29-30
Weight
  decrease, 89. See also Edema
  loss, 834
Well-being, increase. See Physical well-being

Wellbutrin (Wellbutrin SR // bupropion //
    bupropion extended-release), 848
Wernicke's area (sensory speech area), 515f
Western medicine, contrast. *See* Asian medicine
Wheelchair-bound clients, massage (impact),
    251–252
Whiplash, 331
Whirlpools
    definition, 865
    usage, 681
        photograph, 681f
White blood cell (WBC), 577–578
    adhesion, enhancement. *See* Migrating WBC
    count, increase, 89
White muscles. *See* Fast twitch muscles
Womb. *See* Uterus
Women, legs (massage). *See* Pregnant women
Wong-Baker FACES Pain Rating Scale, 206f
Wood
    control. *See* Fire
    correspondences, 776t
    phase, 774
Wool blanket, usage, 678f
Words
    communication, 20
    meaning, 21b
Work, body placement, 118
Work experience. *See* Curriculum vitae
Wound condition, importance, 720
Wraps. *See* Body; Compression wraps; Cover
    wraps; Herbal wraps; Paraffin wraps
Wringing friction, 159

Wrists
    abduction, 321, 323f
    adduction, 321, 323f
    alignment, 147f
    angle, illustration, 118f
    bones, 342–347
    circles, 110
    extension, 321, 322f
    flexion, 321, 322f
    gymnastics, 175t
    movements, 174–175
        muscles, 419f-431f
        muscles, list, 429t
    positioning, 118
Wryneck. *See* Torticollis

X

Xanax (alprazolam), definition, 848
X chromosome, 655
XO female (Turner's syndrome), 655
XXY male (Klinefelter's syndrome), 655

Y

Yang. *See* Yin/Yang
Yawns, 600
    definition, 865
Year of Living Consciously, A (Hendricks), 29
Yellow marrow, 313f
Yin/Yang, 756–758
    relative correspondences, 757t
    symbol, 757
Ylang-ylang, 688

Z

Zahourek, Jon, 386–387
Zang, definition, 865
Zang/fu, 773–774
    definition, 865
Zantac (ranitidine), definition, 848
Zen shiatsu, 756
    principles. *See* Touch
Zill, Robin, 667
Zinc (Zn)
    function, 833
    source, 833
Z-line, 381, 382
Zocor (simvastatin), definition, 848
Zoloft (sertraline), definition, 848
Zona pellucida, illustration, 646
Zone, 698
    definition, 865
    map. *See* Reflexology
    points (addressing), thumb walk (usage), 700f
Zygomatic bone, 467f
Zygomaticus major
    action, 465f
    nerve, 465f
    origins/insertions, 465f
Zygomaticus minor
    action, 465f
    nerve, 465f
    origins/insertions, 465f
Zygote, 218
    division, 653f
Zyrtec (Zyrtec-D // cetirizine), definition, 848